PETERSON'S

JOB
OPPORTUNITIES
HEALTH
AND SCIENCE

COMPANY INFORMATION PROVIDED BY

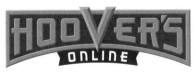

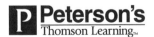
Thomson Learning™

Australia • Canada • Denmark • Japan • Mexico • New Zealand • Philippines
Puerto Rico • Singapore • South Africa • Spain • United Kingdom • United States

About Peterson's

Peterson's is the country's largest educational information/communications company, providing the academic, consumer, and professional communities with books, software, and online services in support of lifelong education access and career choice. Well-known references include Peterson's annual guides to private schools, summer programs, colleges and universities, graduate and professional programs, financial aid, international study, adult learning, and career guidance. Peterson's Web site at petersons.com is the only comprehensive—and most heavily traveled—education resource on the Internet. The site carries all of Peterson's fully searchable major databases and includes financial aid sources, test-prep help, job postings, direct inquiry and application features, and specially created Virtual Campuses for every accredited academic institution and summer program in the U.S. and Canada that offers in-depth narratives, announcements, and multimedia features.

Visit Peterson's Education Center on the Internet (World Wide Web) at www.petersons.com

Copyright © 1999 Peterson's, a division of Thomson Learning. Thomson Learning is a trademark used herein under license.

Previous editions © 1984, 1985, 1986, 1987, 1988, 1989, 1990, 1991, 1992, 1993, 1994, 1995, 1996, 1997, 1998 as *Peterson's Job Opportunities for Health and Science Majors*

Company information provided by Hoover's Online © 1999 by Hoover's, Inc., Austin, Texas

ISSN 1525-206X
ISBN 0-7689-0242-8

Printed in Canada

10 9 8 7 6 5 4 3 2 1

Contents

About This Book

Peterson's *Job Opportunities in Health and Science* offers a wealth of information about 2,000 growing U.S. companies in health- and science-related industries. In this book, you will find information about many companies that are household names and others that may not be familiar to you but are growing and hiring many employees. These companies are located all over the United States, in major metropolitan areas and in out-of-the-way places. They do business in forty-nine industries, including agricultural operations, biomedical and genetic products, chemicals, drugs, fertilizers, food, health maintenance organizations, hospitals, scientific instruments, medical and dental products, pollution control equipment and services, veterinary products and services, and vitamins and nutritional products. Together, these companies employ nearly 6 million people.

About Hoover's Online

The data in this book were provided by Hoover's Online. Hoover's Online is a leading provider of information on nearly 14,000 of the world's largest, fastest-growing, and most influential public and private enterprises. Hoover's Online provides executives, sales and marketing professionals, investors, and job seekers with the information they need to identify and evaluate potential partners, competitors, prospects, investments, and employers. Updated daily by Hoover's staff of more than 100 researchers, writers and editors, Hoover's Online covers a company's history, strategy, officers, competitors, products, operations, and financial health. Hoover's Online also provides links to news, lists, stock quotes, and other features, such as Hoover's Industry Snapshots and Hoover's IPO Central.

What's Inside

Articles

The following articles will help you understand trends that may affect your career, prepare your resume and ace the interview, and develop a highly desirable skill to improve your chances of success.

• Workplace 2000: Health Care

Read how changes in corporate America are affecting today's employment picture. The skills that companies are looking for in employees today and what makes an employee valuable have changed. As a job seeker, are you prepared to take the initiative in your career? Do you thrive on constant change and ambiguity? Can you adjust your sights toward a mobile career path in a global marketplace? Are you willing to keep expanding your knowledge and skills, both technical and interpersonal, to keep yourself employable? Find out what to expect in today's and tomorrow's workplace.

• The World Wide Web—Promises and Pitfalls

It's a new technology—surfing the "Net" to find a job. This article is packed with helpful hints on where to look, what to beware of, and how to get your resume in a Web site that employers will see.

• Researching, Getting, and Keeping Your Ideal Job

This article includes resume and interview advice that can benefit any reader. It can help you identify potential employers; give you resume advice; suggest tips for applying for jobs; provide checklists that will help you before, during, and after interviews; and show you how to convince a potential employer that you would be a valuable employee.

• The Most Desired Job Skill in the World

What is the number one skill that employers look for when hiring new employees? The answer may surprise you. This article tells you what that skill is and how to develop it and use it to your advantage in getting and keeping your desired job.

Company Overviews

The company descriptions provided by Hoover's Online give information about the company's main business function and facts and figures on sales, the company's top three competitors, the company Web site, and other information you need to contact the company or apply for a job, including the company's mailing address, telephone and fax numbers, and name of a human resources contact. The sales and employee figures for each company are for the most recent fiscal year-end available at the time this book went to press in mid-1999.

If you are looking for a job, we strongly recommend that you spend some time focusing your personal goals before jumping into the overviews. Think about the following questions: What kind of job do you want? Where do you want to live? How can you present yourself in the best light? You may want to take a few minutes to review the lists and the job-search article before you peruse the overviews.

Employer-Sponsored Descriptions

Some companies have chosen to supplement the information provided by Hoover's Online to give job seekers additional information about them. You will find these Employer-Sponsored Descriptions in the section following the Company Overviews.

Indexes

Finally, there are indexes in which the companies are listed alphabetically for quick reference and by primary industry and metropolitan area.

How Companies Were Selected for This Book

The 2,000 companies in this book were selected from Hoover's database of nearly 14,000 companies. To be included in this book, an employer had to fall into one of the forty-nine industries that hire people with health and science backgrounds and have had employee growth in the past year.

Whether you prefer to work for a rapidly growing, smaller company that may be just getting started or a larger company that is well established but not growing as rapidly, you'll find plenty of companies from which to choose.

Whether you're looking for information to help you do your job better or looking for a new job, we hope *Job Opportunities in Health and Science* will put you ahead of the competition and help you be successful.

Workplace 2000: Health Care

by Ted Johnson

A great deal of change has occurred in the last few years. It seemed for a while that every day there was news in the health-care industry about mergers and rumors of mergers. Some mergers turned large corporations into giants that do everything from selling major companies their health coverage to laundering hospital linens. Meanwhile, people around the country notice that cities that once had four hospitals now have two; those that had two now have one. Basic health needs once provided by a physician now are provided by a practitioner in a clinic; the physical therapy sessions once conducted in a medical setting are now held in the patient's home.

The public has cast a wary eye on these developments, for there is a perception that health-care companies are attempting to maximize profits at the expense of patient services. But the strongest health-care companies understand that quality care is the most efficient care; that the only way to survive is to focus a talented workforce on the task of improving patient health.

To meet that goal, the health-care industry needs a well-trained, flexible, and creative workforce. It is an industry in which how the patient is handled often has as much an influence on recovery as the treatment itself. It is an industry in which the most successful people may not come from institutions that offer years of advanced technical training in a narrow field. Rather, individuals who can apply new-found skills in a unique way are the ones who may achieve tremendous rewards.

We see examples of this already. Who would have thought fifteen years ago that there would come a day in which health-care companies would employ nurses whose primary role is to teach patients computer skills so they can use that high-tech device to monitor their diabetes?

It is an industry that is constantly evolving. New technologies and drugs will always bring new issues into the field. There is even talk about curing cancer with medication. But one thing is clear: the industry seems to be over the frenzied business affairs of the early 1990s and is focusing its attention on medicine.

"The health-care industry feels the public scorn about its 'for-profit' mentality," says Kevin Lumsdon, managing editor of the industry trade magazine *Hospitals & Health Networks*. "The industry thinks the public sees health care as having gone too far. There are no statistics yet to say real harm has been done to the public good. But there is real skepticism in the public eye, and the quality issues in health care will become a real political football.

"We may soon see consumer protection legislation so that managed care organizations cannot put caps or limits on the amount of care available to a patient," Lumsdon continues. "There will be issues about patients being able to appeal a denial of coverage. For what you see is the public's demand to have more of a consumer say in the quality of health care."

This is a carryover of an era in which the entire health-care industry reformed itself. It was a transformation of such magnitude and power that it went from the boardrooms of billion-dollar companies all the way down to the orderlies in the wards.

"I have been a long-time observer of the health-care industry, and I've never witnessed such rapid, radical, revolutionary transformation," says Dr. David Werdigar, the director of the California Office of Statewide Health Planning and Development. "President Clinton's bill (1994 health-care reform), though it failed legislatively, served as a catalyst for a huge industry to change itself."

Cost Is Everything

The force behind the reform is money. The United States spends too much on its health care.

Like most other industrialized nations in the world, about 5 percent of the U.S. workforce is employed in the health-care industry. *Unlike* other industrialized nations that spend about 5 to 7 percent of their gross national product on health care, the U.S. spends 12 to 13 percent.

What's more, there are estimates that 35 million U.S. citizens (about 15 percent) go without health-care coverage, even though as a nation we spend $1 trillion a year on it.

As a large bulk of the population known as the Baby Boomer generation ages, there will be an increasingly greater demand for health care to meet their needs. That should mean more jobs. But the biggest question facing everyone, from the President of the United States to the CEO of a small regional hospital, is how to pay for it all?

The most obvious trend is managed care, or health maintenance organizations (HMO), which operate by setting the cost of an individual's needs at, say, a monthly fee of $40. If those needs are met for less, that extra money becomes profit for the HMO.

"The economic forces are driving [the industry] toward managed care to control costs," explains Larry Stewart, president of Weatherby Health Care, a national recruiting firm in Norwalk, Connecticut. "The payers [insurance companies] are going to pay for the most economical health care with the same quality."

The effects of this trend are far-reaching. For starters, hospitals will look more and more like large intensive-care units.

"The cost of providing care in that environment is becoming so prohibitive that only the very, very sick will be there," observes Dr. Gene Scott, a vice president for education and organization development at Sutter Health in Sacramento, California.

That will naturally create a need for intensive-care nurses, Scott indicates, but even these people will be subject to the new craze in the industry: cross-training.

TECHNICALLY SPEAKING: TELEMEDICINE

A woman in a rural community is having difficulty giving birth. The nearest neo-natal specialist is 200 miles away, and there is no time to bring the two together. But there is little worry for the woman.

The vital signs of the mother and the baby are being monitored by a specialist on a computer 200 miles away. The specialist is made aware of everything from the baby's blood gases to the amount of oxygen in the delivery room. This allows the specialist to virtually direct the delivery from afar.

That's one example of the pervasive and deep impact the computer is having on the health-care industry. Nearly everyone will have to have a solid knowledge of "information management."

Telecommuting, global linkups, and virtual teaming are already a reality in health care, and it's called Telemedicine.

Medical and financial records are computerized. A day will come, experts say, when the patient will fill out registration forms and make arrangements for payment, via computer, from home.

The impact of high technology on the industry reaches so far that experts foresee no one geographical area becoming a "hot spot" for job growth. Computer linkups will put modernity into the most rural and the most strapped urban medical clinics.

"Hospitals that had trouble recruiting radiologists can now have the best in the business reading their material," says Dr. David Werdigar, director of the Office of Statewide Health Planning for California.

Beverly Campbell, director of health careers education for California's Depart-ment of Education, describes a prototype under development of a "diagnostic" bed for the home. It may become very popular for elderly care. An ill patient lies in the bed, which is laden with diagnostic equipment that automatically analyzes various body functions and transmits the data to a hospital computer, where the patient's records are on file. The computer makes a diagnosis and, in some cases, orders a drug prescription automatically. The medication gets delivered to the patient's door shortly thereafter.

"The patient never leaves home," notes Campbell.

All this equipment, of course, will become more complicated and more expensive.

And Dr. Harry Douglas, vice president for academic affairs for Charles Drew Medical Center in Los Angeles, sees a trend emerging: equipment and instrument repair.

"It's a big field," Douglas observes. "People rely on this equipment, but they don't know how to repair it."

"Even in that hospital environment, where you have narrowly defined jobs, such as respiratory therapist and medical technician, you are going to see a collapsing of those borders," Scott explains. "It will have a positive effect because it will give the jobs more variety."

The age of specialization is over. Today's health-care organizations are begging for the "primary care" physician, one who can provide basic overall medical treatment.

That trend carries over as well to the allied health worker, in and out of hospitals. Physical therapists, medical technicians, and radiologists, among others, are being asked by their employers to expand their expertise into related areas. For instance, physical therapists are often asked to become accredited as occupational therapists, too.

Beverly Campbell, the director of California's Health Careers Education, points out that one study showed that, on average, 46 to 70 hospital workers visit a bedside during a typical three-day stay.

That number is going down. Fewer people, less cost.

Renaissance People

"In the future, workers in health care have to have an overall understanding of how the system works, no matter what profession they are in," maintains Leonard Finocchio, associate director for the Center of Health Professions in San Francisco. "They have to understand all the psychosocial and environmental factors in a patient's condition, such as the effect of poverty. The worker needs to be flexible and multiskilled."

"It'd be best if they had computer training and knowledge of information management," Finocchio adds. "Yet they also have to have a strong foundation in the sciences. More important, they have to be critical thinkers. They are going to be expected to do a lot more than push buttons all day."

Generally speaking, most health-care employees require some higher education and technical training, though the level required varies from position to position. Accordingly, one thing that has to change to meet industry needs is the curriculum in health-care education, says Dr. Harry Douglas, executive vice president of the Charles R. Drew Medical Center in Los Angeles. The founding dean of the school's allied health program, Douglas calls for the "unbundling" of curriculum in schools. For example, there needn't be an anatomy course just for nurses, another just for radiologists, and yet another just for physician assistants. One general anatomy course could meet all those demands.

A solid, basic education is a good starting point for all professions, and that should include liberal arts and sciences and math. "This is the biggest problem: Getting people who don't have the math and literacy skills, so when they go into their health training they struggle because they are learning the technical information as well as trying to get the basic information," Douglas explains.

All of the above applies whether you're already working in health care or just getting started. Experienced health-care workers need to keep upgrading and broadening their knowledge and skills, which could come through additional college courses or through training programs offered by an employer or a professional association. Similarly, those who are in or are returning to college to pursue a health-care career need to take a close look at the curriculum and make sure they'll be getting a broad-based, real-world education (see box, The Nurse Returns).

And speaking of the real world, soon all health-care education will include a class called Cost-Benefit Analysis. Every decision about a patient's care will be judged as to whether it's the most cost-effective method available. Will a worker spend twice as much caring for a patient to get a 10 percent increase in results? The days of "cost is no object" are gone forever.

"You will see more and more people employed in health research services," Werdigar predicts. "These are people who will analyze the cost, quality, and access to health-care services."

The Great Unknown

The merger mania in the industry will leave several giants standing, to be sure. But that doesn't mean there isn't room for smaller, regional companies that give a more personalized touch. There is a large philosophical issue being played out within the industry that pits the business-oriented administrators—the accountants and managers who analyze how much money is spent per patient—against the doctors, who are concerned about patient well-being. More and more doctors are expanding their education to include business practices so they have the training to assume high-level positions and have more say in how patients are treated.

Interestingly, it seems the public understands that these companies have the right to make money. Acceptance depends on quality.

"I don't think people object to the profit motive," says Greg Borzo, business editor at the *American Medical News,* a trade publication for health-care workers. "We've had for-profit hospitals for a long time. Doctors have been profit-oriented for centuries. People object to the restrictions of managed care—the limits on types of coverage or their choice of doctor, or the fact that drugs are available but the health-care companies say they are too expensive."

The companies that do the best will be the ones that are the most responsive to the public's needs, Borzo adds, and pay attention to how they price their services. Companies that evolve into integrated health organizations (IHO), Scott says, may have a better chance of surviving. These days it isn't enough for a hospital to have staff and a place to take care of patients. Many, like Sutter, have to involve the financing arm of the industry. In short, the same people who sell you or your company a health-care plan are the people who provide it.

These organizations produce a layer of administrators whose job is to manage and maintain the quality of the care. "The IHO has mechanisms to help it manage its risk with physicians and its facilities, as well as generate income through its financing arm," explains Scott.

A Job? Aim for the Middle

Nearly all the experts agree, however, that there is an exploding demand for the "mid-level provider."

Two professions that meet these criteria are physician assistant (or physician extender) and nurse practitioner. Both work closely with physicians to do many of the simple but time-consuming tasks once asked of physicians themselves. This has created a demand that, according to the latest data, lists six jobs for every physician assistant or nurse practitioner available.

Why the demand? The quest for cost-effectiveness is forcing managed care groups to reassess how they deliver services. As an example, 60 percent of the case load of one pediatrician consisted of dealing with a common childhood earache. That's something a physician assistant (PA) or nurse practitioner (NP) could easily diagnose and treat. There just isn't a need to pay for all that expensive training of the physician in instances where the quality of the care from a PA or NP would fit the bill.

NPs need a master's degree beyond their nursing degree, which is usually obtained in a hospital setting and often while continuing to work regular shifts. On the other hand, the PA degree can be obtained through a two-year program coupled with work in a hospital setting. A health-care background isn't essential. Viable candidates could be practically anyone with a solid education that includes the requisite science courses in chemistry and biology.

Demand for NPs and PAs is expected to grow dramatically over the next ten years, according to the U.S. Bureau of Labor Statistics. And high demand means good pay: new hires can expect to earn from $52,000 to $70,000 annually. It might be more, because the demand is so great that these job seekers may have competing companies bid on their services. High demand doesn't necessarily correlate, though, with high-density population centers. The pay for these professions may be higher, for example, in Minneapolis than in New York City.

One region of the country isn't really better than any other for these two trained positions, the experts maintain. Looking beyond these positions, there is a need virtually everywhere for trained, highly skilled employees in general—from physicians on down to lab technicians—which is expected to last for at least a decade. "Even at the entry levels, people are expected to have some kind of technical training," Scott reports.

Whether you're looking to switch careers or find your first career, you can count physical therapists (PT) and occupational therapists (OT) among the hottest jobs to consider. An anticipated shortage of these therapists will last until the year 2020, notes Tim Eagleson, vice president of Health Care Resources, a national recruiting firm in Fairfield, Iowa.

The Bureau of Labor Statistics backs him up. "The Labor Department says that even if we recruit all the PT graduates in the next fifteen years, there still will be a vast shortage," Eagleson explains. "It was the second-highest-paying four-year degree in the U.S. (in 1994), right behind certain kinds of engineers."

Just a few years ago, first-year PTs expected to earn $34,000 to $38,000 a year, says Eagleson. Now it's up to $38,000 to $42,000. They could earn almost $60,000 a year after five years of experience. It's a popular crossover field, in that many practicing nurses and technicians re-enter training programs to become accredited in the therapy fields. Physical therapy requires a master's degree to practice, but occupational therapy doesn't. That's why OTs typically earn about $5,000 a year less to start.

Physician, Generalize Thyself

Mel Weinberger of Louisville, Kentucky, is the publisher of *Unique Opportunities*, a national trade publication for the recruitment and retention of physicians. He sees the old patriarchal symbol of American health care—the doctor—getting a rude awakening. They now have bosses. "The biggest change in health care is the growth of physicians as employees," Weinberger comments. "One doctor actually was fired. That never happened before, as long as I can remember."

Physician still ranks as the highest earning profession, according to the Bureau of Labor Statistics, with a median income of about $130,000 a year. But things are changing.

A recent poll of medical school graduates reports that 40 percent of those surveyed preferred to go into a single specialty practice, such as orthopedics or cardiology—not a surprising choice since this is where the most money can be made. Fourteen percent chose to go into a multispecialty group, such as family care or obstetrics/gynecology (Ob/Gyn).

"But only 5.7 percent chose solo practice," Weinberger points out. "It's dead, dead, dead. And those guys in their fifties who are looking to sell their practices end up selling them to hospitals."

However, there is good news—quite good news—when it comes to physicians. No profession may be in greater demand right now than physicians in family practice, pediatrics, internal medicine, and obstetrics. Experts claim this trend could last for a decade. Managed care organizations are looking for these people to meet most of the health-care needs of the populace.

"If you're American-born and American-trained in family practice, you can have your pick of jobs," Weinberger affirms.

"The demand for primary care, family practice, internal medicine and obstetrics/gynecology doctors is so great," Weinberger adds, that "doctors are now free agents, much like athletes." Bett Coffman, who works with Weinberger at *Unique Opportunities*, notes that although specialists make more than general practitioners on average, the rate of pay for doctors practicing in these four fields is growing faster than any other field. In fact, health-care providers need these doctors so much that they bid on the services. Contracts of $350,000 a year are not unheard of.

"There is a great demand for primary care physicians," Coffman emphasizes. "The health-care groups are very competitive, and therefore the prices are going up."

At the same time, it's very, very difficult for a medical school graduate to hang a sign on the street and expect the world to come a callin' to the tune of $350,000 a year. The lone doctor has to pay for a place to practice, a staff, and insurance. Physicians in a managed care organization don't have to worry about those costs. That's the upside. The downside is they may be on a salary, which caps their earnings. And they have to answer to someone who may question their judgment—in other words, they're not the boss.

"Doctors are learning that those bureaucrats are providing a service, which is running a business," Borzo points out. "These people are controlling costs, analyzing services. Those are valuable functions, and, as doctors try to do those tasks themselves, they learn that they are not a waste of time."

Pediatricians in their first year of practice can expect to make anywhere from $80,000 to $130,000. It just depends on where the practice is. The range is similar for first-year internists. The median income for all family practice doctors, as listed in the Medical Group Management Association's 1995 survey, is $122,000. But those at the 90th percentile, which reflects more years of service in the field, make just under $200,000 annually.

NEW AGE, NEW WAYS TO HEAL

Alternative health-care therapies have been around for a long time, but it has been just in the past few years that traditional medical folks have started to give them more acceptance. In response to the thousands of people who now flock to alternative health-care therapists, insurance companies have become more willing to pay for these services. This is a growing trend, confirms Beverly Campbell, director of Health Career Education in California's Department of Education. Treatments based on old wives' tales are becoming more and more legitimate. "The more technically able we are to evaluate what a medication does, the more we see that most medication has a "contra" [or negative] effect," explains Campbell. "Everything has its help side and its bad side as well."

Drinking a concoction of herbs to strengthen one's immunity to allergies, for example, may be more practical for some patients than taking antibiotics.

A degree in herbal therapy does not necessarily guarantee you a position on a staff at a hospital, but health-care workers who accommodate so-called "New-Age" techniques—massage therapy, relaxation techniques, and herbology—can better serve their patients, and that will make them more employable. The emphasis in modern health care is making the patient happy, which also tends to improve the patient's recovery time. Some examples: Nurse practitioners are now being schooled in some "holistic" techniques. Nurses in neonatal care stations, for example, are encouraged to caress and massage their recovering young patients because many studies show that touching improves healing. Another: Rather than undergo a battery of tests and a trial-and-error run of drugs, some patients are discovering that acupuncture is the best way for them to battle severe allergies. And: Acupressure is often included in the rehabilitation schedule of patients who have had surgery, for studies show that this technique brings circulation back to damaged tissue.

"The key to it all," Campbell added, "is that the way the treatment is applied is nearly as important as the treatment itself. Patient satisfaction will be a factor in job success," Campbell said. "The general public does not have a criterion to measure their recovery so they tend to measure it by how nice people are to them. So one thing they teach in schools today is how to be nice to patients."

The roof gets blown off, however, for woman gynecologists. They can earn up to $300,000 early in their careers. "There is a tremendous demand for female gynecologists," Stewart notes. "Hospitals know that certain needs are best met by women, and the demand exceeds the supply."

This isn't the case for some specialists. Weinberger went so far as to say that there is a great chance many anesthesiologists, ophthalmologists, and psychiatrists are looking for work. "Wouldn't it be wise for anesthesiologists to go back to school and get retrained in family practice?" he suggests. "It's very different now. If you viewed the medical profession as stable, it's not. It has changed dramatically."

Go Home

The numbers don't lie. People over the age of 65 in the mid-1990s accounted for 12 percent of the U.S. population. By the year 2040, they will be a whopping 21 percent.

The U.S. is on the verge of having more than 100,000 people over the age of 100, Campbell reports. In the book *Rx 2000*, author Jeffrey Fisher, M.D., predicts that by the year 2050, the outside age for humans could be 150.

The greater the age, the greater the need for health care. The cost of a nursing home may run $130 a day and is expected to rise as the demand increases. And that cost is too high for many of the rising numbers of people who are taking care of their parents. Accordingly, says Campbell, "there is going to be a huge growth in home health care."

Nurses, physical and speech therapists, and nutritionists are but a few of the professions expected to take their expertise to the patient. With the help of computers, they will have immediate access to the patient's records when they're out on a visit. Improved technology also will allow more and more equipment to become mobile, which means more on the diagnostic end can be done outside the hospital (see box, Technically Speaking: Telemedicine).

It's common for many households to have two incomes to meet increased financial burdens. The next trend, therefore, is "adult day care," where the elderly staying with their children are dropped off at a care center in the morning and picked up after work. "This avoids the expensive, and I'd say isolating, part of health care for the elderly," says Werdigar.

In addition, there will be a greater emphasis on "wellness," or preventive medicine and on alternative health care (see box, New Age, New Ways to Heal). Exercise, rehabilitation, and education on proper nutrition will become a regular part of health-care packages. Some insurance companies have even begun to cover the cost of alternative therapies such as acupuncture, herbology, massage, and more.

Forever Learning

The anxiety of finding and then keeping a job does not stop once you are employed. Employees at all levels are having to retrain themselves to meet the needs of their employers. Nurses trained in emergency medicine are being asked to bone up on their skills in surgery techniques. This is called "multi-tasking" or "cross-training." And it's a trend that spells a redefinition—and expansion—of roles in several allied health fields.

For example, in many organizations a radiologist will be expected to do a lot more than take X-rays. That person also will be expected to operate EKG, magnetic resonance imaging (MRI), and nuclear medicine equipment. Instead of 4 technicians (albeit an expert in each), there will be one technician who is competent in all.

This is the main reason why many health care experts do not have the same rosy outlook on the industry's job growth as the Bureau of Labor Statistics. "The incentive in the industry is not to create more jobs," Douglas says, "but to cut costs by reconfiguring the work force."

THE NURSE RETURNS

Kevin Lumsdon, like many health-care experts, came to believe that the traditional role of registered nurses (RN) had been lost to the changing times. Today, an RN is expected to be a manager, a clipboard-holder, or an analyst. The actual duties of patient care were left to personnel with less training, namely Light Vocational Nurses and medical assistants. But recent job trends have forced the managing editor of *Hospitals & Health Networks* to admit he was wrong.

The latest statistics from the Labor Department list RN as the third-highest position in demand through 2006—a position that will have fast growth (about 350,000 more RNs will be needed), high pay (over $30,000 to start), and low unemployment. Only systems analysts and top business executives will be in greater demand.

"One of the things that makes nursing so complicated in terms of employment prospects is that their skills are very broad," says Janet Coffman, associate director for workforce policy at the Pew Health Professions. "In the past few years, as economic pressures became tighter, there was a lot of effort to shift unlicensed nurses into more of the hands-on role in patient care—housekeeping, feeding patients, drawing blood. And that led to RNs being shifted into more of a supervisory role. No one is going back to the old mode, but more registered nurses are being put back into patient care. With the acutely ill, for example, patient status can change hour to hour, and unlicensed personnel do not have the training that RNs do to pick up subtle signs."

The highest-paying nursing jobs by and large will require applicants to have at least a Bachelor of Science (B.S.) degree, which usually comes from a four-year college, as well as training time in wards. This background, Coffman points out, is the wellspring for a great health-care career. "One of the great things about nursing is that the career laddering is so good because nurses have that broad base of knowledge, and they can move up from that into any area."

Demand for nurses will be high nationwide if they have the training. Demand will bring more men into the field, and the pay scale will probably improve for some time. The median annual income for nurses currently ranges from about $33,000 to $44,000, with about 10 percent earning more than $50,000 a year. The key is getting the basic four-year degree and then branching out into whatever specialized field sounds appealing, and that could mean picking up a master's degree—usually a two-year program—to become a nurse practitioner, nurse anesthetist, or nurse midwife. Incomes in those fields accelerate into the $75,000-and-above level quickly.

"They will need to be flexible," Lumsdon says, "but with good training they can market themselves all over the country. It helps if they are willing to move. If they are rooted to one community, then they may have a little harder time earning top dollar."

This trend puts a great deal of pressure on organizations to manage their workers well to ensure that quality care can be given. "When you train someone in all those areas, that person has to do the work to maintain competency in each field," explains Mark Mattes, allied health director of Methodist Health Group in Indianapolis, the largest managed care organization in Indiana.

It also puts a great deal of pressure on the worker. There will be less and less permanence in job status, as well as a constant demand to upgrade services.

"The way to prepare yourself for careers beyond the year 2000 is to see yourself as a renewable career agency," Scott surmises. "That means having the capability to learn. Even though there is a tremendous need for physician assistants and nurse practitioners, to name one field, how they will be used, and where, is likely to be changed in a way no one can predict right now. The real key is to see the benefit of this direction and not get locked into the thought [that] this is what you are for the rest of your life."

Some Things Never Change

For all the advances in technology, for all the radical changes in the basic structure of the industry, health care still comes down to people helping people.

"There needs to be a hands-on practitioner," Stewart notes. "Health care is a vibrant and dynamic industry. It's a be-there kind of activity."

Simply put, the new jobs can be found in two areas: The people who put together the new organizations that will provide health care and the people who do the actual providing.

Organizations are striving to become more flexible to meet the ever-changing, ever-growing needs of the populace. Just about every employee will have an active role in improving the scope and quality of health care.

"That's why its important for more and more people not to get into something with a narrow base," Janet Coffman advises. "It's better to get into something general and then adapt to the marketplace. If a person gets into a narrow technical field, like some forms of imaging, we may develop a way to do it better and less invasively and then that narrow tech field will be gone."

Few industries have changed as much as health care over the last decade. But it is an industry that will always be changing, for technology and research will bring new ways to help the public. In that light, it is an industry that will always need people who are bright enough to see the changes coming, have the know-how to understand how they must adapt, and be creative enough to apply their skills in a challenging, evolving, exciting environment.

Ted Johnson is a freelance writer based in San Ramon, California, who specializes in educational and sports issues.

The World Wide Web— Promises and Pitfalls

by Cristopher J. Maloney

Just when you thought you were doing everything you needed to do to find a wonderful position with the perfect company, someone asks you if you've put your resume on the World Wide Web. Whether you answered "yes," "not yet," or "world-wide-what?," you may be surprised that there is a lot to learn even for seasoned Web wizards. Complete novices will be happy to know that understanding what a job hunter needs to know about the Web is easier than many buzzword-using, keyboard-tapping, computer technocrats might have inadvertently led you to believe. In this article, I'll be discussing the opportunities and risks provided by the Web for job hunters, including what to do and what not to do on the Web with, for example, your resume.

It is impossible to describe in detail exactly what each reader of this book will see on his or her computer when using the Web. Big and small companies provide consumers with dozens of different ways to get connected to the Web (America Online, AT&T, and EarthLink come to mind as just a few of the popular players), and many of these access providers allow their subscribers to use different brands of software within their systems. This article will provide you with insight about the Web and give the wary an understanding of how it all works. I will assume that your access provider and the software you select will make the various steps mentioned obvious once you become a "Web user." In fact, if you are using the Web and you can't figure it out, you have good reason to switch providers or switch software. Using the Web should be EASY!

The Web

The Web allows novices and experts alike to easily and enjoyably navigate many types of information services. It also gives more companies and individuals the opportunity to electronically publish (and distribute more widely) their resource and outreach materials. Millions and millions of users now have access to millions of pages on the Web.

A page on the World Wide Web can contain graphics as well as text. Well-designed Web pages are easy for computer novices to navigate and can be interesting and fun to explore.

The person or company that publishes a Web page can build links on the page that allow you, with the click of your computer's mouse button, to connect to any other page on the World Wide Web. For example, you might use your computer to go to a Web page filled with jobs available at many different companies. This aggregator's page typically allows you to do some type of search by job type and geographic region.

Let's say you want to find a job in St. Louis, Missouri. In the results from a search you may read about a job you really like. Clicking on the name of the company in the job description might take you to more details about the employer and from there you might be invited to link to a Web page operated not by the aggregator but by the headquarters of the hiring company. Once you're on the hiring company's Web site, you might find a link that takes you to a Web site operated by the hiring division.

The aggregator's Web site may be operating out of Princeton, New Jersey, and the hiring company's headquarters could be in Tokyo. Yet, the hiring division (and the computer publishing its Web site) might be in St. Louis. In a matter of seconds, you crossed several mountain ranges, an ocean, and the International Date Line (twice) and all you did was click a button a few times. The Web transcends the boundaries that normally restrict us—time, access to huge sums of travel money, and political borders. Of course, as long as the job isn't too far from where you live, you probably don't care how far or how fast your search took you around the globe.

Get Your Mouse in the Door

Beyond the task of finding a company with a job that matches your interests, it is now easy to regularly visit companies in a way not possible before.

Let's face it, if down the road from your house is a company you have always wanted to work for and you showed up every morning asking if maybe today there was a job opening for you—well, at best you wouldn't be arrested for acting crazy but you certainly wouldn't get hired. But if they have a presence on the World Wide Web, you can stop by the company virtually (no pun intended) every day, every hour if you like. And guess what? Companies love it when people visit their Web sites!

It is probably bad form to show up for an interview if you haven't visited and extensively browsed a would-be employer's Web site. Hiring managers and human resource professionals are pleased to learn that you have followed the company in recent newspaper coverage and can demonstrate knowledge that you might have learned by reading about the company in a book such as this one. Just imagine how pleased they would be if you told them how much you learned from their Web site! Company personnel are typically proud of their Web sites and enjoy discussing them.

You might also feel more comfortable in an interview if you've seen a picture of the hiring manager and learned a bit about his or her history that might be presented in an online biography. Depending on what a company has decided to publish, you might be able to find these things at the company's URL.

Web-Speak: What Is a URL?

URL, or Uniform Resource Locator, is the address of a Web page. It is similar to a phone number. You type a URL into the Web browser software, hit the "Enter" key and your software silently calls another computer on the Web. If the other computer is there (if there aren't any busy signals) then the answering computer "looks" at the URL you entered into your software and determines if you can "speak" to that specific page. The computer you are trying to reach has to determine two things: it has to see if the page exists and, assuming it does, the computer has to check its programming to see if the page is "public" or has restricted access. (Web pages, for example, can be password protected).

This is no more complicated than a high school boy calling his new girlfriend only to have her father answer the telephone. The boy asks, "Is Victoria there, please?" The father asks, "Who is calling, please?" The phone at the girlfriend's house is like the computer with the Web pages, Victoria is like the page, and the father is checking his programming to determine whether his daughter is home and if the caller is granted access.

Of course, instead of answering by saying "Hello," the computer answers by sending instructions to your computer telling it how to display the Web page you requested. On the other hand, Web pages can include audio files that are automatically played by the receiving computer—so don't be surprised if the computer *does* answer by saying "Hello."

Is the Web a Job Hunter's Promised Land?

Not long ago, use of the Web to find a job was pretty much limited to reading postings that, more often than not, only technically oriented people would consider and, not surprisingly, the jobs that could most often be found were typically very technical in nature. In fact, even to this day, many of the jobs posted tend to be for computer programmers, network administrators, and systems analysts.

So, is job hunting on the Web a waste of time for sales and marketing professionals, administrative assistants, teachers, and executives? Not at all!

Job postings on the Web regularly list just about every kind of position that might otherwise be advertised in a local, regional, or national newspaper. So those of you who don't stay up all night learning the latest in programming algorithms will be happy to learn that the jobs you'll find listed on Web pages are not strictly computer related. You are just as likely to find job listings for executive secretary, freelance writer, summer camp counselor, or vice president of sales as you are for computer programmer.

Be Prepared

You are likely to find a place on the Web where you are given the opportunity to fill in a job application or enter your resume. If you can have your word processing software up and running while you're looking for jobs on the Web, it may save you time to cut and paste between the resume on your computer and the Web page you're visiting. This can also help protect you against entering embarrassing spelling errors that you would have corrected using a spellchecker.

Letting the Web Work for You

Have you ever thought, "I bet there is a company out there that would just love to have somebody with my skills. If only they could find me." Well, believe it or not, now they can.

A company that you've never heard of can search Web-based collections of resumes and find *you*.

Where You Shouldn't Put Your Resume On Line

More and more people have been adding something like this at the end of their cover letters and e-mails:

> My resume is available on the World Wide Web at
> http://www.hostingservice.com/~mywebpage/.

Putting your resume on the Web in a resume aggregator's system is probably a very good idea. Intermingling it with a personal Web page, however, can be a very bad idea. Too many personal Web pages are much too personal for the tastes of most employers. Not that there is anything wrong with the Web pages themselves or expressing and supporting your beliefs in a strong and forthright fashion, but when was the last time you started an interview by evangelizing your political, sexual, and religious preferences?

I can't tell you how many times I've heard or read that you can never dress too conservatively during the interview process. My point is, if you're going to invite a potential employer to visit your Web page, dress it conservatively.

Is There Just One Place to Remember?

The list of job and career resources on the Web grows every day. Peterson's, the publisher of this and other career books, also publishes The Education Supersite on the Web. Its URL is www.petersons.com. You can use this site free of charge to search for a job, get tips for preparing your resume, read feature articles, learn about more than 4,000 employers, post your resume (let them find you), e-mail employers, and look for educational opportunities that could improve your readiness for a job or promotion.

It is probably best to think of the Web as a library that gives you access to material and services from a wide range of publishers. Evaluate the publishers. Do they have a history of producing accurate and trusted information? Evaluate the services. Does the service help you? You may find more than one that suits your needs. In the end, the one thing that everyone will agree on is that, clearly, the Web is an important tool for people in the job market.

Researching, Getting, and Keeping Your Ideal Job

How to Track an Industry

Once you have used this book to identify employers you may be interested in, take the time to investigate their industry group. The current financial performance and future prospects of an industry, as a whole, in which you take a job will directly affect your job security, along with your chance for raises and promotions. It is easy to become better informed. Consult with general business magazines such as *Business Week*, *Forbes*, or *Fortune*. They do most of the work for you.

For instance, each year these magazines publish industry-by-industry analyses of the top corporations in the United States. Look for industries that are rated above average in sales growth, profits as a percentage of sales, and growth in the number of employees. Keep in mind that one or two years of bad results for an industry does not necessarily mean the industry is in permanent decline; some industries are more sensitive to short-term economic conditions than others.

How to Track a Company

Once you have checked the overall performance of an industry, you can use the library or your computer to gather more information about a particular company. Perform database searches to look for mention in the press of new products or new contracts, along with comments from industry analysts. You invariably will impress the people who are conducting an interview by informing yourself about their company before you get there. Most interviewees have little or no knowledge of the companies to which they apply. An hour's worth of research time will make you look sharp and prepared and put you in a position to interview *them* while they are interviewing you, *and* you will stand head and shoulders above anyone else applying for the job.

If a company is publicly traded on a stock exchange, you can also take advantage of a good indicator of a company's future performance. Look at the P/E (price to earnings) ratio of companies you are interested in over the last year or so. Compare this ratio with other companies in the same industry. You can find up-to-date figures for most publicly traded companies in the *Wall Street Journal* or *Barron's*. If the P/E of a company in a healthy industry is significantly higher than that of other similar companies, the stock market's judgment is that the near- to mid-term prospects for profitability of that company are good.

Companies that are achieving profitability through sales growth and high profit margins typically will be hiring. The stock market is full of smart people doing their best to judge the prospects of companies year in and year out. They are not always right, of course, but they have more sources of information at their disposal than the average job seeker. Take advantage of them.

The point is that tracking companies takes many different forms. You should study the raw data—the numbers—but look at the intangibles and, especially, at the future.

The Search

In searching for a job, remember that the ideas and techniques that have worked for years still are the most valid and reliable techniques today. Never forget how important a resume is in the job search process. There are plenty of resources you can use to help you create the best resume possible. The idea isn't to dazzle the prospective employer. A good, professional impression will go a long way toward getting you through the interview process and, eventually, to the job offer. Be aware of your appearance and your presentation manner, and play up what you consider your strongest points. A thank-you note after the interview never hurts.

1) Experience counts. Over and over again you will hear that employers are looking for people who already have specific job experience in a given field. If you haven't graduated yet, look into internships or co-op programs. When you hit the job market, you will have a running start.

2) Be wary of growth potential. Despite what you might hear during the interview, the job you first get hired for is often what you are doing ten years later. Do your best to make sure that what you are learning on the job will be of interest to potential future employers. If not, your next job change may be difficult.

3) Use a standard resume format that highlights your applicable experience. The employers who are hiring are receiving large numbers of resumes. Give yourself a better chance of being noticed by using a format that employers are used to reading. They want to see who you worked for, in chronological order, and what you did while you were there.

4) Take advantage of new communications technology. If you have access to the Internet, try posting your resume in an applicable news group or mailing list. Peruse industry-specific computer bulletin boards. Many recent graduates have found jobs this way. The fact that you know how to use today's communications technology highlights one of your skills before you even get an interview.

5) There's no substitute for connections. Begin any job search by talking to ex-classmates and former co-workers. A good reference from someone who knows you and is trusted in the company you are interviewing with counts as much as, and sometimes more than, a great interview. And remember, you can network electronically as well (see tip 4).

6) Personalize your resume and cover letter to fit the job you are looking for. There's nothing wrong with highlighting your applicable experience as much as possible. But, don't go overboard (i.e., don't lie), or you are likely to find yourself living through the "interview from hell."

7) Contact your references in advance. Ask them if they are comfortable with serving as a reference for you. *You* may be almost sure that someone thought the world of you and your work at your last job. Be absolutely certain. There's nothing worse than giving someone as a reference who turns out to be halfhearted about your talents.

8) If it's a choice between money and learning, take learning. Especially when it's early in your career, learning the right set of skills can stand you in good stead for many years to come. Taking a job offer just because of a higher salary might put you into a dead-end specialty within your field.

9) Don't forget sales jobs. No matter what their academic background is, people with good interpersonal skills can make excellent salespeople. If you chose your field as much for the starting salaries as you did for the challenges, consider sales. If you're good at it, you might end up making a better living than your peers who choose traditional jobs.

10) It can be tough out there. Don't give up. If you feel you are up against people with much more experience, sell youth and enthusiasm. If you're up against youth, sell experience. Be active, never lackadaisical, even when you feel down.

When approaching the job market, you'll want to determine what is unique or special about any given company. And you'll want to be aware of some of the major trends driving growth in the industry.

Keeping up with trends—in business, among consumers, in society at large—pays off in a job search focused on rapid-growth companies every bit as much as with corporate giants. It's a useful means of determining whether a company's "unique proposition" makes good business sense and has staying power. If your instincts tell you "that's a smart idea," you just might want to get in touch!

Of course, it isn't always—or only—the brand-spanking-new product or service that dictates success. The "unique proposition" for some companies is simply that they do what they do very well, perhaps in a better or different way than it's been done by competitors for awhile.

In examining the company's "unique proposition," ask about future growth projections and product/service lines. Ask about employee turnover rates. Talk to a few different employees to get their take on the business and day-to-day office life. Discreetly explore sources and adequacy of financing. And definitely get a sense of a company's management style and philosophy. If you pick a winner in the climate that suits you, the opportunity is there for you to grow with the business and make your mark.

Top Skills Employers Look For

No matter what job you hold and what industry you work in, you'll need to be proficient in a number of important skills if you want to prosper in the ever-more-mobile and ever-more-global business world of the next century.

Communication skills: Speaking and writing clearly and persuasively.

Computer literacy: Being adept at accessing, analyzing, and storing data and communicating with other employees via computer.

Flexibility: Having a "go with the flow" mentality that allows you to do different tasks—and even switch jobs—in response to changing business conditions.

Team player: Demonstrating the ability to cooperate and work with others productively to achieve a common goal, putting the needs of the group above your own.

Self-motivation: Getting things done on your own, without having someone else give you guidance and direction on what to do and how to do it.

Cross-cultural skills: Being able to communicate in other languages and understand different cultures.

Making Yourself a Stand-Out Candidate

Getting up to speed on current business trends and deciding what kind of job opportunities you want to tap are important steps in the job-hunting process. Your next task is to communicate that knowledge and your particular assets to potential employers. In other words, you need to build an airtight case for hiring you by letting a company know precisely how you can contribute to its success. This is the time to express your passion and to strut out some new search strategies. And here are some guidelines that could help.

- *Adopt an actor's mentality.* As the old joke goes, how do you get to Carnegie Hall . . . ? Practice. The same theory applies to honing your job-seeking "craft." Be ready for the audition. Don't take rejection personally. Rehearse your lines. Pay attention to the casting director. And use feedback to improve your performance skills.

- *Tailor your tools to your targets.* Sending out hundreds of resumes may feel like an industrious activity, but generic mailings typically get minimal to no results. Of 1,500 successful job seekers surveyed by the *National Business Employment Weekly*, most got in through contacts, only 2 percent through unsolicited mailings.

- *Create your own job security.* Finding a job doesn't mean you will never have to network, trend-track, or update your resume again. Research indicates that most people will work for 10 or more employers over a lifetime. Job security, then, comes not from your current employer but from taking charge of your career and keeping yourself employable.

- *Make change a way of life.* The old order changeth . . . what about you? In a survey of senior managers conducted by EquiPro International, their most frequently cited complaints were about employees accepting the status quo, not taking risks, reacting instead of initiating—in other words, resisting change. As companies live or die based on their ability to manage change, it's fairly obvious that they want to hire people who view change as a challenge and an opportunity.

- *Learn.* The American Society for Training and Development (ASTD) projects that by the year 2000 more than 65 percent of all jobs will require some education beyond high school; 23 million people will be employed in professional and technical jobs—the largest single occupational category—that require ongoing training. The key is to determine the kind of education and training that is valued by your market niche (or one you'd like to enter) at different stages of your career.

- *Upgrade your computer-ease.* The need to be technologically literate is no longer limited to programmers, number crunchers, and data processors. Technology will continue to transform virtually every working environment, affecting how work gets done and, thus, the types of jobs available.

- *Join the team.* Scrap the phrase "it's not in my job description" from your vocabulary. Potential employers want to hear that you're willing to roll up your sleeves and do whatever it takes to get the job done. Any evidence you can offer of your ability to both lead teams and be a good team player will win you points.

- *Get personal.* Whenever possible, present yourself to potential employers either in person or through a person. Resumes and cover letters have their place. But paper is often best used—especially by job seekers who have several years' experience or want to switch fields—to support your image rather than establish it.

- *Get noticed.* Seize every chance to become known or better known (note: this is another activity that shouldn't stop once you land a job). Take an active role in an industry association or a civic group. Publish an article in a trade journal and send "FYI" copies to key contacts and potential employers. Send an item of interest to employers with whom you had a good interview but who weren't hiring at the time. Teach. Give speeches. And always send thank-you letters.

- *Take the scenic route.* One nontraditional way to approach the job market is to become part of the growing contingent workforce—"temporary professionals" or "interim executives" who are matched with needy employers by employment firms that specialize in this area. Assignments are usually specific and short-term (3 to 18 months), which lets you check out different employers and career options and sometimes leads to full-time employment. It tends to work out best if your skills are easily transferable and/or highly specialized and you can handle the uncertainty of when and where you'll be assigned next.

Notes on Resume Design

Your resume is an important tool in the job hunt process. In it, you are trying to give the employer an overview of your work life, your job objective, and your accomplishments—not an easy thing to consolidate onto one piece of paper and a task which could take hours and hours of your time. Find a good resource for advice about writing and designing a resume.

Three things make for a winning resume. First it must be visually inviting. Use a design that is clean, readable, and scannable. Second, it should highlight what you have to offer a particular employer. This may mean modifying your resume for each and every job you apply for. This is easy to do if you have a computer. If you don't, you may want to put your job objective in your cover letter rather than on your resume page. And third, it should highlight your accomplishments, the things that identify you as an outstanding person and employee.

The following is advice on the major points you should consider when creating your resume.

DO strive for consistency in your use of graphic elements. If you capitalized your first job title, subsequent job titles should also be capitalized.

DO use point sizes consistently. For example, using 12-point text and 14-point headings makes good design sense and ensures that your resume won't be misread by a scanner.

DON'T mix typefaces. Choose a typeface with a clean and simple design, e.g., Helvetica, Ariel, Times Roman.

DO make a sophisticated choice when it comes to paper. The color should be white or beige and the finish linen or laid. Keep in mind that using high-quality paper is only important if a person is reviewing your resume. If it is being scanned, plain white paper is the best choice.

DO use the same stock for your cover letter.

DO use black ink. Don't show off by using colors or graphics. Unless you are an expert designer, it will come off as amateurish.

DO print out each resume so that it looks like an original. If you are using a typewriter, make sure the copier you are using is of high quality, such as can be found at a copy shop.

DO keep the design simple and straightforward. If you attempt to be clever or humorous, it may be misinterpreted.

DO proofread the copy several times, and if you are using a computer, use the spell check option every time you make changes or corrections.

DO give it to someone else to read before you print the final version.

DO put your name at the top of each page of your resume.

DON'T include your photograph.

DON'T fold or staple your resume. Send it in an 8½ x 11 envelope and use paper clips.

Quick Tips for Job Search Success

In the four lists that follow, we've provided some proven tips, techniques, and reminders that we're sure will improve even an experienced job seeker's chances of success. You may want to personalize them by adding items based on your own hard-learned lessons from interviews that were less than perfect. Experience is a great teacher and, since you pay dearly for the lessons you learn, you might as well benefit by improving your checklist. It will be invaluable in your future job searches.

We recommend taking the "During the Interview" checklist with you to your job interview. A last-minute glance at it will remind you of the essential things to do to make a terrific first impression.

Checklist #1: Applying for a Job

❑ Thoroughly research the companies you apply to. If, after using this book, you want to delve further to get more information, a good reference librarian can guide you to the best sources for your research, including annual reports, Web sites, trade press articles, and *Who's Who* for information on founders or top executives.

❑ Avoid form letters. Customize your letter to fit each company that you apply to.

❑ Send a query letter without a resume; your intent at this point is to gather information. You can follow up with a tailored resume once you learn more about the qualifications the company is seeking. You can elaborate on the points of your resume during the interview.

❑ Make your approach to the hiring manager. Research the person's name, title, and address and make sure you spell everything correctly in any correspondence.

❑ Don't apply to a company unless you can think of good reasons why you would be a valuable asset to their company. If you can't, they probably won't be able to either.

❑ Give your letter a reasonable amount of time to be delivered to the recipient, then make a call. Be prepared to cite your accomplishments and potential value to the company and the reasons you want to work there.

❑ Be sure your resume is current and that it has no typographical errors. Contact your references now so that you will be ready to provide their names if asked during the interview.

Notes:

Checklist #2: Preparing for the Interview

❑ Ask if you will be interviewing with more than one person. Find out the exact names and titles of all the people who will interview you. Take extra copies of your resume with you.

❑ Find out how long the interview is expected to last. This will help you to determine how much time you have to ask your questions and provide information about yourself.

❑ If you've never been to the company before, make a trial run the day before to see how long it will take to get there. The day of the interview, give yourself plenty of time and get there early.

❑ Make sure your hands, hair, and skin are clean and well-groomed and that your clothes are pressed.

❑ Dress professionally. Minimize accessories and excess baggage. Carry only a small portfolio with copies of your resume and any other materials that demonstrate your skills and accomplishments.

❑ Bring a book or magazine to read, in case you end up waiting for your interviewer. Be judicious in your selection of reading material; comic books would be a poor choice. Remember—everything you say or do makes a statement about who you are.

❑ Prepare a list of questions that you would like to have answered during the interview. If you don't have any questions, it may appear that you are not interested in the job.

❑ Be prepared for the many questions that might be asked of you, even inappropriate ones, and rehearse your responses. If possible, ask a friend to conduct a mock interview with you and focus on difficult questions.

Notes:

Checklist #3: During the Interview

❑ Smile. It will make the interviewer think you are happy and enthusiastic, even if in reality you are nervous.

❑ Shake hands firmly and make eye contact.

❑ Exhibit poise, enthusiasm, and good manners.

❑ Think before you speak. It is perfectly OK to gather your thoughts before you respond to a question.

❑ Speak clearly and confidently and in complete sentences. Avoid using slang expressions—they may make you appear unintelligent and immature.

❑ Listen attentively—sit forward in your chair. Don't interrupt, argue, tell jokes, fidget, chew your nails, or play with your hair or jewelry.

❑ Take notes and check your list of questions to make sure that they have been answered.

❑ It is all right to ask about the salary range if your interviewer has not mentioned it. Don't ask specifics and don't discuss it any further at this stage of the interview process.

❑ Never criticize or complain about your former employer, professors, or anyone for that matter. Nobody else can understand what it was really like at your last job or in the classroom, and you will come across as a disgruntled complainer.

❑ Never lie about your credentials or abilities.

Notes:

Checklist #4: After the Interview

❏ Thank your interviewer (or interviewers) for their time and the opportunity to learn something about their company and the job.

❏ Reiterate your interest in the job if, indeed, you are still interested.

❏ Ask what the time frame is for filling the position and ask if it is OK for you to call your interviewer to check on the status of hiring.

❏ Send a thank-you note the same day or the next day at the latest.

❏ If you haven't heard from the interviewer within a week, make a follow-up call to check on your status.

Notes:

The Most Desired Job Skill in the World

by Paul Dyer

Wh-hat is the number one skill that employers look for when hiring new employees? The answer may surprise you. Certainly, employers evaluate a job candidate's educational background, his or her work-related experience, and the candidate's technical and computer skills. Employees who possess these attributes and skills help an organization achieve its strategic goals. Of course, every organization wants to achieve its goals, so employers try very hard to hire employees who possess these skills. But guess what? None of these things serves as the number one qualification that employers most desire when hiring new employees.

Employers assume that many, if not most, applicants possess enough technical knowledge to do the job. If not, employers are often willing to train employees for those aspects of the work. So what job skills do employers consider most valuable? Numerous recent studies and surveys show that the skills employers most strongly desire relate to *communication*. They want people who can transfer meaning from one human being to another; they want people who can communicate effectively. Not only do communication skills predict a new hire's likelihood of achieving initial success, but employers also promote employees with top-notch communication skills quickly.

As any employer knows, however, finding employees with good communication skills is extraordinarily difficult. One recent survey of personnel interviewers reported that only about half of those interviewing for jobs demonstrated effective communication skills. Employers are looking for skilled communicators at least as hard as you're looking for a job.

Communication Skills and the New Realities

Communication skills were not always at the top of employment recruiters' lists. In a survey conducted in 1975, employers didn't even rate communication skills as one of the top five desired job qualifications. However, just eight years later, a similar survey found that employers rated oral and written communication as the most important of all job qualifications. What changed between 1975 and 1983? A lot. In fact, by the early 1980s a whole new set of rules began to govern the world's economy. These rules continue to intensify through today.

Actions taken by Middle East oil producers on October 16, 1973, signaled profound economic changes that created these new rules. On that date, these producers decided unilaterally to raise the price of oil. The next day, OPEC agreed to cut back oil production voluntarily. Consumers felt the impact of these two actions immediately. The price of oil skyrocketed and long lines formed at gas stations around the world. Although oil prices have greatly moderated since that volatile period, the October 16, 1973, date now holds a historic place in economics. As Harvard's John Kotter has pointed out, this date serves as a point of demarcation: the day the world moved from a U.S.-dominated economy to a global economy. And, oh my, how the rules have changed.

Any organization wishing to find success in the new global economy *must* have few levels of hierarchy and empower employees to work in teams. These teams must make decisions and take action quickly in order to be very responsive to customers' needs. In the modern organization, loose boundaries exist between functions, departments, and even other organizations. More and more companies find success through partnering and joint ventures with other organizations—coming together to meet customer needs, disbanding, and then reforming into some new business arrangement.

These new realities radically changed the way businesses operate: teams, teams, and more teams; very intense global competition; greater focus on quality and customer service; more employee involvement in decision making; and a business pace approaching the speed of light. The world of work is a very dynamic place at the turn of the century! Above all, the global economy's new realities demand employees who communicate very well. As we move into the new millennium, effectively conveying ideas, information, and feelings is much more important than in the old days—even though the old days were only fifteen to twenty years ago.

Communication Defined

Three primary concepts capture the most important practical aspects of communication. First, a skilled communicator must be able to understand clearly (or decode) the messages sent by others. Second, a good communicator must be able to send (or project) messages effectively. Third, people send and receive these messages through one or more of the five senses: seeing, hearing, touching, smelling, and tasting.

How important is it that people accurately and effectively send and receive messages? Sometimes, communication errors present only a minor inconvenience, perhaps with even humorous outcomes. For example, almost all of us have played the "telephone" game. In this game, a group of people sits in a circle. One person begins by whispering a brief story in the ear of the person next to him or her. The person receiving the message then tells the same story to the next person. This communication chain continues until the last person relates the story to the individual who originated the story. The outcome is often hilarious. Participants almost always greatly distort characters' names, event times, and other significant parts of the story's content. While the game is fun, in the real world, this sort of distortion can have grave consequences. Sending the wrong messages or misunderstanding messages sent can drive customers away, create major—sometimes even life-threatening—errors, and destroy teamwork. How important are good communication skills? Once again, in today's business climate they are simply the most important skills of all. And because you're in the midst of a job search, you not only need to possess these skills, you also must be able to demonstrate to a potential employer that you have them.

Speaking Effectively

To speak effectively, you need to speak clearly and concisely both in one-on-one settings and in groups. The goal when you speak in either setting is simple enough: to get your point across. Simple, yes, but ask yourself these three important questions: How do you know when you've achieved this goal? Do you have any speaking habits that interfere with your ability to effectively convey your intended meaning? What can you do to ensure that the message you want to send is indeed the message that is received?

Before you begin speaking, create a brief outline in your mind. Determine the two or three main points you wish to make, and then make them. Throughout your conversation, or during a presentation, you should check for meaning. In other words, ask listeners to summarize what you've said. This will let you know if the listener caught your intended meaning. Confirm the points that are on target and clarify the ones that aren't.

Even though you may feel that you already speak effectively, you may unknowingly possess one or more speaking habits that annoy others. Perhaps you speak too quickly or too slowly. Maybe your speech is too loud or too soft. You may speak too formally or use too much slang. Ask a trusted friend, your spouse, or a respected colleague to provide honest feedback about your speech habits. Regardless of the feedback's content, do not become defensive. Listen carefully and receive it for what it is: a gift that will improve your communication skills. If you identify areas that need improvement, ask a friend or coworker to provide ongoing feedback on those particular areas. It's best if you receive this feedback immediately after you engage in one of the bad habits or after you show noticeable improvement. Here are several other important tips for speaking effectively:

- Make sure you balance your speaking with listening. Nothing is more annoying than participating in a conversation in which one party dominates the discussion by rambling on and on. In casual conversations, do the majority of your speaking in no more than 15- to 45-second chunks. *Very* rarely should your point exceed 1 minute in a one-on-one dialogue.

- Be sure that you understand others' meanings before you respond. Paraphrase their statements, and ask if you are correct. This way you'll be sure you understand, and you'll have a few more seconds to formulate your ideas.

- Build your vocabulary daily. On a sheet of paper, or on index cards, create a *New Words List.* Carry the list with you at all times. Each time you hear or read a word whose meaning is unfamiliar, jot it down on the *New Words List.* Find the word's definition in the dictionary, and then use the word several times the next day. Periodically review the list until the words become a part of your everyday vocabulary.

- Tape record one of your conversations or a presentation. Listen to the tape a few days later. Then identify at least one thing you can do to improve your speaking skills. Share this area with a friend, your spouse, or a colleague, and ask for ongoing feedback as you go about improving.

- To improve your presentation and public speaking skills, consider joining a Toastmasters Club. You can contact Toastmasters on the World Wide Web at www.Toastmasters.org.

- Learn to read nonverbal cues as discussed in the section on the next page.

Listening to Others

This is perhaps the most neglected, and the most important, of all communication competencies. Listening is not sitting quietly as you wait your turn to speak! It is a process that requires active participation and analysis. Listening expert Lyman Steil's four-step listening formula (SIER) serves as a great tool for quickly improving your listening performance.

Sensing. This first step forms the bedrock, the foundation, for listening. When sensing a message, you take in information from others through all of your five senses. Unfortunately, many people rush through this first step (Sensing) and on to steps three and four (Evaluating and Responding). If you fail to sense all of the relative verbal, nonverbal, and other cues, you will destroy the rest of the listening process. Your job during this step is simply to gather information.

Interpreting. Now it's time for you to decode the message. At this point you should not determine whether you agree or disagree with the speaker. You should not yet begin to formulate what you can add to the dialogue. Your essential question during the Interpreting step is, "Do we have shared meaning?" When the speaker finishes talking, you may wish to paraphrase his or her words. Move on in the listening process to the Evaluating step only after the speaker acknowledges, verbally or nonverbally, "Yes, you've got it."

Evaluating. As previously mentioned, poor listeners move much too quickly to this step and then rush on to Responding. By doing so, they very often misinterpret the content of the message. (In addition, poor listening habits can break down relationships. One of the best ways to show people that they matter, that they're important, is to listen. By not taking the time to gather information and to understand clearly the speaker's intended message, poor listeners send another, often unintended message: "You're not valued by me." Obviously, this message undermines relationship building and will lead to further deterioration of the communication process.) Again, to be a great listener, begin your evaluation of the message only after you complete Sensing and Interpreting. You can then determine whether you agree or disagree, what you can add to the dialogue, or if you need more information.

Responding. Notice the word for this step is not "reacting." Responding's roots are in the learning process, whereas reacting comes from emotions. After you take in information through your senses, interpret the message, and evaluate the content, you can decide how best to respond. Here are several other important tips for building effective listening skills:

- Eliminate as many distractions as possible. Find quiet places to conduct dialogues. Don't type, arrange papers, or anything else when on the telephone.

- Encourage others to say more through body language (e.g., smiling, sitting forward in your chair, etc.). Or use a simple statement such as, "Can you say more?"

- Don't interrupt. Listen to *all* of the speaker's words.

- Use open-ended questions or phrases to gather more information, rather than questions that can be answered with a yes or no. For example: "Tell me about," or "how did this occur," or "please explain."

- Use the reflecting technique. Also known as mirroring, this technique allows the listener to reflect the speaker's emotions without agreeing or disagreeing with the content. This technique is especially valuable in situations of conflict. Simply make a short statement that identifies the speaker's emotions and mentions something about the situation. Begin the statement with "you." For example, "You seem upset about not getting the promotion. How can I help?" Or "You appear very excited about winning the award."

- Stay in the *now*. While listening, do not think about the past and do not think about the future. Discipline yourself to actively listen and to focus on the speaker as you gather information. Departures from the *now* are devastating to the listening process.

- Use silence to foster effective communication. During presentations, or in one-on-one conversations, do *not* answer your own questions. After you ask a question, wait; count seconds in your head. Virtually no one can endure the silence for more than 8 to 10 seconds. This is one of the most useful of all communication tips. It takes discipline, but incorporating silence into your communication skills will immediately yield valuable results.

- Use self-disclosure. Share an experience similar to the one the speaker is expressing. Be open, honest, and authentic. Be careful not to engage in one-upmanship.

Nonverbal Communication

Much of the skill in sending and receiving information is unrelated to the content of the message. In other words, it's not just what you say, it's how you say it. Body language such as eye contact, facial expression, movement of the head, and posture all convey meaning. Hand gestures such as a "thumbs up," as well as voice tone, rate of speech, and volume also send powerful messages. Those with good communication skills understand these nonverbal signals and respond to them appropriately.

Nonverbals Observed	Message Sent	Most Likely Reason for the Message
Bill looking around the room during Jane's presentation	This is boring	He was not engaged in active listening

Good communicators also use appropriate nonverbals to help convey the intended message. For example, if you lean forward in your chair, maintain eye contact, and move your head up and down as someone is speaking, you make it clear that the speaker's message is one that you value.

To improve your ability to send and receive nonverbal communication, try this three-week activity. As a first step, keep a record of nonverbal behaviors you observe. On a piece of paper, create three columns with these three headings: Nonverbals Observed; Message Sent; Most Likely Reason for the Message.

During the first week, observe others' communication. During meetings, at restaurants, or in any other setting, make notes in the first column of any nonverbal behaviors you observe. Look for nonverbals such as facial expression, gestures, eye contact, and body posture. In the second column, record the message you think these nonverbal behaviors send. Finally, in the last column, write why you believe the person engaged in the nonverbal behavior.

After the first week, begin to focus on your own communication for one week. Create a second chart with the same three headings. Again, during formal meetings, group or team activities, or one-on-one dialogue, observe and record nonverbals. Note both the nonverbals others display and those you find yourself exhibiting. Again, complete the second and third columns.

At the beginning of the third week, determine the types of messages you'd like to send using nonverbal communication. Create a third chart with the same headings. Each time you *purposely* use a nonverbal, record it in the first column and then complete the last two columns. This exercise will improve your ability to both understand others' nonverbals and effectively manage your own.

In many situations, nonverbal communication skills are more important than verbal or written skills in transferring meaning. As Carol Rudman said in her engaging book *Frames of Reference,* "If your nonverbals contradict your words rather than underline them, people tend to believe the nonverbals as more trustworthy indicators of what you really mean."

Written Communication

Poor writing confuses and annoys the reader. All of us have read documents containing words, words, words . . . and little else. Poorly written e-mails, memos, letters, and reports undermine communication because they fail to transfer meaning. Effective writing is concise, clear, and to the point.

Write from a *you* perspective. Write for your audience, not for yourself. Before you begin writing, ask yourself these two questions: "What does the reader already know? How does the reader feel about me and this subject?" Throughout your writing, maintain a "you" rather than a "me" focus.

Be yourself. Don't try to copy someone else's style. "Write as you speak" serves as a good rule of thumb in business writing. Just be cautious not to become too informal.

Revise and rewrite. The great writer Robert Louis Stevenson once said, "When I say writing, oh believe me, it is rewriting I have chiefly in mind." Of course it takes time and discipline, but *rewriting* dramatically improves writing quality. Here are four good rewriting tips. First, don't procrastinate; begin writing projects early enough to allow time for revisions. Second, after you complete the work, proofread it. Make sure the writing contains no typos, misspellings, or grammatical errors. If writing on a computer, always use the spelling and grammar check. Third, ask someone whose writing you respect and enjoy reading to proof your document. If you're a technical person writing for a nontechnical audience, you should have a nontechnical person proof your materials. Fourth, as soon as possible, seek feedback about what you've written from the readers to whom you sent the information. Find out if you conveyed the message you intended to convey. Then ask, "What could I have done to make this clearer?"

Write clearly. "The potential for adequate coverage of all process factors and elements is somewhat feasible, but unlikely given our capacity limitations and our current functional alignments." Huh? As the writer David Lambuth wrote, "If you have a nail to hit, hit it on the head."

Complex sentences and flowery language will not impress readers. They will, however, stop you from communicating effectively. Put simply, if your readers don't understand your writing, you did not communicate. Along with writing from a "you" perspective, being yourself, and rewriting, here are several ideas to improve your writing clarity.

- Begin writing by outlining the key points and subpoints you wish to communicate.

- Keep your sentence length fairly short: between fifteen and eighteen words.

- Avoid jargon and acronyms. Readers unfamiliar with the terms find this particularly maddening.

- Avoid euphemisms. For example, there are no potholes in Tucson, only "pavement deficiencies."

- Only include as much detail as the reader needs.

- Finally, practice writing in the active voice to add interest and clarity to your writing. Take a look at these two sentences:
  The hiring manager is interested in Jim's job qualifications. (passive voice)
  Jim's job qualifications interest the hiring manager. (active voice)

  The second sentence is much easier to read and understand. To write in the active voice, show the action in the verb rather than in the noun. You can rewrite any passive sentence in the active voice. Here is another example:
  I am excited by this job opportunity.
  This job opportunity excites me.

Writing in the active voice will enhance your ability to communicate with clarity, interest, and power.

Demonstrating Your Communication Skills to Prospective Employers

Of course, if employers want people with good communication skills, you will want to show them that you have these skills. Employers evaluate job applicants' communication skills through three primary avenues: cover letters, resumes, and interview performance. In all three cases, employers evaluate both *content,* what is said or written, and *presentation,* how it is said or written.

In reviewing content, employers look for past achievements that demonstrate applicants' communication skills. Because employers know that past behavior is the best predictor of future behavior, applicants' achievements play an essential role in organizations' hiring decisions. Past leadership positions, speech classes or clubs, writing or speaking awards, or any other achievement requiring communication skills will gain employers' interest. Your cover letters, resume, and interview performance should reflect these past achievements.

My book, *The Ultimate Job Search Survival Guide,* provides detailed "how to" information on identifying and marketing past achievements, preparing professional cover letters and resumes, and achieving peak performance during the interview.

Practice the tips and skills presented here and you'll improve your written and oral communication skills. Improve your communication skills and you will possess the qualities most sought by employers.

Paul L. Dyer is a teacher, consultant, and author of Peterson's The Ultimate Job Search Survival Guide. *You can reach him on the World Wide Web at www.pauldyer.com.*

COMPANY
OVERVIEWS

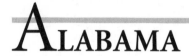

ALABAMA

Alfa Corporation

2108 E. South Blvd., Montgomery, AL 36191

Telephone: 334-288-3900 **Fax:** 334-288-0905 **Other address:** PO Box 11000, Montgomery, AL 36191 **Metro area:** Montgomery, AL **Web site:** http://www.alfains.com **Human resources contact:** Marcia Martin **Sales:** $461 million **Number of employees:** 575 **Number of employees for previous year:** 574 **Industry designation:** Insurance—life **Company type:** Public

Alfa Corporation is a financial services holding company that provides insurance through an arrangement with the Alfa Mutual Companies. About three-fourths of Alfa Corporation's insurance group revenues come from underwriting personal property and casualty insurance; offerings include life, automobile, and fire insurance, as well as coverage for homeowners and farm owners. The firm sells insurance through more than 580 agents in Alabama, Georgia, and Mississippi. Its noninsurance subsidiaries are engaged in consumer financing, real estate sales and investing, and construction.

BioCryst Pharmaceuticals, Inc.

2190 Parkway Lake Dr., Ste. B, Birmingham, AL 35244

Telephone: 205-444-4600 **Fax:** 205-444-4640 **Metro area:** Birmingham, AL **Web site:** http://www.biocryst.com **Human resources contact:** Mike Richardson **Sales:** $7.6 million **Number of employees:** 56 **Number of employees for previous year:** 55 **Industry designation:** Drugs **Company type:** Public **Top competitors:** IDEC Pharmaceuticals Corporation; Genta Incorporated; Immunomedics, Inc.

BioCryst Pharmaceuticals, a development-stage company, uses structure-based drug design to develop small-molecule pharmaceutical products for the treatment of immunological, infectious, and inflammatory diseases. Its lead product inhibits purine nucleoside phosporylase, an enzyme that activates proliferation of pathological T-cells, which can attack healthy cells and tissues; this leads to various conditions, including cutaneous T-cell lymphoma (a severe cancer), psoriasis, transplant rejection, and autoimmune diseases. BioCryst funds its research (in collaboration with the University of Alabama) through agreements with Johnson & Johnson, Torii Pharmaceutical (a subsidiary of Asahi Breweries), and Novartis.

HEALTHSOUTH Corporation

One HealthSouth Pkwy., Birmingham, AL 35243

Telephone: 205-967-7116 **Fax:** 205-969-4719 **Metro area:** Birmingham, AL **Web site:** http://www.healthsouth.com **Human resources contact:** Brandon O. Hale **Sales:** $4 billion **Number of employees:** 56,281 **Number of employees for previous year:** 36,410 **Industry designation:** Hospitals **Company type:** Public **Top competitors:** NovaCare, Inc.; Tenet Healthcare Corporation; Columbia/HCA Healthcare Corporation

HEALTHSOUTH Corporation, the nation's largest provider of rehabilitative health care and outpatient surgery services, has more than 1,800 locations in the US, the UK, and Australia. Patients receive nonemergency surgeries at its outpatient surgery centers, imaging services at its diagnostic centers, and treatments for a wide range of work-related illnesses and injuries at its occupational medicine centers. HEALTHSOUTH contracts with major insurers, managed care plans, and large employers such as Wal-Mart, Goodyear, and Dillard's. The company's aggressive growth includes acquisitions from rivals Columbia/HCA Healthcare and National Surgery Centers.

MedPartners, Inc.

3000 Galleria Tower, Ste. 1000, Birmingham, AL 35244

Telephone: 205-733-8996 **Fax:** 205-733-0704 **Metro area:** Birmingham, AL **Web site:** http:// www.medpartners.com **Human resources contact:** C. Clark Wingfield Jr. **Sales:** $2.6 billion **Number of employees:** 29,256 **Number of employees for previous year:** 20,400 **Industry designation:** Medical practice management **Company type:** Public **Top competitors:** PhyCor, Inc.; Medaphis Corporation; FPA Medical Management, Inc.

This company has partners now, but may not for long. MedPartners is the #1 US physician practice management outfit, ahead of PhyCor and FPA Medical. MedPartners provides management and administration services through long-term contracts (up to 40 years) covering more than 13,500 physicians in 42 states. Touted as a blow for physicians' rights against managed care providers, practice management has proven more difficult and less profitable than originally thought. Accordingly, the company has made plans to leave practice management and build its Caremark prescription benefits and disease management subsidiary. California regulators have seized MedPartners and placed it under Chapter 11 bankruptcy protection.

Protective Life Corporation

2801 Hwy. 280 South, Birmingham, AL 35223

Telephone: 205-879-9230 **Fax:** 205-868-3270 **Other address:** PO Box 2606, Birmingham, AL 35202 **Metro area:** Birmingham, AL **Web site:** http://www.protective.com **Human resources contact:** J. William Hamer Jr. **Sales:** $1.4 billion **Number of employees:** 1,650 **Number of employees for previous year:** 1,300 **Industry designation:** Insurance—life **Company type:** Public **Top competitors:** Jefferson-Pilot Corporation; Conseco, Inc.; Metropolitan Life Insurance Company

Protective Life wants to safeguard your future. Its subsidiaries produce, distribute, and service insurance products as well as investment and retirement plans. The company is organized along three major categories: life insurance (Acquisitions, Individual Life, and West Coast divisions), specialty insurance products (Dental and Consumer Benefits and Financial Institutions divisions), and retirement savings and investment products (Guaranteed Investment Contracts and Investment Products divisions). Protective Life acquires new policies by buying blocks of policies and small to midsized companies.

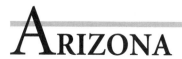

ARIZONA

Arizona Cardinals

8701 S. Hardy Dr., Tempe, AZ 85284

Telephone: 602-379-0101 **Fax:** 602-379-1819 **Other address:** PO Box 888, Phoenix, AZ 85001 **Metro area:** Phoenix, AZ **Web site:** http://www.azcardinals.com **Human resources contact:** Nancy Keenoy **Sales:** $76.9 million (Est.) **Number of employees:** 150 **Industry designation:** Leisure & recreational services **Company type:** Private **Top competitors:** Dallas Cowboys Football Club, Ltd.; Philadelphia Eagles; New York Giants

The Arizona Cardinals, perpetual laggards of the National Football Conference East, have a new strategy: cry havoc and let loose Jake "the Snake" Plummer. In the 1997 season the team finished with a 4-12 record, but rookie quarterback Jake "the Snake" set team records for passing attempts, completions, touchdown passes, and yardage. In the 1998 season, head coach Vince Tobin and "the Snake" put the bite on a number of teams and gave the Cardinals its first playoff win in more than 50 years over divisional rival the Dallas Cowboys. Founded in 1920, the Cardinals called Chicago and St. Louis home before settling in Sun Devil Stadium in Tempe, Arizona.

Arizona Diamondbacks

Bank One Ballpark, 401 E. Jefferson St., Phoenix, AZ 85004

Telephone: 602-462-6500 **Fax:** 602-462-6600 **Metro area:** Phoenix, AZ **Web site:** http://www.azdiamondbacks.com **Human resources contact:** Cheryl Naumann **Number of employees:** 300 **Number of employees for previous year:** 155 **Industry designation:** Leisure & recreational services **Company type:** Private **Top competitors:** San Diego Padres Baseball Club Limited Partnership; Los Angeles Dodgers Inc.; San Francisco Baseball Associates, L.P.

Home run hitters for the Arizona Diamondbacks can make a splash at the team's Bank One Ballpark. The state-of-the-art facility, located in downtown Phoenix, features air-conditioning, a retractable roof, and a swimming pool behind right-center field. Taking the field for the first time in 1998, the expansion team plays in the National League West. Although many young clubs build talent through farm team systems, the Diamondbacks have worked to become instantly competitive by signing veteran free agents such as Matt Williams, Jay Bell, and Randy "Big Unit" Johnson. The club's ownership group is spearheaded by CEO Jerry Colangelo, also owner and CEO of the National Basketball Association's Phoenix Suns.

Forever Living Products International, Inc.

7501 E. McCormick Pkwy. 135 South, Scottsdale, AZ 85038

Telephone: 602-998-8888 **Fax:** 602-905-8451 **Other address:** PO Box 29041, Phoenix, AZ 85038 **Metro area:** Phoenix, AZ **Web site:** http://www.foreverlivingproducts.com **Human resources contact:** Glen B. Banks **Sales:** $1.3 billion (Est.) **Number of employees:** 1,500 **Number of employees for previous year:** 1,360 **Industry designation:** Cosmetics & toiletries **Company type:** Private **Top competitors:** Nature's Sunshine Products, Inc.; Herbalife International, Inc.; Sunrider International

Although Forever Living Products International might not lead to immortality, its aloe vera-based health care products could improve your overall well-being. Founded in 1978, the firm sells an aloe vera juice drink (its first product), as well as products such as tooth gel, shampoo, lotion, deodorant, honey, and nutritional supplements. Owner Rex Maughan also owns 5,000 acres of aloe vera plantations; Aloe Vera of America, an aloe vera processor and packager; and Forever Resorts, a string of 22 resorts located throughout the US, including Dallas-area South Fork Ranch (of "Dallas" TV show fame). Forever Living Products International sells its goods through a worldwide network of independent distributors.

Harlem Globetrotters International, Inc.

400 E. Van Buren St., Ste. 300, Phoenix, AZ 85004

Telephone: 602-258-0000 **Fax:** 602-258-5925 **Metro area:** Phoenix, AZ **Web site:** http://www.harlemglobetrotters.com **Human resources contact:** Barbara Anders **Sales:** $50 million (Est.) **Number of employees:** 75 **Industry designation:** Leisure & recreational services **Company type:** Private

Harlem Globetrotters International, the clown princes of basketball, actually hail from the Chicago area; they played their first game in Hinckley, Illinois, in 1927. Known for their preternatural basketball skills, American flag uniforms, and theme song ("Sweet Georgia Brown"), the team has scored big with fans around the world. The Globetrotters have also scored some important firsts in basketball, including sending Nathaniel "Sweetwater" Clifton to the New York Knicks in 1951 to become the first black player in the NBA. Other notable Harlem Globetrotters include Wilt Chamberlain, Marques Haynes, and Michael "Wild Thing" Wilson, holder of the vertical slam dunk world record at eleven feet, eight inches.

JDA Software Group, Inc.

11811 N. Tatum Blvd., Ste. 2000, Phoenix, AZ 85028

Telephone: 602-404-5500 **Fax:** 602-404-5520 **Metro area:** Phoenix, AZ **Web site:** http://www.jdasoftware.com **Human resources contact:** Judy Wieler **Sales:** $138.5 million **Number of employees:** 683 **Number of employees for previous year:** 387 **Industry designation:** Computers—corporate, professional & financial software **Company type:** Public **Top competitors:** SAP AG; System Software Associates, Inc.; QAD Inc.

JDA Software Group makes software that helps retailers track and analyze inventory and sales. Products include merchandising, financial, and decision-support systems at the corporate level; point-of-sale applications at store level; and logistics and warehouse management systems at the distribution level. JDA's software can also track prices, perform accounting functions, and order more merchandise when inventory is low. The company's salesforce sells directly to a variety of retailers, department and grocery stores, and warehouse operations in more than 30 countries. International sales account for about half of sales.

Managed Care Solutions, Inc.

7600 N. 16th St., Ste. 150, Phoenix, AZ 85020

Telephone: 602-331-5100 **Fax:** 602-331-5911 **Metro area:** Phoenix, AZ **Web site:** http://www.mcsx.com **Human resources contact:** Rita Console **Sales:** $66 million **Number of employees:** 624 **Number of employees for previous year:** 486 **Industry designation:** Health maintenance organization **Company type:** Public **Top competitors:** Tenet Healthcare Corporation; PacifiCare Health Systems, Inc.; Catholic Healthcare West

Managed Care Solutions helps look out for poor and elderly people and people with disabilities. The company operates two HMOs in Arizona: Ventana Health Systems, which serves some 1,200 long-term-care Medicaid patients, and Arizona Health Concepts, which serves some 7,800 acute care Medicaid recipients in two counties. The company also administers HMOs in Hawaii, Michigan, New Mexico, and Texas and holds contracts for indigent care with the County of San Diego and the State of Indiana. It manages on-site clinical services to nursing homes and provides in-home, unskilled services for patients in Arizona. Other programs include contract consulting and feasibility studies.

Medicis Pharmaceutical Corporation

4343 E. Camelback Rd., Ste. 250, Phoenix, AZ 85018

Telephone: 602-808-8800 **Fax:** 602-808-0822 **Metro area:** Phoenix, AZ **Web site:** http://www.medicis.com **Human resources contact:** Adriane Young **Sales:** $77.6 million **Number of employees:** 125 **Number of employees for previous year:** 89 **Industry designation:** Drugs **Company type:** Public **Top competitors:** Glaxo Wellcome plc; Schering-Plough Corporation; American Home Products Corporation

Medicis Pharmaceutical is in the skin trade. The company markets over-the-counter skin products, including Esoterica creams and moisturizers, Theraplex dry skin treatments, Zostrix topical analgesic, Pentrax dandruff shampoo, Occlusal wart treatment, and SalAc face wash. Medicis also sells such prescription and doctor-dispensed products as Dynacin, Theramycin Z, Triaz, and Novacet acne medicines and the anti-itch remedy Zonalon. To save on costs, the company farms out its manufacturing and limits research. Medicis sells primarily to wholesale distributors. It has a joint venture with IMX Pharmaceutical to market psoriasis drugs, and also licenses dermatological products from Hoechst Marion Roussel in the US.

NextHealth, Inc.

16600 N. Lago del Oro Pkwy., Tucson, AZ 85739

Telephone: 520-792-5800 **Fax:** 520-792-5884 **Metro area:** Tucson, AZ **Web site:** http://www.nexthealth.com **Sales:** $26.3 million **Number of employees:** 343 **Number of employees for previous year:** 310 **Industry designation:** Medical services **Company type:** Public **Top competitors:** Magellan Health Services, Inc.; Vail Resorts, Inc.; HEALTHSOUTH Corporation

NextHealth offers psychological treatment ranging from drug rehabilitation to simple stress reduction. The company offers its services through two facilities located northwest of Tucson, near the Santa Catalina Mountains. The 70-bed Sierra Tucson facility offers treatment for substance abuse, behavioral problems, and psychological disorders, including eating disorders. Its Miraval property (with more than 100 beds) offers a vacation alternative, emphasizing emotional growth, stress reduction, and recreation in a resort environment. Entities affiliated with Leon Black control about 38% of NextHealth.

Orthopaedic Biosystems Ltd., Inc.

15990 N. Greenway-Hayden Loop, Ste. 100, Scottsdale, AZ 85260

Telephone: 602-596-4066 **Fax:** 602-596-2180 **Metro area:** Phoenix, AZ **Web site:** http://www.oblinc.com **Human resources contact:** Melody Martin **Sales:** $1.5 million (Est.) **Number of employees:** 19 **Industry designation:** Medical instruments **Company type:** Private

People who've put their shoulders to the wheel once too often may need what Orthopaedic Biosystems offers. It makes suture anchors, which are used to reattach soft tissue to bone, primarily to repair shoulder rotator cuff injuries. The company hopes to expand the anchors' uses to knee, hand, and foot surgery, and it licenses the technology to Mentor for urological applications, and Imcor for use in dental implants. Orthopaedic Biosystems also makes surgical screws and distributes arthroscopic instruments made by T.A.G. Medical Products. The company is developing products to join soft tissues and a remote-surgery knot substitute. Co-founders Ronald Yagoda and Kerry Zang each own about a third of the company.

Osage Systems Group, Inc.

1661 E. Camelback Rd., Ste. 245, Phoenix, AZ 85016

Telephone: 602-274-1299 **Fax:** 602-274-1295 **Metro area:** Phoenix, AZ **Web site:** http://www.osage.com **Sales:** $14.2 million **Number of employees:** 70 **Industry designation:** Computers—services **Company type:** Public

Osage Systems Group (formerly Pacific Rim Entertainment) provides information technology services and support to a wide range of clients, primarily in Arizona, Southern California, and Texas. Its services, which emphasize Sun Microsystems and Oracle products integration, include system architecture and design, product acquisition, configuration and implementation, and operational support throughout the life cycle of its clients' systems. Customers include companies in the semiconductor, manufacturing, and publishing industries, as well as the military. Osage has value added reseller agreements with Sun Microsystems, Oracle, and Cisco Systems, among others.

Pentegra Dental Group, Inc.

2999 N. 44th St., Ste. 650, Phoenix, AZ 85018

Telephone: 602-952-1200 **Fax:** 602-952-0544 **Metro area:** Phoenix, AZ **Web site:** http://www.pentegradental.com **Number of employees:** 3 **Industry designation:** Medical practice management **Company type:** Public **Top competitors:** Monarch Dental Corporation; Castle Dental Centers, Inc.

Pentegra Dental Group wants to manage dental practices across the US and let dentists concentrate on cavities and root canals. It provides clients with billing and collection services, inventory management, purchasing, invoice and payroll processing, patient scheduling, and financial reporting and analysis. Pentegra Dental Group has service agreements with nearly 80 practices that staff about 120 dentists in 26 states. Clients include periodontists, oral surgeons, and pedodontists as well as general dentists. Pentegra's other operations consist of Pentegra, Ltd., a consulting firm, and Napili International, a seminar company.

Phoenix Coyotes Hockey Club

Cellular One Ice Den, 9375 E. Bell Rd., Scottsdale, AZ 85260

Telephone: 602-473-5600 **Fax:** 602-473-5699 **Metro area:** Phoenix, AZ **Web site:** http://www.nhlcoyotes.com/home.shtml **Human resources contact:** Mark Peterson **Sales:** $41.2 million (Est.) **Number of employees:** 120 **Industry designation:** Leisure & recreational services **Company type:** Private **Top competitors:** Dallas Stars L.P.; San Jose Sharks L.P.; Los Angeles Kings

Believe it or not, hockey isn't indigenous to Arizona. Nevertheless, the National Hockey League's Phoenix Coyotes Hockey Club makes the Sunbelt state its home. The Coyotes (formerly the Winnipeg Jets) made their way to Arizona in 1996 after Richard Burke and Steven Gluckstern bought the team and restructured it. The owners also gave the retooled team a new mascot, suggestive of southwestern decor gone terribly awry—Coyote colors include brick red, hunter green, sienna, and purple. In 1998 Gluckstern left to purchase the New York Islanders, leaving Burke as sole owner. The club, which has filled the America West Arena to 97% capacity the past two years, intends to renovate the arena or move to a larger one.

Phoenix Suns

201 E. Jefferson St., Phoenix, AZ 85004

Telephone: 602-379-7900 **Fax:** 602-379-7922 **Other address:** PO Box 1369, Phoenix, AZ 85001 **Metro area:** Phoenix, AZ **Web site:** http://www.nba.com/suns **Human resources contact:** Cheryl Naumann **Sales:** $87 million (Est.) **Number of employees:** 100 **Industry designation:** Leisure & recreational services **Company type:** Private **Top competitors:** Portland Trail Blazers; Seattle SuperSonics; California Sports, Inc.

The Phoenix Suns quietly entered the NBA in 1968, fronted by a group of celebrity investors that included Tony Curtis, Henry Mancini, and Andy Williams. In the early 1970s the Suns rode the wings of Connie "the Hawk" Hawkins, a playground legend previously banned from the NBA amidst betting allegations. Phoenix lost the 1976 NBA title to the Boston Celtics in a series that included a legendary three-overtime loss. It wasn't until 1993 that the Suns reached the finals again, this time with the help of league MVP "Sir Charles" Barkley. (The team lost to the Chicago Bulls.) The team is owned by president and CEO Jerry Colangelo, who also owns the Arizona Diamondbacks baseball team.

quepasa.com, inc.

1 Arizona Center, 400 E. Van Buren, 4th Fl., Phoenix, AZ 85004

Telephone: 602-716-0106 **Metro area:** Phoenix, AZ **Web site:** http://www.quepasa.com **Number of employees:** 34 **Industry designation:** Computers—online services **Company type:** Private **Top competitors:** America Online, Inc.; Yahoo! Inc.; Microsoft Corporation

Here's a search engine for people who prefer surfing "La Red Mundial" to the World Wide Web. The quepasa.com Web site caters to Spanish-speaking Internet users, offering a search engine, news links, free e-mail, and chat rooms all "en Espanol" (although the company does provide an English version of its site as well). quepasa.com also offers links to a variety of subject-related Web sites such as art and culture, entertainment, and sports and recreation. It hopes to garner revenue through advertising and eventually through sales of products and services to its Spanish-speaking clientele. After a planned IPO, Chairman and CEO Jeffrey Peterson will own about 11% of the company.

Rural/Metro Corporation

8401 E. Indian School Rd., Scottsdale, AZ 85251

Telephone: 602-994-3886 **Fax:** 602-481-3328 **Metro area:** Phoenix, AZ **Web site:** http://www.ruralmetro.com **Human resources contact:** Robert B. Hillier **Sales:** $475.6 million **Number of employees:** 12,250 **Number of employees for previous year:** 9,200 **Industry designation:** Medical services **Company type:** Public **Top competitors:** Columbia/HCA Healthcare Corporation; Tenet Healthcare Corporation; American Medical Response

Incoming! Rural/Metro provides ambulance, fire protection, and other safety-related services to municipal, residential, commercial, and industrial customers in the US. The #2 private ambulance service provider in the US (behind American Medical Response), the company responds to emergency calls and offers non-emergency transport between care facilities. Fees collected for ambulance services account for more than 80% of sales. Also the US's #1 private fire service, Rural/Metro provides municipal and commercial firefighting services and trains firefighters for industrial manufacturing facilities. The company provides its services to more than 450 communities in 26 states, Canada, Mexico, and South America.

SalesLogix Corporation

8800 N. Gainey Center Dr., Ste. 200, Scottsdale, AZ 85258

Telephone: 602-368-3700 **Fax:** 602-368-3799 **Metro area:** Phoenix, AZ **Web site:** http://www.saleslogix.com **Human resources contact:** Durlinda Fulkerson **Sales:** $15.6 million (Est.) **Number of employees:** 146 **Industry designation:** Computers—corporate, professional & financial software **Company type:** Private **Top competitors:** The Vantive Corporation; Siebel Systems, Inc.; Microsoft Corporation

SalesLogix is an orderly sort of company. It makes sales automation and customer service software designed primarily for midsized companies. The company's flagship software (SalesLogix) is used by sales professionals to manage and share information about contacts, accounts, and orders. Customer service call centers use SupportLogix to track customer contacts including problem and resolution information. SalesLogix's more than 1,100 customers include technology (Hewlett-Packard), financial services (Paine Webber Group), retail (Tiffany & Co.), telecommunications (MCI WorldCom), and real estate (Del Webb) companies. Investors include Goldman Sachs, Sierra Ventures, and Sigma Partners.

SC&T International, Inc.

15695 N. 83rd Way, Scottsdale, AZ 85260

Telephone: 602-368-9490 **Fax:** 602-607-6801 **Metro area:** Phoenix, AZ **Web site:** http://www.per4mer.com/sct.htm **Human resources contact:** Catherine Copland **Sales:** $4.7 million **Number of employees:** 23 **Number of employees for previous year:** 12 **Industry designation:** Computers—peripheral equipment **Company type:** Public **Top competitors:** Nintendo Co., Ltd.; ThrustMaster, Inc.; Sony Corporation

Kids probably don't know it, but SC&T International might just be their best friend. The company makes sound enhancement products, racing wheels, and game controllers compatible with IBM PCs and SEGA, Nintendo, and Sony PlayStation consoles. Available at retailers such as Best Buy, CompUSA, and Radio Shack, SC&T's products are marketed under the Platinum Sound, Per4mer, Air-Racer, and Hot Wheels names. Among SC&T's offerings is the Air-Racer controller, which responds to the movements of the player's hands and eliminates the use of a thumb pad. Chairman and CEO James Copland and his wife, Catherine (secretary), own 43% of the company.

Styling Technology Corporation

7400 E. Tierra Buena Ln., Scottsdale, AZ 85260

Telephone: 602-609-6000 **Fax:** 602-609-6001 **Metro area:** Phoenix, AZ **Human resources contact:** Kimber Summers **Sales:** $90.4 million **Number of employees:** 195 **Number of employees for previous year:** 101 **Industry designation:** Cosmetics & toiletries **Company type:** Public

Styling Technology develops, produces, and markets professional salon products, including hair, nail, skin, and body care products, salon appliances, and salon wear. The company's customers include beauty and tanning supply distributors, as well as spas, resorts, health and country clubs, beauty salon chains, and hair, nail, and tanning salons. Its products include Body Drench skin care and tanning products, Gena Warm-O-Lotion and Alpha 9 nail care products, and SRC salon appliance products. The merchandise is distributed throughout the US, as well as in Europe, Argentina, Australia, Canada, and New Zealand. Styling Technology has been growing through acquisitions of complementary companies.

Sunquest Information Systems, Inc.

4801 E. Broadway Blvd., Tucson, AZ 85711

Telephone: 520-570-2000 **Fax:** 520-570-2494 **Metro area:** Tucson, AZ **Web site:** http://www.sunquest.com **Human resources contact:** Marsha Morgan **Sales:** $120.8 million **Number of employees:** 899 **Number of employees for previous year:** 828 **Industry designation:** Computers—corporate, professional & financial software **Company type:** Public **Top competitors:** McKesson HBOC, Inc.; IDX Systems Corporation; Shared Medical Systems Corporation

Sunquest Information Systems helps health care providers keep tabs on you. It provides scalable hardware and software for health care information systems used by large and midsized hospitals, clinics, and other health care agencies. Its products integrate equipment; automate laboratory, radiology, and pharmacy processes; and manage high-volume data. The firm's FlexiMed inpatient pharmacy software monitors diagnoses, treatments, inventory, and clinical results. Sunquest, which also provides consulting services, has installed its computer systems at about 1,100 sites in Canada, Europe, Mexico, Saudi Arabia, and the US. Founder and CEO Sidney Goldblatt owns 77% of Sunquest and CFO Nina Dmetruk owns 32%.

Ventana Medical Systems, Inc.

3865 N. Business Center Dr., Tucson, AZ 85705

Telephone: 520-887-2155 **Fax:** 520-887-2558 **Metro area:** Tucson, AZ **Web site:** http://www.ventanamed.com **Human resources contact:** Christopher Payne **Sales:** $47.7 million **Number of employees:** 211 **Number of employees for previous year:** 135 **Industry designation:** Medical instruments **Company type:** Public **Top competitors:** BioGenex Laboratories, Inc.; Thermo Instrument Systems Inc.; Leica AG

Ventana Medical Systems products perform automated processing and microscopic analysis of human tissue for cancer treatment. About 1,200 systems are used in 36 of the 42 principal cancer research centers identified by the National Cancer Institute, including the Mayo Clinic, Johns Hopkins University, and the M.D. Anderson and the Memorial Sloan-Kettering cancer centers. Ventana NexES systems perform multiple tests on a single patient biopsy;TechMate batch processing systems perform high volumes of single tests on multiple patient biopsies. Subsidiary BioTechnology Tools makes tissue processing and slicing products. Ventana sells its instruments and reagents directly in North America, Europe, and Japan.

VIASOFT, Inc.

3033 N. 44th St., Phoenix, AZ 85018

Telephone: 602-952-0050 **Fax:** 602-840-4068 **Metro area:** Phoenix, AZ **Web site:** http://www.viasoft.com **Human resources contact:** Nancy Mattson **Sales:** $113.7 million **Number of employees:** 561 **Number of employees for previous year:** 447 **Industry designation:** Computers—corporate, professional & financial software **Company type:** Public **Top competitors:** Accelr8 Technology Corporation; SEEC, Inc.; International Business Machines Corporation

With the millennium just around the corner, VIASOFT sells year 2000 date conversion products and develops and licenses mainframe software for large customers. Its OnMark 2000 software (about 50% of sales) helps customers address year 2000 problems while giving VIASOFT an entry for sales of its other products. The company's Existing Systems Workbench, an integrated suite of products for IBM-compatible mainframes, lets users manage and redevelop software applications. Customers include large corporations and government agencies. VIASOFT is moving away from year 2000 products and into other software markets.

Zila, Inc.

5227 N. Seventh St., Phoenix, AZ 85014

Telephone: 602-266-6700 **Fax:** 602-234-2264 **Metro area:** Phoenix, AZ **Web site:** http://www.zila.com **Human resources contact:** Janice L. Backus **Sales:** $62.1 million **Number of employees:** 212 **Number of employees for previous year:** 138 **Industry designation:** Drugs **Company type:** Public **Top competitors:** Patterson Dental Company; Del Laboratories, Inc.; DENTSPLY International Inc.

Zila has an oral fixation. Subsidiary Zila Pharmaceuticals sells over-the-counter treatments for mouth sores, chapped lips, and teething pain under the Zilactin name. OraTest, a product to diagnose oral cancer, is approved for sale in several international markets and is awaiting approval from the FDA. Subsidiary Zila Dental Supply offers dentists 20,000 products through telemarketing and direct mail. Subsidiary Cygnus makes intraoral cameras and other dental imaging products. Subsidiary Integrated Dental Technologies sells a Windows-compatible software system for managing dental practices. The company also makes vitamin C and manufactures toluidine, the main ingredient in its cancer tests.

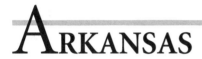

ARKANSAS

Deltic Timber Corporation

210 E. Elm St., El Dorado, AR 71731

Telephone: 870-881-9400 **Fax:** 870-864-6565 **Other address:** PO Box 7200, El Dorado, AR 71731 **Human resources contact:** Carol McKinnon **Sales:** $107 million **Number of employees:** 492 **Number of employees for previous year:** 344 **Industry designation:** Agricultural operations **Company type:** Public **Top competitors:** Georgia-Pacific Group; Louisiana-Pacific Corporation; Weyerhaeuser Company

Deltic Timber grows and harvests timber. The company owns about 370,000 acres of timberland in Arkansas and Louisiana, as well as two mills in Arkansas. Timber is either sold or converted into lumber, which is then sold for use primarily in residential construction. Deltic's other business activities include development of a planned community near Little Rock and farming of cotton, soybeans, corn, and wheat on about 36,000 acres of farmland in northern Louisiana. Deltic also owns 50% of a medium-density fiberboard plant under construction in Arkansas. The company was spun off from Murphy Oil in 1996.

Murphy Oil Corporation

200 Peach St., El Dorado, AR 71731

Telephone: 870-862-6411 **Fax:** 870-864-6373 **Other address:** PO Box 7000, El Dorado, AR 71731 **Web site:** http://www.murphyoilcorp.com **Human resources contact:** Dana Green **Sales:** $1.7 billion **Number of employees:** 1,566 **Number of employees for previous year:** 1,338 **Industry designation:** Oil & gas—exploration & production **Company type:** Public

Murphy Oil explores for oil and natural gas worldwide, refines and markets oil in the US and UK, and conducts Canadian pipeline and crude oil trading operations. Exploration takes place in Bangladesh, Brazil, Canada, China, Denmark, Ecuador, the Falkland Islands, the Faroe Islands, Ireland, Pakistan, Peru, the UK, the US, Venezuela, and the Caspian Sea. The firm also owns and operates US and UK refineries; produces and sells natural gas in Canada, the US, and the UK; and distributes its products under the Murphy USA, SPUR, Murco, and EP brands. It has about 4,600 oil wells and 1,100 gas wells with estimated proved reserves of 220.3 million barrels of oil and 643.6 billion cu. ft. of gas.

Professional Dental Technologies, Inc.

633 Lawrence St., Batesville, AR 72501

Telephone: 870-698-2300 **Fax:** 870-793-5554 **Web site:** http://www.prodentec.com **Human resources contact:** Ernestine Doucet **Sales:** $27.5 million **Number of employees:** 350 **Number of employees for previous year:** 332 **Industry designation:** Medical instruments **Company type:** Public **Top competitors:** The Gillette Company; Conair Corporation; Optiva Corporation

Got plaque buildup? Call Roto-Rooter's cousin, Rota-dent. Professional Dental Technologies' instruments and products diagnose, treat, and prevent dental diseases. Rota-dent (65% of the company's sales) is an electric plaque-removal and teeth-cleaning device used by patients between checkups. Its Pro-Select-3 ultrasonic scaler removes deposits from teeth and roots. Professional Dental also produces voice-activated dental charting software, dental-practice management software, image archiving and cosmetic imaging systems, fluoride rinses and gels, and periodontal probes. The company is controlled by owned by president and CEO William Evans, director Timothy Nolan, and director J. Robert Lemon.

Tyson Foods, Inc.

2210 W. Oaklawn Dr., Springdale, AR 72762

Telephone: 501-290-4000 **Fax:** 501-290-4061 **Metro area:** Fayetteville, AR **Web site:** http://www.tyson.com **Human resources contact:** William P. Jaycox **Sales:** $7.4 billion **Number of employees:** 70,500 **Number of employees for previous year:** 59,400 **Industry designation:** Food—meat products **Company type:** Public **Top competitors:** Gold Kist Inc.; ConAgra, Inc.; Perdue Farms Incorporated

When it comes to pressing its advantage as the nation's #1 poultry producer, Tyson Foods is no chicken. Tyson breeds, processes, and markets chickens and Cornish game hens (chicken accounts for 85% of sales). It also produces tortillas and chips (Mexican Original), seafood, and animal and pet feed, and it raises swine. Tyson sells its products in nearly 60 countries, with food service customers accounting for half of sales. After snapping up embattled meat processor Hudson Foods, Tyson is trimming some fat, exiting noncore operations (pork, seafood) to focus on its poultry business. Senior chairman Don Tyson, son of the founder, owns 44% of the company and controls nearly 90% of the voting power.

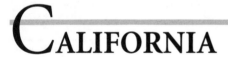

CALIFORNIA

Abgenix, Inc.

7601 Dumbarton Circle, Fremont, CA 94555

Telephone: 510-608-6500 **Fax:** 510-608-6511 **Metro area:** San Francisco, CA **Web site:** http://www.abgenix.com **Human resources contact:** Priti Patel **Sales:** $3.8 million **Number of employees:** 61 **Number of employees for previous year:** 57 **Industry designation:** Drugs **Company type:** Public

Abgenix uses genetically engineered strains of mice to develop antibody therapeutic products for the prevention and treatment of inflammatory and autoimmune disorders, cancer, and transplant-related diseases. The biopharmaceutical company has developed four antibody product candidates through XenoMouse technology (rights acquired through a joint venture with Japan Tobacco). Two candidates undergoing human clinical trials are ABX-CBL to treat transplant-rejection disorders and ABX-IL8 for psoriasis treatment. The company has alliances with Pfizer, Millennium BioTherapeutics, and Schering-Plough Research Institute. Cell Genesys will reduce its share of the company from about 55% to about 40% after the planned IPO.

AboveNet Communications, Inc.

50 W. San Fernando St., Ste. 1010, San Jose, CA 95113

Telephone: 408-367-6666 **Fax:** 408-367-6688 **Metro area:** San Francisco, CA **Web site:** http://www.abovenet.com **Human resources contact:** Barbara Meese **Sales:** $3.4 million **Number of employees:** 71 **Industry designation:** Computers—online services **Company type:** Public **Top competitors:** Exodus Communications, Inc.; Frontier Corporation; Hiway Technologies, Inc.

AboveNet Communications provides outsourced Internet hosting and connectivity services (often dubbed "co-location" or "co-hosting") to companies that depend on the Web to do business. AboveNet combines fault-tolerant facilities in California and Virginia with direct Internet service provider (ISP) access to reduce the number of network connections, or hops, data must make as it is transmitted. Its 300 customers include Supernews (Web discussion and access services, 14% of sales), Liquid Audio (online music delivery), and Internet Gateway (a Canadian ISP). AboveNet markets its services through a direct sales force and through partnerships with value-added resellers, system integrators, and Web hosting services.

ACCPAC International, Inc.

2525 Augustine Dr., Santa Clara, CA 95054

Telephone: 408-562-8400 **Fax:** 408-562-8740 **Metro area:** San Francisco, CA **Web site:** http://www.accpac.com **Human resources contact:** Christine Stell **Sales:** $48.9 million **Number of employees:** 244 **Industry designation:** Computers—corporate, professional & financial software **Company type:** Subsidiary **Top competitors:** Oracle Corporation; Lawson Software; Great Plains Software, Inc.

ACCPAC International develops and markets business management software for small to midsized businesses and for small or home offices. ACCPAC for Windows is the company's accounting software package, available in corporate and small-business versions; it includes applications for financial and operations management. Corporate users have the option to install the company's e.Advantage Server, which enables Internet transactions. Another product, Simply Accounting, is designed to simplify bookkeeping for home office use. ACCPAC International sells its products through a network of value-added resellers, qualified installers, distributors, and others, mostly in the US and Canada.

Active Software, Inc.

3255-1 Scott Blvd., Santa Clara, CA 95054

Telephone: 408-988-0414 **Fax:** 408-988-6607 **Metro area:** San Francisco, CA **Web site:** http://www.activesw.com **Human resources contact:** Andrea Killam **Sales:** $10 million (Est.) **Number of employees:** 75 **Industry designation:** Computers—corporate, professional & financial software **Company type:** Private **Top competitors:** CACI International Inc; Unisys Corporation; Telos Corporation

Active Software doesn't tackle systems integration lying down. Founded in 1995, the company makes systems integration software for combining applications and performing large-scale system upgrades. Its customizable Integration System software stores, queues, and routes events; connects resources; and has tools for system configuration, management, and monitoring. It also offers specific integration programs for customer service, e-commerce, enterprise resource planning, and supply chain management. Active Software has partnerships with industry leaders including Cisco and Sun Microsystems. Founders Jim Green (CEO) and Rafael Bracho (chief technology officer) own the company.

Acuson Corporation

1220 Charleston Rd., Mountain View, CA 94043

Telephone: 650-969-9112 **Fax:** 650-961-4726 **Other address:** PO Box 7393, Mountain View, CA 94039 **Metro area:** San Francisco, CA **Web site:** http://www.acuson.com **Human resources contact:** Charles H. "Chase" Dearborn **Sales:** $455.1 million **Number of employees:** 1,815 **Number of employees for previous year:** 1,777 **Industry designation:** Medical instruments **Company type:** Public **Top competitors:** Elscint Limited; Hologic, Inc.

Acuson is a leading maker of ultrasound imaging equipment used by hospitals, clinics, and other health care facilities for radiological, cardiological, obstetrical/gynecological, and peripheral vascular applications. More than 13,000 of the company's Acuson 128 ultrasound systems have been sold. Other products include the Aspen ultrasound system, based on a new digital architecture; the Sequoia ultrasound system, which offers image clarity competitive with MRI and CAT scans; and the AEGIS system, which stores and manages ultrasound data. About 22% of Acuson's sales are outside the US. Investor and Acuson director Karl Johannsmeier owns about 18% of the company.

ADAC Laboratories

540 Alder Dr., Milpitas, CA 95035

Telephone: 408-321-9100 **Fax:** 408-321-9686 **Metro area:** San Francisco, CA **Web site:** http://www.adaclabs.com **Human resources contact:** Judy Rowe **Sales:** $300.5 million **Number of employees:** 1,031 **Number of employees for previous year:** 880 **Industry designation:** Medical instruments **Company type:** Public **Top competitors:** Royal Philips Electronics; Siemens AG; Elscint Limited

ADAC Laboratories is the US's top manufacturer of medical imaging equipment used in nuclear medicine. The company uses a gamma camera to detect radioisotopes administered to patients to screen for cancer and cardiac disease. The company also provides radiation therapy planning systems, which help cancer treatment centers determine the ideal radiation treatment for each patient. ADAC distributes and refurbishes nuclear medicine systems and computed tomography (or CT scanning) systems made by other companies. ADAC's software segment's products allows companies to archive, integrate, and process patient and laboratory information; the unit accounts for about a quarter of sales.

Adaptec, Inc.

691 S. Milpitas Blvd., Milpitas, CA 95035

Telephone: 408-945-8600 **Fax:** 408-262-2533 **Metro area:** San Francisco, CA **Web site:** http://www.adaptec.com **Human resources contact:** E. J. Tim Harris **Sales:** $1 billion **Number of employees:** 3,276 **Number of employees for previous year:** 2,794 **Industry designation:** Computers—peripheral equipment **Company type:** Public **Top competitors:** Hewlett-Packard Company; Digi International Inc.; Oak Technology, Inc.

Adaptec makes hardware and software that speed data transfer between computers, peripherals, and networks. The company dominates the market for SCSI (small computer system interface) technology, which enables several peripheral devices to connect to one adapter card. Adaptec sells its host adapters, network interface cards, storage controllers, and other systems to Compaq, Dell, IBM, and other makers of computers and peripherals. Its DirectCD software allows data to be written to CD-recordable media. Adaptec has a plant in Singapore and business operations in Asia, Europe, and the US.

ADI Systems, Inc.

2115 Ringwood Ave., San Jose, CA 95131

Telephone: 408-944-0100 **Fax:** 408-944-0300 **Metro area:** San Francisco, CA **Web site:** http://www.adiusa.com **Human resources contact:** Jenny Trankle **Sales:** $1.1 billion (Est.) **Number of employees:** 3,000 **Number of employees for previous year:** 2,500 **Industry designation:** Computers—peripheral equipment **Company type:** Private **Top competitors:** ViewSonic Corporation; NEC Corporation; Sony Corporation

ADI Systems, the North American subsidiary of Taiwan-based color computer monitor magnate ADI Corporation, hopes you look at one of its products every time you turn on a computer. ADI offers models for use at home, in business, and for computer-aided design, graphic design, and multimedia. Founded in 1979, the company prides itself on innovation, pioneering award-winning technology, and its graphics-intensive MicroScan series. ADI also offers the ProVista line for business and home office use. The company sells its products through distributors, manufacturers, and resellers; it also offers technical and customer support over the phone and online.

Advanced Materials Group, Inc.

20211 S. Susana Rd., Rancho Dominguez, CA 90221

Telephone: 310-537-5444 **Fax:** 310-537-4557 **Metro area:** Los Angeles, CA **Web site:** http://www.advmatl.com **Human resources contact:** Suzie Cooley **Sales:** $28.9 million **Number of employees:** 134 **Number of employees for previous year:** 117 **Industry designation:** Chemicals—specialty **Company type:** Public **Top competitors:** Carpenter Co.; Span-America Medical Systems, Inc.; Minnesota Mining and Manufacturing Company

Advanced Materials Group (AMG) has a cushy job. The company converts raw materials such as foam, foil, film, and pressure-sensitive adhesive components into a variety of products, including padding and cushions for helmets, soft luggage, and neck braces. Other offerings include foam inserts and inking felts for computer printer cartridges, car air-conditioner insulators, water and dust seals, and surgical pads. The company's custom manufactured products and components are used in the automotive, electronics, consumer, and medical products markets in the US (91% of sales) and abroad. AMG operates plants in the US (California, Colorado, Oregon, and Texas), Ireland, and Singapore.

Advanced Polymer Systems, Inc.

123 Saginaw Dr., Redwood City, CA 94063

Telephone: 650-366-2626 **Fax:** 650-365-6490 **Metro area:** San Francisco, CA **Web site:** http://www.advancedpolysys.com **Human resources contact:** Shelly Howell **Sales:** $20 million **Number of employees:** 94 **Number of employees for previous year:** 84 **Industry designation:** Medical products **Company type:** Public **Top competitors:** Johnson & Johnson; R.P. Scherer Corporation; Schering-Plough Corporation

Advanced Polymer Systems' patented substances include an improved formula (less irritating to skin) for Retin-A (a leading prescription acne medication), and they are sold worldwide by major companies like Avon and Johnson & Johnson. The company's inventions include its patented Microsponge and Polytrap delivery systems, which use microscopic, sponge-like chemical compounds to ease application of skin care products or to release ingredients (medication). Products in development include Melanin-Microsponge Sunscreen and 5-Fluorouracil, for the potential treatment of precancerous skin conditions.

Adventist Health

2100 Douglas Blvd., Roseville, CA 95661

Telephone: 916-781-2000 **Fax:** 916-783-9909 **Other address:** PO Box 619002, Roseville, CA 95661 **Metro area:** Sacramento, CA **Web site:** http://www.adventisthealth.org **Human resources contact:** Roger Ashley **Sales:** $1.1 billion **Number of employees:** 16,567 **Number of employees for previous year:** 15,351 **Industry designation:** Hospitals **Company type:** Not-for-profit **Top competitors:** Kaiser Foundation Health Plan, Inc.; Tenet Healthcare Corporation; Columbia/HCA Healthcare Corporation

They even stay open on Sundays. Adventist Health is a not-for-profit health care system with strong ties (financially, organizationally, and spiritually) to the Seventh-Day Adventist Church. The West Coast wing of an international organization operating more than 160 Adventist health care operations, Adventist Health runs about 20 Adventist hospitals (with some 2,900 beds), almost 20 home health services facilities, and various other outpatient facilities and hospices in California, Hawaii, Oregon, Utah, and Washington. The organization also works with its own churches and those of other denominations to offer preventative health care such as physical exams, prenatal care, and health education.

Advent Software, Inc.

301 Brannan St., San Francisco, CA 94107

Telephone: 415-543-7696 **Fax:** 415-543-5070 **Metro area:** San Francisco, CA **Web site:** http://www.advent.com **Human resources contact:** Lisa Ebersole **Sales:** $71 million **Number of employees:** 481 **Number of employees for previous year:** 325 **Industry designation:** Computers—corporate, professional & financial software **Company type:** Public **Top competitors:** DST Systems, Inc.; The Thomson Corporation; SunGard Data Systems Inc.

Decisions, decisions. Advent Software is a leading provider of software products that automate and integrate the investment management process. Its flagship product, Axys, helps customers decide about and track investments. Other products include Rex (automated reconciliation of multiple bank accounts), Moxy (trading and order management), Qube (client contact management), and WebView (Internet investment tracking). Customers include investment advisers, brokerage firms, banks, and universities. Through acquisitions, the company now also offers software for charitable organizations. Advent licenses its products to more than 4,500 institutions in more than 20 countries, representing about 25,000 users.

Affymetrix, Inc.

3380 Central Expwy., Santa Clara, CA 95051

Telephone: 408-731-5000 **Fax:** 408-481-0422 **Metro area:** San Francisco, CA **Web site:** http://www.affymetrix.com **Human resources contact:** Karen Hayes **Sales:** $52 million **Number of employees:** 321 **Number of employees for previous year:** 242 **Industry designation:** Instruments—scientific **Company type:** Public **Top competitors:** Abbott Laboratories; The Perkin-Elmer Corporation; Nycomed Amersham plc

Affymetrix's GeneChip system identifies, analyzes, and manages complex genetic information. Variations in a gene's normal sequence and expression can signal hereditary and environmental diseases such as cystic fibrosis and cancer. Identifying these variations may provide the key to a cure or help assess the effectiveness of a treatment. GeneChip analyzes large amounts of genetic material; the firm's software determines a sample's nucleic sequence in minutes. The technology also can be used to monitor drug resistance in HIV patients. Affymetrix serves clients in the genomics (study of genes) industry and diagnostic markets. Glaxo Wellcome owns almost 40% of the company.

Agouron Pharmaceuticals, Inc.

10350 N. Torrey Pines Rd., Ste. 100, La Jolla, CA 92037

Telephone: 619-622-3000 **Fax:** 619-622-3298 **Metro area:** San Diego, CA **Web site:** http://www.agouron.com **Human resources contact:** Pat Moses **Sales:** $466.5 million **Number of employees:** 991 **Number of employees for previous year:** 708 **Industry designation:** Drugs **Company type:** Public **Top competitors:** Abbott Laboratories; Glaxo Wellcome plc; Merck & Co., Inc.

Agouron Pharmaceuticals develops drugs to treat cancer, viral diseases, and immuno-inflammatory diseases, including HIV, the common cold, cytomegalovirus infection, herpes, and hepatitis C. The company uses technology based on the molecular structure of proteins to create synthetic drugs for specific purposes. Its first commercial product, Viracept, is a protease inhibitor drug designed to treat the virus that causes AIDS. Other products under development include treatments for solid tumors and other conditions associated with cancer. Agouron is being acquired by Warner-Lambert, which is hoping to use Agouron to boost its development pipeline.

Alaris Medical, Inc.

10221 Wateridge Circle, San Diego, CA 92121

Telephone: 619-458-7000 **Fax:** 619-458-7760 **Metro area:** San Diego, CA **Web site:** http://www.alarismed.com **Human resources contact:** James Runchey **Sales:** $380.1 million **Number of employees:** 2,588 **Number of employees for previous year:** 1,356 **Industry designation:** Medical products **Company type:** Public **Top competitors:** Baxter International Inc.; Fresenius Medical Care Aktiengesellschaft; Abbott Laboratories

Alaris Medical makes intravenous infusion therapy systems, periodic patient-monitoring equipment, and related accessories. Its infusion pumps deliver fluids—generally pharmaceuticals or nutritionals—to patients in hospitals or alternate-care sites. The company's proprietary disposable administration sets, which consist of a plastic pump interface and tubing, can only be used with its pumps. Other Alaris Medical products measure patient respiration, pulse, and blood pressure. Alaris Medical was known as Advanced Medical prior to its 1996 acquisition of IVAC. Chairman Jeffrey Picower owns nearly 80% of the company.

Alliance Imaging, Inc.

1065 N. PacifiCenter Dr., Ste. 200, Anaheim, CA 92806

Telephone: 714-688-7100 **Fax:** 714-688-3388 **Metro area:** Los Angeles, CA **Web site:** http://www.allianceimaging.com **Human resources contact:** Christi Braun **Sales:** $86.5 million **Number of employees:** 613 **Number of employees for previous year:** 383 **Industry designation:** Medical instruments **Company type:** Public

Alliance Imaging provides comprehensive magnetic resonance imaging (MRI) services to hospitals and other health care providers. The company's MRI services include providing imaging equipment, equipment maintenance and upgrades, support technicians, day-to-day operation management, educational and marketing support, and insurance. Its MRI services are provided on a mobile, shared-user basis and on a full-time basis to single customers. Alliance Imaging targets small to medium-sized hospitals, clinics, multiphysician groups, and health maintenance organizations. Apollo Management owns 84% of Alliance.

Alliance Pharmaceutical Corp.

3040 Science Park Rd., San Diego, CA 92121

Telephone: 619-558-4300 **Fax:** 619-558-3625 **Metro area:** San Diego, CA **Web site:** http://www.allp.com **Human resources contact:** Carole McWilson **Sales:** $21.2 million **Number of employees:** 284 **Number of employees for previous year:** 213 **Industry designation:** Biomedical & genetic products **Company type:** Public **Top competitors:** Baxter International Inc.; Abbott Laboratories; Merck & Co., Inc.

Alliance Pharmaceutical is bubbling with hope for its products. The company uses perfluorochemical technology to develop medical imaging and therapeutic products. Three products in advanced stages of development are Imagent, an agent that enhances ultrasound images of blood flow abnormalities; Oxygent, a temporary oxygen carrier that reduces or eliminates the need for blood transfusions during elective surgery; and LiquiVent, a pulmonary drug used to treat patients with acute respiratory failure. The company is also developing alternative drug delivery systems using foams, gels, microemulsions, and other agents. Joint development partners include Schering and VIA Medical.

Alpha Microsystems

2722 S. Fairview St., Santa Ana, CA 92704

Telephone: 714-957-8500 **Fax:** 714-957-8705 **Metro area:** Los Angeles, CA **Web site:** http://www.alphamicro.com **Human resources contact:** Michelle Duggin **Sales:** $19.3 million **Number of employees:** 263 **Number of employees for previous year:** 191 **Industry designation:** Computers—services **Company type:** Public **Top competitors:** Computer Horizons Corp.; Cambridge Technology Partners (Massachusetts), Inc.; Control Data Systems, Inc.

For Alpha Microsystems, hardware equaled nowhere. The firm abandoned its hardware roots to provide consulting, maintenance, networking, and other information technology services. The support, directed primarily at the Internet and corporate intranet markets, accounts for almost 70% of sales. The company also makes online business tracking software (AlphaCONNECT), which captures formatted data from Internet sources on public and private companies and converts it for use in word processing, spreadsheet, and other office applications. Alpha Microsystems continues to acquire small firms to expand its product line.

AltaVista Company

529 Bryant St., Palo Alto, CA 94301

Telephone: 650-617-3400 **Fax:** 650-617-3441 **Metro area:** San Francisco, CA **Web site:** http://www.altavista.com **Human resources contact:** Lyn Christensen **Sales:** $30 million **Number of employees:** 80 **Industry designation:** Computers—online services **Company type:** Subsidiary **Parent company:** Digital Equipment Corporation **Top competitors:** Excite, Inc.; Lycos, Inc.; Yahoo! Inc.

AltaVista has a different view these days. The company, a subsidiary of Compaq Computer, manages the AltaVista high-speed search engine for locating information on the Internet. The engine lets users find data by typing in key words, asking questions, or perusing through subject categories. Long respected by the computer cognoscenti for its performance, AltaVista is expanding beyond its search mode roots. Compaq, hoping to ride the profitable market for Internet stocks and take the subsidiary public, continues to add content and services to AltaVista's Web home page such as e-mail, instant language translation, and electronic commerce to reshape the site as a premier Internet destination.

American Protective Services, Inc.

7770 Pardee Ln., Oakland, CA 94621

Telephone: 510-568-0276 **Fax:** 510-430-1130 **Metro area:** San Francisco, CA **Web site:** http://www.apsinc.com **Human resources contact:** Thomas A. Sutak **Sales:** $390 million (Est.) **Number of employees:** 18,000 **Number of employees for previous year:** 16,400 **Industry designation:** Protection—safety equipment & services **Company type:** Private **Top competitors:** Borg-Warner Security Corporation; Pinkerton's, Inc.; Wackenhut Corporation

There's no such thing as financial security or job security, but at least there's personal security. American Protective Services (APS) provides security services for business and industrial customers. The company's services—including on-site security guards, background checks, and security audits—are offered through some 85 full-service branch offices across North America. Its customers include hospitals, casinos, nuclear plants, banks, and high-rise office buildings. The IPSA International division specializes in security consulting and executive protection. APS was founded in 1945 by Thomas H. Keating, father of chairman Thomas W. Keating, to provide security on ships and docks in San Francisco Bay.

American Shared Hospital Services

4 Embarcadero Center, Ste. 3620, San Francisco, CA 94111

Telephone: 415-788-5300 **Fax:** 415-788-5660 **Metro area:** San Francisco, CA **Web site:** http://www.ashs.com **Human resources contact:** Shirley Tunic **Sales:** $35.2 million **Number of employees:** 344 **Number of employees for previous year:** 325 **Industry designation:** Medical services **Company type:** Public

American Shared Hospital Services provides mobile and shared diagnostic imaging services and respiratory therapy contract management services to more than 200 hospitals, medical centers, and medical offices in 23 states. American Shared is selling its magnetic resonance imaging (MRI), computed axial tomography scanning (CT), ultrasound, and nuclear medicine business, its respiratory therapy services business, and its cardiac catheterization laboratory to Alliance Imaging. The company will be left with its 81% stake in GK Financing LLC, which provides Gamma Knife radiosurgery services to major medical centers.

American Vanguard Corporation

4695 MacArthur Ct., Newport Beach, CA 92660

Telephone: 949-260-1200 **Fax:** 949-260-1201 **Metro area:** Los Angeles, CA **Sales:** $67 million **Number of employees:** 200 **Number of employees for previous year:** 195 **Industry designation:** Chemicals—specialty **Company type:** Public **Top competitors:** Aceto Corporation; Crompton & Knowles Corporation; FMC Corporation

American Vanguard makes specialty chemicals to protect the health of animals, crops, and humans. Subsidiary AMVAC Chemical's products include pesticides, plant growth regulators, and soil fumigants in liquid, powder, and granular forms. Subsidiary GemChem sells the company's chemicals nationally to the agriculture, cosmetic, nutritional, and pharmaceutical industries. American Vanguard also markets its products through a subsidiary in the UK and through import/export brokers. Customers include Novartis, ConAgra, Sumitomo Chemical, and Terra Industries. Co-chairmen Herbert Kraft and Glenn Wintemute each own about 25% of the company.

Amgen Inc.

One Amgen Center Dr., Thousand Oaks, CA 91320

Telephone: 805-447-1000 **Fax:** 805-447-1010 **Metro area:** Los Angeles, CA **Web site:** http://wwwext.Amgen.com **Human resources contact:** Edward F. Garnett **Sales:** $2.6 billion **Number of employees:** 5,500 **Number of employees for previous year:** 5,308 **Industry designation:** Biomedical & genetic products **Company type:** Public **Top competitors:** Merck & Co., Inc.; Glaxo Wellcome plc; Novartis AG

The biggest of the biotech big'uns, Amgen makes and markets therapeutic products for hematopoiesis (blood cell production), inflammation and autoimmunity, neurobiology, and soft-tissue repair. Anti-anemia drug EPOGEN and immune system stimulator NEUPOGEN account for more than 90% of sales, while a third drug, INFERGEN, has FDA approval as a treatment for hepatitis C. The company spends nearly one-fourth of its sales on research and development. Amgen has research and marketing alliances with several companies, including Hoffman-La Roche, Johnson & Johnson, and Kirin, the Japanese brewer that also operates a fast-growing pharmaceuticals unit.

Amylin Pharmaceuticals, Inc.

9373 Towne Centre Dr., San Diego, CA 92121

Telephone: 619-552-2200 **Fax:** 619-552-2212 **Metro area:** San Diego, CA **Web site:** http://www.amylin.com **Human resources contact:** Suzanne S. Burgess **Sales:** $16.2 million **Number of employees:** 278 **Number of employees for previous year:** 214 **Industry designation:** Drugs **Company type:** Public

Diabetes is a stubborn disease, as Amylin Pharmaceuticals has discovered. The company develops therapies for treating diabetes and associated disorders based on the hormone amylin, which is believed to play an important role in the regulation of metabolism. The firm is developing the drug exendin as a treatment for type two diabetes. However, its leading drug candidate, pramlintide, has not performed well in clinical trials and Johnson & Johnson, a provider of key financial assistance for the drug's commercial development, has withdrawn its support. Amylin is scaling back on drug trials, delaying its filing for FDA approval, selling off its Cabrillo Laboratories division, and letting go 75% of its workforce.

Anacomp, Inc.

12365 Crosthwaite Circle, Poway, CA 92064

Telephone: 619-679-9797 **Fax:** 619-748-9482 **Metro area:** San Diego, CA **Web site:** http://www.anacomp.com **Human resources contact:** Wally Boehm **Sales:** $499 million **Number of employees:** 3,400 **Number of employees for previous year:** 2,700 **Industry designation:** Computers—peripheral equipment **Company type:** Public **Top competitors:** Bell & Howell Company; Micrographic Technology Corp.; Imation Corp.

Anacomp understands data pack rats. The company is a world leader in providing information storage services and products. It operates more than 75 service bureaus worldwide, furnishing document storage and management services to clients in such industries as banking and insurance. Anacomp uses storage technologies that include computer-output-to-microfilm, microfiche, rewriteable CDs, electronic document management and document imaging, and computer output for the Internet and corporate intranets. The company also manufactures information storage systems and sells storage media. Anacomp markets its products and services in more than 65 countries. About a third of its sales are to customers outside the US.

Anaheim Angels Baseball Club, Inc.

2000 Gene Autry Way, Anaheim, CA 92806

Telephone: 714-940-2000 **Fax:** 714-940-2205 **Metro area:** Los Angeles, CA **Web site:** http://www.angelsbaseball.com **Human resources contact:** Jenny Price **Sales:** $62.6 million **Number of employees:** 150 **Industry designation:** Leisure & recreational services **Company type:** Subsidiary **Top competitors:** The Athletics Investment Group; Texas Rangers Baseball; The Seattle Mariners Professional Baseball Organization

The Anaheim Angels Baseball Club is praying Mo Vaughn helps it move on to glory. After finishing three games behind the American League West champ Texas Rangers in 1998, Anaheim made the former Boston Red Sox slugger and league MVP the highest-paid non-pitcher in baseball, at $13.3 million a year. The team was formed in 1960 by actor Gene Autry (died 1998). In 1996 Walt Disney bought 25% of the team (with an option to buy the rest), giving it a new name (it was the California Angels for more than 30 years) and a renovated and renamed ballpark, Edison International Field. Although they have yet to play in a World Series, the Angels have fielded such greats as pitcher Nolan Ryan and second baseman Rod Carew.

Anergen, Inc.

301 Penobscot Dr., Redwood City, CA 94063

Telephone: 415-361-8901 **Fax:** 650-361-8958 **Metro area:** San Francisco, CA **Web site:** http://www.biospace.com/b2/company_profile.cfm?CompanyID=1278 **Human resources contact:** Charon Spencer **Sales:** $5.8 million **Number of employees:** 72 **Number of employees for previous year:** 65 **Industry designation:** Biomedical & genetic products **Company type:** Subsidiary

Anergen, a subsidiary of Corixa, develops treatments for autoimmune diseases. With its trademark AnergiX drug, the company seeks to treat multiple sclerosis, rheumatoid arthritis, insulin-dependent diabetes, myasthenia gravis (a neuromuscular disease causing muscle weakness and possible death), and inflammatory bowel disease. Anergen is also developing AnervaX for treating rheumatoid arthritis and insulin-dependent diabetes. Both AnergiX and AnervaX are in clinical tests. Anergen is collaborating with pharmaceutical firm N. V. Organon to produce a treatment for rheumatoid arthritis.

ANSYS Diagnostics, Inc.

25200 Commercentre Dr., Lake Forest, CA 92630

Telephone: 949-770-9381 **Fax:** 949-768-0311 **Metro area:** Los Angeles, CA **Web site:** http://www.ansysinc.com **Human resources contact:** Linda Merrill **Sales:** $19 million (Est.) **Number of employees:** 241 **Industry designation:** Medical services **Company type:** Private **Top competitors:** Lab Holdings, Inc.; Biosite Diagnostics Incorporated; Diagnostic Products Corporation

For all those employers who get a little TesTy about their workers' drug use, ANSYS Diagnostics makes TesTcup and TesTstik—self-contained, disposable, on-site tests that can detect up to five different illegal substances in blood, tissue, urine, and other samples. (The products are made by Roche Diagnostic Systems.) Other products include ON-SITE Alcohol (which takes only about two minutes to detect ethanol in saliva or urine) and a line of specialty laboratory and research products, which are used by scientists to extract a substance from a liquid for analysis and to isolate nucleic acids. After the planned IPO, entities associated with venture capitalist Ronald Hall will own about 45% of the company.

Aradigm Corporation

26219 Eden Landing Rd., Hayward, CA 94545

Telephone: 510-783-0100 **Fax:** 510-783-0410 **Metro area:** San Francisco, CA **Human resources contact:** Norma Milligin **Sales:** $17.5 million **Number of employees:** 148 **Number of employees for previous year:** 92 **Industry designation:** Drugs **Company type:** Public

Aradigm helps the medicine go down better for people who swoon at the sight of a needle. Aradigm develops and produces handheld electronic inhalers—pulmonary drug-delivery systems that calibrate airflow and dosage—designed to reduce the need for injections and improve the effectiveness of drugs. The company's SmartMist system enhances delivery of asthma medications by administering drugs according to the patient's breathing to make dosage more exact than is possible with manually activated inhalers. Through agreements with SmithKline Beecham and Novo Nordisk, Aradigm is adapting its patented drug-delivery technology for pain management and diabetes treatment.

Ariba Technologies, Inc.

1314 Chesapeake Terrace, Sunnyvale, CA 94089

Telephone: 408-543-3800 **Fax:** 408-543-3900 **Metro area:** San Francisco, CA **Web site:** http://www.ariba.com **Sales:** $23 million (Est.) **Number of employees:** 100 **Industry designation:** Computers—corporate, professional & financial software **Company type:** Private **Top competitors:** Intelisys Electronic Commerce LLC; Commerce One, Inc.; Clarus Corporation

Ariba Technologies is ORMed to the teeth. Founded in 1996, the startup provides Operating Resource Management (ORM) products that help large corporations track and manage office equipment and supply purchases over the Internet and corporate intranets. Ariba's e-commerce software links client offices with suppliers. Its customers include Bristol-Myers Squibb, Chevron, Cisco Systems, and Federal Express. Ariba is the brainchild of co-founder and CEO Keith Krach, a Harvard wunderkind who at age 26 served as General Motors' youngest VP. The market noticed Ariba from the start, partly as a result of Krach's finding the right backing (venture capitalists) and gathering a savvy team of seasoned executives.

Artecon, Inc.

6305 El Camino Real, Carlsbad, CA 92009

Telephone: 760-931-5500 **Fax:** 408-944-1200 **Metro area:** San Diego, CA **Web site:** http://www.artecon.com **Human resources contact:** Carroll Schultz **Sales:** $66.3 million **Number of employees:** 287 **Number of employees for previous year:** 219 **Industry designation:** Computers—peripheral equipment **Company type:** Public **Top competitors:** Ciprico Inc.; Procom Technology, Inc.; Overland Data, Inc.

Artecon (formed through a reverse merger with Storage Dimensions) makes third-party computer data storage systems for such clients as Sun Microsystems, Motorola, AT&T, and Lockheed Martin. The company's disk and tape storage systems (including proprietary software and industry-standard hardware) for PCs, networks, and workstations are sold under such brands as Lynx, Sphinx, MEGAFLEX, RAIDFlex, and AerREAL. Artecon's telecommunications division offers systems integration services in addition to telecommunications storage products. Chairman William Sauey owns 25% of Artecon, which sells its products directly and through resellers. Artecon is consolidating its operations and reducing its workforce to cut costs.

Arterial Vascular Engineering, Inc.

3576 Unocal Place, Santa Rosa, CA 95403

Telephone: 707-525-0111 **Fax:** 707-525-0114 **Metro area:** San Francisco, CA **Web site:** http://www.avei.com **Human resources contact:** Becky Daly **Sales:** $387.6 million **Number of employees:** 2,177 **Number of employees for previous year:** 869 **Industry designation:** Medical instruments **Company type:** Subsidiary **Top competitors:** Medtronic, Inc.; Johnson & Johnson; Guidant Corporation

Arterial Vascular Engineering (AVE), a Medtronic subsidiary, has been unstinting in its attention to coronary stents. AVE makes the GFX and Micro Stent II stent systems as well as percutaneous transluminal coronary angioplasty (PTCA) balloon catheters. Its stents—expandable steel-mesh tubes—are used during angioplasty and other procedures that clear clogged arteries; after the surgery, the stents stay in place to prop arteries open. The company also makes Bridge stents for the kidneys and pelvic area. AVE has customers in the US, Japan, and about 40 other countries; foreign sales account for about 35% of sales.

ArthroCare Corporation

595 N. Pastoria Ave., Sunnyvale, CA 94086

Telephone: 408-736-0224 **Fax:** 408-736-0226 **Metro area:** San Francisco, CA **Web site:** http://www.arthrocare.com **Human resources contact:** Gwen Taylor **Sales:** $24.6 million **Number of employees:** 108 **Number of employees for previous year:** 79 **Industry designation:** Medical instruments **Company type:** Public **Top competitors:** Johnson & Johnson; United States Surgical Corporation; Smith & Nephew plc

With the wave of a wand, ArthroCare makes tissue disappear. The company's proprietary technology uses radio frequency energy to remove soft tissue from the body. Lead product ArthroCare Electrosurgery System 2000 lets surgeons use specialized wands to focus the energy and minimize damage to nearby healthy tissue, simultaneously sealing small bleeding vessels. Initially used in arthroscopic procedures to repair knees, shoulders, and other joints, the electrosurgery system product line has been expanded to include equipment used in ear, nose, and throat procedures (marketed by Xomed); myocardial revascularization procedures (marketed by a Boston Scientific subsidiary); and cosmetic and dermatology procedures.

ARV Assisted Living, Inc.

245 Fischer Ave., Ste. D-1, Costa Mesa, CA 92626

Telephone: 714-751-7400 **Fax:** 714-751-1743 **Metro area:** Los Angeles, CA **Web site:** http://www.arvi.com **Human resources contact:** Laura J. Loda **Sales:** $128.6 million **Number of employees:** 2,600 **Number of employees for previous year:** 2,200 **Industry designation:** Nursing homes **Company type:** Public

ARV Assisted Living operates about 60 assisted-living facilities for the elderly in 10 states, including California, Texas, and Florida. Residents live in private or semiprivate rooms or suites, eat in a communal setting, and have access to housekeeping services. ARV offers 24-hour care, assistance with personal hygiene and medication administration, and other services for those who need them. About 95% of revenues come from residents who pay for services with their own funds or through private insurance. An affiliate of investment bank Lazard Freres owns a 40% stake in the company. ARV owns 14 of the facilities it operates, and it leases others from a Lazard Freres subsidiary, Kapson Senior Quarters.

Aspect Development, Inc.

1300 Charleston Rd., Mountain View, CA 94043

Telephone: 650-428-2700 **Fax:** 650-968-4335 **Metro area:** San Francisco, CA **Web site:** http://www.aspectdv.com **Human resources contact:** Jill Beckman-Donley **Sales:** $86.4 million **Number of employees:** 536 **Number of employees for previous year:** 300 **Industry designation:** Computers—corporate, professional & financial software **Company type:** Public

Aspect Development's software helps electronics and other high-tech and industrial manufacturers manage information about components and suppliers. Its products allow companies including Honeywell, IBM, Texas Instruments, and Lucent Technologies search for, organize, and compare the design and other technical information of some three million components. Aspect Development generates most of its revenues from its VIP reference database and Explore client/server software. Other products include Krakatoa, software that helps customers create and maintain online catalogs. Aspect Development sells through offices in North America, Europe, and Asia, as well as through agreements with SAP, Baan, and Digital Equipment.

The Athletics Investment Group

7677 Oakport St., Ste. 200, Oakland, CA 94621

Telephone: 510-638-4900 **Fax:** 510-562-1633 **Metro area:** San Francisco, CA **Web site:** http://www.oaklandathletics.com **Human resources contact:** Eleanor Yee **Sales:** $56.4 million (Est.) **Number of employees:** 70 **Industry designation:** Leisure & recreational services **Company type:** Private **Top competitors:** Anaheim Angels Baseball Club, Inc.; Texas Rangers Baseball; The Seattle Mariners Professional Baseball Organization

Oakland Athletics fans know all about extreme sports—the baseball club is perpetually at the top or at the bottom of the standings. The team has won 15 American League pennants, but it has also finished last a record 28 times. Oakland is the club's third home, having also played in Philadelphia (where Connie Mack managed for 50 years) and Kansas City. The A's have won nine World Series; the team last won the big show in 1989 behind the power hitting of Jose Canseco and Mark McGwire ("The Bash Brothers"). San Francisco Bay area businessmen Steve Schott and Ken Hofmann bought the team in 1995 from the Haas family (owner of Levi Strauss), but Schott and Hoffman have since put the A's up for sale.

At Home Corporation

425 Broadway St., Redwood City, CA 94063

Telephone: 650-569-5000 **Fax:** 650-569-5100 **Metro area:** San Francisco, CA **Web site:** http://www.home.net **Human resources contact:** Leilani T. Gayles **Sales:** $48 million **Number of employees:** 570 **Number of employees for previous year:** 329 **Industry designation:** Computers—online services **Company type:** Public **Top competitors:** Microsoft Corporation; U S WEST, Inc.; Time Warner Inc.

At Home means business. It uses cable TV systems to provide high-speed Internet and other online services to consumers (@Home) and businesses (@Work), with network technology capable of delivering data about a hundred times faster than traditional telephone modems. At Home, which teams with cable operators to market and provide its services, has partnerships that give it access to about 50 million North American homes passed by cable. AT&T Broadband & Internet Services (formerly TCI) holds a 40% stake. Other investors include US cable operators Cablevision, Comcast, and Cox. The firm has agreed to buy Excite, the #2 Internet directory.

audiohighway.com

20600 Mariani Ave., Cupertino, CA 95014

Telephone: 408-255-5301 **Fax:** 408-255-5591 **Metro area:** San Francisco, CA **Web site:** http://www.audiohighway.com **Sales:** $4,000 **Number of employees:** 15 **Industry designation:** Computers—online services **Company type:** Public **Top competitors:** broadcast.com inc.; Yahoo! Inc.; America Online, Inc.

audiohighway.com offers online access to a more than 3,500 audio titles, including news, music, and comedy programs as well as books, sports updates, and self-help courses. The company's AudioCast system allows users to download selected programs from its Web site and then play them. In addition, users can listen to broadcasts in real time through Microsoft's NetShow software. audiohighway.com's content is provided by National Public Radio, "Newsweek," and Dow Jones, among other sources. The company generates its sales through advertising, but it has also launched an e-commerce site that sells computers and premium audio content (such as training seminars). CEO Nathan Schulhof owns 10% of the company.

Aurora Biosciences Corporation

11010 Torreyana Rd., San Diego, CA 92121

Telephone: 619-452-5000 **Fax:** 619-452-5723 **Metro area:** San Diego, CA **Web site:** http://www.aurorabio.com **Human resources contact:** Pamela Fritz **Sales:** $26.5 million **Number of employees:** 102 **Number of employees for previous year:** 50 **Industry designation:** Drugs **Company type:** Public **Top competitors:** CombiChem, Inc.; Repligen Corporation; Endogen, Inc.

Aurora Biosciences develops and sells drug-discovery technologies and services. Along with such collaborators as Bristol-Myers Squibb, Eli Lilly, and Merck, Aurora Biosciences is developing a system using fluorescent assay technologies and ultra-high throughput screening systems (UHTSS) to allow researchers to overcome many limitations of traditional drug-discovery processes. The UHTSS is expected to be operational by the year 2000. Many of Aurora Biosciences' tests are designed to be performed with living mammalian cells to better model human disease processes. The company has an exclusive license from Lidak Pharmaceuticals to sell a fluorescent reporter, which measures unbound free fatty acid levels.

Autodesk, Inc.

111 McInnis Pkwy., San Rafael, CA 94903

Telephone: 415-507-5000 **Fax:** 415-507-5100 **Metro area:** San Francisco, CA **Web site:** http://www.autodesk.com **Human resources contact:** Stephen McMahon **Sales:** $740.2 million **Number of employees:** 2,470 **Number of employees for previous year:** 2,044 **Industry designation:** Computers—engineering, scientific & CAD-CAM software **Company type:** Public **Top competitors:** Parametric Technology Corporation; Unigraphics Solutions Inc.; Dassault Systemes S.A.

One of the world's largest PC software companies, Autodesk is a leading supplier of computer-aided design (CAD) automation software. The company sells a family of CAD products including AutoCAD, AutoCAD LT, AutoSketch, and AutoCAD Designer, available in nearly 20 languages. Its flagship AutoCAD product is used primarily by architects and mechanical engineers to perform design, modeling, drafting, mapping, and rendering. Design automation software accounts for most of Autodesk's sales, but the company also develops design software for multimedia and for home improvement. Its Discreet Logic division develops software and systems for visual effects and editing.

Autologic Information International, Inc.

1050 Rancho Conejo Blvd., Thousand Oaks, CA 91320

Telephone: 805-498-9611 **Fax:** 805-499-1167 **Metro area:** Los Angeles, CA **Web site:** http://www.autologic.com **Human resources contact:** Amy Daniels **Sales:** $87.6 million **Number of employees:** 433 **Number of employees for previous year:** 410 **Industry designation:** Computers—peripheral equipment **Company type:** Public **Top competitors:** Tekgraf, Inc.; Scitex Corporation Ltd.; ECRM Incorporated

Autologic Information International (aii) hasn't perished, it's helping to publish. The company makes image setting publishing equipment and software. Its products include laser imaging systems, workflow management software (Ad Manager), and interface products (which let different prepress hardware systems communicate). aii also makes laser cinema recorders, which transfer computer images directly onto film (used in the movies "Armageddon" and "Titanic"). Subsidiary Xitron sells similar prepress products to the lower-end market. aii targets high-volume, deadline-sensitive printing operations. Volt Information Sciences, a provider of technical personnel and support, owns 59% of the company.

Avant! Corporation

46871 Bayside Pkwy., Fremont, CA 94538

Telephone: 510-413-8000 **Fax:** 510-413-8080 **Metro area:** San Francisco, CA **Web site:** http://www.avanticorp.com **Human resources contact:** Linda Gunther **Sales:** $227.1 million **Number of employees:** 701 **Number of employees for previous year:** 444 **Industry designation:** Computers—engineering, scientific & CAD-CAM software **Company type:** Public **Top competitors:** Synopsys, Inc.; Cadence Design Systems, Inc.; Mentor Graphics Corporation

Avant! (pronounced ah-VON-tee) develops integrated circuit design automation (ICDA) software products that enable IC designers to solve design problems. The company produces IC layout and verification software for high-density, high-performance IC designs. Products designed with these tools include microprocessors, high-end graphics chips, application-specific standard products, and complex application-specific ICs. Avant! believes its products reduce IC manufacturing costs by reducing IC die size and the number of iterations required to complete a design. Since 1995 Avant! has been battling a code-theft suit filed by rival Cadence Design Systems, and several company executives have also been indicted.

Avigen, Inc.

1201 Harbor Bay Pkwy., Ste. 1000, Alameda, CA 94502

Telephone: 510-748-7150 **Fax:** 510-748-7155 **Metro area:** San Francisco, CA **Web site:** http://www.avigen.com **Human resources contact:** Sandy Delph **Sales:** $100,000 **Number of employees:** 44 **Number of employees for previous year:** 38 **Industry designation:** Biomedical & genetic products **Company type:** Public **Top competitors:** Chiron Corporation; Novartis AG; Vical Incorporated

Development-stage Avigen uses viruses as a vector of attack. One of the company's therapies uses adeno-associated virus, a nonpathogenic human virus, to deliver therapeutic genes to cells that need treatment. Avigen believes this type of therapy may effectively treat various cancers, anemia, hemophilia, and metabolic diseases. The company hopes another of its therapies, which facilitates DNA delivery to chromosomes, may be useful in the treatment of such blood-related diseases as sickle-cell anemia and HIV. Neither technology has reached the production stage. Johns Hopkins University is among the organizations with which Avigen has licensing agreements.

Aviron

297 N. Bernardo Ave., Mountain View, CA 94043

Telephone: 650-919-6500 **Fax:** 650-919-6610 **Metro area:** San Francisco, CA **Web site:** http://www.aviron.com **Human resources contact:** Theresa Williamson **Sales:** $700,000 **Number of employees:** 100 **Number of employees for previous year:** 70 **Industry designation:** Drugs **Company type:** Public

Aviron, a development-stage biopharmaceutical company, develops vaccines based on live virus attenuation techniques and genetic-engineering technologies. The company has undertaken Phase III clinical trials for its leading vaccine, an intranasal spray (FluMist) for flu prevention. Aviron's intranasal vaccine for croup is in Phase II clinical trials, and its subunit vaccine for mononucleosis, developed in collaboration with SmithKline Beecham, is in Phase I clinical trials in Europe. The company is also researching and developing vaccines for diseases caused by cytomegalovirus, herpes simplex 2, and respiratory syncytial virus. American Home Products is licensing Aviron's nasal-spray flu vaccine.

Axiohm Transaction Solutions, Inc.

15070 Avenue of Science, San Diego, CA 92128

Telephone: 619-451-3485 **Fax:** 619-451-3573 **Metro area:** San Diego, CA **Web site:** http://www.dhtech.com **Human resources contact:** Geri Westberg **Sales:** $231 million **Number of employees:** 1,513 **Number of employees for previous year:** 925 **Industry designation:** Computers—peripheral equipment **Company type:** Public **Top competitors:** Seiko Epson Corporation; Printronix, Inc.; Zebra Technologies Corporation

Axiohm Transaction Solutions (known as DH Technology before merging with Axiohm SA) is a leading maker of transaction printers and ancillary products used to output such documents as airline and lottery tickets and banking and sales receipts. Its product line includes thermal and impact printers, printer mechanisms, and magnetic-stripe and smart-card readers. The company also is developing a presence in the market for bar code printers. It sells worldwide to manufacturers such as NCR, which accounts for about a third of sales. Company co-chairmen Patrick Dupuy and Gilles Gibier (the founders of Axiohm SA) each own 27% of Axiohm Transaction Solutions.

AXYS Pharmaceuticals, Inc.

180 Kimball Way, South San Francisco, CA 94080

Telephone: 650-829-1000 **Fax:** 650-829-1001 **Metro area:** San Francisco, CA **Web site:** http://www.axyspharm.com/index.html **Human resources contact:** Robb Anderson **Sales:** $47.4 million **Number of employees:** 395 **Number of employees for previous year:** 160 **Industry designation:** Drugs **Company type:** Public **Top competitors:** Titan Pharmaceuticals, Inc.; CombiChem, Inc.; Genelabs Technologies, Inc.

AXYS Pharmaceuticals, the product of the merger of Arris Pharmaceutical and Sequana Therapeutics, tests innumerable small-molecule chemical compounds in a search for leads for new drugs. With the help of large pharmaceutical partners, the company is attempting to develop new treatments for respiratory, nervous, cardiovascular, and metabolic disorders, as well as infectious diseases, osteoporosis, and cancer. The company is able to test a great number of compounds with the potential to become future pharmaceuticals by using its proprietary database software and robotic testing equipment.

BackWeb Technologies, Inc.

2077 Gateway Place, Ste. 500, San Jose, CA 95110

Telephone: 408-933-1700 **Fax:** 408-933-1800 **Metro area:** San Francisco, CA **Web site:** http://www.backweb.com **Human resources contact:** Sowji Reddy **Number of employees:** 140 **Number of employees for previous year:** 20 **Industry designation:** Computers—online services **Company type:** Private **Top competitors:** PointCast Incorporated; Marimba, Inc.; Intuit Inc.

BackWeb Technologies' rap is that it wants you to push it—p-push it real fast. Founded in 1995, the company makes communications acceleration software based on push technology for the Web, intranets, and extranets. Its customizable software, which helps organizations manage sales, human resources, software distribution, e-commerce, and other tasks, can set up broadcast channels that download preferred data directly to users without delays or interruptions. BackWeb Sales Accelerator (designed for sales chains) organizes customer information, industry news, pricing strategies, and other data into pop-up text, graphics, audio, and/or video files. Customers include Compaq, Cisco Systems, and AT&T.

BARRA, Inc.

2100 Milvia St., Berkeley, CA 94704

Telephone: 510-548-5442 **Fax:** 510-548-4374 **Metro area:** San Francisco, CA **Web site:** http://www.barra.com. **Human resources contact:** Carmel Galvin **Sales:** $137.4 million **Number of employees:** 696 **Number of employees for previous year:** 504 **Industry designation:** Computers—corporate, professional & financial software **Company type:** Public **Top competitors:** Merrill Lynch & Co., Inc.; FactSet Research Systems Inc.; Primark Corporation

BARRA is doing its best to make the lives of portfolio managers and brokers a little easier. The company's customers pay annual subscription fees of $10,000 to $30,000 to access BARRA's risk and valuation models. The models focus on equities, bonds, and derivatives. BARRA also offers consulting and risk management services, investment data products, and indexing services (it has teamed with Standard & Poor's to develop several indexes). BARRA also owns 50% of asset management firm Symphony Asset Management and 50% of the Portfolio System For Institutional Trading (POSIT), a computerized trading system for institutional investors. BARRA has more than 1,200 customers in more than 30 countries.

Benton Oil and Gas Company

1145 Eugenia Place, Ste. 200, Carpinteria, CA 93013

Telephone: 805-566-5600 **Fax:** 805-566-5610 **Metro area:** Los Angeles, CA **Web site:** http://www.bentonoil.com **Human resources contact:** Jennifer J. Young **Sales:** $112.1 million **Number of employees:** 71 **Number of employees for previous year:** 55 **Industry designation:** Oil & gas—exploration & production **Company type:** Public

Benton Oil and Gas is an independent firm that develops and produces oil and gas properties primarily in Venezuela and Russia. It also has holdings in China, Jordan, Senegal, and the US. The company targets new reserves in foreign locations deemed risky by other firms; it also seeks out underdeveloped existing oil and gas fields where new drill zones might improve production. Benton Oil and Gas has estimated proved reserves of about 121,000 barrels of oil equivalent. Venezuela's PDVSA Petroleo y Gas represents more than 90% of the company's annual revenues.

Bergen Brunswig Corporation

4000 Metropolitan Dr., Orange, CA 92868

Telephone: 714-385-4000 **Fax:** 714-385-1442 **Metro area:** Los Angeles, CA **Web site:** http://www.bergenbrunswig.com **Human resources contact:** Carol E. Scherman **Sales:** $17.1 billion **Number of employees:** 5,400 **Number of employees for previous year:** 5,100 **Industry designation:** Drugs & sundries—wholesale **Company type:** Public **Top competitors:** McKesson HBOC, Inc.; AmeriSource Health Corporation; Cardinal Health, Inc.

Bergen Brunswig is the third-largest wholesale pharmaceutical distributor in the US, behind McKesson HBOC and Cardinal Health. The company distributes drugs and medical-surgical supplies to a wide variety of customers, including hospitals and managed care facilities, and provides over-the-counter medications, beauty products, and sundries to drugstores. The company also assists its small retailers in the Good Neighbor Pharmacy program. It distributes from about 64 locations in 29 states. Government opposition has ended Bergen Brunswig's agreement to be bought by Cardinal Health.

Biex, Inc.

6693 Sierra Ln., Ste. F, Dublin, CA 94568

Telephone: 925-556-0300 **Fax:** 925-556-0800 **Metro area:** San Francisco, CA **Web site:** http://www.biex.com **Human resources contact:** Edgar A. Luce **Number of employees:** 85 **Number of employees for previous year:** 28 **Industry designation:** Medical products **Company type:** Private

Biex identifies women at risk of spontaneous preterm labor and delivery of pregnancies. Its SalEst system measures the hormone estriol in saliva to predict early deliveries and thereby reduce the costs and mortality rates associated with them. Saliva samples are taken using Biex's proprietary collection kit, either in a doctor's office or at home by a patient; samples go to a lab for analysis. Biex says that clinical trials indicate that SalEst is more accurate in identifying risk than is the most common predictive method currently in use. Biex is preparing SalEst's commercial launch (aimed at physicians and third-party payors) and plans to form alliances with pharmaceutical and other firms.

Biomagnetic Technologies, Inc.

9727 Pacific Heights Blvd., San Diego, CA 92121

Telephone: 619-453-6300 **Fax:** 619-453-4913 **Metro area:** San Diego, CA **Human resources contact:** Lisa Scott **Sales:** $2.8 million **Number of employees:** 59 **Number of employees for previous year:** 58 **Industry designation:** Medical instruments **Company type:** Public **Top competitors:** General Electric Company; Shimadzu Corporation; Siemens AG

Biomagnetic Technologies quantifies your magnetism. The company's Magnes magnetic source imaging (MSI) systems measure magnetic fields in the body to provide information about the functions of the brain, heart, and other organs without the invasiveness of surgery or magnetic resonance imaging (MRI). The company is exploring new applications for its systems (especially to evaluate epilepsy), which are marketed to large hospitals and medical research laboratories. Magnes MSI systems are installed at more than 20 facilities in Austria, France, Germany, Japan, and the US. Chairman Enrique Maso owns about 30% of the company; director Martin Egli owns about another quarter.

Biopool International, Inc.

6025 Nicolle St., Ste. A, Ventura, CA 93003

Telephone: 805-654-0643 **Fax:** 805-654-0681 **Metro area:** Los Angeles, CA **Human resources contact:** Bobbie Jones **Sales:** $15 million **Number of employees:** 117 **Number of employees for previous year:** 114 **Industry designation:** Medical products **Company type:** Public **Top competitors:** Meridian Diagnostics, Inc.; Bio-Reference Laboratories, Inc.; i-STAT Corporation

Take a dip in the Biopool! The company makes in vitro diagnostic products for testing blood clotting and bleeding disorders, evaluating risk factors for cardiovascular diseases, and detecting drug abuse. Biopool markets its more than 150 products to hospitals, clinics, labs, and blood banks in more than 50 countries. These products, made in California, Pennsylvania, and Sweden, are also distributed by such companies as Allegiance, and are sold to original equipment manufacturers. Biopool International has product development alliances with such companies as Bayer, Ortho Diagnostic Systems (a Johnson & Johnson subsidiary), and Sigma Diagnostics (a Sigma-Aldrich subsidiary).

Bio-Rad Laboratories, Inc.

1000 Alfred Nobel Dr., Hercules, CA 94547

Telephone: 510-724-7000 **Fax:** 510-741-5817 **Metro area:** San Francisco, CA **Web site:** http://www.bio-rad.com **Human resources contact:** Richard J. Anderson **Sales:** $441.9 million **Number of employees:** 2,675 **Number of employees for previous year:** 2,650 **Industry designation:** Medical instruments **Company type:** Public **Top competitors:** Epitope, Inc.; ChemTrak Incorporated

Bio-Rad Laboratories makes and sells life-science research products, systems for clinical diagnostics, and analytical instruments worldwide. The company offers more than 5,000 products to government agencies, private industry, universities, and hospital laboratories. Bio-Rad makes products to separate chemical and biological substances and to analyze, identify, and purify their components. In addition, the company makes automated test systems and test kits and services FT-IR spectrometer systems and semiconductor-manufacturing instruments. The company has acquired key assets of Chiron Diagnostics and other companies to expand its product line in diagnostic controls, imaging services, and semiconductor products.

Biosite Diagnostics Incorporated

11030 Roselle St., San Diego, CA 92121

Telephone: 619-455-4808 **Fax:** 619-455-4815 **Metro area:** San Diego, CA **Web site:** http://www.biosite.com/ **Human resources contact:** Laura Weatherford **Sales:** $34.4 million **Number of employees:** 216 **Number of employees for previous year:** 176 **Industry designation:** Medical products **Company type:** Public **Top competitors:** Roche Holding Ltd; Abbott Laboratories; Dade Behring

Biosite Diagnostics makes truth serum in a specimen cup. The company's diagnostic products include Triage Panel for Drugs of Abuse (Triage DOA), a single-sample urine test that identifies commonly abused drugs. Biosite also makes Triage Cardiac Panel and Triage Meter Panel for diagnosing heart disease, as well as Triage C. Difficile for detecting an intestinal bug. It is developing diagnostic products for congestive heart failure and sepsis, for detecting certain bacterial and parasitic infections, and for determining the drug dosages. Biosite has strategic relationships with Novartis and Scios, among others, and distributes Triage DOA in the US through Curtin Matheson Scientific.

Bright Light Technologies, Inc.

915 Cole St., Ste. 338, San Francisco, CA 94117

Telephone: 415-905-5595 **Fax:** 415-905-5188 **Metro area:** San Francisco, CA **Web site:** http://www.brightlight.com **Human resources contact:** Valerie Hansen **Number of employees:** 20 **Industry designation:** Computers—online services **Company type:** Private

Bright Light Technologies wants to cook spam's goose by pitting people and computers against unwanted e-mail, or "spam." Its Bright Mail service starts with decoy e-mail accounts designed to receive spam, which is forwarded to human component BLOC (The Bright Light Operations Center), where messages are evaluated for content and structure. Message analysts issue new rules to the firm's Spam Wall software, which is updated continuously and transmitted to users. The firm targets Internet service providers, businesses, and individuals. Users include AT&T Worldnet, EarthLink Network, and Concentric. Bright Light Technologies was created by CEO and owner Sunil Paul, formerly with spam-beleaguered America Online.

BroadVision, Inc.

585 Broadway, Redwood City, CA 94063

Telephone: 650-261-5100 **Fax:** 650-261-5900 **Metro area:** San Francisco, CA **Web site:** http://www.broadvision.com **Human resources contact:** Sharon Haag **Sales:** $50.9 million **Number of employees:** 188 **Number of employees for previous year:** 147 **Industry designation:** Computers—online services **Company type:** Public **Top competitors:** ConnectInc.com; Open Market, Inc.; America Online, Inc.

BroadVision wants to facilitate Web commerce. Its BroadVision One-To-One software lets companies design their own Web sites to maximize potential for online sales and marketing. One-To-One allows users to manage online transactions involving ordering and payment, order fulfillment, billing, customer service, and other activities. It also lets users collect, track, and manage information about Web site visitors and use the resulting profiles to customize content. Customers include Prodigy Services Company and Olivetti Telemedia. The company has offices in the US, Asia, and Europe. The Asia/Pacific region and Europe account for about 50% of sales. CEO Pehong Chen owns around 28% of BroadVision.

Brown and Caldwell

3480 Buskirk Ave., Ste. 150, Pleasant Hill, CA 94523

Telephone: 925-937-9010 **Fax:** 925-937-9026 **Metro area:** San Francisco, CA **Web site:** http://www.brownandcaldwell.com **Human resources contact:** Chris Dorr **Sales:** $110 million (Est.) **Number of employees:** 900 **Number of employees for previous year:** 760 **Industry designation:** Pollution control equipment & services **Company type:** Private **Top competitors:** Malcolm Pirnie, Inc.; Philip Services Corp.; EMCON

Brown and Caldwell is headed straight to the gutter—to clean it up. The employee-owned firm provides environmental consulting and engineering services to industrial, governmental, and utility clients. Brown and Caldwell designs and builds water, wastewater, and solid-waste systems; provides watershed and stormwater management services; and engineers and repairs pipelines. The company also offers such services as soil and groundwater remediation, underground storage-tank installation, risk assessment, and customized data management systems. Founded in 1947, Brown and Caldwell has offices in 18 US states as well as in Argentina and Canada.

Cadence Design Systems, Inc.

2655 Sealy Ave., Bldg. 5, San Jose, CA 95134

Telephone: 408-943-1234 **Fax:** 408-943-0513 **Metro area:** San Francisco, CA **Web site:** http://www.cadence.com **Human resources contact:** Ron Kirchenbaur **Sales:** $1.2 billion **Number of employees:** 3,945 **Number of employees for previous year:** 3,190 **Industry designation:** Computers—engineering, scientific & CAD-CAM software **Company type:** Public **Top competitors:** IKOS Systems, Inc.; Synopsys, Inc.; Avant! Corporation

Cadence Design Systems is the world's leading provider of electronic design automation (EDA) software, which is used to design integrated circuits (ICs) and electronic systems such as telephones, fax machines, and computers. Core products include Allegro, a board layout tool; Virtuoso, for custom IC layout and library development; and integrated layout analysis tools for board-level design and verification. Cadence also designs components, including ICs and software, for electronics companies and offers consulting and training services. Since 1995 Cadence has been embroiled in a code-theft suit against #2 EDA firm Avant! (Avant! executives have been indicted.) About 45% of Cadence's sales are outside the US.

Caere Corporation

100 Cooper Ct., Los Gatos, CA 95032

Telephone: 408-395-7000 **Fax:** 408-354-2743 **Metro area:** San Francisco, CA **Web site:** http://www.caere.com **Human resources contact:** Claire Brown **Sales:** $65.8 million **Number of employees:** 295 **Number of employees for previous year:** 293 **Industry designation:** Optical character recognition **Company type:** Public **Top competitors:** National Computer Systems, Inc.; FileNET Corporation; Xerox Corporation

Caere has a cure for tired typists. The firm continues to wage a battle with Xerox to be the world's #1 developer of optical character recognition products—software and hardware used to scan text into a machine-readable form for databases, spreadsheets, and word processing. Caere's products include the OmniPage, M/Series, and WordScan lines. The company also makes electronic forms software and document management tools. Caere makes much of its money bundling its software with scanners made by other manufacturers, including Hewlett-Packard. It sells its products through distributors, superstores, mail order, and the Internet. Distributor Ingram Micro accounts for nearly 25% of Caere's sales.

California Cooperative Creamery

621 Western Ave., Petaluma, CA 94952

Telephone: 707-763-1931 **Fax:** 707-778-2343 **Metro area:** San Francisco, CA **Web site:** http://www.cal-gold.com **Human resources contact:** Julie Marchman **Sales:** $485 million **Number of employees:** 285 **Industry designation:** Food—dairy products **Company type:** Cooperative **Top competitors:** California Milk Producers; Dairy Farmers of America; Darigold Inc.

No doubt the cows producing milk for the California Cooperative Creamery are udderly proud of their work. The cooperative consists of about 500 dairy farmers in Northern California, the California Central Valley, and Nevada. The farmers and cows also churn out butter, cheese, and nonfat dairy milk. The cooperative has four manufacturing facilities and distributes its products under the California Gold Dairy Products label. Its facilities produce about 200,000 pounds of cheese daily. In 1997 the cooperative joined with Dairyman's Creamery Cooperative Association of Tulare to form the largest cheese plant on the West Coast. The cooperative was founded in 1913.

California Pacific Medical Center

3700 California St., 1st Fl., San Francisco, CA 94120

Telephone: 415-563-4321 **Fax:** 415-885-8686 **Other address:** PO Box 7999, San Francisco, CA 94120 **Metro area:** San Francisco, CA **Web site:** http://www.cpmc.org **Human resources contact:** Cecilia Conte **Sales:** $308.5 million **Number of employees:** 3,650 **Number of employees for previous year:** 2,517 **Industry designation:** Hospitals **Company type:** Not-for-profit

Leave a kidney in San Francisco? If you did, chances are you got a new one at California Pacific Medical Center, a private, not-for-profit complex with campuses in the heart of hospital-heavy San Francisco. The hospital is well known for its specialty care offerings, including obstetrics and gynecology, neurosciences and pediatrics, neurosciences and orthopedics, and organ transplantation. The 938-bed facility is also a center for professional education and basic biomedical, clinical, and behavioral research. It is acquiring the 341-bed Davies Medical Center, which specializes in microsurgery and HIV care. California Pacific is part of the Sutter Health not-for-profit regional health care system.

Calypte Biomedical Corporation

1440 Fourth St., Berkeley, CA 94710

Telephone: 510-526-2541 **Fax:** 510-526-5381 **Metro area:** San Francisco, CA **Web site:** http://www.calypte.com **Human resources contact:** Nancy Yu **Sales:** $1 million **Number of employees:** 50 **Number of employees for previous year:** 38 **Industry designation:** Drugs **Company type:** Public **Top competitors:** Abbott Laboratories; Epitope, Inc.; Johnson & Johnson

Fear of needles need not stop you from getting tested for HIV infection. Calypte Biomedical's urine-based HIV-1 test is touted as having several benefits over blood tests and has received FDA approval for use in professional laboratories. The company hopes to receive approval for over-the-counter sales as well. Calypte is also working on urine-based diagnostic tests for other sexually-transmitted diseases (chlamydia, HIV-2, syphilis, herpes). In addition, the company owns 44% of Pepgen Corporation, which is developing an oral interferon product to treat multiple sclerosis. Calypte Biomedical is buying Cambridge Biotech, with which it has been jointly marketing its products.

CAM Data Systems, Inc.

17520 Newhope St., Ste. 100, Fountain Valley, CA 92708

Telephone: 714-241-9241 **Fax:** 714-241-9893 **Metro area:** Los Angeles, CA **Web site:** http://www.camdata.com **Human resources contact:** Linh Vo **Sales:** $18.8 million **Number of employees:** 161 **Number of employees for previous year:** 145 **Industry designation:** Computers—corporate, professional & financial software **Company type:** Public **Top competitors:** JDA Software Group, Inc.; HNC Software Inc.; NCR Corporation

CAM Data Systems helps small retailers win at the track. The company makes turnkey point-of-sale equipment and software systems that help retailers track sales and inventory, provide accounting and sales reports, and identify winning and losing merchandise. The company provides software and hardware, installs and services the systems, and furnishes technical support and on-site training. Its Profit$ system provides color and size inventory tracking capabilities to apparel and shoe retailers; the CAM system helps durable goods retailers with reorderable inventory. CAM Data Systems sells its products directly throughout the US.

Cardiac Pathways Corporation

995 Benecia Ave., Sunnyvale, CA 94086

Telephone: 408-737-0505 **Fax:** 408-737-1700 **Metro area:** San Francisco, CA **Web site:** http://www.cardiac.com **Human resources contact:** Allison Herd **Sales:** $2.4 million **Number of employees:** 127 **Number of employees for previous year:** 112 **Industry designation:** Medical instruments **Company type:** Public **Top competitors:** Medtronic, Inc.; Johnson & Johnson; Boston Scientific Corporation

Cardiac Pathways gets to the heart of the matter with its heart rhythm diagnostic and treatment products. The company's diagnostic mapping systems and minimally invasive systems treat abnormally rapid heart rhythms (tachyarrhythmias), which can cause palpitations and cardiac arrest. Its arrhythmia mapping systems are designed to quickly locate the source of tachyarrhythmias. Cardiac Pathway's nonsurgical technique for treatment neutralizes heart tissue that causes dangerous heart rhythms. The company is also developing diagnostic and treatment products for ventricular tachycardia and atrial fibrillation, two other types of abnormal heart rhythms. Cardiac Pathways' products are sold around the world.

Cardima, Inc.

47266 Benicia St., Fremont, CA 94538

Telephone: 510-354-0300 **Fax:** 510-657-4476 **Metro area:** San Francisco, CA **Web site:** http://www.cardima.com **Human resources contact:** Senja Stevig **Sales:** $2.5 million **Number of employees:** 115 **Number of employees for previous year:** 101 **Industry designation:** Medical instruments **Company type:** Public **Top competitors:** Johnson & Johnson; C. R. Bard, Inc.; Boston Scientific Corporation

Cardima makes catheters and microcatheters to use in the diagnosis and treatment of cardiac arrhythmias. The company's microcatheters, which include the Cardima Pathfinder AF and the Tracer VT, diagnose an arrhythmia by locating its origin (mapping), then restore normal heart rhythms by isolating and destroying the arrhythmia-causing tissue. Two of the company's mapping products have received FDA approval and are being marketed in the US; others have received marketing approval in Europe and Japan. Most products are still in the testing phase, but Cardima also currently makes and sells Venaport LR guiding catheters. The company is a 1992 spinoff from Target Therapeutics (now part of Boston Scientific).

CardioDynamics International Corporation

6175 Nancy Ridge Dr., Ste. 300, San Diego, CA 92121

Telephone: 619-535-0202 **Fax:** 619-535-0055 **Metro area:** San Diego, CA **Web site:** http://www.cardiodynamics.com **Human resources contact:** Heather Hejmanowsky **Sales:** $2.1 million **Number of employees:** 48 **Number of employees for previous year:** 38 **Industry designation:** Medical products **Company type:** Public **Top competitors:** Medical Graphics Corporation; Abbott Laboratories; Baxter International Inc.

There's a new beat sounding in heart monitors. CardioDynamics International's BioZ System, Portable BioZ, and BioZ.com devices give doctors a low-risk, noninvasive way to gather cardiac data (such as contraction strength and pumping capability) previously collected with a catheter inserted in the pulmonary artery. The digital system measures cardiac activity by passing an electric current through the aorta. Applications include cardiac evaluation, high-risk pregnancies or deliveries, and sports medicine. CardioDynamics hopes to benefit from cost-containment trends in the health care industry. Co-chairman Allen Paulson owns about 40% of the company.

CardioGenesis Corporation

540 Oakmead Pkwy., Sunnyvale, CA 94086

Telephone: 408-328-8500 **Fax:** 408-328-8515 **Metro area:** San Francisco, CA **Web site:** http://www.cardiogenesis.com **Sales:** $3.1 million **Number of employees:** 81 **Number of employees for previous year:** 57 **Industry designation:** Medical instruments **Company type:** Subsidiary **Top competitors:** Eclipse Surgical Technologies, Inc.; PLC Systems Inc.

CardioGenesis, a subsidiary of Eclipse Surgical Technologies, makes proprietary systems, including disposable components, to treat patients suffering from angina. The company developed Transmyocardial Revascularization, a new technique that uses laser energy to create channels in oxygen-deprived regions of the heart muscle. Patients remain conscious during the procedures, which are minimally invasive. CardioGenesis has installed about 45 systems worldwide, including more than a dozen in the United States. The company is conducting clinical trials in the United States of additional related systems.

CardioThoracic Systems, Inc.

10600 N. Tantau Ave., Cupertino, CA 95014

Telephone: 408-342-1700 **Fax:** 408-342-1717 **Metro area:** San Francisco, CA **Web site:** http://www.cardioth.com **Human resources contact:** Debbie Sheets **Sales:** $16.1 million **Number of employees:** 147 **Number of employees for previous year:** 126 **Industry designation:** Medical instruments **Company type:** Public **Top competitors:** Medtronic, Inc.; Heartport, Inc.; Guidant Corporation

CardioThoracic Systems (CTS) has its heart in the right place, developing new techniques for minimally invasive direct coronary bypass (MIDCAB) surgery. Involving only 3"-4" incisions and special rib-spreading and platform devices, CTS's MIDCAB technique eliminates the need for heart-lung machines, speeds recovery time, and cuts costs by about half. Other developments include the Access MV System and OPCAB (Off-Pump Coronary Artery Bypass) Midline Multi-Vessel System, which enable greater efficacy in multi-vessel, beating-heart bypass surgery. Through its CORriculum program, CTS has trained over 1,000 surgeons, nurses, and anesthesiologists at 370 bypass centers to use the company's techniques.

Catalytica, Inc.

430 Ferguson Dr., Mountain View, CA 94043

Telephone: 650-960-3000 **Fax:** 650-960-0127 **Metro area:** San Francisco, CA **Web site:** http://www.catalytica-inc.com **Human resources contact:** John M. Hart **Sales:** $375.2 million **Number of employees:** 1,400 **Number of employees for previous year:** 1,165 **Industry designation:** Pollution control equipment & services **Company type:** Public

Catalytica is a specialty chemical and combustion systems company. Its Catalytica Combustion Systems subsidiary works with precious metals firm Tanaka to develop and market catalytic combustors; it also works with turbine manufacturers such as General Electric to make the XONON Flameless Combustion system, which reduces or eliminates toxins created by utilities' natural gas turbines. The firm's Catalytica Pharmaceuticals unit conducts research and development with drug manufacturer Pfizer. Catalytica also produces active chemicals in bulk and drugs in individual dosage form for companies worldwide, including Glaxo Wellcome, a top pharmaceutical maker. Morgan Stanley Capital Partners III owns 32% of Catalytica.

C-ATS Software Inc.

1870 Embarcadero Rd., Palo Alto, CA 94303

Telephone: 650-321-3000 **Fax:** 650-321-3050 **Metro area:** San Francisco, CA **Web site:** http://www.cats.com **Human resources contact:** Jill Kulick **Sales:** $18.5 million **Number of employees:** 110 **Number of employees for previous year:** 103 **Industry designation:** Computers—corporate, professional & financial software **Company type:** Subsidiary

It's the C-ATS meow in financial risk management. A subsidiary of management software provider Misys, C-ATS Software makes software designed to model changing financial situations around the globe, such as fluctuating currency exchange and interest rates, and to evaluate investment options. Its three product lines—C-ATALYST, CARMA, and FiCAD—produce forecasts, simulations, reports and graphics. Most programs operate on UNIX workstations and PCs and are used by securities firms, fund managers, corporations, and insurance companies. Clients outside the US account for 80% of sales. The C-ATS Consulting Services division offers CARMA implementation and customer support.

CBT Group PLC

1005 Hamilton Ct., Menlo Park, CA 94025

Telephone: 650-614-5900 **Fax:** 650-614-5901 **Metro area:** San Francisco, CA **Web site:** http://www.cbtsys.com **Human resources contact:** Cynthia A. McCaffrey **Sales:** $162.2 million **Number of employees:** 702 **Number of employees for previous year:** 481 **Industry designation:** Computers—corporate, professional & financial software **Company type:** Public **Top competitors:** Harcourt General, Inc.; Gartner Group, Inc.; Knowledge Universe, L.L.C.

Employees expecting a day outside the office for computer training may be disappointed: CBT Group enables staff to train at their desks using their own computers. Subsidiary CBT Systems provides a computer-based library of software containing more than 625 titles for client/server, Internet/intranet, and mainframe technologies. The self-paced software runs on networked and stand-alone PCs. The company has agreements to co-develop training software with Microsoft and Oracle (among other companies), and its library covers products from IBM and Intel. Each course is between four and eight hours long. Subsidiaries CBTWeb and CBTWeb Plus help businesses offer similar courses over the Internet or on intranets.

CCL Plastic Packaging

2501 W. Rosecrans Ave., Los Angeles, CA 90059

Telephone: 310-635-4444 **Fax:** 310-635-3877 **Metro area:** Los Angeles, CA **Human resources contact:** Fabian Botero **Sales:** $59.4 million **Number of employees:** 600 **Number of employees for previous year:** 450 **Industry designation:** Rubber & plastic products **Company type:** Subsidiary **Top competitors:** Owens-Illinois, Inc.; Rotonics Manufacturing Inc.; Triple S Plastics, Inc.

CCL Plastic Packaging, formerly SEDA Specialty Corporation, keeps the lid on specialty plastic packaging components for the personal care, food and beverage, industrial and household chemical, and pharmaceutical industries. Products include lined and unlined plastic caps and closures and flexible plastic tubes, as well as custom products. The company's plastic screw caps are designed to prevent leaks, spoilage, and tampering; its plastic tubes are used for lotions, shampoos, foodstuffs, and household chemicals. CCL Plastic Packaging is part of CCL Industries' container division, and the parent sees it as the cornerstone of plans for growth.

Cellegy Pharmaceuticals, Inc.

1065 E. Hillsdale Blvd., Ste. 418, Foster City, CA 94404

Telephone: 650-524-1600 **Fax:** 650-524-1616 **Metro area:** San Francisco, CA **Web site:** http://www.cellegy.com **Sales:** $800,000 **Number of employees:** 30 **Number of employees for previous year:** 26 **Industry designation:** Drugs **Company type:** Public

Cellegy Pharmaceuticals is developing prescription pharmaceuticals, consumer skin care products, and transdermal drug-delivery technologies. The company expects its products to treat such medical and cosmetic problems as male andropause, debilitating chronic skin diseases, dermatitis, acne, rosacea, severe dry skin, wrinkles and other sun damage, and hemorrhoids. The company, which has not yet completed development of any of its products, has entered into licensing agreements with Neutrogena for its azelaic acid and metabolic moisturizer technologies and with Glaxo Wellcome for Glylorin, its ichthyosis (extremely scaly skin) treatment. Glylorin is in the late stages of clinical testing.

Celtrix Pharmaceuticals, Inc.

3055 Patrick Henry Dr., Santa Clara, CA 95054

Telephone: 408-988-2500 **Fax:** 408-450-4700 **Metro area:** San Francisco, CA **Sales:** $700,000 **Number of employees:** 87 **Number of employees for previous year:** 73 **Industry designation:** Biomedical & genetic products **Company type:** Public

Celtrix Pharmaceuticals, a development-stage pharmaceutical company, is placing its bets on SomatoKine, a DNA-derived protein complex that may have uses in regenerating muscle, bone, and other tissue lost due to trauma, disease, and aging. SomatoKine has finished Phase II clinical trials to study its effects on muscle loss after hip surgery. The complex is also being studied for possible uses in repairing severely burned tissue and in preventing muscle loss attributable to such wasting diseases as AIDS and cancer. By agreement with Celtrix Pharmaceuticals, The Green Cross Corporation has the rights to develop and commercialize SomatoKine in Japan as a treatment for osteoporosis.

Centaur Pharmaceuticals, Inc.

484 Oakmead Pkwy., Sunnyvale, CA 94086

Telephone: 408-822-1600 **Fax:** 408-481-1601 **Metro area:** San Francisco, CA **Web site:** http://www.centpharm.com **Human resources contact:** Lucy O. Day **Sales:** $11.8 million (Est.) **Number of employees:** 90 **Industry designation:** Drugs **Company type:** Private **Top competitors:** NeoTherapeutics, Inc.; Cortex Pharmaceuticals, Inc.; Amgen Inc.

Centaur Pharmaceuticals is developing and testing nitrone-related therapeutics (NRTs) to treat strokes and illnesses like Parkinson's disease, AIDS dementia, and Alzheimer's disease. These conditions all involve oxidative stress—the formation of cell-damaging oxygen agents called free radicals—which Centaur hopes to neutralize through its oral and intravenous treatments, now in clinical and preclinical trials. Centaur Pharmaceuticals is also trying to determine whether its NRT technology can be used to treat arthritis, multiple sclerosis, ophthalmic disorders, and other conditions. The firm has a research and marketing pact with Astra AB for its stroke and Alzheimer's treatments.

Centura Software Corporation

975 Island Dr., Redwood Shores, CA 94065

Telephone: 650-596-3400 **Fax:** 650-596-4900 **Metro area:** San Francisco, CA **Web site:** http://www.centurasoft.com **Human resources contact:** Sandra Sanchez **Sales:** $53.5 million **Number of employees:** 204 **Number of employees for previous year:** 180 **Industry designation:** Computers—corporate, professional & financial software **Company type:** Public **Top competitors:** BMC Software, Inc.; Oracle Corporation; Sybase, Inc.

Centura Software (formerly Gupta Corporation) makes tools that help large companies build global computer networks or Internet software applications. The company designs databases (SQLBase), connectivity products (SQLHost), and development tools (Centura and SQLWindows). Software development teams in large corporations such as UPS, Automatic Data Processing, and Deutsche Bank use its products. The company continues to position its products to be Web- and mobile computing-capable. Investor group Crossroads Capital Partners owns almost 40% of Centura.

The Cerplex Group, Inc.

1382 Bell Ave., Irvine, CA 92168

Telephone: 949-754-5300 **Fax:** 949-754-5492 **Metro area:** San Diego, CA **Web site:** http:// www.cerplex.com **Human resources contact:** Robert P. Dunce **Sales:** $66.4 million **Number of employees:** 1,350 **Number of employees for previous year:** 260 **Industry designation:** Computers—services **Company type:** Public **Top competitors:** Pomeroy Select Integration Solutions, Inc.; PC Service Source, Inc.; DecisionOne Holdings Corp.

Cerplex has a surplus of services. The Cerplex Group (formerly Aurora Electronics) repairs computer, telecommunications, and electronic office equipment for manufacturers. The company services products ranging from laptops, hubs, and modems to ATMs and pay phones. It performs repairs, conversions, and upgrades through depot repair facilities. Cerplex also distributes spare parts for the computer industry. The company offers materials management services including inventory management and electronic materials recycling and remarketing. Customers include Rank Xerox and British Telecommunications (17% and 11% of sales, respectively). Venture capital firm Welsh, Carson, Anderson & Stowe owns 67% of the company.

Cerus Corporation

2525 Stanwell Dr., Ste. 300, Concord, CA 94520

Telephone: 925-603-9071 **Fax:** 925-603-9099 **Metro area:** San Francisco, CA **Human resources contact:** Debra Hall **Sales:** $2.9 million **Number of employees:** 83 **Number of employees for previous year:** 76 **Industry designation:** Biomedical & genetic products **Company type:** Public

Cerus develops blood-pathogen inactivation systems intended to improve the safety of blood transfusions. The company's systems involve the use of its proprietary small-molecule compounds to prevent pathogens, such as viruses and bacteria, from replicating in blood. Its systems are also designed to inhibit leukocyte activity that is responsible for adverse immune and other transfusion-related reactions. All of Cerus' products are in clinical trials or preclinical development. Cerus has a marketing agreement with Baxter Healthcare, which has invested about $15 million in Cerus' research and owns about 16% of the company's stock.

Chevron Chemical Company

6001 Bollinger Canyon Rd., San Ramon, CA 94583

Telephone: 925-842-1000 **Fax:** 925-842-5775 **Metro area:** San Francisco, CA **Web site:** http:// www.chevron.com/about/petrochem/main.html **Human resources contact:** R.W. Culbertson **Sales:** $3.5 billion **Industry designation:** Chemicals—specialty **Company type:** Subsidiary

Chevron subsidiary Chevron Chemical Company (CCC) makes and markets industrial chemicals in 80 countries. The company produces a range of petrochemicals, including benzene, cumene, cyclohexane, paraxylene, ethylene, normal alpha olefins (NAOs), propylene, polyethylene, styrene, and polystyrene, through its U.S. Chemicals division and its International Group. CCC is a top maker of NAOs and a leading producer of linear and low-density polyethylene, high-density polyethylene, and polyethylene pipe. The company's Oronite division, a market leader in deposit-control gasoline additives, sells lubricant and fuel additives worldwide. The division has additive plants in Brazil, France, Japan, Singapore, and the US.

Cholestech Corporation

3347 Investment Blvd., Hayward, CA 94545

Telephone: 510-732-7200 **Fax:** 510-732-7227 **Metro area:** San Francisco, CA **Web site:** http:// www.cholestech.com **Sales:** $21.7 million **Number of employees:** 141 **Number of employees for previous year:** 107 **Industry designation:** Medical products **Company type:** Public **Top competitors:** Roche Holding Ltd; Abbott Laboratories; Johnson & Johnson

You might not want to know your cholesterol level, but Cholestech is going to tell you anyway with its proprietary blood diagnostic test. The company sells its Cholestech LDX system worldwide to hospitals, managed care organizations, and companies for employee wellness programs. It also has a distribution agreement with McKesson HBOC and an agreement with Health Management Services to test Wal-Mart shoppers' cholesterol levels at selected US stores. The system features a telephone-sized electronic analyzer and disposable test cassettes that let users perform combinations of tests in five minutes or less, using just a drop of whole blood. It also measures glucose and lipids to assess cardiac and diabetes risks.

ChromaVision Medical Systems, Inc.

33171 Paseo Cerveza, San Juan Capistrano, CA 92675

Telephone: 949-443-3355 **Fax:** 949-443-3366 **Metro area:** Los Angeles, CA **Web site:** http://
www.chromavision.com **Human resources contact:** Leslie Waters **Sales:** $100,000 **Number of
employees:** 56 **Number of employees for previous year:** 39 **Industry designation:** Medical
instruments **Company type:** Public

ChromaVision Medical Systems develops and makes the ChromaVision Automated Cellular Imaging System
(ChromaVision ACIS), a programmable blood-screening system for identifying abnormal cells. Its microscope can
scan up to 100 patient samples at once. The system's computer identifies as few as one affected cell in 120 million
(chemical reagents change the color of abnormal cells), counts the abnormal cells, makes a digital image of them,
and records the data. The instrument awaits FDA approval for commercial medical use. ChromaVision Medical
Systems' technology can be used to screen for Down's Syndrome and may be adapted for virus and cancer
detection. Safeguard Scientifics owns 26% of the firm.

Circon Corporation

6500 Hollister Ave., Santa Barbara, CA 93117

Telephone: 805-685-5100 **Fax:** 805-968-8174 **Metro area:** Santa Barbara, CA **Web site:** http://
www.circoncorp.com **Human resources contact:** Jon St. Clair **Sales:** $160 million **Number of
employees:** 1,204 **Number of employees for previous year:** 1,177 **Industry designation:**
Medical instruments **Company type:** Subsidiary **Top competitors:** Johnson & Johnson; Stryker
Corporation; Boston Scientific Corporation

Circon, a subsidiary of Maxxim Medical, produces endoscopes and miniature video systems for medical
applications. Circon's endoscope systems allow doctors to see internal tissue (stomach, lungs, kidney, bladder,
uterus) and perform minimally invasive surgery and other procedures; the systems include video cameras and light
sources. Endoscopic surgery reduces the cost of procedures and lessens the need for postoperative hospitalization.
The firm, with facilities in North America and Europe, also makes other types of medical devices and systems,
including those used in gynecological surgery.

Clarify Inc.

2125 O'Nel Dr., San Jose, CA 95131

Telephone: 408-573-3000 **Fax:** 408-573-3001 **Metro area:** San Francisco, CA **Web site:** http://
www.clarify.com **Human resources contact:** Laraine Sanford **Sales:** $130.5 million **Number of
employees:** 488 **Number of employees for previous year:** 405 **Industry designation:**
Computers—corporate, professional & financial software **Company type:** Public **Top competitors:** Siebel
Systems, Inc.; Remedy Corporation; The Vantive Corporation

Need help keeping your ducks in a row? Clarify makes software that automates front-office functions such as help
desk and customer sales and service. ClearSales manages leads, generates quotes, and forecasts sales. Telemarketers
and customer service departments use ClearCallCenter to route calls to the agents most suitable for a customer's
needs and to identify selling opportunities (through call scripting). ClearHelpDesk tracks tasks across groups,
monitors service agreements, and tracks support costs. Other products track service contracts and manage repair
centers. CommCenter is specifically designed for telecommunications customer service. Customers include General
Electric, Microsoft, and Sprint.

Clontech Laboratories, Inc.

1020 E. Meadow Circle, Palo Alto, CA 94303

Telephone: 650-424-8222 **Fax:** 650-424-1088 **Metro area:** San Francisco, CA **Web site:** http://
www.clontech.com **Sales:** $47.8 million (Est.) **Number of employees:** 312 **Industry designation:**
Medical services **Company type:** Private **Top competitors:** Becton, Dickinson and Company; The
Perkin-Elmer Corporation; Abbott Laboratories

Clontech Laboratories didn't make Dolly, but its products can help get into her genes. The firm sells more than
1,500 kits and other biological products to help research scientists identify and analyze genes, gene expression, and
protein interactions. Clontech sells its tests and other products mainly to government and academic institutions and
biotechnology and pharmaceutical firms. Clontech sometimes works with other firms to create new products, such
as its cDNA microarray project with Molecular Dynamics. The company markets its products in more than 30
countries via units in Germany, Japan, and the UK. Founder and CEO Kenneth Fong owns 75% of Clontech;
venture capital firm Summit Ventures owns the rest.

The Clorox Company

1221 Broadway, Oakland, CA 94612

Telephone: 510-271-7000 **Fax:** 510-832-1463 **Metro area:** San Francisco, CA **Web site:** http://www.clorox.com **Human resources contact:** Janet M. Brady **Sales:** $2.7 billion **Number of employees:** 6,600 **Number of employees for previous year:** 5,500 **Industry designation:** Soap & cleaning preparations **Company type:** Public **Top competitors:** The Procter & Gamble Company; Colgate-Palmolive Company; S.C. Johnson & Son, Inc.

Brands cannot live by bleach alone. Best known for its namesake bleach (#1 in the world), The Clorox Company makes a host of laundry and cleaning products (Pine-Sol, Soft Scrub), insecticides (Combat), cat litter (Fresh Step), car-care products (Armor All), and charcoal briquettes (Kingsford). Many of the company's brands lead their markets. Its 1999 acquisition of First Brands strengthened Clorox in such areas as cat litter and car care and helped the company diversify into plastic wraps with market leader Glad. Clorox sells its products in more than 80 countries; growing international sales account for about 20% of its total. Chemical giant Henkel owns 30% of the company.

CMD Technology, Inc.

19 Morgan, Irvine, CA 92618

Telephone: 949-454-0800 **Fax:** 949-455-1656 **Metro area:** Los Angeles, CA **Web site:** http://ftp.cmd.com **Human resources contact:** Fran Richardson **Sales:** $50 million (Est.) **Number of employees:** 200 **Industry designation:** Computers—peripheral equipment **Company type:** Private **Top competitors:** Adaptec, Inc.; Ciprico Inc.; Photonics Corporation

Founded in 1986, CMD Technology makes chips for interfacing computer peripherals and storing data. Its semiconductor unit offers SCSI (small computer system interface), RAID (redundant array of independent disks), and IDE chips that are ultimately used to connect dozens of peripherals to PCs with little hassle. The firm's storage unit offers OEMs, systems integrators, and resellers a line of controllers (including the high-performance Viper-brand family of RAID products) for PCs, workstations, LANs, and mid-range systems. CMD's semiconductor products support such applications as video/multimedia, document imaging, high-speed networking, and online connectivity. Clients include Dell, Compaq, and Gateway.

CNET, Inc.

150 Chestnut St., San Francisco, CA 94111

Telephone: 415-395-7800 **Fax:** 415-395-9205 **Metro area:** San Francisco, CA **Web site:** http://www.cnet.com **Human resources contact:** Heather McGaughy **Sales:** $56.4 million **Number of employees:** 581 **Number of employees for previous year:** 372 **Industry designation:** Computers—online services **Company type:** Public **Top competitors:** International Data Group; Wired Digital, Inc.; ZDNet Group

CNET feeds the public's appetite for high-tech, providing programming and information relating to computers, the Internet, and digital technologies via the World Wide Web and television. CNET operates a range of Web sites including cnet.com (its central site), shareware.com, search.com, snap.com (in which television network NBC owns a 60% interest) and news.com. It produces "TV.COM," the first nationally syndicated TV series about the Internet, as well as "CNET Central, The Web," and "The New Edge," which are carried on the USA Network and the Sci-Fi Channel. CNET receives over three-fourths of its sales from its Internet operations (primarily advertisements).

Cohesion Technologies, Inc.

2500 Faber Place, Palo Alto, CA 94303

Telephone: 650-354-4300 **Fax:** 650-856-0533 **Metro area:** San Francisco, CA **Web site:** http://www.cohesiontech.com **Sales:** $2 million **Number of employees:** 73 **Number of employees for previous year:** 69 **Industry designation:** Medical products **Company type:** Public **Top competitors:** Anika Therapeutics, Inc.; Integra LifeSciences Corporation; Focal, Inc.

For Cohesion Technologies, healing is a sticky business. Spun off from Collagen Aesthetics (formerly Collagen Corporation) in 1998, the firm is developing products to prevent internal wounds from leaking blood and other vital fluids into the body cavity. Its CoStasis sealant (made in part from cow collagen) mixes with a patient's plasma to form a clot over bleeding tissue. The company's CoSeal forms a reabsorbable seal over an internal surgical wound. One of the firm's products—bone-graft substitute Collagraft—is sold on the market by a Bristol-Myers Squibb subsidiary. Other products in development include CoStop, another healing adhesive designed to prevent painful internal tissue adhesions.

Collateral Therapeutics, Inc.

9360 Towne Centre Dr., San Diego, CA 92121

Telephone: 619-824-6500 **Fax:** 619-824-6563 **Metro area:** San Diego, CA **Sales:** $5.4 million **Number of employees:** 27 **Industry designation:** Biomedical & genetic products **Company type:** Public **Top competitors:** Repligen Corporation; Vical Incorporated

Collateral Therapeutics develops nonsurgical gene therapy products for treatment of various cardiovascular diseases and as an alternative to coronary bypass surgery and angioplasty. Products are in various stages of research, development, and trials and include treatments for coronary artery disease, peripheral vascular disease, congestive heart failure, and post-heart-attack muscle regeneration. Support for product development, manufacturing, and marketing is generated through strategic partners such as Schering. Collateral has research licenses with universities including the University of California and New York University. CEO Jack Reich owns about 12% of the company; VP H. Kirk Hammond owns about 15%.

CombiChem, Inc.

9050 Camino Santa Fe, San Diego, CA 92121

Telephone: 619-530-0484 **Fax:** 619-530-9998 **Metro area:** San Diego, CA **Web site:** http://www.combichem.com/home.html **Human resources contact:** Bobbie Bosley **Sales:** $15.1 million **Number of employees:** 73 **Number of employees for previous year:** 56 **Industry designation:** Drugs **Company type:** Public

CombiChem helps accelerate pharmaceutical and biotechnology companies' drug discovery process. Its computerized Discovery Engine process targets likely drug candidates by searching its libraries for hypothetical drug compounds. Its Virtual Library holds computational representations of about 500 billion drug-like molecules and its Universal Informer Library is a computer-designed collection of about 10,000 physical compounds to find molecular structures that match hypothetical drug compounds. The company is collaborating with Novartis to discover pesticides for crops and has drug discovery agreements with Teijin Limited, Roche Bioscience, Sumitomo Pharmaceuticals, ImClone Systems, and Athena Neurosciences.

Compass Plastics & Technologies Inc.

15730 S. Figueroa St., Gardena, CA 90248

Telephone: 323-770-8771 **Fax:** 310-523-9859 **Metro area:** Los Angeles, CA **Sales:** $44 million **Number of employees:** 471 **Number of employees for previous year:** 285 **Industry designation:** Rubber & plastic products **Company type:** Public **Top competitors:** Lynch Corporation; Summa Industries; McKechnie plc

Compass Plastics & Technologies keeps its bearings by making injection-molded plastic parts for electronics manufacturers. Through subsidiaries AB Plastics and M.O.S. Plastics, Compass makes housings for computer monitors, televisions, and electronic keyboards. Its main customers include Sony (a customer since 1972), Hewlett Packard, Apple Computer, and Matsushita. Compass Plastics also paints and assembles mechanical and electronic components. The company has an agreement to acquire Gumsung Plastics, USA. Director Christopher Mills owns about 20% of the company.

CompuMed, Inc.

1230 Rosecrans Ave., Ste. 1000, Manhattan Beach, CA 90266

Telephone: 310-643-5106 **Fax:** 310-536-6128 **Metro area:** Los Angeles, CA **Web site:** http://www.compumed.net **Human resources contact:** Foo Dang **Sales:** $1.8 million **Number of employees:** 28 **Number of employees for previous year:** 26 **Industry designation:** Medical services **Company type:** Public **Top competitors:** Lunar Corporation; Norland Medical Systems, Inc.; Hologic, Inc.

CompuMed develops systems that diagnose and monitor cardiovascular disease and osteoporosis. The company primarily provides computerized electrocardiograms (ECGs) and ECG interpretations to some 1,000 health care providers and institutions across the US. CompuMed is seeking distributors for its OsteoGram software, which monitors osteoporosis by analyzing bone density. A device to monitor osteoporosis—the OsteoView—is in the works. The company conducts bone-density research through agreements with the University of Massachusetts and Varian Imaging Products. CompuMed is seeking development partners for its Detoxahol product, designed to lower blood-alcohol levels in inebriated people.

Computer Motion, Inc.

130-B Cremona Dr., Goleta, CA 93117

Telephone: 805-968-9600 **Fax:** 805-685-9277 **Metro area:** Santa Barbara, CA **Web site:** http://www.computermotion.com **Human resources contact:** Georgia Kruip **Sales:** $10.6 million **Number of employees:** 146 **Number of employees for previous year:** 94 **Industry designation:** Medical instruments **Company type:** Public

Computer Motion makes robotic and computerized surgical equipment. Founded to conduct robotics research for NASA, the National Science Foundation, and the US Navy, the company's primary product, AESOP, is a voice-controlled, robotic endoscope positioning system used in minimally invasive surgical procedures. FDA-approved AESOP holds the endoscope (here a small surgical camera), and responds to the surgeon's verbal commands. The company is also testing ZEUS, a three-armed version of AESOP, and has been granted FDA market clearance for HERMES, which coordinates movements with several surgical devices. These systems are designed to centralize operating-room activities under the voice control of the surgeon.

Concentric Network Corporation

10590 N. Tantau Ave., Cupertino, CA 95014

Telephone: 408-342-2800 **Fax:** 408-342-2810 **Metro area:** San Francisco, CA **Web site:** http://www.concentric.com **Human resources contact:** Frederick J. Schreiber **Sales:** $82.8 million **Number of employees:** 569 **Number of employees for previous year:** 387 **Industry designation:** Computers—services **Company type:** Public **Top competitors:** AT&T Broadband & Internet Services; MCI WorldCom, Inc.; America Online, Inc.

Concentric Network offers a full round of Internet and networking services. The company provides Web hosting, local Internet dial-up and remote access, Internet telephony and videoconferencing, and virtual private networks (enterprise networks with hardware leased from a third party, in this case Concentric). Its customers include corporations such as Microsoft's WebTV Networks (one-third of sales), AT&T, and 3Com; consumers; and small businesses. Rock star David Bowie's BowieNet Internet service uses Concentric's technology. The company has teamed with Telecom Italia (which owns about 10% of Concentric through a subsidiary) to offer the MondoNet global Internet protocol-based network.

Connetics Corp.

3400 W. Bayshore Rd., Palo Alto, CA 94303

Telephone: 650-843-2800 **Fax:** 650-843-2899 **Metro area:** San Francisco, CA **Web site:** http://www.connetics.com **Human resources contact:** Rebecca Gardener **Sales:** $7.5 million **Number of employees:** 84 **Number of employees for previous year:** 72 **Industry designation:** Drugs **Company type:** Public **Top competitors:** Vertex Pharmaceuticals Incorporated; Osiris Therapeutics, Inc.; Chiroscience Group plc

"When immune systems go haywire" isn't a Fox special; it's Connetics Corp.'s niche. The company specializes in treatments for autoimmune diseases involving connective tissues, including dermatitis, scleroderma, multiple sclerosis, and rheumatoid arthritis. Its ConXn product (based on relaxin, a natural substance that promotes connective tissue remodeling) is in trials for treatment of scleroderma, a thickening of skin and organs. Other drugs include highly potent topical corticosteroids for dematological conditions, gamma interferon, and a TCR peptide vaccine. Connetics acquires promising drug treatments from other drug companies, including SmithKline Beecham and Genentech, to further develop and market them.

Consumer Net Marketplace, Inc.

1900 Los Angeles Ave., 2nd Fl., Simi Valley, CA 93065

Telephone: 805-520-7170 **Fax:** 805-520-7211 **Metro area:** Los Angeles, CA **Web site:** http://www.cnmnetwork.com **Human resources contact:** Olivia Salyer **Sales:** $30,000 (Est.) **Number of employees:** 64 **Number of employees for previous year:** 52 **Industry designation:** Computers—online services **Company type:** Private **Top competitors:** America Online, Inc.; Yahoo! Inc.; iMALL, Inc.

Consumer Net Marketplace is bringing a little roadside shopping to the information highway. As an Internet service provider (ISP), the company brings businesses and consumers together by providing both business and individual users such services as dial-up Internet access, dedicated connectivity, and Web creation and hosting. The ISP also owns and operates an Internet shopping mall hosting more than 1,200 businesses and offers proprietary software enabling customers to make secure commercial transactions over the Internet. After Consumer Net Marketplace's planned IPO, founder and CEO Fredrick Rice will own about half of the company.

The Cooper Companies, Inc.

10 Faraday, Irvine, CA 92618

Telephone: 949-597-4700 **Fax:** 949-597-0662 **Metro area:** Los Angeles, CA **Web site:** http://www.coopercos.com **Human resources contact:** Lorie Ferguson **Sales:** $147.2 million **Number of employees:** 1,900 **Number of employees for previous year:** 1,400 **Industry designation:** Medical products **Company type:** Public **Top competitors:** Johnson & Johnson; Wesley Jessen VisionCare, Inc.; Bausch & Lomb Incorporated

Count on The Cooper Companies to come through with such health care products as contact lenses, gynecological instruments, and disposable medical products. Subsidiary CooperVision (about 80% of sales) makes specialty contact lenses, including soft toric (for astigmatism), spherical (for myopia), disposable, and colored lenses. Subsidiary CooperSurgical specializes in handheld instruments, surgical instruments, and accessories for the OB-GYN market. In 1998 Cooper discontinued operations of its Hospital Group of America, and announced it would sell most of the group's properties (which included three psychiatric hospitals and 17 supporting outpatient clinics) to Universal Health Services.

CORE INC.

18881 Von Karman Ave., Ste. 1750, Irvine, CA 92612

Telephone: 949-442-2100 **Fax:** 949-442-2102 **Metro area:** Los Angeles, CA **Human resources contact:** Sara Tague **Sales:** $45.6 million **Number of employees:** 925 **Number of employees for previous year:** 870 **Industry designation:** Medical practice management **Company type:** Public

CORE's core has changed. The company has made the transition from evaluating patient care utilization for managed health care providers to managing disability programs for large companies such as Bell Atlantic Corporation, General Electric, and Motorola. CORE repositioned itself because profits were elusive in the intensely competitive health care utilization field. The company made the change through a series of acquisitions in 1998, including the workers compensation assets of Transcend Services, Inc.; Disability Reinsurance Management Services, Inc.; and Social Security Disability Consultants & Disability Services, Inc.

COR Therapeutics, Inc.

256 E. Grand Ave., South San Francisco, CA 94080

Telephone: 650-244-6800 **Fax:** 650-244-9208 **Metro area:** San Francisco, CA **Web site:** http://www.corr.com **Human resources contact:** Lynn Hughes **Sales:** $42 million **Number of employees:** 321 **Number of employees for previous year:** 182 **Industry designation:** Drugs **Company type:** Public **Top competitors:** Eli Lilly and Company

COR Therapeutics develops pharmaceutical products for the treatment and prevention of severe cardiovascular disease. INTEGRILIN, its core product, has been recommended by the FDA's Cardiovascular and Renal Drugs Advisory Committee for use with coronary angioplasty; it has not yet received FDA approval of the drug for treatment of acute coronary syndromes. Schering-Plough, which has a marketing agreement with COR Therapeutics, has filed for approval of INTEGRILIN in Europe for the treatment of unstable angina, myocardial infarction, and coronary angioplasty. COR Therapeutics is also evaluating other products, including one intended to treat deep vein thrombosis and pulmonary embolism.

CorVel Corporation

2010 Main St., Ste. 1020, Irvine, CA 92614

Telephone: 949-851-1473 **Fax:** 949-851-1469 **Metro area:** Los Angeles, CA **Web site:** http://www.corvel.com **Human resources contact:** Sharon O'Connor **Sales:** $141.7 million **Number of employees:** 2,200 **Number of employees for previous year:** 1,900 **Industry designation:** Medical practice management **Company type:** Public **Top competitors:** Value Health, Inc.; Mutual Risk Management Ltd.; Concentra Managed Care, Inc.

CorVel Corporation has corv-ed out a niche providing workers' compensation medical cost containment and managed care services. The company's services include automated medical fee auditing, early intervention, utilization review, medical case management, vocational rehabilitation services, and independent medical examinations. CorVel provides its services to insurance companies, third-party administrators, and corporations, thus helping them manage the medical costs and monitor the quality of care associated with workers' compensation claims. Computer networking company ENStar owns nearly 25% of CorVel.

Coulter Pharmaceutical, Inc.

550 California Ave., Ste. 200, Palo Alto, CA 94306

Telephone: 650-849-7500 **Fax:** 650-849-7530 **Metro area:** San Francisco, CA **Web site:** http://www.coulterpharm.com **Human resources contact:** Kay Slocum **Sales:** $34.3 million **Number of employees:** 137 **Number of employees for previous year:** 66 **Industry designation:** Drugs **Company type:** Public

Development-stage Coulter Pharmaceutical is using conjugated antibodies, tumor-activated peptide drugs, and other technologies to develop new treatments for cancer. The company's lead candidate, Bexxar, is in late-phase clinical trials for use in treating non-Hodgkin's lymphoma; if approved by the FDA, the drug could become the first radioimmunotherapy cancer treatment OK'd in the US. Coulter Pharmaceutical is also developing a new version of doxorubicin, an antibiotic used to treat some solid-tumor cancers. The firm plans to directly market and sell its products in the US, and to use marketing partners, such as SmithKline Beecham, to market its products internationally.

CRL Network Services, Inc.

1 Kearny St., Ste. 1450, San Francisco, CA 94108

Telephone: 415-837-5300 **Fax:** 415-392-9000 **Metro area:** San Francisco, CA **Web site:** http://www.crl.com **Sales:** $11.7 million (Est.) **Number of employees:** 59 **Industry designation:** Computers—online services **Company type:** Private **Top competitors:** PSINet Inc.; UUNET WorldCom; Concentric Network Corporation

CRL Network Services thinks of itself as a top-drawer—make that top-tier—Internet service provider (ISP). As a Tier 1 ISP, CRL uses its own facilities-based Internet backbone to provide connectivity and Web hosting services to small and medium-sized businesses. It offers dial-up and dedicated access, WAN and Ethernet services, and specialty services such as security (firewalls), remote access management, and network integration. The company has 30 points of presence (POPs) in US metropolitan areas. Clients include Office Depot, Southwest Airlines, the US Department of Commerce, and the Federal Reserve Board. Chairman and CEO James Couch, who founded CRL in 1983, owns the company.

CV Therapeutics, Inc.

3172 Porter Dr., Palo Alto, CA 94304

Telephone: 650-812-0585 **Fax:** 650-858-0390 **Metro area:** San Francisco, CA **Human resources contact:** Diane Larson **Sales:** $2.6 million **Number of employees:** 62 **Number of employees for previous year:** 44 **Industry designation:** Drugs **Company type:** Public

CV Therapeutics discovers, develops, and commercializes novel, small-molecule drugs to treat chronic cardiovascular diseases. Through its expertise in the area of molecular cardiology, the company has developed drugs including CVT-124, which has potential applications in the treatment of edema associated with congestive heart failure and in the prevention and treatment of acute renal failure. The target market for CVT-124 includes patients who have not responded well to diuretics. Another of its drugs is ranolazine, a compound that was licensed from Roche subsidiary Syntex and has been developed for the treatment of angina. It is collaborating with Incyte on a gene database for cardiovascular biology.

Cypress Bioscience, Inc.

4350 Executive Dr., Ste. 325, San Diego, CA 92121

Telephone: 619-452-2323 **Fax:** 619-452-1222 **Metro area:** San Diego, CA **Sales:** $2.7 million **Number of employees:** 39 **Number of employees for previous year:** 36 **Industry designation:** Medical products **Company type:** Public **Top competitors:** Baxter International Inc.

Cypress Bioscience makes medical devices to treat some types of immune system diseases; it is also developing therapies for treating blood platelet disorders. FDA-approved PROSORBA column, the company's flagship product, pumps blood through a cylinder of Protein A to remove certain antibodies from a patient's plasma and thus treat an autoimmune-related bleeding disorder. Cypress Bioscience is seeking additional FDA approval to market the PROSORBA column as a rheumatoid arthritis treatment. The company is also developing Cyplex, infusible platelet membranes that can replace platelet transfusions. Cyplex has a longer shelf life than donated platelets and does not transmit viruses.

Cypros Pharmaceutical Corporation

2714 Loker Ave. West, Carlsbad, CA 92008

Telephone: 760-929-9500 **Fax:** 760-929-8038 **Metro area:** San Diego, CA **Web site:** http://www.cypros.com **Human resources contact:** Fredric I. Storch **Sales:** $3.4 million **Number of employees:** 42 **Number of employees for previous year:** 39 **Industry designation:** Drugs **Company type:** Public

Cypros Pharmaceutical develops, acquires, and markets acute-care drugs for use in hospitals. The company sells Glofil and Inulin, which are intravenous drugs that assess kidney functions, and Ethamolin, which treats esophageal bleeding associated with liver disease and hypertension. It is launching two burn/wound care products (Neoflo and Sildaflo). Drugs in development include Ceresine and Cordox; both may be useful in the treatment of disorders related to impaired blood flow, which starves cells of oxygen. CPC-111 may also have applications in bypass surgery and sickle-cell anemia treatment, and Ceresine has the potential to minimize tissue damage associated with head injuries and strokes.

Dairyman's Cooperative Creamery Association

400 S. M St., Tulare, CA 93274

Telephone: 559-687-8287 **Fax:** 559-685-6911 **Metro area:** Bakersfield, CA **Human resources contact:** Sue Brown **Sales:** $691.8 million **Number of employees:** 530 **Number of employees for previous year:** 525 **Industry designation:** Food—dairy products **Company type:** Division **Top competitors:** Foremost Farms USA; Dairy Farmers of America; Darigold Inc.

Dairyman's Cooperative Creamery is an udder story. The cooperative, which runs the nation's largest single dairy-processing facility, produces nonfat and whole milk powder, yogurt, cheese, cream cheese, and butter through joint ventures with packagers and marketers of those products. The cooperative is a division of Land O'Lakes, the nation's second-largest dairy co-op. Started with a single plant in 1909, the association has produced butter for Land O'Lakes since 1983 and became part of the larger co-op in 1998. The 240 members of Dairyman's Cooperative Creamery run dairies in California's Tulare, Kings, and Fresno Counties.

Delta Dental Plan of California

100 First St., San Francisco, CA 94105

Telephone: 415-972-8300 **Fax:** 415-972-8366 **Metro area:** San Francisco, CA **Web site:** http://www.deltadentalca.org **Human resources contact:** Sandra J. Boros **Sales:** $2.3 billion **Number of employees:** 2,115 **Number of employees for previous year:** 1,960 **Industry designation:** Insurance—accident & health **Company type:** Not-for-profit **Top competitors:** PacifiCare Health Systems, Inc.; WellPoint Health Networks Inc.; Pacific Mutual Holding Company

Delta Dental Plan of California is one of the nation's largest dental insurers, providing coverage through health maintenance organizations, preferred provider plans, and government programs such as California's Denti-Cal. A not-for-profit organization, the company is a member of the Delta Dental Plans Association and has affiliates nationwide. The company serves more than 10 million enrollees in California. Non-government clients account for about half of its California participants. Delta Dental also has more than one million members outside California. More than two-thirds of the nation's dentists and more than 90% of California's dentists participate in Delta Dental's programs.

Dental/Medical Diagnostic Systems, Inc.

200 N. Westlake Blvd., Ste. 202, Westlake Village, CA 91362

Telephone: 805-381-2700 **Fax:** 805-374-1966 **Metro area:** Los Angeles, CA **Web site:** http://www.dmdcorp.com **Human resources contact:** Robyn Pope **Sales:** $19.2 million **Number of employees:** 79 **Number of employees for previous year:** 57 **Industry designation:** Medical instruments **Company type:** Public **Top competitors:** Patterson Dental Company; Henry Schein, Inc.; DENTSPLY International Inc.

Dental/Medical Diagnostic Systems (DMDS) knows that sometimes the best way to get people to brush their teeth is to show 'em in full, living color their unsightly plaque buildup. To accomplish this feat, the company makes the TeliCam II and TeliCam Elite, intraoral camera systems that capture, store, display, and print full-color images of teeth, gums, and other parts of the mouth. In addition to its imaging technology, DMDS markets the Apollo 95E, a tooth whitening system made by BriteSmile (formerly Ion Laser Technology) that doesn't use lasers. The company is developing a digital X-ray system, which reduces radiation and eliminates time-consuming film development, with Suni Imaging Microsystems.

DepoMed, Inc.

1170 B Chess Dr., Foster City, CA 94404

Telephone: 650-513-0990 **Fax:** 650-513-0999 **Metro area:** San Francisco, CA **Sales:** $800,000 **Number of employees:** 17 **Number of employees for previous year:** 8 **Industry designation:** Drugs **Company type:** Public **Top competitors:** Penwest Pharmaceuticals Co.; Kos Pharmaceuticals, Inc.; ALZA Corporation

DepoMed, a development stage company, engineers oral drug delivery systems. The company's Gastric Retention system is designed to enable drugs to remain undigested in the stomach for longer periods of time, thus increasing efficacy while reducing dosage. The Reduced Irritation system reduces stomach irritation caused by ingestion of certain drugs. DepoMed funds its research through collaborative agreements with companies such as Bristol-Myers Squibb and R.W. Johnson Pharmaceutical Research, a subsidiary of Johnson & Johnson; DepoMed is independently developing a calcium supplement and an aspirin product that would incorporate its delivery systems. Chairman John Shell owns about one-fourth of DepoMed.

Dey, Inc.

2751 Napa Valley Corporate Dr., Napa, CA 94558

Telephone: 877-666-1534 **Fax:** 707-224-9264 **Metro area:** San Francisco, CA **Human resources contact:** Amelia Villegas **Sales:** $219.8 million (Est.) **Number of employees:** 663 **Industry designation:** Drugs **Company type:** Private

Dey helps people breathe easy. The company makes prescription drugs for the treatment of respiratory diseases and allergies. Its premeasured unit dose inhalation products include treatments for asthma and chronic obstructive pulmonary disease. Its Dey-Pak sodium chloride solution products are used in tracheal care and to dilute concentrated inhalation solutions. Dey markets EpiPen autoinjectors, used by patients to self-administer epinephrine for allergic reactions. The company sells its products directly to physicians, institutional purchasers, wholesalers, pharmacies, and HMOs. Lipha Americas, an affiliate of Merck KGaA, will reduce its stake in Dey to 84% after the planned IPO.

Diagnostic Products Corporation

5700 W. 96th St., Los Angeles, CA 90045

Telephone: 323-776-0180 **Fax:** 323-776-0204 **Metro area:** Los Angeles, CA **Web site:** http://www.dpcweb.com **Human resources contact:** Ava Sedgwick **Sales:** $196.6 million **Number of employees:** 1,601 **Number of employees for previous year:** 1,467 **Industry designation:** Medical products **Company type:** Public **Top competitors:** Chiron Corporation; Abbott Laboratories; Becton, Dickinson and Company

Diagnostic Products Corporation (DPC) is one of the world's leading independent makers of immunodiagnostic kits that detect minute amounts of allergens, drugs, or hormones in human and animal tissues. Traditionally testing has been conducted through radioimmunoassay (RIA) test kits, but since demand for such products (which use radioisotopes) has declined because of environmental concerns, the company has added nonisotopic tests, including a fully automated testing system called IMMULITE (60% of sales). DPC makes more than 400 kinds of test kits, which detect disease, allergies, or substance abuse, for sale in more than 100 countries, primarily to hospitals and laboratories.

Dionex Corporation

1228 Titan Way, Sunnyvale, CA 94086

Telephone: 408-737-0700 **Fax:** 408-739-8437 **Other address:** PO Box 3603, Sunnyvale, CA 94088 **Metro area:** San Francisco, CA **Web site:** http://www.dionex.com **Human resources contact:** Debbie Sedgwick **Sales:** $150.5 million **Number of employees:** 715 **Number of employees for previous year:** 685 **Industry designation:** Instruments—scientific **Company type:** Public **Top competitors:** The Perkin-Elmer Corporation; Waters Corporation; Hewlett-Packard Company

Thirsty? Whether it's water, milk, beer, or coffee, Dionex's analytical instruments make sure it's contaminant-free. Chemists in the food and beverage, biotechnology, electronics, and petrochemicals industries use the company's chromatography systems to isolate and quantify individual components of complex chemical mixtures. Dionex's instruments can be used for ion chromatography (separating and identifying charged molecules), high-performance liquid chromatography (separating and identifying biological molecules such as amino acids and proteins), and sample extraction. Dionex operates its own sales network in the US and 10 other countries. About half of its sales are outside North America.

Directed Electronics, Inc.

2560 Progress St., Vista, CA 92083

Telephone: 760-598-6200 **Fax:** 760-598-6400 **Metro area:** San Diego, CA **Web site:** http://www.directed.com **Human resources contact:** Kristen Fullerton **Sales:** $79 million (Est.) **Number of employees:** 170 **Number of employees for previous year:** 150 **Industry designation:** Protection—safety equipment & services **Company type:** Private **Top competitors:** LoJack Corporation; Code-Alarm, Inc.; Winner International

Ever wonder who designed the auto alarm that seems to have a mind of its own? Most likely it was Directed Electronics, the world's #1 designer of auto security systems. The firm has designed a programmable computerized alarm system, as well as a remote system that starts a car at a predetermined time or by the push of a button. A Taiwanese manufacturer produces about 30 models of car alarms (Viper, Python, Sidewinder, and more) for the firm. Directed Electronics also makes car audio equipment—speakers, subwoofers, amplifiers, and related installation tools. President and CEO Darrell Issa and his wife, Katherine, own the firm, which was founded in 1982.

Documentum, Inc.

5671 Gibraltar Dr., Pleasanton, CA 94588

Telephone: 925-463-6800 **Fax:** 925-463-6850 **Metro area:** San Francisco, CA **Web site:** http://www.documentum.com **Human resources contact:** Ana Recio **Sales:** $123.8 million **Number of employees:** 616 **Number of employees for previous year:** 388 **Industry designation:** Computers—corporate, professional & financial software **Company type:** Public **Top competitors:** FileNET Corporation; PC DOCS Group International Inc.; Computron Software, Inc.

Documentum is a leading maker of software that lets a global company's employees share, manage, and update documents through computer networks and intranets. With Documentum's Enterprise Document Management System suite, manufacturers can provide new product information at once to all of its employees, and design teams can see their latest changes. Documentum continues a strategy of expanding its products into new markets and tailoring them accordingly; the company sells to process manufacturing, discrete manufacturing, finance, utility, and government entities. Documentum was spun off from Xerox, which owns 10% of the company.

DriveSavers

400 Bel Marin Keys Blvd., Novato, CA 94949

Telephone: 415-382-2000 **Fax:** 415-883-0780 **Metro area:** San Francisco, CA **Web site:** http://www.drivesavers.com **Human resources contact:** Jaynie Greer **Sales:** $4 million (Est.) **Number of employees:** 20 **Industry designation:** Computers—services **Company type:** Private **Top competitors:** Comdisco, Inc.; ONTRACK Data International, Inc.; Strategia Corporation

DriveSavers throws out life preservers for lost data. Founded in 1989, the company rescues data lost or corrupted by user errors, computer malfunctions, viruses, and natural disasters (fire, flood, or mudslide). It is authorized to open most companies' hardware without voiding the warranty and can save from most operating systems and rotating media (hard drives, floppies, CD-ROMs). Standard turnaround is 24-48 hours, but the company also offers DataExpress service, which transmits recovered data over high-speed, secured transmission lines. DriveSavers has saved the day for rocker Sting, writers of "The Simpsons," and the "Star Wars" remake. Founders Jay Hagan and Scott Gaidano own the company.

DSP Group, Inc.

3120 Scott Blvd., Santa Clara, CA 95054

Telephone: 408-986-4300 **Fax:** 408-986-4323 **Metro area:** San Francisco, CA **Web site:** http://www.dspg.com **Human resources contact:** Judy Siljander **Sales:** $63.9 million **Number of employees:** 105 **Number of employees for previous year:** 91 **Industry designation:** Computers—corporate, professional & financial software **Company type:** Public **Top competitors:** Lucent Technologies Inc.; Texas Instruments Incorporated

DSP Group gets its name from the digital signal processors (DSP) and related software it develops. The company's DSP integrated circuits convert light, sound, and speech wave forms into digital values for digital speech products used in multimedia PCs, telecommunications, consumer telephony, and consumer electronics. Telephone answering devices are a major end use for DSP Group's products. Microsoft, Panasonic, Samsung, and Sony are among the companies that use DSP Group products in their offerings. DSP Group has operations in California and Israel, as well as sales offices in Paris and Tokyo.

Dunn-Edwards Corporation

4885 E. 52nd Place, Los Angeles, CA 90040

Telephone: 323-771-3330 **Fax:** 323-771-4440 **Metro area:** Los Angeles, CA **Web site:** http://www.dunnedwards.com **Human resources contact:** Jack Slagle **Sales:** $238 million (Est.) **Number of employees:** 1,570 **Number of employees for previous year:** 1,550 **Industry designation:** Paints & related products **Company type:** Private **Top competitors:** The Sherwin-Williams Company; Benjamin Moore & Co.; Kelly-Moore Paint Company, Inc.

Dunn-Edwards manufactures paints, varnishes, lacquers, enamels, and paint-related products, including wall-coverings, brushes, and rollers. Operating in the southwestern part of the US, the company maintains more than 50 retail outlets, while its New Mexico subsidiary adds more than a dozen stores to its chain. Owned lock, stock, and bucket by the Arthur Edwards family, Dunn-Edwards does more than just add color to homes and buildings. After the 1992 Los Angeles riots damaged many of its stores, the company's employees established its Unity in the Community program to train South-Central L.A. residents in the painting industry and help them find jobs.

Dura Pharmaceuticals, Inc.

7475 Lusk Blvd., San Diego, CA 92121

Telephone: 619-457-2553 **Fax:** 619-457-2555 **Metro area:** San Diego, CA **Web site:** http://www.durapharm.com **Human resources contact:** Yolanda Jackson **Sales:** $199.2 million **Number of employees:** 942 **Number of employees for previous year:** 644 **Industry designation:** Drugs **Company type:** Public **Top competitors:** Rhone-Poulenc S.A.; Astra AB; Glaxo Wellcome plc

Dura Pharmaceuticals markets specialty respiratory prescription pharmaceuticals. The company's products are sold in the US to treat patients suffering from asthma, hay fever, chronic obstructive pulmonary disease, the common cold, and related respiratory complaints. Dura Pharmaceuticals typically acquires the products it sells from other makers, but the company is developing Spiros, a proprietary pulmonary dry-powder drug-delivery system that doesn't require forceful inhalation (it is being reviewed by the Food and Drug Administration). Dura Pharmaceuticals markets to allergists, pulmonologists, pediatricians, general physicians, and insurers.

EarthLink Network, Inc.

3100 New York Dr., Pasadena, CA 91107

Telephone: 626-296-2400 **Fax:** 626-296-2470 **Metro area:** Los Angeles, CA **Web site:** http://www.earthlink.net **Human resources contact:** Michael Ihde **Sales:** $175.9 million **Number of employees:** 807 **Number of employees for previous year:** 621 **Industry designation:** Computers—online services **Company type:** Public **Top competitors:** MCI WorldCom, Inc.; AT&T Corp.; America Online, Inc.

The name is EarthLink, but with losses shrinking and subscribership soaring, this company's on Cloud Nine. Earthlink Network is one of the world's largest Internet service providers, with 815,000 subscribers throughout the US and Canada. Its Network TotalAccess software package works with third-party browsers through telephone or cable modems, ISDN lines, or frame relay connections. Services include e-mail, business and personal Web sites, ISDN services, and an Internet shopping mall and gaming service. Earthlink, which provides Internet access from 1,400 points through EarthLink Sprint Internet, focuses on forming promotion partnerships with media and consumer products companies. Sprint owns 28% of the firm.

Eclipse Surgical Technologies, Inc.

1049 Kiel Ct., Sunnyvale, CA 94089

Telephone: 408-747-0120 **Fax:** 408-747-0215 **Metro area:** San Francisco, CA **Human resources contact:** Luanna Cracolice **Sales:** $12 million **Number of employees:** 123 **Number of employees for previous year:** 113 **Industry designation:** Medical instruments **Company type:** Public **Top competitors:** Johnson & Johnson; PLC Systems Inc.; United States Surgical Corporation

Eclipse Surgical Technologies will leave a hole in your heart and not feel a pang of guilt. The company's laser and fiber-optic systems are used for transmyocardial revascularization and percutaneous transluminal myocardial revascularization, procedures that use a laser to cut channels through the heart muscle into the heart chamber to help circulation in advanced cardiac patients. Its Eclipse TMR 2000 system, which is composed of fiber-optic and laser surgical tools on a powered base unit, has been approved for sale in the US by the FDA. Chairman and CEO Douglas Murphy-Chutorian owns about 30% of the company.

Eco Soil Systems, Inc.

10890 Thornmint Rd., Ste. 200, San Diego, CA 92127

Telephone: 619-675-1660 **Fax:** 619-592-7642 **Metro area:** San Diego, CA **Web site:** http://www.ecosoil.com **Human resources contact:** Peg Barber **Sales:** $82.4 million **Number of employees:** 126 **Number of employees for previous year:** 66 **Industry designation:** Fertilizers **Company type:** Public **Top competitors:** The Scotts Company; Terra Industries Inc.; LESCO, Inc.

Eco Soil Systems messes around with microbes. The company's Bioject microbe-fermentation system is designed to help control soil, crop, and turf problems and is used primarily on golf courses. Its microorganisms are intended to replace or complement chemical pesticides and fertilizers to help reduce the negative environmental effect of chemicals on the soil. Expanding to include agriculture, Eco Soil markets through direct sales, independent dealers, and distributors. Other products include CleanRack (water-treatment system) and CalJect and SoluJect (inject nonbiological soil agents into irrigation systems). Eco Soil also sells traditional chemical fertilizers, pesticides, and other turf-maintenance products.

Eltron International, Inc.

41 Moreland Rd., Simi Valley, CA 93065

Telephone: 805-579-1800 **Fax:** 805-579-1808 **Metro area:** Los Angeles, CA **Web site:** http://www.eltron.com **Human resources contact:** Bruce Beebe **Sales:** $105 million **Number of employees:** 486 **Number of employees for previous year:** 409 **Industry designation:** Computers—peripheral equipment **Company type:** Subsidiary **Top competitors:** Bull Run Corporation; Datamax International Corporation; Axiohm Transaction Solutions, Inc.

Eltron International, a Zebra Technologies subsidiary, makes direct thermal and thermal transfer bar code printers, plastic card printers, software, specialized print engines, related accessories, and supplies. The company's bar code printers are used for retail inventory accounting, laboratory specimen processing, airline ticketing, package tracking, and identification cards. Eltron's plastic card printers create photographic images more quickly and cheaply than traditional photography and can be used for identification cards and driver's licenses. VARs, OEMs, and distributors from more than 80 countries sell Eltron products to such clients as UPS, which accounts for about 24% of sales.

EMCON

400 S. El Camino Real, Ste. 1200, San Mateo, CA 94402

Telephone: 650-375-1522 **Fax:** 650-375-0763 **Metro area:** San Francisco, CA **Web site:** http://www.emconinc.com **Human resources contact:** Barry Langford **Sales:** $130 million **Number of employees:** 1,088 **Number of employees for previous year:** 972 **Industry designation:** Pollution control equipment & services **Company type:** Public

Wiping away industrial clients' little spills, EMCON is the "quicker picker-upper" for solid and hazardous waste, providing transfer, disposal, and storage services. A leader in the design, construction, and remediation of waste facilities throughout the world, EMCON has two operating divisions. The Professional Services Division includes facility, solid-waste, and site restoration services; the Operations and Construction Division offers related services such as landfill construction and the operation and maintenance of existing landfills. Joint venture ET Environmental builds solid-waste transfer stations and provides other environmental services. EMCON operates in the Americas, East Asia, and the Middle East.

ENDOcare, Inc.

7 Studebaker, Irvine, CA 92618

Telephone: 949-595-4770 **Fax:** 949-595-4766 **Metro area:** Los Angeles, CA **Web site:** http://www.ecare.org/ **Human resources contact:** Christine Concepcion **Sales:** $2.1 million **Number of employees:** 39 **Number of employees for previous year:** 31 **Industry designation:** Medical products **Company type:** Public **Top competitors:** EDAP TMS S.A.; Urologix, Inc.; VidaMed, Inc.

ENDOcare won't freeze your butt off, but it does the next best thing to treat prostate cancer and urological dysfunctions. Focusing on benign prostate hyperplasia (BPH) and prostate cancer, the company makes minimally invasive medical devices using either heat or cold to remove enlarged prostate tissue or cancer cells. Its CRYOcare cryosurgical system freezes malignant cells and reduces recovery time and complications in treating both prostate and liver cancer. Its Horizon Temporary Stent uses a heated tube to treat BPH. Other products include Prolase, a laser catheter, and Urolop and Vaporbar disposable electrodes. ENDOcare has hired former US senator Bob Dole to help advertise its products.

EndoSonics Corporation

2870 Kilgore Rd., Rancho Cordova, CA 95670

Telephone: 916-638-8008 **Fax:** 916-638-8112 **Metro area:** Sacramento, CA **Web site:** http://www.endosonics.com **Human resources contact:** Oti M. Wooster **Sales:** $44.1 million **Number of employees:** 350 **Number of employees for previous year:** 300 **Industry designation:** Medical instruments **Company type:** Public **Top competitors:** Hewlett-Packard Company; Johnson & Johnson; Schneider SA

EndoSonics makes imaging catheters that help cardiologists clear nasty plaque from clogged hearts. Its intravascular ultrasound (IVUS) imaging system uses digital technology to provide ultrasound images showing blood flow, the thickness of a vessel wall, and a 3-D representation of an artery. The IVUS system also features a fluoroscopic window that lets users view both ultrasound and angiography images simultaneously. Used in balloon angioplasty, the company's IVUS imaging catheters work with the imaging system to provide ultrasound images and to clear the blocked artery. About 65% of the company's sales are in Europe and Japan. EndoSonics and Cordis are developing a catheter/angioballoon.

En Pointe Technologies, Inc.

100 N. Sepulveda Blvd., 19th Fl., El Segundo, CA 90245

Telephone: 310-725-5200 **Fax:** 310-725-5240 **Metro area:** Los Angeles, CA **Web site:** http://www.enpointe.com **Human resources contact:** Robert Chilman **Sales:** $567.7 million **Number of employees:** 633 **Number of employees for previous year:** 434 **Industry designation:** Computers—services **Company type:** Public **Top competitors:** ENTEX Information Services, Inc.; Dell Computer Corporation; CHS Electronics, Inc.

Computer reseller En Pointe Technologies helps its customers reach their peak. Operating a "virtual warehouse" using its En Pointe Information Connection (EPIC) software, En Pointe steers clear of physical inventories and relies on allied distributors to fill customer orders. The company makes more than 60% of its purchases through Ingram Micro and InaCom, and it offers services such as technical support and network design. Customers can also purchase equipment via the Firstsource.com Web site operated by subsidiary Purchase Pointe. Co-founder, chairman, and CEO Attiazaz "Bob" Din and his family (including his wife, En Pointe co-founder and director Naureen Din) own about a third of En Pointe.

Excite, Inc.

555 Broadway, Redwood City, CA 94063

Telephone: 650-568-6000 **Fax:** 650-568-6030 **Metro area:** San Francisco, CA **Web site:** http://corp.excite.com **Human resources contact:** Elizabeth M. Berecz **Sales:** $154.1 million **Number of employees:** 711 **Number of employees for previous year:** 434 **Industry designation:** Computers—online services **Company type:** Public **Top competitors:** Yahoo! Inc.; Infoseek Corporation; Lycos, Inc.

Excite is the #2 World Wide Web search and delivery service (behind Yahoo!). Its services include shopping, entertainment, chat channels, and geographic search aids (City.Net). The company's other services include the WebCrawler search and directory tool, and Excite Communities, which provides e-mail and other services. The Excite engine provides search capabilities based on proper name, keyword, phrase, concept, or Boolean logic. About 20 million people use Excite each month. Key partners include America Online, which sold WebCrawler to Excite and owns about 12% of the company; and Intuit, which owns 10%. At Home Corporation, a provider of high-speed Internet access via cable TV, has agreed to acquire Excite.

Exodus Communications, Inc.

2831 Mission College Blvd., Santa Clara, CA 95054

Telephone: 408-346-2200 **Fax:** 408-346-2201 **Metro area:** San Francisco, CA **Web site:** http://www.exodus.net **Human resources contact:** Robert Helms **Sales:** $52.7 million **Number of employees:** 472 **Number of employees for previous year:** 220 **Industry designation:** Computers—online services **Company type:** Public **Top competitors:** AboveNet Communications, Inc.; Cable & Wireless plc; MCI WorldCom, Inc.

Exodus Communications tries to be the perfect host. Founded by Indian immigrants K. B. Chandrasekhar (chairman) and B. V. Jagadeesh, the company offers services (such as server hosting and Internet connectivity) that let businesses outsource the management of their Internet sites. Exodus has eight Internet Data Centers where clients store their servers in secure vaults. In addition to providing storage space, the company furnishes services such as maintenance and network connections. Its clients include CBS Sports, eBay, and MSN Hotmail. Exodus is expanding its geographic penetration and security services offerings through acquisitions.

FemRx, Inc.

1221 Innsbruck Dr., Sunnyvale, CA 94089

Telephone: 408-752-8580 **Fax:** 408-752-8590 **Metro area:** San Francisco, CA **Web site:** http://www.femrx.com **Human resources contact:** Virginia Sutherst **Sales:** $1.6 million **Number of employees:** 69 **Number of employees for previous year:** 56 **Industry designation:** Medical instruments **Company type:** Subsidiary **Top competitors:** Conceptus, Inc.; Johnson & Johnson

FemRx makes surgical devices and systems for treating gynecological disorders. The company's STAR System and Flo-Stat System are used in a minimally invasive procedure it calls OPERA, or outpatient endometrial resection/ ablation. OPERA offers an alternative to hysterectomies for patients suffering from abnormal uterine bleeding. A gynecologist uses STAR's resectoscope to collect samples, surgically remove the endometrial lining, and coagulate the uterine cavity. Flo-Stat monitors and regulates fluids used in the procedure. The firm's Diva product removes large tissue masses such as fibroids. FemRx is a subsidiary of Johnson & Johnson.

Fitness Holdings, Inc.

5020 Franklin Dr., Pleasanton, CA 94588

Telephone: 925-416-3100 **Fax:** 925-416-3147 **Metro area:** San Francisco, CA **Web site:** http://www.24hourfitness.com **Human resources contact:** Elaine Montaine **Sales:** $261.9 million (Est.) **Number of employees:** 11,500 **Industry designation:** Leisure & recreational services **Company type:** Private

Fitness Holdings owns and operates more than 170 fitness centers under the name 24 Hour Fitness. It offers aerobic, cardiovascular, and weight lifting services to its 1.6 million members. About 50 of its facilities also feature such amenities as squash, racquetball, and basketball courts, swimming pools, steam and sauna rooms, and whirlpools. Its 24 Hour Fitness centers (the majority of which are actually open 24 hours a day) are located in California (about 100 locations), Colorado, Hawaii, Idaho, Nebraska, Nevada, Oregon, and Texas. Fitness Holdings intends to continue to expand by opening and acquiring additional facilities. Investment partnership McCown De Leeuw & Co. owns 55% of the company.

Foundation Health Systems, Inc.

21600 Oxnard St., Woodland Hills, CA 91367

Telephone: 818-676-6775 **Fax:** 818-676-8591 **Metro area:** Los Angeles, CA **Web site:** http://www.fhs.com **Human resources contact:** Karin D. Mayhew **Sales:** $7.1 billion **Number of employees:** 15,200 **Number of employees for previous year:** 3,825 **Industry designation:** Health maintenance organization **Company type:** Public **Top competitors:** Kaiser Foundation Health Plan, Inc.; UnitedHealth Group; Aetna Inc.

Foundation Health Systems (formed from the merger of Health Systems International and Foundation Health Corporation) provides managed health care and other medical coverage to more than six million members in more than 20 states. Three health plan divisions cover California and other western states, as well as southwestern and northeastern states. Through its subsidiaries, Foundation Health offers HMOs, preferred provider networks, administration of government health contracts (Medicare, Medicaid, CHAMPUS, and Veterans Administration), life insurance, and other specialty services (such as dental and vision services).

Fountain View, Inc.

11900 W. Olympic Blvd., Los Angeles, CA 90064

Telephone: 310-571-0351 **Fax:** 310-571-0364 **Metro area:** Los Angeles, CA **Sales:** $67.9 million (Est.) **Number of employees:** 5,900 **Industry designation:** Nursing homes **Company type:** Private **Top competitors:** ARV Assisted Living, Inc.; Sun Healthcare Group, Inc.; Mariner Post-Acute Network, Inc.

Fountain View doesn't give its elderly clients the fountain of youth, but the nursing facility operator does help them live their lives more comfortably. The company operates 44 skilled nursing facilities and six assisted living centers in Arizona, Southern California, and Texas. The centers provide subacute specialty care, including dialysis, chemotherapy, tracheotomy and ventilator care, and blood transfusions. Through its subsidiary Locomotion Therapy, Fountain View offers occupational, physical, and speech therapy to both affiliated and unaffiliated health care facilities. Investment firm Heritage Partners owns about half of the company.

FPA Medical Management, Inc.

3636 Nobel Dr., Ste. 200, San Diego, CA 92122

Telephone: 619-453-1000 **Fax:** 619-453-0951 **Metro area:** San Diego, CA **Web site:** http://www.fpamm.com **Human resources contact:** Judy Baum **Sales:** $1.2 billion **Number of employees:** 4,700 **Number of employees for previous year:** 4,000 **Industry designation:** Medical practice management **Company type:** Public **Top competitors:** MedPartners, Inc.

FPA Medical Management is a physician practice management firm that partners with doctors, hospitals, and other medical providers. FPA's affiliated professional corporations organize and manage physician practices that contract with HMOs and other health plans to provide services to their enrollees. FPA is affiliated with about 22,000 physicians and provides services to more than one million enrollees in 13 states, including California, Florida, and New York. It also serves emergency departments in about 20 states. FPA's rapid growth has coincided with eyebrow-raising financial practices that came to a head in 1998 when the company was named in a rash of shareholder lawsuits and filed for bankruptcy protection.

Genentech, Inc.

One DNA Way, South San Francisco, CA 94080

Telephone: 650-225-1000 **Fax:** 650-225-6000 **Metro area:** San Francisco, CA **Web site:** http://www.gene.com **Human resources contact:** Judy Heyboer **Sales:** $1.1 billion **Number of employees:** 3,389 **Number of employees for previous year:** 3,242 **Industry designation:** Biomedical & genetic products **Company type:** Public **Top competitors:** Amgen Inc.; Chiron Corporation; Glaxo Wellcome plc

Try on some designer genes. Genentech, the world's #1 biotech firm, makes genetically engineered drugs. Products include Herceptin (breast cancer), Activase (post-heart-attack blood-clot-busters), Protropin and Nutropin (human growth hormones), and Pulmozyme (a cystic fibrosis treatment). Other products include Actimmune (interferon); the antibody Rituxan, made in collaboration with IDEC Pharmaceuticals; and many other products in development. Genentech receives royalties for hepatitis B vaccines, bovine growth hormones, and its first product, Humulin (human insulin). The company sells seven drugs in the US; Hoffman-La Roche handles foreign sales. Swiss drug giant Roche Holding owns about 66% of the company.

Genetronics Biomedical Ltd.

11199 Sorrento Valley Rd., San Diego, CA 92121

Telephone: 619-597-6006 **Fax:** 619-597-0119 **Metro area:** San Diego, CA **Web site:** http://www.genetronics.com **Human resources contact:** Rayne Romaine **Sales:** $3.7 million **Number of employees:** 85 **Industry designation:** Biomedical & genetic products **Company type:** Public **Top competitors:** ALZA Corporation; Alkermes, Inc.; Matrix Pharmaceutical, Inc.

Genetronics Biomedical is electrifying patients with its therapies. The firm focuses on electroporation, an infusion therapy that uses electricity to open cell membranes, letting drugs or genes enter. Its MedPulser treats Kaposi's sarcoma and cancers of the head, neck, liver, pancreas, and skin without the debilitating side effects of traditional treatments. Electroporation is also used in vascular therapy, injecting heparin or other pulmonary drugs directly into vascular tissue. Genetronics is applying its technology to the development of a painless drug-delivery system with uses in pediatric medicine and erectile dysfunction treatment. It has a licensing agreement with Johnson & Johnson.

Gentle Dental Service Corporation

222 N. Sepulveda Blvd., Ste. 740, El Segundo, CA 90245

Telephone: 310-765-2400 **Fax:** 310-765-2459 **Metro area:** Los Angeles, CA **Web site:** http://www.wwide.com/gentle **Human resources contact:** Steven M. Wolfe **Sales:** $43.4 million **Number of employees:** 898 **Number of employees for previous year:** 137 **Industry designation:** Medical practice management **Company type:** Subsidiary

Gentle Dental Service, a subsidiary of InterDent, sells practice management services to over 250 affiliated dentists in 70 offices throughout California, Hawaii, Idaho, Oregon, and Washington. The company—like others in this growing industry—provides facilities, equipment, and proprietary software to its members and takes care of payroll, accounting, insurance, and personnel matters. For its services, which also include advertising and marketing, the company receives reimbursement of expenses plus 15-30% of dentists' net revenues. InterDent acquired Gentle Dental in 1999.

GeoCities

1918 Main St., Ste. 300, Santa Monica, CA 90405

Telephone: 310-664-6500 **Fax:** 310-664-6520 **Metro area:** Los Angeles, CA **Web site:** http://www.geocities.com **Human resources contact:** Kelly L. Boyer **Sales:** $18.4 million **Number of employees:** 114 **Industry designation:** Computers—online services **Company type:** Public **Top competitors:** Lycos, Inc.; WhoWhere; Microsoft Corporation

GeoCities is a pioneer in the world of Web-based community sites. Its 40 themed neighborhoods (WallStreet, CapitolHill) allow three million member "homesteaders" (users) to interact with others on their areas of interest. The company provides free disk space and publishing tools to create personal Web pages. About 90 companies advertise on the GeoCities site. Through partnerships, GeoCities also offers CDs, credit cards, and books. Advertising by software marketer Surplus Direct/Egghead accounts for about 12% of sales. CMGI and SOFTBANK Holdings presently own 30% and 22% of GeoCities, respectively. Internet giant Yahoo! has agreed to acquire the company.

Geron Corporation

230 Constitution Dr., Menlo Park, CA 94025

Telephone: 650-473-7700 **Fax:** 650-473-7701 **Metro area:** San Francisco, CA **Web site:** http://www.geron.com **Human resources contact:** Elaine Hamilton **Sales:** $6.8 million **Number of employees:** 97 **Number of employees for previous year:** 89 **Industry designation:** Drugs **Company type:** Public

If Geron could turn back time, it would make a lot of money. The company (which takes its name from the Greek word for old man) conducts research on the aging process, focusing on telomeres, structures that act as a molecular "clock" for cellular aging, and telomerase, an enzyme that seems to prolong the cellular lifespan. By creating a telomerase inhibitor, Geron hopes to allow the telomeres of a cancerous cell to continue aging and eventually die. Its research has applications to skin aging, osteoporosis, and Alzheimer's disease. Geron has research collaborations with the research groups at Johns Hopkins and University of Wisconsin that discovered a method for culturing human stem cells.

Gilead Sciences, Inc.

333 Lakeside Dr., Foster City, CA 94404

Telephone: 650-574-3000 **Fax:** 650-573-4800 **Metro area:** San Francisco, CA **Web site:** http://www.gilead.com **Human resources contact:** Jennifer Brogel **Sales:** $32.6 million **Number of employees:** 293 **Number of employees for previous year:** 289 **Industry designation:** Biomedical & genetic products **Company type:** Public **Top competitors:** Amgen Inc.; Agouron Pharmaceuticals, Inc.; Hoffmann-La Roche, Inc.

Gilead Sciences discovers and develops new human therapeutics based on nucleotides, the building blocks of genes. The company's research and development efforts encompass three interrelated programs: small-molecule antivirals, cardiovascular therapeutics, and genetic code blockers. Gilead's research focuses on treatments for viral infections such as HIV and hepatitis B, cardiovascular disease, and cancer. Gilead has developed a compound that cures influenza in laboratory animals within a day; the company began testing the drug on humans in 1998.

Golden State Warriors

1011 Broadway, Oakland, CA 94607

Telephone: 510-986-2200 **Fax:** 510-986-2202 **Metro area:** San Francisco, CA **Web site:** http://www.nba.com/warriors **Human resources contact:** Erica Brown **Sales:** $48 million (Est.) **Number of employees:** 100 **Industry designation:** Leisure & recreational services **Company type:** Private **Top competitors:** Phoenix Suns; Seattle SuperSonics; California Sports, Inc.

After four consecutive years of losing seasons, the Golden State Warriors are gaining a reputation for choking both on and off the court. The team first hit the professional basketball courts in 1946 as the Philadelphia Warriors, a charter member of the old Basketball Association of America (BAA). Following a stint in San Francisco, the team became the Golden State Warriors in 1971. The Warriors won the NBA championship in 1975. The team's most notable event during the 1990s has been the 1997 choking assault of the head coach by Latrell Sprewell (who was then suspended and later traded to the New York Knicks in 1999). Owned by Chris Cohan, the team plays in Oakland Coliseum Arena.

GoTo.com, Inc.

130 W. Union St., Pasadena, CA 91103

Telephone: 818-244-6897 **Fax:** 626-535-2701 **Metro area:** Los Angeles, CA **Web site:** http://www.goto.com **Human resources contact:** Bonnie Robb **Number of employees:** 38 **Industry designation:** Computers—online services **Company type:** Private **Top competitors:** America Online, Inc.; Excite, Inc.; Yahoo! Inc.

GoTo.com helps find the needle in that gargantuan haystack known as the World Wide Web. The company's free online search service attracts more than 2.5 million unique visitors a month. It emphasizes simplicity, foregoing e-mail, chat rooms, and other services to focus only on search functions. Unlike other search engines, GoTo.com generates advertising revenue not through banner or other site-placed ads, but by allowing Web sites such as Barnesandnoble.com and 800-Florals to purchase levels of placement and exposure in the set of search results. The company was founded in 1997 by Idealab , which develops Internet businesses.

Harmonic Inc.

549 Baltic Way, Sunnyvale, CA 94089

Telephone: 408-542-2500 **Fax:** 408-542-2522 **Metro area:** San Francisco, CA **Web site:** http://www.harmonic-lightwaves.com **Human resources contact:** Anne Lynch **Sales:** $83.9 million **Number of employees:** 293 **Number of employees for previous year:** 253 **Industry designation:** Fiber optics **Company type:** Public

Harmonic Lightwaves develops, makes, and sells integrated fiber-optic transmission equipment for hybrid fiber/coaxial cable, satellite, and wireless TV networks. Products include optical transmitters and node receivers, return-path transmitters and receivers, and network management and high-speed data delivery hardware and software that enable high-speed Internet connection, videos on demand, and other interactive services. The firm sells its products worldwide through a direct-sales force and distributors to such clients as Cox Communications, AT&T Broadband & Internet Services (the former TCI), and Time Warner. Foreign sales make up about 60% of revenues.

Healtheon Corporation

4600 Patrick Henry Dr., Santa Clara, CA 95054

Telephone: 408-876-5000 **Fax:** 408-876-5010 **Metro area:** San Francisco, CA **Web site:** http://www.healtheon.com **Human resources contact:** Debra Machado **Sales:** $13.4 million **Number of employees:** 379 **Industry designation:** Computers—corporate, professional & financial software **Company type:** Public **Top competitors:** McKesson HBOC, Inc.; Shared Medical Systems Corporation; National Data Corporation

Healtheon's software and services enable health care information, both medical and administrative, to be exchanged over the Internet, saving time, money—and even lives. The company is building a system to automate such tasks as HMO enrollment, referrals, data retrieval, and claims processing for use by insurers, doctors, pharmacies, and consumers. Managed care provider Beech Street and the Brown & Toland physician networks account for about 90% of sales. Healtheon's shareholders include chairman and co-founder James Clark, who also co-founded Silicon Graphics and Netscape; United HealthCare; and SmithKline Beecham.

Health Systems Design Corporation

1330 Broadway, Oakland, CA 94612

Telephone: 510-763-2629 **Fax:** 510-763-2081 **Metro area:** San Francisco, CA **Web site:** http://www.hsdc.com **Human resources contact:** Gaye Kelly **Sales:** $25.9 million **Number of employees:** 161 **Number of employees for previous year:** 139 **Industry designation:** Computers—corporate, professional & financial software **Company type:** Public **Top competitors:** Computer Sciences Corporation; Sunquest Information Systems, Inc.; McKesson HBOC, Inc.

This company doesn't design gyms. Health Systems Design (HSD) makes managed care information systems software for HMOs, insurance providers, and physicians. Its flagship DIAMOND software suite manages data about providers, employer groups, contracts, referrals, and health care services. The data is used to create reports, manage costs, and ensure accurate reimbursements and proper risk pool accounting. HSD also offers services such as implementation, training, support, and modification. Customers include Kaiser Permanente (20% of sales), Covation Health Services (11%), and Blue Cross/Blue Shield of North Carolina (8%). Co-founders Richard Auger (chairman) and Catherine Roth together own 41% of the company.

Herman Goelitz, Inc.

2400 N. Watney Way, Fairfield, CA 94533

Telephone: 707-428-2800 **Fax:** 707-423-4436 **Metro area:** San Francisco, CA **Web site:** http://www.jellybelly.com **Sales:** $100 million (Est.) **Industry designation:** Food—confectionery **Company type:** Private **Top competitors:** Hershey Foods Corporation; Tootsie Roll Industries, Inc.; Mars, Inc.

The label on a pair of jeans tells you something about the product, but have you ever scanned a jelly bean for a brand name? Herman Goelitz—better known as the maker of Jelly Belly, "The original gourmet jelly bean" —prints the Jelly Belly logo on every one of the more than one million jelly beans it produces hourly at its California and Illinois facilities. Jelly Belly candies debuted in 1976 and account for about 70% of the company's sales, come in more than 40 flavors, and are exported to about 35 countries. Other products include candy corns, chocolate candies, gummies, licorice, and nuts. Herman Goelitz is owned and run by descendants of Gustav and Albert Goelitz, who founded the company in 1869.

Hill Physicians Medical Group, Inc.

2401 Crow Canyon, Ste. 130, San Ramon, CA 94583

Telephone: 925-838-6101 **Fax:** 925-820-8252 **Metro area:** San Francisco, CA **Human resources contact:** Nancy Staffieri **Sales:** $189.6 million (Est.) **Number of employees:** 345 **Number of employees for previous year:** 298 **Industry designation:** Health care—outpatient & home **Company type:** Private

Hill Physicians Medical Group, an independent practice association (IPA), has more than 330,000 HMO members, about 2,500 physicians, and more than 20 hospitals providing managed health care services in the Bay Area, Sacramento, and Shasta regions of Northern California. In addition to primary-care and specialty physician services, the group provides mental and behavioral health treatment to its members through Pathmakers (formerly Pacific Applied Psychology Associates), and offers a Health Education Program with classes taught by multidisciplinary health professionals. Hill Physicians Medical Group is managed by PriMed Management.

HMT Technology Corporation

1055 Page Ave., Fremont, CA 94538

Telephone: 510-490-3100 **Fax:** 510-623-9642 **Metro area:** San Francisco, CA **Web site:** http://www.hmtt.com **Human resources contact:** Phyllis Ziakas **Sales:** $356.2 million **Number of employees:** 2,248 **Number of employees for previous year:** 1,211 **Industry designation:** Computers—peripheral equipment **Company type:** Public **Top competitors:** Fuji Electric Co., Ltd.; Hoya Corporation; Showa Denko K.K.

HMT Technology is a film buff of a different type. The firm makes thin-film disks for high-capacity hard drives. Its products, most of which are 3-1/2" disks, are used in high-end PCs, network servers, and workstations. HMT designs its disks for drives with a variety of storage capacities and to meet a range of design- and performance-related requirements. The company sells most of its products to the Asian subsidiaries of US companies. Nearly 29% of its sales are to Iomega. Three other customers—Maxtor, Western Digital, and Samsung—account for 23%, 19%, and 16% of sales, respectively.

HNC Software Inc.

5930 Cornerstone Ct. W., San Diego, CA 92121

Telephone: 619-546-8877 **Fax:** 619-452-6524 **Metro area:** San Diego, CA **Web site:** http://www.hncs.com **Human resources contact:** Laurel Jones **Sales:** $178.6 million **Number of employees:** 706 **Number of employees for previous year:** 385 **Industry designation:** Computers—corporate, professional & financial software **Company type:** Public **Top competitors:** Fair, Isaac and Company, Incorporated; NeuralTech, Inc.; JDA Software Group, Inc.

HNC Software is hard to beat when it comes to predictive client/server software for decision-making applications. The company's software detects debit and credit card fraud, manages merchant risk, automates lending decisions and home valuations, and manages retail inventories. The company's products are primarily used by the retail, banking, and insurance industries, but HNC is seeking to expand its product line through acquisitions of companies with related products. HNC's Aptex subsidiary has formed a partnership with Infoseek to create an Internet document analyzer, and its Retek Information Systems has joined clothier Brooks Brothers to design an inventory-management linking system for retailers' intranets.

Hollis-Eden Pharmaceuticals, Inc.

9333 Genesee Ave., Ste. 110, San Diego, CA 92121

Telephone: 619-587-9333 **Fax:** 619-558-6470 **Metro area:** San Diego, CA **Human resources contact:** Candice Byrne **Sales:** $100,000 **Number of employees:** 14 **Number of employees for previous year:** 9 **Industry designation:** Drugs **Company type:** Public

Hollis-Eden Pharmaceuticals is a development-stage pharmaceutical company focusing on drugs for the treatment of infectious diseases such as HIV and AIDS, hepatitis B and C, and malaria. The company's initial products, Inactivin and Reversionex (currently under development), strive to inhibit HIV replication, strengthen the immune system, and reduce the viral load of infected patients. Hollis-Eden is also researching drugs that allow the human body to better tolerate mismatched organ and tissue transplants. The company uses outside contractors to manufacture its products. Founder and CEO Richard Hollis owns about 40% of the company.

HS Resources, Inc.

One Maritime Plaza, 15th Fl., San Francisco, CA 94111

Telephone: 415-433-5795 **Fax:** 415-433-5811 **Metro area:** San Francisco, CA **Web site:** http://www.hsresources.com **Human resources contact:** Annette Montoya **Sales:** $214.2 million **Number of employees:** 260 **Number of employees for previous year:** 233 **Industry designation:** Oil & gas—exploration & production **Company type:** Public

HS Resources is an independent oil and gas acquisition, exploration, and production company. The firm operates primarily in the Rocky Mountain areas of Colorado, Montana, and Wyoming, as well as in portions of Arkansas, Louisiana, Mississippi, New Mexico, Oklahoma, and Texas. HS Resources owns interests in about 5,400 wells, of which the company operates about 60%. HS Resources has proved reserves of about 45 million barrels of oil and about 750 billion cu. ft. of gas. The company maintains offices in Denver; Evans, Colorado; Houston; San Francisco; and Tulsa, Oklahoma. To focus on its Gulf Coast and Rocky Mountain operations, it sold its HSRTW, Inc., to Questar Corporation.

Hyperion Solutions Corporation

1344 Crossman Ave., Sunnyvale, CA 94089

Telephone: 408-744-9500 **Fax:** 408-744-0400 **Metro area:** San Francisco, CA **Web site:** http://www.hyperion.com **Sales:** $82.2 million **Number of employees:** 420 **Number of employees for previous year:** 252 **Industry designation:** Computers—corporate, professional & financial software **Company type:** Public **Top competitors:** Microsoft Corporation; System Software Associates, Inc.; Oracle Corporation

Hyperion has made a hyperactive jump in the corporate data analysis market. Hyperion Solutions, formed by the 1998 merger of financial management specialist Hyperion Software and data analysis firm Arbor Software, makes software and development tools that let big businesses access and process voluminous amounts of data for strategic planning. Hyperion continues to partner with leading manufacturers such as IBM and Fujitsu in efforts to expand its product line and international presence. More than 20% of Hyperion's sales come from outside the US.

Hyseq, Inc.

670 Almanor Ave., Sunnyvale, CA 94086

Telephone: 408-524-8100 **Fax:** 408-524-8141 **Metro area:** San Francisco, CA **Web site:** http://www.hyseq.com **Sales:** $9.6 million **Number of employees:** 195 **Number of employees for previous year:** 169 **Industry designation:** Biomedical & genetic products **Company type:** Public **Top competitors:** Human Genome Sciences, Inc.; Affymetrix, Inc.; Incyte Pharmaceuticals, Inc.

Hyseq's slice of life is the development of gene-based products and tests using its proprietary DNA array technology. The human genetics industry has created a market for Hyseq's patented sequencing by hybridization (SBH) process, which is the fastest and cheapest method in the race to identify and analyze gene functions. This research could lead to more effective treatments for diabetes and AIDS. The company's HyX Platform includes DNA probes, robots, and software. Hyseq has teamed with Perkin-Elmer to develop the Hychip DNA Module, with University of California-San Francisco to research genes that cause cardiovascular and metabolic disorders, and with Chiron to develop therapeutics and vaccines.

ICN Pharmaceuticals, Inc.

3300 Hyland Ave., Costa Mesa, CA 92626

Telephone: 714-545-0100 **Fax:** 714-641-7215 **Metro area:** Los Angeles, CA **Web site:** http://www.icnpharm.com **Human resources contact:** Jack L. Sholl **Sales:** $838.1 million **Number of employees:** 15,744 **Number of employees for previous year:** 12,784 **Industry designation:** Drugs **Company type:** Public **Top competitors:** Glaxo Wellcome plc; Novartis AG; Merck & Co., Inc.

ICN Pharmaceuticals makes drugs, research chemicals, and diagnostic products. Led by flamboyant CEO Milan Panic, who briefly served as prime minister of his native Yugoslavia, the company sells about 70 antibacterial products. Its leading product is a broad-spectrum antiviral agent, ribavirin, which is marketed in the US, Canada, and most of Europe under the name Virazole, and is used to treat viral infections such as herpes, influenza, chicken pox, hepatitis, and HIV. Virazole has been used in the US and Europe on hospitalized infants and young children with severe lower-respiratory infections, but it has received US approval as a treatment for hepatitis C.

ICU Medical, Inc.

951 Calle Amanecer, San Clemente, CA 92673

Telephone: 949-366-2183 **Fax:** 949-366-8368 **Metro area:** Los Angeles, CA **Web site:** http://www.icumed.com **Human resources contact:** Janice Rough **Sales:** $39.8 million **Number of employees:** 222 **Number of employees for previous year:** 130 **Industry designation:** Medical products **Company type:** Public **Top competitors:** Baxter International Inc.; Becton, Dickinson and Company; Abbott Laboratories

ICU Medical designs, manufactures, and markets disposable medical devices used to protect health care workers and patients from the accidental spread of infectious diseases, such as HIV and hepatitis B. The company's primary products are intravenous (IV) connection devices designed to prevent needlesticks and accidental disconnections (its CLAVE needleless IV connector accounts for nearly 70% of sales). It also makes devices that protect against contact with potentially infectious body fluids during enteral feeding and gastric lavage (stomach pumping) procedures. Subsidiary Budget Medical Products makes custom IV sets that incorporate the CLAVE system.

IDEC Pharmaceuticals Corporation

11011 Torreyana Rd., San Diego, CA 92121

Telephone: 619-550-8500 **Fax:** 619-550-8751 **Metro area:** San Diego, CA **Human resources contact:** Connie L. Matsui **Sales:** $87 million **Number of employees:** 365 **Number of employees for previous year:** 339 **Industry designation:** Drugs **Company type:** Public

IDEC Pharmaceuticals develops therapies for the treatment of cancer and autoimmune and inflammatory diseases. The company's only approved product, Rituxan, is a monoclonal antibody used in the treatment of B-cell non-Hodgkin's lymphomas. IDEC has an agreement with Genentech to develop and market the drug, which has received regulatory approval in the US and Switzerland. Genentech is still waiting for approval by the Food and Drug Administration for its Rituxan manufacturing facilities. Both companies entered into a licensing agreement with Zenyaku Kogyo to market the drug in Japan.

IKOS Systems, Inc.

19050 Pruneridge Ave., Cupertino, CA 95016

Telephone: 408-255-4567 **Fax:** 408-366-8699 **Metro area:** San Francisco, CA **Web site:** http://www.ikos.com **Human resources contact:** Donna Antosiak **Sales:** $40.9 million **Number of employees:** 256 **Number of employees for previous year:** 219 **Industry designation:** Computers—engineering, scientific & CAD-CAM software **Company type:** Public **Top competitors:** Cadence Design Systems, Inc.; Mentor Graphics Corporation; Synopsys, Inc.

IKOS Systems is a high-tech circuit rider. The firm designs and manufactures hardware and software systems for the simulation and emulation of integrated circuits (ICs) and IC-based electronic systems. Its Voyager hardware and software systems are used by IC designers to simulate complex IC designs. The company also provides consulting and support for its customers. IKOS markets its products to the communications, semiconductor, multimedia, computer, aerospace, and consumer electronics industries through a direct sales force and distributors. Customers include Lucent Technologies (13% of sales) and chip makers Texas Instruments, Motorola, and STMicroelectronics.

Immersion Corporation

2158 Paragon Dr., San Jose, CA 95131

Telephone: 408-467-1900 **Fax:** 408-467-1901 **Metro area:** San Francisco, CA **Web site:** http://www.immerse.com **Sales:** $4.2 million (Est.) **Number of employees:** 33 **Number of employees for previous year:** 25 **Industry designation:** Computers—peripheral equipment **Company type:** Private **Top competitors:** ThrustMaster, Inc.; Logitech International SA; Labtec Inc.

Since 1992, Immersion has been pushing, jostling, and pulling its way into the joystick market. Its I-FORCE standard helps games bump, pull, push, and otherwise manhandle players with up to a pound of force, simulating G-forces from sharp turns, gun recoil, linebacker tackles, car collisions, and explosions. Products include joysticks, the FEELit mouse, and medical simulators featuring the squish of surgery. Immersion's MicroScribe hardware makes 3-D models with spatial geometric information from real objects and digitally represents them on screen for the entertainment, engineering, architecture, and medical industries. Logitech has a 10% stake in the firm, which licenses its technology to other companies.

The Immune Response Corporation

5935 Darwin Ct., Carlsbad, CA 92008

Telephone: 760-431-7080 **Fax:** 760-431-8636 **Metro area:** San Diego, CA **Web site:** http://www.imnr.com **Human resources contact:** Lisa Gonzalez **Sales:** $17.7 million **Number of employees:** 156 **Number of employees for previous year:** 143 **Industry designation:** Biomedical & genetic products **Company type:** Public

Immune Response is a development-stage company whose primary project is an injectable immune-based therapy called REMUNE, which is designed to slow or stop the progression of HIV infections into AIDS. The company is also developing and testing therapeutic products for other autoimmune conditions—psoriasis, rheumatoid arthritis, multiple sclerosis, and some types of cancer. Immune Response is developing a technology to deliver gene therapy to liver cells as a treatment for such diseases as hemophilia A and hepatitis B. REMUNE is in Phase III clinical trials for FDA approval; Agouron Pharmaceuticals has agreed to market the drug. Other treatments are also in testing, but none have yet been brought to market.

Impulse! Buy Network, Inc.

433 Airport Blvd., 1st Fl., Burlingame, CA 94010

Telephone: 650-401-2288 **Fax:** 650-401-2289 **Metro area:** San Francisco, CA **Web site:** http://www.impulsebuy.net **Human resources contact:** Ali Baghdad **Number of employees:** 25 **Industry designation:** Computers—online services **Company type:** Private **Top competitors:** CMGI, Inc.; USWeb/CKS; DoubleClick Inc.

You think spending money is easy now? Get a load of Impulse! Buy Network's double-click purchase strategy. The company teams with merchants on a variety of Web sites through which customers can buy brand-name goods at discount prices, simply by clicking on a banner ad. Impulse! Buy Network has inked deals with more than 50 merchants (including Hammacher Schlemmer, J. Crew, Packard Bell, and The Sharper Image) and distributes ads to heavy-hitting Web sites such as Yahoo , Intellipost, and iVillage. Yahoo! and Japan's SOFTBANK own stakes in the company.

Incyte Pharmaceuticals, Inc.

3174 Porter Dr., Palo Alto, CA 94304

Telephone: 650-855-0555 **Fax:** 650-855-0572 **Metro area:** San Francisco, CA **Web site:** http://www.incyte.com **Human resources contact:** Kristina Hathaway **Sales:** $134.8 million **Number of employees:** 867 **Number of employees for previous year:** 676 **Industry designation:** Biomedical & genetic products **Company type:** Public **Top competitors:** Genzyme Corporation; Human Genome Sciences, Inc.; Gene Logic Inc.

Incyte Pharmaceuticals incites war against diseases with its databases of information on human, animal, plant, and microorganism genes. Its LifeSeq database links biological data with proprietary genetic information to aid drug discovery. Incyte also produces the LifeSeq FL (full-length gene), LifeSeq Atlas (gene mapping), PathoSeq (microbial gene sequence), and PhytoSeq (crop plant gene sequence) databases. Subsidiary Synteni provides microarrays for drug firms and other clients; Incyte Genetics is mapping the human genome. Its diaDexus joint venture with SmithKline Beecham creates tests using genetic data to detect disease. Its alliance with CV Therapeutics is developing a cardiovascular gene database.

Indus International, Inc.

60 Spear St., San Francisco, CA 94105

Telephone: 415-904-5000 **Fax:** 415-904-4949 **Metro area:** San Francisco, CA **Web site:** http://www.indusgroup.com **Human resources contact:** Robert Pocsik **Sales:** $195.5 million **Number of employees:** 1,037 **Number of employees for previous year:** 896 **Industry designation:** Computers—corporate, professional & financial software **Company type:** Public

Indus International, formed by the merger of The Indus Group and TSW International, is the world's largest provider of enterprise asset management software and support services. Through its PassPort and MPAC software lines, Indus provides systems for efficiently managing labor, materials, inventory, purchasing, regulations, documentation, and finance. Partnerships with Oracle and PeopleSoft enable Indus to make its software compatible with other business information software. The company sells software licenses, services, and maintenance to a variety of industries and public-sector concerns. Warburg, Pincus Investors and chairman Robert Felton own 35% and 26% of the company, respectively.

Influence, Inc.

71 Stevenson St., Ste. 1120, San Francisco, CA 94105

Telephone: 415-546-7700 **Fax:** 415-546-7744 **Metro area:** San Francisco, CA **Web site:** http://www.influencemedical.com **Human resources contact:** Clare Hartley **Sales:** $1.1 million (Est.) **Number of employees:** 106 **Number of employees for previous year:** 76 **Industry designation:** Medical products **Company type:** Private **Top competitors:** MedCare Technologies, Inc.; UroMed Corporation; Advanced UroScience, Inc.

With Influence, you don't always have to go with the flow. With operations in Israel, the US, Germany, and the UK, Influence develops products for the diagnosis and treatment of urinary incontinence, including diagnostic tools, remote-controlled catheter systems, and surgical tools. Its surgical procedure products (including In-Tac, In-Fast, and Straight-In) are used in minimally invasive procedures for bladder neck surgery in women; its Repose surgical system is used to treat sleep apnea and snoring. The company also makes the In-Flow remote-controlled catheter for women. After a planned IPO, Influence will develop more ear, nose, and throat products.

Infoseek Corporation

1399 Moffett Park Dr., Sunnyvale, CA 94089

Telephone: 408-543-6000 **Fax:** 408-734-9350 **Metro area:** San Francisco, CA **Web site:** http://www.infoseek.com **Human resources contact:** Patty Bustos **Sales:** $50.7 million **Number of employees:** 319 **Number of employees for previous year:** 171 **Industry designation:** Computers—online services **Company type:** Public **Top competitors:** America Online, Inc.; Yahoo! Inc.; Lycos, Inc.

Infoseek doesn't want you to pass GO on your way to the Internet. By joining forces with The Walt Disney Company, Infoseek has evolved from a simple search engine to the operator of the GO Network, a gateway to the Internet combining Infoseek's search and directory services with several Disney-related Web sites (Disney.com, ESPN.com). The GO Network is among Media Metrix's top five Web properties and boasts an audience of more than 20 million visitors each month. Infoseek still operates the Infoseek Web site, but it is hoping to draw visitors to the GO Network and may eventually reroute all Infoseek visitors directly there. Almost 90% of the company's revenue comes from advertising. Disney owns 43% of Infoseek.

Inhale Therapeutic Systems Inc.

150 Industrial Rd., San Carlos, CA 94070

Telephone: 650-631-3100 **Fax:** 650-631-3150 **Metro area:** San Francisco, CA **Web site:** http://www.inhale.com **Human resources contact:** Yvonne Gherug **Sales:** $21.8 million **Number of employees:** 205 **Number of employees for previous year:** 147 **Industry designation:** Medical products **Company type:** Public

Inhale Therapeutic Systems hopes to help patients breathe a little easier by offering them an alternative to medication injections—the firm is developing a deep-lung drug delivery system for existing macromolecule drugs, which are currently delivered by injection. Inhale is developing inhalants to treat diabetes, osteoporosis, Paget's disease, asthma, emphysema, infertility, hepatitis, multiple sclerosis, and other illnesses. Several of the drugs are in clinical trial. The company plans to formulate, make, and package the drug powders and to subcontract manufacture of the delivery devices. Inhale has collaborative agreements with such firms as Eli Lilly, Hoechst Marion Roussel, and Pfizer.

InnerDyne, Inc.

1244 Reamwood Ave., Sunnyvale, CA 94089

Telephone: 408-745-6010 **Fax:** 408-745-6570 **Metro area:** San Francisco, CA **Human resources contact:** Linda Blevins **Sales:** $17.6 million **Number of employees:** 128 **Number of employees for previous year:** 119 **Industry designation:** Medical products **Company type:** Public **Top competitors:** Johnson & Johnson; United States Surgical Corporation

InnerDyne develops and markets products that utilize its proprietary radial dilation technology in minimally invasive surgery. The company's first commercial product, The Step, incorporates that technology to enable surgeons to enter a patient's body by creating a small puncture wound that can be dilated. The Step device provides access to the abdominal cavity and aids in the visualization and treatment of target areas while minimizing tissue trauma. Other proprietary systems developed by InnerDyne include biocompatible coatings to help deliver pharmaceuticals to specific areas in the body and a thermal ablation system to treat excessive uterine bleeding.

InSight Health Services Corp.

4400 MacArthur Blvd., Ste. 800, Newport Beach, CA 92660

Telephone: 949-476-0733 **Fax:** 949-851-4488 **Metro area:** Los Angeles, CA **Web site:** http://www.InSightHealth.com **Human resources contact:** Cecilia A. Gusastaferro **Sales:** $114.3 million **Number of employees:** 850 **Number of employees for previous year:** 624 **Industry designation:** Medical services **Company type:** Public **Top competitors:** US Diagnostic Inc.; Syncor International Corporation; Medical Resources, Inc.

With its MRI and computed tomography imaging equipment, InSight Health Services knows what evil lurks within the hearts, brains, and pancreases of men. The company offers diagnostic services to hospitals and HMOs through more than 100 imaging centers, including 57 mobile MRI units. It also has conventional X-ray, mammogram, ultrasound, and nuclear medicine equipment. InSight's Gamma Knife center uses high dosages of focused radiation to irradiate brain lesions. The company also provides such related services as marketing, scheduling, and billing. Its facilities are located in 28 states with a strong presence in California, Texas, the East Coast, and the Midwest. General Electric owns nearly 60% of InSight.

InSite Vision Incorporated

965 Atlantic Ave., Alameda, CA 94501

Telephone: 510-865-8800 **Fax:** 510-865-5700 **Metro area:** San Francisco, CA **Web site:** http://www.insitevision.com **Human resources contact:** Sherry Flodin **Sales:** $100,000 **Number of employees:** 48 **Number of employees for previous year:** 47 **Industry designation:** Drugs **Company type:** Public **Top competitors:** Allergan, Inc.; Novartis AG; Pharmacia & Upjohn, Inc.

InSite Vision licenses ophthalmic products and technologies developed by academic institutions, runs preclinical and clinical tests, and establishes partnerships with pharmaceutical companies to complete development and to sell its products. A dry-eye treatment made by CIBA Vision Ophthalmics, called AquaSite, is made with InSite's DuraSite eyedrop-based delivery technology. The company is developing a genetic-based glaucoma test with the San Francisco branch of the University of California and the University of Connecticut Health Center. InSite also has licensed an inserter device for retinal treatment from the University of Rochester. The company does not make or market its products.

Integrated Surgical Systems, Inc.

1850 Research Park Dr., Davis, CA 95616

Telephone: 530-792-2600 **Fax:** 530-792-2690 **Metro area:** Sacramento, CA **Web site:** http://www.robodoc.com **Human resources contact:** Monica Neuman **Sales:** $4.9 million **Number of employees:** 84 **Number of employees for previous year:** 64 **Industry designation:** Medical instruments **Company type:** Public

Integrated Surgical Systems' computer-guided robotics are used in orthopedic and neurosurgery. The ROBODOC Surgical Assistant System provides precise total hip replacements and has been used in more than 2,000 surgeries in Europe (but still awaits FDA approval). The FDA-approved ORTHODOC Presurgical Planner turns computed tomography scan data into 3-D images for planning hip replacements. NeuroMate (also FDA-approved) has been used in more than 1,500 neurosurgeries in France and Japan. IBM, which helped develop the underlying technology, owns more than 40% of Integrated Surgical Systems. John Kapoor, chairman of drugmaker Akorn, owns about 20%.

International Microcomputer Software, Inc.

75 Rowland Way, Novato, CA 94945

Telephone: 415-257-3000 **Fax:** 415-257-3565 **Metro area:** San Francisco, CA **Web site:** http://www.imsisoft.com **Human resources contact:** Thalia Thiesen **Sales:** $62.5 million **Number of employees:** 338 **Number of employees for previous year:** 215 **Industry designation:** Computers—engineering, scientific & CAD-CAM software **Company type:** Public **Top competitors:** Corel Corporation; Lernout & Hauspie Speech Products N.V.; Autodesk, Inc.

International Microcomputer Software, Inc. (IMSI) doesn't shrink your PC. The company makes business productivity, computer-aided design, utility, and visual content software. Its software (including TurboCAD, WinDelete, and MasterClips) expands basic PC functions with features including precision drawing, project management, and voice recognition. The company also sells mouse input devices and software that enables recipe and menu planning. IMSI sells its software directly and through retailers and distributors worldwide. It primarily targets small to midsized businesses and consumers. Customers include Ingram Micro (20% of sales) and Tech Data. The company has sold its Family Heritage software line.

International Network Services

1213 Innsbruck Dr., Sunnyvale, CA 94089

Telephone: 408-542-0100 **Fax:** 408-542-0101 **Metro area:** San Francisco, CA **Web site:** http://www.ins.com **Human resources contact:** Steven R. Umphreys **Sales:** $169.7 million **Number of employees:** 1,353 **Number of employees for previous year:** 813 **Industry designation:** Computers—services **Company type:** Public **Top competitors:** Andersen Consulting; InaCom Corp.

The INS that people invite into their workplace is International Network Services, a computer networking consultant for "FORTUNE" 1000 companies. INS helps its customers design a network, choose the proper equipment (although it is not a reseller), install the system, and monitor its performance. Through its EnterprisePRO service, INS provides also intranet management to clients. The company serves its customers, including MCI WorldCom, AT&T, and PCS Group (Sprint PCS), from offices across the US and in Canada, the Netherlands, and the UK. Founder and chairman Donald McKinney owns a third of INS. Networking equipment giant Cisco also has a minority stake in the company.

International Remote Imaging Systems, Inc.

9162 Eton Ave., Chatsworth, CA 91311

Telephone: 818-709-1244 **Fax:** 818-700-9661 **Metro area:** Los Angeles, CA **Web site:** http://www.proiris.com **Human resources contact:** Carla Torres **Sales:** $27.5 million **Number of employees:** 159 **Number of employees for previous year:** 129 **Industry designation:** Medical instruments **Company type:** Public **Top competitors:** Applied Imaging Corp.; Vysis, Inc.; Hycor Biomedical Inc.

The Yellow IRIS and the White IRIS aren't diseased flowers, but they could be used to detect diseases in people. International Remote Imaging Systems (IRIS), using its patented slideless Automated Intelligent Microscopy technology, manufactures the Yellow IRIS automated urinalysis workstation, the PowerGene family of genetic analyzers, and has developed the White IRIS leukocyte differential analyzer. These systems automate the steps in microscope analysis and certain tests performed by hospitals and other laboratories. IRIS also makes urine analysis test strips, supplies for its systems, and, through subsidiary StatSpin, a variety of other small instruments and laboratory supplies.

Interpore International, Inc.

181 Technology Dr., Irvine, CA 92618

Telephone: 949-453-3200 **Fax:** 949-453-3225 **Metro area:** Los Angeles, CA **Web site:** http://www.interpore.com **Human resources contact:** Sharon Evans **Sales:** $30.2 million **Number of employees:** 120 **Number of employees for previous year:** 85 **Industry designation:** Medical products **Company type:** Public

Interpore International manufactures synthetically produced bone repair material for use in the orthopedic, oral, and maxillofacial markets under its Pro Osteon name. Pro Osteon is derived from marine coral, which is converted into an implant material that provides a structure for new bone growth. Interpore International also makes the IP200, which is an implant used to replace bone in periodentistry, oral, and craniofacial surgery. The company's subsidiary, Cross Medical Products, is a spinal-implant device supplier.

Intraware, Inc.

25 Orinda Way, Orinda, CA 94563

Telephone: 925-253-4500 **Fax:** 925-253-4584 **Metro area:** San Francisco, CA **Web site:** http://www.intraware.com **Human resources contact:** Joanie Creger **Sales:** $38.4 million **Number of employees:** 126 **Industry designation:** Computers—corporate, professional & financial software **Company type:** Public **Top competitors:** Programmer's Paradise, Inc.; pcOrder.com, Inc.; En Pointe Technologies, Inc.

Hoping to narrow the chasm between software vending and the IT professional, Intraware wants to be a go-between. Through its Web site, the company offers an array of services permitting software vendors to display their wares and IT professionals to check them out. Among its primary services are its IT Knowledge Center (software evaluation tools for IT professionals), intraware.shop (online software procurement services), and SubscribNet (through which IT pros can monitor software updates and licenses). About 25 vendors, including Netscape (now part of America Online) and Sun Microsystems, offer their products via Intraware's services. The company's 1,700 customers include IT professionals from AT&T and Oracle.

Intuitive Surgical, Inc.

1340 W. Middlefield Rd., Mountain View, CA 94043

Telephone: 650-237-7000 **Fax:** 650-526-2060 **Metro area:** San Francisco, CA **Web site:** http://www.intuitivesurgical.com **Human resources contact:** Michael Lau **Number of employees:** 109 **Number of employees for previous year:** 100 **Industry designation:** Medical instruments **Company type:** Private **Top competitors:** Heartport, Inc.; Computer Motion, Inc.; Boston Scientific Corporation

With technology befitting "Star Trek'"s USS "Enterprise," Intuitive Surgical has developed an integrated system of software, hardware, mechanics, and optics that allows doctors to operate on patients while seated at a remote console. The surgeon views the procedure in 3-D, manipulating instrument handles. A computer faithfully reproduces the doctor's hand movements in real-time, precise microsurgery performed by tiny electromechanical arms and instruments inserted in the patient's body through small puncture incisions. The system aims to provide more control than minimally invasive surgery and to reduce the trauma of traditional open surgery. Initially, Intuitive Surgical will market to cardiac surgery hospitals.

InVision Technologies, Inc.

7151 Gateway Blvd., Newark, CA 94560

Telephone: 510-739-2400 **Fax:** 510-739-6400 **Metro area:** San Francisco, CA **Web site:** http://www.invision-tech.com **Human resources contact:** Gail Sines **Sales:** $63.3 million **Number of employees:** 265 **Number of employees for previous year:** 194 **Industry designation:** Protection—safety equipment & services **Company type:** Public **Top competitors:** Vivid Technologies, Inc.; Thermedics Inc.; L-3 Communications Holdings, Inc.

A deterrent to would-be terrorists, InVision Technologies has more than 100 explosives detection units installed in civilian airports worldwide. Its main product, the CTX 5000, scans more than 300 checked bags per hour. InVision's second-generation version, the CTX 5500, scans even faster and can accommodate larger luggage. The company has enjoyed a virtual monopoly, as it has been the only firm sanctioned by the Federal Aviation Administration (FAA) to provide bomb scanning equipment in US airports, but the FAA is allowing competitors to enter the market. InVision is adapting its equipment to scan carry-on luggage and to detect drugs and mail bombs. Investor Eugenio Rendo owns 35% of the company.

Isis Pharmaceuticals, Inc.

2292 Faraday Ave., Carlsbad, CA 92008

Telephone: 760-931-9200 **Fax:** 760-931-9639 **Metro area:** San Diego, CA **Web site:** http://www.isip.com **Human resources contact:** Patricia Lowenstam **Sales:** $39.2 million **Number of employees:** 346 **Number of employees for previous year:** 338 **Industry designation:** Drugs **Company type:** Public **Top competitors:** Hybridon, Inc.

Isis Pharmaceuticals discovers and develops drugs through the use of antisense technology, which targets disease-causing proteins before they are produced. Isis focuses on the treatment of infectious and inflammatory diseases and cancers. Its flagship product, Vitravene, treats cytomegalovirus retinitis in AIDS patients and is distributed worldwide by CIBA Vision, the eye care division of Novartis. Through co-development agreements with Boehringer Ingelheim and Novartis, Phase II clinical trials continue for the treatment of psoriasis, rheumatoid arthritis, ulcerative colitis, renal transplant rejection, and tumors. Isis also collaborates with Merck and Zeneca.

Javelin Systems, Inc.

17891 Cartwright Rd., Irvine, CA 92614

Telephone: 949-440-8000 **Fax:** 949-440-8057 **Metro area:** Los Angeles, CA **Web site:** http://www.jvln.com **Human resources contact:** Sherie Sellers **Sales:** $29.6 million **Number of employees:** 165 **Number of employees for previous year:** 35 **Industry designation:** Computers—peripheral equipment **Company type:** Public **Top competitors:** MicroTouch Systems, Inc.; MICROS Systems, Inc.; NCR Corporation

Javelin Systems is piercing its way into the touch screen computer industry. The company's point-of-sale computers, which are targeted toward restaurants and retailers, can capture orders and transmit the information directly to corporate headquarters for use in inventory management and sales analysis. Among Javelin's offerings are the Javelin-HHT 40, a wireless handheld system, and the Javelin-LC, an eight-inch square model. The company also offers related installation, maintenance, and network support services. Having secured a contract to serve as one of five companies supplying 13,000 McDonald's restaurants with point-of-sale computers, Javelin Systems is well on its way to touch screen computer ubiquity.

Jenner Biotherapies, Inc.

2010 Crow Canyon Place, Ste. 100, San Ramon, CA 94583

Telephone: 925-824-3150 **Fax:** 925-824-3151 **Metro area:** San Francisco, CA **Web site:** http://www.jennerbio.com **Human resources contact:** Anthony E. Maida III **Number of employees:** 10 **Number of employees for previous year:** 5 **Industry designation:** Drugs **Company type:** Private **Top competitors:** Intracel Corporation; Genzyme Molecular Oncology; CEL-SCI Corporation

Jenner Technologies, a development stage company, is working on drugs and drug delivery systems to treat various cancers and side effects related to chemotherapy. The company's research involves both development of cancer vaccines and macrophage activation, which prompts the immune system to attack tumors and also alleviates side effects of chemotherapy. Jenner's lead product, ACT, stimulates macrophages to destroy cancer cells, and is currently undergoing clinical trials funded by the National Cancer Institute. Other products, Onco Vax-P and Onco Vax-CL, are being developed as vaccines for prostrate, colorectal, and other cancers. Jenner has licenses with Novartis and Eli Lilly.

John Paul Mitchell Systems

9701 Wilshire Blvd., Beverly Hills, CA 90212

Telephone: 310-276-7957 **Fax:** 805-298-0390 **Metro area:** Los Angeles, CA **Sales:** $185 million (Est.) **Number of employees:** 100 **Number of employees for previous year:** 89 **Industry designation:** Cosmetics & toiletries **Company type:** Private **Top competitors:** L'Oreal; Helene Curtis Industries, Inc.; Revlon, Inc.

John Paul Mitchell Systems markets more than 35 different hair care products in 29 countries. From pomades to shampoos, all come in the company's signature white bottles with distinctive black lettering. John Paul Mitchell Systems was founded in Hawaii in 1980 by John Paul "J.P." DeJoria and Paul Mitchell. After escaping bankruptcy, the company succeeded with products such as "awapuhi" shampoo made from Hawaiian ginger root. Chairman and CEO DeJoria, with his black ponytail and beard (as seen in the company's commercials), once rode with the Hell's Angels and is married to a former Playboy centerfold. He has also raced his own solar-powered race car in Australia's Pentax World Solar Challenge.

JTS Corporation

166 Baypointe Pkwy., San Jose, CA 95134

Telephone: 408-468-1800 **Fax:** 408-468-1801 **Metro area:** San Francisco, CA **Human resources contact:** Pat Dorr **Sales:** $145.9 million **Number of employees:** 6,500 **Number of employees for previous year:** 1,300 **Industry designation:** Computers—peripheral equipment **Company type:** Public **Top competitors:** Fujitsu Limited; Seagate Technology, Inc.

JTS Corporation manufactures computer disk drives. The company is concentrating solely on the sales of its Champion family of 3-1/2" drives. Its drives are sold through resellers, but the company's main focus is on providing them for PC manufacturers to use as hard drives for midrange desktop PCs. JTS has abandoned production of its 3" drives for portable computers because of a lack of industrywide acceptance. JTS has sold the assets of its Atari game division (the former reigning king of the video game empire) to toymaker Hasbro. JTS manufactures its products in Madras, India.

Kaiser Foundation Health Plan, Inc.

One Kaiser Plaza, Oakland, CA 94612

Telephone: 510-271-5910 **Fax:** 510-271-6493 **Metro area:** San Francisco, CA **Web site:** http://www.kaiserpermanente.org **Human resources contact:** James B. Williams **Sales:** $14.5 billion **Number of employees:** 100,000 **Number of employees for previous year:** 90,000 **Industry designation:** Health maintenance organization **Company type:** Not-for-profit **Top competitors:** PacifiCare Health Systems, Inc.; WellPoint Health Networks Inc.; Aetna Inc.

No longer the master of the HMO world, not-for-profit Kaiser Foundation Health Plan is still the largest managed health care company in the US, with more than nine million members in 19 states and the District of Columbia. It sponsors the Permanente Medical Groups, associations of doctors that provide medical care to Kaiser health plan subscribers under the Kaiser Permanente name. The company has more than 10,000 group-practice physicians; it also runs a network of Kaiser Foundation hospitals. Kaiser is facing skyrocketing costs and stiff competition from commercial providers of managed care.

Kanakaris Communications, Inc.

29350 Pacific Coast Hwy., Ste. 12, Zuma Beach Terrace, Malibu, CA 90265

Telephone: 310-589-2767 **Fax:** 310-589-2632 **Metro area:** Los Angeles, CA **Web site:** http://www.kanakaris.com **Sales:** $235,000 **Number of employees:** 12 **Industry designation:** Computers—online services **Company type:** Public **Top competitors:** broadcast.com inc.; Organic Online, Inc.; USWeb/CKS

Kanakaris Communications hopes the Web is synonymous with profits. The firm provides a variety of Internet-based services ranging from Web page design, content development, and Web hosting, to electronic commerce, downloadable music sites, and online advertising. Through its flagship site, NetBooks.com, customers can download books or publish their own works electronically. In addition, subsidiary Desience offers a variety of technology products and services, including the design, manufacture, and installation of computers and peripherals for corporations and government agencies. Nelson Vazquez owns 33% of the firm.

KeraVision, Inc.

48630 Milmont Dr., Fremont, CA 94538

Telephone: 510-353-3000 **Fax:** 510-353-3030 **Metro area:** San Francisco, CA **Web site:** http://www.keravision.com/main.html **Human resources contact:** Linda Schott **Sales:** $400,000 **Number of employees:** 108 **Number of employees for previous year:** 95 **Industry designation:** Medical products **Company type:** Public **Top competitors:** Autonomous Technologies Corporation; Chiron Corporation; Summit Technology, Inc.

KeraVision might have done wonders for Mr. Magoo—and in less than 15 minutes. The firm has developed a product to correct myopia (Intacs) and is working on treatments for farsightedness and astigmatism. Intacs reshapes the curvature of the cornea, eliminating the need for glasses or contact lenses. The Intacs implants, two half-circles of super-thin acrylic material, are inserted between layers of corneal tissue in a brief outpatient procedure. Although the arcs are considered permanent implants, the surgery is reversible. Intacs, which is awaiting final FDA approval, already sells in Canada, France, and Germany. KeraVision is buying Transcend Therapeutics.

Kingston Technology Company

17600 Newhope St., Fountain Valley, CA 92708

Telephone: 714-435-2600 **Fax:** 714-435-2699 **Metro area:** Los Angeles, CA **Web site:** http://www.kingston.com **Human resources contact:** Daniel Hsu **Sales:** $1 billion **Number of employees:** 663 **Number of employees for previous year:** 547 **Industry designation:** Computers—peripheral equipment **Company type:** Subsidiary **Parent company:** SOFTBANK CORP. **Top competitors:** Cisco Systems, Inc.; Micron Technology, Inc.; Samsung Group

Kingston Technology is the world's leading maker of memory boards used to increase the capacity and speed of computers and printers; it also makes storage peripherals, processor upgrades, networking equipment, and housings for storage products. The company sells its products worldwide through more than 3,000 distributors and resellers. The management of Kingston Technology is known for being equitable—founders John Tu and David Sun sold 80% of the company to Japanese computer conglomerate SOFTBANK for $1.5 billion and then forked over $100 million in employee bonuses.

Komag, Incorporated

1704 Automation Pkwy., San Jose, CA 95131

Telephone: 408-576-2000 **Fax:** 408-944-9255 **Metro area:** San Francisco, CA **Web site:** http://www.komag.com **Human resources contact:** Elizabeth A. Lamb **Sales:** $328.9 million **Number of employees:** 4,738 **Number of employees for previous year:** 4,101 **Industry designation:** Computers—peripheral equipment **Company type:** Public **Top competitors:** HMT Technology Corporation; Fuji Electric Co., Ltd.; International Business Machines Corporation

With more than 340 million disks under its belt, Komag is the leading independent maker of magnetic thin-film disks used in computer hard drives. The company's products—which spin at up to 10,000 rpm—are scanned by magnetic heads to record or retrieve information for desktop computers, network file servers, workstations, and other computer systems. Disk drive makers Western Digital, Maxtor, Seagate, Quantum, and IBM together account for more than 95% of Komag's sales. The company, which is battling a prolonged slump in the disk drive industry, operates manufacturing facilities in Japan, Malaysia, and the US. More than 50% of Komag's products are manufactured in the Far East.

La Jolla Pharmaceutical Company

6455 Nancy Ridge Dr., San Diego, CA 92121

Telephone: 619-452-6600 **Fax:** 619-452-6893 **Metro area:** San Diego, CA **Web site:** http://www.ljpc.com **Human resources contact:** Kimberly Ellstrom **Sales:** $8.6 million **Number of employees:** 109 **Number of employees for previous year:** 101 **Industry designation:** Drugs **Company type:** Public **Top competitors:** Anergen, Inc.; Immunex Corporation; Vertex Pharmaceuticals Incorporated

Development-stage La Jolla Pharmaceutical Company researches and develops specific therapeutics for the treatment of autoimmune and inflammatory diseases. Therapies currently available for these disorders address only the disease symptoms or suppress the entire immune system and often have severe side effects. The company is developing Toleragens, a proprietary therapy that blocks processes underlying the disease while leaving the balance of the immune system intact. The company is also conducting clinical trials of its lead compound for lupus, LJP 394, and is exploring the use of Toleragens to fight arterial blood clots and hemolytic disease, a fetal condition caused by Rh incompatibility between mother and child.

Landec Corporation

3603 Haven Ave., Menlo Park, CA 94025

Telephone: 650-306-1650 **Fax:** 650-368-9818 **Metro area:** San Francisco, CA **Web site:** http://www.landec.com **Human resources contact:** Cathy Wooten **Sales:** $33.5 million **Number of employees:** 175 **Number of employees for previous year:** 162 **Industry designation:** Chemicals—plastics **Company type:** Public **Top competitors:** Monsanto Company; E. I. du Pont de Nemours and Company; The Dow Chemical Company

Landec's specialty polymer products don't turn into pumpkins at midnight, but the changes are nearly as sudden and much more practical. Its unique polymers change physical characteristics when exposed to even slight temperature changes. Landec serves the food processing, agricultural, industrial, and medical industries. Its Intellicoat seed coating is designed to allow early planting of crop seeds by preventing germination until warm weather arrives. The Intellipac permeable membrane allows oxygen and carbon dioxide to enter and escape from sealed packages, keeping fresh-cut produce fresher. Landec also makes flexible QuickCast splints and casts, which are easy to apply, remold, and remove.

Launch Media, Inc.

2700 Pennsylvania Ave., Santa Monica, CA 90404

Telephone: 310-526-4300 **Fax:** 310-526-4400 **Metro area:** Los Angeles, CA **Web site:** http://www.launch.com **Sales:** $5 million (Est.) **Number of employees:** 73 **Industry designation:** Computers—online services **Company type:** Private **Top competitors:** Wenner Media; Viacom Inc.; TCI Music, Inc.

You can really take off with Launch Media's Web site, the place for music news, reviews, and interviews. Launch's proprietary content, which covers all musical genres except classical, is targeted at the much-coveted 12-34 year-old population. The company offers free online access to personalized music information for some one million registered users. It also offers services such as free homepages, online chat, and instant messaging. In addition, the company publishes "Launch," a monthly music CD-ROM featuring song samples and video clips. Launch Media generates about 60% of sales through advertising and the remainder through subscription fees and merchandising.

Leiner Health Products Inc.

901 E. 233rd St., Carson, CA 90745

Telephone: 310-835-8400 **Fax:** 310-835-6615 **Metro area:** Los Angeles, CA **Human resources contact:** John Kelly **Sales:** $502.1 million (Est.) **Number of employees:** 1,683 **Industry designation:** Vitamins & nutritional products **Company type:** Private **Top competitors:** Bayer AG; American Home Products Corporation; Bristol-Myers Squibb Company

Whether you're looking for prevention or a cure, Leiner Health Products has a pill for you. The firm is a top manufacturer of vitamins (including its own brand, Your Life), minerals, supplements, and over-the-counter drugs sold primarily under private labels. Leiner Health Products makes more than 500 nutritional products such as vitamins C and E (accounting for 36% of sales, excluding sales of Canadian subsidiary Vita Health). Its more than 100 pharmaceuticals include cold medicines and analgesics. The company's products are sold at more than 50,000 US supermarkets, drugstores, and other outlets, including Wal-Mart (which accounts for one-fourth of sales). Chairman Charles Baird owns 86% of the company.

Lifeguard, Inc.

PO Box 5506, San Jose, CA 95150

Telephone: 408-943-9400 **Fax:** 408-383-4259 **Metro area:** San Francisco, CA **Web site:** http://www.lifeguard.com **Sales:** $328.2 million (Est.) **Number of employees:** 507 **Number of employees for previous year:** 474 **Industry designation:** Health maintenance organization **Company type:** Private

It's not "Baywatch"; it's health care. Lifeguard operates health plans serving 220,000 members in 25 California counties. Plans include an HMO with multiple benefit levels; out-of-area plans for members living outside the network of more than 10,000 doctors and 100 hospitals; and Lifeguard for Seniors, a federally approved Medicare supplement. The network offers preventative health education through employer outreach programs and targeted interventions, as well as acupuncture and pharmacy management. Lifeguard participates in the Health Insurance Plan of California, an insurance purchasing pool for businesses that offers plans for groups as small as two employees.

Ligand Pharmaceuticals Incorporated

10275 Science Center Dr., San Diego, CA 92121

Telephone: 619-550-7500 **Fax:** 619-550-7506 **Metro area:** San Diego, CA **Web site:** http://www.ligand.com **Human resources contact:** William Pettit **Sales:** $17.7 million **Number of employees:** 345 **Number of employees for previous year:** 329 **Industry designation:** Drugs **Company type:** Public **Top competitors:** IDEC Pharmaceuticals Corporation; AXYS Pharmaceuticals, Inc.; Agouron Pharmaceuticals, Inc.

Ligand Pharmaceuticals develops small-molecule drugs used to regulate hormone-activated intracellular receptors (IRs). IRs help regulate the genetic processes affecting many diseases, including certain cancers and cardiovascular and skin diseases. Ligand's anti-cancer treatment Panretin gel has received FDA approval; other products in various stages of development include Targetrin for cancer, Kaposi's sarcoma, and psoriasis; Androgen Antagonists for prostate cancer and hirsutism; and Androgen Agonists, a hormone-replacement therapy. Subsidiary Seragen develops treatments for cancer and skin diseases. About 65% of Ligand's revenues come from research pacts and development projects with other drug makers.

LJL BioSystems, Inc.

404 Tasman Dr., Sunnyvale, CA 94089

Telephone: 408-541-8787 **Fax:** 408-541-8786 **Metro area:** San Francisco, CA **Web site:** http://www.ljlbio.com **Human resources contact:** Cheryl Harrah **Sales:** $4.4 million **Number of employees:** 73 **Number of employees for previous year:** 49 **Industry designation:** Biomedical & genetic products **Company type:** Public **Top competitors:** Nycomed Amersham plc; Aurora Biosciences Corporation; The Perkin-Elmer Corporation

LJL BioSystems is accelerating the drug discovery process with its high-throughput screening (HTS) instruments and fluorescence-based assay technologies. The company began selling its first HTS product, the Analyst, in 1998; the Analyst allows users to perform cellular and biochemical assays in multiple detection formats on up to 384 samples at a time. LJL Biosystems' proprietary FLARe technology (licensed from FluorRx, Inc.) uses long-lived fluorescent reagents; its first reagent, TKX, is designed for use with the Analyst. The company also makes clinical diagnostic products for original equipment manufacturers. Spousal co-founders Lev Leytes (CEO) and Galina Leytes (EVP) own about one-third of LJL BioSystems.

Logistix

48021 Warm Springs Blvd., Fremont, CA 94539

Telephone: 510-656-8000 **Fax:** 510-438-9486 **Metro area:** San Francisco, CA **Web site:** http://www.logistix.com **Human resources contact:** Ruth Belmar **Sales:** $320 million (Est.) **Number of employees:** 2,000 **Number of employees for previous year:** 1,800 **Industry designation:** Computers—services **Company type:** Private

Logistix works behind the scenes for big-name hardware and software makers. The company provides supply-chain management services, including the manufacture, packaging, distribution, testing, repair, and support of hardware and software for such companies as Adobe, Apple, Microsoft, Sun Microsystems, and Hewlett-Packard. Other services include duplicating disks and CD-ROMs, providing call-center support, and managing licensing and royalties. The company has facilities in the US and Ireland, typically near its clients' plants. Logistix has an alliance with CyberSource to provide inventory management and secure e-commerce services. Logistix's owners, Marta and Steve Weinstein, founded the company in 1974.

Longs Drug Stores Corporation

141 N. Civic Dr., Walnut Creek, CA 94596

Telephone: 925-937-1170 **Fax:** 925-210-6886 **Metro area:** San Francisco, CA **Web site:** http://www.longs.com **Human resources contact:** Leslie C. Anderson **Sales:** $3.3 billion **Number of employees:** 17,300 **Number of employees for previous year:** 16,500 **Industry designation:** Retail—drugstores **Company type:** Public **Top competitors:** Walgreen Co.; Rite Aid Corporation; Wal-Mart Stores, Inc.

Longs Drug Stores wants to be known for being short on hassle and long on service. A leading drugstore chain, with more than 380 stores in the western US and Hawaii, Longs prides itself on customer service (it even has pink-coated consultants dedicated to beauty products). Long known for giving store managers autonomy to select merchandise, the company has centralized some decisions on product displays and inventory levels to boost profits. Pharmaceutical products account for about a third of sales; most of the rest comes from cosmetics, food, greeting cards, over-the-counter health products, and photofinishing. The Long family owns about 20% of the firm; employees own about 20%.

LookSmart Ltd.

487 Bryant St., San Francisco, CA 94107

Telephone: 415-597-4850 **Fax:** 415-597-4860 **Metro area:** San Francisco, CA **Web site:** http://www.looksmart.com **Sales:** $3 million (Est.) **Industry designation:** Computers—online services **Company type:** Private **Top competitors:** Yahoo! Inc.; Lycos, Inc.; Infoseek Corporation

Internet publisher LookSmart provides the World Wide Web's largest editorially reviewed Website database. Its integrated search engine offers keyword matches and then distributes online content into about 20,000 subject categories. Whether accessed from www.looksmart.com or through an AltaVista or HotBot search, LookSmart is a reliable provider of quality matches—editors review every site and attempt to exclude violent or pornographic listings. Evan Thornley and Tracey Ellery (who are married) started the company in 1996 with funding from Reader's Digest, but later bought back its holdings. In 1998 Netscape (now part of AOL) added LookSmart as one of the six search engines included on its NetSearch browser function.

Los Angeles Clippers

3939 S. Figueroa St., Los Angeles Sports Arena, Los Angeles, CA 90037

Telephone: 213-748-0500 **Fax:** 213-745-0494 **Metro area:** Los Angeles, CA **Web site:** http://www.nba.com/clippers **Human resources contact:** Pablo Garcia **Sales:** $39.3 million (Est.) **Number of employees:** 90 **Industry designation:** Leisure & recreational services **Company type:** Private **Top competitors:** California Sports, Inc.; Phoenix Suns; Seattle SuperSonics

The Los Angeles Clippers are pinning their hopes on the seven-foot one-inch frame of the Kandi Man. The team is looking to Michael Olowokandi, the Nigerian-born center and first overall pick in the 1998-99 NBA draft, to pull them out of the Western Conference's Pacific Division cellar. The Clippers first joined the league in 1970 as the Buffalo Braves and were coached by hall-of-famer Dolph Schayes, later selected as one of the NBA's 50 greatest players of all time. In 1978 the team moved to San Diego and changed its name. In 1984 owner Donald Sterling took the team to Los Angeles. Notable players who have worn Clippers jerseys include World B. Free, Bill Walton, Danny Manning, and Dominique Wilkins.

Los Angeles Kings

3900 W. Manchester Blvd., Inglewood, CA 90305

Telephone: 310-419-3160 **Fax:** 310-673-8927 **Other address:** PO Box 17013, Inglewood, CA 90308 **Metro area:** Los Angeles, CA **Web site:** http://www.lakings.com **Human resources contact:** Margaret Castaneda **Sales:** $38.5 million (Est.) **Number of employees:** 75 **Industry designation:** Leisure & recreational services **Company type:** Private **Top competitors:** Dallas Stars L.P.; San Jose Sharks L.P.; Phoenix Coyotes Hockey Club

The Los Angeles Kings have yet to wear the crown. The team, which took the ice in 1967, wasn't considered royalty for most of its first 20 years—until it acquired Canadian hockey great Wayne Gretzky. He energized the franchise, which took its first division title but failed to win the Stanley Cup. Gretzky was traded in 1996. The Kings are owned by Denver billionaire Philip Anschutz and Los Angeles developer Edward Roski, who are hoping to revive interest in the team with big-name talent. The two are also building Staples Center, a basketball and hockey arena that will open in downtown Los Angeles in 1999.

The MacNeal-Schwendler Corporation

815 Colorado Blvd., Los Angeles, CA 90041

Telephone: 213-258-9111 **Fax:** 213-259-3838 **Metro area:** Los Angeles, CA **Web site:** http://www.macsch.com **Human resources contact:** Richard Lander **Sales:** $125.4 million **Number of employees:** 700 **Number of employees for previous year:** 627 **Industry designation:** Computers—engineering, scientific & CAD-CAM software **Company type:** Public **Top competitors:** Structural Dynamics Research Corporation; Parametric Technology Corporation; ANSYS, Inc.

The MacNeal-Schwendler Corporation (MSC) is a leading worldwide provider of mechanical computer-aided engineering software. Software products (about 77% of sales) include the modular MSC/NASTRAN (a basic analytical tool) and MSC/PATRAN (a pre- and post-processor for engineering analysis). Engineers use the software to simulate design functions, see if designs work, and assure they can be made. MSC also offers products for solving such problems as high-speed impacts, noise, and vibrations. Services include consulting, training, customization, integration, and systems reengineering. Clients come from the aerospace (about 39% of sales), industrial (28%), automotive (26%), computer, and electronics markets.

Marketplace.net, Inc.

888 Saratoga Ave., Ste. 1, San Jose, CA 95129

Telephone: 408-261-4680 **Fax:** 408-261-4685 **Metro area:** San Francisco, CA **Web site:** http://www.stockmaster.com **Human resources contact:** Leslie Torrance **Sales:** $1.5 million (Est.) **Number of employees:** 10 **Number of employees for previous year:** 3 **Industry designation:** Computers—online services **Company type:** Private **Top competitors:** Bridge Information Systems, Inc.; Reuters Group PLC; Bloomberg L.P.

Marketplace.net shells out the skinny on publicly traded stocks and mutual funds over its StockMaster Web site. The company offers individual investors free access to 15- to 20-minute delayed quotes and performance charts, historical data, SEC filings, news, and message boards. Its subscription services include company and industry profiles. StockMaster, which notches about a million visitors per month, also funnels up-to-date and historical stock data to companies for use on their Web sites. The company is owned by founder and CEO Mark Torrance, who established the service as a hobby while attending the Massachusetts Institute of Technology in 1993.

MarketWatch.com, Inc.

825 Battery St., San Francisco, CA 94111

Telephone: 415-733-0500 **Fax:** 415-392-1972 **Metro area:** San Francisco, CA **Web site:** http://cbs.marketwatch.com **Human resources contact:** Helen Presser **Sales:** $7 million **Number of employees:** 51 **Industry designation:** Computers—online services **Company type:** Public **Top competitors:** TheStreet.com, Inc.; Dow Jones & Company, Inc.; Yahoo! Inc.

MarketWatch.com's Web site is a smorgasbord of financial information, featuring news, stock quotes, critical analysis, and other information (most of which is updated throughout the day). The site features free information, but the company also offers two subscription packages that feature more detailed financial analysis. The company's staff of more than 40 reporters provides original content; the Web site also incorporates information from third parties such as the Associated Press, Hoover's, and Reuters. MarketWatch.com gets 68% of its revenues from advertisers. Television network CBS and Data Broadcasting Corporation each own about 38% of the company.

Maxicare Health Plans, Inc.

1149 S. Broadway St., Los Angeles, CA 90015

Telephone: 213-765-2000 **Fax:** 213-765-2670 **Metro area:** Los Angeles, CA **Web site:** http://www.maxicare.com **Human resources contact:** Charmaine Hancock **Sales:** $735.2 million **Number of employees:** 540 **Number of employees for previous year:** 490 **Industry designation:** Health maintenance organization **Company type:** Public **Top competitors:** Anthem Insurance Companies, Inc.; PacifiCare Health Systems, Inc.; Foundation Health Systems, Inc.

Maxicare Health Plans is cutting to cure … itself. Looking for a buyer for its Carolina operations, the HMO has already agreed to sell its Wisconsin operations to Managed Health Services Insurance and has sold its Illinois operations to a subsidiary of First American Group. Maxicare's subsidiaries, Maxicare Life, Health Insurance, and HealthAmerica, also operate in California, Indiana, and Louisiana. The company offers group, Medicaid, and Medicare HMO policies; PPO insurance; exclusive provider organization insurance; group life and accident policies; administrative services; and wellness programs. Maxicare also offers pharmacy programs including benefit design, claims processing, and mail-order services.

Maxim Pharmaceuticals, Inc.

8899 University Center Ln., Suite 400, San Diego, CA 92122

Telephone: 619-453-4040 **Fax:** 619-453-5005 **Metro area:** San Diego, CA **Web site:** www.maxim.com **Human resources contact:** Kathryn Harr **Sales:** $200,000 **Number of employees:** 53 **Number of employees for previous year:** 23 **Industry designation:** Drugs **Company type:** Public **Top competitors:** SmithKline Beecham Corporation; Immunex Corporation; AVANIR Pharmaceuticals

Development-stage Maxim Pharmaceuticals is maximizing its product line. The company's Maxamine is in clinical trials for use in the treatment of skin cancer and leukemia, with possible additional applications in the treatment of renal cancer and hepatitis C. Maxim believes Maxamine protects and stimulates immune system cells while destroying cancerous cells. It is also designed to let the patient self-administer the drug at home. Maxim Pharmaceuticals is also developing MaxVax, a mucosal delivery system for vaccines targeting respiratory, gastrointestinal, and sexually transmitted diseases; and MaxDerm, a topical treatment for cold sores, canker sores, shingles, and burns.

McKesson HBOC, Inc.

McKesson Plaza, One Post St., San Francisco, CA 94104

Telephone: 415-983-8300 **Fax:** 415-983-7160 **Metro area:** San Francisco, CA **Web site:** http://www.mckhboc.com **Human resources contact:** E. Christine Rumsey **Sales:** $20.9 billion **Number of employees:** 13,700 **Number of employees for previous year:** 13,300 **Industry designation:** Drugs & sundries—wholesale **Company type:** Public **Top competitors:** AmeriSource Health Corporation; Bergen Brunswig Corporation; Cardinal Health, Inc.

First, you get your pills. Next, you need some water. McKesson HBOC delivers both, along with the technology to help your doctor track your medication. McKesson HBOC was formed when McKesson, North America's top distributor of pharmaceuticals and health care products, bought HBO & Company (HBOC), the world leader in health care information systems and technology. Other subsidiaries distribute medical and surgical products to the health care industry and distribute bottled water (Sparkletts, Alhambra, Crystal). McKesson HBOC is the US's #3 bottled-water supplier, behind Nestle and Suntory. Prior to the HBOC purchase employees owned about 21% of McKesson through profit-sharing.

Meade Instruments Corp.

6001 Oak Canyon, Irvine, CA 92620

Telephone: 949-451-1450 **Fax:** 949-451-1460 **Metro area:** Los Angeles, CA **Web site:** http://www.meade.com **Human resources contact:** Kristen Sumwalt **Sales:** $59.9 million **Number of employees:** 305 **Number of employees for previous year:** 236 **Industry designation:** Instruments—scientific **Company type:** Public **Top competitors:** Canon Inc.; Minolta Co., Ltd.; Nikon Corporation

Meade Instruments has been opening windows to the universe for more than 25 years. The world's top manufacturer of telescopes, it owns 70% of the market for high-end instruments and about 40% of the low-end market. Meade's Schmidt-Cassegrain telescopes are popular among universities, scientific laboratories, and aerospace companies, though amateur astronomers are the company's primary customers. Stargazers can spend as much as $15,000 on one of the 40 types of telescopes Meade sells through its network of 500 authorized dealers, including Service Merchandise and the Nature Company (which account for 14% and 12% of sales, respectively). Meade also sells binoculars and related supplies to keep things in focus.

Medstone International, Inc.

100 Columbia, Ste. 100, Aliso Viejo, CA 92656

Telephone: 949-448-7700 **Fax:** 949-448-7882 **Metro area:** Los Angeles, CA **Web site:** http://www.medstone.com **Human resources contact:** Grant Lenning **Sales:** $23.8 million **Number of employees:** 82 **Number of employees for previous year:** 77 **Industry designation:** Medical instruments **Company type:** Public **Top competitors:** Dornier GmbH; EDAP TMS S.A.; Siemens AG

Since the spinoff of ENDOcare (maker of urological-treatment equipment and devices), Medstone International is focusing on developing its lithotripsy business. The company's lithotripters create shockwaves that travel through fluid, then into a patient's body, where they disintegrate kidney stones; the firm also creates software that governs the procedure. Medstone offers lithotripsy services in the US and internationally; it uses mobile units to take the procedure to more than 90 US sites each year. In a joint effort with Novartis, the company is seeking FDA approval for using its lithotripter and a drug to noninvasively treat gallstones. It is also investigating shockwave therapy for orthopedic applications.

Megabios Corp.

863-A Mitten Rd., Burlingame, CA 94010

Telephone: 650-697-1900 **Fax:** 650-652-1990 **Metro area:** San Francisco, CA **Web site:** http://www.megabios.com **Human resources contact:** Michael Coyne **Sales:** $8.1 million **Number of employees:** 79 **Number of employees for previous year:** 63 **Industry designation:** Biomedical & genetic products **Company type:** Public **Top competitors:** Introgen Therapeutics, Inc.; Genzyme Corporation; Genentech, Inc.

Megabios is mutating. The development-stage company—formerly focused on developing inhalable or injectable gene therapy delivery systems—has purchased fledgling biotech firm GeneMedicine; the combined company will change its name to Valentis. GeneMedicine brings to the marriage its work on therapeutic proteins designed to correct or modulate muscle, blood, inflammatory, cardiovascular, metabolic, and other disorders; its Interleukin-2 (being developed in partnership with a Roche subsidiary) is being eyed for use against head and neck cancer. The combined company also has alliances with such major drugmakers as Glaxo Wellcome, Eli Lilly, Merck, and Pfizer.

Memorial Health Services Inc.

2801 Atlantic Ave., Long Beach, CA 90801

Telephone: 562-933-9700 **Fax:** 562-933-1266 **Metro area:** Los Angeles, CA **Human resources contact:** Patti Ossen **Sales:** $519.9 million **Number of employees:** 7,500 **Number of employees for previous year:** 7,028 **Industry designation:** Hospitals **Company type:** Not-for-profit **Top competitors:** Columbia/HCA Healthcare Corporation; Catholic Healthcare West; Tenet Healthcare Corporation

Memorial Health Services (MHS) is a not-for-profit corporation that owns four hospitals in Southern California: Anaheim Memorial Medical Center, Long Beach Memorial Medical Center (which includes Miller Children's Hospital), Orange Coast Memorial Medical Center, and Saddleback Memorial Medical Center. The facilities offer a full spectrum of medical services along with specialty clinics and centers. MHS has a ten-year contract to provide medical care for PacifiCare Health Systems's HMO, PacifiCare of California. The company also has a stake in for-profit National Healthcare Services.

Mentor Corporation

5425 Hollister Ave., Santa Barbara, CA 93111

Telephone: 805-681-6000 **Fax:** 805-967-3013 **Metro area:** Santa Barbara, CA **Web site:** http://www.mentorcorp.com **Human resources contact:** Ramona E. Schwab **Sales:** $215.3 million **Number of employees:** 1,612 **Number of employees for previous year:** 1,403 **Industry designation:** Medical products **Company type:** Public **Top competitors:** INAMED Corporation; C. R. Bard, Inc.; Pfizer Inc

Whether you want to pump it up or slim it down, Mentor's got something for you. The company makes breast implants (known in the trade as mammary prostheses), tissue expanders, facial implants, and penile implants (for the treatment of impotence). Mentor is also working to market an ultrasonic liposuction device for kinder, gentler removal of unwanted fat. The company produces incontinence products (including disposable catheters, leg bags, and odor eliminators) and ophthalmology products used in cataract and glaucoma surgery (intraocular lenses, coagulators, and surgical instruments). Plastic surgery products account for about half of Mentor's sales.

Micro Therapeutics, Inc.

1062 Calle Negocio #F, San Clemente, CA 92673

Telephone: 949-361-0616 **Fax:** 949-361-0210 **Metro area:** Los Angeles, CA **Sales:** $4.2 million **Number of employees:** 123 **Number of employees for previous year:** 84 **Industry designation:** Medical instruments **Company type:** Public **Top competitors:** Boston Scientific Corporation; Medtronic, Inc.; Cook Group Inc.

Micro Therapeutics is coming on like clot busters! The company's minimally invasive medical instruments are used to diagnose and treat vascular diseases and neurovascular brain disorders. Micro Therapeutics' catheters, infusion wires, and other products are used to dissolve blood clots in arteries, veins, and hemodialysis access grafts. Its neurovascular products include infusion microcatheters and a liquid embolic system used to treat aneurysms. Subsidiary Genyx Medical is eyeing gynecological applications. Micro Therapeutics has alliances with such companies as Guidant and Abbott to distribute its products in North America, Europe, and the Pacific Rim. Venture capital firm Menlo Ventures owns 31% of the firm.

Mighty Ducks of Anaheim

2695 Katella Ave., Anaheim, CA 92806

Telephone: 714-704-2700 **Fax:** 714-940-2953 **Metro area:** Los Angeles, CA **Web site:** http://www.mightyducks.com **Human resources contact:** Jenny Price **Sales:** $49.6 million **Number of employees:** 50 **Industry designation:** Leisure & recreational services **Company type:** Subsidiary **Parent company:** The Walt Disney Company **Top competitors:** Phoenix Coyotes Hockey Club; Los Angeles Kings; Dallas Stars L.P.

The Mighty Ducks of Anaheim took the ice in 1993 when The Walt Disney Company decided it wanted a National Hockey League (NHL) team, and they have been scoring in and out of the rink ever since. In its first year the team, whose name was inspired by the popularity of Walt Disney's hit film "The Mighty Ducks," tied an NHL record for the most wins (33) by an expansion franchise. The Mighty Ducks also went on to become one of the NHL's top merchandise sellers. Steven Brill, screenwriter of the team's namesake film, is suing Disney for a 5% stake in all merchandise sales related to the Mighty Ducks, who play their home games at the Arrowhead Pond arena.

MiniMed Inc.

12744 San Fernando Rd., Sylmar, CA 91342

Telephone: 818-362-5958 **Fax:** 818-364-2246 **Metro area:** Los Angeles, CA **Web site:** http://www.minimed.com **Human resources contact:** Linda Whitney **Sales:** $138.6 million **Number of employees:** 891 **Number of employees for previous year:** 485 **Industry designation:** Medical products **Company type:** Public **Top competitors:** Chronimed Inc.; Transworld HealthCare, Inc.; PolyMedica Corporation

MiniMed is the #1 maker of external insulin pumps and related disposables for the treatment of diabetes. The firm's pumps deliver hundreds of tiny infusions of insulin, thus replacing the need for injections and its implantable insulin pumps are approved for sale in Europe. MiniMed also makes glucose monitors; its new glucose sensor (the first with continuous measurements) awaits FDA approval. The firm has alliances to retool its pumps to deliver drugs that treat high blood pressure (with United Therapeutics) and HIV (with Trimeris). MiniMed acquired Home Medical Supply, whose pharmacies allow MiniMed to distribute prescription drugs as well as its own products. CEO Alfred Mann owns 35% of MiniMed.

MobiNetix Systems, Inc.

500 Oakmead Pkwy., Sunnyvale, CA 94086

Telephone: 408-524-4200 **Fax:** 408-524-4299 **Metro area:** San Francisco, CA **Web site:** http://www.mobinetix.com **Human resources contact:** Stephanie Schweizer **Sales:** $11 million **Number of employees:** 60 **Number of employees for previous year:** 45 **Industry designation:** Computers—peripheral equipment **Company type:** Public **Top competitors:** IVI Checkmate Corp.; VeriFone, Inc.; NCR Corporation

MobiNetix Systems has eliminated business on a handshake, yet doesn't mind if you refuse to sign on the dotted line. The company formerly known as PenUltimate offers touch screens and personal digital assistants (PDAs) for the retail, health care, insurance, financial services, and identification and security industries. MobiNetix also offers application software and transaction devices for the card authorization terminal and PDA markets. Its top clients (IBM, Federated, Fujitsu) are good for 68% of sales. Subsidiary PenWare offers point-of-transaction systems and electronic signature capture devices such as the clipboards used by UPS delivery drivers worldwide.

ModaCAD, Inc.

1954 Cotner Ave., Los Angeles, CA 90025

Telephone: 310-312-9826 **Fax:** 310-751-2120 **Metro area:** Los Angeles, CA **Web site:** http://www2.modacad.com **Human resources contact:** Deirdre Abbott **Sales:** $7.8 million **Number of employees:** 86 **Number of employees for previous year:** 52 **Industry designation:** Computers—engineering, scientific & CAD-CAM software **Company type:** Public

ModaCAD develops design software for the apparel, textile, and home furnishings industries, among others. The ModaDESIGN PRO software suite is the flagship of the company's CAD (computer-aided design) products for business. ModaCAD also has designs on the e-commerce arena with its virtual-sample software; uses include interactive kiosks where customers see customized furniture—with fabric and finish options—on-screen in a 3-D environment. ModaCAD and Intel are partnering to bring similar technology to the fashion industry. Broderbund has licensed ModaCAD's consumer software for do-it-yourself decorators. Founder and chairman Joyce Freedman and her husband Lee (CFO) own about 26% of the company.

Molecular Biosystems, Inc.

10070 Barnes Canyon Rd., San Diego, CA 92121

Telephone: 619-452-0681 **Fax:** 619-812-7600 **Metro area:** San Diego, CA **Web site:** http://www.mobi.com **Human resources contact:** Laura Gross **Sales:** $6.2 million **Number of employees:** 148 **Number of employees for previous year:** 140 **Industry designation:** Medical products **Company type:** Public **Top competitors:** Nycomed Amersham plc; Schering AG; Mallinckrodt Inc.

Molecular Biosystems makes ultrasound imaging agents used in assessing heart function. The company's Optison agent—made in part from albumin, a naturally-occurring protein found in blood—contains microspheres designed to reflect sound waves during sonography, thus allowing a clearer picture of blood flow and surrounding tissue. The FDA has approved Optison for use in assessing heart function, and the company is testing it for use in other organs. It is also testing Oralex, an orally administered agent that facilitates imaging of internal organs. Molecular Biosystems currently generates its revenues from collaborative agreements with larger companies like Mallinckrodt and Chugai Pharmaceutical.

Molecular Devices Corporation

1311 Orleans Dr., Sunnyvale, CA 94089

Telephone: 408-747-1700 **Fax:** 408-747-3601 **Metro area:** San Francisco, CA **Web site:** http://www.moldev.com **Human resources contact:** Janice Dahlin **Sales:** $47.8 million **Number of employees:** 164 **Number of employees for previous year:** 146 **Industry designation:** Medical instruments **Company type:** Public **Top competitors:** Thermo BioAnalysis Corporation; Bio-Rad Laboratories, Inc.; Bio-Tek Instruments, Inc.

Molecular Devices Corporation makes bioanalytical measurement systems designed to make the process of developing drugs efficient and cost effective. Scientists and other researchers worldwide use the company's products, which incorporate instruments, software, and disposable test kits, for such applications as pharmaceutical research, clinical development, manufacturing, and quality control. Foreign buyers account for about 40% of total product sales. Molecular Device's product line includes MAXline Microplate Readers, which measures light absorption; cell analysis products; and the Threshold System, which measures contaminants in biopharmaceuticals. Kopp Investment Advisors owns about 25% of the company.

Molecular Dynamics, Inc.

928 E. Arques Ave., Sunnyvale, CA 94086

Telephone: 408-773-1222 **Fax:** 408-773-8343 **Metro area:** San Francisco, CA **Web site:** http://www.mdyn.com **Human resources contact:** Paulette Cabral **Sales:** $55.7 million **Number of employees:** 286 **Number of employees for previous year:** 238 **Industry designation:** Instruments—scientific **Company type:** Subsidiary **Top competitors:** Hitachi, Ltd.; Fuji Photo Film Co., Ltd.; Bio-Rad Laboratories, Inc.

Molecular Dynamics, which is a subsidiary Amersham Pharmacia Biotech (a joint venture of Nycomed Amersham and Pharmacia & Upjohn), makes high-performance instruments that analyze gene DNA makeup. Its PhosphorImager (more than half of sales) records digital images of DNA in a computer for quantitative analysis. A similar device, FluorImager SI, replaces the use of radioactive labeling substances with a fluorescent gel. Molecular markets its products worldwide to government and academic gene researchers and to pharmaceutical companies. It is part of a long-term $63 million government-funded project (along with Affymetrix, Inc.) to develop miniaturized DNA diagnostic systems.

Molecular Simulations Incorporated

9685 Scranton Rd., San Diego, CA 92121

Telephone: 619-458-9990 **Fax:** 619-458-0136 **Metro area:** San Diego, CA **Web site:** http://www.msi.com **Human resources contact:** Gina Gonzalez **Sales:** $56.7 million **Number of employees:** 300 **Number of employees for previous year:** 268 **Industry designation:** Computers—engineering, scientific & CAD-CAM software **Company type:** Subsidiary **Top competitors:** Tripos, Inc.; Simulations Plus, Inc.; Quintiles Transnational Corp.

How many guinea pigs are out of work because of Molecular Simulations Incorporated (MSI)? MSI makes software that lets researchers simulate, at the molecular level, the physical properties and behavior of the products they're developing. Its Cerius2 suite features modules that align molecules for comparison, predict behaviors of mixtures, and simulate behaviors of compounds over time. Insight II provides a 3-D environment for simulations, and WebLab brings research teams together over the Internet or a corporate intranet. MSI also offers contract research and collaborative R&D services on a per-project basis. MSI primarily targets the biotechnology, chemical, petrochemical, and pharmaceutical industries.

Mpath Interactive, Inc.

665 Clyde Ave., Mountain View, CA 94043

Telephone: 650-429-3900 **Fax:** 650-429-3911 **Metro area:** San Francisco, CA **Web site:** http://www.mpath.com **Sales:** $8 million (Est.) **Number of employees:** 111 **Industry designation:** Computers—online services **Company type:** Private **Top competitors:** ZDNet Group; Sony Corporation; SEGA Enterprises, Ltd.

Mpath feels your pain and allows you to inflict it on others via the Internet. Mpath Interactive operates www.Mplayer.com, an interactive Web site where users can play online interactive games like Cyberstrike 2 and Dominion Storm against fellow Web denizens. The company offers more than 80 games to choose from: some are free, but others require the game's CD. If cybersmashing isn't your style, Mpath offers HearMe.com, which provides live audio chat rooms as well as On Stage (virtual music concerts without the high ticket prices or the pervasive smell of marijuana). Its Mpath Foundation unit also creates online communities for third parties using its POP.X technology.

MTI Technology Corporation

4905 E. La Palma Ave., Anaheim, CA 92807

Telephone: 714-970-0300 **Fax:** 714-693-2202 **Metro area:** Los Angeles, CA **Web site:** http://www.mti.com **Human resources contact:** Kathie Nichols **Sales:** $200 million **Number of employees:** 562 **Number of employees for previous year:** 511 **Industry designation:** Computers—peripheral equipment **Company type:** Public **Top competitors:** Sun Microsystems, Inc.; EMC Corporation; International Business Machines Corporation

MTI Technology is the attic in your house of data. The firm is a provider of high-performance data storage products and services. Storage is the backbone of MTI's business, and its products include storage servers and RAID (redundant array of independent disks) storage subsystems (about 60% of sales), tape library systems, database accelerators, and software. Its clients include Compaq, Hoffmann-La Roche, investment management specialist FMR, and Lockheed Martin. About a quarter of the company's sales come from Europe. Chairman Raymond Noorda, former CEO of Novell, owns about half of MTI.

Nanogen, Inc.

10398 Pacific Center Ct., San Diego, CA 92121

Telephone: 619-546-7700 **Fax:** 619-546-7718 **Metro area:** San Diego, CA **Web site:** http://www.nanogen.com **Sales:** $7.6 million **Number of employees:** 132 **Number of employees for previous year:** 90 **Industry designation:** Biomedical & genetic products **Company type:** Public **Top competitors:** Merck & Co., Inc.; Affymetrix, Inc.; ONCOR, Inc.

Development-stage company Nanogen combines microelectronics with molecular biology to identify and test samples containing charged molecules. Using microchips, Nanogen's system allows molecules to be identified and analyzed as they move around designated sites on the chips, depending on their positive or negative charge. Nanogen believes its system will have uses in medical diagnostics, biomedical research, genomics, genetic testing, and drug discoveries. The company is establishing corporate alliances with biotechnology companies such as Becton Dickinson, Hoechst, and Elan to commercialize products using its proprietary microchip technology.

Natrol, Inc.

21411 Prairie St., Chatsworth, CA 91311

Telephone: 818-739-6000 **Fax:** 818-739-6001 **Metro area:** Los Angeles, CA **Web site:** http://www.natrol.com **Human resources contact:** Marcelo Aguilera **Sales:** $68.2 million **Number of employees:** 185 **Industry designation:** Vitamins & nutritional products **Company type:** Public

Natrol produces more than 145 dietary supplements, including vitamins, herbs, weight-control products, and hormones. Under the Natrol name, the company sells its products throughout the US to grocery stores and supermarkets, drug and retail chains, and health food stores. Its main products include Ester-C vitamin C and Kavatrol, an herbal kava formula used as a calming aid. The company also owns a bulk-ingredient business that supplies dehydrated vegetable products to other companies. It makes most of its products at its California facility and advertises its products nationally through a variety of media. The Balbert Family Trust owns 49% of the company.

Natural Alternatives International, Inc.

1185 Linda Vista Dr., San Marcos, CA 92069

Telephone: 760-744-7340 **Fax:** 760-744-9589 **Metro area:** San Diego, CA **Web site:** http://www.nai-online.com **Human resources contact:** Jo Phillippe **Sales:** $67.9 million **Number of employees:** 128 **Number of employees for previous year:** 110 **Industry designation:** Vitamins & nutritional products **Company type:** Public **Top competitors:** General Nutrition Companies, Inc.; NBTY, Inc.; Rexall Sundown, Inc.

How totally alternative! Natural Alternatives International (NAI) makes vitamins and other nutritional supplements for the private-label market. It assists its clients by offering for free a variety of services (such as graphic design, brochures, and foreign product registration) to help them market NAI-made vitamins under their own brand names. NAI does not charge its customers for these supplemental services. Clients include Nu Skin International, NSA International (which together account for more than half of sales), Bally Total Fitness, NordicTrack, and Jenny Craig International. Mother/son founding team Marie and Mark LeDoux together own about 25% of the company and serve as chair and CEO, respectively.

NeoMagic Corporation

3260 Jay St., Santa Clara, CA 95054

Telephone: 408-988-7020 **Fax:** 408-988-7032 **Metro area:** San Francisco, CA **Web site:** http://www.neomagic.com **Human resources contact:** Kennneth Murray **Sales:** $240.5 million **Number of employees:** 162 **Number of employees for previous year:** 86 **Industry designation:** Computers—peripheral equipment **Company type:** Public **Top competitors:** Intel Corporation; Trident Microsystems, Inc.; ATI Technologies Inc.

NeoMagic's multimedia accelerators (the MagicGraph and MagicMedia families) facilitate complex displays combining graphics, video, and audio on notebook computers. The fabless company (NeoMagic outsources its manufacturing and assembly work) designs an accelerator for entry-level laptops and other models with enough power for full-motion video, added colors, and 3-D effects. NeoMagic's proprietary technology, called MagicWare, combines analog circuits, complex logic, and memory circuits on a single chip. The company's customer list includes most of the laptop makers. More than 80% of NeoMagic's sales are to locations outside the US.

NeoTherapeutics, Inc.

157 Technology Dr., Irvine, CA 92618

Telephone: 949-788-6700 **Fax:** 949-788-6706 **Other address:** PO Box 57052, Irvine, CA 92619 **Metro area:** Los Angeles, CA **Web site:** http://www.neotherapeutics.com **Human resources contact:** Shelton K. Stern **Sales:** $100,000 **Number of employees:** 33 **Number of employees for previous year:** 27 **Industry designation:** Drugs **Company type:** Public

NeoTherapeutics develops drugs to treat degenerative conditions of the central nervous system such as stroke, spinal cord injuries, Parkinson's disease, and memory loss associated with Alzheimer's disease and aging. The company's patented technology is based on tiny synthetic molecules that encourage nerve cell regrowth and prevent degeneration. NeoTherapeutic believes that its AIT-082 (NEOTROFIN) is the first orally active drug for nerve regeneration to be clinically tested on humans. The company also is working on treatments for dementia, depression, and migraine headaches. Members of the Glasky family own about 25% of the company.

NETCOM On-Line Communication Services, Inc.

2 N. Second St., Plaza A, San Jose, CA 95113

Telephone: 408-881-2000 **Fax:** 408-881-3250 **Metro area:** San Francisco, CA **Web site:** http://www.netcom.com **Human resources contact:** Barrie Stone **Sales:** $160.7 million **Number of employees:** 800 **Number of employees for previous year:** 759 **Industry designation:** Computers—online services **Company type:** Subsidiary **Top competitors:** AT&T Corp.; MCI WorldCom, Inc.; America Online, Inc.

NETCOM On-Line Communication Services, a subsidiary of local and long-distance phone service provider ICG Communications, provides Internet connections and bundled services to residential and business customers. Along with its individual productivity, business connectivity, and Web-hosting products, NETCOM offers 24-hour customer support and high-speed connectivity. It has local access numbers in more than 360 locations across Canada, the UK, and the US. The company, which has about 560,000 subscribers, is focusing its attention on business customers, moving from flat-rate pricing to a tiered structure, and disconnecting customers who take up more than their fair share of the unlimited access service.

Network Appliance, Inc.

2770 San Tomas Expwy., Santa Clara, CA 95051

Telephone: 408-367-3000 **Fax:** 408-367-3151 **Metro area:** San Francisco, CA **Web site:** http://www.netapp.com **Human resources contact:** Chris Carlton **Sales:** $166.2 million **Number of employees:** 450 **Number of employees for previous year:** 265 **Industry designation:** Computers—peripheral equipment **Company type:** Public **Top competitors:** Sun Microsystems, Inc.; Auspex Systems, Inc.

Just because you can't see computer files in cyberspace doesn't mean that they don't need to be filed. Network Appliance takes care of this problem with its NetCache software and NetApp suite of network storage servers, or "filers." These products are designed for high-traffic, data-intensive networks typically used by Internet service providers and corporate intranets. Equipment features include quick installation (about fifteen minutes), few system commands (only 40), high-powered ONTAP operating system, fibre channel support, and SecureShare simultaneous access by users from all Windows, UNIX, and Web platforms. Customers include Yahoo , AOL, Motorola, Siemens, and UK's #1 ISP, Demon Internet.

Neurex Corporation

3760 Haven Ave., Menlo Park, CA 94025

Telephone: 650-853-1500 **Fax:** 650-853-1538 **Metro area:** San Francisco, CA **Web site:** http://www.neurex.com **Human resources contact:** Sandy Cooper **Sales:** $2.4 million **Number of employees:** 140 **Number of employees for previous year:** 75 **Industry designation:** Biomedical & genetic products **Company type:** Subsidiary

Pharmaceutical company Neurex, a subsidiary of Irish drug delivery systems maker Elan, focuses on the treatment of pain and cardiorenal and neurological diseases. The company's first product, Corlopam, controls high blood-pressure associated with surgery and treats malignant hypertension. Ziconotide, in clinical development, is intended for severe pain management for terminal AIDS and cancer patients. The drug is also being developed for treatment of brain damage caused by closed head trauma, coronary bypass surgery, and stroke. The company develops and markets its products by allying with companies such as biomedical specialist Medtronic and drug giant Warner-Lambert.

Neurocrine Biosciences, Inc.

3050 Science Park Rd., San Diego, CA 92121

Telephone: 619-658-7600 **Fax:** 619-658-7602 **Metro area:** San Diego, CA **Web site:** http://www.neurocrine.com **Human resources contact:** Judy Michelle **Sales:** $16 million **Number of employees:** 108 **Number of employees for previous year:** 103 **Industry designation:** Drugs **Company type:** Public **Top competitors:** Elan Corporation, plc; Biogen, Inc.; Teva Pharmaceutical Industries Limited

For Neurocrine Biosciences, it's all chemical. The development-stage company uses biotechnology to develop treatments for diseases of the central nervous and immune systems. Neurocrine Biosciences bases its research on the molecular relationships among the body's central nervous, immune, and endocrine systems. The firm is developing treatments for anxiety, depression, and substance abuse (with research partner, Johnson & Johnson subsidiary Janssen Pharmaceutica); multiple sclerosis (with Novartis); obesity and Alzheimer's disease (with Eli Lilly); and other neurodegenerative diseases. Neurocrine Biosciences' Canadian subsidiary, Neuroscience Pharma, is also developing treatments for Alzheimer's disease.

North American Scientific, Inc.

20200 Sunburst St., Chatsworth, CA 91311

Telephone: 818-734-8600 **Fax:** 818-734-8606 **Metro area:** Los Angeles, CA **Web site:** http://www.nasi.net **Human resources contact:** David King **Sales:** $5.8 million **Number of employees:** 35 **Number of employees for previous year:** 15 **Industry designation:** Medical products **Company type:** Public **Top competitors:** Imagyn Medical Technologies, Inc.; Theragenics Corporation; Implant Sciences Corporation

Business is hot for North American Scientific. The company makes low-level radiation sources and standards (sealed radioactive devices) that health care providers, environmental monitoring companies, and researchers use to test and adjust the accuracy of their radiological equipment. North American Scientific has also moved into providing radioactive seeds for brachytherapy (a treatment that involves implanting radioactive material in cancer patients to target tumors) that are marketed through Mentor Corporation (a key partner and customer) under the IoGold trade name. The company's brachytherapy seeds are currently approved for treatment of prostate cancer. The firm is acquiring Theseus Medical Imaging.

Oacis Healthcare Holdings Corp.

100 Drake's Landing Rd., Ste. 100, Greenbrae, CA 94904

Telephone: 415-925-0121 **Fax:** 415-925-4610 **Metro area:** San Francisco, CA **Web site:** http://www.oacis.com **Human resources contact:** Jay Allen **Sales:** $27.5 million **Number of employees:** 194 **Number of employees for previous year:** 172 **Industry designation:** Computers—corporate, professional & financial software **Company type:** Subsidiary **Top competitors:** Shared Medical Systems Corporation; Cerner Corporation; McKesson HBOC, Inc.

Send your camel to tech-ed. Oacis Healthcare Holdings makes medical hardware and software. Its Oacis system functions as an electronic medical database that collects clinical, financial, and demographic data from multiple departments throughout a hospital or integrated health care system. The patient-based database can then be reviewed and updated instantaneously by physicians, nurses, and other clinicians. The system, which can be purchased as a package or in modules, is sold direct in North America and through distributors elsewhere. Oacis also performs such services as project planning, hardware integration, database configuration, testing, and training. Science Applications International owns the company.

Oakland Raiders

1220 Harbor Bay Pkwy., Alameda, CA 94502

Telephone: 510-864-5000 **Fax:** 510-864-5134 **Metro area:** San Francisco, CA **Web site:** http://www.raiders.com **Sales:** $78.3 million (Est.) **Number of employees:** 90 **Industry designation:** Leisure & recreational services **Company type:** Private **Top competitors:** The Denver Broncos Football Club; Seattle Seahawks; Kansas City Chiefs

The Oakland Raiders lives up to its name. The NFL team is known for hard hitting on the field and the "Just win, baby" slogan of owner Al Davis. Davis quickly discards coaches who displease him (Mike Shanahan walked the plank and is now coach of the Super Bowl champion Denver Broncos) and can alienate fans (the Bay Area saw the team move to Los Angeles for 12 years). The team has cultivated an outlaw image since Davis took control in 1963. Famous for hellraisers such as quarterback Ken Stabler and legendary coach John Madden, the team has won three Super Bowls and gone to the playoffs 18 times. The Raiders faltered and recovered while in LA, only to falter again since its mid-1990s' return to Oakland.

Ocular Sciences, Inc.

475 Eccles Ave., South San Francisco, CA 94080

Telephone: 650-583-1400 **Fax:** 650-583-9017 **Metro area:** San Francisco, CA **Human resources contact:** Terence M. Fruth **Sales:** $151.9 million **Number of employees:** 1,438 **Number of employees for previous year:** 1,167 **Industry designation:** Medical products **Company type:** Public **Top competitors:** Novartis AG; Johnson & Johnson; Bausch & Lomb Incorporated

Ocular Sciences' income is disposable in a sense: The company makes soft contact lenses. Weekly and monthly disposable lenses account for about three-quarters of sales. Other lines include annual replacement and specialty lenses such as toric (for astigmatism), bifocal, and tinted lenses. Unlike many competitors that have established brand names with the public, Ocular Sciences sells to private optical practices and retailers worldwide. Brands include Hydron, Clinasoft, Mediflex, Edge, Ultraflex, and Procon, but the firm also produces private-label lenses for other customers. Most of Ocular Sciences' products are made in Puerto Rico and the UK. Founder John Fruth owns 23% of the company.

OnDisplay

2682 Bishop Dr., Ste. 215, San Ramon, CA 94583

Telephone: 925-355-3200 **Fax:** 925-355-3222 **Metro area:** San Francisco, CA **Web site:** http://www.ondisplay.com **Number of employees:** 50 **Industry designation:** Computers—corporate, professional & financial software **Company type:** Private **Top competitors:** Prologic Management Systems, Inc.; ConnectInc.com; Open Market, Inc.

Many firms developing innovative Web technologies are on display, but few take center stage. OnDisplay, however, is doing just that as a startup that develops, makes, and sells software for managing e-commerce (online trade). Its flagship CenterStage software translates online data such as Web site pages and e-mail (even if the data is seemingly incompatible), and organizes it in more accessible, easy-to-use formats. OnDisplay's software automates purchasing, accounting, distribution, and other business tasks to speed business-to-business transactions. Customers include Office Depot and drug company McKesson HBOC. Chief technology officer Trung Dung and CEO Mark Pine own the firm, which they founded in 1996.

Organic Online, Inc.

510 Third St., Ste. 540, San Francisco, CA 94107

Telephone: 415-284-6888 **Fax:** 415-284-6891 **Metro area:** San Francisco, CA **Web site:** http://www.organic.com **Human resources contact:** David Lopez **Sales:** $140 million (Est.) **Number of employees:** 350 **Number of employees for previous year:** 200 **Industry designation:** Computers—online services **Company type:** Private **Top competitors:** USWeb/CKS; fine.com International Corporation; Modem Media.Poppe Tyson, Inc.

Organic Online is planting seeds of e-commerce in the fertile soil of the Internet. Co-founded in 1993 by Matthew Nelson, Jonathan Nelson, and Brian Behlendorf, Organic specializes in helping companies develop their online presence. The company offers its clients Web site design and hosting services and e-commerce development tools, as well as advertising and marketing strategies, public relations services, and research services. It caters to a variety of high-profile clients, including Starbucks, barnesandnoble.com, and Music Boulevard. Organic has offices in Chicago, New York City, San Francisco, and Brazil. It is largely employee-owned, but advertising giant Omnicom Group holds a minority stake.

OrthAlliance, Inc.

23848 Hawthorne Blvd., Ste. 200, Torrance, CA 90505

Telephone: 310-791-5656 **Fax:** 310-791-5660 **Metro area:** Los Angeles, CA **Human resources contact:** Paul H. Hayase **Sales:** $74.4 million **Number of employees:** 700 **Number of employees for previous year:** 565 **Industry designation:** Medical practice management **Company type:** Public **Top competitors:** Orthodontic Centers of America, Inc.; Apple Orthodontix, Inc.; Monarch Dental Corporation

OrthAlliance manages a network of almost 70 orthodontic practices with 180 offices in 18 states, primarily in the South, West, and Midwest. The company generally acquires certain operating assets of the practice and employs all non-professional employees. OrthAlliance provides administration and management services, including billing, inventory procurement, financial reporting, employee training, and employee recruitment. OrthAlliance, which went public in 1997, also provides capital for the development and growth of allied practices. The company continues to grow through acquisitions and expansions.

Otis Spunkmeyer Inc.

14490 Catalina St., San Leandro, CA 94577

Telephone: 510-357-9836 **Fax:** 510-357-5680 **Metro area:** San Francisco, CA **Human resources contact:** Steve Ricks **Sales:** $186 million (Est.) **Industry designation:** Food—confectionery **Company type:** Private **Top competitors:** Archway Cookies, Inc.; Keebler Foods Company; RJR Nabisco Holdings Corp.

Cookie eaters know that Otis Spunkmeyer's products are more appetizing than its name. The company, founded in 1977 by Kenneth Rawlings and named by his 12-year-old daughter, makes frozen cookie dough, frozen baked muffins, bagels, and gourmet coffee. Otis Spunkmeyer delivers its products to convenience stores, grocery stores, and other retail shops, where the goods are baked in countertop ovens provided by the company. With about 60 distribution centers in the US, Mexico, and the UK, the company plans to add pastries, rugelah, and miniature cakes to its product line. Investment firm First Atlantic Capital bought a 60% stake in the company in 1999; Otis Spunkmeyer's managers are among its other shareholders.

OZ Interactive, Inc.

525 Brannan St., 4th Fl., San Francisco, CA 94107

Telephone: 415-536-0500 **Fax:** 415-536-0536 **Metro area:** San Francisco, CA **Web site:** http://www.oz.com **Sales:** $6 million (Est.) **Number of employees:** 75 **Industry designation:** Computers—online services **Company type:** Private **Top competitors:** blaxxun interactive; Worlds Inc.; REALAX Software AG

OZ Interactive's hardware and software whirl computer users away to 3-D virtual reality environments, like Ozone, where they can assume an identity (called an "avatar"); personalize its looks; and move, speak, and interact with others in real time. Founded in 1990 by Gudjon Gudjonsson and Skuli Morgensen, OZ plans to work with large media firms to co-develop environments and characters that will facilitate collaborative efforts. OZ is gearing the use of its technology to entertainment (virtual concerts and gaming sites), education (distance learning), and business communications (virtual product galleries and employee chat lounges). Ericsson uses OZ's products in its 3-D virtual product showcase.

Pacer Technology

9420 San Anita Ave., Rancho Cucamonga, CA 91730

Telephone: 909-987-0550 **Fax:** 909-987-0490 **Metro area:** Los Angeles, CA **Web site:** http://www.pacertech.com **Human resources contact:** Helen Komroek **Sales:** $31.9 million **Number of employees:** 130 **Number of employees for previous year:** 98 **Industry designation:** Chemicals—specialty **Company type:** Public **Top competitors:** Dexter Corporation; Imperial Chemical Industries PLC; H.B. Fuller Company

Adhesive and sealant maker Pacer Technology has a firm bond with its customers in the consumer, automotive, and industrial markets. Primary products of Pacer's consumer division include Super Glue, modeling glue, and manicure products Gem and Mr. Mustache. Its PRO SEAL adhesives and sealants are used for body and engine parts and trim applications. The company also sells its sticky stuff to industrial markets that include aerospace, electronics, and maintenance repair applications. Pacer sells its products worldwide through its own sales force and through independent distributors. Subsidiary Pacer Tech Ltd. markets the company's products in Europe.

Pacific Biometrics, Inc.

25651 Atlantic Ocean Dr., Ste. A-1, Lake Forest, CA 92630

Telephone: 949-455-9724 **Fax:** 949-588-2788 **Metro area:** Los Angeles, CA **Web site:** http://www.pacbio.com **Human resources contact:** Tanya Mills **Number of employees:** 37 **Number of employees for previous year:** 31 **Industry designation:** Medical products **Company type:** Public **Top competitors:** Metra Biosystems, Inc.; Hologic, Inc.; Lunar Corporation

Just sweat or spit and you won't get cut. Pacific Biometrics wants to steer patients away from surgery with its noninvasive diagnostic products for chronic diseases. The company's Osteopatch (based on its Sweatpatch device) uses perspiration to measure signs of osteoporosis; its SalivaSac allows the osmotic collection of saliva without contamination, and is used to detect diabetes. Pacific Biometrics' laboratory in Seattle includes a Centers for Disease Control-designated cholesterol reference method network laboratory, which provides contract research and clinical trial development. The company's revenues come primarily from short-term laboratory contracts with pharmaceutical firms and research organizations.

Pacific Mutual Holding Company

700 Newport Center Dr., Newport Beach, CA 92660

Telephone: 949-640-3011 **Fax:** 949-640-7614 **Other address:** PO Box 9000, Newport Beach, CA 92658 **Metro area:** Los Angeles, CA **Web site:** http://www.pacificlife.com **Human resources contact:** Anthony J. Bonno **Sales:** $2.6 billion **Number of employees:** 3,422 **Number of employees for previous year:** 2,750 **Industry designation:** Insurance—life **Company type:** Mutual company **Top competitors:** Transamerica Corporation; Metropolitan Life Insurance Company; The Prudential Insurance Company of America

Life insurance is Pacific Mutual Holding's stock-in-trade. The firm is the mutual holding company that owns Pacific LifeCorp, a stock company whose primary subsidiary, Pacific Life, is the largest California-based life insurance outfit. Pacific Life offers fixed and variable life insurance policies, annuities, and pension plans; other subsidiaries manage health plans (PM Group Life) and provide real estate advice (PMRealty Advisors). Through Pacific Mutual Distributors, the company markets such investment products as fixed and variable annuities, mutual funds, and index funds. With operations both in the US and the UK, Pacific Mutual also owns almost a third of PIMCO Advisors, a major investment management firm.

Pacific Pharmaceuticals, Inc.

6730 Mesa Ridge Rd., Ste. A, San Diego, CA 92121

Telephone: 619-550-3900 **Fax:** 619-550-3929 **Metro area:** San Diego, CA **Web site:** http://www.pacificpharm.com **Sales:** $300,000 **Number of employees:** 7 **Number of employees for previous year:** 6 **Industry designation:** Biomedical & genetic products **Company type:** Public **Top competitors:** DUSA Pharmaceuticals, Inc.; Pharmacyclics, Inc.; Miravant Medical Technologies

Pacific Pharmaceuticals has seen the light. Not only did it change its name from the unpronounceable Xytronyx, the company is developing a photodynamic immunotherapy technology based on light-activated drugs. Other technologies and products include gene-based products that enhance the effectiveness of chemotherapy in brain cancer patients, a disposable periodontal tissue monitor to diagnose periodontitis, and a group of printing dyes that brighten when exposed to ultraviolet light. Pacific Pharmaceuticals is a subsidiary of Procept, a company engaged in the development of anti-infectives and immunosuppressants.

Pandesic LLC

440 Potrero Ave., Sunnyvale, CA 94086

Telephone: 408-616-1900 **Fax:** 408-616-1910 **Metro area:** San Francisco, CA **Web site:** http://www.pandesic.com **Human resources contact:** Stella Begonia **Number of employees:** 25 **Industry designation:** Computers—corporate, professional & financial software **Company type:** Joint venture **Top competitors:** Internet Commerce Corporation; Open Market, Inc.; BroadVision, Inc.

Pandesic wants to be pandemic. The company, a joint venture formed in 1997 between Intel and SAP, develops and sells systems to small- and medium-sized companies so they can do commerce on the Web. The systems consist of SAP's finance, shipping, inventory, and other business process software; Intel-based PC servers; and support services. Pandesic charges a small up-front fee, then takes a percentage (sometimes as much as 6%) of a customer's monthly sales. The company is limiting international expansion to concentrate on US sales, and continues to ally with manufacturers like Compaq, Hewlett-Packard, and Citibank to develop security and other specific aspects of Web commerce.

Penederm Incorporated

320 Lakeside Dr., Foster City, CA 94404

Telephone: 650-358-0100 **Fax:** 650-358-0101 **Metro area:** San Francisco, CA **Web site:** http://www.penederm.com **Human resources contact:** Margaret O'Neill **Sales:** $9 million **Number of employees:** 52 **Number of employees for previous year:** 39 **Industry designation:** Drugs **Company type:** Subsidiary

Penederm, a subsidiary of generic drug maker Mylan Laboratories, makes dermatological drugs. Its prescription drugs treat acne (Avita) and several types of skin fungus (Mentax). Penederm is also developing treatments for inflammatory fungal conditions, nail fungus, and psoriasis, and it makes over-the-counter sunscreens (DuraScreen), skin lotions, and fungus treatments. The company's products use its patented TopiCare Delivery Compounds that deposit and hold drugs and skin care agents on targeted levels of the skin. TopiCare is also sold as an ingredient to cosmetic firms. Penederm sells its prescription drugs to dermatologists in the US, and its nonprescription drugs through partners in the US and abroad.

PeopleSoft, Inc.

4440 Rosewood Dr., Pleasanton, CA 94588

Telephone: 925-694-3000 **Fax:** 925-694-2699 **Metro area:** San Francisco, CA **Web site:** http://www.peoplesoft.com **Human resources contact:** Larry Butler **Sales:** $1.3 billion **Number of employees:** 4,452 **Number of employees for previous year:** 2,490 **Industry designation:** Computers—corporate, professional & financial software **Company type:** Public **Top competitors:** Oracle Corporation; Baan Company N.V.; SAP AG

Only "people people" need apply. PeopleSoft, which delivered the market's first network-based human resource software, is a leading designer of applications for managing company operations across computer networks. (Germany-based SAP is #1.) Primary products include PeopleSoft HRMS (human resources), PeopleSoft Financials, PeopleSoft Manufacturing, and PeopleSoft Distribution. Other products include Red Pepper (inventory planning) and PeopleTools (development and reporting software). The company also develops industry-specific software for the transportation and utility markets, among others. PeopleSoft sells its products worldwide. Co-founder, chairman, and CEO Dave Duffield owns about 20% of the company.

Perclose, Inc.

199 Jefferson Dr., Menlo Park, CA 94025

Telephone: 650-473-3100 **Fax:** 650-473-3110 **Metro area:** San Francisco, CA **Web site:** http://www.perclose.com **Human resources contact:** Jean Munson **Sales:** $10.6 million **Number of employees:** 198 **Number of employees for previous year:** 132 **Industry designation:** Medical products **Company type:** Public **Top competitors:** American Home Products Corporation; Datascope Corp.; C. R. Bard, Inc.

Sure, you could lie still for several hours after your angioplasty or angiography, waiting for a blood clot to form over the little hole in your artery. Or your doctor could use one of Perclose's suture-based closure devices to surgically repair the catheterization site and get you back on your feet (and off the hospital's meter) in no time. Perclose sells its Prostar system (for balloon angioplasty, stenting, and atherectomy procedures) and Techstar system (for diagnostic procedures for vascular diseases of the lower legs) in Europe, Japan, and the US. It is developing the Heartflo Anastomosis System, a system for sewing up arterial grafts. Chairman John Simpson owns nearly 18% of the company.

Pharmacyclics, Inc.

995 E. Arques Ave., Sunnyvale, CA 94086

Telephone: 408-774-0330 **Fax:** 408-774-0340 **Metro area:** San Francisco, CA **Web site:** http://www.pcyc.com **Human resources contact:** Colleen DeGeorge **Sales:** $3.5 million **Number of employees:** 63 **Number of employees for previous year:** 46 **Industry designation:** Drugs **Company type:** Public **Top competitors:** Medical Resources, Inc.; Mallinckrodt Inc.; QLT PhotoTherapeutics Inc.

Pharmacyclics rides herd on the development of drugs that enhance radiation therapy, chemotherapy, and photodynamic therapy by localizing in cancer cells. These drugs, which are activated by light, chemicals, or X-rays, may help treat cancer, atherosclerosis, and other diseases. The firm also researches drugs to improve diagnostic imaging, to which end it has licensing agreements with The University of Texas, ophthalmic firm E-Z-EM, and imaging agent experts Nycomed Amersham and Alcon Laboratories. The National Cancer Institute is funding clinical trials for Gd-Tex, a radiation sensitizer. All drugs are in the research and development stage; company revenues come from licenses, grants, and contracts.

PharmaPrint Inc.

4 Park Plaza, Ste. 1900, Irvine, CA 92614

Telephone: 949-794-7778 **Fax:** 949-794-7777 **Metro area:** Los Angeles, CA **Web site:** http://www.pharmaprint.com **Sales:** $100,000 **Number of employees:** 24 **Number of employees for previous year:** 12 **Industry designation:** Drugs **Company type:** Public **Top competitors:** Shaman Pharmaceuticals, Inc.; Xenova Group plc; AyurCore, Inc.

PharmaPrint is a developmental stage company that makes pharmaceutical drugs out of herbal medicines. The company finds the active compounds in unregulated herbal medicines and uses them to make standardized drugs that can be tested, submitted for FDA approval, and prescribed in precise doses. Its technology was developed at the University of Southern California by Dr. Tasneem A. Khwaja, the company founder and a 20% shareholder. PharmaPrint has an agreement to make herbal supplements for American Home Products under the Centrum brand name. The company also is developing drugs to treat prostate enlargement, mild depression, and motion sickness.

Photonics Corporation

1515 Centre Pointe Dr., Milpitas, CA 95035

Telephone: 408-942-4000 **Fax:** 408-942-4027 **Metro area:** San Francisco, CA **Sales:** $5.6 million **Number of employees:** 29 **Number of employees for previous year:** 18 **Industry designation:** Computers—peripheral equipment **Company type:** Public **Top competitors:** Adaptec, Inc.; Intel Corporation; SIIG, Inc.

Photonics (also known as DTC Data Technology, or DTC) produces device controllers for computers. After acquiring DTC, Photonics licensed its original infrared LAN products business to Moldat Wireless Technologies and began taking advantage of DTC's name recognition in the controller market. The company's products control the flow of data between a computer's CPU and peripherals such as disk drives, CD-ROMs, modems, printers, and scanners. Products include controllers for SCSI (small computer systems interface), Integrated Device Electronics (IDE), Enhanced IDE, and parallel input/output (IO). Photonics markets to resellers, distributors, and original equipment manufacturers.

Photo Research, Inc.

9731 Topanga Canyon Place, Chatsworth, CA 91311

Telephone: 818-341-5151 **Fax:** 818-341-7070 **Metro area:** Los Angeles, CA **Web site:** http://www.photoresearch.com **Human resources contact:** Terri Thomas **Industry designation:** Instruments—scientific **Company type:** Subsidiary **Parent company:** Excel Technology, Inc. **Top competitors:** OSI Systems, Inc.; Advanced Photonix, Inc.; EG&G, Inc.

Photo Research helps find the color in your life. The company, a subsidiary of Excel Technology, makes precision instruments and related software for measuring color and light. Its Spectra SpotMeter helps engineers design products that emit light, such as aircraft and automotive instrument panels, headlights and taillights, motion picture screens, and flat-panel displays. Its handheld, battery-powered LITEMATE enables users to measure luminance in rooms. Photo Research also offers support services including consulting, training, maintenance, and calibration of its products. The company primarily targets the automotive, aerospace, R&D, and motion picture markets.

PIER 39 L.P.

Beach & The Embarcadero Sts., San Francisco, CA 94133

Telephone: 415-705-5500 **Fax:** 415-981-8808 **Metro area:** San Francisco, CA **Web site:** http://pier39.com **Human resources contact:** Bobbi Degl'Innocenti **Sales:** $145 million (Est.) **Number of employees:** 200 **Industry designation:** Leisure & recreational services **Company type:** Private

Situated at Beach Street and The Embarcadero on San Francisco's waterfront, PIER 39 is one of the city's most popular attractions, offering more than 100 stores and 10 full-service restaurants with views of the Bay. In addition, the company's Blue & Gold Fleet runs cruises and ferries on the Bay, offers tours of Alcatraz, and shows films about San Francisco at its Cinemax Theater. PIER 39 also houses the UnderWater World aquarium, and the world-famous California sea lions at K-Dock. The complex, which attracts more than 10 million visitors annually, is open year-round. Founded in 1978, PIER 39 is owned by Chicago-based developer Moor & South.

Pilot Network Services, Inc.

1080 Marina Village Pkwy., Alameda, CA 94501

Telephone: 510-433-7800 **Fax:** 510-433-7809 **Metro area:** San Francisco, CA **Web site:** http://www.pilot.net **Sales:** $11.3 million **Number of employees:** 102 **Industry designation:** Computers—services **Company type:** Public **Top competitors:** ISS Group, Inc.; Check Point Software Technologies Ltd.; AXENT Technologies, Inc.

Pilot Network Services earns its wings keeping hackers out of corporate networks. The company provides such Internet security services as secure access, hosting, electronic commerce, and extranet services. For a fixed monthly fee, Pilot Network continuously manages and monitors Internet traffic to customer networks, allowing the company to respond quickly to security threats. Its Dynamic Security Infrastructure includes a proprietary multilayered defensive architecture combined with its Network Security Centers, which are located in New York, Chicago, Los Angeles, and San Francisco. Customers include the American Stock Exchange (AMEX), E-Stamp, PeopleSoft, Playboy Enterprises, and PR Newswire.

Pinkerton's, Inc.

4330 Park Terrace Dr., Westlake Village, CA 91361

Telephone: 818-706-6800 **Fax:** 800-706-5512 **Metro area:** Los Angeles, CA **Web site:** http://www.pinkertons.com **Human resources contact:** Sally R. Phillips **Sales:** $1 billion **Number of employees:** 48,000 **Number of employees for previous year:** 47,000 **Industry designation:** Protection—safety equipment & services **Company type:** Subsidiary **Top competitors:** Wackenhut Corporation; Borg-Warner Security Corporation; Pittston Brink's Group

Pinkerton's is watching you. A leading US security and investigation firm with offices worldwide, Pinkerton's provides security personnel and consulting services; it also performs background checks, employee screenings, and general, undercover, and specialized investigations. Most of its revenue (90%) is generated by security officers, who are used by hospitals, government, special-events promoters, and industrial and commercial customers for security, access and traffic control, theft prevention, and related services. Pinkerton's consulting leg conducts on-site security-system design and analysis and provides global-risk assessments of terrorist and political activities. Sweden's Securitas owns the company.

Platinum Software Corporation

195 Technology Dr., Irvine, CA 92618

Telephone: 949-453-4000 **Fax:** 949-453-4091 **Metro area:** Los Angeles, CA **Web site:** http://www.platsoft.com **Human resources contact:** Nancy Orr **Sales:** $98.5 million **Number of employees:** 624 **Number of employees for previous year:** 440 **Industry designation:** Computers—corporate, professional & financial software **Company type:** Public **Top competitors:** Baan Company N.V.; SAP AG; PeopleSoft, Inc.

Platinum helps companies manage their green and gold. Platinum Software develops enterprise resource planning software products that help businesses handle everything from payables and receivables to inventories, budgets, purchasing, distribution, and foreign currency transactions. Subsidiary DataWorks makes manufacturing management software. Focusing on midsized firms and divisions of large companies, Platinum's customers include financial, insurance, education, hospitality, and technology firms. Platinum, which generates more than 70% of its sales in the US, sells its software primarily through telesales and resellers.

PMR Corporation

501 Washington St., 5th Fl., San Diego, CA 92103

Telephone: 619-610-4001 **Fax:** 619-610-4184 **Metro area:** San Diego, CA **Web site:** http://pmrcorp.com **Human resources contact:** Heidi Anderson **Sales:** $67.5 million **Number of employees:** 818 **Number of employees for previous year:** 434 **Industry designation:** Medical practice management **Company type:** Public **Top competitors:** Health Management Associates, Inc.; Tenet Healthcare Corporation; Magellan Health Services, Inc.

Pass the Prozac. PMR Corporation develops and manages outpatient programs for people with mental disorders such as schizophrenia and manic depression. The company manages about 60 outpatient programs in 23 states throughout the US and operates four substance abuse rehabilitation programs in California. PMR provides case management services to community mental health centers in Tennessee and has formed a specialty pharmacy joint venture with Counsel Corporation subsidiary Stadtlander. San Diego-based health care provider ScrippsHealth accounts for about 14% of sales. PMR scuttled its plans to purchase Behavioral Healthcare Corporation but has agreed to a joint venture on an outpatient project.

PointCast Incorporated

501 Macara Ave., Sunnyvale, CA 94086

Telephone: 408-990-7000 **Fax:** 408-990-0080 **Metro area:** San Francisco, CA **Web site:** http://www.pointcast.com **Human resources contact:** Brian Taffe **Sales:** $18 million (Est.) **Number of employees:** 267 **Number of employees for previous year:** 196 **Industry designation:** Computers—online services **Company type:** Private **Top competitors:** Data Broadcasting Corporation; NewsEdge Corporation; America Online, Inc.

PointCast's Network Client software (downloadable from the Internet) delivers information straight to desktop computers. The leading supplier of so-called push information on the Internet, the company pointcasts selectable channels, including company information (some of which is provided by Hoover's), news, sports, and weather, to users' computers. PointCast combines aspects of TV broadcasting with the online advantages of user-personalized, up-to-the-minute information. The company offers a range of online publications, including "Money" and "Time." PointCast's ad-supported information is displayed on idle computer screens (instead of a screen-saver) and is free of charge.

Portal Software, Inc.

20883 Stevens Creek Blvd., Cupertino, CA 95014

Telephone: 408-343-4400 **Fax:** 408-343-4401 **Metro area:** San Francisco, CA **Web site:** http://www.portal.com **Human resources contact:** Annette D. Surtees **Sales:** $26.7 million (Est.) **Number of employees:** 242 **Industry designation:** Computers—corporate, professional & financial software **Company type:** Private **Top competitors:** LHS Group Inc.; Saville Systems PLC; Amdocs Limited

Portal Software is a gateway to understanding Internet service. The company (formerly Portal Information Network), which began as an Internet service provider, makes customer management and billing software for providers of Internet-based services. Its Infranet product automates such tasks as user authorization, activity tracking, and billing. It enables immediate service activation and lets subscribers access real-time information about their accounts. Portal also offers consulting, maintenance, and training services. Customers include BellSouth, CyberCash, and UUNET WorldCom. Director Arthur Patterson (through Accel Partners) and founder and CEO John Little own 31% and 28% of the company, respectively.

Preview Travel, Inc.

747 Front St., San Francisco, CA 94111

Telephone: 415-439-1200 **Fax:** 415-421-4982 **Metro area:** San Francisco, CA **Web site:** http://www.previewtravel.com **Human resources contact:** Ken Farber **Sales:** $14 million **Number of employees:** 181 **Number of employees for previous year:** 169 **Industry designation:** Computers—online services **Company type:** Public **Top competitors:** The SABRE Group Holdings, Inc.; Pegasus Systems, Inc.; Microsoft Corporation

Through its Web site, Preview Travel operates a full-service travel agency offering one-stop shopping for a variety of travel services. It also operates America Online's travel service and a co-branded travel Web site with Excite, and it handles travel reservations for search engine Lycos. Preview Travel participates in several travel-related projects with companies such as American Airlines Vacations, CNET's SNAP , MasterCard International, Royal Caribbean International, and USA TODAY. Its News Travel Network division syndicates news insert series ("Dr. Dean Edell's Medical Reports") to local TV stations and produces programming ("Globe-Trotter") for broadcast, cable, and in-flight markets.

Primedex Health Systems, Inc.

1516 Cotner Ave., Los Angeles, CA 90025

Telephone: 310-478-7808 **Fax:** 310-445-2980 **Metro area:** Los Angeles, CA **Human resources contact:** Ruth Villiger-Wilson **Sales:** $58.8 million **Number of employees:** 437 **Number of employees for previous year:** 410 **Industry designation:** Medical services **Company type:** Public **Top competitors:** US Diagnostic Inc.; Medical Resources, Inc.; Syncor International Corporation

Primedex Health Systems captures the true aura of Californians. Through its RadNet Management and Diagnostic Imaging Services subsidiaries, Primedex owns and and manages about 30 California facilities that offer magnetic resonance imaging (MRI), ultrasound, mammography, diagnostic radiology, and similar services. The company also owns a cancer therapy center. Medical services at these facilities are provided by Beverly Radiology Medical Group, which is almost wholly-owned by Primedex CEO Howard Berger. Berger also owns more than one-fourth of Primedex. Primedex, which was formerly controlled by penny stock promoter Robert E. Brennan, has considering putting itself up for sale.

Printrak International Inc.

1250 N. Tustin Ave., Anaheim, CA 92807

Telephone: 714-238-2000 **Fax:** 714-666-1055 **Metro area:** Los Angeles, CA **Web site:** http://www.printrakinternational.com **Human resources contact:** Jan Peterson **Sales:** $71.9 million **Number of employees:** 417 **Number of employees for previous year:** 287 **Industry designation:** Protection—safety equipment & services **Company type:** Public **Top competitors:** Digital Biometrics, Inc.; Identix Incorporated; The National Registry, Inc.

Printrak International has sticky fingers—on file. The company sells real-time, automated fingerprint-identification systems in 26 countries. Biometric technology translates the finger's loops and whorls into a map for identification from a database. Its Digital Justice Solution system integrates fingerprint input from a hard copy or live-scan, remote workstations and central sites, mugshot searches, and database systems. Printrak can link 911 dispatchers, responding officers, investigators, booking officers, jailers, and supervisors. Clients include the FBI, Scotland Yard, and the Royal Canadian Mounted Police, and more than 200 other law enforcement agencies. CEO Richard Giles owns about 53% of the company.

Printronix, Inc.

17500 Cartwright Rd., Irvine, CA 92623

Telephone: 949-863-1900 **Fax:** 949-660-8682 **Other address:** PO Box 19559, Irvine, CA 92623 **Metro area:** Los Angeles, CA **Web site:** http://www.printronix.com **Human resources contact:** Juli A. Mathews **Sales:** $170.4 million **Number of employees:** 922 **Number of employees for previous year:** 866 **Industry designation:** Computers—peripheral equipment **Company type:** Public **Top competitors:** Zebra Technologies Corporation; Lexmark International Group, Inc.; Hewlett-Packard Company

Printronix makes printers that print just about everything except money—from reports with graphics to bar code labels to jewelry tags and plastic membership cards. A leading maker of high-speed industrial printers, Printronix produces line matrix printers for heavy-duty jobs such as invoicing, continuous-form printing, and bar code labels, plus laser and thermal printers for business and industrial applications. Products are sold primarily to manufacturers and resellers; IBM accounts for about a quarter of Printronix's sales. The company has operations in Singapore and the Netherlands and sales offices throughout Europe. Founder and chairman Robert Kleist owns 18% of Printronix.

Procom Technology, Inc.

2181 Dupont Dr., Irvine, CA 92612

Telephone: 949-852-1000 **Fax:** 949-261-7380 **Metro area:** Los Angeles, CA **Web site:** http://www.procom.com **Human resources contact:** Atashe Aydin **Sales:** $111.9 million **Number of employees:** 308 **Number of employees for previous year:** 246 **Industry designation:** Computers—peripheral equipment **Company type:** Public **Top competitors:** NEC Corporation; Meridian Data, Inc.; Storage Technology Corporation

CD-ROM-based computer storage products are Procom Technology's biggest line, but the company also makes RAID (redundant arrays of independent disks) and tape backup subsystems, and hard disk drive upgrade packages. The company's products are sold through computer resellers, value-added resellers, and distributors to corporations, financial institutions, and government agencies. Procom's four founders—chairman and CEO Alex Razmjoo and EVPs Frank Alaghband, Nick Shahrestany, and Alex Aydin—own about 60% of the company. Procom has offices in Canada, Europe, and the US, and sells its products worldwide.

Prolong International Corporation

6 Thomas, Irvine, CA 92618

Telephone: 949-587-2700 **Fax:** 949-587-2707 **Metro area:** Los Angeles, CA **Web site:** http://www.prolong.com **Human resources contact:** Donna Raddack **Sales:** $35 million **Number of employees:** 57 **Number of employees for previous year:** 43 **Industry designation:** Chemicals—specialty **Company type:** Public **Top competitors:** Burmah Castrol plc; WD-40 Company; First Brands Corporation

A holding company, Prolong International makes and sells high-performance lubricants through its Prolong Super Lubricant subsidiary. The company's products are sold to the consumer automotive market as engine lubricants and as fuel and transmission treatments. Prolong lubricants are based on a patented formula referred to as anti-friction metal treatment (AFMT), an additive that the company believes can be adapted for use as a lubricant in the industrial, governmental, and military markets. The company sells its products through automotive retailers and direct-response infomercials. Prolong has more than 200 distributors in Africa, Asia, and North and South America.

Prospect Medical Holdings, Inc.

515 S. Flower St., Ste. 1640, Los Angeles, CA 90071

Telephone: 213-629-2185 **Fax:** 213-629-2272 **Metro area:** Los Angeles, CA **Web site:** http://www.prospectmedical.com **Human resources contact:** Pam Powell **Sales:** $50 million (Est.) **Number of employees:** 261 **Industry designation:** Medical practice management **Company type:** Private **Top competitors:** FPA Medical Management, Inc.; MedPartners, Inc.; PhyCor, Inc.

The prospect of prosperity keeps pulling Prospect Medical Holdings toward physician practice management. The company provides personnel, claims, case management, and data collection services to nearly 1,400 specialists, as well as some 350 primary care physicians, through subsidiaries Prospect Medical Systems and Sierra Medical Group, both of which operate in Southern California. The company runs 11 medical and six administrative offices. Founded in 1993 as Med-Search to manage a single practice, the company grew slowly until it was acquired by Prospect Medical Systems in 1996. Since then, it has grown primarily through acquisitions.

Protection One, Inc.

6011 Bristol Pkwy., Culver City, CA 90230

Telephone: 310-342-6300 **Fax:** 310-649-1385 **Metro area:** Los Angeles, CA **Web site:** http://www.protectionone.com **Human resources contact:** Michele Manning **Sales:** $421.1 million **Number of employees:** 852 **Number of employees for previous year:** 814 **Industry designation:** Protection—safety equipment & services **Company type:** Public **Top competitors:** Ameritech Corporation; Tyco International Ltd.; Pittston Brink's Group

Protection One is the #2 security-monitoring company in the US, behind Tyco International, which owns ADT. Protection One has more than 1.5 million subscribers in 48 states. In addition to monitoring home alarm systems and dispatching assistance when needed, it also provides enhanced services such as patrol services, paging, and two-way voice equipment. The company participates in joint ventures and other strategic alliances (such as co-marketing arrangements with Oregon utility and former parent PacifiCorp and home builder Kaufman & Broad). Electric and gas utility Western Resources, which sold its alarm operations to Protection One in 1997, owns 82% of the company.

Protein Design Labs, Inc.

2375 Garcia Ave., Mountain View, CA 94043

Telephone: 650-903-3700 **Fax:** 650-903-3730 **Metro area:** San Francisco, CA **Web site:** http://www.pdl.com **Human resources contact:** Vernetta Wilson **Sales:** $30.8 million **Number of employees:** 217 **Number of employees for previous year:** 208 **Industry designation:** Biomedical & genetic products **Company type:** Public **Top competitors:** Celltech plc

If your body starts fighting you, Protein Design Labs hopes to help you fight right back—the firm develops human and humanized monoclonal antibodies to prevent and treat autoimmune diseases, inflammatory conditions, viral infections, cancers, and other conditions. Protein Design Labs has FDA approval for Zenapax, which fights kidney transplant rejection. Zenapax, which has also been approved for use in Switzerland, is licensed to drug giant Roche. Protein Design Labs, which has several other compounds in preclinical stages and in human clinical trials, has a collaborative agreement with Eli Lilly & Company and a cross-license agreement with Genentech.

ProtoSource Corporation

2800 28th St., Ste. 170, Santa Monica, CA 90405

Telephone: 310-314-9801 **Fax:** 310-452-5115 **Metro area:** Los Angeles, CA **Web site:** http://www.protosource.com **Human resources contact:** Raymond J. Meyers **Sales:** $900,000 **Number of employees:** 21 **Number of employees for previous year:** 14 **Industry designation:** Computers—online services **Company type:** Public **Top competitors:** CompuServe Interactive Services, Inc.; AT&T Corp.; America Online, Inc.

Even though the beach is more than 150 miles away, ProtoSource gets residents of central California up and surfing. Through its ProtoSource Network, the Internet service provider offers online access to about 3,400 residential, business, and government agency customers in Fresno and six nearby communities. In addition to monthly fee-based Internet access, ProtoSource offers computer network consulting, intranet design, and Web site design and hosting services. ProtoSource, formerly a developer of agribusiness software, plans to grow through acquisitions of other Internet services companies in central California.

QAD Inc.

6450 Via Real, Carpinteria, CA 93013

Telephone: 805-684-6614 **Fax:** 805-684-9998 **Metro area:** Los Angeles, CA **Web site:** http://www.qad.com **Human resources contact:** Barry R. Anderson **Sales:** $193.3 million **Number of employees:** 917 **Number of employees for previous year:** 786 **Industry designation:** Computers—corporate, professional & financial software **Company type:** Public **Top competitors:** i2 Technologies, Inc.; Baan Company N.V.; System Software Associates, Inc.

QAD isn't God, but it is a maker of resource planning software for global manufacturing companies. The company's primary product, MFG/PRO, is a software package designed to streamline the manufacturing process in the electronics, food and beverage, automotive, medical, and packaged goods industries. MFG/PRO helps manage accounts payable, inventory, repetitive manufacturing, and purchasing, and it schedules everything from work orders to procurement. The company gets most of its revenue from licensing MFG/PRO to more than 4,000 customers (including Lucent, PepsiCo, and Ford) in over 80 countries. Founder, chairman, and president Pamela Meyer Lopker and her husband, CEO Karl Lopker, own about two-thirds of QAD.

QuadraMed Corp.

80 E. Sir Francis Drake Blvd., Ste. 2A, Larkspur, CA 94939

Telephone: 415-461-7725 **Fax:** 415-461-7785 **Metro area:** San Francisco, CA **Web site:** http://www.quadramed.com **Human resources contact:** Mark Slippy **Sales:** $44.9 million **Number of employees:** 754 **Number of employees for previous year:** 171 **Industry designation:** Computers—corporate, professional & financial software **Company type:** Public **Top competitors:** National Data Corporation; ENVOY Corporation; Health Management Systems, Inc.

QuadraMed and its subsidiaries develop financial and decision-making software for health care providers. Its QuanTIM suite of products uses electronic data interchange to give clients access to information used to manage claims, track payer contracts, and facilitate reimbursement. EZ CAP software gives providers up-to-date information on assigned enrollees. Three-quarters of QuadraMed's revenues are from product licenses; the rest comes from support services (business office outsourcing, reimbursement consulting). Some 80% of the acquisitive firm's 3,200 customers are hospitals; others include home health care agencies, physicians groups, and insurers.

Quality Resorts of America, Inc.

11707 Fair Oaks Blvd., Ste. 210, Fair Oaks, CA 95628

Telephone: 916-967-9812 **Fax:** 916-967-0469 **Metro area:** Sacramento, CA **Web site:** http://www.rv4fun.com/aboutqra.html **Human resources contact:** Susan Bienias **Sales:** $3.8 million **Number of employees:** 75 **Number of employees for previous year:** 70 **Industry designation:** Leisure & recreational services **Company type:** Public **Top competitors:** Hyatt Corporation; Trendwest Resorts, Inc.; Fairfield Communities, Inc.

Quality Resorts of America operates four membership-based resorts in Northern California: Redwood Trails, Lighthouse Marina, River Grove Resort, and Klamath Cove Resort. Guests bring their own sleeping equipment (RVs, tents) or rent equipment at the resorts. Resort amenities include horseback riding, swimming, nature trails and hiking, water skiing, fishing, and hunting. Most of the company's sales come from membership sales (from $2,995 to $6,995) and membership dues (about $300 a year), which allow guests unlimited visits of up to 15 days. Additional sales are generated by rental units and storage fees, among other resort operations. The Brindle family owns about 50% of Quality Resorts.

Quidel Corporation

10165 McKellar Ct., San Diego, CA 92121

Telephone: 619-552-1100 **Fax:** 619-453-4338 **Metro area:** San Diego, CA **Web site:** http://www.quidel.com **Human resources contact:** Kellie Fontes **Sales:** $45.7 million **Number of employees:** 312 **Number of employees for previous year:** 290 **Industry designation:** Medical products **Company type:** Public **Top competitors:** Abbott Laboratories; SmithKline Beecham plc; Becton, Dickinson and Company

Quidel susses out disease—it makes point-of-care diagnostic products for infectious diseases, allergies, and autoimmune disorders; strep throat tests account for more than 30% of sales. Other products test for mononucleosis, chlamydia, and the ulcer-causing "H. pylori" bacteria. Quidel's over-the-counter products include ovulation predictors and pregnancy tests (Conceive, Q-Test, and Rapid-Vue brands); together, consumer and professional-use pregnancy tests make up more than 35% of sales. A direct sales force and a distributor network sell Quidel's tests to doctors and labs, as well as to retail drugstores. Quidel has a pact with Glaxo Wellcome to develop flu and herpes tests.

Quote.com, Inc.

850 N. Shoreline Blvd., Mountain View, CA 94043

Telephone: 650-930-1000 **Fax:** 650-930-1111 **Metro area:** San Francisco, CA **Web site:** http://www.quote.com **Sales:** $12 million (Est.) **Number of employees:** 100 **Number of employees for previous year:** 75 **Industry designation:** Computers—online services **Company type:** Private **Top competitors:** MarketWatch.com, Inc.; Yahoo! Inc.; Intuit Inc.

Quote.com provides financial information to more than 300,000 subscribers through its Web site. The company's offerings include real-time stock quotes, business and industry news, earnings reports, and company profiles. It also allows customers to track multiple portfolios and price trends, analyze market or industry movements, and receive daily e-mail updates. In addition, businesses can integrate Quote.com's financial information into their own Web sites. The company receives its news and information from Standard & Poor's, Reuters, and PR Newswire, among other information providers. Founded in 1993, Quote.com is funded by three venture capital firms and an investment research company.

Randall Foods, Inc.

4901 S. Boyle Ave., Vernon, CA 90058

Telephone: 323-587-2383 **Fax:** 323-586-1587 **Metro area:** Los Angeles, CA **Human resources contact:** Evelynn Cherne **Sales:** $284.2 million (Est.) **Number of employees:** 633 **Number of employees for previous year:** 475 **Industry designation:** Food—meat products **Company type:** Private **Top competitors:** Foster Poultry Farms Inc.; Tyson Foods, Inc.; ConAgra, Inc.

Few chickens ever die of old age. Poultry processor Randall Foods processes poultry in Texas and Louisiana and transports it for sales to West Coast stores, mainly in Arizona, California, Nevada, and Utah. The firm fought in California's "fresh chicken" labeling wars in the mid-1990s, lobbying to allow its long-haul chicken to be sold as fresh alongside "never-frozen" birds from in-state producers. Randall Foods plucked new business from an old plant in 1997, buying an abandoned Louisiana poultry processing plant from rival ConAgra. Randall Foods also processes and distributes other meats and seafood. CEO Stan Bloom owns the company.

Raster Graphics, Inc.

3025 Orchard Pkwy., San Jose, CA 95134

Telephone: 408-232-4000 **Fax:** 408-232-4101 **Metro area:** San Francisco, CA **Web site:** http://www.rgi.com **Human resources contact:** Lynne Reynolds **Sales:** $54.7 million **Number of employees:** 218 **Number of employees for previous year:** 155 **Industry designation:** Computers—peripheral equipment **Company type:** Subsidiary

Raster Graphics makes digital color printers for BIG projects. The company's Digital ColorStation (DCS) is used to make point-of-purchase displays, vinyl and cloth banners, trade show exhibit graphics, billboards, courtroom graphics, and backlit signs. DCS can print materials up to 52 inches wide and 100 feet long. Raster Graphics sells its printers to color photo labs, reprographic houses, graphic arts service bureaus, exhibit builders, screen printers, and in-house print shops. Raster Graphics also sells specialized printer ink and makes image processing software used in its printers and third-party printers. The company is a subsidiary of photofinishing equipment maker Gretag Imaging Holding AG.

Raytel Medical Corporation

2755 Campus Dr., Ste. 200, San Mateo, CA 94403

Telephone: 650-349-0800 **Fax:** 650-349-8850 **Metro area:** San Francisco, CA **Web site:** http://www.raytel.com **Human resources contact:** Dennis Conroy **Sales:** $107.6 million **Number of employees:** 849 **Number of employees for previous year:** 827 **Industry designation:** Health care—outpatient & home **Company type:** Public **Top competitors:** In Home Health, Inc.; Medtronic, Inc.; St. Jude Medical, Inc.

Raytel? Pray tell. Raytel Medical provides diagnostic and therapeutic services for patients with cardiovascular disease, including pacemaker monitoring, cardiac event detection, Holter monitoring, and magnetic resonance imaging (MRI). The company manages two hospital-based heart centers (in California and Texas) along with a handful of physician practices, cardiovascular diagnostic facilities, and hospital-based cardiac catheterization laboratories. Raytel serves about 200,000 patients annually, of whom about 50,000 receive heart-monitoring services. Its Raytel Imaging Network consists of some 475 independent imaging centers in the Mid-Atlantic states, including five centers managed by the company.

Red Brick Systems, Inc.

485 Alberto Way, Los Gatos, CA 95032

Telephone: 408-399-3200 **Fax:** 408-399-3277 **Metro area:** San Francisco, CA **Web site:** http://www.redbrick.com **Human resources contact:** Peggy J. DeLeon **Sales:** $43.3 million **Number of employees:** 291 **Number of employees for previous year:** 248 **Industry designation:** Computers—corporate, professional & financial software **Company type:** Subsidiary **Top competitors:** Sybase, Inc.; International Business Machines Corporation; Oracle Corporation

Red Brick Systems, a subsidiary of Informix, makes high-performance data management software for UNIX and Windows NT systems. Its flagship Red Brick Warehouse and related connectivity software and administration tools create a system of data analysis, storage, and regeneration accessible through private networks and the Internet. The software suite incorporates load processing, query processing, and data management, which are the major components of a data warehouse. Red Brick sells its products through hardware partnerships, software providers, systems integrators, and value-added resellers in more than 20 countries. Customers include AT&T, Healthsource, General Mills, PepsiCo, and Tandy Corporation.

Research Engineers, Inc.

22700 Savi Ranch Pkwy., Yorba Linda, CA 92887

Telephone: 714-974-2500 **Fax:** 714-974-4771 **Metro area:** Los Angeles, CA **Web site:** http://www.reiusa.com **Human resources contact:** Clara Young **Sales:** $12.3 million **Number of employees:** 102 **Number of employees for previous year:** 93 **Industry designation:** Computers—engineering, scientific & CAD-CAM software **Company type:** Public **Top competitors:** Intergraph Corporation; Structural Dynamics Research Corporation; Landmark Graphics Corporation

Research Engineers' products give shape to great ideas. The company makes stand-alone and network-based civil and mechanical engineering software for worldwide markets including architecture, transportation, and utilities. The company's software integrates modeling, analysis, design drafting, and reporting. Its structural analysis and design software (including STAAD and FabriCAD) is available in eight international languages. Research Engineers also makes other Windows-based software (Stardyne, Civilsoft, and Visual Solid) for mechanical, civil, and pipe engineers. Customers include Exxon, NASA, and Siemens. Chairman and CEO Amrit Das owns 32% of the company.

ResMed Inc.

10121 Carroll Canyon Rd., San Diego, CA 92131

Telephone: 619-689-2400 **Fax:** 619-880-1618 **Metro area:** San Diego, CA **Web site:** http://www.resmed.com **Human resources contact:** Nancy Silva **Sales:** $66.5 million **Number of employees:** 373 **Number of employees for previous year:** 270 **Industry designation:** Medical products **Company type:** Public **Top competitors:** Respironics, Inc.; Mallinckrodt Inc.; Non-Invasive Monitoring Systems, Inc.

Need a full night's rest? ResMed makes devices that help diagnose and treat obstructive sleep apnea, a disorder characterized by restricted breathing and disrupted sleep. The company's flow generators (continuous and variable positive airway pressure—CPAP and VPAP—systems) administer air through nasal masks to keep patients' airways open. ResMed also makes head harnesses, masks, and other accessories, including humidifiers, replacement air filters, and carry bags for portable systems. While ResMed makes its products primarily in Australia, the company sells them in North America (52% of sales), Europe (35%) and around the world.

ReSound Corporation

220 Saginaw Dr., Seaport Centre, Redwood City, CA 94063

Telephone: 650-780-7800 **Fax:** 650-367-0675 **Metro area:** San Francisco, CA **Web site:** http://www.resound.com **Human resources contact:** Joseph E. Black **Sales:** $123.4 million **Number of employees:** 1,041 **Number of employees for previous year:** 974 **Industry designation:** Medical products **Company type:** Public **Top competitors:** Symphonix Devices, Inc.; Bausch & Lomb Incorporated; Telex Communications, Inc.

More than 890,000 people worldwide can tell how good hearing-device manufacturer ReSound's name sounds. Its In-the-Ear, Behind-the-Ear, In-the-Canal, and Completely-in-the-Canal hearing aids are programmed to adjust continuously to the acoustic environment and the individual client's range of hearing. Through a strategic alliance with AudioLogic and GN Danavox A/S, the company is developing a digital signal processing platform for future generations of hearing devices. ReSound is also working with Motorola to address hearing impairment and communications markets. Its products are distributed through more than 6,300 authorized outlets in more than 35 countries.

RiboGene, Inc.

26118 Research Rd., Hayward, CA 94545

Telephone: 510-732-5551 **Fax:** 510-732-7741 **Metro area:** San Francisco, CA **Human resources contact:** Jan Ivy **Sales:** $3 million **Number of employees:** 26 **Industry designation:** Drugs **Company type:** Public **Top competitors:** ICN Pharmaceuticals, Inc.; Amgen Inc.; Agouron Pharmaceuticals, Inc.

RiboGene identifies and develops potential drug candidates for the treatment of infectious diseases caused by bacterial, fungal, and viral infections. The development stage company is focusing its drug discovery on compounds that inhibit or interfere with pathogen-specific translation mechanisms. RiboGene is developing two antibacterial candidates with partner Dainippon Pharmaceutical and focuses its antiviral research on two hepatitis C treatments. It also has research agreements with Trega Biosciences, Pharmacopeia, ArQule, and Georgia State University, and additional licensing agreements with the University of Washington and McGill University. Abbott Laboratories owns about 12% of RiboGene.

Royale Energy, Inc.

7676 Hazard Center Dr., Ste. 1500, San Diego, CA 92108

Telephone: 619-297-8505 **Fax:** 619-297-0438 **Metro area:** San Diego, CA **Web site:** http://www.royl.com **Sales:** $9.1 million **Number of employees:** 13 **Number of employees for previous year:** 11 **Industry designation:** Oil & gas—exploration & production **Company type:** Public **Top competitors:** Fan Energy Inc.; Delta Petroleum Corporation; Key Production Company, Inc.

Royale Energy wants to rule in Northern California's Sacramento and San Joaquin basins, where the company concentrates its exploration and production efforts. Royale Energy operates 51 wells and has 16.3 billion cu. ft. of natural gas reserves in Northern California. The company also owns leasehold interests in Texas and Oklahoma; overall, its proved reserves consist of 16.9 million cu. ft. of natural gas and 4,700 barrels of oil. Through their Royale Petroleum holding company, CEO Donald Hosmer and CFO Stephen Hosmer (sons of chairman Harry Hosmer), own 32% of Royale Energy.

Sacramento Kings

One Sports Pkwy., Sacramento, CA 95834

Telephone: 916-928-0000 **Fax:** 916-928-6912 **Metro area:** Sacramento, CA **Web site:** http://www.nba.com/kings **Sales:** $51.9 million (Est.) **Number of employees:** 80 **Industry designation:** Leisure & recreational services **Company type:** Private **Top competitors:** Phoenix Suns; California Sports, Inc.; Seattle SuperSonics

The Sacramento Kings have been dethroned for almost half a century now. The franchise was founded in 1948 and won the NBA title in 1951 as the Rochester Royals. The club was known as the Cincinnati Royals, the Kansas City-Omaha Kings, and the Kansas City Kings before moving to Sacramento in 1985. Playing under coach Bob Cousy in 1972-73, guard Nate "Tiny" Archibald was the first NBA player to lead the league in both scoring (34 points) and assists (11.4). Other luminary Kings have included Bob Davies, Maurice Stokes, Oscar Robertson, Jack Twyman, and Sam Lacey, and coaches Cotton Fitzsimmons and Bill Russell. A limited partnership led by Jim Thomas owns the club.

SafeGuard Health Enterprises, Inc.

505 N. Euclid St., Anaheim, CA 92803

Telephone: 714-778-1005 **Fax:** 714-758-4383 **Other address:** PO Box 3210, Anaheim, CA 92803 **Metro area:** Los Angeles, CA **Human resources contact:** Hal Nutter **Sales:** $95.4 million **Number of employees:** 358 **Number of employees for previous year:** 307 **Industry designation:** Medical practice management **Company type:** Public

SafeGuard Health Enterprises offers US employers a variety of dental care benefit programs. It provides dental benefits to some 1.2 million employees of approximately 5,500 governmental, private sector, and multiple employer trust customers. Employers can choose from its dental HMO, PPO, or standard indemnity plans. SafeGuard's managed dental care plans (SafeGuard Health Plans, SafeGuard Dental Plans, and American Dental Corporation plans) provide a panel of about 14,000 independent dental offices with about 16,000 dentists. The company's primary operations are in California, Colorado, Florida, Missouri, and Texas. It also owns SafeHealth Life Insurance, which writes dental indemnity insurance in 16 states.

Safeskin Corporation

12671 High Bluff Dr., San Diego, CA 92130

Telephone: 619-794-8111 **Fax:** 619-350-2378 **Metro area:** San Diego, CA **Web site:** http://www.safeskin.com **Human resources contact:** Robert Zabaronick **Sales:** $237.1 million **Number of employees:** 5,341 **Number of employees for previous year:** 4,100 **Industry designation:** Medical & dental supplies **Company type:** Public **Top competitors:** Allegiance Corporation; Pacific Dunlop Limited; Maxxim Medical, Inc.

Please turn your head and cough. Safeskin is the top maker of disposable latex examination gloves for the US medical market and is one of the world's leading makers of powder-free (70% of sales) gloves. All of its medical gloves are hypoallergenic; its powder-free gloves also avoid the skin irritation that some people experience when using powdered gloves. The company also makes synthetic and sterile surgical gloves. It sells its gloves to dentists, clinics, and other caregivers, as well as to high-tech and industrial markets; 60% of end users are acute care facilities. Sales to medical supply distributors McKesson General Medical and Owens & Minor account for 22% and about 20% of sales, respectively.

Sage Software, Inc.

56 Technology South, Irvine, CA 92618

Telephone: 949-753-1222 **Fax:** 949-753-1859 **Metro area:** Los Angeles, CA **Web site:** http://www.sota.com **Human resources contact:** Kelly Henry **Sales:** $64 million **Number of employees:** 460 **Number of employees for previous year:** 420 **Industry designation:** Computers—corporate, professional & financial software **Company type:** Subsidiary **Top competitors:** Timeline, Inc.; Great Plains Software, Inc.; Lawson Software

Call it number crunching in a box. Sage Software (formerly State of the Art)—the US subsidiary of UK-based Sage Group—provides accounting and financial management software, support, and services. The firm's Acuity Financials accounting software is designed for large businesses (up to 1,000 employees), its MAS 90 line of software is geared for medium companies, and its BusinessWorks line is designed for smaller firms that need software with more functionality than is available in off-the-shelf accounting products. The company markets its products through accountants as well as resellers.

San Diego Chargers Football Co.

4020 Murphy Canyon Rd., San Diego, CA 92123

Telephone: 619-874-4500 **Fax:** 619-292-2760 **Other address:** PO Box 609609, San Diego, CA 92160 **Metro area:** San Diego, CA **Web site:** http://www.chargers.com **Sales:** $82.5 million (Est.) **Industry designation:** Leisure & recreational services **Company type:** Private **Top competitors:** The Denver Broncos Football Club; Seattle Seahawks; Kansas City Chiefs

The San Diego Chargers Football Co. started in 1959 as the Los Angeles Chargers. The team almost went back to LA in 1997, after plans to remodel its stadium were delayed. The $78 million remodeling of Jack Murphy Stadium added 11,500 seats and expanded parking facilities. QUALCOMM paid $18 million to have the stadium renamed Qualcomm Stadium. Work on the facility was completed in time for the 1998 Super Bowl to be held there, and the Chargers have signed an agreement to stay in San Diego until 2020. Owner Alex Spanos bought the National Football League team in 1984. Spanos got his start selling sandwiches to migrant workers. He also owns apartment-building concern A.G. Spanos Companies.

SanDisk Corporation

140 Caspian Ct., Sunnyvale, CA 94089

Telephone: 408-542-0500 **Fax:** 408-542-0503 **Metro area:** San Francisco, CA **Web site:** http://www.sandisk.com **Human resources contact:** Marianne Jackson **Sales:** $135.8 million **Number of employees:** 477 **Number of employees for previous year:** 445 **Industry designation:** Computers—peripheral equipment **Company type:** Public **Top competitors:** Samsung Group; Catalyst Semiconductor, Inc.; Toshiba Corporation

SanDisk is a leading maker of flash memory storage devices, integrated circuits that retain data when power is off (other memory chips lose stored data as soon as power is disconnected). The company's products include removable and embedded memory cards, used in such products as Eastman Kodak's digital cameras and mobile communication devices made by Nokia and Siemens. SanDisk has sales offices in Germany, Hong Kong, Japan, and the US. Exports account for nearly 60% of its sales. Computer storage products maker Seagate Technology owns about 25% of the company.

San Francisco Baseball Associates, L.P.

3Com Park at Candlestick Point, San Francisco, CA 94124

Telephone: 415-468-3700 **Fax:** 415-330-2725 **Metro area:** San Francisco, CA **Web site:** http://www.sfgiants.com **Human resources contact:** Joyce Thomas **Sales:** $69.8 million **Number of employees:** 140 **Number of employees for previous year:** 137 **Industry designation:** Leisure & recreational services **Company type:** Partnership **Top competitors:** Colorado Rockies Baseball Club; Los Angeles Dodgers Inc.; San Diego Padres Baseball Club Limited Partnership

San Francisco Baseball Associates, known as the San Francisco Giants, started out in 1883 as the New York City Gothams. Renamed the Giants two years later, it was the premier National League team for 25 years, winning 10 pennants and three World Series championships. In 1958 the Giants joined the former Brooklyn Dodgers as transplants to the West Coast. Willie Mays suited up for the Giants for 15 years, becoming the third-greatest home run hitter in history and arguably the best all-around player ever. The Giants won the 1962 World Series over the powerhouse New York Yankees, and lost to the Oakland A's in the 1989 "Bay Bridge Series" that was postponed for 10 days after an earthquake devastated the Bay Area.

Sangstat Medical Corporation

1505 Adams Dr., Menlo Park, CA 94025

Telephone: 650-328-0300 **Fax:** 650-328-8892 **Metro area:** San Francisco, CA **Human resources contact:** Pat Donchin **Sales:** $19.7 million **Number of employees:** 112 **Number of employees for previous year:** 75 **Industry designation:** Medical instruments **Company type:** Public **Top competitors:** Novartis AG

SangStat Medical offers a broad spectrum of about a dozen therapeutic and monitoring product candidates to improve the outcome of organ transplants. The company's products include SangCya, a generic form of cyclosporine, an anti-rejection drug; CELSIOR, which preserves organ viability prior to transplantation; sHLA-STAT Class I, which improves the early diagnosis of acute-rejection episodes; Thymoglobulin, an antibody that prevents graft rejection in kidney transplants; and Sang-35, a form of cyclosporine (awaiting FDA approval). SangStat bought IMTIX, from which it licensed many of its products, in 1998 from Rhone-Poulenc Group.

San Jose Sharks L.P.

San Jose Arena, 525 W. Santa Clara St., San Jose, CA 95113

Telephone: 408-287-7070 **Fax:** 408-999-5797 **Other address:** PO Box 1240, San Jose, CA 95113 **Metro area:** San Francisco, CA **Web site:** http://www.sj-sharks.com **Human resources contact:** Carol Ross **Sales:** $49.2 million (Est.) **Number of employees:** 130 **Industry designation:** Leisure & recreational services **Company type:** Private **Top competitors:** Dallas Stars L.P.; Los Angeles Kings; Phoenix Coyotes Hockey Club

The San Jose Sharks began play in the National Hockey League in 1991 after co-owners George and Gordon Gund agreed to sell their Minnesota North Stars franchise in exchange for an expansion team. Playing in San Jose Arena, the team made it into the playoffs for the first time in 1994 after only three years in the league. All-stars who have skated for the San Jose Sharks include right wing Owen Nolan, goalie Arturs Irbe, and defenseman Sandis Ozolinsh. The not-for-profit Sharks Foundation provides assistance and support to youth and community organizations throughout the Bay Area.

Scheid Vineyards Inc.

13470 Washington Blvd., Ste. 300, Marina del Rey, CA 90292

Telephone: 310-301-1555 **Fax:** 310-301-1569 **Metro area:** Los Angeles, CA **Human resources contact:** Viola Charo **Sales:** $17.5 million **Number of employees:** 75 **Number of employees for previous year:** 63 **Industry designation:** Agricultural operations **Company type:** Public **Top competitors:** Beringer Wine Estates Holdings, Inc.; The Wine Group; The Robert Mondavi Corporation

Scheid Vineyards operates nearly 6,000 acres of wine grape vineyards in Monterey and San Benito counties, California. Of its total acres, about 1,700 are managed for others and more than 4,000 are managed for its own products. Cabernet Sauvignon, Chenin Blanc, Merlot, Gewurtztraminer, Chardonnay, and Sauvignon Blanc are among the 14 varieties of premium grapes grown on its properties. About 90% of its production is sold to two customers: Canandaigua Brands and Diageo's International Distillers and Vintners North America. These customers' labels include Beaulieu Vineyard, Glen Ellen, Blossom Hill, Inglenook, Paul Masson, and Taylor California Cellars. CEO Alfred Scheid owns more than half of the company.

Scios Inc.

2450 Bayshore Pkwy., Mountain View, CA 94043

Telephone: 650-966-1550 **Fax:** 650-968-2438 **Metro area:** San Francisco, CA **Web site:** http://www.sciosinc.com **Human resources contact:** Lauretta Cesario **Sales:** $73.7 million **Number of employees:** 350 **Number of employees for previous year:** 335 **Industry designation:** Biomedical & genetic products **Company type:** Public **Top competitors:** Glaxo Wellcome plc; Merck & Co., Inc.; Novartis AG

Scios is a biopharmaceutical company that develops protein-based drugs and other acute illness treatments. Its products, which are in various stages of research, development, and trials, include Natrecor BNP, for acute congestive heart failure (awaiting FDA approval); Fiblast, which enhances wound healing; Insulinotropin, for Type II diabetes; and a potential treatment for Alzheimer's disease. Scios has joint development agreements with biopharmaceutical companies such as Abbott Labs and Eli Lilly to research and market its products. It also has an agreement with SmithKline Beecham to co-promote the latter's antidepressant Paxil.

SEGA of America Inc.

255 Shoreline Dr., Ste. 200, Redwood City, CA 94065

Telephone: 650-508-2800 **Fax:** 650-802-3622 **Metro area:** San Francisco, CA **Web site:** http://www.sega.com **Human resources contact:** Mike Killeen **Industry designation:** Computers—peripheral equipment **Company type:** Subsidiary **Parent company:** SEGA Enterprises, Ltd. **Top competitors:** Nintendo Co., Ltd.; Sony Corporation; Broderbund Software, Inc.

SEGA of America can't stop daydreaming of being #1. The subsidiary of SEGA Enterprises develops and markets television-based video game consoles and related software and is anticipating the 1999 US release of SEGA's brand-new, 128-bit console, Dreamcast, which will feature a built-in modem and 3-D graphics. SEGA is retiring its disappointing 32-bit SegaSaturn system, which lost out to Sony's PlayStation and the Nintendo 64. It also makes Pico, an electronic learning aid for children between the ages of 3 and 7. In 1998 SEGA of America announced a workforce reduction of 30% following the SegaSaturn game system's loss of market share and in anticipation of the release of Dreamcast.

Seminis, Inc.

1905 Lirio Ave., Saticoy, CA 93004

Telephone: 805-647-1572 **Fax:** 805-647-8963 **Metro area:** Los Angeles, CA **Web site:** http://www.seminis.com **Human resources contact:** Tom Stevenson **Sales:** $428.4 million **Number of employees:** 3,000 **Industry designation:** Agricultural operations **Company type:** Subsidiary **Top competitors:** Pioneer Hi-Bred International, Inc.; Monsanto Company; DEKALB Genetics Corporation

Seminis doesn't put up with any bad seeds. A subsidiary of Mexican agricultural giant Empresas la Moderna (ELM), Seminis is the world's largest producer of fruit and vegetable seeds, with about 8,000 seed varieties and about 25% of the world market. Some of its seeds are genetically engineered to be disease and insect resistant, thereby reducing dependence on chemicals and producing higher crop yields. The company sells seeds (under primary brands Asgrow, Petoseed, and Royal Sluis) in more than 120 countries. About 12% of sales are used for research. Formed in 1994, Seminis has grown by acquiring other seed companies. ELM will retain control of the company after Seminis' planned IPO.

Sepragen Corporation

30689 Huntwood Ave., Hayward, CA 94544

Telephone: 510-476-0650 **Fax:** 510-476-0655 **Metro area:** San Francisco, CA **Web site:** http://www.sepragen.com **Human resources contact:** Linda Misko **Sales:** $1.6 million **Number of employees:** 22 **Number of employees for previous year:** 21 **Industry designation:** Instruments—scientific **Company type:** Public **Top competitors:** Pharmacia & Upjohn, Inc.; United States Filter Corporation; APV PLC

Sepragen's motives are pure. Its liquid-processing equipment, based on innovative radial flow chromatography (separating a substance into its basic chemical components), is used by pharmaceutical firms (more than 90% of sales), food and beverage makers, and the waste management industry. Applications include purifying biological drugs, de-bittering citrus juice, improving infant formula, and separating toxins from waste. Sepragen products include liquid chromatography columns (specially coated tubes) and chromatography workstations. CEO Vinit Saxena, who invented the company's original technology, owns 21% of Sepragen. Michael Schneider, head of waste recycler Romic Environmental Technologies, owns 22%.

SeraCare, Inc.

1925 Century Park East, Ste. 1970, Los Angeles, CA 90067

Telephone: 310-772-7777 **Fax:** 310-772-7770 **Metro area:** Los Angeles, CA **Human resources contact:** Jerry L. Burdick **Sales:** $12.3 million **Number of employees:** 386 **Number of employees for previous year:** 164 **Industry designation:** Medical products **Company type:** Public

SeraCare collects and processes human blood plasma for use in such medical products as treatments for hemophilia, blood-typing tests, diagnostic kits, and immune globulins (used to strengthen the immune system after exposure to such diseases as hepatitis and rabies). SeraCare operates 17 plasma collection centers in 12 states. The centers draw blood from paid donors, extract plasma from the blood, return red blood cells to the donors, and then sell the plasma to firms that turn it into usable products. SeraCare also collects specialty plasmas, such as the tetanus antibody. SeraCare emerged from Chapter 11 bankruptcy protection in 1996 with a yen for acquisition.

SIBIA Neurosciences, Inc.

505 Coast Blvd. South, Ste. 300, La Jolla, CA 92037

Telephone: 619-452-5892 **Fax:** 619-452-9279 **Metro area:** San Diego, CA **Web site:** http://www.sibia.com **Human resources contact:** Lynn Alba **Sales:** $7 million **Number of employees:** 111 **Number of employees for previous year:** 106 **Industry designation:** Drugs **Company type:** Public **Top competitors:** Neurocrine Biosciences, Inc.; Cambridge NeuroScience, Inc.; Athena Neurosciences, Inc.

SIBIA Neurosciences is working to discover and develop small-molecule drugs that will treat such central nervous system disorders as Alzheimer's disease, Parkinson's disease, and schizophrenia. None of the company's proposed pharmaceutical products have completed trials, but SIBIA Neurosciences has developed proprietary drug-discovery technologies it uses to identify new drug candidates; these are also licensed to other drug makers (Novartis, Merck, and more). Other sources for SIBIA Neurosciences' research funding include collaborative agreements with such companies as Bristol-Myers Squibb, Meiji Seika Kaisha, and Eli Lilly. The Salk Institute founded SIBIA in 1981 and owns one-fifth of it.

Siebel Systems, Inc.

1855 S. Grant St., San Mateo, CA 94402

Telephone: 650-295-5000 **Fax:** 650-295-5111 **Metro area:** San Francisco, CA **Web site:** http://www.siebel.com **Human resources contact:** Les Cundall **Sales:** $391.5 million **Number of employees:** 473 **Number of employees for previous year:** 213 **Industry designation:** Computers—corporate, professional & financial software **Company type:** Public **Top competitors:** Baan Company N.V.; The Vantive Corporation; Trilogy Software, Inc.

Siebel Systems hits the sale on the head. The company is a leading provider of sales automation and customer service software. Its main product, Siebel Sales Enterprise, offers client information and decision support across a corporation's worldwide computer network. Glaxo Wellcome, Prudential Insurance, and Lucent Technologies are listed among Siebel's global clientele. The company continues to expand its product breadth and industry presence through acquisitions. President and CEO Thomas Siebel owns 28% of Siebel Systems; Andersen Consulting owns 8%.

Signal Pharmaceuticals, Inc.

5555 Oberlin Dr., San Diego, CA 92121

Telephone: 619-558-7500 **Fax:** 619-558-7513 **Metro area:** San Diego, CA **Web site:** http://www.electriciti.com/signal **Human resources contact:** Lori Cain **Sales:** $7.6 million (Est.) **Number of employees:** 82 **Industry designation:** Drugs **Company type:** Private **Top competitors:** Merck & Co., Inc.; Sanofi; Glaxo Wellcome plc

Drug discovery company Signal Pharmaceuticals is identifying drugs that regulate genes and the production of disease-causing proteins. The company maps gene-regulating pathways in cells in an effort to identify molecular targets that activate or deactivate genes. By identifying these genes, the company hopes to develop treatments that can selectively regulate their activation. Signal's drug discovery programs concern autoimmune and inflammatory disorders, bone metabolism, neurological and cardiovascular diseases, cancer, and viral infections. The company has collaborative discovery agreements with Nippon Kayaku, DuPont Pharmaceuticals, and affiliates of Ares-Serono, Roche, and Akzo Nobel.

SIMS Communications, Inc.

18001 Cowan, Stes. C&D, Irvine, CA 92614

Telephone: 949-724-9094 **Fax:** 949-261-0323 **Metro area:** Los Angeles, CA **Human resources contact:** Bruce S. Schames **Sales:** $1 million **Number of employees:** 38 **Number of employees for previous year:** 36 **Industry designation:** Medical services **Company type:** Public **Top competitors:** ARDIS Telecom and Technologies, Inc.; On-Point Technology Systems, Inc.; Maxxis Group, Inc.

SIMS Communications markets medical software, machines that vend videos and phone cards, and kiosks that connect consumers directly with medical equipment merchandisers. The company's MedCard division offers an electronic system for medical benefits verification and third-party insurance claims billing. Its One Medical Service unit installs catalog kiosks and point-of-sale terminals in pharmacies and medical facilities so customers can order home medical equipment directly from vendors. Its Moviebar subsidiary rents movies via vending machines in hotels, while Link International Technologies provides vending machines that dispense prepaid activated long distance calling cards.

Simulation Sciences Inc.

601 Valencia Ave., Ste. 100, Brea, CA 92823

Telephone: 714-579-0412 **Fax:** 714-579-0236 **Metro area:** Los Angeles, CA **Web site:** http://www.simsci.com **Human resources contact:** Daniel T. Nichols **Sales:** $60.6 million **Number of employees:** 368 **Number of employees for previous year:** 260 **Industry designation:** Computers—engineering, scientific & CAD-CAM software **Company type:** Subsidiary **Top competitors:** Gensym Corporation; ICARUS International, Inc.; Aspen Technology, Inc.

Simulation Sciences, a subsidiary of UK-based BTR Siebe, makes analytical software that simulates chemical processes, including distillation, fluid flow, and heat transfer, and the physical configuration of a plant. The software is used primarily in the oil and gas industry, but chemical companies and construction companies also use it. Plant engineers utilize Simulation Sciences' software to optimize production runs by determining such factors as manufacturing trade-offs, amounts of energy used, and the most efficient use of materials. Customers include Chevron, Allied Signal, Hoechst, and Unocal.

SMART Modular Technologies, Inc.

4305 Cushing Pkwy., Fremont, CA 94538

Telephone: 510-623-1231 **Fax:** 510-623-1434 **Metro area:** San Francisco, CA **Web site:** http://www.smartm.com **Human resources contact:** Phyllis Pineda **Sales:** $714.7 million **Number of employees:** 831 **Number of employees for previous year:** 636 **Industry designation:** Computers—peripheral equipment **Company type:** Public **Top competitors:** Solectron Corporation; Kingston Technology Company; Micron Technology, Inc.

SMART's smarts are in computer components. SMART Modular Technologies is a top US maker of PC cards, embedded computers, and memory modules. The company offers more than 500 products for computer, networking, and telecommunications manufacturers. Customers include Compaq (more than 60% of sales), Cisco, and Hewlett-Packard. SMART's market advantage is its fast product turnaround for customers. The company has manufacturing facilities in California, Malaysia, Puerto Rico, and Scotland. CEO Ajay Shah and VP Lata Krishnan (husband and wife co-founders of SMART) together own nearly a fourth of the company; co-founder and director Mukesh Patel owns 15%.

Somnus Medical Technologies, Inc.

285 N. Wolfe Rd., Sunnyvale, CA 94086

Telephone: 408-773-9121 **Fax:** 408-773-9137 **Metro area:** San Francisco, CA **Web site:** http://www.somnus.com **Human resources contact:** Michael Garey **Sales:** $7.4 million **Number of employees:** 78 **Number of employees for previous year:** 63 **Industry designation:** Medical products **Company type:** Public **Top competitors:** Mallinckrodt Inc.; Respironics, Inc.; ResMed Inc.

Somnus Medical Technologies, a modern-day Morpheus for those afflicted with certain sleep disorders (as well as for their bedmates), makes medical devices to treat upper airway disorders such as snoring, obstructive sleep apnea, and enlarged turbinates (the soft tissue in the nasal cavity). The company's somnoplasty system tightens tissue in the upper airway using radiofrequency technology combined with needle electrodes that deliver thermal energy to obstructed areas. The company is developing a direct sales force to market its products in the US and Canada and has an exclusive three-year distribution arrangement with Medtronic, which will distribute its products in Asia, Australia, and Europe.

Spiros Development Corporation II, Inc.

7475 Lusk Blvd., San Diego, CA 92121

Telephone: 619-457-2553 **Fax:** 619-457-2555 **Metro area:** San Diego, CA **Sales:** $222,000 **Number of employees:** 3 **Industry designation:** Drugs **Company type:** Public **Top competitors:** Glaxo Wellcome plc; Astra AB; Rhone-Poulenc Rorer Inc.

Not that anybody would blame an asthma sufferer for the hole in the ozone layer . . . . but Spiros Development's inhaler is designed to deliver anti-asthma drugs without the use of chlorofluorocarbons (CFCs). The company was spun off from Dura Pharmaceuticals in 1997 to fund development of the dry-powder inhaler, which the company hopes will replace traditional metered-dose inhalers. The Spiros inhaler principally addresses respiratory conditions, such as asthma and chronic obstructive pulmonary disease. Dura Pharmaceuticals, which retains a controlling interest in Spiros Development, will make and market the inhaler and any other products which gain FDA approval.

The Sports Club Company, Inc.

11100 Santa Monica Blvd., Ste. 300, Los Angeles, CA 90025

Telephone: 310-479-5200 **Fax:** 310-479-8350 **Metro area:** Los Angeles, CA **Human resources contact:** Charla Peterson **Sales:** $81.9 million **Number of employees:** 2,250 **Number of employees for previous year:** 2,100 **Industry designation:** Leisure & recreational services **Company type:** Public **Top competitors:** Bally Total Fitness Holding Corporation; Fitness Holdings, Inc.

The Sports Club Company operates highbrow sports and fitness clubs in Southern California, Las Vegas, and New York City. The company owns and operates two types of clubs, differentiated primarily by the level of amenities and services provided, diversity of facilities available, and fees charged. The four Sports Clubs locations (two in metropolitan Los Angeles and one each in New York City and Las Vegas) have been developed as urban country clubs, complete with such amenities as valet parking, squash courts, in-club restaurants, and poolside juice bars. The company's nine Southern California Spectrum Clubs, designed as smaller-scale Sports Clubs, have fewer recreational and social facilities.

STAAR Surgical Company

1911 Walker Ave., Monrovia, CA 91016

Telephone: 626-303-7902 **Fax:** 626-303-2962 **Metro area:** Los Angeles, CA **Web site:** http://www.staar.com **Human resources contact:** Laurie Fowler **Sales:** $55.1 million **Number of employees:** 270 **Number of employees for previous year:** 269 **Industry designation:** Medical products **Company type:** Public

STAAR Surgical makes products for minimally invasive ophthalmic surgical procedures. Its products, which are awaiting FDA approval in the US, are sold in Canada, China, Europe, South Africa, and South America. Its leading products include foldable intraocular lenses, which replace natural lenses removed in cataract surgery, and the Glaucoma Wick, which is inserted into the eye of a glaucoma sufferer as a long-term treatment. Other products include implantable contact lenses for vision correction, and STAARVISC solution, used during the implantation procedure for intraocular and implantable contact lenses. Independent sales representatives and medical distributors market the company's products.

SteriGenics International, Inc.

4020 Clipper Ct., Fremont, CA 94538

Telephone: 510-770-9000 **Fax:** 510-770-1499 **Metro area:** San Francisco, CA **Web site:** http://www.sterigenics.com **Human resources contact:** Linda Gruehl **Sales:** $47 million **Number of employees:** 321 **Number of employees for previous year:** 275 **Industry designation:** Medical services **Company type:** Public **Top competitors:** Griffith Micro Science International, Inc.; Cyclopss Corporation; Isomedix, Inc.

SteriGenics provides contract sterilization services. Although the sterilization of medical products (including needles, scalpels, and cotton gauze) has accounted for some 80% of its business, SteriGenics also treats nonmedical products, including spices, herbs, cosmetics, and food-packaging materials, and the company plans to expand these services. The company uses gamma irradiation, a faster method than conventional fumigation, to sterilize products at its 12 facilities in six states; it also operates one electron beam facility. SteriGenics leases MiniCell sterilization units to companies needing high-volume sterilization.

SUGEN, Inc.

230 E. Grand Ave., South San Francisco, CA 94080

Telephone: 650-553-8300 **Fax:** 650-553-8301 **Metro area:** San Francisco, CA **Web site:** http://www.sugen.com **Human resources contact:** Dorian Rinella **Sales:** $14.9 million **Number of employees:** 189 **Number of employees for previous year:** 160 **Industry designation:** Biomedical & genetic products **Company type:** Public **Top competitors:** AVAX Technologies, Inc.; ImClone Systems Incorporated; OSI Pharmaceuticals, Inc.

SUGEN develops small-molecule drugs that target cellular signal transduction pathways; variations in these pathways are present in cancer, diabetes, and other disorders. SUGEN's drugs are intended to signal molecules that function as enzymatic switches to turn on and off specific pathways. Products in development include SU101 for treating brain, prostate, and other cancers; SU5416 for treating solid tumors; and SU5271 for treating psoriasis. SUGEN's research and development partners include Zeneca, ASTA Medica, Allergan, and Taiho. Founder and CEO Stephen Evans-Freke and director Jeremy Curncock Cook each own about 5% of the company; Zeneca owns nearly 20%.

Summa Industries

21250 Hawthorne Blvd., Ste. 500, Torrance, CA 90503

Telephone: 310-792-7024 **Fax:** 310-792-7079 **Metro area:** Los Angeles, CA **Web site:** http://www.Summalndustries.com **Human resources contact:** Paul A. Walbrun **Sales:** $85.7 million **Number of employees:** 675 **Number of employees for previous year:** 357 **Industry designation:** Rubber & plastic products **Company type:** Public **Top competitors:** Parker Hannifin Corporation; Aeroquip-Vickers, Inc.; National Service Industries, Inc.

Summa Industries never met a plastic component it didn't like. The acquisitive company's subsidiaries make a range of plastics components for the lighting and materials-handling industries, among others. Subsidiary LexaLite makes plastic lighting components and KVP/Falcon Plastic Belting makes parts for conveyor belts used in food processing. Manchester Plastics fabricates plastic sheet products, Ny-Glass Plastics makes plastic precision- and custom-molded parts for electronics and telecommunications products, and Agricultural Products makes products used in irrigation. The company has sold GST Industries, its nonplastics operation. Summa has facilities in California, Florida, Michigan, Oklahoma, and Tennessee.

Sunkist Growers, Inc.

14130 Riverside Dr., Sherman Oaks, CA 91423

Telephone: 818-986-4800 **Fax:** 818-379-7405 **Other address:** PO Box 7888, Van Nuys, CA 91409 **Metro area:** Los Angeles, CA **Web site:** http://www.sunkist.com **Human resources contact:** John R. McGovern **Sales:** $1.1 billion **Number of employees:** 875 **Number of employees for previous year:** 813 **Industry designation:** Agricultural operations **Company type:** Cooperative **Top competitors:** Chiquita Brands International, Inc.; Orange-co, Inc.; Dole Food Company, Inc.

Perhaps the US enterprise least susceptible to an outbreak of scurvy, Sunkist Growers is a cooperative owned by 6,500 citrus farmers in California and Arizona. Sunkist markets fresh oranges, lemons, grapefruit, and tangerines in the US and overseas. Fruit that doesn't meet fresh market standards is sent to the co-op's Processed Products division, where it's turned into juices and oils for use in food products. The Sunkist brand is one of the most recognized names in the US; through licensing agreements, the name appears on dozens of beverages and other products, from flowers to fruit rolls, in more than 50 countries. About one-fourth of Sunkist's sales come from outside the US, mainly Japan and Hong Kong.

Sunrider International

1625 Abalone Ave., Torrance, CA 90501

Telephone: 310-781-3808 **Fax:** 310-222-9273 **Metro area:** Los Angeles, CA **Web site:** http://www.sunrider.com **Human resources contact:** Gary Morris **Sales:** $700 million (Est.) **Number of employees:** 200 **Number of employees for previous year:** 163 **Industry designation:** Vitamins & nutritional products **Company type:** Private **Top competitors:** Nu Skin USA, Inc.; Nature's Sunshine Products, Inc.; Herbalife International, Inc.

Sunrider International markets a variety of health and beauty products made from herbs and herbal extracts, including Sunrider nutritional products and SunSmile and Kandesn personal-care products. Sunrider sells its products, which are made in China, Singapore, Taiwan, and the US, through multilevel marketing via some one million independent distributors in more than 25 countries. Owners Tei Fu Chen and Oi-Lin Chen (husband and wife: he studied pharmacy; she's a medical doctor) started the company in 1982. The couple paid $93 million to the IRS in 1997 for charges of conspiracy, tax evasion, and smuggling in connection with Sunrider's operations.

Sunrise Medical Inc.

2382 Faraday Ave., Ste. 200, Carlsbad, CA 92008

Telephone: 760-930-1500 **Fax:** 760-930-1575 **Metro area:** San Diego, CA **Web site:** http://www.sunrisemedical.com **Human resources contact:** Roberta C. Baade **Sales:** $657.2 million **Number of employees:** 4,400 **Number of employees for previous year:** 4,254 **Industry designation:** Medical products **Company type:** Public **Top competitors:** Invacare Corporation; Graham-Field Health Products, Inc.; Medline Industries, Inc.

Sunrise Medical makes medical products used in institutional and home care settings. The company is the #2 US maker of wheelchairs and accessories behind Invacare; its models include ultralight and sporting wheelchairs under the Quickie brand name. Sunrise also makes bathing and lifting products, home respiratory devices (under the DeVilbiss and PulseDose brands), health care beds and furniture, speech communication devices, and therapeutic mattresses. The company manufactures its products in Europe and North America and distributes to more than 100 countries. It has consolidated its operations into three business units: Home Healthcare Group, Continuing Care Group, and Sunrise Medical Europe.

SuperGen, Inc.

2 Annabel Ln., Ste. 220, San Ramon, CA 94583

Telephone: 925-327-0200 **Fax:** 925-327-7347 **Metro area:** San Francisco, CA **Web site:** http://www.supergen.com **Human resources contact:** Christina Wang **Sales:** $3 million **Number of employees:** 54 **Number of employees for previous year:** 46 **Industry designation:** Drugs **Company type:** Public **Top competitors:** Bristol-Myers Squibb Company; Immunex Corporation; Amgen Inc.

Pharmaceutical company SuperGen focuses on acquiring rights to late-stage drug research and development in order to avoid the risks and costs of bringing new products to market. SuperGen owns marketing rights to several approved anticancer drugs. It is developing generic drugs and enhanced versions of existing drugs patented by other companies; these include treatments for leukemia, breast cancer, Hodgkin's disease, and ovarian cancer. SuperGen also owns the rights to an antiobesity drug and is working on drugs to treat anemia related to chemotherapy, radiotherapy, and kidney disease. Larry Ellison (chairman of software giant Oracle) owns 17% of the SuperGen.

Superior National Insurance Group, Inc.

26601 Agoura Rd., Calabasas, CA 91302

Telephone: 818-880-1600 **Fax:** 818-880-8615 **Metro area:** Los Angeles, CA **Web site:** http://www.superior.com **Human resources contact:** Curtis H. Carson **Sales:** $153.6 million **Number of employees:** 410 **Number of employees for previous year:** 355 **Industry designation:** Insurance—accident & health **Company type:** Public **Top competitors:** Zenith National Insurance Corp.; American International Group, Inc.

Ah, the sweet sound of Californians coming up lame on the job. Well, maybe the sound isn't so sweet, but the fear of hearing it has made Superior National Insurance Group the Golden State's largest workers' compensation specialist. Through its Superior National and Superior Casualty insurance subsidiaries, the firm sells workers' comp policies in California (95% of premiums) and Arizona. Superior National focuses on smaller accounts and low-risk industries. Other company subsidiaries provide data processing, vocational rehabilitation, legal, and paralegal services in-house. The firm is controlled by entities associated with Insurance Partners LP, including Centre Re, Keystone Inc., and Chase Manhattan Bank.

SVG-Tinsley

3900 Lakeside Dr., Richmond, CA 94806

Telephone: 510-222-8110 **Fax:** 510-223-4534 **Metro area:** San Francisco, CA **Human resources contact:** Ahmad Zimi **Sales:** $17.4 million **Number of employees:** 113 **Number of employees for previous year:** 104 **Industry designation:** Instruments—scientific **Company type:** Subsidiary **Top competitors:** BMC Industries, Inc.; Precision Optics Corporation, Inc.; Optical Coating Laboratory, Inc.

SVG-Tinsley (formerly Tinsley Laboratories) designs and produces precision lenses and mirrors used by cinematographers and professional photographers, in large-scale telescopes, and for pilot training and advanced avionics. Sales to the US government account for about 30% of the company's sales, while about 20% of revenues come from foreign sales. Customers include aerospace and defense firms, color television tube makers, and universities. Through a joint agreement, SVG-Tinsley is working with NASA, SEMATECH, and Silicon Valley Group Lithography to develop products designed for space exploration and semiconductor production. The company is a subsidiary of Silicon Valley Group.

Symphonix Devices, Inc.

3047 Orchard Pkwy., San Jose, CA 95134

Telephone: 408-232-0710 **Fax:** 408-232-0720 **Metro area:** San Francisco, CA **Web site:** http://www.symphonix.com **Sales:** $600,000 **Number of employees:** 61 **Number of employees for previous year:** 45 **Industry designation:** Medical products **Company type:** Public **Top competitors:** Siemens AG; Bausch & Lomb Incorporated; Royal Philips Electronics

Symphonix Devices is bringing a symphony of sound to people suffering from moderate to severe hearing loss. The development-stage company makes semi-implantable and implantable hearing devices called soundbridges. Marketed to ear, nose, and throat surgeons, its Vibrant hearing device directly drives the three small bones of the middle ear through a rice grain-sized floating mass transducer (FMT) attached to a bone in the middle ear. The FMT converts sound into mechanical vibrations and enhances the natural movement of the middle ear's bones. The company has distribution agreements with Newmedic, Gaes, Biocord, Biomedical Technology, and Danaflex to distribute the Vibrant line throughout the European Union.

Synbiotics Corporation

11011 Via Frontera, San Diego, CA 92127

Telephone: 619-451-3771 **Fax:** 619-451-5719 **Metro area:** San Diego, CA **Web site:** http://www.synbiotics.com **Sales:** $31.4 million **Number of employees:** 135 **Number of employees for previous year:** 104 **Industry designation:** Veterinary products & services **Company type:** Public **Top competitors:** Schering-Plough Corporation; Pfizer Inc; IDEXX Laboratories, Inc.

Concerned with the conditions of cats, cows, and canines, Synbiotics provides rapid and laboratory diagnostic products for the animal health care industry. The company makes and/or distributes test kits for feline leukemia and immunodeficiency virus, feline and canine heartworm disease, and canine brucellosis and hip dysplasia. The company also sells diagnostic products for horses and cows, markets vaccines, and is developing a canine pregnancy test. Started in 1982 to develop therapies for human diseases, Synbiotics is now one of a few biotech companies focusing solely on the less demanding animal health care market. About three-quarters of the company's sales occur in North America.

Syncor International Corporation

6464 Canoga Ave., Woodland Hills, CA 91367

Telephone: 818-737-4000 **Fax:** 818-737-4898 **Metro area:** Los Angeles, CA **Web site:** http://www.syncor.com **Human resources contact:** Sheila H. Coop **Sales:** $449 million **Number of employees:** 2,900 **Number of employees for previous year:** 2,281 **Industry designation:** Drugs **Company type:** Public

Syncor International compounds, dispenses, and distributes radiopharmaceutical products to clinics and hospitals through a network of almost 120 US and 13 foreign nuclear pharmacy service centers. Through a joint venture and subsidiaries, Syncor owns and operates almost 50 medical imaging centers in 11 states and Puerto Rico. Its imaging centers provide diagnostic services such as MRIs, nuclear imaging, X-rays, ultrasounds, and mammography. The company also makes iodine capsules and markets imaging cold kits, isotopes, medical reference sources, and other nuclear and pharmacy equipment and accessories. Syncor International's foreign centers are located in Asia, Mexico, the Pacific, and South Africa.

Target Therapeutics, Inc.

47201 Lakeview Blvd., Fremont, CA 94538

Telephone: 510-440-7700 **Fax:** 510-440-7894 **Metro area:** San Francisco, CA **Web site:** http://www.tget.com **Human resources contact:** Robert G. MacLean **Sales:** $69.8 million **Number of employees:** 402 **Number of employees for previous year:** 317 **Industry designation:** Medical & dental supplies **Company type:** Subsidiary **Parent company:** Boston Scientific Corporation **Top competitors:** Becton, Dickinson and Company; Guidant Corporation; Johnson & Johnson

Target Therapeutics, a subsidiary of Boston Scientific, develops and markets specialized disposable and implantable medical devices and components. The company makes disposable microcatheters, guide wires, microcoils, and angioplasty products used to reach disease sites throughout the body via the circulatory system. The company's products help doctors perform pinpoint procedures, such as the treatment of diseased, ruptured, or blocked blood vessels in the brain that are responsible for stroke, by threading the devices through small blood vessels to the treatment site.

Tejon Ranch Co.

4436 Lebec Rd., Lebec, CA 93243

Telephone: 805-327-8481 **Fax:** 805-248-2318 **Other address:** PO Box 1000, Lebec, CA 93243 **Metro area:** Bakersfield, CA **Web site:** http://www.tejon.com **Sales:** $52.9 million **Number of employees:** 88 **Number of employees for previous year:** 52 **Industry designation:** Agricultural operations **Company type:** Public **Top competitors:** King Ranch, Inc.; Koch Industries, Inc.; Bartlett and Company

One of the nation's largest ranches, Tejon Ranch raises cattle and farm crops such as nuts and wine grapes. Located on 270,000 contiguous acres in Southern California, the company raises stocker cattle (those it buys at low weight, fattens on range forage, and sells) and conducts commercial cow-calf operations (wherein the herd is replenished by its own offspring and excess numbers are sold commercially). Tejon Ranch also offers its location for movie shoots, raises quarter horses for competitive events, and leases land for oil, gas, and mineral production.

Teknowledge Corporation

1810 Embarcadero Rd., Palo Alto, CA 94303

Telephone: 650-424-0500 **Fax:** 650-493-2645 **Metro area:** San Francisco, CA **Web site:** http://www.teknowledge.com **Sales:** $11.1 million **Number of employees:** 71 **Industry designation:** Computers—corporate, professional & financial software **Company type:** Public **Top competitors:** Perceptronics, Inc.; IntelliCorp, Inc.; Trilogy Software, Inc.

Teknowledge's software is a bit-fueled philosopher, teaching computers the art of reason. The company provides government entities with expert systems and knowledge processing applications. What that means is artificial intelligence (AI); Teknowledge has been a key advocate in using AI to solve real-world business problems since it was spawned in the early 1980s at the storied Stanford University computer science labs. Teknowledge products apply AI and its human expertise emulation to tutor, sell, plan, and assess. The company continues to expand beyond its federal parameters by applying its technology to the Internet and focusing on e-commerce applications.

Tenet Healthcare Corporation

3820 State St., Santa Barbara, CA 93105

Telephone: 805-563-7000 **Fax:** 805-563-7070 **Metro area:** Santa Barbara, CA **Web site:** http://www.tenethealth.com **Human resources contact:** Alan R. Ewalt **Sales:** $9.9 billion **Number of employees:** 116,800 **Number of employees for previous year:** 105,000 **Industry designation:** Hospitals **Company type:** Public **Top competitors:** Columbia/HCA Healthcare Corporation; Kaiser Foundation Health Plan, Inc.; Daughters of Charity National Health System

Tenet Healthcare Corporation is the nation's #2 hospital chain (after Columbia/HCA). The company owns or operates more than 120 hospitals in 18 states. Tenet also owns a hospital in Barcelona, Spain. In addition, subsidiaries own or operate clinics, HMOs, a PPO, home health care programs, long-term-care facilities, a managed care insurance company, medical office buildings, outpatient surgery centers, and rehabilitation and specialty hospitals. Tenet also provides management and administrative services for independent physicians or groups. The company has a strategic partnership with MedPartners, which will create the largest health care network in Southern California.

TeraStor Corporation

2310 N. First St., San Jose, CA 95131

Telephone: 408-914-4000 **Fax:** 408-914-4008 **Metro area:** San Francisco, CA **Web site:** http://www.terastor.com **Human resources contact:** Ann Reeves **Number of employees:** 120 **Number of employees for previous year:** 110 **Industry designation:** Computers—peripheral equipment **Company type:** Private **Top competitors:** Imation Corp.; Seagate Technology, Inc.; Quantum Corporation

TeraStor has a new breed of storage devices waiting to take on the Earth. The development-stage company has designed the Near Field Recording mass storage products, which combine characteristics of hard drives and magneto-optical technologies. These rewritable disk drives have a higher storage capacity than optical disk drives and most tape drives, and will sport lower prices. They can be used in servers, storage subsystems, and workstations, and are designed for backups, archiving large amounts of data, and creating multimedia content. Mitsumi Electric has signed on to manufacture TeraStor's products, which are targeted at OEMs, system integrators, and VARs. Investors include Quantum and Winfield Capital.

Tetra Tech, Inc.

670 N. Rosemead Blvd., Pasadena, CA 91107

Telephone: 626-351-4664 **Fax:** 626-351-5291 **Metro area:** Los Angeles, CA **Web site:** http://www.tetratech.com **Human resources contact:** Richard A. Lemmon **Sales:** $382.9 million **Number of employees:** 3,600 **Number of employees for previous year:** 2,262 **Industry designation:** Pollution control equipment & services **Company type:** Public **Top competitors:** Roy F. Weston, Inc.; The IT Group, Inc.; Black & Veatch

Tetra Tech brings a technical touch to other companies' problems with its engineering and consulting services. The company operates in three areas: resource management, telecommunications, and infrastructure. Activities include groundwater cleanup, environmental restoration, and watershed management. Telecommunications services include securing sites and building infrastructure for broadband and wireless telecom networks. Tetra Tech also constructs government buildings and wastewater treatment facilities. Nearly half of the company's business comes from contracts with US government agencies.

THERMOGENESIS CORP.

3146 Gold Camp Dr., Rancho Cordova, CA 95670

Telephone: 916-858-5100 **Fax:** 916-858-5199 **Metro area:** Sacramento, CA **Web site:** http://www.thermogenesis.com **Human resources contact:** Nancy Allardyce **Sales:** $4.4 million **Number of employees:** 89 **Number of employees for previous year:** 85 **Industry designation:** Biomedical & genetic products **Company type:** Public **Top competitors:** LifeCell Corporation; Mallinckrodt Inc.; Harris Corporation

THERMOGENESIS makes blood run cold ... really cold. The company makes equipment that harvests, freezes, and thaws blood components such as clotting proteins, hormones, enzymes, and progenitor and stem cells from blood in umbilical cords and placentas. Its core line of products are rapid blood-plasma freezers and thawers that it sells to blood banks, blood transfusion centers, and hospitals throughout the US and in more than 30 other countries. The equipment can also be used to freeze biologic material such as sperm, ova, and heart valves. The company itself may also be feeling the chill; recurring losses and heavy debts have raised doubts that it can continue as a going concern.

Think3

2880 Lakeside Dr., Ste. 250, Santa Clara, CA 95054

Telephone: 408-987-2200 **Fax:** 408-727-0237 **Metro area:** San Francisco, CA **Web site:** http://www.cadlab.com **Human resources contact:** Todd Gomes **Sales:** $20 million (Est.) **Number of employees:** 250 **Industry designation:** Computers—engineering, scientific & CAD-CAM software **Company type:** Private **Top competitors:** Parametric Technology Corporation; Structural Dynamics Research Corporation; Autodesk, Inc.

Eureka! Think3's not only got it, it's gold. Eureka Gold is a leading mechanical computer-aided design software suite that enables 2-D and 3-D drafting, surfacing, solid modeling, and assembly. Engineers at Toyota and Peugeot use Eureka, which has a mid-range price tag starting at $12,000. Also available from Think3 is TeamManager, a project management program. After marketing almost exclusively in Europe since its founding in 1979, Think3 is expanding its sales worldwide through value-added resellers. Joe Costello, former CEO of Cadence Design Systems and the big cheese at Think3, held a contest in 1998 to change the company's name from Cad.Lab.

ThirdAge Media, Inc.

585 Howard St., San Francisco, CA 94105

Telephone: 415-267-4600 **Fax:** 415-908-6909 **Metro area:** San Francisco, CA **Web site:** http://www.thirdagemedia.com **Human resources contact:** Dionne Sharrow **Number of employees:** 50 **Industry designation:** Computers—online services **Company type:** Private **Top competitors:** America Online, Inc.; Yahoo! Inc.; AARP

ThirdAge Media knows that surfing the Net isn't just for the young—it's also for the young at heart. Through its thirdage.com Web site, older adults can plug in to the Internet and view information on topics ranging from health to technology to romance. Boasting 600,000 visitors each month, the Web site also offers free e-mail, personal homepages, and chat rooms centering on themes such as comparative religions, crafts, and online dating. In addition to its Web site, ThirdAge Media offers a syndicated news service and participates in research programs. CEO Mary Furlong founded the company in 1996. Investors in ThirdAge Media include US West Interactive Services Group.

Thoratec Laboratories Corporation

6035 Stoneridge Dr., Pleasanton, CA 94588

Telephone: 925-847-8600 **Fax:** 925-847-8574 **Metro area:** San Francisco, CA **Web site:** http://www.thoratec.com **Human resources contact:** Michelle Crawford **Sales:** $17 million **Number of employees:** 138 **Number of employees for previous year:** 108 **Industry designation:** Medical products **Company type:** Public **Top competitors:** ABIOMED, Inc.; World Heart Corporation; Thermo Cardiosystems Inc.

Suffering from a broken heart? Thoratec's there for the rebound. The company makes artificial heart devices for patients awaiting a heart transplant. Its lead product, the FDA-approved Ventricular Assist Device (VAD), uses a blood pump, a console to activate the pump, and tubes connecting the pump to the heart. The pump is worn outside the body, allowing its use by small patients. Thoratec developed Thoralon, a strong, flexible material that doesn't cause adverse reactions, and uses it in all the company's products. The firm is also testing Thoralon for replacement blood vessels in heart bypass surgery and for blood-vessel grafts for hemodialysis patients (a use approved in Canada and other countries).

Ticketmaster Group, Inc.

8800 Sunset Blvd., West Hollywood, CA 90069

Telephone: 310-360-6000 **Fax:** 310-360-0207 **Metro area:** Los Angeles, CA **Web site:** http://www.ticketmaster.com **Human resources contact:** Michael Castro **Sales:** $341 million **Number of employees:** 6,355 **Number of employees for previous year:** 5,330 **Industry designation:** Leisure & recreational services **Company type:** Subsidiary **Top competitors:** ETM Entertainment Network; Prologue Systems; SFX Entertainment, Inc.

Ticketmaster Group is the leading provider of automated ticketing services worldwide. The company provides client venues and promoters with ticket inventory control and management, a distribution network, and marketing and support services. It generates revenues primarily by adding service charges to tickets sold through phone orders and independent sales outlets at locations apart from entertainment venue box offices. The company also publishes the monthly entertainment magazine "Live!" USA Networks, parent of Ticketmaster Group, plans to fold the ticketing giant into its latest venture, USA/Lycos Interactive Networks, a merger of Internet portal Lycos with its 61%-owned Ticketmaster Online-CitySearch.

Ticketmaster Online-CitySearch, Inc.

790 E. Colorado Blvd., Ste. 200, Pasadena, CA 91101

Telephone: 626-405-0050 **Fax:** 626-405-9929 **Metro area:** Los Angeles, CA **Web site:** http://www.ticketmaster.com **Sales:** $40.2 million **Number of employees:** 581 **Industry designation:** Computers—online services **Company type:** Public **Top competitors:** Microsoft Corporation; ETM Entertainment Network; America Online, Inc.

Barry Diller has done it again. The chairman of USA Networks merged Ticketmaster Online with online cultural guide CitySearch (purchased by USA in 1998) to create Ticketmaster Online-CitySearch (USA Networks retained a 61% interest). Not content with that feat, Diller has agreed to merge Ticketmaster Online-CitySearch with Lycos to create an e-commerce titan, USA/Lycos Interactive Networks (USA Networks will own 61%). But the deal could fall apart because of the refusal of several Lycos shareholders to support the merger. The firm offers tickets, merchandise, and listings of community goings-on, news, and sports. American Express and film director Steven Spielberg own minority interests in the company.

Tier Technologies, Inc.

1350 Treat Blvd., Ste. 250, Walnut Creek, CA 94596

Telephone: 925-937-3950 **Fax:** 925-937-3752 **Metro area:** San Francisco, CA **Web site:** http://www.tier.com **Human resources contact:** Stephen McCarty **Sales:** $57.7 million **Number of employees:** 569 **Number of employees for previous year:** 231 **Industry designation:** Computers—services **Company type:** Public **Top competitors:** BrightStar Information Technology Group, Inc.; Whittman-Hart, Inc.; Computer Horizons Corp.

Tier Technologies keeps computer systems in line with the times. The company provides information technology services such as consulting; software engineering; and systems development, integration, and migration. Tier also designs applications for data warehousing, e-commerce, and the Internet. When designing systems, the company identifies and uses viable applications within the user's existing system. It primarily targets large businesses and government organizations. Customers include Humana (27% of sales), the State of Missouri (20%), and Unisys (11%). James Bildner (chairman and CEO) and William Barton (president and chief technology officer) control 63% of the company's voting power.

Titan Pharmaceuticals, Inc.

400 Oyster Point Blvd., Ste. 505, South San Francisco, CA 94080

Telephone: 650-244-4990 **Fax:** 650-244-4956 **Metro area:** San Francisco, CA **Web site:** http://www.titanpharm.com **Human resources contact:** Leslie Marinai **Sales:** $17.5 million **Number of employees:** 28 **Number of employees for previous year:** 10 **Industry designation:** Biomedical & genetic products **Company type:** Public **Top competitors:** Eli Lilly and Company; Johnson & Johnson; Diacrin, Inc.

Drugs for cancer, Parkinson's disease, "and" schizophrenia? Development-stage Titan Pharmaceuticals thinks big. The biopharmaceutical firm identifies and acquires new drug technology for development. Iloperidon, its flagship drug candidate, is in trials for schizophrenia and related diseases. Other development projects include treatments for Parkinson's and other neurological disorders, and for lung, pancreatic, colorectal, skin, and other cancers. Titan Pharmaceuticals is also developing gene-therapy cancer treatments. It operates through subsidiaries Ingenex (gene-based therapies), ProNeura (implantable drug delivery technology for central nervous system disorders), and Theracell (cell-based therapy).

Total Renal Care Holdings, Inc.

21250 Hawthorne Blvd., Ste. 800, Torrance, CA 90503

Telephone: 310-792-2600 **Fax:** 310-792-8928 **Metro area:** Los Angeles, CA **Web site:** http://www.totalrenal.com **Human resources contact:** Marie Ficarella **Sales:** $1.2 billion **Number of employees:** 8,830 **Number of employees for previous year:** 3,125 **Industry designation:** Medical services **Company type:** Public **Top competitors:** Gambro AB; Renal Care Group, Inc.; Fresenius Medical Care Aktiengesellschaft

Kidney caregiver Total Renal Care Holdings is the third-largest US chain of dialysis centers, trailing Fresenius Medical Care and Gambro Healthcare Patient Services. Its Total Renal Care centers provide dialysis and related services to patients suffering from chronic kidney failure. It operates more than 430 outpatient dialysis centers in more than 30 states, Washington, DC, Puerto Rico, Argentina, Guam, Italy, and the UK. The firm also provides dialysis services to about 280 hospitals, runs a pharmacy and two Total Renal Research labs, and provides home-based dialysis and pre- and postoperative kidney transplant care. The company continues to grow via acquisitions.

Trega Biosciences, Inc.

3550 General Atomics Ct., San Diego, CA 92121

Telephone: 619-410-6500 **Fax:** 619-410-6501 **Metro area:** San Diego, CA **Web site:** http://www.trega.com **Human resources contact:** Delise West **Sales:** $10.8 million **Number of employees:** 108 **Number of employees for previous year:** 87 **Industry designation:** Drugs **Company type:** Public

Trega, formerly Houghten Pharmaceuticals, works to speed the discovery of new drugs using combinatorial chemistry to search for new small-molecule drug therapies. The company has discovered a family of proprietary compounds that are being tested for the treatment of diabetes, obesity, and cancer. Its strategy is to collaborate with other companies while also conducting internal drug research. Trega has several corporate partnerships, including agreements with health and consumer products maker Procter & Gamble, drug makers Novo Nordisk and Novartis, and biotechnology firm Immunex.

Troy Group, Inc.

2331 S. Pullman St., Santa Ana, CA 92705

Telephone: 949-250-3280 **Fax:** 949-250-8972 **Metro area:** Los Angeles, CA **Web site:** http://www.troygroup.com **Human resources contact:** Laurel Toland **Sales:** $40 million (Est.) **Number of employees:** 150 **Industry designation:** Computers—peripheral equipment **Company type:** Private **Top competitors:** Check Technology Corporation; International Business Machines Corporation; The Standard Register Company

Don't try to imitate at home what the Troy Group does in the marketplace. The company helps users print and distribute financial documents (checks, money orders, payment coupons, and deposit and withdrawal slips) with its magnetic ink character recognition (MICR) products and accessories. Its products, including laser and impact printers, toners, and ribbons, are sold directly to large and midsized businesses and through dealers and resellers. Troy Group sells check printing systems to the US Treasury and manufactures MICR toner cartridges for Hewlett-Packard's LaserJet printers. After Troy's planned IPO, CEO and co-founder Patrick Dirk and his wife, Mary, will own about 60%.

Two Dog Net, Inc.

337 Preston Ct., Livermore, CA 94550

Telephone: 925-447-0226 **Fax:** 925-447-5567 **Metro area:** San Francisco, CA **Web site:** http://www.twodog.net **Sales:** $50,000 (Est.) **Number of employees:** 8 **Industry designation:** Computers—online services **Company type:** Private **Top competitors:** America Online, Inc.; The Walt Disney Company; The Learning Company, Inc.

Parents of Web-surfing toddlers may want to add a couple dogs to the family. Two Dog Net, a development-stage company, plans to provide kid-safe Web services for children ages three to 14. Its TwoDogNet Web site will offer educational content, secure e-mail and chat rooms, a Web magazine, and children's products. The site will also feature a search engine that allows users to visit only preapproved sites (no pornography, violence, or other adult content). Two Dog Net's proprietary technology will allow parents to add or remove Web sites from the approved list and to customize content for different age groups. CEO Nasser Hamedani and his family own 80% of the company.

UCSF Stanford Health Care

5 Thomas Mellon Circle, San Francisco, CA 94134

Telephone: 415-353-4500 **Fax:** 415-353-4520 **Metro area:** San Francisco, CA **Web site:** http://www.ucsfstanford.org **Human resources contact:** Felix R. Barthelemy **Sales:** $1.3 billion (Est.) **Number of employees:** 12,500 **Number of employees for previous year:** 5,500 **Industry designation:** Hospitals **Company type:** Private **Top competitors:** Columbia/HCA Healthcare Corporation; Catholic Healthcare West; Sutter Health

With hospitals ranking in the nation's top 10, UCSF Stanford Health Care isn't hurting. The organization was formed by the 1997 merger of the medical operations of the University of California at San Francisco and Stanford University, each of which owns half of the organization. The system consists of UCSF/Mount Zion Medical Center, UCSF Medical Center, Stanford Hospital and Clinics, Lucile Salter Packard Children's Hospital at Stanford, and the schools' combined clinical practices. The universities' schools of medicine are not affiliated with the system. UCSF Stanford and BMJ Publishing have purchased the "Western Journal of Medicine," the official journal of the California Medical Association.

Unigen Corporation

45388 Warm Springs Blvd., Fremont, CA 94539

Telephone: 510-668-2088 **Fax:** 510-661-2788 **Metro area:** San Francisco, CA **Web site:** http://www.unigen.com **Human resources contact:** Pamela Morgan **Sales:** $350 million (Est.) **Number of employees:** 100 **Number of employees for previous year:** 80 **Industry designation:** Computers—peripheral equipment **Company type:** Private

Is your computer acting forgetful? Maybe it's time for a memory upgrade. Unigen manufactures and sells more than 1,500 types of memory modules to upgrade desktop and portable PCs, workstations, servers, and printers. Its parts are compatible with computers made by Apple, Compaq, Intel, Sun Microsystems, Toshiba, and IBM. The company's RAMhunter search tool helps customers determine which memory module is needed for their particular computer or printer. Unigen offers technical support and works with its customers to design specific modules for their systems. Clients include original equipment manufacturers, distributors, and resellers.

UroQuest Medical Corporation

173 Constitution Dr., Menlo Park, CA 94025

Telephone: 650-463-5180 **Fax:** 650-463-5181 **Metro area:** San Francisco, CA **Web site:** http://www.uroquest.com **Sales:** $17.6 million **Number of employees:** 278 **Number of employees for previous year:** 267 **Industry designation:** Medical products **Company type:** Public

UroQuest Medical's products are designed to help men and women manage urological disorders such as leakage and inability to empty the bladder. Its internal On-Command catheter lets a patient use magnets to control urine flow. On-Command is meant to reduce the restricted movement, medical problems, and discomfort associated with other treatments such as diapers, penile clamps, and external catheters. The On-Command catheter for men is in US clinical trials, and the company is studying the feasibility of the device for women. Its BMT Inc. subsidiary manufactures On-Command catheters and makes silicone-based devices for airway and voice problems. Warburg, Pincus Investors, L.P., owns about 25% of UroQuest Medical's stock.

USA Biomass Corporation

52300 Enterprise Way, Coachella, CA 92236

Telephone: 760-398-9520 **Fax:** 760-398-9530 **Metro area:** Los Angeles, CA **Web site:** http://www.usabiomass.com **Human resources contact:** Robin Swanson **Sales:** $2 million **Number of employees:** 98 **Number of employees for previous year:** 70 **Industry designation:** Agricultural operations **Company type:** Public

USA Biomass (formerly AMCOR Capital), through its subsidiaries, grows grapes, develops real estate, and performs natural waste recycling—a new business segment that is stirring up interest in the firm, thanks to a California law that requires local governments to recycle 50% of all natural waste, such as leaves and tree branches, by 2000. Subsidiary TransPacific has tree maintenance and biomass recycling contracts with numerous California cities and counties, as well as with commercial concerns. The company's other operations include vertically integrated table grape production in California's Coachella Valley, as well as a golf course and an adjacent 1,350-acre residential development near San Antonio.

USCS International, Inc.

2969 Prospect Park Dr., Rancho Cordova, CA 95670

Telephone: 916-636-4500 **Fax:** 916-636-4530 **Metro area:** Sacramento, CA **Web site:** http://www.uscs.com **Human resources contact:** Calvin R. "Randy" Gorrell **Sales:** $299.3 million **Number of employees:** 2,067 **Number of employees for previous year:** 2,038 **Industry designation:** Computers—corporate, professional & financial software **Company type:** Subsidiary **Top competitors:** CSG Systems International, Inc.; Moore Corporation Limited

USCS International, a subsidiary of DST Systems, makes customer-management software and provides bill-processing services for communications, financial services, utilities, and other companies. Its software manages customer functions such as account setup, order processing, and support for cable TV, phone, and direct-broadcast satellite companies in more than 20 countries and in several languages. Clients include Ameritech, AT&T, and Federal Express. USCS International turns clients' electronic data into customer billing statements and offers statement-based marketing and advertising, as well as single billing for multiservice charges.

U.S. Home & Garden Inc.

655 Montgomery St., Ste. 830, San Francisco, CA 94111

Telephone: 415-616-8111 **Fax:** 415-616-8110 **Metro area:** San Francisco, CA **Human resources contact:** Lynda G. Gustafson **Sales:** $67.1 million **Number of employees:** 210 **Number of employees for previous year:** 123 **Industry designation:** Fertilizers **Company type:** Public **Top competitors:** Monsanto Company; American Home Products Corporation; The Scotts Company

U.S. Home & Garden helps your plants grow and protects them from perils such as insects and animals. The company's Easy Gardener subsidiary makes lawn and garden products, including weed trimmer replacement parts (Weed Wizard) and specialty fencing. The company's biggest seller is its landscape fabric—a mesh material that assists plant growth but prevents weeds (sold under WeedBlock, Landmaster, and other labels). Other products include plant food (Jobe's plant food spikes, Ross tree root feeders), lawn edging (Emerald Edge, Plasti-Chain), and animal repellents. Its Golden West Agri-Products subsidiary makes chemicals for farms and orchards. Insiders own about 30% of the company.

USWeb/CKS

2880 Lakeside Dr., Ste. 300, Santa Clara, CA 95054

Telephone: 408-987-3200 **Fax:** 408-986-6701 **Metro area:** San Francisco, CA **Web site:** http://www.uswebcks.com **Human resources contact:** Linda Keala **Sales:** $228.6 million **Number of employees:** 527 **Number of employees for previous year:** 316 **Industry designation:** Computers—online services **Company type:** Public **Top competitors:** Cambridge Technology Partners (Massachusetts), Inc.; Modem Media.Poppe Tyson, Inc.; Organic Online, Inc.

USWeb/CKS (formerly USWeb) offers Internet, intranet, and extranet services to medium-sized and large companies such as Apple, Barnes & Noble, Blue Cross, Charles Schwab, Levi's, and Harley-Davidson. With about 60 offices in the US and Europe, the company provides its clients with advice on the best uses of the Web for advertising, marketing, and improving business processes. USWeb/CKS is the result of a 1998 acquisition of CKS by USWeb. The deal was a move by both companies towards providing their clients with one-stop shopping for Web-based communication and advertising services.

Varian, Inc.

3120 Hansen Way, Palo Alto, CA 94304

Telephone: 650-213-8000 **Metro area:** San Francisco, CA **Web site:** www.varianinc.com **Sales:** $557.8 million **Number of employees:** 3,033 **Industry designation:** Instruments—scientific **Company type:** Public **Top competitors:** Hewlett-Packard Company; Jeol Ltd.; Thermo Electron Corporation

Varian makes toys for supergeeks. The company, a spinoff of high-tech firm Varian Associates, is a leading manufacturer of scientific instruments and equipment, including chromatography and optical spectroscopy systems for chemical analysis, nuclear magnetic resonance spectroscopy systems used in medical and materials research, vacuum pumps, helium leak detectors, and commercial and industrial gauges. Varian also provides contract manufacturing of printed wiring assemblies and electronic subassemblies. The company has factories in Australia, Italy, the Netherlands, and the US. About 45% of its sales are outside North America. Varian was formed in 1999 when Varian Associates split into three public companies.

Varian Medical Systems, Inc.

3100 Hansen Way, Palo Alto, CA 94304

Telephone: 650-493-4000 **Fax:** 650-424-5358 **Metro area:** San Francisco, CA **Web site:** http://www.varian.com/vms **Human resources contact:** Jack McCarthy **Sales:** $1.4 billion **Number of employees:** 6,900 **Number of employees for previous year:** 6,500 **Industry designation:** Medical instruments **Company type:** Public **Top competitors:** General Electric Company; Siemens AG; Toshiba Corporation

Varian is varyin' (its name). Formerly Varian Associates, Varian Medical Systems (VMS) has a new name after the spinoff of Varian, Inc. (analytical instruments) and Varian Semiconductor Equipment Associates in 1999. VMS operates in two divisions: Its oncology unit (76% of sales) makes linear accelerators (used in both medical and industrial settings), simulators, brachytherapy systems, and data management systems. Its X-ray products unit makes X-ray tubes (used in radiology, CT scans, mammography, and other applications) and imaging subsystems, which (used for image intensification). VMS's Ginzton Technology Center is focused on new developments in brachytherapy, digital X-ray imaging, and biotechnologies.

Veronex Technologies, Inc.

1508 Brookhollow Dr., Ste. 363, Santa Ana, CA 92705

Telephone: 714-668-0100 **Fax:** 714-668-0680 **Metro area:** Los Angeles, CA **Web site:** http://www.veronex.com **Human resources contact:** Desaree Peterson **Sales:** $132,000 **Industry designation:** Computers—corporate, professional & financial software **Company type:** Public **Top competitors:** Thinking Tools, Inc.; MERANT plc; CPS Systems, Inc.

Once primarily a natural resources developer, Veronex Technologies (formerly International Veronex Resources) now also produces and supports software for developing and deploying networked applications, solving the year 2000 problem, and creating databases. Clients use its I/Nova Tool Set (which evaluates source codes from multiple programs) for systems engineering and reengineering once they've performed analyses of their outdated systems. The software helps users examine such items as input and output, inventory, and data codes. It also assists with locating and correcting data problems associated with the year 2000. Cede & Co. owns 49% of the firm, which still explores for gas.

Veterinary Centers of America, Inc.

3420 Ocean Park Blvd., Ste. 1000, Santa Monica, CA 90405

Telephone: 310-392-9599 **Fax:** 310-392-9263 **Metro area:** Los Angeles, CA **Web site:** http://www.vcai.com **Human resources contact:** Nanette Duff-Sullivan **Sales:** $281 million **Number of employees:** 3,036 **Number of employees for previous year:** 2,178 **Industry designation:** Veterinary products & services **Company type:** Public

With almost 160 animal hospitals in 26 states, Veterinary Centers of America operates one of the largest full-service animal hospital networks in the country as well as one of the largest veterinary laboratory networks. Its hospitals account for more than 70% of sales and provide services from basic pet wellness (routine exams, vaccinations, neutering, and dental care) to specialty surgeries such as orthopedics for birds. More than 13,000 animal hospitals in 49 states use its 15 veterinary diagnostic laboratories' services, including tests on blood, urine, and tissue samples. The company owns a 50% interest (with Heinz Pet Products) in pet-food maker Vet's Choice and invests in Veterinary Pet Insurance.

Vical Incorporated

9373 Towne Centre Dr., Ste. 100, San Diego, CA 92121

Telephone: 619-453-9900 **Fax:** 619-646-1150 **Metro area:** San Diego, CA **Web site:** http://www.vical.com **Human resources contact:** Sue Bacino **Sales:** $5.9 million **Number of employees:** 101 **Number of employees for previous year:** 89 **Industry designation:** Biomedical & genetic products **Company type:** Public

Vical discovers and develops gene-based drugs for the treatment and prevention of cancer, infectious diseases, and metabolic disorders. Introduced directly into targeted cells, Vical's gene therapy treatments stimulate the production of proteins that selectively correct and modulate disease conditions. All of its products (including ALLOVECTIN-7, a treatment for melanoma and head and neck tumors, and VAXID, a drug for non-Hodgkin's B-cell lymphoma) are in clinical trial, research, or preclinical phases. Vical's corporate partners include Merck, Pasteur Merieux Connaught, Rhone-Poulenc Rorer, and Genzyme; its institutional partners include the University of Michigan and the Wisconsin Alumni Research Foundation.

ViewSonic Corporation

381 Brea Canyon Rd., Walnut, CA 91789

Telephone: 909-444-8800 **Fax:** 909-869-7958 **Metro area:** Los Angeles, CA **Web site:** http://www.viewsonic.com **Human resources contact:** Joanne Thielen **Sales:** $826 million (Est.) **Number of employees:** 675 **Number of employees for previous year:** 600 **Industry designation:** Computers—peripheral equipment **Company type:** Private **Top competitors:** Proxima Corporation; TeleVideo, Inc.; ADI Systems, Inc.

ViewSonic, founded by James Chu in 1987 as Keypoint Technology, makes color computer monitors. Its Professional series is designed for such high-end applications as computer-assisted design, desktop publishing, and graphic design. Its Graphics series is for slightly less-demanding graphics applications and office automation, and the E2 series is for small business and personal use. ViewSonic also makes multimedia monitors, SVGA and LCD projectors, and calibration kits for monitor color matching. ViewSonic operates in Canada, China, France, Germany, Japan, Taiwan, the UK, and the US, selling its displays through mail-order and Internet companies, computer dealers, and other resellers.

Viking Components

30200 Avenida de las Banderas, Rancho Santa Margarita, CA 92688

Telephone: 949-643-7255 **Fax:** 949-643-7250 **Metro area:** Los Angeles, CA **Web site:** http://www.vikingcomponents.com **Human resources contact:** Susie Lewis **Sales:** $253 million (Est.) **Number of employees:** 450 **Number of employees for previous year:** 385 **Industry designation:** Computers—peripheral equipment **Company type:** Private

Truly a memorable company, Viking Components sells memory upgrades and related equipment for PCs. It makes more than 2,000 memory modules to upgrade a wide variety of systems. Other products include internal fax modems for desktop computers, modems and special low-power memory cards for portable computers, and tiny smart cards that provide a memory boost to electronic equipment (such as digital cameras and laptops). The company has offices in Colorado, Illinois, New York, Utah, and Singapore and production facilities in the US and Ireland. Viking Components was founded in 1988 by owner Glen McCusker.

VIVUS, Inc.

605 E. Fairchild Dr., Mountain View, CA 94043

Telephone: 650-934-5200 **Fax:** 650-934-5389 **Metro area:** San Francisco, CA **Web site:** http://www.vivus.com **Human resources contact:** John C. Meyer **Sales:** $74.7 million **Number of employees:** 233 **Number of employees for previous year:** 107 **Industry designation:** Medical products **Company type:** Public **Top competitors:** Pharmacia & Upjohn, Inc.; Pfizer Inc; Imagyn Medical Technologies, Inc.

VIVUS develops and makes therapeutic systems for impotence. The company's Medicated Urethral System for Erection (MUSE) is a noninvasive system that delivers topical pharmaceuticals via the urethra. The company's first product, MUSE, is a small, single-use disposable plastic applicator that dispenses the drug alprostadil shortly after administration. The company was steadily building a public presence and market share when it was hit by Pfizer's anti-impotence pill Viagra, which became the fastest-selling medication in history within two weeks of its 1998 release. Reeling, VIVUS is weighing its options, including a possible sale of the company .

Voxel

26081 Merit Circle, Ste. 117, Laguna Hills, CA 92653

Telephone: 949-348-3200 **Fax:** 949-348-8665 **Metro area:** Los Angeles, CA **Web site:** http://www.voxel.com **Sales:** $100,000 **Number of employees:** 38 **Number of employees for previous year:** 24 **Industry designation:** Medical products **Company type:** Public

Voxel's story breaks down in Chapter 7. Currently operating under Chapter 7 bankruptcy, the company is being acquired by Holographic Dimensions. Voxel's proprietary Digital Holography System produces 3-D X-rays of internal anatomical structures. The system, which includes the Voxcam, Voxbox, and Voxfilm, can record up to 200 cross-sectional, two-dimensional computed tomography (CT) or magnetic resonance (MR) images and use them to render an accurate, 3-D replica of a portion of the patient's anatomy. The 3-D images have potential applications in medical diagnosis and in surgical planning. Voxel is developing a commercial version of its system to bring to market.

Vyrex Corporation

2159 Avenida de la Playa, La Jolla, CA 92037

Telephone: 619-454-4446 **Fax:** 619-459-9522 **Metro area:** San Diego, CA **Human resources contact:** Steven J. Kemper **Sales:** $100,000 **Number of employees:** 21 **Number of employees for previous year:** 10 **Industry designation:** Drugs **Company type:** Public **Top competitors:** Bionutrics, Inc.; Hauser, Inc.; Pure World, Inc.

Biotech company Vyrex researches antioxidants to develop cures for respiratory, cardiovascular, and anti-inflammatory disorders. The development-stage company is working on Vantox, an antioxidant inhaler for asthma, and Panavir, which is designed to prevent the HIV virus from attaching to cells. The company has also developed a proprietary research method, CD-Tagging, which aids in identifying and analyzing gene function. Vyrex is moving into the nutritional supplement market and has an agreement with Uncle Ben's to develop a line of Wellness Foods. Through an agreement with Retired Persons Services, Vyrex plans to market nutritional supplements for the AARP. Chairman and CEO Sheldon Hendler owns 42% of Vyrex.

Wahlco Environmental Systems, Inc.

3600 W. Segerstrom Ave., Santa Ana, CA 92704

Telephone: 714-979-7300 **Fax:** 714-979-2309 **Metro area:** Los Angeles, CA **Web site:** http://www.wahlco.com **Human resources contact:** Anne L. Anderson **Sales:** $49.7 million **Number of employees:** 425 **Number of employees for previous year:** 354 **Industry designation:** Pollution control equipment & services **Company type:** Subsidiary **Top competitors:** Badger Meter, Inc.

Wahlco Environmental Systems, a subsidiary of former rival Thermatrix, makes and markets air pollution control and power plant efficiency equipment for electric utilities, independent power producers, and industrial manufacturers worldwide. The company's flow diverters, dampers, fabric and metallic expansion joints, hydraulic equipment, piping systems, and related services account for almost 80% of revenues. Wahlco also provides mechanical plant installation services and rents equipment. The company has subsidiaries in the UK and the US. Its principal export markets are in Asia, Canada, and Europe.

Walker Interactive Systems, Inc.

303 Second St., San Francisco, CA 94107

Telephone: 415-495-8811 **Fax:** 415-957-1711 **Metro area:** San Francisco, CA **Web site:** http://www.walker.com **Human resources contact:** Wallace E. Breitman **Sales:** $101.4 million **Number of employees:** 539 **Number of employees for previous year:** 520 **Industry designation:** Computers—corporate, professional & financial software **Company type:** Public **Top competitors:** SAP AG; PeopleSoft, Inc.; Hyperion Solutions Corporation

Walker Interactive Systems' financial software does everything except slash actual costs—that's your problem. The company provides financial, operational, and analytic software for corporations, universities, and government agencies that use multisite networked computers. The software helps entities do planning, budgeting, forecasting, consolidation, and performance management. The majority of Walker Interactive's licensing sales come from its Tamaris line of business and financial software, which it sells directly to organizations in the US, the UK, and the Asia/Pacific region. Walker Interactive also offers maintenance and consulting services. International business accounts for more than 30% of sales.

Watson Pharmaceuticals, Inc.

311 Bonnie Circle, Corona, CA 91720

Telephone: 909-270-1400 **Fax:** 909-270-1096 **Metro area:** Los Angeles, CA **Web site:** http://www.watsonpharm.com **Human resources contact:** Sally Lillard **Sales:** $556.1 million **Number of employees:** 1,020 **Number of employees for previous year:** 515 **Industry designation:** Drugs—generic **Company type:** Public **Top competitors:** Novartis AG; Glaxo Wellcome plc; Merck & Co., Inc.

The drug's afoot. Watson Pharmaceuticals makes generic and branded drugs, focusing on niche pharmaceuticals. It offers generic versions of brand-name products such as cardiovascular drugs Lopressor and Inderal, analgesics Vicodin and Lortab, and asthma drugs Proventil and Ventolin. Watson's branded drugs are focused primarily in dermatology (acne drugs), women's health (contraceptives and hormone regulators), and neuropsychiatry (epilepsy drugs), but it also makes antihypertensives Dilacor XR (the company's top seller) and Microzide. Watson has grown its branded business through acquisitions and plans further expansion via joint ventures. It owns half of Somerset Pharmaceuticals and ANCIRC Pharmaceuticals.

WD-40 Company

1061 Cudahy Place, San Diego, CA 92110

Telephone: 619-275-1400 **Fax:** 619-275-5823 **Metro area:** San Diego, CA **Web site:** http://www.wd40.com **Human resources contact:** Mary Rudy **Sales:** $144.4 million **Number of employees:** 167 **Number of employees for previous year:** 166 **Industry designation:** Chemicals—specialty **Company type:** Public **Top competitors:** The Lubrizol Corporation; The Dow Chemical Company; Burmah Castrol plc

WD-40 Company aims to make things slicker than the hands of a bacon-eatin' politician. The company's namesake petroleum-based product (90% of sales) is used as a lubricant, rust preventative, penetrant, and moisture displacer. Most US households have a can of WD-40, which is sold through retail outlets and industrial distributors in more than 150 countries. The company also makes 3-IN-ONE Oil, a drip oil lubricant, and T.A.L. 5, an extra-strength synthetic lubricant. International sales account for more than 40% of total revenues. WD-40 has operations in Australia, Canada, Malaysia, the UK, and the US. To expand its line of products that help the handyman, the company is buying the Lava soap line from Block Drug.

WebTV Networks, Inc.

1250 Charleston Rd., Mountain View, CA 94043

Telephone: 650-614-5500 **Fax:** 650-326-5277 **Metro area:** San Francisco, CA **Web site:** http://webtv.net **Human resources contact:** Raquel Cariasl **Sales:** $9.8 million **Number of employees:** 500 **Number of employees for previous year:** 249 **Industry designation:** Computers—online services **Company type:** Subsidiary **Top competitors:** America Online, Inc.; WorldGate Communications, Inc.; uniView Technologies Corporation

"Baywatch" puts surfing on TV; WebTV lets TVs do the surfing. A subsidiary of Microsoft, WebTV (founded by three former Apple employees) provides Internet access and other services, such as e-mail, through a set-top receiver device. Licensees like Mitsubishi, Philips, and Sony make WebTV set-top boxes; WebTV's revenues come from these licensing fees, subscriptions to the service, and advertising sales. Most of its 500,000 subscribers are over 40 years old and do not own a personal computer. WebTV Plus lets users watch TV and surf the Internet simultaneously, print Web pages, and go to Web sites related to program subjects by clicking on an on-screen icon. WebTV for Windows connects PCs to the service.

WellPoint Health Networks Inc.

21555 Oxnard St., Woodland Hills, CA 91367

Telephone: 818-703-4000 **Fax:** 818-703-2848 **Metro area:** Los Angeles, CA **Web site:** http://www.wellpoint.com **Human resources contact:** Tom Van Berkem **Sales:** $6.5 billion **Number of employees:** 10,100 **Number of employees for previous year:** 6,600 **Industry designation:** Health maintenance organization **Company type:** Public **Top competitors:** Foundation Health Systems, Inc.; PacifiCare Health Systems, Inc.; Kaiser Foundation Health Plan, Inc.

WellPoint Health Networks, the #2 health insurer in California (after Kaiser Permanente), serves about 30 million members nationally through HMOs, PPOs, and specialty networks such as dental and mental health plans. The company operates as Blue Cross of California in its home state, where some two-thirds of its medical care members reside, and as UNICARE elsewhere. WellPoint also sells life insurance through subsidiary WellPoint Life Insurance and workers' compensation services through subsidiary UNICARE Financial. The company is a care contractor for Medi-Cal, California's Medicaid program, and provides third-party administration for self-insured businesses.

Western Fiberglass, Inc.

1555 Copperhill Pkwy., Santa Rosa, CA 95403

Telephone: 707-523-2050 **Fax:** 707-523-2046 **Metro area:** San Francisco, CA **Web site:** http://www.westernfg.com **Human resources contact:** Sue Lilo **Sales:** $3.4 million (Est.) **Number of employees:** 21 **Number of employees for previous year:** 20 **Industry designation:** Glass products **Company type:** Private **Top competitors:** Ameron International Corporation; Geneva Steel Company; A. O. Smith Corporation

Western Fiberglass has insulated itself from market volatility by expanding its offerings. Initially focused on fiberglass, it makes equipment for use in the aerospace, automotive, petroleum, and food-processing markets, among others. Its flex-pipe systems are used in applications that include gas-station construction, pumping gas into and out of underground storage tanks, and handling hazardous-waste materials, as well as applications in the food service industry. Western Fiberglass also makes sumps, seals, and related items. Industrial customers also use its pipes, catch basins, and vessel linings, and other products including epoxies and extrusions. President Michael Lewis and his family own the company.

Who? Vision Systems, Inc.

100 N. Pointe Dr., Lake Forest, CA 92630

Telephone: 949-837-5353 **Fax:** 949-837-5355 **Metro area:** Los Angeles, CA **Web site:** http://www.whovision.com **Human resources contact:** Linda Duffy **Number of employees:** 37 **Industry designation:** Protection—safety equipment & services **Company type:** Private **Top competitors:** Identix Incorporated; The National Registry, Inc.; Diebold, Incorporated

Prepare to forget your mother's maiden name, because Who? Vision Systems is bringing fingerprint identification out of the Bat Cave and into your everyday life. From the bank to the video store, the firm hopes to create a brave new world where fingerprints provide a cheaper, more secure alternative to traditional security devices such as PIN numbers and personal details. TactileSense, the firm's proprietary biometric technology allows fingerprinting sensors to be imbedded in everyday devices such as computer keyboards. The sensors generate high-resolution images of your fingertip, which are converted into digital images and matched against a computer record. Safeguard Scientifics owns over 35% of the firm.

Wilbur-Ellis Company

345 California St., Ste. 27, San Francisco, CA 94104

Telephone: 415-772-4000 **Fax:** 415-772-4011 **Metro area:** San Francisco, CA **Web site:** http://www.wilbur-ellis.com **Human resources contact:** Ofelia Lee **Sales:** $900 million (Est.) **Number of employees:** 2,100 **Number of employees for previous year:** 1,900 **Industry designation:** Chemicals—specialty **Company type:** Private **Top competitors:** Agway Inc.; Agrium Inc.; Transammonia, Inc.

With respect to the children's song, the farmer spends as much time with the products supplied by Wilbur-Ellis as he does in the dell. The company distributes animal feed, fertilizer, insecticides, seed, gear boxes, and machinery through more than 100 outlets in North America and about 20 international offices (it has an equity interest in about a third of its suppliers). Its Connell Brothers subsidiary handles international sales in Asia and Africa. Wilbur-Ellis also provides consulting and other agriculture-related services. Founded in 1921 by Brayton Wilbur Sr. and Floyd Ellis as a fish-oil supplier, the company is now managed by Brayton Wilbur Jr.

Wilshire Technologies, Inc.

5861 Edison Place, Carlsbad, CA 92008

Telephone: 760-929-7200 **Fax:** 760-929-6949 **Metro area:** San Diego, CA **Human resources contact:** Christine Murphy **Sales:** $3.8 million **Number of employees:** 19 **Number of employees for previous year:** 18 **Industry designation:** Medical & dental supplies **Company type:** Public **Top competitors:** Johnson & Johnson; Baxter International Inc.; Kimberly-Clark Corporation

Now that it's gotten its breast implant business off its chest, Wilshire Technologies is cleaning up by supplying disposable products for clean rooms. Its engineered polymer products—including gloves, swabs, and wipes—help microelectronics, semiconductor, and disk drive makers keep their clean rooms free of contamination. Wilshire Technologies sells its products under such names as DuraCLEAN, PolyDERM, and UltraSOLV. The company sells its products directly and through distributors such as VWR Scientific Products (one-third of sales). Predecessor Wilshire Foam Products, whose medical products included breast implants, has been named in numerous lawsuits (that business has been sold).

Women.com Networks, Inc.

1820 Gateway Dr., Ste. 100, San Mateo, CA 94404

Telephone: 650-378-6500 **Fax:** 650-378-6599 **Metro area:** San Francisco, CA **Web site:** http://www.women.com **Human resources contact:** Tiffany Chelsvig **Number of employees:** 200 **Industry designation:** Computers—online services **Company type:** Joint venture **Top competitors:** Oxygen Media, Inc.; Lifetime Television; iVillage Inc.

A joint venture between The Hearst Corporation and Women.com? Looks like a yin-yin situation. The new company, Women.com Networks, combined Women.com's professional mom-on-the-go ethos with the more domestic editorial fare of Hearst's HomeArts.com. Together these two sites reach a larger audience than any other women's Web site, more than four million women a month—grave news for popular sites like iVillage and Oxygen Media. Women.com's content includes horoscopes and home economics tips (HomeArts.com) as well as business tips, financial planning links (Women.com), and other female-centered clicks. Hearst and Women.com Networks each own 50% of the new joint venture.

Women First HealthCare, Inc.

12220 El Camino Real, Ste. 400, San Diego, CA 92130

Telephone: 619-509-1171 **Fax:** 619-509-1353 **Metro area:** San Diego, CA **Web site:** http://www.womenfirst.com **Human resources contact:** Robert L. Jones **Sales:** $4.8 million (Est.) **Number of employees:** 116 **Industry designation:** Drugs **Company type:** Private **Top competitors:** Duramed Pharmaceuticals, Inc.; Novogen Limited; American Home Products Corporation

Menopause giving you pause? Well, now there's Women First HealthCare to help ease the transition. The company distributes pharmaceuticals, self-care products, and educational materials to women in midlife through a mail-order catalog and via Internet retailer As We Change (aswechange.com). Pharmaceuticals include Ortho-Est, an estrogen replacement drug offered through an agreement with Johnson & Johnson subsidiary Ortho-McNeil, and Provochol, a cholesterol reducer licensed for distribution from Bristol-Myers Squibb. Self-care products include skin moisturizers, nutritional supplements, and personal lubricants. Chairman Edward Calesa owns more than 40% of the company; Johnson & Johnson owns about 15%.

XOMA Ltd.

2910 Seventh St., Berkeley, CA 94710

Telephone: 510-644-1170 **Fax:** 510-644-0539 **Metro area:** San Francisco, CA **Web site:** http://www.xoma.com **Human resources contact:** Victoria Campbell **Sales:** $6.3 million **Number of employees:** 167 **Number of employees for previous year:** 160 **Industry designation:** Biomedical & genetic products **Company type:** Public

XOMA, a biopharmaceutical company, develops products to treat infections, immunologic and inflammatory disorders, and infectious complications caused by injury and surgery. It is focusing on developing products that utilize a bactericidal/permeability-increasing protein, a white blood cell protein that is known to kill certain bacteria, neutralize endotoxins, and inhibit new blood vessel growth. Its Neuprex drug is in clinical trials for treating bacterial infections and trauma- and surgery-related complications. The company is also developing a topical treatment for infections and diseases of the cornea, as well as fungicidal compounds. XOMA is working with Genentech to develop an antibody product to treat psoriasis.

Xoom.com, Inc.

300 Montgomery St., Ste. 300, San Francisco, CA 94104

Telephone: 415-445-2525 **Fax:** 415-445-2526 **Metro area:** San Francisco, CA **Web site:** http://xoom.com **Sales:** $8.3 million **Number of employees:** 95 **Number of employees for previous year:** 39 **Industry designation:** Computers—online services **Company type:** Public **Top competitors:** GeoCities; theglobe.com, inc.; WhoWhere

Xoom.com is an Internet-based direct-marketing company. It offers a variety of free services, including e-mail, chat rooms, and home pages, to attract cybersurfers to its community Web site. Xoom.com sends advertisements, retail offers, and newsletters to its members via e-mail on a weekly basis and offers an online travel service in conjunction with Camelot International. The offers include Xoom.com's proprietary and third-party products, such as computer software, consumer electronics, and clip art. The company, which generates sales from advertising and electronic commerce, has created co-branded Web sites with Phillips Publishing, "USA Today," and ZDNet. Chairman Chris Kitze owns 32% of the company.

Yahoo! Inc.

3420 Central Expwy., Santa Clara, CA 95051

Telephone: 408-731-3300 **Fax:** 408-731-3301 **Metro area:** San Francisco, CA **Web site:** http://www.yahoo.com **Human resources contact:** Beth Haba **Sales:** $203.3 million **Number of employees:** 803 **Number of employees for previous year:** 386 **Industry designation:** Computers—online services **Company type:** Public **Top competitors:** Lycos, Inc.; America Online, Inc.; Excite, Inc.

Drawing 30 million visitors to its Web site each month, Yahoo! can lay claim to the top spot among Internet portals. The company also boasts about 3,800 advertisers (banner ads bring in the bulk of Yahoo!'s revenue) and stands apart as one of the few Internet players operating in the black. The Web site features items such as e-mail, chat rooms, news, and stock quotes. The company is looking to diversify its revenue stream via e-commerce and sponsorships, and pending acquisitions of GeoCities and broadcast.com will extend its reach into personal Web pages and Web-based audio and video. Internet investor SOFTBANK owns 28% of Yahoo!; founders and "chief Yahoo s" David Filo and Jerry Yang, about 11% each.

ZDNet Group

650 Townsend St., San Francisco, CA 94103

Telephone: 415-551-4500 **Fax:** 415-551-4605 **Metro area:** San Francisco, CA **Web site:** http://www.zdnet.com **Human resources contact:** Pam Harbidge **Sales:** $32.2 million **Number of employees:** 304 **Industry designation:** Computers—online services **Company type:** Public **Top competitors:** CNET, Inc.; International Data Group; CMP Media Inc.

ZDNet Group is Ziff-Davis' entry into the online derby. Part of Ziff-Davis, the #1 US computer magazine publisher, ZDNet offers an online community where visitors can access a wide range of information. zdnet.com features more than 25 channels where Web surfers can find games, financial tips, and more than 800 news stories each month. The site also includes more than 30,000 consumer product reviews and some 12,000 downloadable computer programs. ZDNet offers readers links to Ziff-Davis magazines (such as "PC Magazine"), and members can access bulletin boards, chat rooms, e-mail, and online forums. ZDNet trades separately as a tracking stock. Ziff-Davis owns 84% of the company.

Zip2 Corporation

444 Castro St., Ste. 101, Mountain View, CA 94041

Telephone: 650-429-4400 **Fax:** 650-429-4500 **Metro area:** San Francisco, CA **Web site:** http://www.zip2.com **Human resources contact:** Lyn Christensen **Sales:** $5 million (Est.) **Number of employees:** 150 **Number of employees for previous year:** 90 **Industry designation:** Computers—online services **Company type:** Private **Top competitors:** Yahoo! Inc.; America Online, Inc.; Ticketmaster Online-CitySearch, Inc.

Zip2 provides newspapers and other media companies with customized online business directories, entertainment guides, auto- and home-finder guides, and other community-specific Web sites. The company provides customized Web development packages to which newspaper customers can add editorial content; customers maintain their own Web site guides. Zip2 receives licensing fees and percentages of advertising revenues generated by clients from their guides. The company's 160 customers include Knight Ridder and A.H. Belo as well as individual newspapers in the Hearst, Times Mirror, and Scripps Howard chains. Alta Vista, Compaq's Internet search engine subsidiary, is buying Zip2.

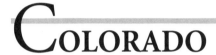

COLORADO

Air Methods Corporation

7301 S. Peoria, Englewood, CO 80112

Telephone: 303-792-7400 **Fax:** 303-790-0499 **Metro area:** Denver, CO **Web site:** http://www.airmethods.com **Human resources contact:** Judy Goebel **Sales:** $48.7 million **Number of employees:** 438 **Number of employees for previous year:** 329 **Industry designation:** Medical services **Company type:** Public **Top competitors:** Rowan Companies, Inc.; CHC Helicopter Corporation; Proflight Medical Response, Inc.

Air Methods provides emergency medical air transportation services through its Flight Services Division to hospitals in 15 states. The company, which also franchises its services to Brazil's Unimed Air, operates a fleet of more than 35 helicopters and six airplanes equipped with medical interiors that serve as intensive care units. The company also designs, services, and installs medical and other specialized interiors in aircraft owned by third parties, including commercial and government clients, and installs aerospace systems for nonmedical functions such as navigation, environmental control, and structural and electrical equipment. Subsidiary Mercy Air Service operates five helicopters in Southern California.

American Coin Merchandising, Inc.

5660 Central Ave., Boulder, CO 80301

Telephone: 303-444-2559 **Fax:** 303-443-2264 **Metro area:** Denver, CO **Web site:** http://www.skill-crane.com **Sales:** $97.7 million **Number of employees:** 798 **Number of employees for previous year:** 487 **Industry designation:** Leisure & recreational services **Company type:** Public **Top competitors:** WMS Industries Inc.; Play By Play Toys & Novelties, Inc.; International Game Technology

Thanks to American Coin Merchandising, Inc. (ACMI), kids all over the US are begging their parents for change. ACMI is the leading operator of coin-operated skill-crane games in the country, with more than 11,500 machines (operating under the SugarLoaf Toy Shoppes, SugarLoaf Treasure Shoppes, SugarLoaf Fun Shoppes, and SugarLoaf Beanie Bag Shoppes names) located in retailers throughout the US and in British Columbia. Depending upon the machine, players pay 25 or 50 cents to finesse a crane and grab items such as stuffed animals, watches, and jewelry from inside the enclosed display area. ACMI also operates kiddie rides in supermarkets and mass merchandisers and bulk vending equipment (toys, gumballs).

Applied Films Corporation

9586 I-25 Frontage Rd., Longmont, CO 80504

Telephone: 303-774-3200 **Fax:** 303-678-9275 **Metro area:** Denver, CO **Human resources contact:** Deb Hasler **Sales:** $53 million **Number of employees:** 296 **Number of employees for previous year:** 232 **Industry designation:** Glass products **Company type:** Public **Top competitors:** Asahi Glass Company, Limited; Nippon Sheet Glass Company, Limited; Applied Materials, Inc.

Applied Films provides thin-film coated glass for the flat-panel display industry, which includes liquid crystal displays used in laptop computers, cellular phones, calculators, and other electronic devices. It purchases thin glass from suppliers and then coats it with silicon dioxide and indium tin oxide. The company also sells thin-film-coating equipment to makers of information content displays. Applied Films markets its products in the US and China through an internal sales force and in China, Japan, South Korea, and Taiwan through outside sales representatives. Co-founder and chairman Cecil Van Alsburg and co-founder and VP John Chapin own about 17% of Applied Films each.

BI Incorporated

6400 Lookout Rd., Boulder, CO 80301

Telephone: 303-218-1000 **Fax:** 303-218-1250 **Metro area:** Denver, CO **Web site:** http://www.bi.com **Human resources contact:** Karen Mahoney **Sales:** $61.4 million **Number of employees:** 824 **Number of employees for previous year:** 742 **Industry designation:** Protection—safety equipment & services **Company type:** Public **Top competitors:** Ameritech Corporation; Cornell Corrections, Inc.; Wackenhut Corrections Corporation

Thanks to BI, felons can wear bangles and feel safe—because they are not in prison. BI makes electronic monitoring bracelets and systems used by corrections agencies to administer home arrest programs. The company's BI Home Escort monitoring system includes a radio transmitter worn on the offender's ankle. BI also provides supervisory services for misdemeanor and felony probationers. The company, which supervises more than 40,000 offenders nationwide, is expanding its community correction (probation monitoring) operations as a key part of its growth strategy. BI is selling its Correctional Information Systems software unit.

Birner Dental Management Services, Inc.

3801 E. Florida Ave., Ste. 508, Denver, CO 80210

Telephone: 303-691-0680 **Fax:** 303-691-0889 **Metro area:** Denver, CO **Human resources contact:** Teresa J. Cooper **Sales:** $21.7 million **Number of employees:** 356 **Number of employees for previous year:** 317 **Industry designation:** Medical practice management **Company type:** Public **Top competitors:** Monarch Dental Corporation

Birner Dental Management Services, which acquires and develops dental-practice networks, is a company that leaves its dentists smiling. The firm frees dentists of their administrative duties by providing management services—marketing, equipment supply, patient scheduling, staffing, recruiting, training of non-dental personnel, billing, and negotiating with managed care organizations. Birner Dental manages 35 offices in Colorado and New Mexico, the majority of which it operates under the Perfect Teeth name. Some locations offer special services such as orthodontics, oral surgery, and periodontics.

Booth Creek Ski Holdings, Inc.

1000 S. Frontage Rd. West, Ste. 100, Vail, CO 81657

Telephone: 970-476-4030 **Fax:** 970-479-0291 **Other address:** PO Box 129, Truckee, CA 96160 **Web site:** http://www.boothcreek.com **Human resources contact:** Laura B. Moriarty **Sales:** $104.9 million (Est.) **Number of employees:** 6,254 **Number of employees for previous year:** 5,118 **Industry designation:** Leisure & recreational services **Company type:** Private **Top competitors:** Vail Resorts, Inc.; Intrawest Corporation; American Skiing Company

Your last resort is probably owned by Booth Creek Ski Holdings. With eight ski resort complexes, 11 separate resorts, and some 9,000 acres of ski terrain, Booth Creek is one of the US's largest ski companies. The company focuses on midsized regional resorts near major skiing populations, such as Boston (Waterville Valley, Mt. Cranmore), Los Angeles (Bear Mountain), San Francisco (Northstar-at-Tahoe, Sierra-at-Tahoe), and Seattle (Summit at Snoqualmie). It also owns the Grand Targhee resort in Wyoming. The company encourages customer loyalty and increased visitation through two frequent-skier programs, Vertical Plus and Vertical Value. CEO George Gillett, former owner of the Vail Associates ski company, owns 34% of Booth Creek.

Catholic Health Initiatives

1999 Broadway, Ste. 2605, Denver, CO 80202

Telephone: 303-298-9100 **Fax:** 303-298-9690 **Metro area:** Denver, CO **Web site:** http://www.mercyrose.org/chi.html **Human resources contact:** Michael Fordyce **Sales:** $4.5 billion **Number of employees:** 44,000 **Industry designation:** Hospitals **Company type:** Not-for-profit **Top competitors:** Beverly Enterprises, Inc.; Tenet Healthcare Corporation; Columbia/HCA Healthcare Corporation

Giant not-for-profit Catholic Health Initiatives (CHI) is an amalgamation of three Catholic health care systems (Catholic Health Corporation of Omaha, Nebraska; Franciscan Health System of Aston, Pennsylvania; and Sisters of Charity Health Care Systems of Cincinnati). CHI, sponsored by 11 different congregations, serves more than 70 communities in 22 states spanning the western, Rocky Mountain, upper-midwestern, central-midwestern, southeastern, and eastern regions. It operates more than 60 hospitals and about 50 long-term-care facilities. Many administrative functions have been centralized in Cincinnati.

CET Environmental Services, Inc.

7670 S. Vaughn Ct., Ste. 130, Englewood, CO 80112

Telephone: 303-708-1360 **Fax:** 303-708-1349 **Metro area:** Denver, CO **Web site:** http://www.cetenvironmental.com **Human resources contact:** Liane Downing **Sales:** $54.2 million **Number of employees:** 350 **Number of employees for previous year:** 250 **Industry designation:** Pollution control equipment & services **Company type:** Public

CET Environmental Services provides complete turnkey services for environmental remediation, water and wastewater treatment, and emergency responses to hazardous spills. Remediation services include health-risk and environmental assessments; storage tank management; facility decontamination, demolition, and site restoration; and remedial design, construction, operation, and maintenance. CET Environmental Services has emergency response agreements with such customers as Exxon, Conoco, and Texaco. Its subsidiary Water Quality Management builds and maintains municipal and industrial treatment plants. CET Environmental has locations throughout the southern and western US and in Latin America.

Colorado Avalanche

1635 Clay St., Denver, CO 80204

Telephone: 303-893-6700 **Fax:** 303-575-1920 **Metro area:** Denver, CO **Web site:** http://www.coloradoavalanche.com **Human resources contact:** Cheryl Miller **Sales:** $53.2 million **Number of employees:** 44 **Industry designation:** Leisure & recreational services **Company type:** Subsidiary **Top competitors:** Northwest Sports Enterprises Ltd.; Edmonton Oilers Hockey Club; Calgary Flames Limited Partnership

The Rocky Mountain air must agree with the NHL's Colorado Avalanche. The team, which began in 1979 as the Quebec Nordiques, won the Stanley Cup in 1996, its inaugural year in Colorado. The Avalanche seem to be succeeding where a string of other professional hockey teams (Denver Falcons, Denver Mavericks, and Colorado Rockies) have failed; TV and radio broadcasts are breaking records, and some 3,000 fans are on a waiting list for season tickets. Ascent Entertainment, which owns the Avalanche as well as the NBA's Denver Nuggets, is building its teams a new $140 million arena. The Pepsi Center is scheduled for completion in 1999.

Colorado MEDtech, Inc.

6175 Longbow Dr., Boulder, CO 80301

Telephone: 303-530-2660 **Fax:** 303-581-1010 **Metro area:** Denver, CO **Web site:** http://www.cmed.com **Human resources contact:** Frances Reel **Sales:** $47.3 million **Number of employees:** 410 **Number of employees for previous year:** 245 **Industry designation:** Medical products **Company type:** Public **Top competitors:** SeaMED Corporation; Arthur D. Little, Inc.; Analogic Corporation

Colorado MEDtech (CMED) isn't all talk. Through subsidiaries RELA and Novel Biomedical, CMED makes equipment for a variety of health care and medical device companies. Novel Biomedical specializes in custom-designed devices, primarily catheters. Erbtec Engineering makes components for medical imaging applications, and CMED's Respiratory Product division develops respiratory equipment. Its BioMed Y2K readies hospitals' medical and administrative equipment for the year 2000. GE Medical Systems and Gen-Probe each account for about 25% of the company's sales. The company has four plants in Colorado and Minnesota.

Colorado Rockies Baseball Club

2001 Blake St., Denver, CO 80205

Telephone: 303-292-0200 **Fax:** 303-312-2116 **Metro area:** Denver, CO **Web site:** http://www.coloradorockies.com **Human resources contact:** Elizabeth Stecklein **Sales:** $116.6 million (Est.) **Number of employees:** 200 **Industry designation:** Leisure & recreational services **Company type:** Private **Top competitors:** San Francisco Baseball Associates, L.P.; Los Angeles Dodgers Inc.; San Diego Padres Baseball Club Limited Partnership

Playing in Denver, even the smallest bunt is a mile high (above sea level). The Colorado Rockies Baseball Club began rounding the bases in 1993 as one of Major League Baseball's first expansion teams since 1969. They have been setting records ever since, aided in part by hitter-friendly Coors Field, where a single becomes a home run in the rarified air. The team has one of the highest attendance rates in baseball; it drew a record 4.5 million fans during its first season. The Rockies also reached the playoffs in 1995 becoming the first expansion team to make the postseason before its eighth year. The team is owned by a group of investors that includes Coors Brewing and Denver Publishing.

Coram Healthcare Corporation

1125 17th St., Ste. 2100, Denver, CO 80202

Telephone: 303-292-4973 **Fax:** 303-298-0043 **Metro area:** Denver, CO **Web site:** http://www.coram-healthcare.com **Human resources contact:** Vito Ponzio **Sales:** $526.5 million **Number of employees:** 3,600 **Number of employees for previous year:** 2,800 **Industry designation:** Health care—outpatient & home **Company type:** Public **Top competitors:** In Home Health, Inc.; Lincare Holdings Inc.; Apria Healthcare Group Inc.

Coram Healthcare Corporation has put its heart in home health care. It is one of the largest providers of infusion therapy services at patients' homes and other outpatient settings. It operates about 100 branches in more than 40 states and one in Canada and offers a range of services that include anti-infective, chemotherapy, pain management, nutrition, women's health, and other therapies. Coram also offers a mail-order pharmacy and a resource network for HMOs. In addition, it is building patient care programs in AIDS, asthma, and other fields. After an aggressive period of expansion that left it deeply in debt, Coram has bounced back with new contracts and acquisitions.

CSG Systems International, Inc.

7887 E. Belleview, Ste. 1000, Englewood, CO 80111

Telephone: 303-796-2850 **Fax:** 303-796-2878 **Metro area:** Denver, CO **Web site:** http://www.csgsys.com **Human resources contact:** Paul Shaddock **Sales:** $236.6 million **Number of employees:** 1,328 **Number of employees for previous year:** 1,141 **Industry designation:** Computers—corporate, professional & financial software **Company type:** Public **Top competitors:** USCS International, Inc.; Convergys Corporation

CSG Systems International's software automates customer service and billing transactions for cable TV, direct broadcast satellite, online services, and other telecommunications companies. Its Communications Control System sets up, activates, and supports customer accounts and performs order processing, invoicing, production and mailing, reporting, and marketing analysis. CSG Systems' clients serve more than 20 million US customers. Its Bytel subsidiary provides customer service and billing software to cable TV and telephone companies in the UK. CSG Systems' sales staff markets directly to its clients, including Time Warner, AT&T's cable unit (formerly TCI), Prodigy Communications, and MediaOne Group.

The Denver Broncos Football Club

13655 Broncos Pkwy., Englewood, CO 80112

Telephone: 303-649-9000 **Fax:** 303-649-9354 **Metro area:** Denver, CO **Web site:** http://www.denverbroncos.com **Human resources contact:** Sheila Thomas **Sales:** $76.3 million (Est.) **Number of employees:** 89 **Industry designation:** Leisure & recreational services **Company type:** Private **Top competitors:** Kansas City Chiefs; Oakland Raiders; Seattle Seahawks

To many fans in orange and blue, the Denver Broncos' back-to-back 1998 and 1999 Super Bowl victories over the Green Bay Packers and the Atlanta Falcons eased the pain of four previous Super Bowl defeats. Broncos owner Pat Bowlen knows little about losing: Since he bought the team in 1984, the Broncos have won five AFC titles and kept alive a string of home-game sellouts that stretches back 28 years. In 1998 the City of Denver released the Broncos from their Mile High Stadium lease (which expires in 2018) on the provision the club stays in Denver for at least 25 years. Voters later approved a referendum to build the club a new $360 million stadium.

Denver Nuggets

1635 Clay St., Denver, CO 80204

Telephone: 303-893-6700 **Fax:** 303-575-1920 **Metro area:** Denver, CO **Web site:** http://www.nba.com/nuggets **Human resources contact:** Cheryl Miller **Sales:** $37.8 million (Est.) **Number of employees:** 100 **Industry designation:** Leisure & recreational services **Company type:** Private **Top competitors:** Utah Jazz; San Antonio Spurs, Ltd.; Minnesota Timberwolves

The Denver Nuggets franchise originated in the American Basketball Association in 1967. It brought the ABA's high-scoring style into the NBA when the two leagues merged in 1976. Led by Alex English, the team set the all-time record for single-season scoring average in 1981-82. The club has struggled during most of the 1990s as a revolving door to managers, coaches, and players, and its attendance has been in decline. During the 1997-98 season, the team finished just two wins ahead of the worst record in NBA history. Ascent Entertainment, which owns the Nuggets and the NHL's Colorado Avalanche, is building the new $165 million Pepsi Center arena for its teams.

Evergreen Resources, Inc.

1401 17th St., Ste. 1200, Denver, CO 80202

Telephone: 303-298-8100 **Fax:** 303-298-7800 **Metro area:** Denver, CO **Web site:** http://www.evergreen-res.com **Human resources contact:** Annette Sasin **Sales:** $19.1 million **Number of employees:** 64 **Number of employees for previous year:** 43 **Industry designation:** Oil & gas—exploration & production **Company type:** Public

Evergreen Resources explores, develops, operates, and buys oil and gas properties. Its principal operations consist of developing and expanding its wholly owned coalbed methane project in Colorado's Raton Basin; these holdings cover about 129,000 acres. Evergreen Resources has 95 natural gas wells in Colorado; the firm has estimated proved reserves of 224 billion cu. ft. Gas is transported through company-owned gathering systems to Colorado Interstate Gas pipelines. Customers Natural Gas Transmission Services, Enserco Energy, and Aquila Energy account for 80% of sales. Internationally, Evergreen Resources owns or has interests in projects in Chile, the Falkland Islands, and the UK.

Fan Energy Inc.

1801 Broadway, Ste. 720, Denver, CO 80202

Telephone: 303-296-6600 **Fax:** 303-296-2433 **Metro area:** Denver, CO **Number of employees:** 1 **Industry designation:** Oil & gas—exploration & production **Company type:** Private

Fan Energy is an early-stage energy exploration firm with a focus on acquiring and holding oil and natural gas properties. The company has a 25% working interest in two exploratory prospects in California's Sacramento Basin. After reviewing 3-D seismic data on most of the 30,000 acres in the prospects, Fan Energy participated in an initial exploratory well—a dry hole. The company plans to drill additional exploratory or development wells at the North California sites. Following the planned IPO, chairman George Fancher Jr. (a veteran of more than three decades in the oil industry) will reduce his stake in the company to as low as approximately 23%.

Foreland Corporation

12596 W. Bayaud Ave., Ste. 300, Lakewood, CO 80228

Telephone: 303-988-3122 **Fax:** 303-988-3234 **Metro area:** Denver, CO **Web site:** http://www.foreland.com **Sales:** $2.3 million **Number of employees:** 17 **Number of employees for previous year:** 16 **Industry designation:** Oil & gas—exploration & production **Company type:** Public

Call it crazy, but oil exploration company Foreland hunts elephants in Nevada. Those "elephants," however, refer to as-yet-undiscovered oil reserves of more than 100 million barrels. Foreland discovered the Ghost Ranch and Deadman Creek oil fields in Nevada's Great Basin area using 3-D seismic techniques for development drilling and exploration. The firm has an agreement to buy the refining and transportation businesses of Petro Source Corporation. After the purchase, Foreland will be able to refine, process, and distribute its own oil products. Foreland has estimated proved reserves of 2.5 million barrels.

Forest Oil Corporation

1600 Broadway, Ste. 2200, Denver, CO 80202

Telephone: 303-812-1400 **Fax:** 303-812-1602 **Metro area:** Denver, CO **Web site:** http://www.forestoil.com **Human resources contact:** Kathy Davis **Sales:** $321.8 million **Number of employees:** 274 **Number of employees for previous year:** 267 **Industry designation:** Oil & gas—exploration & production **Company type:** Public **Top competitors:** Apache Corporation; Plains Resources Inc.; Mitchell Energy & Development Corp.

Forest Oil explores for oil and natural gas and acquires and develops oil and natural gas properties in the Gulf of Mexico, the western US, and Canada. The company specializes in increasing production in existing fields. Forest Oil produces over 31 billion cu. ft. of natural gas and more than one billion barrels of oil per year. Approximately 18% of its sales are to oil and gas giant Enron, with which it has a sales pact. Forest is focused on acquiring domestic reserves, increasing production from existing fields, and exploring for additional reserves. Billionaire Philip Anschutz's Anschutz Corporation owns 40% of the company.

4Front Technologies, Inc.

5650 Greenwood Plaza Blvd., Ste. 107, Englewood, CO 80111

Telephone: 303-721-7341 **Fax:** 303-220-1818 **Metro area:** Denver, CO **Web site:** http://www.ffst.com **Sales:** $148.9 million **Number of employees:** 726 **Number of employees for previous year:** 367 **Industry designation:** Computers—services **Company type:** Public **Top competitors:** Atos; Cap Gemini S.A.; Computer Sciences Corporation

The British are .coming, the British are .coming. 4Front Technologies provides networking and other computer services to corporations and government agencies, primarily in the UK but increasingly in other parts of Europe. 4Front's services include system integration, hardware maintenance, and help desk support. The growing company supplies a broad range of system components from manufacturers such as IBM, Seagate, and Sony. It publishes business software, including Shortlands, an accounting tool used by the construction industry, and Pharaoh, an asset- and property-management product used by health trusts and municipalities. Other 4Front clients include DuPont, Fujitsu, and the UK Ministry of Defense.

Hach Company

5600 Lindbergh Dr., Loveland, CO 80538

Telephone: 970-669-3050 **Fax:** 970-669-2932 **Other address:** PO Box 389, Loveland, CO 80539 **Metro area:** Denver, CO **Web site:** http://www.hach.com **Human resources contact:** Randall A. Peterson **Sales:** $128.1 million **Number of employees:** 955 **Number of employees for previous year:** 875 **Industry designation:** Instruments—scientific **Company type:** Public **Top competitors:** Thermo Instrument Systems Inc.; Osmonics, Inc.; Ionics, Incorporated

Hach Company is an expert at the dirty pool. The company makes water testing kits and scientific instruments, including laboratory instruments and process analyzers that measure the chemical content and other properties of water. Its products, which include spectrophotometers, process turbidimeters, and pH controllers, are used in the US and abroad to help companies and governments ensure water quality. Subsidiary Environmental Test Systems makes testing materials primarily for pools and spas. Co-founder and chairman Kathryn Hach-Darrow—whose son Bruce Hach is CEO—owns 54% of the family business.

Hauser, Inc.

5555 Airport Blvd., Boulder, CO 80301

Telephone: 303-443-4662 **Fax:** 303-441-5800 **Metro area:** Denver, CO **Web site:** http://www.hauser.com **Human resources contact:** Peg Bundgaard **Sales:** $32 million **Number of employees:** 320 **Number of employees for previous year:** 314 **Industry designation:** Drugs **Company type:** Public **Top competitors:** NaPro BioTherapeutics, Inc.; Bristol-Myers Squibb Company; Xechem International, Inc.

Mother Nature is Hauser's #1 supplier. The company makes nutraceuticals (all-natural dietary supplements), natural flavor extracts, and natural food ingredients marketed under the NaturEnhance brand name. The natural products unit accounts for close to 45% of Hauser's sales. Hauser Laboratories and Shuster Laboratories, the company's technical services units, research and develop new products and extracting processes for the pharmaceutical, medical device, and natural products industries. These activities account for another 45% of Hauser's sales. The company's pharmaceuticals unit focuses on supplying paclitaxel, a cancer drug derived from the Pacific yew tree, to pharmaceutical companies around the world.

Heska Corporation

1825 Sharp Point Dr., Fort Collins, CO 80525

Telephone: 970-493-7272 **Fax:** 970-484-9505 **Metro area:** Denver, CO **Web site:** http://www.heska.com **Human resources contact:** Diane McCoy **Sales:** $39.8 million **Number of employees:** 533 **Number of employees for previous year:** 475 **Industry designation:** Veterinary products & services **Company type:** Public **Top competitors:** Virbac Corporation

If you lie down with dogs, you could get up with fleas—but not if veterinary products maker Heska prevents the problem. The firm develops and makes diagnostic products, vaccines, and pharmaceuticals for domestic animals. Products include treatments for fleas, allergies, skin problems, heartworms, dental hygiene, viral infections, thyroid problems, arthritis, and cancer. Heska operates veterinary diagnostic labs in Colorado and the UK (Bloxham Laboratories), and it owns Diamond Animal Health, which makes its products along with third-party manufacturers. Additionally, the company has research and development (Bayer; Ralston Purina), marketing (Eisai; Novartis), and manufacturing (Novartis) partnerships.

High Speed Access Corp.

4100 E. Mississippi Ave., Denver, CO 80246

Telephone: 303-256-2000 **Fax:** 303-256-2001 **Metro area:** Denver, CO **Web site:** http://www.hsacorp.net **Human resources contact:** Susan Francke **Sales:** $337,000 (Est.) **Number of employees:** 156 **Industry designation:** Computers—online services **Company type:** Private **Top competitors:** WorldGate Communications, Inc.; OneMain.com, Inc.; SoftNet Systems, Inc.

High Speed Access contracts with cable-TV operators to provide fast-paced Internet service in places where the pace of living is a little slower. The company targets so-called exurban markets (where cable systems pass less than 100,000 homes), offering Internet access via both high-speed cable modems and standard dial-up service. It serves more than 5,000 customers (including 2,800 cable modem users) in 14 markets in 11 states. Microsoft co-founder Paul Allen's Vulcan Ventures owns 54% of High Speed Access, and Vulcan's Charter Communications cable unit has agreed to give the company rights to at least 750,000 homes passed. Kentucky investment group Broadband Solutions owns 37% of High Speed Access.

Horizon Organic Holding Corporation

6311 Horizon Ln., Longmont, CO 80503

Telephone: 303-530-2711 **Fax:** 303-530-2714 **Metro area:** Denver, CO **Web site:** http://www.horizonorganic.com **Human resources contact:** Liz Balles **Sales:** $49.4 million **Number of employees:** 138 **Number of employees for previous year:** 117 **Industry designation:** Food—dairy products **Company type:** Public **Top competitors:** Organic Valley/CROPP Cooperatives; H.P. Hood, Inc.

Milking a growing demand for organic foods, Horizon Organic produces certified organic milk, cheese, and other dairy products. Horizon, the #1 organic brand in the US, distributes its milk nationwide through its network of organic milk producers and processors, including two company-owned organic dairy farms in Idaho and Maryland. Horizon is focusing its marketing efforts on Denver, Los Angeles, New York, San Francisco, and other cities where demand for chemical-free food is high. The company's 40 products are sold by more than 5,000 supermarkets, specialty retailers, and natural foods stores. Horizon also owns the Juniper Valley Farms brand of organic dairy products. Suiza Foods owns 12% of the company.

Image Guided Technologies, Inc.

5710-B Flatiron Pkwy., Boulder, CO 80301

Telephone: 303-447-0248 **Fax:** 303-447-3905 **Metro area:** Denver, CO **Web site:** http://www.imageguided.com **Human resources contact:** Jill Worsham **Sales:** $5.7 million **Number of employees:** 118 **Number of employees for previous year:** 28 **Industry designation:** Instruments—scientific **Company type:** Public

Image Guided Technologies' products let surgeons make the kindest cut and manufacturers check the smallest nut. IGT makes 3-D optical devices that are used in minimally invasive, image-guided surgery and in product inspecting. Its FlashPoint optical localizer shows doctors the location of surgical instruments inside a patient's body via a computer screen, and its related Pixsys system lets manufacturers perform quality-control checks. In addition, IGT makes surgical instruments, as well as implants used in orthopedic, cardiovascular, and dental procedures. The company markets to original equipment manufacturers, and its localizers account for about 80% of sales.

ImageMatrix Corporation

400 S. Colorado Blvd., Ste. 500, Denver, CO 80246

Telephone: 303-399-3700 **Fax:** 303-399-1554 **Metro area:** Denver, CO **Web site:** http://www.image-matrix.com **Human resources contact:** Pat Milstein **Sales:** $5.1 million **Number of employees:** 48 **Number of employees for previous year:** 39 **Industry designation:** Computers—corporate, professional & financial software **Company type:** Public **Top competitors:** FileNET Corporation; Perot Systems Corporation; Optika, Inc.

ImageMatrix provides productivity and customer service systems to HMOs, dental and insurance providers, and other health care organizations. The company's systems combine its proprietary software with third-party hardware, peripherals, and other software modules. ImageMatrix software, the licensing of which accounts for about 58% of sales, features CaptureMatrix (for digitally converting claims), ClaimMatrix (for processing claims), and ServiceMatrix (for customer service uses). The company also offers installation, design, integration, maintenance, and training services. ImageMatrix plans to merge with MindWorks, which produces document management software for workgroups.

Isonics Corporation

5906 McIntyre St., Golden, CO 80403

Telephone: 303-279-7900 **Fax:** 303-279-7300 **Metro area:** Denver, CO **Web site:** http://www.isonics.com **Human resources contact:** Paul J. Catuna **Sales:** $6.8 million **Number of employees:** 38 **Number of employees for previous year:** 11 **Industry designation:** Chemicals—specialty **Company type:** Public

Isonics develops products based on ultrapure, enriched stable isotopes for use in the energy, medical, and pharmaceutical industries. The company provides most of the world's supply of isotopically depleted zinc (DZ), which is used to prevent corrosion and reduce cracking in nuclear power plants. An isotope enrichment plant in Russia is integral to the processing of Isonics products. General Electric (GE) developed the application of DZ and, combined with DZ sales to end users, accounts for a majority of sales. Isonics also develops carbon-13 for use in diagnostic testing kits. Founders and GE veterans James Alexander and Boris Rubizhevsky own about 35% and 30% of the company, respectively.

J.D. Edwards & Company

1 Technology Way, Denver, CO 80237

Telephone: 303-334-4000 **Fax:** 303-334-4678 **Metro area:** Denver, CO **Web site:** http://www.jdedwards.com **Sales:** $934 million **Number of employees:** 4,950 **Number of employees for previous year:** 3,577 **Industry designation:** Computers—corporate, professional & financial software **Company type:** Public **Top competitors:** Oracle Corporation; SAP AG; Baan Company N.V.

J.D. Edwards wants to command the voyages of your enterprise. The company is a leading maker of enterprise resource planning (ERP) software. Its OneWorld software manages and stores data from a company's manufacturing, finance, distribution, and human resources operations, among others. OneWorld unifies IBM mainframe, UNIX, and Windows NT systems on a network and incorporates customized applications for industries such as construction, engineering, energy, and chemicals. The company's WorldSoftware offers the same ERP functions for IBM AS/400 systems. J.D. Edwards markets its software through 50 offices worldwide. Billionaire co-founder and chairman Edward McVaney owns 32% of the company.

Key Production Company, Inc.

707 17th St., Ste. 3300, Denver, CO 80202

Telephone: 303-295-3995 **Fax:** 303-295-3494 **Metro area:** Denver, CO **Web site:** http://www.keyproduction.com **Human resources contact:** Sharon Pope **Sales:** $37.4 million **Number of employees:** 61 **Number of employees for previous year:** 56 **Industry designation:** Oil & gas—exploration & production **Company type:** Public **Top competitors:** KCS Energy, Inc.; Unit Corporation; HS Resources, Inc.

Key Production is trying to open doors to oil and gas in 14 US states. The exploration and production company concentrates on the Anadarko Basin of Oklahoma, California, the Rocky Mountain region, North Texas, and the Gulf Coast. Key Production has proved reserves of 68 billion cu. ft. of natural gas and six million barrels of oil. The company has working interests in nearly 2,000 oil and gas wells and owns 298,000 acres of developed and undeveloped land. Key Production has exploration rights on an additional 107,000 acres as part of a joint venture with EEX.

Meteor Industries, Inc.

216 16th St., Ste. 730, Denver, CO 80202

Telephone: 303-572-1135 **Fax:** 303-572-1803 **Metro area:** Denver, CO **Sales:** $118.4 million **Number of employees:** 320 **Number of employees for previous year:** 273 **Industry designation:** Oil refining & marketing **Company type:** Public

Meteor Industries distributes fuels and also owns and operates convenience stores through its subsidiaries in the western US. The company conducts its petroleum marketing and convenience store business through its Hillger Oil, Graves Oil & Butane, and Flieschli Oil subsidiaries. It distributes gasoline, diesel, lubricants, and propane to truck stops, gas stations, convenience stores, commercial fleet distribution centers, mining companies, and utilities. It has distribution agreements with Phillips Petroleum, Conoco, Exxon Lubricants, Diamond Shamrock, and Fina Oil. It owns or has leasehold interests in 20 retail outlets and nine cardlock facilities, which offer 24-hour access to fuel through debit cards.

NAVIDEC, Inc.

14 Inverness Dr., Bldg. F, Ste. 116, Englewood, CO 80112

Telephone: 303-790-7565 **Fax:** 303-790-8845 **Metro area:** Denver, CO **Web site:** http://www.navidec.com **Human resources contact:** Cindy Barnard **Sales:** $8.6 million **Number of employees:** 51 **Number of employees for previous year:** 37 **Industry designation:** Computers—services **Company type:** Public **Top competitors:** Open Market, Inc.; Online System Services, Inc.; autobytel.com inc.

Web navigators use NAVIDEC's products. The company designs and implements Web sites for e-commerce and order placement, and develops marketing tools such as interactive kiosks. NAVIDEC provides computer and network infrastructure and software, and resells and installs high-tech systems and components from third-party manufacturers such as AT&T, Sybase, and Tektronix. Customers include Destination Hotels and Resorts, the Colorado Avalanche hockey team, Live Entertainment, and PRIMESTAR. NAVIDEC's newest venture, Wheels, is an online car-shopping service the company developed and operates in Colorado and Oregon. CEO Ralph Armijo owns 24% of the company.

NxTrend Technology, Inc.

5555 Tech Center Dr., Colorado Springs, CO 80919

Telephone: 719-590-8940 **Fax:** 719-528-1465 **Metro area:** Colorado Springs, CO **Web site:** http://www.nxtrend.com **Human resources contact:** Glenn Goldberg **Sales:** $58 million (Est.) **Number of employees:** 325 **Number of employees for previous year:** 287 **Industry designation:** Computers—corporate, professional & financial software **Company type:** Private **Top competitors:** J.D. Edwards & Company; System Software Associates, Inc.; Prophet 21, Inc.

NxTrend Technology hopes to set the next trend. Founded in 1979, the company (formerly R&D Systems) makes distribution management software for the electrical supply, plumbing, HVAC, building materials, and industrial supply markets. Its UNIX- and Windows NT-based software packages (including Trend, WDS-II, and SHIMS) perform such applications as inventory management, order processing, warehouse logistics, and strategic analysis for wholesale distributors. Customers include Missouri Valley Electric, Briggs Weaver, and Inland Diesel. NxTrend, which has shown a profit every year of its existence, is owned by co-founder and chairman Guy Lammle and venture capital funds Summit Partners and TA Associates.

Online System Services, Inc.

1800 Glenarm Place, Ste. 800, Denver, CO 80202

Telephone: 303-296-9200 **Fax:** 303-295-3584 **Metro area:** Denver, CO **Web site:** http://www.ossinc.net **Human resources contact:** Kim Castillo **Sales:** $1.6 million **Number of employees:** 54 **Number of employees for previous year:** 42 **Industry designation:** Computers—online services **Company type:** Public **Top competitors:** NetGravity, Inc.; BroadVision, Inc.; Open Market, Inc.

With love from i2u. Online System Services' (OSS) i2u software products and services turn broadband operators (cable TV firms) into high-speed Internet service providers. Its turnkey systems (hardware, software, and training) facilitate expansion into the Internet service provider market. Its i2u Foundation software enables broadband operators to create complex Web sites (personal home pages, business directories, online forums) where users generate and update the site's content. OSS also provides e-commerce and banking products and services. The company, whose customers include American Telecasting and RE/MAX International, has exited the general Web site development and health care information businesses.

Optical Security Group, Inc.

535 16th St., Ste. 920, Denver, CO 80202

Telephone: 303-534-4500 **Fax:** 303-534-1010 **Metro area:** Denver, CO **Web site:** http://www.opticalsecurity.com **Sales:** $9.8 million **Number of employees:** 80 **Number of employees for previous year:** 57 **Industry designation:** Protection—safety equipment & services **Company type:** Public **Top competitors:** American Bank Note Holographics, Inc.; APi Group, Inc.; HoloPak Technologies, Inc.

Optical Security Group sells holograms for hockey, foils for football, and labels for licenses. The company makes security labels, laminates, foils, holograms, and microdots and threads used to combat counterfeiters. Businesses and government agencies use the products to authenticate licenses, permits, credit cards, event tickets, checks, and labels. National Football League licensees represent 25% of revenues, and the National Hockey League, World Championship Wrestling, and American Express are also customers. Optical Security has offices in Europe, the UK, and the US, but also sells in Asia and South America. The firm is exiting its non-security operations. CEO Richard Bard owns about 25% of the company.

Optika, Inc.

7450 Campus Dr., 2nd Fl., Colorado Springs, CO 80920

Telephone: 719-548-9800 **Fax:** 719-531-7915 **Metro area:** Colorado Springs, CO **Web site:** http://www.optika.com **Human resources contact:** Les Brown **Sales:** $18.5 million **Number of employees:** 173 **Number of employees for previous year:** 168 **Industry designation:** Computers—corporate, professional & financial software **Company type:** Public **Top competitors:** Inso Corporation; Vignette Corporation; Dataware Technologies, Inc.

Optika (formerly Optika Imaging Systems) makes scalable, customizable software for managing e-commerce and graphics. Its client/server-based FilePower suite enables users to perform such functions as image management, storage and retrieval, output to laserdisc, and image development. The company's eMedia software, which is being test-marketed, helps users manage e-commerce transactions among themselves, their customers, and their suppliers. Optika also offers support, maintenance, training, and consulting services. Clients include Citibank, Home Depot, MCI, Walt Disney, and Coca-Cola.

OraLabs Holding Corp.

2901 S. Tejon St., Englewood, CO 80110

Telephone: 303-783-9499 **Fax:** 303-783-5759 **Metro area:** Denver, CO **Human resources contact:** Emile "Red" Jordan **Sales:** $6.8 million **Number of employees:** 80 **Number of employees for previous year:** 65 **Industry designation:** Drugs & sundries—wholesale **Company type:** Public

OraLabs produces health and beauty care products. The company's diverse line of goods includes sun-block lip balm and cold and sore throat sprays, but is best known for its Ice Drops line of breath-freshening liquid drops. OraLabs also operates as a private-label contractor, producing personal care products for such companies as Rite-Aid and Sally's Beauty Supply. Its products are found at checkout counters in more than 50,000 US retail stores and in 25 international markets. Chairman and CEO Gary H. Schlatter owns 80% of the company's stock.

Prima Energy Corporation

1801 Broadway, Ste. 500, Denver, CO 80202

Telephone: 303-297-2100 **Fax:** 303-297-7708 **Metro area:** Denver, CO **Web site:** http://www.primaenergy.com **Human resources contact:** Nancy Hewitt **Sales:** $30.1 million **Number of employees:** 88 **Number of employees for previous year:** 76 **Industry designation:** Oil & gas—exploration & production **Company type:** Public

Prima Energy explores for, develops, trades, produces, and markets crude oil and natural gas from about 370 wells in Colorado's Wattenberg Field area, the Texas Panhandle, and Wyoming's Powder River and Wind River Basins. In addition to selling gas and oil (about 46% of revenues), the firm operates oil and gas properties, acquires oil and gas leases, and provides oilfield services such as supplying completion rigs, offering trucking, and renting pumps, tanks, and other equipment. The firm has estimated proved reserves of more than 63 billion cu. ft. of natural gas and 3.4 million barrels of oil.

Pro-Dex, Inc.

1401 Walnut St., Ste. 540, Boulder, CO 80302

Telephone: 303-443-6136 **Fax:** 303-443-2770 **Metro area:** Denver, CO **Web site:** http://www.PDEX.com **Human resources contact:** Jim Patton **Sales:** $22.6 million **Number of employees:** 141 **Number of employees for previous year:** 138 **Industry designation:** Medical & dental supplies **Company type:** Public **Top competitors:** Block Drug Company, Inc.; Young Innovations, Inc.; Patterson Dental Company

Fighting for teeth, justice, and the American way, dental product maker Pro-Dex is gunning for the Cavity Creeps. Through subsidiary Challenge Products, the company offers such preventive dental wares as fluoride gel and rinses under the brands Perfect Choice, Dual-XTM, and Dentalite. Distribution subsidiary Biotrol International markets dental products for Challenge and other manufacturers, but Challenge has marketing agreements with other firms. Micro Motors makes miniature pneumatic motors and handpieces for use in dental, medical, and industrial applications. Oregon Micro Systems specializes in motion-control circuit boards for medical testing equipment. VC Ronald Goss owns about 30% of Pro-Dex.

Proformance Research Organization, Inc.

5335 W. 48th Ave., Denver, CO 80212

Telephone: 303-458-1000 **Fax:** 303-458-6454 **Metro area:** Denver, CO **Web site:** http://www.proform-golf.com **Human resources contact:** Lou Royston **Sales:** $119,000 (Est.) **Number of employees:** 28 **Industry designation:** Leisure & recreational services **Company type:** Private **Top competitors:** The Arnold Palmer Golf Company

If you want to swing hard, Proformance Research Organization (PRO) will show you how. Formerly known as World Associates, the company has seven schools located near golf courses in Arizona, California, Colorado, Florida, Iowa, Nevada, and New York; the schools offer two- to five-day intensive golf instruction programs. PRO also operates two golf Learning Centers, which cater to local residents seeking hourly instruction. In addition to running its schools, PRO sells videotapes and booklets, and it markets golf clubs, bags, hats, and accessories for Fila. William Leary, a former pro football player for the Denver Broncos, founded PRO in 1993. The company filed to go public in August 1998.

Renaissance Entertainment Corporation

275 Century Circle, Ste. 102, Louisville, CO 80027

Telephone: 303-664-0300 **Fax:** 303-444-8365 **Metro area:** Denver, CO **Web site:** http://www.recfair.com/fair **Sales:** $14.2 million **Number of employees:** 37 **Industry designation:** Leisure & recreational services **Company type:** Public

Living the fantasy life, Renaissance Entertainment operates five Renaissance Faires in the US. Each recreates a 16th century English village, featuring craft shops, food vendors, jugglers, jousting, and other pageantry. The events typically last bewteen six and nine weekends a year. Its Faires draw more than 700,000 visitors annually in the Chicago; Los Angeles; San Francisco; New York City; and Washington, DC metropolitan areas. Renaissance Entertainment markets its Faires as family entertainment through multimedia advertising and joint sponsorships with companies such as Eastman Kodak, Hyatt, and Coca-Cola.

Rhythms NetConnections Inc.

6933 S. Revere Pkwy., Englewood, CO 80112

Telephone: 303-476-4200 **Fax:** 303-476-4201 **Metro area:** Denver, CO **Web site:** http://www.rhythms.net **Sales:** $528,000 (Est.) **Number of employees:** 220 **Industry designation:** Computers—online services **Company type:** Private **Top competitors:** GTE Corporation; At Home Corporation; Qwest Communications International Inc.

Without missing a beat, Rhythms NetConnections provides Internet access and remote network connections with speedy digital subscriber line (DSL) technology. The firm's packet-based network, which uses local telephone lines, allows simultaneous access for many users on one connection. Rhythms NetConnections maintains about 650 DSL-equipped phone lines for businesses and service providers in 10 metropolitan markets, including Chicago, New York, and San Francisco; the firm is under contract to supply another 9,000 lines. Rhythms NetConnections has marketing agreements with Cisco Systems, MCI WorldCom, and Microsoft. CEO Catherine Hapka, who formerly ran U S West's data networking business, owns 10% of the company.

Rocky Mountain Internet, Inc.

1099 18th, Ste. 3000, Denver, CO 80202

Telephone: 303-672-0700 **Fax:** 303-672-0711 **Metro area:** Denver, CO **Web site:** http://www.rmii.com **Human resources contact:** July Kozacik **Sales:** $6.1 million **Number of employees:** 72 **Number of employees for previous year:** 29 **Industry designation:** Computers—online services **Company type:** Public **Top competitors:** ICG Communications, Inc.; GTE Corporation; Qwest Communications International Inc.

Coloradoans can send a Rocky Mountain "Hi" online via Rocky Mountain Internet (RMI). The company offers dedicated and dial-up Internet access through points-of-presence (POPs) in nine Colorado cities (representing more than 85% of the state's population). RMI also offers Web development and hosting, systems integration, network management, and e-commerce support. Through a contract with PSI Net, RMI offers dedicated and dial-up Internet services to customers in PSI Net's 400 POPs worldwide. RMI also offers Internet Protocol (IP) long-distance telephony to residents of Denver, Boulder, and Colorado Springs.

St. Mary Land & Exploration Company

1776 Lincoln St., Ste. 1100, Denver, CO 80203

Telephone: 303-861-8140 **Fax:** 303-861-0934 **Metro area:** Denver, CO **Web site:** http://www.stmaryland.com **Human resources contact:** Margo Whittemore **Sales:** $78.7 million **Number of employees:** 110 **Number of employees for previous year:** 103 **Industry designation:** Oil & gas—exploration & production **Company type:** Public **Top competitors:** Pioneer Natural Resources Company; Apache Corporation; Mitchell Energy & Development Corp.

St. Mary Land & Exploration isn't afraid to travel: The oil and gas exploration and production company spreads its operations over five areas in the US: the midcontinent, the ArkLaTex region, south Louisiana, the Williston Basin in North Dakota and Montana, and the Permian Basin in West Texas and New Mexico. The company has estimated proved reserves of 11.5 million barrels of oil and nearly 200 billion cu. ft. of natural gas. St. Mary Land & Exploration also has a 37% interest in Summo Minerals Corporation, a North American copper mining company.

Specialty Care Network, Inc.

44 Union Blvd., Ste. 600, Lakewood, CO 80228

Telephone: 303-716-0041 **Fax:** 303-716-1298 **Metro area:** Denver, CO **Web site:** http://www.scneti.com **Human resources contact:** Carolyn Paschall **Sales:** $79.2 million **Number of employees:** 841 **Number of employees for previous year:** 219 **Industry designation:** Medical practice management **Company type:** Public

Specialty Care Network is a musculoskeletal physician practice management company. The company is affiliated with about 20 practices in 11 states including Pennsylvania, New Jersey, New York, Texas, Georgia, Maryland, and Florida. The company has more than 160 affiliated physicians who are trained in many musculoskeletal disciplines, including orthopedics, joint replacement surgery, sports medicine, spinal care, hand and upper extremity care, foot and ankle care, and physiatry. Specialty Care Network also manages an outpatient surgery center and an outpatient magnetic resonance imaging (MRI) center.

Storage Technology Corporation

2270 S. 88th St., Louisville, CO 80028

Telephone: 303-673-5151 **Fax:** 303-673-4444 **Metro area:** Denver, CO **Web site:** http://www.stortek.com **Human resources contact:** Laurie N. Dodd **Sales:** $2.3 billion **Number of employees:** 8,700 **Number of employees for previous year:** 8,300 **Industry designation:** Computers—peripheral equipment **Company type:** Public **Top competitors:** EMC Corporation; Hitachi, Ltd.; International Business Machines Corporation

When your database gets too big, Storage Technology (StorageTek) has a solution. The company makes information storage systems, including disk drives, tape libraries, and corporate network backup and recovery software products for customers in 40 countries. Its products are sold to major corporations and government agencies such as Chase Manhattan, Ameritech, and the US Postal Service. StorageTek also makes network connectivity and security tools. The company has entered into a strategic agreement with tape drive rival IBM, which is selling StorageTek's mainframe online products worldwide. StorageTek has also formed strategic alliances with Compaq, Hewlett-Packard, and other computer manufacturers.

Triumph Fuels Corporation

1493 Hwy. 6 & 50, Fruita, CO 81521

Telephone: 970-858-0300 **Fax:** 970-858-9626 **Human resources contact:** Jackie Leopold **Sales:** $270 million (Est.) **Number of employees:** 311 **Industry designation:** Oil refining & marketing **Company type:** Private

Triumph Fuels Corporation distributes and markets branded and unbranded refined petroleum products—gasoline, diesel fuel, and lubricants—to commercial and retail customers in the Southwest. The company also sells gas on consignment; provides direct fueling for vehicles, ships, and locomotives at automated and semi-automated facilities; and owns or operates 19 SuperMart gasoline stations. Triumph Fuels, which operates in Colorado, Texas, and Utah, is expanding through the acquisition and consolidation of other independent wholesalers. The firm has marketing agreements with BP Amoco, Chevron, Diamond Shamrock, Phillips, Shell, and Texaco. Director David Horvitz owns nearly 65% of the company.

United States Exploration, Inc.

1560 Broadway, Ste. 1900, Denver, CO 80202

Telephone: 303-863-3550 **Fax:** 303-863-1932 **Metro area:** Denver, CO **Human resources contact:** Murray N. Brooks **Sales:** $2 million **Number of employees:** 26 **Number of employees for previous year:** 19 **Industry designation:** Oil & gas—exploration & production **Company type:** Public

The deceptively named United States Exploration does not explore for oil and gas—it just owns the reserves. The company operates through several wholly owned subsidiaries, including Argas, which maintains gas-gathering systems in Kansas; Five Star Petroleum, which holds oil and gas leases in Oklahoma; and US Gas Gathering, which operates a gathering system and holds gas leases. US Exploration outsources drilling to contractors. The company's strategy of growth through acquisition has not faltered even in the wake of management shake-ups. Dale Jensen owns about 25% of the company.

Verio Inc.

8005 S. Chester St., Ste. 200, Englewood, CO 80112

Telephone: 303-645-1900 **Fax:** 303-792-5644 **Metro area:** Denver, CO **Web site:** http://www.verio.com **Human resources contact:** Deb Mayfield Gahan **Sales:** $120.7 million **Number of employees:** 853 **Industry designation:** Computers—online services **Company type:** Public **Top competitors:** GTE Corporation; PSINet Inc.; UUNET WorldCom

With a huge wad of cash from a host of venture-capital firms and an IPO, Verio is buying regional and local Internet service providers (ISPs) across the US. It owns or has majority stakes in more than 35 business-oriented providers across the US. Verio is buying ISPs with a large number of dedicated accounts (business accounts with direct lines to the provider) and is marketing to business and institutional subscribers. The firm's customers include General Electric, Microsoft, Princeton University, and Ziff-Davis. Brooks Fiber Properties, a unit of MCI WorldCom, owns approximately 17% of Verio.

Connecticut

Alexion Pharmaceuticals, Inc.

25 Science Park, Ste. 360, New Haven, CT 06511

Telephone: 203-776-1790 **Fax:** 203-772-3655 **Metro area:** New York, NY **Human resources contact:** Edith Huzar **Sales:** $5 million **Number of employees:** 69 **Number of employees for previous year:** 51 **Industry designation:** Biomedical & genetic products **Company type:** Public **Top competitors:** Chiron Corporation; Abbott Laboratories; Immunex Corporation

Oh, rats! Alexion Pharmaceuticals' xenotransplantation products aren't ready for humans yet, but the firm nonetheless made a splash by curing spinal injuries in rodents with genetically altered cells from pigs. US Surgical partners with Alexion in its work on transplantation across species lines. Alexion's other development projects include C5 Complement Inhibitor drugs (designed to prevent disease-causing cells from forming, to treat complications related to cardiovascular surgery and such autoimmune disorders as lupus and rheumatoid arthritis) and Apogen therapeutics (designed to destroy disease-causing cells, to treat multiple sclerosis, diabetes, and other conditions).

Arch Chemicals, Inc.

501 Merritt 7, Norwalk, CT 06856

Telephone: 203-229-2900 **Fax:** 203-229-3213 **Metro area:** New York, NY **Web site:** http://www.archchemicals.com **Human resources contact:** Mark A. Killian **Sales:** $862.8 million **Number of employees:** 3,000 **Number of employees for previous year:** 2,950 **Industry designation:** Chemicals—specialty **Company type:** Public **Top competitors:** Great Lakes Chemical Corporation; Rohm and Haas Company; Sumitomo Chemical Company, Limited

An archenemy of dandruff and dirty swimming pools, Arch Chemicals operates worldwide in three business segments. Its performance chemicals unit is a leading supplier of biocides used in antidandruff shampoos. Its other products include hydrazine propellants that are used on most of the world's satellites. Arch Chemical's water chemicals business is a leading maker of hypochlorite pool sanitizers. The microelectronic chemicals sector provides advanced photoresists, wet process chemicals, and chemical management services to the semiconductor industry. The company has operations in Africa, Asia, Europe, and North and South America. Arch Chemicals was spun-off from Olin in early 1999.

ATMI, Inc.

7 Commerce Dr., Danbury, CT 06810

Telephone: 203-794-1100 **Fax:** 203-792-8040 **Metro area:** New York, NY **Web site:** http://www.atmi.com **Human resources contact:** Phyllis Banucci **Sales:** $97.9 million **Number of employees:** 455 **Number of employees for previous year:** 376 **Industry designation:** Pollution control equipment & services **Company type:** Public **Top competitors:** Ebara Corporation; EMCORE Corporation

ATMI, Inc. (formerly Advanced Technology Materials) makes materials and equipment for the semiconductor industry. Its Advanced Delivery & Chemical Systems unit (45% of sales) makes chemicals and delivery systems for the chemical vapor deposition (CVD) process that coats the surface of semiconductor wafers with a thin insulating film. Subsidiary EcoSys makes dry-chemical, liquid, and oxidation scrubbers designed to control the environmental hazards associated with the CVD process. ATMI's Epitronics unit provides CVD processing of bare wafers that are not yet part of integrated circuits. The company sells its products in North America, Europe, and Asia directly and through manufacturers' representatives.

@plan.inc

3 Landmark Sq., Ste. 400, Stamford, CT 06901

Telephone: 203-961-0340 **Fax:** 203-964-0136 **Metro area:** New York, NY **Web site:** http://www.webplan.net **Human resources contact:** Nancy A. Lazaros **Sales:** $3.1 million (Est.) **Number of employees:** 19 **Industry designation:** Computers—services **Company type:** Private **Top competitors:** Excite, Inc.; ACNielsen Corporation; Media Metrix, Inc.

Internet advertisers, ad agencies, and online retailers are clamoring to get data on Web site usage, and @plan.inc is ready to give them the inside scoop. By visiting the @plan.inc Web site, the company's more than 250 clients can access its proprietary systems and get the skinny on attributes (lifestyle information, product preferences, demographic data) of Web site visitors. @plan.inc's data is collected by The Gallup Organization from a sample of about 40,000 Web users. The company counts broadcast.com, Modem Media.Poppe Tyson, Preview Travel, and Saatchi & Saatchi among its customers. Directors W. Patrick Ortale and Donald M. Johnston own about 45% and 27% of the company, respectively.

ChiRex Inc.

300 Atlantic St., Ste. 402, Stamford, CT 06901

Telephone: 203-351-2300 **Fax:** 203-425-9996 **Metro area:** New York, NY **Web site:** http://www.chirex.com/ **Sales:** $119.7 million **Number of employees:** 630 **Number of employees for previous year:** 587 **Industry designation:** Drugs **Company type:** Public **Top competitors:** Roberts Pharmaceutical Corporation; Alusuisse Lonza Group Ltd.; Laporte plc

ChiRex performs contract manufacturing of pharmaceutical and other chemical products for such drug-industry heavyweights as Sanofi (which accounts for more than one-third of Chirex's sales), Glaxo Wellcome, and SmithKline Beecham. Clients hire ChiRex to support and supplement their in-house development and manufacturing operations. ChiRex offers a host of related services (product analysis, documentation, hazard evaluation, and more). Nearly all the products it develops are covered by secrecy agreements that restrict naming the customer, drug, or its indications. The company, which went public in 1996, makes more than 50 different products, 90% of which are pharmaceutical.

Cognitronics Corporation

3 Corporate Dr., Danbury, CT 06810

Telephone: 203-830-3400 **Fax:** 203-830-3405 **Metro area:** New York, NY **Web site:** http://www.cognitronics.com **Human resources contact:** Janet Freund **Sales:** $28.9 million **Number of employees:** 96 **Number of employees for previous year:** 94 **Industry designation:** Computers—peripheral equipment **Company type:** Public **Top competitors:** Brooktrout Technology, Inc.; Lucent Technologies Inc.; Active Voice Corporation

Cognitronics makes telephone announcement systems and other voice processing products. Its passive announcers are used by telecommunications and telephone companies to give callers information about network conditions or procedures. Its intelligent announcers provide call forwarding and caller identification. Cognitronics also makes central office grade announcement systems, fixed application systems that provide voice processing, hold music and messages, and interactive voice response, fax, and voice mail. Other products include interactive voice response, fax, voice mail, voice-activated dialing, prepaid debit card, audiotex, and other features.

Command Systems, Inc.

76 Batterson Park Rd., Farmington, CT 06032

Telephone: 860-409-2000 **Fax:** 860-409-2099 **Metro area:** Hartford, CT **Web site:** http://www.commandsys.com **Human resources contact:** Deb Leavitt **Sales:** $35.2 million **Number of employees:** 334 **Number of employees for previous year:** 293 **Industry designation:** Computers—services **Company type:** Public **Top competitors:** IMRglobal Corp.; SunGard Data Systems Inc.; PRT Group Inc.

Command Systems helps financial services companies take command of their information technology problems. The company provides application development and implementation, network design, Internet/intranet development, backup and recovery, year 2000 remediation, and education and training. Command offers support services primarily through offices in the US. Workers in India develop software and perform year 2000 system upgrades. Command resells hardware and software from industry leaders that include Compaq, Hewlett-Packard, Oracle, and Microsoft. Chairman and CEO Edward Caputo owns 52% of the company.

CuraGen Corporation

555 Long Wharf Dr., 11th Fl., New Haven, CT 06511

Telephone: 203-401-3330 **Fax:** 203-401-3333 **Metro area:** New York, NY **Web site:** http://www.curagen.com **Human resources contact:** Jannine Malicki **Sales:** $9.3 million **Number of employees:** 303 **Number of employees for previous year:** 168 **Industry designation:** Biomedical & genetic products **Company type:** Public **Top competitors:** Human Genome Sciences, Inc.; Millennium Pharmaceuticals, Inc.; Incyte Pharmaceuticals, Inc.

CuraGen Corporation wants to cura genetic afflictions. Using proprietary genomics-based research tools, the company focuses on improving agricultural seed production and developing new drugs for such conditions as heart disease, cancer, and diabetes. CuraGen's discovery processes include SeqCalling, a database that can quickly generate coding sequences of a sample's genetic makeup, and GeneCalling, which creates an expression of genetic differences between healthy and diseased samples. Its PathCalling process identifies how proteins interact and is being used to identify possible drug treatments for diseases. CuraGen has alliances with Glaxo Wellcome, Pioneer Hi-Bred International, Genetech, Biogen, and Dupont.

Dexter Corporation

One Elm St., Windsor Locks, CT 06096

Telephone: 860-292-7675 **Fax:** 860-292-7673 **Metro area:** Hartford, CT **Web site:** http://www.dexelec.com **Human resources contact:** Lawrence McClure **Sales:** $1.2 billion **Number of employees:** 5,000 **Number of employees for previous year:** 4,800 **Industry designation:** Chemicals—specialty **Company type:** Public **Top competitors:** H.B. Fuller Company; The Valspar Corporation; Minnesota Mining and Manufacturing Company

A maker of specialty materials for the aerospace, electronics, food packaging, and medical industries, Dexter is the oldest company listed on the NYSE. Aerospace products include adhesives used in aircraft construction. The electronics division makes epoxy molding materials for the protection, packaging, and assembly of electronic and electrical components. In addition, the company is a magnate of magnets: It makes more permanent magnets and assemblies than any other company in the US. Life Technologies (in which Dexter owns 71%) produces culture media, animal serum, and reagent supplements products used to grow and study cells. Dexter has sold its food packaging unit to Valspar.

DIANON Systems, Inc.

200 Watson Blvd., Stratford, CT 06497

Telephone: 203-381-4000 **Fax:** 203-381-4079 **Metro area:** New York, NY **Web site:** http://www.dianon.com **Human resources contact:** Theresa Fereira **Sales:** $62.2 million **Number of employees:** 502 **Number of employees for previous year:** 429 **Industry designation:** Medical services **Company type:** Public **Top competitors:** Quest Diagnostics Incorporated; Laboratory Corporation of America Holdings; SmithKline Beecham plc

Doctors throughout the US send blood, tissue, cell, and urine samples to DIANON Systems for testing and diagnosis. DIANON Systems' two anatomical pathology and clinical chemistry laboratories can test for nearly all types of cancers and many chronic and genetic diseases. The company purchases or licenses new diagnostic technologies from test developers, then markets its services to about 50,000 physicians in oncology, urology, dermatology, gynecology, and gastroenterology. DIANON Systems also has a program that assists developers in commercializing new tests. Director G. S. Beckwith Gilbert owns nearly 27% of the company.

Electronic Retailing Systems International, Inc.

488 Main Ave., Norwalk, CT 06851

Telephone: 203-849-2500 **Fax:** 203-849-2501 **Metro area:** New York, NY **Web site:** http://www.ersi.com **Human resources contact:** Virginia Menz **Sales:** $3.8 million **Number of employees:** 122 **Number of employees for previous year:** 89 **Industry designation:** Computers—peripheral equipment **Company type:** Public **Top competitors:** Telepanel Systems Inc.; NCR Corporation; International Business Machines Corporation

Don't try to put a label on Electronic Retailing Systems International (ERS), the company whose ShelfNet system replaces paper price tags on store shelves with small, easily updated LCD units. ERS's new wireless ShelfNet system is taking the place of its original wired system. ShelfNet combines software, a microwave transmitter, antennas, and shelf-mounted, battery-operated LCD units. Five types of shelf units are offered to accommodate various fixture types, such as freezers. ShelfNet software installs on a PC or store processors and ties into the check-out scanner system for accurate pricing. Customers include A&P and Kmart. Systems may be purchased or leased under the company's Save-As-You-Go plan.

FactSet Research Systems Inc.

One Greenwich Plaza, Greenwich, CT 06830

Telephone: 203-863-1500 **Fax:** 203-863-1501 **Metro area:** New York, NY **Web site:** http://www.factset.com **Human resources contact:** Daniel A. Viens **Sales:** $78.9 million **Number of employees:** 265 **Number of employees for previous year:** 193 **Industry designation:** Computers—online services **Company type:** Public **Top competitors:** IDD Information Services; Track Data Corporation; Datastream Systems, Inc.

FactSet provides more than 100 databases of online financial information from more than 30 sources, including EDGAR SEC filings, Compustat, Interactive Data, and First Call. Subscribers can manipulate and analyze data ranging from federal securities filings to historical financial statistics using FactSet's proprietary software. Users pay a monthly fixed fee for access to the services, or they pay in the form of commissions on securities transactions directed to the firm's FactSet Data Systems unit. FactSet has offices in Hong Kong, London, Sydney, Tokyo, and the US. Chairman and CEO Howard Wille and president and chief technology officer Charles Snyder each own about 20% of the company.

FlexiInternational Software, Inc.

2 Enterprise Dr., Shelton, CT 06484

Telephone: 203-925-3040 **Fax:** 203-925-3044 **Metro area:** New York, NY **Web site:** http://www.flexi.com **Human resources contact:** Rosemarie Ferraro **Sales:** $30.2 million **Number of employees:** 139 **Number of employees for previous year:** 138 **Industry designation:** Computers—corporate, professional & financial software **Company type:** Public **Top competitors:** Oracle Corporation; PeopleSoft, Inc.; SAP AG

FlexiInternational Software crunches numbers with its sophisticated financial and accounting software. The company's Flexi line of software (FlexiFinancials, FlexiInfoSuite, and FlexiTools) provides a complete array of financial applications, a family of reporting and workflow applications, and tools for customization and development. Products can be fully integrated or used on a stand-alone basis. FlexiInternational Software's products support technologies such as the Internet and corporate intranets. The company has nine sales offices in the US and one in the UK. Its customers include banks, insurance companies, and health care and technology organizations.

Hartford Life, Inc.

200 Hopmeadow St., Simsbury, CT 06089

Telephone: 860-843-7716 **Fax:** 860-843-3528 **Metro area:** Hartford, CT **Web site:** http://www.thehartford.com **Human resources contact:** Ann M. de Raismes **Sales:** $5.8 billion **Number of employees:** 4,000 **Number of employees for previous year:** 3,727 **Industry designation:** Insurance—life **Company type:** Public **Parent company:** The Hartford Financial Services Group Inc. **Top competitors:** Massachusetts Mutual Life Insurance Company; American General Financial Group; John Hancock Mutual Life Insurance Company

Oh, dear, we need to save for our retirement. Hartford Life is the top seller of individual annuities in the US. The company offers a wide variety of variable and adjustable annuities and other retirement savings products, including such high-profile mutual fund families as Wellington, Putnam, and Dean Witter Morgan Stanley. It also provides individual life insurance and employee benefits products, including group life and disability insurance. Hartford sells its products through independent agents, securities brokers, and banks. The Hartford Financial Services Group, a property/casualty company that spun off Hartford Life, owns 81% of the company.

Hexcel Corporation

2 Stamford Plaza, 281 Tresser Blvd., Stamford, CT 06901

Telephone: 203-969-0666 **Fax:** 203-358-3993 **Metro area:** New York, NY **Web site:** http://www.hexcel.com **Human resources contact:** Jim Conzen **Sales:** $1.1 billion **Number of employees:** 5,597 **Number of employees for previous year:** 5,013 **Industry designation:** Chemicals—fibers **Company type:** Public **Top competitors:** Cade Industries, Inc.; Zoltek Companies, Inc.; Cytec Industries Inc.

The first footprints on the moon didn't come from Neil Armstrong, but from Hexcel. A maker of advanced composite materials, Hexcel made the footpads on the Apollo ll lunar module. Hexcel's fibers and fabrics are now used to make printed circuit boards, window blinds, and bullet-resistant vests. Its composite materials also are used in snowboards, golf clubs, and athletic shoes. Engineered products by Hexcel go into aircraft components, overhead storage compartments, and lavatories. The commercial aerospace industry accounts for 64% of sales. Hexcel operates manufacturing facilities in the US and Europe. Ciba Specialty Chemicals Holding of Switzerland owns almost half of the company.

International Telecommunication Data Systems, Inc.

225 High Ridge Rd., Stamford, CT 06905

Telephone: 203-329-3300 **Fax:** 203-323-1314 **Metro area:** New York, NY **Web site:** http://www.itds.com **Human resources contact:** Susan Vickers **Sales:** $115.5 million **Number of employees:** 539 **Number of employees for previous year:** 188 **Industry designation:** Computers—corporate, professional & financial software **Company type:** Public **Top competitors:** LHS Group Inc.; ALLTEL Corporation; Cincinnati Bell Inc.

International Telecommunication Data Systems (ITDS) builds and services flexible billing systems for the cellular telephone industry and for other wireless and satellite telecommunication providers. The company's software enables clients to offer many features to cellular phone customers at different rates, then use the billing information for marketing and sales plans. ITDS's products are also used for service activation, credit analysis, collections, and inventory management. The systems support the two predominant cellular protocols (AMPS and GSM) and are used to provide service to more than a million subscribers. Customers include Aliant Communications, Nextel, and MCI WorldCom.

Lexington Healthcare Group, Inc.

1577 New Britain Ave., Farmington, CT 06052

Telephone: 860-674-2700 **Fax:** 860-674-5900 **Metro area:** Hartford, CT **Human resources contact:** David O. Bond **Sales:** $58.3 million **Number of employees:** 1,294 **Number of employees for previous year:** 1,200 **Industry designation:** Nursing homes **Company type:** Public **Top competitors:** Beverly Enterprises, Inc.; Sun Healthcare Group, Inc.; Mariner Post-Acute Network, Inc.

Some senior citizens find their old Kentucky home not in the Bluegrass State, but in one of Lexington Healthcare Group's nursing and sub-acute care homes in Connecticut and Massachusetts; the firm owns or manages 11 facilities. Subsidiary Balz Medical Services provides medical supplies, linens, nutritional supplements, and similar supplies to affiliated and nonaffiliated nursing homes. Professional Relief Nurses offers nursing and related services to homebound patients, hospitals, and other care facilities. Acquisitive Lexington Healthcare also has joint ventures that offer rehabilitation, pharmacy, and psychological services to nursing homes. Chairman and CEO Jack Friedler owns about half of the company.

Lifecodes Corporation

550 West Ave., Stamford, CT 06902

Telephone: 203-328-9500 **Fax:** 203-328-9599 **Metro area:** New York, NY **Web site:** http://www.lifecodes.com **Human resources contact:** Kelly Knobel **Sales:** $22.8 million (Est.) **Number of employees:** 170 **Number of employees for previous year:** 75 **Industry designation:** Biomedical & genetic products **Company type:** Private **Top competitors:** Laboratory Corporation of America Holdings; Affymetrix, Inc.; Abbott Laboratories

Lifecodes can read the bar codes that make you who you are. The company provides DNA testing services, including paternity testing, forensic identification, and transplant compatibility testing. The acquisitive company also makes and sells DNA testing products, including reagents and DNA probes, which are sold as standardized test kits. Subsidiary Cellmark regularly provides forensic DNA identification and expert DNA testimony in criminal cases nationwide (think O. J. and JonBenet). Lifecodes' transplant tests identify genetic sequencing in DNA; this helps to determine whether a donor's bone marrow or organ transplant will be rejected by the recipient. The firm provides services in the US and Europe.

Life Re Corporation

969 High Ridge Rd., Stamford, CT 06905

Telephone: 203-321-3000 **Fax:** 203-329-8635 **Metro area:** New York, NY **Human resources contact:** Donna McCabe **Sales:** $645.8 million **Number of employees:** 128 **Number of employees for previous year:** 123 **Industry designation:** Insurance—life **Company type:** Subsidiary

Life Re, a subsidiary of Swiss Reinsurance, provides reinsurance for life and health risks in the US and Canada. The company and subsidiary TexasRe Life Insurance, which in turn owns Life Reassurance Corporation of America, cover a portfolio of group life, group health, special risk insurance, and ordinary life insurance products, including term, universal, and whole life. Life Re reinsures mortality and morbidity risks associated with life insurance products. Life Re also reinsures investment-related risks for universal life products. The company writes reinsurance on a direct basis with primary life insurance companies and does not write primary insurance or surplus relief reinsurance.

Loctite Corporation

10 Columbus Blvd., Hartford, CT 06106

Telephone: 860-520-5000 **Fax:** 860-520-5073 **Metro area:** Hartford, CT **Web site:** http://www.loctite.com **Human resources contact:** Bruce Vakiener **Sales:** $788.9 million **Number of employees:** 4,725 **Number of employees for previous year:** 4,300 **Industry designation:** Chemicals—specialty **Company type:** Subsidiary **Parent company:** Henkel KGaA **Top competitors:** Imperial Chemical Industries PLC; Borden, Inc.; H.B. Fuller Company

It's always a sticky situation for Loctite, a leading maker of super glue (cyanoacrylates). The company sells its sealants, adhesives, and coatings for the auto aftermarket, industrial markets and retail sale in more than 80 countries in Europe, Asia, and the Americas. Loctite's products help "keep things together" in a diverse lineup of items that include compact disc players, computers, cosmetics, airplanes, automobiles, syringes, speakers, and vacuum cleaners. The company is a wholly owned subsidiary of Henkel KGaA, a German manufacturer of chemicals, detergents, adhesives, and cosmetics. Loctite is selling its automotive aftermarket business to Automotive Performance Group.

MacDermid, Incorporated

245 Freight St., Waterbury, CT 06702

Telephone: 203-575-5700 **Fax:** 203-575-5630 **Metro area:** Waterbury, CT **Web site:** http://www.macd.com **Human resources contact:** Gary St. Pierre **Sales:** $314.1 million **Number of employees:** 1,200 **Number of employees for previous year:** 1,086 **Industry designation:** Chemicals—specialty **Company type:** Public **Top competitors:** Engelhard Corporation; OM Group, Inc.; LeaRonal, Inc.

Called "Clan MacDermid" by its management, this specialty chemicals company (founded by a Scotsman) has grown bigger than several pairs of britches. MacDermid makes more than 1,000 proprietary chemical compounds used in metal and plastics finishing, electronics, and graphic arts. Its products are used to activate, polish, electroplate, strip, and coat metal surfaces, among other applications. MacDermid also offers horizontal processing equipment used in the production of printed circuit boards and distributes others' chemicals. It has operations in 19 countries. Chairman Emeritus Harold Leever and his family, including son and CEO Daniel, own about 21% of MacDermid.

Magellan Petroleum Corporation

149 Durham Rd., Oak Park, Unit 31, Madison, CT 06443

Telephone: 203-245-7664 **Metro area:** New York, NY **Web site:** http://www.magpet.com **Sales:** $15.3 million **Number of employees:** 34 **Number of employees for previous year:** 33 **Industry designation:** Oil & gas—exploration & production **Company type:** Public **Top competitors:** Santos Ltd; Canada Southern Petroleum Ltd.; Woodside Petroleum Ltd.

Magellan Petroleum has gone around the world to explore and develop oil and gas reserves. It operates primarily through its majority-owned Magellan Petroleum Australia Limited (MPAL), a publicly traded Australian company. MPAL's chief assets are its interests in the Mereenie oil and gas field and the Palm Valley gas field in the Amadeus Basin in Australia's Northern Territory. It has proved reserves of 85 billion cu. ft. of natural gas and 915,000 barrels of oil. MPAL's main customer is the Northern Territory's Power and Water Authority. MPAL and Magellan Petroleum also own interests in oil and gas properties in Tapia Canyon, California; the Gladden Basin, Belize; and the southeastern Yukon Territory, Canada.

netValue Holdings, Inc.

1960 Bronson Rd., Bldg. 2, Fairfield, CT 06430

Telephone: 203-319-7000 **Fax:** 203-254-9815 **Metro area:** New York, NY **Web site:** http://www.netvalueinc.com **Human resources contact:** Craig Zalinsky **Number of employees:** 23 **Industry designation:** Computers—online services **Company type:** Public **Top competitors:** Super Coups Network; Money Mailer Holdings Inc.; Catalina Marketing Corporation

Why wait for the Sunday paper for a chance to clip coupons? netValue Holdings provides bargain hunters the opportunity to print coupons directly from the Internet. Through the development-stage company's primary product, CouponsOnline, consumer goods manufacturers, retailers, and other businesses can offer coupons and promotional items from their Web sites. The company also offers AisleManager, which provides additional features (sorting, multiple printing, bulk loading) for high-volume users of CouponsOnline. A shakeup in management has caused netValue Holdings to put IPO plans on hold.

Neurogen Corporation

35 NE Industrial Rd., Branford, CT 06405

Telephone: 203-488-8201 **Fax:** 203-483-8651 **Metro area:** New York, NY **Web site:** http://www.neurogen.com **Human resources contact:** Christina Marks **Sales:** $11.1 million **Number of employees:** 148 **Number of employees for previous year:** 130 **Industry designation:** Drugs **Company type:** Public

Neurogen Corporation is a developmental stage pharmaceuticals company. The company discovers and develops therapeutic products that treat psychiatric and neurological disorders by regulating nerve cell communications in the brain. Specifically, Neurogen believes it can capitalize on advances in molecular biology, medicinal chemistry, and neurobiology to produce a new generation of psychotherapeutics for treating anxiety, psychosis, epilepsy, dementia, sleep and stress disorders, obesity, and depression. The company has a collaborative research agreement with pharmaceutical company Pfizer to develop antianxiety drug NGD-91, which Pfizer intends to market as a treatment for anxiety in household pets.

Novametrix Medical Systems Inc.

5 Technology Dr., Wallingford, CT 06492

Telephone: 203-265-7701 **Fax:** 203-284-0753 **Other address:** PO Box 690, Wallingford, CT 06492 **Metro area:** New York, NY **Web site:** http://www.novametrix.com **Human resources contact:** Lorraine Tagliatela **Sales:** $31.6 million **Number of employees:** 200 **Number of employees for previous year:** 189 **Industry designation:** Medical instruments **Company type:** Public **Top competitors:** Vital Signs, Inc.; Allied Healthcare Products, Inc.; Mallinckrodt Inc.

Novametrix Medical Systems' products let medical personnel keep tabs on patients in operating rooms and intensive-care units; the company's monitors and sensors are also used in outpatient clinics, nursing homes, and other health care facilities. Among the company's products are noninvasive, continuous monitors and sensors that measure exhaled carbon dioxide levels, determine blood oxygen levels, and monitor oxygen and carbon dioxide levels through the skin. Other monitors measure pressure, flow, and volume in patients' airways and lungs. Novametrix Medical Systems assembles its products from components made by third parties and sells them in more than 75 countries.

Open Solutions Inc.

300 Winding Brook Dr., Glastonbury, CT 06033

Telephone: 860-652-3155 **Fax:** 860-652-3156 **Metro area:** Hartford, CT **Web site:** http://www.opensolutions.com **Human resources contact:** Lauren Wright **Sales:** $6.6 million (Est.) **Number of employees:** 121 **Industry designation:** Computers—corporate, professional & financial software **Company type:** Private **Top competitors:** Electronic Data Systems Corporation; Fiserv, Inc.; ALLTEL Corporation

Processing problems? Open Solutions' software supports deposits and loans, teller functions, home-based Internet banking, and platform automation for midsized banks and credit unions. The company makes OSI System software that is also used for third-party functions such as check processing, automated teller machine transactions, and general ledger applications. Open Solutions sells its software through its direct sales force, primarily to banks and credit unions in the Northeast. The cost of the OSI System ranges from about $140,000 to $1.5 million. The company also provides training and support services for its software.

The Perkin-Elmer Corporation

761 Main Ave., Norwalk, CT 06859

Telephone: 203-762-1000 **Fax:** 203-762-6000 **Metro area:** New York, NY **Web site:** http://www.perkin-elmer.com **Human resources contact:** Rafael Garofalo **Sales:** $1.5 billion **Number of employees:** 7,188 **Number of employees for previous year:** 5,685 **Industry designation:** Instruments—scientific **Company type:** Public **Top competitors:** Bio-Rad Laboratories, Inc.; Waters Corporation; Incyte Pharmaceuticals, Inc.

If you are exploring the latest frontiers, Perkin-Elmer has some of the tools you may need. The firm makes life science systems (60% of sales) for use in AIDS research, in crime labs, and for mapping human genes. Its products are used in the pharmaceutical, food, environmental testing, agriculture, biotechnology, and chemical manufacturing industries. The company also makes analytical instruments such as gas and liquid chromatographs, spectrometers, and laboratory information management systems, but it is selling that division to screening instrument maker EG&G Inc. Joint venture Celera Genomics is developing gene and related medical information. About 60% of the company's sales come from outside the US.

Phoenix Home Life Mutual Insurance Company

One American Row, Hartford, CT 06102

Telephone: 860-403-5000 **Fax:** 860-403-5855 **Other address:** PO Box 5056, Hartford, CT 06102 **Metro area:** Hartford, CT **Web site:** http://www.phl.com **Human resources contact:** Ann Cowen **Sales:** $3.6 billion **Number of employees:** 4,138 **Number of employees for previous year:** 3,972 **Industry designation:** Insurance—life **Company type:** Mutual company **Top competitors:** Metropolitan Life Insurance Company; The Prudential Insurance Company of America; New York Life Insurance Company

Phoenix Home Life Mutual Insurance Company, formed in the 1992 merger of Phoenix Mutual and Home Life, is one of the top 10 US mutual life insurance firms. Owned by 3.3 million policyholders, the firm sells individual and group insurance and annuities, employee benefit programs, reinsurance, and such investment products as mutual funds and variable annuities. Through publicly traded Phoenix Investment Partners, the firm offers investment management services; other subsidiaries sell trust services (Phoenix Charter Oak Trust), real estate (Phoenix Realty Group), and administrative services (Financial Administrative Services). Property/casualty insurer American Phoenix is being sold to Hilb, Rogal and Hamilton.

Playtex Products, Inc.

300 Nyala Farms Rd., Westport, CT 06880

Telephone: 203-341-4000 **Fax:** 203-341-4260 **Metro area:** New York, NY **Web site:** http://www.playtexproductsinc.com **Human resources contact:** Frank M. Sanchez **Sales:** $669.6 million **Number of employees:** 1,945 **Number of employees for previous year:** 1,640 **Industry designation:** Cosmetics & toiletries **Company type:** Public **Top competitors:** Evenflo Company, Inc.; Unilever PLC; The Procter & Gamble Company

Messy kids are great for Playtex Products. The infant- and personal care company makes Playtex Spill-Proof cups (#1 with 70% of the market), disposable nursers, hard bottles, and pacifiers, as well as the Diaper Genie diaper disposal system. Its largest brand is Playtex tampons, which generate 40% of sales. The company makes Woolite rug and upholstery cleaner, household and industrial gloves under the names Playtex Living and Handsaver, Banana Boat and BioSun sunblock and suntan lotion, and Tek toothbrushes. Playtex operates about 20 manufacturing and distribution facilities in Canada, Puerto Rico, and the US. Chairman Robert Haas owns 33% of the company; investors led by banker Richard Blum own 20%.

PrimeEnergy Corporation

One Landmark Sq., Stamford, CT 06901

Telephone: 203-358-5700 **Fax:** 203-358-5786 **Metro area:** New York, NY **Human resources contact:** Virginia Crowe **Sales:** $28.6 million **Number of employees:** 173 **Number of employees for previous year:** 169 **Industry designation:** Oil & gas—exploration & production **Company type:** Public **Top competitors:** The Houston Exploration Company; Cabot Oil & Gas Corporation; Venus Exploration, Inc.

PrimeEnergy hopes to keep the pump primed with its oil and gas exploration and production activities, which take place primarily in Texas, Oklahoma, and West Virginia. Its PrimeEnergy Management unit is the managing general partner in 51 oil and gas limited partnerships. Through subsidiaries Prime Operating and Eastern Oil Well Service, PrimeEnergy operates more than 1,700 oil and gas wells in which the company and its affiliates hold interests. Subsidiary Southwest Oilfield Construction provides site preparation and construction services for PrimeEnergy and third parties. CEO Charles Drimal owns 23% of the company, which has proved reserves of 1.4 million barrels of oil and 16.7 billion cu. ft. of gas.

Reunion Industries, Inc.

62 Southfield Ave., One Stamford Landing, Stamford, CT 06902

Telephone: 203-324-8858 **Fax:** 203-967-3923 **Metro area:** New York, NY **Human resources contact:** Richard L. Evans **Sales:** $97.3 million **Number of employees:** 1,074 **Number of employees for previous year:** 1,060 **Industry designation:** Rubber & plastic products **Company type:** Public **Top competitors:** Siegel-Robert Inc.; International Smart Sourcing, Inc.; Plastronics Plus

If plastics and grapes can come together in a business plan, then Reunion Industries is aptly named. The company, through Oneida Rostone, makes precision plastic components for makers of business machines, telecommunications and computer equipment, and recreational products. The company is also engaged in the production of wine grapes in the Napa Valley. From 1992 to 1997 Reunion also worked in oil and gas exploration and production, before it attempted to sell its Reunion Energy unit to Bargo Energy. Bargo successfully sued Reunion for breach of contract in 1998, a move that scuttled the sale. Industrial parts maker Chatwins Group owns 38% of Reunion.

Scan-Optics, Inc.

169 Progress Dr., Manchester, CT 06040

Telephone: 860-645-7878 **Fax:** 860-645-7995 **Metro area:** Hartford, CT **Web site:** http://www.scanoptics.com **Human resources contact:** Marianna C. Emanuelson **Sales:** $54 million **Number of employees:** 339 **Number of employees for previous year:** 324 **Industry designation:** Optical character recognition **Company type:** Public **Top competitors:** BancTec, Inc.; Symbol Technologies, Inc.; National Computer Systems, Inc.

Scan-Optics has moved from a simple scan operation to a full-fledged information laundering company. The company makes data processing and image scanning systems used to process health care, government, and order forms; shareholder proxies; automobile registrations; credit card slips; time cards; and other documents. The company's customers include health care organizations, subscriptions and catalog fulfillment companies, government agencies, manufacturers, and financial institutions. Scan-Optics also offers services, which account for about one-quarter of revenues. Japanese office equipment distributor Toyo Officemation accounts for 39% of sales.

SS&C Technologies, Inc.

80 Lamberton Rd., Windsor, CT 06095

Telephone: 860-298-4500 **Fax:** 860-298-4900 **Metro area:** Hartford, CT **Web site:** http://www.ssctech.com **Human resources contact:** Rodly Millet **Sales:** $69.8 million **Number of employees:** 457 **Number of employees for previous year:** 318 **Industry designation:** Computers—corporate, professional & financial software **Company type:** Public **Top competitors:** SunGard Data Systems Inc.; DST Systems, Inc.; State Street Corporation

SS&C Technologies makes software that helps clients analyze and manage large amounts of complex investment information. Its programs let users organize and price assets and liabilities, manage asset and mortgage loan portfolios, and process orders on an automated basis. The firm sells its software to insurance companies, government agencies, banks, asset managers, and other financial services organizations throughout the world. Customers include Citibank, The Bank of New York, Scudder Kemper Investments, and Liberty Mutual Group. SS&C also provides consulting services in conjunction with its products. Founder and CEO William Stone owns about a third of the company.

Titan Sports, Inc.

1241 E. Main St., Titan Towers, Stamford, CT 06905

Telephone: 203-352-8600 **Fax:** 203-353-2808 **Metro area:** New York, NY **Web site:** http://www.wwf.com **Human resources contact:** Matt DeLuca **Sales:** $500 million (Est.) **Number of employees:** 300 **Industry designation:** Leisure & recreational services **Company type:** Private **Top competitors:** Time Warner Inc.; National Basketball Association; National Football League

Are you ready to rumble? If so, Titan Sports has the action you need. The company owns the World Wrestling Federation (WWF), which produces and promotes wrestling matches around the country. It also produces the popular "Raw is War" program for USA Networks as well as pay-per-view events. The company, founded in 1982 to promote the WWF, licenses merchandise based on its characters, who include Stone Cold Steve Austin, The Undertaker, and Kane. In addition, Titan Sports has purchased the Las Vegas-based Debbie Reynolds Hotel & Casino; it plans to convert the property into a wrestling-themed casino. Chairman Vince McMahon's grandfather founded the WWF in 1963. The McMahon family owns Titan Sports.

Tosco Corporation

72 Cummings Point Rd., Stamford, CT 06902

Telephone: 203-977-1000 **Fax:** 203-964-3187 **Metro area:** New York, NY **Web site:** http://www.tosco.com **Human resources contact:** Wanda Williams **Sales:** $12 billion **Number of employees:** 26,200 **Number of employees for previous year:** 24,300 **Industry designation:** Oil refining & marketing **Company type:** Public **Top competitors:** The Southland Corporation; Ultramar Diamond Shamrock Corporation; Sunoco, Inc.

Tosco is the US's leading independent oil refiner and petroleum marketer, ahead of Ultramar Diamond Shamrock and Sunoco. The company owns Circle K (the #2 convenience store chain in the US) and is the leading operator of company-controlled convenience stores. It operates more than 5,200 US stores, including about 2,500 Circle K outlets located primarily in the Sunbelt. Other retail stores operate under the BP, 76, and Exxon brand names. Tosco has eight refineries in California, New Jersey, Pennsylvania, and Washington. The company is beginning polypropylene production in a joint venture with Union Carbide.

TSI International Software Ltd.

45 Danbury Rd., Wilton, CT 06897

Telephone: 203-761-8600 **Fax:** 203-762-9677 **Metro area:** New York, NY **Web site:** http://www.tsisoft.com **Human resources contact:** Ann Curry **Sales:** $45.3 million **Number of employees:** 298 **Number of employees for previous year:** 173 **Industry designation:** Computers—corporate, professional & financial software **Company type:** Public **Top competitors:** Active Software, Inc.; BEA Systems, Inc.; New Era of Networks, Inc.

TSI International Software wants your data to come together ... right now. The company's interfacing software integrates seemingly disparate applications within an organization and from external businesses. Its flagship Mercator line integrates data between applications and creates complete data transformations, while its Trading Partner software lets customers communicate with business partners through direct connections, value-added networks, or the Internet. TSI also supports its legacy KEY/MASTER data entry software, and offers support services. Customers include General Motors, Citibank, IBM, and Nestle. In 1999 TSI bought Braid Group, one of the UK's leading financial-transaction software firms.

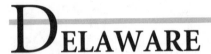

DELAWARE

Christiana Care Corporation

501 W. 14th St., Wilmington, DE 19801

Telephone: 302-733-1000 **Fax:** 302-733-1313 **Metro area:** Philadelphia, PA **Web site:** http://www.christianacare.org **Human resources contact:** Ben Shaw **Sales:** $616 million (Est.) **Number of employees:** 8,500 **Industry designation:** Hospitals **Company type:** Private **Top competitors:** Catholic Health East; Helix/Medlantic; Bon Secours Health System, Inc.

Christiana Care hopes its patients are patient with all of the company's name changes. Formerly the Medical Center of Delaware (with several other operational unit names melded into it), the integrated health care network serves patients in Delaware and surrounding areas of Pennsylvania, Maryland, and New Jersey. The company's Wilmington and Christiana hospitals—which together have 1,000 beds—serve more than 35,000 patients annually. The network, which offers managed-care plans, also includes family practice, preventive medicine, physical therapy, extended care, home health care, and other services. The network sponsors a residency program and is affiliated with other local and regional hospitals.

ICI Americas Inc.

Concord Plaza, 3411 Silverside Rd., Wilmington, DE 19850

Telephone: 302-887-3000 **Fax:** 302-887-1367 **Metro area:** Philadelphia, PA **Web site:** http://www.icinorthamerica.com **Human resources contact:** D.I. Hartnett **Number of employees:** 23,443 **Industry designation:** Chemicals—diversified **Company type:** Subsidiary **Parent company:** Imperial Chemical Industries PLC **Top competitors:** M. A. Hanna Company; Spartech Corporation; Cabot Corporation

ICI Americas cooks a witch's brew of useful chemicals. A subsidiary of the ICI Group, ICI Americas is one of the largest chemical companies in the US. ICI Americas' nearly 100 facilities churn out concoctions such as coatings, polyester, explosives, tioxide, acrylics, polyurethane, fragrances, and food products. The coating division makes popular brands of paints, such as Glidden and Devoe, for sale at company-owned (nearly 500) and independent paint stores. It also makes adhesives (Liquid Nails), caulks, and sealants. ICI Americas, like its parent, is selling and buying assets to move from the bulk chemical sector to the lighter specialty segment of the chemical industry.

Strategic Diagnostics Inc.

111 Pencader Dr., Newark, DE 19702

Telephone: 302-456-6789 **Fax:** 302-456-6770 **Other address:** PO Box 14063, Research Triangle Park, NC 27709 **Metro area:** Philadelphia, PA **Web site:** http://www.sdix.com **Sales:** $15.7 million **Number of employees:** 107 **Number of employees for previous year:** 105 **Industry designation:** Pollution control equipment & services **Company type:** Public

Strategic Diagnostics produces immunoassay-based test kits for water quality management, food safety monitoring, crop seed production, and assessment and remediation of contaminated waste sites. Formerly EnSys Environmental Products, the company sells more than 150 types of tests, including those sold under the D TECH, EnSys RIS, RaPID Assay, and EnviroGard brand names. Strategic Diagnostics sells its products to the water quality, industrial testing, and agricultural markets in North and South America, Europe, and Asia. The company also markets its Macra test kit to assess the risk for coronary heart disease.

Townsends Incorporated

Rte. 24 East, Millsboro, DE 19966

Telephone: 302-934-9221 **Fax:** 302-934-3121 **Other address:** PO Box 468, Millsboro, DE 19966 **Web site:** http://www.townsends.com **Human resources contact:** Allison Derickson **Sales:** $530 million (Est.) **Number of employees:** 4,800 **Number of employees for previous year:** 4,500 **Industry designation:** Food—meat products **Company type:** Private **Top competitors:** Gold Kist Inc.; Tyson Foods, Inc.; ConAgra, Inc.

Townsends has a few more feathers in its cap than poultry processing. In addition to producing fresh chicken products (whole birds, parts, boneless breasts, and roasters), the diversified food company refines soybean oil for condiments and produces a line of prepared foods including entrees, desserts, and 30 kinds of soups. John G. Townsend Jr. founded Townsends in the 1890s as a lumber business (his grandson is chairman and CEO). The first vertically integrated poultry company in the US, Townsends has operations in Arkansas, Delaware, Maryland, and North Carolina, and sells its products through major chains and distributors in the US and foreign markets, particularly Asia.

DISTRICT OF COLUMBIA

American Security Inc.

1701 Pennsylvania Ave. NW, Ste. 400, Washington, DC 20006

Telephone: 202-879-2689 **Metro area:** Washington, DC **Sales:** $4,000 (Est.) **Number of employees:** 1 **Industry designation:** Protection—safety equipment & services **Company type:** Private **Top competitors:** Borg-Warner Security Corporation; The Kroll-O'Gara Company; Pinkerton's, Inc.

There's no security like American Security, and company founder David Gladstone believes that the citizens of the land of the free are willing to pay for it. American Security, which is planning to become a national consolidator in the fragmented security industry, has set its sights on acquiring companies engaged in the investigations, consulting, and information aspects of the security market. Gladstone is chairman of American Capital Strategies, a buyout and specialty finance firm, and he has participated in more than 300 company purchases or financings. He owns 15% of American Security.

CAIS Internet, Inc.

1255 22nd St. NW, 4th Fl., Washington, DC 20037

Telephone: 202-715-1300 **Fax:** 202-463-7190 **Metro area:** Washington, DC **Web site:** http://www.cais.com **Human resources contact:** Leslie Harpold **Sales:** $5.3 million (Est.) **Number of employees:** 109 **Industry designation:** Computers—online services **Company type:** Private **Top competitors:** WorldGate Communications, Inc.; 3Com Corporation; uniView Technologies Corporation

CAIS Internet plays with jacks. Plugged into phone lines in apartments and hotels, the jacks are equipped with patented OverVoice technology that creates local area networks (LANs), allowing Internet connections for multiple dwellers. Users can chat on the phone and the Internet at the same time. CAIS has OverVoice connections in about 1,900 apartments and 1,900 hotel rooms and an agreement for a nationwide rollout with Hilton. CAIS also markets digital subscriber line service (high-speed Internet access over phone lines) with Covad Communications and Bell Atlantic (mainly in Washington, DC), as well as dedicated access service to Internet service providers and Web site hosting.

Complete Wellness Centers, Inc.

725 Independence Ave. SE, Washington, DC 20003

Telephone: 202-543-6800 **Fax:** 202-543-5360 **Metro area:** Washington, DC **Web site:** http://www.completewellness.com **Human resources contact:** Dan Holmes **Sales:** $8.8 million **Number of employees:** 400 **Number of employees for previous year:** 147 **Industry designation:** Medical practice management **Company type:** Public **Top competitors:** American HealthChoice, Inc.; HealthTech International, Inc.; Jenny Craig, Inc.

Complete Wellness Centers wants to get physical. The company's subsidiaries develop and manage about 140 integrated medical centers comprised of traditional health care providers such as physicians and physical therapists, and alternative health care providers such as chiropractors, acupuncturists, and massage therapists. Complete Wellness also offers Nutri/System weight loss programs and Smokenders smoking cessation programs. In addition to its patient wellness centers (more than 95% of its sales), the company has two subsidiaries offering administrative services to medical and chiropractic clinics (Complete Billing) and HMOs (Optimum Health Services). Complete Wellness Centers operates across the US.

The Union Labor Life Insurance Company

111 Massachusetts Ave. NW, Washington, DC 20001

Telephone: 202-682-0900 **Fax:** 202-682-7932 **Metro area:** Washington, DC **Human resources contact:** Rick Silas **Sales:** $496 million (Est.) **Number of employees:** 1,426 **Number of employees for previous year:** 1,425 **Industry designation:** Insurance—life **Company type:** Private

The Union Labor Life Insurance Company (ULLICO) is an insurance and financial-services holding company owned by labor unions and related companies. Founded in 1925, the firm serves organized employers, individual union members, and jointly managed trust funds. Its subsidiaries include Union Labor Life Insurance, ULLICO Casualty, Trust Fund Advisors (services for managed trust funds), AMI Capital (multifamily mortgage loans), Zenith Administrators (third-party benefits administrator), and Financial Freedom Senior Funding (reverse mortgages for senior citizens). The company's "J for Jobs" program finances union-built commercial real estate projects.

Washington Wizards

601 F St. NW, Washington, DC 20001

Telephone: 202-661-5000 **Fax:** 202-661-5101 **Metro area:** Washington, DC **Web site:** http://www.nba.com/wizards **Human resources contact:** Kim Whittington **Sales:** $76.5 million (Est.) **Number of employees:** 100 **Industry designation:** Leisure & recreational services **Company type:** Private **Top competitors:** New Jersey Nets; New York Knickerbockers; Miami Heat

As one of the older teams in the NBA, the Washington Wizards know it takes more than magic to win a championship. The team began as the Chicago Packers in 1961, then moved to Baltimore to become the Bullets in 1963. Owner Abe Pollin (who also owns the Washington Capitals hockey team) bought the team in 1964, which became the Washington Bullets in 1974. Led by MVP Wes Unseld (now in the front office), the Bullets won their first and only NBA championship in 1978. Pollin changed the team's name in 1997 as part of an antiviolence campaign. With stars like Rod Strickland and Juwan Howard, the Wizards work their basketball magic in Washington's new MCI Center.

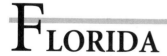

FLORIDA

AAA

1000 AAA Dr., Heathrow, FL 32746

Telephone: 407-444-7000 **Fax:** 407-444-7380 **Metro area:** Orlando, FL **Web site:** http://www.aaa.com **Human resources contact:** Carol Droessler **Sales:** $2.8 billion **Number of employees:** 37,000 **Industry designation:** Leisure & recreational services **Company type:** Not-for-profit

This isn't your father's AAA. The not-for-profit organization (formerly the American Automobile Association) still offers its trademark emergency roadside service to some 30 million stranded motorists yearly, but it has expanded its offerings in recent years to include various financial services as well. AAA Financial Services Corporation offers credit cards, personal loans, vehicle financing, and leasing and deposit services. AAA also sells insurance, operates travel agencies, publishes tour books and maps, and performs public services. Founded in 1902 by nine auto clubs, AAA has grown to include 100 clubs and about 1,000 US and Canadian offices. The organization has about 40 million members.

Amazon Herb Company

1002 Jupiter Park Ln., Ste. 1, Jupiter, FL 33458

Telephone: 561-575-7663 **Fax:** 561-575-7935 **Metro area:** West Palm Beach, FL **Web site:** http://www.rainforestbio.com **Human resources contact:** Connie Lynch **Sales:** $2.5 million (Est.) **Number of employees:** 10 **Number of employees for previous year:** 8 **Industry designation:** Vitamins & nutritional products **Company type:** Private **Top competitors:** Rexall Sundown, Inc.; Herbalife International, Inc.; Sunrider International

Amazon Herb sees green in South America's trees. Under the name Rainforest Bio-Energetics, the company sells herbs and herbal extracts (such as una de gato, a vine bark) through a multilevel marketing network of about 8,000 independent distributors. The company buys raw materials grown primarily in Peru, contracts with third parties to make its products, and packages them under its own label for sale in the US. About 40% of its raw materials are sold to other manufacturers for private-label products. Founded by CEO John Easterling in 1990, the company donates 10% of its net profits for rain forest preservation. After Amazon Herb's planned IPO, Easterling will own 54.5% of the company.

American Bankers Insurance Group, Inc.

11222 Quail Roost Dr., Miami, FL 33157

Telephone: 305-253-2244 **Fax:** 305-252-6947 **Metro area:** Miami, FL **Web site:** http://www.abig.com **Human resources contact:** Phillip Sharkey **Sales:** $1.6 billion **Number of employees:** 3,265 **Number of employees for previous year:** 2,943 **Industry designation:** Insurance—life **Company type:** Public

American Bankers Insurance Group (ABIG) sells wholesale credit-related specialty insurance. Financial institutions, credit card companies, retailers, and automobile and manufactured-housing dealers then retail these policies to consumers. Products include property insurance (on items ranging from mobile homes to appliances), as well as life, unemployment, and disability insurance. Subsidiaries include American Bankers Insurance Company of Florida and American Bankers Life Assurance Co. of Florida, Caribbean American Property Insurance Co., American Reliable Insurance, and Bankers American Life Assurance. In 1998 merger plans with consumer services giant Cendant fell apart, but in 1999 Fortis plans to buy ABIG.

AmeriPath, Inc.

7289 Garden Rd., Ste. 200, River Beach, FL 33404

Telephone: 561-845-1850 **Fax:** 561-845-2498 **Metro area:** West Palm Beach, FL **Web site:** http://www.ameripath.com **Human resources contact:** Stephen V. Fuller **Sales:** $177.3 million **Number of employees:** 1,346 **Number of employees for previous year:** 994 **Industry designation:** Medical practice management **Company type:** Public **Top competitors:** Sheridan Healthcare, Inc.; Medical Manager Corporation; DIANON Systems, Inc.

AmeriPath, the US's largest anatomic pathology practice management company, manages 17 physician practices through subsidiaries and affiliations in eight states in the South and Midwest. Its network of over 130 physicians provides anatomic pathology services, which involve the diagnosis of diseases through the examination of cells and tissues, in both outpatient and hospital laboratories. The company manages the nonmedical aspects of all the practices, including payroll and staffing services, equipment supply, and financial reporting and administration. AmeriPath continues to develop its regional network of practices through acquisitions.

Andrx Corporation

4001 SW 47th Ave., Ste. 201, Fort Lauderdale, FL 33314

Telephone: 954-584-0300 **Fax:** 954-327-5283 **Metro area:** Miami, FL **Web site:** http://www.andrx.com **Human resources contact:** Ann Scarpati **Sales:** $247.1 million **Number of employees:** 527 **Number of employees for previous year:** 384 **Industry designation:** Medical products **Company type:** Public **Top competitors:** Elite Pharmaceuticals, Inc.; Biovail Corporation International

Andrx specializes in timed-release drug delivery systems. The company is developing generic versions of timed-release brand name drugs like Dilacor and Cardizem (both for hypertension and angina). Its version of Dilacor, its first product, is being marketed as Diltia. Andrx is also developing its own brand name versions of existing drugs, using the its timed-release technology. While awaiting FDA approval of its products, the company relies on revenues from its Anda subsidiary, a generic drug distributor. Andrx is a 50% partner in ANCIRC Pharmaceuticals, which develops timed-release bioequivalent drugs. Germany's Hoechst, which makes Cardizem, is paying Andrx $40 million a year not to market its version.

Armor Holdings, Inc.

13386 International Pkwy., Jacksonville, FL 32218

Telephone: 904-741-5400 **Fax:** 904-741-5407 **Metro area:** Jacksonville, FL **Web site:** http://www.armorholdings.com **Human resources contact:** Jennifer Gouin **Sales:** $97.2 million **Number of employees:** 2,834 **Number of employees for previous year:** 1,830 **Industry designation:** Protection—safety equipment & services **Company type:** Public **Top competitors:** Group 4 Securitas (International) BV; Wackenhut Corporation; Pinkerton's, Inc.

Its finances aren't bullet-proof, but many of its products are. Armor Holdings provides security products and services worldwide. Under the name American Body Armor & Equipment, it makes such items as bullet- and projectile-resistant clothing, bomb-disposal suits, and letter-bomb suppression packages. Subsidiary NIK Public Safety produces portable narcotic identification kits, restraints, evidence tape, and other law enforcement paraphernalia. Subsidiary Defense Technology makes nonlethal devices including rubber bullets, pepper sprays, and flameless expulsion grenades. Armor Holdings' Federal Laboratories unit makes MACE spray. The company also offers security consultancy services and installs alarm systems.

Autonomous Technologies Corporation

2800 Discovery Dr., Orlando, FL 32826

Telephone: 407-384-1600 **Fax:** 407-384-1699 **Metro area:** Orlando, FL **Web site:** http://www.autonomous.com **Human resources contact:** Roz Palmiere **Sales:** $200,000 **Number of employees:** 88 **Number of employees for previous year:** 62 **Industry designation:** Medical instruments **Company type:** Public **Top competitors:** Coherent, Inc.; VISX, Incorporated; Summit Technology, Inc.

Autonomous Technologies, which is being acquired by Summit Technology, applies the missile-tracking technology it developed for the Pentagon's "Star Wars" program to attack a new enemy: nearsightedness. The company is developing equipment for photorefractive keratectomy (PRK) laser surgery in which a weak laser beam removes tiny layers of tissue and sculpts the cornea to improve sight. First-generation systems for PRK surgery required that patients' eyes remain still, but the Autonomous LADARVision system is designed to track a patient's slightest involuntary eye movement. The company is in a partnership with CIBA Vision, a subsidiary of Swiss drug maker Novartis, to commercialize its technology.

Baptist Health Systems of South Florida

6855 Red Rd., Coral Gables, FL 33143

Telephone: 305-273-2555 **Fax:** 305-273-2556 **Metro area:** Miami, FL **Web site:** http://www.baptisthealth.net **Human resources contact:** Carl Gustafson **Sales:** $1 billion **Number of employees:** 7,503 **Number of employees for previous year:** 7,200 **Industry designation:** Hospitals **Company type:** Not-for-profit **Top competitors:** HEALTHSOUTH Corporation; Catholic Health East; Columbia/HCA Healthcare Corporation

Baptist Health Systems of South Florida is a not-for-profit health care organization comprised of five hospitals in the Miami area. A provider for about 30 health plans, Baptist Health offers a wide range of services including a comprehensive cancer program, pediatric services, addiction treatment, outpatient services, and home care. With more than 1,000 hospital beds and about 1,000 physicians, Baptist Health was lined up to merge with Catholic organization Mercy Health System of Miami; the deal was called off in 1998 when Baptist Health refused to stop offering abortions at one of its hospitals.

Bentley Pharmaceuticals, Inc.

2 Urban Center, Ste. 400, Tampa, FL 33609

Telephone: 813-281-0961 **Fax:** 813-282-8941 **Metro area:** Tampa-St. Petersburg, FL **Web site:** http://www.bentleypharm.com **Human resources contact:** Terri Kaiser **Sales:** $15.2 million **Number of employees:** 141 **Number of employees for previous year:** 122 **Industry designation:** Drugs **Company type:** Public **Top competitors:** Merck & Co., Inc.; Medeva PLC; Schering-Plough Corporation

Bentley Pharmaceuticals makes, licenses, and distributes drugs primarily in Spain. The company's pharmaceuticals (including Belmazol, Controlvas, Belmalax, Loperamida, Finedal, Lactoliofil, Acyclovir and Senioral) treat cardiovascular, gastrointestinal, respiratory and neurological problems, as well as infectious diseases and obesity. Additionally, the company sells disposable linens to emergency care providers and ambulance services in the US. Bentley sold its French Chimos/LBF subsidiary after sales significantly dropped. The company is expanding into South America and other European markets outside Spain.

BMJ Medical Management, Inc.

4800 N. Federal Hwy., Ste. 101E, Boca Raton, FL 33431

Telephone: 561-391-1311 **Fax:** 561-391-1389 **Metro area:** West Palm Beach, FL **Web site:** http://www.bmji.com **Human resources contact:** Meg Finnegan **Sales:** $37 million **Number of employees:** 845 **Number of employees for previous year:** 555 **Industry designation:** Medical practice management **Company type:** Public

BMJ Medical Management provides medical practice management services to physicians involved in musculoskeletal care. It provides nonmedical management, administrative, and development services including billing, payroll, legal services, and marketing. The company is affiliated with about 30 physician practices comprising more than 180 physicians, the majority of whom are orthopedic surgeons, in Arizona, California, Florida, New Jersey, Pennsylvania, and Texas. BMJ, like the rest of the physician practice management industry, is working to pull out of a slump by establishing ancillary services (including ambulatory surgery centers, physical therapy centers, MRI facilities, and mobile units) to boost revenues.

Cardiac Control Systems, Inc.

3 Commerce Blvd., Palm Coast, FL 32164

Telephone: 904-445-5450 **Fax:** 904-445-7226 **Metro area:** Daytona Beach, FL **Web site:** http://www.ccspace.com **Human resources contact:** Janice Cormier **Sales:** $5.9 million **Number of employees:** 51 **Industry designation:** Medical products **Company type:** Public **Top competitors:** Sulzer Medica Ltd.; Guidant Corporation; Medtronic, Inc.

Cardiac Control Systems helps keeps hearts beating and blood flowing with its implantable cardiac pacing systems, which consist of single- and dual-chamber pacemakers, electrode leads, and external equipment for programming and monitoring. Pacemakers electrically stimulate the hearts of patients with arrhythmia and other heart conditions, restoring rhythmic contractions and circulation. The company's newest system—designed to reduce complications—requires only one electrode lead to be implanted. Cardiac Control sells its systems to hospitals and physicians; it also sells components to original equipment manufacturers.

CDSI Holdings Inc.

100 SE Second St., Miami, FL 33131

Telephone: 305-579-8000 **Fax:** 305-579-8022 **Metro area:** Miami, FL **Web site:** http://www.PC411.com **Human resources contact:** Patricia Freitas **Sales:** $100,000 **Number of employees:** 8 **Number of employees for previous year:** 4 **Industry designation:** Computers—online services **Company type:** Public

CDSI Holdings (formerly PC411) is moving from an industry that's smoking to the smoking industry. CDSI, which had focused solely on its PC411 online directory service, has shifted its primary business to marketing remote-controlled cigarette-vending machines, designed to curb underage smoking. Only authorized operators (typically cashiers) can control the dispensing of cigarettes from the machines. The company sold PC411, which provides online directory services, including about 110 million US and Canadian residence and business telephone numbers, addresses, and zip codes, to Digital Asset Management (DAM) in 1998. As part of the deal, CDSI acquired 42% of DAM. New Valley Corporation owns about 67% of CDSI.

Coast Dental Services, Inc.

2502 Rocky Point Dr. North, Ste. 1000, Tampa, FL 33607

Telephone: 813-288-1999 **Fax:** 813-281-9284 **Metro area:** Tampa-St. Petersburg, FL **Sales:** $34.5 million **Number of employees:** 455 **Number of employees for previous year:** 190 **Industry designation:** Medical practice management **Company type:** Public

Coast Dental Services develops and manages a network of general dentistry practices located in Atlanta and several cities in Florida. The company's more than 90 dental centers utilize a uniform operating model. Each dental center focuses on nonspecialized dental products and procedures, particularly low-cost basic dental service. Centralized management and administrative duties allow dentists to focus on patient care and see more patients each week. Coast Dental also facilitates the training of the dentists and hygienists at each dental center. Coast Dental's centers are staffed by 85 dentists and have served more than 500,000 patients.

COLLEGIS, Inc.

2300 Maitland Center Pkwy., Ste. 340, Maitland, FL 32751

Telephone: 407-660-1199 **Fax:** 407-660-8040 **Metro area:** Orlando, FL **Web site:** http://www.collegis.com **Human resources contact:** Bob Cominsky **Sales:** $22.8 million (Est.) **Number of employees:** 388 **Industry designation:** Computers—services **Company type:** Private

COLLEGIS teaches universities the three R's—resource development, remote learning, and recruiting. The company provides information technology (IT) services for higher education institutions nationwide. COLLEGIS typically targets colleges and universities with IT personnel budgets of more than $1 million. New Jersey's Brookdale Community College, one of the company's more than 35 clients, accounts for 13.5% of sales. COLLEGIS' services include installing and managing computer networks, training, technical staffing, strategic planning, Internet implementation, and online course design. The company plans to expand its sales force and partner with software vendors to broaden its reach.

Comprehensive Care Corporation

4200 W. Cypress, Ste. 300, Tampa, FL 33607

Telephone: 813-876-5036 **Fax:** 813-872-1561 **Metro area:** Tampa-St. Petersburg, FL **Human resources contact:** Lucinda Figueroa **Sales:** $46.1 million **Number of employees:** 347 **Number of employees for previous year:** 303 **Industry designation:** Health care—outpatient & home **Company type:** Public **Top competitors:** Horizon Health Corporation; Magellan Health Services, Inc.; Integra, Inc.

Comprehensive Care provides psychiatric and substance abuse services for managed health care providers through its Comprehensive Behavioral Care (CompCare) subsidiary. Most services are provided under capitation agreements, in which providers pay the company a fixed monthly fee. Comprehensive Care provides its services in 10 states and Puerto Rico at facilities under contract with the company. Managed care agreements account for more than 80% of operating revenues. The company has nine contracts with PCA, a subsidiary of Humana. Comprehensive Care is currently seeking new contracts to replace those in Puerto Rico that will expire in 1999.

CompScript, Inc.

1225 Broken Sound Pkwy., Boca Raton, FL 33481

Telephone: 561-994-8585 **Fax:** 561-994-6104 **Metro area:** West Palm Beach, FL **Human resources contact:** Mary Ann Falzone **Sales:** $50.6 million **Number of employees:** 365 **Number of employees for previous year:** 332 **Industry designation:** Medical practice management **Company type:** Subsidiary **Top competitors:** Chronimed Inc.; Express Scripts, Inc.; MIM Corporation

CompScript's prescription scripts aren't complimentary. (They have to be able to rake in the dough for parent Omnicare "somehow.") The company offers pharmacy management services to more than 25,000 residents of long-term care facilities in Alabama, Florida, Louisiana, Mississippi, and Ohio. CompScript has seven pharmacy locations in those states. In addition to pharmacy management, CompScript offers infusion therapy, consulting services, and a mail prescription service for patients with long-term needs. Part of a series of Omnicare acquisitions in 1998, CompScript bolsters its parent company's position in the southeastern US.

Computer Management Sciences, Inc.

8133 Baymeadows Way, Jacksonville, FL 32256

Telephone: 904-737-8955 **Fax:** 904-737-6376 **Metro area:** Jacksonville, FL **Web site:** http://www.cmsx.com **Human resources contact:** Rusty Bozman **Sales:** $90.2 million **Number of employees:** 736 **Number of employees for previous year:** 533 **Industry designation:** Computers—services **Company type:** Subsidiary **Top competitors:** Electronic Data Systems Corporation; International Business Machines Corporation; Computer Sciences Corporation

Can we get a little service? Computer Management Sciences, a subsidiary of Computer Associates International, provides information technology consulting and custom software development. Through a network of branch offices and systems outsourcing centers across the US, the company renders a range of technical support, strategic planning, systems integration, database administration, and training services to clients such as Xerox, Dow Jones, and DaimlerChrysler. Computer Management Sciences' consulting services include enterprise planning and designing information systems and reengineering business processes. The company also offers software application design, development, and implementation services.

Concord Camera Corp.

4000 Hollywood Blvd., Ste.650-N, Hollywood, FL 33021

Telephone: 954-331-4200 **Fax:** 954-981-3055 **Metro area:** Miami, FL **Web site:** http://www.concordcam.com **Sales:** $102.7 million **Number of employees:** 157 **Number of employees for previous year:** 140 **Industry designation:** Photographic equipment & supplies **Company type:** Public **Top competitors:** Fuji Photo Film Co., Ltd.; Eastman Kodak Company; Konica Corporation

Smile! You've been caught by Concord Camera. The company makes conventional and single-use 35 mm and Advanced Photo System cameras, as well as 110 film cartridges. Its products are made in China, and more than 65% of sales are to original equipment manufacturers. Concord's top three customers are Kodak, Imation, and Agfa. About half of sales are made to customers in the US, including retailers such as Wal-Mart; cameras are distributed worldwide through sales offices in Canada, China, France, Germany, Hong Kong, Japan, Panama, and the UK. Concord sells its cameras under such trade names as Concord, Keystone, Fun Shooter, and Le Clic in the US and Argus in other parts of the world, as well as private labels.

Continucare Corporation

100 SE Second St., 36th Fl., Miami, FL 33131

Telephone: 305-350-7515 **Fax:** 305-350-9830 **Metro area:** Miami, FL **Human resources contact:** Marina DeMaio **Sales:** $64.3 million **Number of employees:** 300 **Number of employees for previous year:** 200 **Industry designation:** Health care—outpatient & home **Company type:** Public **Top competitors:** Metropolitan Health Networks, Inc.; Sheridan Healthcare, Inc.; FPA Medical Management, Inc.

Continucare offers a continuum of outpatient health care services through its network of physicians, outpatient clinics, rehab centers, home health care agencies, diagnostic imaging centers, and labs. Based in Florida and concentrating its operations there (about 95% of its sales come from the Sunshine State), the company provides health care to several HMOs (including Humana and Foundation Health Systems) from about 300 locations. Continucare continues to add to its web of health care providers via acquisitions. The company has moved away from behavioral health to concentrate on other services.

Correctional Services Corporation

1819 Main St., Ste. 1000, Sarasota, FL 34236

Telephone: 941-953-9199 **Fax:** 941-953-9198 **Metro area:** Sarasota, FL **Web site:** http://www.correctionalservices.com **Human resources contact:** Vikki Schmidt **Sales:** $58.6 million **Number of employees:** 1,730 **Number of employees for previous year:** 1,265 **Industry designation:** Protection—safety equipment & services **Company type:** Public **Top competitors:** Prison Realty Corporation; Cornell Corrections, Inc.; Wackenhut Corporation

When this landlord comes calling, the tenants are always home. Correctional Services develops and manages private correctional and detention facilities in nine US states and Puerto Rico. It has 35 contracts to manage secure facilities (prisons, juvenile detention centers and boot camps, and illegal alien processing centers) and non-secure facilities (half-way houses). It also offers inmate programs such as substance abuse treatment and behavioral modification counseling. The firm markets its services to local, state, and federal government agencies. It will gain some 3,000 housed students with its purchase of Youth Services International, a juvenile-offender facility operator.

CRYO-CELL International, Inc.

3165 McMullen Booth Rd., Bldg. 5, Clearwater, FL 33761

Telephone: 727-723-0333 **Fax:** 727-723-0444 **Metro area:** Tampa-St. Petersburg, FL **Web site:** http://www.cryo-cell.com **Human resources contact:** Gerald F. Maass **Sales:** $331,000 **Number of employees:** 14 **Number of employees for previous year:** 11 **Industry designation:** Medical products **Company type:** Public **Top competitors:** Cryomedical Sciences, Inc.; THERMOGENESIS CORP.; CryoLife, Inc.

After you cut the cord, CRYO-CELL International would like to store it. The company's CCEL cryopreservation unit is designed to store umbilical cord blood stem cells (bone marrow's key ingredient), sperm, and cancerous tumors upon which doctors can perform tests. The CCEL unit uses a computer to insert and retrieve specimens preserved in liquid nitrogen while protecting other specimens from room-temperature air. Through its Lifespan cell-bank program, CRYO-CELL provides its technology and equipment to medical facilities. CRYO-CELL has hired several media firms to produce infomercials and videotapes about its products and services.

Datamax International Corporation

4501 Parkway Commerce Blvd., Orlando, FL 32808

Telephone: 407-578-8007 **Fax:** 407-578-8377 **Metro area:** Orlando, FL **Web site:** http://www.datamaxcorp.com **Human resources contact:** David Rogers **Sales:** $120 million (Est.) **Number of employees:** 565 **Number of employees for previous year:** 537 **Industry designation:** Computers—peripheral equipment **Company type:** Private **Top competitors:** NCR Corporation; International Imaging Materials, Inc.; Zebra Technologies Corporation

Business is black and white for Datamax International. The company makes products for bar coding and automatic identification labeling, including software, thermal printers, and related products such as label-verification systems and thermal transfer ribbons. Datamax's products create labels that are used, in conjunction with bar code scanners, to track merchandise, prices, and inventory, as well as tools and equipment. Subsidiary Pioneer Labels makes custom labels, tickets, and tags. Sales in some 90 foreign countries, including China (for which the company designed a system with 14,000 Chinese characters), account for more than 30% of Datamax's sales. The company has postponed its planned IPO.

Dental Care Alliance, Inc.

1343 Main St., 7th Fl., Sarasota, FL 34236

Telephone: 941-955-3150 **Fax:** 941-366-9615 **Metro area:** Sarasota, FL **Web site:** http://www.dentalcarealliance.com **Human resources contact:** Tracy Crawford **Sales:** $7.9 million **Number of employees:** 84 **Number of employees for previous year:** 76 **Industry designation:** Medical practice management **Company type:** Subsidiary **Top competitors:** Castle Dental Centers, Inc.; Monarch Dental Corporation; Coast Dental Services, Inc.

Dental Care Alliance takes a bite out of the dental practice management market. The firm, a subsidiary of InterDent, provides management and licensing services to more than 30 dental practices in Florida and Michigan. Dental Care Alliance's management services include nondental personnel hiring and administration, patient scheduling, quality assurance, financial assistance, and billing. Its licensing services include marketing, advertising, and purchasing. The company plans to add more practices within its service areas. Dental Care Alliance was incorporated in 1996 as the successor to the businesses of Golden Care Holdings and InterDent acquired the firm in 1999.

Eckerd Corporation

8333 Bryan Dairy Rd., Largo, FL 33777

Telephone: 727-395-6000 **Fax:** 727-395-7934 **Metro area:** Tampa-St. Petersburg, FL **Web site:** http://www.eckerd.com **Human resources contact:** Dennis Cuff **Sales:** $6.1 billion **Number of employees:** 53,800 **Number of employees for previous year:** 46,700 **Industry designation:** Retail—drugstores **Company type:** Subsidiary **Parent company:** J. C. Penney Company, Inc. **Top competitors:** Walgreen Co.; CVS Corporation; Rite Aid Corporation

Eckerd welcomes the pill-popping public. The nation's #4 drugstore chain, Eckerd has more than 2,900 stores in 24 states, primarily in the Northeast, Southeast, and Southwest. Its primary focus is the sale of prescription and over-the-counter drugs; it also sells merchandise such as books and magazines, cosmetics, food, fragrances, greeting cards, and toys. A major player in the photofinishing business, the chain features overnight photo services in all stores and photos-in-an-hour Express Photo labs in nearly 600 stores. Eckerd, like other pharmacies, has benefited from managed care prescription sales, which account for more than 75% of its prescription revenues. Eckerd is a subsidiary of J. C. Penney.

Eclipsys Corporation

777 E. Atlantic Ave., Ste. 200, Delray Beach, FL 33483

Telephone: 561-243-1440 **Fax:** 561-243-9390 **Metro area:** West Palm Beach, FL **Web site:** http://www.eclipsnet.com **Human resources contact:** Mark Green **Sales:** $170.7 million **Number of employees:** 1,406 **Number of employees for previous year:** 997 **Industry designation:** Computers—corporate, professional & financial software **Company type:** Public **Top competitors:** IDX Systems Corporation; McKesson HBOC, Inc.; Shared Medical Systems Corporation

Eclipsys markets its health care information software to large hospitals, integrated health care delivery networks, and academic medical centers. The company's software includes its Sunrise-brand suites, which assists in clinical management, patient information access management, patient financial management, and data warehousing and analysis. Eclipsys also provides outsourcing, remote processing, and networking services. It has strategic relationships with Partners HealthCare System for research, development, and testing of its products. Eclipsys sells its products in North America, Europe, and Asia.

Exactech, Inc.

4613 NW Sixth St., Gainesville, FL 32609

Telephone: 352-377-1140 **Fax:** 352-378-2617 **Metro area:** Gainesville, FL **Web site:** http://www.hawkassociates.com/exactech **Human resources contact:** Betty Petty **Sales:** $24 million **Number of employees:** 57 **Number of employees for previous year:** 45 **Industry designation:** Medical products **Company type:** Public **Top competitors:** Pfizer Inc; Bristol-Myers Squibb Company; DePuy, Inc.

Orthopedic implant device maker Exactech's joints aren't the kind you hang out "in" —they're the kind you hang out "on." Hospitals, surgeons, and clinics worldwide use the company's hip and knee devices to replace joints that have deteriorated because of injury or disease. Exactech makes a number of knee and hip replacement systems to fit physicians' preferences and patients' needs; its computerized ACCUMATCH Implant Selection System helps physicians select the appropriate hip system. Products are sold through independent dealers and distributors in the US and in eight other countries. Foreign sales account for nearly 20% of revenues. Chairman and CEO William Petty and his family own about 40% of Exactech.

Exigent International, Inc.

1225 Evans Rd., Melbourne, FL 32904

Telephone: 407-952-7550 **Fax:** 407-952-7555 **Metro area:** Melbourne, FL **Web site:** http://www.xgnt.com **Human resources contact:** David Miller **Sales:** $35.7 million **Number of employees:** 299 **Number of employees for previous year:** 291 **Industry designation:** Computers—services **Company type:** Public **Parent company:** Software Technology **Top competitors:** Logicon, Inc.; Datron Systems Incorporated; Integral Systems, Inc.

Exigent International's software keeps tabs on satellites and airline luggage, both of which often seem lost in space. Its Software Technology subsidiary makes satellite tracking and control software primarily for the US government (65% of sales), as well as for aerospace and defense contractors (including Lockheed Martin and Motorola). Its software provides launch support, data analysis, mission tracking, and operations simulation. Its flagship OS/COMET suite is used in the Iridium global communications system and the Navstar Global Positioning System. Subsidiary FotoTag makes baggage and passenger tracking systems for airlines and airports. Exigent International sells its products directly and through VARs.

FARO Technologies, Inc.

125 Technology Park, Lake Mary, FL 32746

Telephone: 407-333-9911 **Fax:** 407-333-4181 **Metro area:** Orlando, FL **Web site:** http://www.faro.com **Human resources contact:** Sharon Trowbridge **Sales:** $27.5 million **Number of employees:** 190 **Number of employees for previous year:** 111 **Industry designation:** Computers—engineering, scientific & CAD-CAM software **Company type:** Public **Top competitors:** MetaCreations Corporation; Real 3D, Inc.; Immersion Corporation

Corporate spies may be out of business. FARO Technologies' 3-D digitizers create digital representations of 3-D objects in a process called reverse engineering. Its portable FAROArm, consisting of a moveable armature and laptop, is used to take measurements, perform inspections by comparing objects against digital prototypes, and to study competitors' products. More than 20 FAROArm models are used by customers in the aerospace, automotive, and equipment industries. Two makers of athletic shoes—NIKE and Reebok—are FARO customers. An Air Force contractor has used FAROArm to measure and reconstruct a jet fighter cockpit. The company has offices in the US and Europe.

FDP Corp.

2140 S. Dixie Hwy., Miami, FL 33133

Telephone: 305-858-8200 **Fax:** 305-854-6305 **Metro area:** Miami, FL **Web site:** http://www.fdpcorp.com **Human resources contact:** Carol Sweeny **Sales:** $40.9 million **Number of employees:** 440 **Number of employees for previous year:** 380 **Industry designation:** Computers—corporate, professional & financial software **Company type:** Public **Top competitors:** Policy Management Systems Corporation; ALLIED Group, Inc.; DST Systems, Inc.

FDP makes policy management EZ.. Its Home Office Systems division makes software used by life insurance companies and other financial institutions to process life insurance, pensions, and annuity products. Products sold through its Agency Partner division let agents market and manage interest-sensitive and other life insurance policies. FDP also makes sales illustration software. Its Pension Partner division's software assists life insurance agents, third-party administrators, and others in administering benefit, contribution, and cafeteria plans. Founder and CEO Michael Goldberg and his wife, Cindy, own 50% of the company, which computer software and services company SunGard Data Systems is buying.

FinancialWeb.com, Inc.

201 Park Place, Ste. 321, Altamonte Springs, FL 32701

Telephone: 407-834-4443 **Fax:** 407-834-3870 **Metro area:** Orlando, FL **Web site:** http://www.axxessinc.com **Human resources contact:** Kevin A. Lichtman **Sales:** $68,977 **Number of employees:** 11 **Industry designation:** Computers—online services **Company type:** Public **Top competitors:** Market Guide Inc.; The Dun & Bradstreet Corporation; Reuters Group PLC

FinancialWeb.com (formerly Axxess) publishes a family of Web sites dedicated to financial information. The company is in a development stage, and its new moniker is the latest in a series of names that dates back to the company's founding in 1983. FinancialWeb.com offers 17 Web sites that contain financial editorial content, charts, investor news, securities data, stock quotes, and other financial data. To date the company has relied on private equity investments and loans, but it plans to generate revenues from advertising now that its sites are up and running.

The Florida Marlins

2267 NW 199th Ave., Miami, FL 33056

Telephone: 305-626-7400 **Fax:** 305-626-7428 **Metro area:** Miami, FL **Web site:** http://www.flamarlins.com **Human resources contact:** Ruby Mattei **Sales:** $88.2 million (Est.) **Number of employees:** 160 **Number of employees for previous year:** 102 **Industry designation:** Leisure & recreational services **Company type:** Private **Top competitors:** The Philadelphia Phillies; The Atlanta Braves; Metropolitan Baseball Club Inc.

The Florida Marlins came out swinging in 1993 as one of Major League Baseball's first National League expansion teams in almost 25 years. The team rose to success quickly; in 1997 it defeated the Cleveland Indians to bring home a World Series championship. The bright times didn't last long in the Sunshine State: former team owner Wayne Huizenga proceeded to gut the championship team in order to drastically lower payroll. The next season the team posted the worst record ever (54-108) for a defending World Series team. In 1998 Huizenga sold the team to John Henry, a multimillionaire commodities trader.

Florida Panthers Holdings, Inc.

450 E. Las Olas Blvd., Fort Lauderdale, FL 33301

Telephone: 954-712-1300 **Fax:** 954-627-5051 **Metro area:** Miami, FL **Web site:** http://www.flpanthers.com **Sales:** $296.2 million **Number of employees:** 3,587 **Number of employees for previous year:** 3,060 **Industry designation:** Leisure & recreational services **Company type:** Public **Top competitors:** Club Mediterranee S.A.; ClubCorp International, Inc.; Westin Hotels & Resorts Worldwide

Through its subsidiaries, Florida Panthers Holdings owns the Florida Panthers hockey team and manages sports arenas, but most of its sales come from its seven luxury resorts (six of which are in Florida). The Florida Panthers play their home games at the National Car Rental Center, an arena the company developed and manages. Chairman Wayne Huizenga has controlling interest of Florida Panthers Holdings; he also owns the Miami Dolphins and National Car Rental. To help build popularity for the Panthers, the company runs two Florida ice rinks— Incredible Ice and Gold Coast. Florida Panthers Holdings also owns 78% of Decoma Miami Associates, which operates the Miami Arena (home court for the NBA's Miami Heat).

Forcenergy Inc

2730 SW Third Ave., Ste. 800, Miami, FL 33129

Telephone: 305-856-8500 **Fax:** 305-856-4300 **Metro area:** Miami, FL **Web site:** http://www.forcenergy.net **Human resources contact:** Frank Angerame **Sales:** $281.7 million **Number of employees:** 275 **Number of employees for previous year:** 204 **Industry designation:** Oil & gas—exploration & production **Company type:** Public

Forcenergy forces energy—in the form of oil and natural gas—out of the ground. The independent gas and oil firm (which has sought bankruptcy protection) develops oil and natural gas properties and produces oil from about 500 wells in the Gulf of Mexico. Focusing its drilling activities on a relatively small area allows Forcenergy to use its experience in the region to maximize drilling success and minimize finding and development costs. It is developing fields at Cook Inlet, Alaska; it owns interests in 3,200 producing onshore oil and gas wells in the Appalachian, Gulf Coast, Permian Basin, and Rocky Mountain regions of the US; and it has stakes in undeveloped oil fields in Australia and West Africa.

Fountain Pharmaceuticals, Inc.

7279 Bryan Dairy Rd., Largo, FL 33777

Telephone: 727-548-0900 **Fax:** 727-546-5909 **Metro area:** Tampa-St. Petersburg, FL **Web site:** http://www.fountainpharm.com **Human resources contact:** Francis J. Werner **Sales:** $1.5 million **Number of employees:** 16 **Number of employees for previous year:** 7 **Industry designation:** Biomedical & genetic products **Company type:** Public **Top competitors:** L'Oreal; Pfizer Inc; Advanced Polymer Systems, Inc.

Fountain Pharmaceuticals has a very small sphere of influence. The company develops "cosmeceuticals" based on its proprietary drug-delivery technology: microscopic spheres carry chemical formulations that are released when applied to the skin. The company develops sunscreens, lotions, and moisturizers under the Octazome, LyphaZone, and Daylong brands and licenses the technology to other companies, including Nycomed Amersham and Spirig AG. The company is pursuing potential medical applications, including burn care and topical steroids, for its technology. Director Joseph Schuchert owns 45% of the company.

French Fragrances, Inc.

14100 NW 60th Ave., Miami Lakes, FL 33014

Telephone: 305-818-8000 **Fax:** 305-818-8010 **Metro area:** Miami, FL **Web site:** http://www.frenchfragrances.com **Human resources contact:** Errol Spence **Sales:** $309.6 million **Number of employees:** 190 **Number of employees for previous year:** 170 **Industry designation:** Cosmetics & toiletries **Company type:** Public

Something sweet is in the air at French Fragrances. The company manufactures, distributes, and markets perfume, cologne, eau de toilette, body spray, after-shave, and scented bath and body products for men and women. French Fragrances distributes its products to more than 31,000 department stores, mass merchandisers, drugstores, and cosmetics stores in the US. The company markets about 160 brands and has exclusive rights to manufacture and market fragrances bearing fashionable names such as Halston, Geoffrey Beene, and Benetton. French Fragrances also owns J.P. Fragrances, another distributor of perfumes and colognes. Chairman Rafael Kravec owns about 20% of the company's stock.

Genetic Vectors, Inc.

5201 NW 77th Ave., Ste. 100, Miami, FL 33166

Telephone: 305-716-0000 **Fax:** 305-716-0001 **Metro area:** Miami, FL **Web site:** http://www.gvec.com **Human resources contact:** Sandra Chiong **Sales:** $100,000 **Number of employees:** 9 **Number of employees for previous year:** 5 **Industry designation:** Biomedical & genetic products **Company type:** Public **Top competitors:** Epoch Pharmaceuticals, Inc.; IDEXX Laboratories, Inc.; Xenometrix, Inc.

Development-stage Genetic Vectors is spoiling to knock out contamination in the biopharmaceutical as well as the food, brewing, and wine industries. Its initial product, the EpiDNA Picogram Assay, is a nonradioactive three-hour test designed to help biopharmaceutical manufacturers meet FDA quality guidelines. The kit tests for DNA and RNA to identify traces of biological impurities. Genetic Vectors has temporarily withdrawn EpiDNA from the market so it can improve its sensitivity. The company is also developing products that will determine the presence of yeast strains in wine and other foods and beverages that cause spoilage. Former parent Nyer Medical Group owns about 40% of the company.

George E. Warren Corporation

605 17th St., Vero Beach, FL 32960

Telephone: 561-778-7100 **Fax:** 561-778-7171 **Metro area:** Melbourne, FL **Human resources contact:** Martin Paris **Sales:** $2.6 billion (Est.) **Number of employees:** 24 **Number of employees for previous year:** 23 **Industry designation:** Oil refining & marketing **Company type:** Private **Top competitors:** Exxon Corporation; The Williams Companies, Inc.; Columbia Energy Group

If you need to unload a little liquid natural gas, let George do it. George E. Warren Corporation is a refiner and major private wholesale distributor of liquid natural gas and other petroleum products in the southeastern US. It was founded in Boston as a coal and oil distributor by George E. Warren in 1907; it moved to Florida in the early 1990s. The company, which distributes its products by tank trucks and pipeline, has eight refining facilities in Port Everglades and Tampa, Florida; Venice, Louisiana; Greenville and Hattiesburg, Mississippi; Monument, New Mexico; and Galena and Bellville, Texas. Its products include propane, propylene, ethylene, gasoline, and heating oil. President Thomas Corr owns the company.

Golden Bear Golf, Inc.

11780 US Hwy. 1, North Palm Beach, FL 33408

Telephone: 561-626-3900 **Fax:** 561-626-4104 **Metro area:** West Palm Beach, FL **Web site:** http://www.nicklaus.com/gbg **Human resources contact:** Sandy Gurman **Sales:** $63.6 million **Number of employees:** 528 **Number of employees for previous year:** 459 **Industry designation:** Leisure & recreational services **Company type:** Public **Top competitors:** The Arnold Palmer Golf Company; Family Golf Centers, Inc.; Ashworth, Inc.

Golden Bear Golf is a golf products and services company that includes 14 instruction centers, course construction and renovation, and the licensing of golf-related apparel and other products. The company offers its products and services in 35 countries, primarily under the brand names Nicklaus, Jack Nicklaus, and Golden Bear. Golden Bear Golf went into the fiscal rough in 1998 when falsified records at Paragon Construction, its golf course construction subsidiary, compelled it to restate 1997's losses at $24.7 million (as opposed to $2.9 million). Golfing great Jack Nicklaus controls the company.

Grand Court Lifestyles, Inc.

2650 N. Military Trail, Ste. 350, Boca Raton, FL 33431

Telephone: 561-997-0323 **Fax:** 561-997-5424 **Metro area:** West Palm Beach, FL **Web site:** http://www.grandcourtlifestyles.com **Human resources contact:** Kathy Warzecha **Sales:** $41.8 million **Number of employees:** 1,900 **Number of employees for previous year:** 1,500 **Industry designation:** Nursing homes **Company type:** Public **Top competitors:** Life Care Centers of America; Emeritus Assisted Living; ARV Assisted Living, Inc.

Grand Court Lifestyles owns and manages a portfolio of adult retirement apartments. The company, which focuses on private pay rather than Medicare tenants, operates more than 45 facilities containing an aggregate of some 6,400 units in 12 Sunbelt and Midwestern states. It also operates one nursing home. Grand Court residents can opt for independent or assisted living, with services such as meals, housekeeping, transportation, and rehabilitation. Revenues are obtained from sales of limited partnership interests in the communities, tenant fees, and property management contracts. The company has aggressive growth plans. CEO John Luciani and COO Bernard Rodin each own about 42% of the company.

Health Management Associates, Inc.

5811 Pelican Bay Blvd., Ste. 500, Naples, FL 34108

Telephone: 941-598-3131 **Fax:** 941-597-5794 **Web site:** http://www.hma-corp.com **Human resources contact:** Frederick L. Drow **Sales:** $1.1 billion **Number of employees:** 15,000 **Number of employees for previous year:** 10,000 **Industry designation:** Hospitals **Company type:** Public **Top competitors:** Quorum Health Group, Inc.; Province Healthcare Company; Community Health Systems, Inc.

Even Ma and Pa Kettle need a little doctorin'. Health Management Associates (HMA) operates more than 30 hospitals, including four psychiatric centers, in rural areas of 11 states in the southeastern and southwestern US. HMA has grown by annually acquiring a small number of financially ailing hospitals with good turnaround potential in growing markets. It cuts costs while upgrading the facility and equipment and recruiting medical specialists, garnering business from patients formerly forced to travel to receive medical treatment. Its consolidation strategy allows HMA to save money on administrative and purchasing costs.

Hi-Rise Recycling Systems, Inc.

16255 NW 54th Ave., Miami, FL 33014

Telephone: 305-624-9222 **Fax:** 305-594-4228 **Metro area:** Miami, FL **Web site:** http://www.hiri.com **Human resources contact:** Bradley A. Hacker **Sales:** $31.2 million **Number of employees:** 375 **Number of employees for previous year:** 87 **Industry designation:** Pollution control equipment & services **Company type:** Public **Top competitors:** Wastequip, Inc.; Zodiac SA; United Dominion Industries Limited

Revenues are in the chute for Hi-Rise Recycling Systems, Inc., which sells, installs and maintains automated recycling systems for multi-story buildings. The company's proprietary systems allows residents to separate their recyclables and trash using their existing or retrofit trash chutes. Hi-Rise Recycling's Wilkinson subsidiary is one of the oldest US chute companies, and Wilkinson Compactors is a major compactor manufacturer. The firm's Hesco Sales subsidiary makes containers and recycling equipment, such as vertical and horizontal balers. Hi-Rise Recycling's core geographic markets are New York City, Toronto, and south and west Florida.

Hitsgalore.com Inc.

4707 140th Ave. North, Ste. 107, Clearwater, FL 33762

Telephone: 727-530-4800 **Fax:** 727-530-4707 **Metro area:** Tampa-St. Petersburg, FL **Web site:** http://www.hitsgalore.com **Sales:** $1.5 million **Number of employees:** 4 **Industry designation:** Computers—online services **Company type:** Public **Top competitors:** Yahoo! Inc.; Lycos, Inc.; Infoseek Corporation

Hitsgalore.com is the renamed and refocused Systems Communications. The company, which went public in a blank check offering in 1988, is cashing in on the World Wide Web: It changed its name to Hitsgalore.com in 1999 following a reverse merger with an Internet search engine company and is exiting the health care data analysis business. Its National Solutions Corporation subsidiary—which hires subcontractors to perform health care cost containment and case management for large corporations—will be spun off into a separate company, International Healthcare Solutions. Hitsgalore.com, which features a business-to-business search engine, was launched in 1998.

IMRglobal Corp.

26750 US Hwy. 19 North, Ste. 500, Clearwater, FL 33761

Telephone: 727-797-7080 **Fax:** 727-791-8152 **Metro area:** Tampa-St. Petersburg, FL **Web site:** http://www.imr.com **Human resources contact:** John Nyhan **Sales:** $158.3 million **Number of employees:** 2,500 **Number of employees for previous year:** 1,535 **Industry designation:** Computers—services **Company type:** Public **Top competitors:** Keane, Inc.; Computer Horizons Corp.; CIBER, Inc.

IMRglobal (formerly Information Management Resources) provides application software and transitional outsourcing services to large businesses, primarily in the financial, retail, insurance, and utility industries. Services include software development, application maintenance, legacy system transitions, and year 2000 conversions, which account for more than 50% of sales. The company runs its services on a fixed-price, fixed-time basis and subcontracts employees as needed. Its software facilities in India and Ireland help control costs and enable the company to offer its services around the clock via satellite communications. IMRglobal has operations in Australia, Canada, Japan, the UK, and the US.

Integrated Spatial Information Solutions, Inc.

13119 Professional Dr., Ste. 200, Jacksonville, FL 32225

Telephone: 904-220-4747 **Fax:** 904-220-4741 **Metro area:** Jacksonville, FL **Human resources contact:** Frederick G. Beisser **Sales:** $8.1 million **Number of employees:** 86 **Number of employees for previous year:** 84 **Industry designation:** Computers—engineering, scientific & CAD-CAM software **Company type:** Public **Top competitors:** Environmental Systems Research Institute Inc.; Logicon, Inc.; Analytical Surveys, Inc.

Integrated Spatial Information Solutions (formerly DCX) wants its customers to know where they stand—literally. Through its PlanGraphics subsidiary, the company designs geographic information systems (GIS) for government entities, utility companies, and commercial customers. PlanGraphics offers advisory, data integration, and implementation services, and its systems are used in applications such as environmental remediation, land management, mineral exploration, and military planning. Integrated Spatial Information Solutions also serves as a reseller of satellite imagery through an agreement with Space Imaging EOSAT. Customers include Qwest Communications, Raytheon, and the US Army Corps of Engineers.

Intelligent Life Corporation

11811 US Hwy. 1, Ste. 101, North Palm Beach, FL 33408

Telephone: 561-627-7330 **Fax:** 561-627-7335 **Metro area:** West Palm Beach, FL **Web site:** http://www.bankrate.com **Sales:** $3.8 million (Est.) **Number of employees:** 120 **Industry designation:** Computers—online services **Company type:** Private **Top competitors:** Bridge Information Systems, Inc.; Reuters Group PLC; The McGraw-Hill Companies, Inc.

Intelligent life exists on the financial planet. Intelligent Life provides consumer banking, credit, and personal finance information to magazines and newspapers. It makes its findings available through its Bankrate.com Web site, its "Bank Rate Monitor" publication, and about 60 distribution partners such as America Online and Money.com. Intelligent Life's content covers domestic and foreign markets and provides data regarding credit cards, mortgage loans, checking accounts, auto loans, ATM fees, and yields on savings accounts. The company is also introducing new Web sites targeted at women, college students, Spanish-speakers, and minorities. Chairman Peter Morse owns about 55% of the company.

Intelligent Medical Imaging, Inc.

4360 Northlake Blvd., Ste. 214, Palm Beach Gardens, FL 33410

Telephone: 561-627-0344 **Fax:** 561-627-0409 **Metro area:** West Palm Beach, FL **Web site:** http://www.imii.com/home.html **Human resources contact:** Barbara Stellner **Sales:** $3.8 million **Number of employees:** 127 **Number of employees for previous year:** 87 **Industry designation:** Medical instruments **Company type:** Public **Top competitors:** International Remote Imaging Systems, Inc.; NeoPath, Inc.; Neuromedical Systems, Inc.

Intelligent Medical Imaging makes the MICRO21, an automated microscope system that hospitals, medical laboratories, and medical researchers use as a diagnostic tool. A technician loads the system with up to 100 prepared slides, pushes start, and lets the system's "visual artificial intelligence" software analyze the samples. The product is FDA-approved for several analytical procedures and has many more potential uses. The system is designed to have lower operating costs, greater accuracy, and better analytical capabilities than manual microscopic procedures.

International Speedway Corporation

1801 W. International Speedway Blvd., Daytona Beach, FL 32114

Telephone: 904-254-2700 **Fax:** 904-947-6791 **Metro area:** Daytona Beach, FL **Web site:** http://www.daytonausa.com/isc.shtml **Human resources contact:** Rick Thompson **Sales:** $187.4 million **Number of employees:** 440 **Number of employees for previous year:** 395 **Industry designation:** Leisure & recreational services **Company type:** Public **Top competitors:** Speedway Motorsports, Inc.; Championship Auto Racing Teams, Inc.; Dover Downs Entertainment, Inc.

Vroom! Vroom! Vroom! Punch it, Jeb! International Speedway Corporation (ISC) promotes more than 80 motorsports events annually. The firm owns and operates such racing venues as the Daytona International Speedway (home of the Daytona 500), Talladega Superspeedway, Darlington Raceway, and Tucson Raceway Park. Admissions account for about 50% of revenues; most of the rest comes from broadcasting rights, advertising, and other racing-related sales. ISC's motorsports theme park, DAYTONA USA, offers interactive exhibits, theaters, and memorabilia. The France family owns about two-thirds of the company and controls the National Association for Stock Car Auto Racing (NASCAR).

Jacksonville Jaguars

One ALLTEL Stadium Place, Jacksonville, FL 32202

Telephone: 904-633-6000 **Fax:** 904-633-6050 **Metro area:** Jacksonville, FL **Web site:** http://www.jaguarsnfl.com **Human resources contact:** Kelli Bohn **Sales:** $66.8 million (Est.) **Number of employees:** 110 **Industry designation:** Leisure & recreational services **Company type:** Private **Top competitors:** Baltimore Ravens; Tennessee Titans Inc.; Pittsburgh Steelers

The Jacksonville Jaguars have really pounced on their competition, becoming one of the most successful expansion teams in NFL history. In 1995 the Jaguars began play as the league's 30th expansion team, and since then they have made the playoffs three times, including a 1997 appearance in the AFC Championship game (which they lost to the New England Patriots). The team is led by quarterback Mark Brunell and coached by Tom Coughlin. Touchdown Jacksonville , a group formed in 1989 to bring pro football to the city, was awarded the franchise in 1993. It also negotiated to split the cost of a new stadium with the city that year. Wayne Weaver, part owner of Shoe Carnival, owns a majority interest in the team.

JLM Industries, Inc.

8675 Hidden River Pkwy., Tampa, FL 33637

Telephone: 727-632-3300 **Fax:** 727-632-3301 **Metro area:** Tampa-St. Petersburg, FL **Web site:** http://www.jlmgroup.com **Human resources contact:** Nancy Sylvester **Sales:** $305.7 million **Number of employees:** 170 **Number of employees for previous year:** 161 **Industry designation:** Chemicals—specialty **Company type:** Public

JLM Industries is sticking to its business. The firm's acetone and phenol are used in adhesives, coatings, plastics, solvents, and other products around the world. JLM Industries has a plant near Chicago and another (a joint venture with GE and a CITGO affiliate) in Indiana. Most of the production from the Indiana plant is earmarked for GE; JLM buys the rest and distributes it, along with propylene and other commodity chemicals. Customers include manufacturers and other chemical companies. JLM Industries owns or co-owns terminals and storage facilities in North Carolina and Texas; it also operates in Europe, South America, and Asia. President and CEO John Macdonald owns more than 60% of the company.

Just Like Home, Inc.

2440 Tamiami Tr. N., Nokomis, FL 34275

Telephone: 941-966-3636 **Fax:** 941-966-6678 **Metro area:** Sarasota, FL **Web site:** http://www.justlikehome.com **Sales:** $2.5 million **Number of employees:** 140 **Number of employees for previous year:** 116 **Industry designation:** Nursing homes **Company type:** Public

Just Like Home may not be home sweet home, but it does offer a home away from home. The firm's assisted-living facilities, which each house between 16 and 45 residents, provide care for elderly clients who are frail or mentally impaired and require some assistance. The company offers such services as housekeeping, laundry, meal preparation, exercise programs, transportation, and administering medication. In addition, the firm provides aides to elderly clients who live at home and need help with personal care, housekeeping, cooking, shopping, or transportation. CEO and president John Robenalt and VP Elizabeth Conard own 36% of the firm, which owns or manages nine Florida facilities with more than 189 beds.

Kos Pharmaceuticals, Inc.

1001 Brickell Bay Dr., 25th Fl., Miami, FL 33131

Telephone: 305-577-3464 **Fax:** 305-577-4596 **Metro area:** Miami, FL **Web site:** http://www.kospharm.com/ **Human resources contact:** Arthur W. Brinkmann **Sales:** $13 million **Number of employees:** 447 **Number of employees for previous year:** 237 **Industry designation:** Drugs **Company type:** Public **Top competitors:** Warner Chilcott Public Limited Company; Sheffield Pharmaceuticals, Inc.; Forest Laboratories, Inc.

Named after the Greek isle where Hippocrates founded medicine, Kos Pharmaceuticals develops drugs to treat chronic cardiovascular and respiratory diseases. The company's cardiovascular product NIASPAN (the first drug of its kind approved by the FDA) lowers harmful cholesterol through controlled-release formulations containing niacin. The company is also developing aerosolized inhalation products for asthma and other respiratory diseases. Kos Pharmaceuticals has agreements with Fuisz Technologies for the development of products used to treat disorders such as angina pectoris and hypertension. The company makes and markets its own products. Chairman Michael Jaharis owns half of Kos Pharmaceuticals.

Lincare Holdings Inc.

19337 US 19 North, Ste. 500, Clearwater, FL 33758

Telephone: 727-530-7700 **Fax:** 727-532-9692 **Metro area:** Tampa-St. Petersburg, FL **Web site:** http://www.lincare.com **Human resources contact:** Mark Schuetzler **Sales:** $487.4 million **Number of employees:** 4,200 **Number of employees for previous year:** 3,500 **Industry designation:** Medical services **Company type:** Public **Top competitors:** Apria Healthcare Group Inc.; RoTech Medical Corporation; Coram Healthcare Corporation

Lincare Holdings, with more than 140,000 customers in 39 states, is one of the nation's largest providers of oxygen and other respiratory therapy services to in-home patients. The company provides its services through more than 300 offices to patients who suffer from obstructive pulmonary diseases such as emphysema, chronic bronchitis, or asthma and who require supplemental oxygen or other respiratory therapy services. Lincare Holdings provides and services such products as home oxygen equipment (oxygen concentrators and liquid oxygen systems), nebulizers, apnea monitors, continuous positive airway pressure devices, noninvasive bi-level ventilation, and ventilators.

Maxxim Medical, Inc.

10300 49th St. North, Clearwater, FL 33762

Telephone: 727-561-2100 **Fax:** 727-561-2180 **Metro area:** Tampa-St. Petersburg, FL **Web site:** http://www.maxximmedical.com **Human resources contact:** Suzanne R. Garon **Sales:** $522.5 million **Number of employees:** 4,068 **Number of employees for previous year:** 3,958 **Industry designation:** Medical & dental supplies **Company type:** Public **Top competitors:** Allegiance Corporation; Isolyser Company, Inc.; Johnson & Johnson

Cleanliness is Maxxim's axiom. Maxxim Medical makes sterile medical specialty products and disposables; it is tops in the non-latex glove market. The Case Management division (producing about three-fourths of sales) sells custom procedure trays (it's #2 behind Allegiance), infection-control apparel, and other surgical products. Its Argon Medical unit makes disposable products such as guidewires, needles, catheters, and high-pressure syringes, as well as procedure trays. Subsidiary Circon produces endoscopes and miniature video systems for medical use. The Maxxim Medical Europe division distributes medical products throughout that continent. Maxxim's maximum leader, Kenneth Davidson, plays a mean guitar.

Medical Industries of America, Inc.

1903 S. Congress Ave., Ste. 400, Boynton Beach, FL 33426

Telephone: 561-737-2227 **Fax:** 561-737-5008 **Metro area:** West Palm Beach, FL **Sales:** $4.5 million **Number of employees:** 133 **Number of employees for previous year:** 54 **Industry designation:** Medical services **Company type:** Public **Top competitors:** Apria Healthcare Group Inc.; PhyCor, Inc.; Integrated Health Services, Inc.

When the pope needs stand-by air ambulance service, he calls on Medical Industries of America. Not only does the company's Global Air Rescue provide air transport to critical care patients, but its other subsidiaries also offer a variety of health care options, primarily to doctors and hospitals in Florida. Ivanhoe Medical Systems offers sleep disorder diagnostic services, while Heart Labs of America has mobile labs for performing cardiac catheterization. Other subsidiaries include Florida Physicians Internet, PRN of North Carolina, Care America Integrated Health Services, Your Good Health Network of Florida and Pharmacy Care Specialists.

Medical Manager Corporation

3001 N. Rocky Point Dr. East, Ste. 100, Tampa, FL 33607

Telephone: 813-287-2990 **Fax:** 813-289-6420 **Metro area:** Tampa-St. Petersburg, FL **Web site:** http://www.medicalmanager.com **Human resources contact:** Trish Donavon **Sales:** $135.9 million **Number of employees:** 1,152 **Number of employees for previous year:** 809 **Industry designation:** Medical practice management **Company type:** Public **Top competitors:** Health Systems Design Corporation; Sunquest Information Systems, Inc.; Health Management Systems, Inc.

Medical Manager provides practice-management information systems to health care service providers. The company's primary software product, The Medical Manager, includes clinical, financial, administrative, and patient-information applications used by physicians, practice-management organizations, and managed-care organizations. The scalable software also facilitates the processing of claims, and promotes more effective communication between medical providers. The Medical Manager software is marketed nationwide by a network of sales subsidiaries; client support services are also available. Medical Manager went public in 1997 to consolidate several firms engaged in the software's development and distribution.

Medical Technology Systems, Inc.

12920 Automobile Blvd., Clearwater, FL 34622

Telephone: 727-576-6311 **Fax:** 727-579-8067 **Metro area:** Tampa-St. Petersburg, FL **Human resources contact:** Peter Benjamin **Sales:** $24.1 million **Number of employees:** 275 **Number of employees for previous year:** 225 **Industry designation:** Medical products **Company type:** Public **Top competitors:** McKesson HBOC, Inc.; Shared Medical Systems Corporation; Cardinal Health, Inc.

Medical Technology Systems, through three subsidiaries, provides medication-dispensing systems and other products and services primarily to nursing home pharmacies. Its dispensing systems division (which accounts for more than half of sales) uses specialized machines to fill disposable punch cards with a 30-day supply of medication. The company also sells prescription labels, automated dispensing systems, and software for charting medication records. One subsidiary provides clinical laboratory services, such as blood and tissue analysis. Most company subsidiaries went briefly into Chapter 11 in 1996. Chairman and CEO Todd E. Siegel controls the company.

Medicore, Inc.

2337 W. 76th St., Hialeah, FL 33016

Telephone: 305-558-4000 **Fax:** 305-825-0961 **Metro area:** Miami, FL **Sales:** $38.9 million **Number of employees:** 524 **Number of employees for previous year:** 321 **Industry designation:** Medical products **Company type:** Public

Medicore's subsidiaries make electronic and electromechanical products and provide medical services and supplies. The company's Techdyne subsidiary does contract manufacturing of printed circuit boards (PCBs), cables, and electromechanical assemblies for computer OEMs such as IBM (about 20% of sales), EMC, and Motorola. After its acquisition of PCB maker Lytton, PCBs are now 26% of Techdyne's business. Techdyne also makes and distributes medical disposables (exam gloves, bandages, swabs), and blood lancets under the names Medi-Lance and Lady Lite. Subsidiary Dialysis Corporation of America provides outpatient dialysis services at three locations in Pennsylvania.

Metropolitan Health Networks, Inc.

5100 Town Center Circle, Ste. 560, Boca Raton, FL 33486

Telephone: 561-416-9484 **Fax:** 561-416-9487 **Metro area:** West Palm Beach, FL **Web site:** http://www.metcare.com **Human resources contact:** Amy Pacey **Sales:** $14 million **Number of employees:** 138 **Number of employees for previous year:** 108 **Industry designation:** Health care—outpatient & home **Company type:** Public **Top competitors:** Physician Health Corporation; SunStar Healthcare, Inc.; Continucare Corporation

Metropolitan Health Networks operates an integrated health-care delivery network in South Florida's Dade, Broward, and Palm Beach counties. The network's physician practices provide both primary and specialized care. Through its Metcare Diagnostic Services subsidiary, the company provides such services as radiology, magnetic resonance imaging (MRI), ultrasound, and other diagnostic techniques. Subsidiary MetBilling Group provides information systems management and billing services to network members. The highly acquisitive company establishes contracts and affiliations with medical groups it doesn't buy outright.

Miami Dolphins Limited

7500 SW 30th St., Davie, FL 33314

Telephone: 954-452-7000 **Fax:** 954-452-7027 **Metro area:** Miami, FL **Web site:** http://dolphinsendzone.com/home.html **Sales:** $103.1 million (Est.) **Number of employees:** 169 **Industry designation:** Leisure & recreational services **Company type:** Private **Top competitors:** New England Patriots; New York Jets Football Club, Inc.; Buffalo Bills, Inc.

The vultures are circling, according to Jimmy Johnson, coach of the NFL's Miami Dolphins. Johnson was hired by Miami to recreate the "Dallas miracle." (He led the Cowboys from a 1-15 season in 1989 to a Super Bowl win in 1993.) But after three seasons in Miami, the results of his efforts differ little from Don Shula's in his last years there—good but not great. Johnson's performance may have him watching over his shoulder for vultures, but as the youngest team in pro football, Miami has the potential to drop-kick all rivals. H. Wayne Huizenga owns the team, Pro Player (formerly Joe Robbie) Stadium, and the Florida Panthers NHL team. He sold the Florida Marlins (1997 World Series champs) in 1998.

Miami Heat

SunTrust International Center, One SE Third Ave., Ste. 2300, Miami, FL 33131

Telephone: 305-577-4328 **Fax:** 305-372-0802 **Metro area:** Miami, FL **Web site:** http://www.nba.com/heat **Human resources contact:** Lynn Margulies **Sales:** $50 million (Est.) **Number of employees:** 95 **Number of employees for previous year:** 87 **Industry designation:** Leisure & recreational services **Company type:** Private **Top competitors:** New Jersey Nets; New York Knickerbockers; Washington Wizards

The Miami Heat joined the National Basketball Association (NBA) in 1988 as an expansion team. After seven straight disappointing seasons, the team finally took off when head coach and club president Pat Riley took the helm. Riley, who led the "Showtime"-era Los Angeles Lakers of the 1980s to four championships, brought Miami to a franchise-best 61-21 record in only two years of leadership. Although Riley's Heat have become ubiquitous playoff contenders, they have yet to sizzle their way to the NBA finals. Mickey Arison, CEO of Carnival Corporation, and his family own the Miami Heat.

National Diagnostics, Inc.

755 W. Brandon Blvd., Brandon, FL 33511

Telephone: 813-661-9501 **Fax:** 813-681-6159 **Metro area:** Tampa-St. Petersburg, FL **Human resources contact:** Vicky Simmons **Sales:** $9.9 million **Number of employees:** 118 **Number of employees for previous year:** 113 **Industry designation:** Medical services **Company type:** Public **Top competitors:** Medical Resources, Inc.; Syncor International Corporation; Raytel Medical Corporation

National Diagnostics provides diagnostic imaging services through several outpatient centers in Florida. The company offers magnetic resonance imaging (MRI), computed tomography (CT), ultrasound, nuclear medicine, general radiology and fluoroscopy, and mammography services through four fixed sites and mobile facilities. Roughly half of National Diagnostics revenues come from its primary facility in Brandon, Florida. The company has agreed to merge with American Enterprise Solutions, with National Diagnostics owning about 12% of the merged companies. National Diagnostics will be the surviving entity but will change its name to American Enterprise Solutions.

NeoMedia Technologies, Inc.

2201 Second St., Ste. 600, Fort Myers, FL 33901

Telephone: 941-337-3434 **Fax:** 941-337-3668 **Metro area:** Fort Myers, FL **Web site:** http://www.neom.com **Human resources contact:** John Mantica **Sales:** $23.5 million **Number of employees:** 87 **Number of employees for previous year:** 59 **Industry designation:** Computers—services **Company type:** Public

NeoMedia Technologies may dream of leading the emerging field of intelligent documents, but the company pays its bills as a computer systems integrator. NeoMedia operates in four areas: document management, legacy-to-open-system conversions (migration), year 2000 compliance, and intelligent document systems (which turn printed materials into the equivalent of floppy disks). Document management and equipment reselling provide nearly 80% of revenues; the rest come from year 2000 and migrations operations, including its ADAPT/2000 date-correction software. NeoMedia's hopes are pinned on its proprietary software, sales of which doubled in 1997 to about 10%. Founder Charles Fritz owns about 25% of the company.

North Broward Hospital District

303 SE 17th St., Fort Lauderdale, FL 33316

Telephone: 954-355-5100 **Fax:** 954-355-4966 **Metro area:** Miami, FL **Web site:** http://www.nbhd.org **Human resources contact:** Harolynn Lanza **Sales:** $476.5 million **Number of employees:** 6,779 **Number of employees for previous year:** 6,615 **Industry designation:** Hospitals **Company type:** Government-owned **Top competitors:** Bon Secours Health System, Inc.; Catholic Health East; Columbia/HCA Healthcare Corporation

Government-owned North Broward Hospital District is the largest public hospital system in Florida. It serves Broward County with four hospitals (Broward General, North Broward, Coral Springs, and Imperial Point medical centers), and a host of community-based centers. Broward General features an American Sleep Disorders Association-accredited lab and the Chris Evert Women and Children's Center. Other facilities include a Neurological Institute (at North Broward) and a sports medicine program (at Coral Springs). The system also includes the Children's Diagnostic and Treatment Center, Clinica de las Americas, and two Family Health Place centers.

Noven Pharmaceuticals, Inc.

11960 SW 144th St., Miami, FL 33186

Telephone: 305-253-5099 **Fax:** 305-251-1887 **Metro area:** Miami, FL **Human resources contact:** Carolyn D. Donaldson **Sales:** $21.8 million **Number of employees:** 190 **Number of employees for previous year:** 146 **Industry designation:** Medical products **Company type:** Public **Top competitors:** Sano Corporation; Cygnus, Inc.; Minnesota Mining and Manufacturing Company

Noven Pharmaceuticals develops transdermal drug delivery systems. Products include drug delivery systems for motion sickness, angina, and nicotine withdrawal. The company's systems utilize an adhesive patch containing medication that is administered through the skin and into the blood stream over an extended period of time. Noven has developed and patented small, thin, solid-state, multilaminate transdermal drug delivery systems that can be adapted to deliver many different kinds of drugs. It is developing products for applications including dental pain management, antifungal therapy, asthma, and anxiety disorders. Noven has received FDA approval for its Combipatch, a hormone replacement for menopausal women.

Ocean Bio-Chem, Inc.

4041 SW 47th Ave., Fort Lauderdale, FL 33314

Telephone: 954-587-6280 **Fax:** 954-587-2813 **Metro area:** Miami, FL **Sales:** $12.8 million **Number of employees:** 73 **Number of employees for previous year:** 48 **Industry designation:** Soap & cleaning preparations **Company type:** Public

Ocean Bio-Chem makes and markets a variety of maintenance and appearance products for boats, recreational vehicles, and aircraft under the Star Brite brand name. The marine line consists of vinyl protectants, teak cleaners and teak oils, hull cleaners, and other related products. The recreational line includes detergents, polishes, fabric cleaners, and antifreeze. In addition, the company makes polishes and cleaners for aircraft. Ocean Bio-Chem's products are sold through national retail chains and specialized marine retailers; Wal-Mart and West Marine account for about 25% of the company's sales. President and CEO Peter Dornau owns more than 55% of Ocean Bio-Chem.

Omega Research, Inc.

8700 W. Flagler St., Ste. 250, Miami, FL 33174

Telephone: 305-551-9991 **Fax:** 305-551-2240 **Metro area:** Miami, FL **Web site:** http://www.omegaresearch.com **Human resources contact:** Leona Bodie **Sales:** $28.2 million **Number of employees:** 177 **Number of employees for previous year:** 139 **Industry designation:** Computers—corporate, professional & financial software **Company type:** Public

Omega Research makes investment analysis software for Windows operating systems. Omega's TradeStation is a professional software package that evaluates trading goals, compares historical data, and recommends a course of action by pager if the customer is not in front of the computer. The company's OptionStation software enables professional investors who are not options experts to take a position in the options market based on risk and the customer profile. SuperCharts generates analyses in a chart format that allows individuals to draw trend lines, identify patterns, and perform historical analysis. Co-CEOs William and Ralph Cruz own approximately 40% of the company.

Optimum Health Services, Inc.

17757 US 19 North, Ste. 350, Clearwater, FL 33764

Telephone: 727-536-9956 **Fax:** 727-536-2246 **Metro area:** Tampa-St. Petersburg, FL **Web site:** http://www.optimum-health.net **Human resources contact:** David A. Sherwin **Sales:** $1,000 (Est.) **Number of employees:** 14 **Industry designation:** Health maintenance organization **Company type:** Private

Optimum Health Services is out to optimize choice in health care. In addition to its traditional physician network, the Florida managed care company provides clients with a list of credentialed holistic care providers. Optimum Health Services concentrates on disease management protocols for wellness, and includes wellness products (such as SMOKENDERS and Nutri/Systems) as well as access to fitness centers in its program. It focuses on drawing holistically inclined physicians into its provider network. Optimum Health Services' network includes almost 3,000 provider locations. The company's owner, Complete Wellness Centers, is spinning off Optimum Health Services.

Orange-co, Inc.

2020 US Hwy. 17 South, Bartow, FL 33831

Telephone: 941-533-0551 **Fax:** 941-533-6357 **Other address:** PO Box 2158, Bartow, FL 33831 **Metro area:** Lakeland, FL **Human resources contact:** Paul Mabry **Sales:** $118.9 million **Number of employees:** 350 **Number of employees for previous year:** 340 **Industry designation:** Agricultural operations **Company type:** Public **Top competitors:** Tropicana Products, Inc.; Lykes Bros. Inc.; The Coca-Cola Company

You'd be surprised if Orange-co didn't deal with oranges. The firm grows, processes, packages, and markets citrus products. It owns almost 14,000 acres of citrus groves in Florida and provides management services (including caretaking, harvesting, and marketing) for nearly 3,000 acres of groves owned by others. Orange-co processes bulk frozen concentrated orange and grapefruit juices, not-from-concentrate juices, and citrus by-products at its Florida, plant. It also makes non-citrus juice-based drinks and concentrated liquid tea and coffee. Orange-co's products are sold to major food service companies, dairies, and other industrial users. Chairman and CEO Ben Hill Griffin owns more than 50% of Orange-co.

Orlando Magic

2 Magic Place, 8701 Maitland Summit Blvd., Orlando, FL 32810

Telephone: 407-916-2400 **Fax:** 407-916-2810 **Other address:** PO Box 95, Orlando, FL 32802 **Metro area:** Orlando, FL **Web site:** http://www.nba.com/magic **Human resources contact:** Lorisse Garcia **Sales:** $63.7 million (Est.) **Number of employees:** 122 **Number of employees for previous year:** 110 **Industry designation:** Leisure & recreational services **Company type:** Private **Top competitors:** New Jersey Nets; New York Knickerbockers; Miami Heat

An NBA team and subsidiary of RDV Sports, the Orlando Magic first dribbled onto the court in 1989. Unlike most expansion teams, the Magic struggled for only a short time in its infancy. The team drafted Goliath-like center Shaquille O'Neal in 1992 and instantly became a serious NBA competitor. In 1995 the Magic, behind the talents of O'Neal and guard Anfernee "Penny" Hardaway, made the NBA finals, but the team was swept by the Houston Rockets. Orlando experienced two big losses in 1996: It was crushed in the playoffs by the Chicago Bulls, and O'Neal left in favor of a free-agent contract with the Los Angeles Lakers. Rich DeVos, co-founder of Amway, owns the team.

The Orlando Predators Entertainment, Inc.

20 N. Orange Ave., Ste. 101, Orlando, FL 32801

Telephone: 407-648-4444 **Fax:** 407-648-8101 **Metro area:** Orlando, FL **Sales:** $2.7 million **Number of employees:** 46 **Number of employees for previous year:** 41 **Industry designation:** Leisure & recreational services **Company type:** Public **Top competitors:** Orlando Magic; Tampa Bay Buccaneers; National Football League

Orlando Predators Entertainment owns and operates the Orlando Predators professional arena football team of the Arena Football League (AFL). The company sells tickets to Predators' home games, advertising and promotions to team sponsors, and Predators merchandise (athletic clothing, including sweatshirts, T-shirts, jackets, and caps). It also derives revenues from the sale of local and regional broadcast rights to Predators' games, its share of contracts with national broadcast organizations, and expansion team fees paid through the AFL. Chairman William Meris owns more than half the company.

Orthodontic Centers of America, Inc.

5000 Sawgrass Village Circle, Ste. 25, Ponte Vedra Beach, FL 32082

Telephone: 904-280-4500 **Fax:** 904-273-5554 **Metro area:** Jacksonville, FL **Web site:** http://www.ocai.com **Human resources contact:** Damien Leone **Sales:** $171.3 million **Number of employees:** 1,721 **Number of employees for previous year:** 1,287 **Industry designation:** Medical practice management **Company type:** Public **Top competitors:** Castle Dental Centers, Inc.; Apple Orthodontix, Inc.; OrthAlliance, Inc.

Brace yourself: Orthodontic Centers of America (OCA) is a dental practice management firm aiming to take a bite out of the nationwide market. In return for a fee, OCA provides capital financing for developing, acquiring, and consolidating orthodontic practices and also manages business and marketing aspects. The company's proprietary office design and patient scheduling system maximize efficiency and allow each orthodontist to see many more patients per day. OCA serves more than 230 orthodontists working in approximately 415 centers in about 40 states across the US. The company's centers treat about 130,000 patients every year.

Orthodontix, Inc.

2222 Ponce de Leon Blvd., Ste. 300, Coral Gables, FL 33134

Telephone: 305-446-8661 **Fax:** 305-445-0563 **Metro area:** Miami, FL **Web site:** http://www.orthodontix.com **Human resources contact:** Helaine Clein **Number of employees:** 220 **Industry designation:** Medical practice management **Company type:** Public **Top competitors:** Apple Orthodontix, Inc.; Omega Orthodontics, Inc.; OrthAlliance, Inc.

Orthodontix doesn't straighten teeth, but it does try to straighten the business sides of orthodontics practices. The company provides nonorthodontic staff and generally owns the equipment and assets used in the practice. Practice management services include billing, purchasing, payroll, employee benefits, advertising, and financial and productivity reporting and analysis. The company provides these services through agreements with professional associations of orthodontists who use the services. The company has service agreements with about 30 orthodontists in 40 offices in a dozen states.

Paradise, Inc.

1200 Dr. Martin Luther King Jr. Blvd., Plant City, FL 33566

Telephone: 813-752-1155 **Fax:** 813-754-3168 **Metro area:** Tampa-St. Petersburg, FL **Sales:** $22 million **Number of employees:** 275 **Number of employees for previous year:** 200 **Industry designation:** Food—confectionery **Company type:** Public **Top competitors:** Dole Food Company, Inc.; United Foods, Inc.; Fresh Del Monte Produce Inc.

Regardless of your feelings toward fruitcake, Paradise supplies the candied fruit that makes this holiday treat possible. Although the company sells its candied fruit to commercial bakers and institutional users, more than 75% of its sales are to retail outlets that cater to the home baking market. Candied fruit brand names include Pennant and Mor-Fruit. In addition, Paradise grows and sells fresh and frozen strawberries to commercial and institutional users and repackages edible nuts. The company also produces molded-plastic containers for its own products and third parties. The Gordon family owns nearly 40% of the company.

Pediatrix Medical Group, Inc.

1455 Northpark Dr., Fort Lauderdale, FL 33326

Telephone: 954-384-0175 **Fax:** 954-384-7657 **Metro area:** Miami, FL **Web site:** http://www.pediatrix.com **Human resources contact:** Diane E. Schnitzer **Sales:** $185.4 million **Number of employees:** 939 **Number of employees for previous year:** 570 **Industry designation:** Medical practice management **Company type:** Public **Top competitors:** Medaphis Corporation; MedPartners, Inc.; Columbia/HCA Healthcare Corporation

Managing doctors isn't child's play. Pediatrix Medical Group is the leading contract manager of hospital-based neonatal and pediatric intensive care units (NICUs and PICUs). The company manages, staffs, and administers units and takes care of billing and reimbursement. The company has been growing quickly through the acquisition of neonatal, pediatric, and perinatal physician practices, developing regional networks in Denver, Phoenix, Southern California, and Texas (but its full range of operations encompasses more than 250 physicians in 20 states and Puerto Rico). In addition, Pediatrix actively markets itself directly to physician groups through telemarketing and advertising.

Phoenix International Ltd., Inc.

500 International Pkwy., Heathrow, FL 32746

Telephone: 407-548-5100 **Fax:** 407-548-5295 **Metro area:** Orlando, FL **Web site:** http://www.phoenixint.com **Human resources contact:** Barbara Brescia **Sales:** $25.9 million **Number of employees:** 368 **Number of employees for previous year:** 216 **Industry designation:** Computers—corporate, professional & financial software **Company type:** Public

Phoenix International integrates financial information and transaction processing in its client-server software, used by more than 120 customers worldwide. Its Phoenix System, compatible with a variety of platforms, is scalable and year 2000 compliant. The software performs system administration, nightly processing, and budgeting, as well as general ledger, teller, and investment functions. It also tracks individual account activity, assesses trends, produces reports, and conducts market reviews. Phoenix International offers trade and global payment software for international clients. The firm's customers include mid-market financial institutions in the US, as well as foreign retail-oriented institutions.

PhyMatrix Corp.

777 S. Flagler Dr., Phillips Point, Ste 1000E, West Palm Beach, FL 33401

Telephone: 561-655-3500 **Fax:** 561-833-7175 **Metro area:** West Palm Beach, FL **Web site:** http://www.phymatrix.com **Human resources contact:** Faye Traeger **Sales:** $346.5 million **Number of employees:** 2,960 **Number of employees for previous year:** 1,055 **Industry designation:** Medical practice management **Company type:** Public

PhyMatrix is planning to divest its medical practice management operations in favor of the less-crowded clinical trials site management business. For now, however, it has management contracts to provide administrative services to some 350 physicians in the US, which generate about 45% of sales. The company also operates ancillary medical centers, such as those for imaging, radiation therapy, and ambulatory surgery (also 45% of sales). Through its DASCO subsidiaries, PhyMatrix provides consulting services to medical facility development projects. Chairman Abraham Gosman, who has related interests in nursing home operator CareMatrix and real estate investment trust Meditrust, owns 25% of PhyMatrix.

Prestige Cosmetics Corporation

1441 W. Newport Center Dr., Deerfield Beach, FL 33442

Telephone: 954-480-9202 **Fax:** 954-480-9220 **Metro area:** West Palm Beach, FL **Human resources contact:** Maral Cappotto **Sales:** $30 million (Est.) **Number of employees:** 128 **Number of employees for previous year:** 101 **Industry designation:** Cosmetics & toiletries **Company type:** Private **Top competitors:** The Procter & Gamble Company; L'Oreal; Revlon, Inc.

You can't buy taste or class, but Prestige is easier to come by. Prestige Cosmetics makes cosmetics under the Prestige and Prestige Studio Make-Up brand names, as well as under private labels for retailers. Its products include lipstick, cosmetic pencils, lip gloss, powder, eye shadow, blush, concealers, mascara, foundation, and nail polish. Prestige markets its products to mass-merchandisers (including Sears and Wal-Mart), drugstores, and supermarkets in the US and 27 other countries. It operates a plant in Florida and distribution facilities in Australia, Canada, and Italy. After its planned IPO, co-founders and brothers Jacques and Gabriel Cohen will own about 36% and 25% of the company, respectively.

Priority Healthcare Corporation

285 W. Central Pkwy., Altamonte Springs, FL 32714

Telephone: 407-869-7001 **Fax:** 800-862-6208 **Metro area:** Orlando, FL **Web site:** http://www.priorityhealthcare.com **Human resources contact:** Barbara J. Luttrell **Sales:** $275.6 million **Number of employees:** 145 **Number of employees for previous year:** 135 **Industry designation:** Drugs & sundries—wholesale **Company type:** Public

Priority Healthcare Corporation distributes specialty pharmaceuticals and related medical supplies. Its Priority Healthcare Distribution division provides overnight distribution of environmentally sensitive pharmaceuticals to oncologists and dialysis centers nationwide. The Priority Pharmacy Services division, which serves individuals, ships prefilled syringes to about 1,500 customers, including those suffering from hepatitis, melanoma, cancer, and HIV. Formed in 1994 as a subsidiary of drug wholesaler Bindley Western Industries (which spun off its 82% stake to shareholders in 1999), Priority Healthcare specializes in alternative site distribution.

ProxyMed, Inc.

2501 Davie Rd., Ste. 230, Fort Lauderdale, FL 33317

Telephone: 954-473-1001 **Fax:** 954-473-0620 **Metro area:** Miami, FL **Web site:** http://www.proxymed.com **Human resources contact:** Bennett Marks **Sales:** $37.8 million **Number of employees:** 324 **Number of employees for previous year:** 154 **Industry designation:** Medical services **Company type:** Public **Top competitors:** National Data Corporation; ENVOY Corporation

ProxyMed provides electronic transaction services to doctors and others in the health care industry over its ProxyNet online network. Its software programs ProxyScript and PreScribe automate pharmacy management and prescription ordering via the Internet. ClinScan enables doctors to place lab orders and receive results online. The system also handles payor claims processing. In addition, the company provides pharmacy services for long-term-care facilities and offers full-scale Internet access. ProxyMed has been on an acquisitions binge, snapping up companies that broaden its range of services in an effort to provide one-stop-shopping convenience to its customers.

PSS World Medical, Inc.

4345 Southpoint Blvd., Jacksonville, FL 32216

Telephone: 904-332-3000 **Fax:** 904-332-3205 **Metro area:** Jacksonville, FL **Web site:** http://www.pssd.com **Human resources contact:** Jean Collins **Sales:** $1.3 billion **Number of employees:** 4,000 **Number of employees for previous year:** 2,600 **Industry designation:** Medical & dental supplies **Company type:** Public **Top competitors:** Bergen Brunswig Corporation; Allegiance Corporation; Owens & Minor, Inc.

Psst—need drugs fast? PSS World Medical provides same-day distribution of medical supplies, equipment, and pharmaceuticals to office-based physicians and nursing homes. PSS World Medical's distribution facilities serve more than 100,000 clients nationwide. PSS also distributes radiographic and other imaging equipment. The company distributes medical supplies in Belgium, France, Germany, Luxembourg, and the Netherlands from three European distribution sites. PSS has an exclusive distribution contract with Abbott Laboratories for practices with fewer than 25 doctors. Formerly known as Physician Sales & Service, the company became PSS Worldwide Medical when it acquired Gulf South Medical Supply.

Radiation Therapy Services, Inc.

1850 Boy Scout Dr., Ste. A-101, Fort Myers, FL 33907

Telephone: 941-931-7275 **Fax:** 941-931-7380 **Metro area:** Fort Myers, FL **Web site:** http://www.rtsx.com **Human resources contact:** Debbie Guild **Sales:** $39 million (Est.) **Number of employees:** 400 **Number of employees for previous year:** 317 **Industry designation:** Health care—outpatient & home **Company type:** Private **Top competitors:** Catholic Health East; Baptist Health Systems of South Florida; Cancer Treatment Holdings, Inc.

Radiation Therapy Services operates a network of 21 freestanding and hospital-based radiation therapy centers, including 15 in Florida, four in New York, and two in Nevada. The company offers a wide variety of radiation therapy services, ranging from basic external beam therapy to hyper-accurate and ultra-powerful stereotactic radiosurgery used for inoperable brain tumors. The company plans to use proceeds from its planned IPO to pay off debt, expand its network in its current markets, enter such new markets as the Maryland area, and acquire existing businesses as part of a consolidation strategy.

Regional Capital Management Corporation

1635D Royal Palm Dr., Gulfport, FL 33707

Telephone: 727-381-6226 **Fax:** 727-345-6325 **Metro area:** Tampa-St. Petersburg, FL **Number of employees:** 1 **Industry designation:** Nursing homes **Company type:** Private **Top competitors:** Beverly Enterprises, Inc.; Mariner Post-Acute Network, Inc.; Extendicare Inc.

Startup Regional Capital Management plans to develop, build, and operate assisted-living centers, with a focus on suburban areas in the Southeast; the company plans to use proceeds from the planned IPO to kick off its two initial development projects in Florida. The locally managed properties will offer on-site medical services, recreation activities, meals, housekeeping, and other services. Founder and sole officer Thomas Minkoff will reduce his ownership from 66% to 28% after the planned IPO. Minkoff has a background in real estate development and in the home health care industry.

Renex Corp.

2100 Ponce de Leon Blvd., Ste. 950, Coral Gables, FL 33134

Telephone: 305-448-2044 **Fax:** 305-448-1154 **Metro area:** Miami, FL **Human resources contact:** Nadine Lewis **Sales:** $37.8 million **Number of employees:** 284 **Number of employees for previous year:** 262 **Industry designation:** Medical services **Company type:** Public **Top competitors:** Renal Care Group, Inc.; Fresenius Medical Care Aktiengesellschaft; Gambro AB

Renex provides dialysis and ancillary services to about 1,100 patients suffering from chronic kidney failure. The company provides its services at 18 outpatient dialysis facilities in Florida, Georgia, Louisiana, Massachusetts, Mississippi, Missouri, New Jersey, and Pennsylvania. It also operates staff-assisted home hemodialysis programs in St. Louis and Tampa and provides inpatient dialysis services at 12 hospitals. Each facility has between eight and 21 dialysis stations featuring state-of-the-art equipment, as well as TVs and VCRs for patient entertainment. The company continues to grow through acquisitions, the development of new facilities, and alliances with hospitals and managed care organizations.

Rexall Sundown, Inc.

6111 Broken Sound Pkwy. NW, Boca Raton, FL 33487

Telephone: 561-241-9400 **Fax:** 561-995-0197 **Metro area:** West Palm Beach, FL **Web site:** http://www.rexallsundown.com **Human resources contact:** Nancy May **Sales:** $530.7 million **Number of employees:** 1,300 **Number of employees for previous year:** 820 **Industry designation:** Vitamins & nutritional products **Company type:** Public **Top competitors:** General Nutrition Companies, Inc.; Perrigo Company; Herbalife International, Inc.

The sun has yet to set on leading vitamin maker Rexall Sundown, which makes herbal supplements, homeopathic remedies, personal care goods, and weight control products, as well as multivitamin formulas, individual vitamins, and mineral products. Altogether the firm has some 1,000 products. More than half its sales come from such mass-market retailers as Kmart and Wal-Mart. It also sells through mail order and direct network sales (its Rexall Showcase International has 100,000 independent distributors). Founder and chairman Carl DeSantis and his family own about half the firm, which is the US distributor for Cellasene (dubbed the "Viagra of cellulite" for the clamor it has caused among seekers of thinner thighs).

Rica Foods, Inc.

95 Merrick Way, Ste. 507, Coral Gables, FL 33134

Telephone: 305-476-1757 **Fax:** 305-476-1760 **Metro area:** Miami, FL **Sales:** $103.7 million **Number of employees:** 3,000 **Number of employees for previous year:** 1,990 **Industry designation:** Food—meat products **Company type:** Public **Top competitors:** Pilgrim's Pride Corporation; ConAgra, Inc.; Tyson Foods, Inc.

Be it egg or nugget form, it's Chicken down the hatch with Rica Foods. It is Costa Rica's largest poultry producer through its Pipasa and As de Oros subsidiaries. It markets whole chickens; sausage, nuggets, and other processed products; animal feed; and eggs. The company supplies chicken to McDonald's, Burger King, Subway, and other restaurants as well as to supermarkets and food service clients in Central America. It also operates 36 As de Oros fried chicken restaurants and exports chicken to Asia. Formerly Costa Rica International, the company acquired its poultry operations in 1996 and changed its name accordingly. Chairman, president, and CEO Calixto Chaves (Pipasa's founder) owns 44%.

RoTech Medical Corporation

4506 L. B. McLeod Rd., Ste. F, Orlando, FL 32811

Telephone: 407-841-2115 **Fax:** 407-841-9318 **Metro area:** Orlando, FL **Human resources contact:** Veronica Royce **Sales:** $422.7 million **Industry designation:** Health care—outpatient & home **Company type:** Subsidiary **Top competitors:** American HomePatient, Inc.; Apria Healthcare Group Inc.; Coram Healthcare Corporation

Breathe deeply and repeat after us: RoTech Medical Corporation is a subsidiary of postacute care provider Integrated Health Services that provides comprehensive home health care and primary care physician services to patients in 40 states. The company operates about 700 home health care locations, primarily in nonurban areas. RoTech provides respiratory therapy products and services (mostly bottled oxygen) and home infusion services (antibiotics, enteral nutrition, hydration therapy, pain management, and chemotherapy). RoTech also rents and sells medical equipment. Oxygen services for Medicaid patients accounts for about 50% of sales.

Sheridan Healthcare, Inc.

4651 Sheridan St., Ste. 400, Hollywood, FL 33021

Telephone: 954-987-5822 **Fax:** 954-987-8359 **Metro area:** Miami, FL **Human resources contact:** Karen Winselman **Sales:** $113 million **Number of employees:** 770 **Number of employees for previous year:** 680 **Industry designation:** Medical practice management **Company type:** Public

Sheridan Healthcare, which is being taken private, is a physician practice management company. About 190 of its physicians (anesthesiologists, neonatologists, pediatricians, obstetricians, and ER physicians) provide specialist services at 35 medical facilities in Florida, New York, Ohio, Pennsylvania, Texas, Virginia, and West Virginia. The company also provides support services such as billing, malpractice risk management, and collections. In addition to its hospital-based services, Sheridan owns or manages the practices of almost 60 office-based physicians at some 30 locations in Florida and Texas.

Smith-Gardner & Associates, Inc.

1615 S. Congress Ave., Delray Beach, FL 33445

Telephone: 561-265-2700 **Fax:** 561-265-2566 **Metro area:** West Palm Beach, FL **Web site:** http://www.smithgardner.com **Human resources contact:** Marilyn Baumler **Sales:** $18.7 million **Number of employees:** 249 **Industry designation:** Computers—corporate, professional & financial software **Company type:** Public **Top competitors:** Open Market, Inc.; InterWorld Corporation; Pandesic LLC

Smith-Gardner & Associates makes software and hardware for businesses that perform high-volume catalog, e-commerce, mail-order, and wholesale sales. Its scalable MACS software can process up to 200,000 transactions daily and help clients advertise; perform marketing analyses; and manage inventory, shipping, and accounting. Add-on options manage tasks such as ordering, customer service, billing, telemarketing, and assembly. Smith-Gardner's WebOrder helps with Internet transactions. The firm offers support, consulting, installation, and training services. Customers include Cyberian Outpost, Egghead.com, and Nordstrom. Co-founders and co-chairmen Allan Gardner and Wilburn Smith each own 20% of the company.

SportsLine USA, Inc.

6340 NW Fifth Way, Fort Lauderdale, FL 33309

Telephone: 954-351-2120 **Fax:** 954-351-9175 **Metro area:** Miami, FL **Web site:** http://www.cbs.sportsline.com **Human resources contact:** Randall Hafer **Sales:** $30.6 million **Number of employees:** 303 **Number of employees for previous year:** 202 **Industry designation:** Computers—online services **Company type:** Public **Top competitors:** America Online, Inc.; The Walt Disney Company; Time Warner Inc.

SportsLine USA operates the cbs.sportsline.com Web site, which provides real-time sports news. The service covers sporting events, teams, and players and includes photos, audio and video clips, and original Internet broadcast programs. Other SportsLine Web sites provide information on sports superstars such as Wayne Gretzky and Shaquille O'Neal and odds and information on major sporting events (vegasinsider.com). Advertising accounts for more than half of SportsLine's sales; subscriptions, content licensing, and the sales of sports-themed merchandise account for the remainder. An affiliation with CBS provides SportsLine with free advertising during CBS's TV sports broadcasts.

The Stephan Co.

1850 W. McNab Rd., Fort Lauderdale, FL 33309

Telephone: 954-971-0600 **Fax:** 954-971-0636 **Metro area:** Miami, FL **Sales:** $27.1 million **Number of employees:** 206 **Number of employees for previous year:** 156 **Industry designation:** Cosmetics & toiletries **Company type:** Public **Top competitors:** The Procter & Gamble Company; Unilever; Revlon, Inc.

From shampoos to shaving lotions, Stephan has helped make primping possible for more than 100 years. The company makes and sells hair care and personal care products in the US and Canada via retail stores and mail order; it also distributes products to salons. Subsidiaries include Foxy Products, Old 97, Williamsport Barber and Beauty Corp., Stephan & Co., Scientific Research Products, Trevor Sorbie of America, and Stephan Distributing. The company sells products under brands such as Stephan, Cashmere Bouquet (talc), Quinsana Medicated (talc), Balm Barr, Stretch Mark, Protein 29, and Wildroot. Stephan is buying cleaning product maker and equipment distributor Rex Chemical.

Sterile Recoveries, Inc.

28100 US Hwy. 19 North, Ste. 201, Clearwater, FL 33761

Telephone: 727-726-4421 **Fax:** 727-726-8959 **Metro area:** Tampa-St. Petersburg, FL **Human resources contact:** Karen A. Reber **Sales:** $52.3 million **Number of employees:** 1,025 **Number of employees for previous year:** 774 **Industry designation:** Medical & dental supplies **Company type:** Public **Top competitors:** Owens & Minor, Inc.; Allegiance Corporation; Maxxim Medical, Inc.

Sterile Recoveries provides hospital and surgical centers with reusable surgical products such as gowns, towels, and basins that it sorts, sterilizes, and packages at eight regional facilities. Its daily pick-up and delivery service offers a cost-effective alternative to in-house recovery programs. The firm also offers disposable accessory packs for surgical procedures. Customers in 20 states include more than 300 hospitals and surgery centers such as Duke University Medical Center, Henry Ford Hospital, and Johns Hopkins Medical Hospital. Through agreements with VHA and Health Services Corporation of America, Sterile Recoveries serves approximately 2,600 health care organization and hospital members.

Sunterra Corp.

1781 Park Center Dr., Orlando, FL 32835

Telephone: 407-532-1000 **Fax:** 407-532-1141 **Metro area:** Orlando, FL **Web site:** http://www.sigr.com **Human resources contact:** Vickie Brownie **Sales:** $450 million **Number of employees:** 6,500 **Number of employees for previous year:** 4,150 **Industry designation:** Leisure & recreational services **Company type:** Public **Top competitors:** Marriott International, Inc.; Silverleaf Resorts, Inc.; Trendwest Resorts, Inc.

Sunterra can take you to some of the sunniest places on earth. Formerly Signature Resorts, Sunterra is one of the world's largest time-share vacation companies, with more than 80 resort locations in North America, Europe, Mexico, and the Caribbean. Approximately 200,000 families own vacation interests in one of the company's resorts, entitling them to a one-week stay at a resort as well as "vacation points," which may be redeemed at any participating resort location. Sunterra also offers financing to its owners and develops and manages resort properties. It markets properties under its Sunterra Resorts name and, through licencing agreements, the Embassy Vacation Resorts and Westin Vacation Club Resorts names.

Tampa Bay Buccaneers

One Buccaneer Place, Tampa, FL 33607

Telephone: 813-870-2700 **Fax:** 813-878-0813 **Metro area:** Tampa-St. Petersburg, FL **Web site:** http://www.nfl.com/buccaneers/index.html **Sales:** $76.8 million (Est.) **Number of employees:** 160 **Industry designation:** Leisure & recreational services **Company type:** Private **Top competitors:** Detroit Lions; Minnesota Vikings Football Club; The Green Bay Packers, Inc.

The National Football League's Tampa Bay Buccaneers have a new strategy—winning! Founded in 1976, the team snapped a streak of 14 consecutive losing seasons by making it to the playoffs in 1997 under new coach Tony Dungy. (The team went 8-8 the following season.) Those bay winds are blowing in other changes as well. Led by financier Malcolm Glazer, who purchased the Bucs in 1995, the team has a new logo, new colors, and new front-office management, as well as a new stadium (Raymond James Stadium). As part of the nation's most-watched sports league, the Bucs expect to get $74 million a year from a new NFL TV contract. The team's day-to-day operations are handled by Glazer's two sons.

Tampa Bay Devil Rays

Tropicana Field, One Tropicana Dr., St. Petersburg, FL 33705

Telephone: 727-825-3137 **Fax:** 727-825-3111 **Metro area:** Tampa-St. Petersburg, FL **Web site:** http://www.devilray.com **Number of employees:** 120 **Industry designation:** Leisure & recreational services **Company type:** Private **Top competitors:** New York Yankees; Toronto Blue Jays Baseball Club; The Boston Red Sox

Even though 1998 was their inaugural season, baseball's Tampa Bay Devil Rays didn't lose 100 games. The club, which plays its home games at Tropicana Field, finished 63-99, aided by such well-known veterans as Wade Boggs and Fred McGriff. In some respects, the club did better than its owners, a consortium of six general and nine limited partners: one owner was sentenced to jail, two were accused of shady campaign contributions, and another lost his job as CEO at Danka Industries. This calamity made managing partner and CEO Vincent Naimoli (who owns about 17% of the Devil Rays) look like a saint, who cursed out several reporters and angered community leaders with other inflammatory comments.

Tampa Bay Lightning

401 Channelside Dr., Tampa, FL 33602

Telephone: 813-229-2658 **Fax:** 813-229-3350 **Metro area:** Tampa-St. Petersburg, FL **Web site:** http://www.tampabaylightning.com **Human resources contact:** Willie Van Der Merwe **Sales:** $41.9 million (Est.) **Number of employees:** 75 **Industry designation:** Leisure & recreational services **Company type:** Private **Top competitors:** Florida Panthers Holdings, Inc.; Washington Capitals; Carolina Hurricanes Hockey Club

When the Tampa Bay Lightning first struck the ice for the 1992-93 NHL season, some hockey fans wondered how the cold-clime pastime would do in sunny Florida. The Lightning subsequently set an all-time record for regular season attendance for a hockey game: 27,227. The team played in nonhockey arenas such as the Expo Hall for the first few years and then moved into its own home in downtown Tampa in 1996. In 1998 Art Williams, a Palm Beach insurance maven, bought the team for $117 million. However Williams, after owning the team for less than a year, sold the Lightning to an investment group led by Michigan billionaire William Davidson. The group also owns the NBA's Detroit Pistons

Technical Chemicals and Products, Inc.

3341 SW 15th St., Pompano Beach, FL 33069

Telephone: 954-979-0400 **Fax:** 954-979-0009 **Metro area:** Miami, FL **Web site:** http://www.techchem.com **Human resources contact:** Jerry Foster **Sales:** $6.2 million **Number of employees:** 64 **Number of employees for previous year:** 62 **Industry designation:** Medical products **Company type:** Public **Top competitors:** Becton, Dickinson and Company; Cygnus, Inc.; Selfcare, Inc.

From a "+" or a "-" to a complete overhaul of operations, Technical Chemicals and Products, Inc. (TCPI) knows change. The company is switching gears from making to developing tests and other products that can be used in physicians' offices, patients' homes, or other locations. TCPI makes about 50 products, including tests for pregnancy, cholesterol, infectious diseases, blood glucose levels, and drug use. TCPI has marketing agreements with other companies, including Amway, and it sells its products through private, discount, and supermarket labels. The company is developing transdermal drug-delivery systems through its Pharmetrix Division. President and CEO Jack Aronowitz owns about 45% of TCPI.

Technisource, Inc.

1901 W. Cypress Creek Rd., Ste. 401, Fort Lauderdale, FL 33309

Telephone: 954-493-8601 **Fax:** 954-493-8603 **Metro area:** Miami, FL **Web site:** http://www.tsi.net **Human resources contact:** Mike Gallagher **Sales:** $105.7 million **Number of employees:** 1,073 **Industry designation:** Computers—services **Company type:** Public **Top competitors:** Andersen Consulting; International Business Machines Corporation; Computer Sciences Corporation

Techie personnel firm Technisource provides information technology (IT) staffers through 20 offices in the US and Canada. The company maintains a database of more than 100,000 IT professionals offering more than 40,000 skills, including system and software design and development, documentation, training, resource planning, help-desk support, Internet and intranet development, systems administration, and year 2000 compliance. Among the company's 200 clients are such major corporations as Motorola (21% of sales), Rockwell (15%), AT&T, and General Motors. Co-founders Joseph Collard and James Robertson own nearly 70% of the company.

The Ultimate Software Group, Inc.

3111 Stirling Rd., Fort Lauderdale, FL 33312

Telephone: 954-266-1000 **Fax:** 954-266-1300 **Metro area:** Miami, FL **Web site:** http://www.ultimatesoftware.com **Human resources contact:** Vivian Maza **Sales:** $43.3 million **Number of employees:** 322 **Number of employees for previous year:** 265 **Industry designation:** Computers—corporate, professional & financial software **Company type:** Public **Top competitors:** PeopleSoft, Inc.; SAP AG; Oracle Corporation

The Ultimate Software Group markets its human resource management and payroll software primarily to midsized companies in a variety of industries including manufacturing, health care, and finance. Its UltiPro HRMS/Payroll software integrates human resource and payroll capabilities with embedded Internet technology, employee self-service capabilities, and Cognos Corporation's tools for data analysis and custom report generation. Ultimate Software also provides implementation, training, customer support, and maintenance services. The company markets its products through direct sales and a network of strategic partners. Customers include The Florida Marlins, Telemundo Group, US Filter, and Winn-Dixie Stores.

Uniroyal Technology Corporation

2 N. Tamiami Trail, Ste. 900, Sarasota, FL 34236

Telephone: 941-361-2100 **Fax:** 941-361-2131 **Metro area:** Sarasota, FL **Web site:** http://www.uniroyaltech.com **Human resources contact:** Martin J. Gutfreund **Sales:** $220.6 million **Number of employees:** 1,160 **Number of employees for previous year:** 1,100 **Industry designation:** Chemicals—diversified **Company type:** Public **Top competitors:** NS Group, Inc.; Ashland Inc.; Minnesota Mining and Manufacturing Company

Love the feel and look of Naugahyde? Then thank Uniroyal Technology. Naugahyde, vinyl-covered fabric, is the most well-known of this company's coated-fabric products. Through its high-performance plastics division, Uniroyal also makes Royalite thermoplastic products and Polycast acrylic sheets and rods for use in a range of applications, including aviation (windshields) and security (bulletproof shields). The firm also makes specialty adhesives, primarily for the construction market. Its optoelectronics division makes light-emitting diodes. Director Thomas Russell owns about 13% of the company, and chairman and CEO Howard Curd and the US Environmental Protection Agency each own about 7% of Uniroyal.

US Diagnostic Inc.

777 S. Flagler Dr., Ste. 1201 East, West Palm Beach, FL 33401

Telephone: 561-832-0006 **Fax:** 561-833-8391 **Metro area:** West Palm Beach, FL **Web site:** http://www.usdl.com **Sales:** $195.7 million **Number of employees:** 1,487 **Number of employees for previous year:** 1,300 **Industry designation:** Medical services **Company type:** Public

US Diagnostic is one of the nation's leading providers of outpatient radiology services. It owns and operates freestanding and hospital-affiliated diagnostic imaging facilities and clinical laboratories, primarily outside major metropolitan areas. The company offers services including X-ray and fluoroscopy, ultrasound, and CT testing at 120 fixed-site centers in 18 states. Locations include Bluefield, Virginia; Columbus, Georgia; Lafayette, Louisiana; Santa Fe, New Mexico; and Sherman Oaks, California. US Diagnostic also performs services to 40 hospitals and manages 19 additional facilities.

Viragen, Inc.

865 SW 78th Ave., Ste. 100, Plantation, FL 33324

Telephone: 954-233-8746 **Fax:** 954-233-1414 **Metro area:** Miami, FL **Web site:** http://www.viragen.com **Human resources contact:** Maria Rios **Sales:** $1.1 million **Number of employees:** 41 **Number of employees for previous year:** 33 **Industry designation:** Drugs **Company type:** Public **Top competitors:** Schering-Plough Corporation; Genentech, Inc.; Glaxo Wellcome plc

Viragen is no buttinsky. The development-stage company works with human interferons, which it hopes to use to treat AIDS, herpes, hepatitis B and C, and multiple sclerosis. Produced in white blood cells, interferons do exactly what their name suggests: they interfere with the growth of malignant cancer cells and such foreign substances as viruses. Viragen has developed but not yet received FDA or European Union approval for Omniferon, an injectable form of human interferon. The company has white blood cell supply agreements with The American Red Cross, America's Blood Centers, the Scottish National Blood Transfusion Service, and German Red Cross blood blanks. Viragen has facilities in Florida and Scotland.

Vision Twenty-One, Inc.

7209 Bryan Dairy Rd., Largo, FL 33777

Telephone: 727-545-4300 **Fax:** 888-324-2862 **Metro area:** Tampa-St. Petersburg, FL **Web Site:** http://www.vision21.com **Human resources contact:** Lynn Heckler **Sales:** $56.3 million **Number of employees:** 711 **Number of employees for previous year:** 539 **Industry designation:** Medical practice management **Company type:** Public **Top competitors:** Omega Health Systems, Inc.; Physicians Resource Group, Inc.; Sight Resource Corporation

Vision Twenty-One provides management and administrative services to a network of optometrists, ophthalmologists, ambulatory surgical centers, and retail optical centers in about 25 states (more than 4,400 clinics and surgical centers with more than 5,800 affiliated providers). The company handles the non-professional aspects of each participating business, while the on-site doctors or managing professionals focus on patient care and professional employee concerns. Vision Twenty-One contracts with insurance companies and HMOs to provide eye care services; it also operates a buying group through its Block Vision subsidiary.

Vistana, Inc.

8801 Vistana Centre Dr., Orlando, FL 32821

Telephone: 407-239-3100 **Fax:** 407-239-3111 **Metro area:** Orlando, FL **Web site:** http://www.vistanainc.com **Human resources contact:** Joy Theis **Sales:** $233.7 million **Number of employees:** 3,227 **Number of employees for previous year:** 1,984 **Industry designation:** Leisure & recreational services **Company type:** Public **Top competitors:** Cendant Corporation

Vistana develops and operates time-share resorts in the US. It sells vacation ownership interests in these resorts. The company runs six properties (three in Florida, two in Colorado, and one in Arizona), with a total of 1,660 units. Vistana is developing four more resorts in South Carolina, Florida, and Arizona. Through a joint venture with Sun International Hotels, the firm is developing a vacation ownership resort in the Bahamas. Vistana is also the exclusive sales and marketing agent for The Christie Lodge in Avon, Colorado. The company has a base of more than 65,000 vacation ownership interests. Co-CEOs Jeffrey Adler and Raymond Gellein (also chairman) own about 26% and 28% of the company, respectively.

Visual Edge Systems Inc.

2424 N. Federal Hwy., Ste. 100, Boca Raton, FL 33431

Telephone: 561-750-7559 **Fax:** 561-750-7299 **Metro area:** West Palm Beach, FL **Web site:** http://www.theshark.com **Human resources contact:** Kelly Finley **Sales:** $2.6 million **Number of employees:** 52 **Number of employees for previous year:** 22 **Industry designation:** Leisure & recreational services **Company type:** Public

Visual Edge Systems' personalized "One-On-One With Greg Norman" videotapes digitally combine footage of the golfer's swing with a synchronized split-screen comparison to professional golfer Greg Norman's swing. Its six "One-On-One" tapes include lessons for basic golf fundamentals, senior golfers, and lower-handicap players. The tapes are sold to event organizers and golf courses as promotional and teaching tools. The firm plans to produce other videos for the short game, sand play, and putting. Through an exclusive agreement, Cadillac offers a free One-On-One golf lesson with a test drive. Marion Interglobal, Ltd owns almost 50% of Visual Edge Systems.

Wackenhut Corporation

4200 Wackenhut Dr., Ste. 100, Palm Beach Gardens, FL 33140

Telephone: 561-622-5656 **Fax:** 561-691-6736 **Metro area:** Miami, FL **Web site:** http://www.wackenhut.com **Human resources contact:** Sandra Nusbaum **Sales:** $1.8 billion **Number of employees:** 70,000 **Number of employees for previous year:** 56,000 **Industry designation:** Protection—safety equipment & services **Company type:** Public **Top competitors:** Borg-Warner Security Corporation; Prison Realty Corporation; Pinkerton's, Inc.

Wackenhut provides security to commercial, industrial, and governmental customers; through subsidiary Wackenhut Corrections, it also manages more than 40 correctional facilities with some 30,000 beds. The company touts its Custom Protection Officer program, which provides specially trained security personnel. Special services include executive protection, crash-fire-rescue services, airport security, nuclear power plant security, and investigations. Wackenhut also provides food, laundry, and janitorial services for prisons; through another subsidiary it offers employee leasing. The firm operates in 48 states and 50 countries. Founder George Wackenhut controls the company.

Wackenhut Corrections Corporation

4200 Wackenhut Dr., Ste. 100, Palm Beach Gardens, FL 33410

Telephone: 561-622-5656 **Fax:** 561-691-6736 **Metro area:** West Palm Beach, FL **Web site:** http://www.wackenhut.com/wcc/wccindex.htm **Human resources contact:** Sandra Nusbaum **Sales:** $311.8 million **Number of employees:** 6,301 **Number of employees for previous year:** 4,182 **Industry designation:** Protection—safety equipment & services **Company type:** Public **Top competitors:** Cornell Corrections, Inc.; Prison Realty Corporation; UK Detention Services, Ltd.

The second-largest developer and operator of private prisons in the US (after Prison Realty), Wackenhut Corrections manages private correctional and detention facilities in the US, the UK, and Australia. (It is the market leader overseas.) Wackenhut Corrections has contracts to manage more than 40 facilities. Its services include prison design, construction, consulting, and rehabilitative and educational programs. Wackenhut Corrections operates prisons under contract for federal, state, and local governments. Security firm Wackenhut Corp. owns 54% of Wackenhut Corrections.

World Fuel Services Corporation

700 S. Royal Poinciana Blvd., Ste. 800, Miami Springs, FL 33166

Telephone: 305-884-2001 **Fax:** 305-883-0186 **Metro area:** Miami, FL **Web site:** http://www.wfscorp.com **Human resources contact:** Ileana Garcia **Sales:** $801.7 million **Number of employees:** 364 **Number of employees for previous year:** 267 **Industry designation:** Oil refining & marketing **Company type:** Public **Top competitors:** Safety-Kleen Corp.; Caltex Petroleum Corporation; Mercury Air Group, Inc.

Fill 'er up and check the oil while you're at it. World Fuel Services is an aviation and marine fueling services company and one of the leading recyclers of used oil in the US. Through its subsidiaries the company provides fueling and logistics services to small to midsized air carriers, cargo and charter carriers, and private aircraft at more than 1,100 airports around the world. Subsidiary Trans-Tec provides fueling services to marine vessels in more than 1,100 ports in over 150 countries. Another subsidiary, International Petroleum, collects and recycles nonhazardous used oil, wastewater, and petroleum-contaminated liquids. Recycled oil products are sold to commercial and industrial customers.

Xomed Surgical Products, Inc.

6743 Southpoint Dr. North, Jacksonville, FL 32216

Telephone: 904-296-9600 **Fax:** 904-296-9666 **Metro area:** Jacksonville, FL **Web site:** http://www.xomed.com **Human resources contact:** Bud Stevens **Sales:** $91.4 million **Number of employees:** 724 **Number of employees for previous year:** 513 **Industry designation:** Medical instruments **Company type:** Public **Top competitors:** Smith & Nephew plc

Xomed Surgical Products knows the ear, nose, and throat (ENT) market. The company is the market leader in surgical products for ENT specialists—Xomed makes everything from high-tech tissue-removal systems and minimally-invasive endoscopy instruments to implantable monitoring systems and disposables. The company sells its products in the US through its own sales force and abroad through a network of distributors. Xomed has formed an alliance to market ArthroCare's ENTec tissue-removal products. Warburg, Pincus Investors owns about 45% of the company.

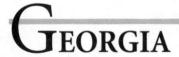

GEORGIA

American Megatrends, Inc.

6145-F Northbelt Pkwy., Norcross, GA 30071

Telephone: 770-246-8600 **Fax:** 770-246-8790 **Metro area:** Atlanta, GA **Web site:** http://www.ami.com **Human resources contact:** Dora Johnson **Sales:** $100 million (Est.) **Number of employees:** 400 **Industry designation:** Computers—peripheral equipment **Company type:** Private **Top competitors:** Phoenix Technologies Ltd.; SystemSoft Corporation; Diamond Multimedia Systems, Inc.

American Megatrends survives on gut feelings. The company provides core computer technologies, including Basic Input/Output Systems (AMIBIOS), which convey information between a computer's hardware and operating systems; motherboards; RAID (redundant array of independent disks) controllers, which boost performance and recovery; and system management hardware and software. Founded in 1985, the company sells its products to manufacturers such as Dell Computer, Compaq Computer, and Hewlett-Packard, and to resellers and integrators. The engineer-heavy (about half of its employees) company continues to increase its global growth. Founder and president Subramonian Shankar, an India native, owns American Megatrends.

American Software, Inc.

470 E. Paces Ferry Rd. NE, Atlanta, GA 30305

Telephone: 404-261-4381 **Fax:** 404-264-5514 **Metro area:** Atlanta, GA **Web site:** http://www.amsoftware.com **Human resources contact:** Chad Been **Sales:** $107.5 million **Number of employees:** 701 **Number of employees for previous year:** 610 **Industry designation:** Computers—corporate, professional & financial software **Company type:** Public **Top competitors:** i2 Technologies, Inc.; Manugistics Group, Inc.; System Software Associates, Inc.

From sea to shining sea American Software's products work to organize and integrate the various functions of midsized businesses, including financial, production, purchasing, and order fulfillment. The company's Intelliprise enterprise resource planning software is designed for use by large businesses. Other products let far-flung offices work together over the Internet. Through subsidiaries, American performs systems integration, Web hosting, and high-volume e-mail management services. American Software also owns 84% of supply chain management software maker Logility. Co-founders James Edenfield (CEO) and Thomas Newberry (Newberry) control 73% of the company's voting power.

The Atlanta Braves

521 Capitol Ave. SW, Atlanta, GA 30312

Telephone: 404-577-9100 **Fax:** 404-614-1391 **Other address:** PO Box 4064, Atlanta, GA 30302 **Metro area:** Atlanta, GA **Web site:** http://www.atlantabraves.com **Human resources contact:** Lisa Stricklin **Sales:** $119.6 million **Industry designation:** Leisure & recreational services **Company type:** Subsidiary **Top competitors:** The Philadelphia Phillies; Metropolitan Baseball Club Inc.; Montreal Baseball Club Inc.

The Atlanta Braves always seem to be in the playoffs (the club has a record seven consecutive postseason appearances) and on the television. Media baron Ted Turner is responsible for both phenomena—he bought the Braves in 1976 with the idea of televising games on his fledgling cable superstation, TBS. The move brought stability and national exposure to the team. The Braves won the National League championship four times in the 1990s and won the 1995 World Series. Formed in 1871, the team called Boston and Milwaukee home before moving to Atlanta in 1966. In 1998 the Braves lost the pennant race to the San Diego Padres. Turner Broadcasting, part of media giant Time Warner, owns the team.

Atlanta Falcons

One Falcon Place, Suwanee, GA 30024

Telephone: 770-945-1111 **Fax:** 770-271-1221 **Metro area:** Atlanta, GA **Web site:** http://www.atlantafalcons.com **Sales:** $77.6 million (Est.) **Industry designation:** Leisure & recreational services **Company type:** Private **Top competitors:** New Orleans Saints; St. Louis Rams Football Company; San Francisco 49ers

The NFL's Atlanta Falcons have become true birds of prey. Under former Denver Broncos coach Dan Reeves, the Falcons gained glory in 1998-99, winning only its second division title in more than 30 years and advancing to its first Super Bowl. The team was crushed in the big game by the defending champ Denver Broncos. The franchise, valued at $191 million, was awarded to Rankin Smith in 1965 for a record $8.5 million. He brought the spotlight to his team in 1992 with the building of the Georgia Dome, a stadium with more than 71,000 seats; the stadium hosted the 1994 Super Bowl and is scheduled to host another in 2000. Smith died in 1997, leaving ownership of the franchise with the Smith family.

Bull Run Corporation

4370 Peachtree Rd. NE, Atlanta, GA 30319

Telephone: 404-266-8333 **Fax:** 404-261-9607 **Metro area:** Atlanta, GA **Sales:** $29.8 million **Number of employees:** 134 **Number of employees for previous year:** 123 **Industry designation:** Computers—peripheral equipment **Company type:** Public **Top competitors:** Axiohm Transaction Solutions, Inc.; Printronix, Inc.; IVI Checkmate Corp.

You won't find this company in Pamplona, but you might find its products printing out hospital bills for people who run with the bulls. Bull Run is the parent of Datasouth, which makes heavy-duty dot matrix and thermal printers and portable and desktop printers used to print items such as hospital bills, airline tickets, and labels. Through other subsidiaries and affiliates, Bull Run owns interests in 10 TV stations, three daily newspapers, and a sporting goods maker, and provides promotional and event management services to universities and athletic conferences. The SABRE Group accounts for more than 30% of sales. CEO Robert Prather and chairman Mack Robinson control nearly 25% of the company.

Carson, Inc.

64 Ross Rd., Savannah Industrial Park, Savannah, GA 31405

Telephone: 912-651-3400 **Fax:** 912-651-3471 **Metro area:** Savannah, GA **Web site:** http://www.carsonproductsco.com **Human resources contact:** Allena Lee-Brown **Sales:** $150.7 million **Number of employees:** 988 **Number of employees for previous year:** 698 **Industry designation:** Cosmetics & toiletries **Company type:** Public **Top competitors:** Revlon, Inc.; Alberto-Culver Company; Soft Sheen Products Inc.

If your beauty routine involves products called Dark & Lovely, Excelle, Beautiful Beginnings, Posner, Afro Sheen, Let's Jam, or Magic Shave, you must be a Carson customer. Carson makes hair-care and beauty products for consumers of African descent. The company sells more than 70 products—including hair relaxers and texturizers, hair color, shaving, and hair-maintenance products—to customers in more than 60 countries. Carson sold its Cutex nail polish remover business in order to focus on ethnic products. Growth is expected from sales efforts in Africa, Brazil, and the Caribbean. Director Vincent Wasik controls about 80% of the company's stock.

Centennial HealthCare Corporation

400 Perimeter Center Terrace, Ste. 650, Atlanta, GA 30346

Telephone: 770-698-9040 **Fax:** 770-395-9776 **Metro area:** Atlanta, GA **Web site:** http://www.centennialhc.com **Human resources contact:** Wesley Dedman **Sales:** $304.3 million **Number of employees:** 10,100 **Number of employees for previous year:** 8,300 **Industry designation:** Nursing homes **Company type:** Public

Centennial HealthCare provides long-term health care services to the elderly and other patients at about 90 skilled nursing facilities throughout the US. Services provided by the company include nursing and support, housekeeping, laundry, dietary, recreational, and social services. Centennial also provides specialty services such as rehabilitation therapy, respiratory therapy, infusion therapy, wound care, and other subacute services. The company operates through its subsidiaries with nursing facilities in 18 states, primarily in North Carolina, Indiana, and Michigan. Welsh, Carson, Anderson & Stowe called off its acquisition of the company.

Cerulean Companies, Inc.

3350 Peachtree Rd. NE, Atlanta, GA 30326

Telephone: 404-842-8423 **Fax:** 404-842-8010 **Metro area:** Atlanta, GA **Web site:** http://www.cerulean-companies.com **Human resources contact:** Jim Burns **Sales:** $1.3 billion (Est.) **Number of employees:** 2,494 **Number of employees for previous year:** 2,325 **Industry designation:** Insurance—accident & health **Company type:** Private **Top competitors:** The Prudential Insurance Company of America; Aetna Inc.; UnitedHealth Group

Cerulean Companies has the Blues in Georgia—Blue Cross and Blue Shield. Cerulean, which has agreed to be acquired by WellPoint Health Networks, was formed as the holding company for Georgia Blue when it became a for-profit company in 1996. Through three subsidiaries (HMO Georgia, Greater Georgia Life Insurance, and Group Benefits of Georgia) Georgia Blue offers a variety of insurance plans, including HMOs, preferred provider organizations, point-of-service network plans, and group life, indemnity, accidental death, and disability insurance. It also operates five community health partnership networks. Founded in 1937, Georgia Blue has more than 750,000 insurance contracts with about 1.6 million members.

Clarus Corporation

3950 Johns Creek Ct., Ste. 100, Suwanee, GA 30024

Telephone: 770-291-3900 **Fax:** 770-291-3999 **Metro area:** Atlanta, GA **Web site:** http://www.claruscorp.com **Human resources contact:** Arthur G. Walsh Jr. **Sales:** $41.6 million **Number of employees:** 343 **Number of employees for previous year:** 223 **Industry designation:** Computers—corporate, professional & financial software **Company type:** Public **Top competitors:** PeopleSoft, Inc.; Lawson Software; Oracle Corporation

Clarus is helping clear things up. The company (formerly SQL Financials International) makes Web-based finance and human resources software for automating such functions as accounting; analysis and reporting; e-commerce management; and personnel, benefits, and payroll management. The company's software, including CLARUS Financials and CLARUS HRMS, enables users to personalize and configure applications without complex programming. Clarus also provides software support services such as implementation and maintenance, training, and upgrading. Its more than 300 customers include First Data, MasterCard International, and T. Rowe Price Associates.

ClientLink, Inc.

3025 Windward Plaza, Ste. 200, Alpharetta, GA 30202

Telephone: 770-663-3900 **Fax:** 770-663-8987 **Metro area:** Atlanta, GA **Web site:** http://www.clientlink.com **Human resources contact:** Barbara Snyderman **Sales:** $9 million **Number of employees:** 120 **Number of employees for previous year:** 91 **Industry designation:** Computers—corporate, professional & financial software **Company type:** Subsidiary **Top competitors:** Computer Sciences Corporation; Andersen Consulting; Perot Systems Corporation

ClientLink, a subsidiary of CompuCom Systems, provides information technology design, development, and implementation services. The company's client/server and Internet/intranet services include customized information management systems, data collection systems, and Web site development. ClientLink specializes in developing systems for businesses that process large amounts of data in areas such as financial services, inventory management, and sales commission calculation. The company's customers include Gillette, Hewlett-Packard, Honda of America, and MCI WorldCom. CompuCom, which is planning to spin the company off in 1998, will hold some 60% of ClientLink after the planned IPO.

CompDent Corporation

100 Mansell Ct. East, Ste. 400, Roswell, GA 30076

Telephone: 770-998-8936 **Fax:** 770-998-6871 **Metro area:** Atlanta, GA **Web site:** http://www.compdent.com **Human resources contact:** Karen Mitchell **Sales:** $173.3 million **Number of employees:** 600 **Number of employees for previous year:** 460 **Industry designation:** Medical practice management **Company type:** Public

CompDent is a dental HMO that provides full-service dental benefits to employers and other business organizations as well as individuals. The company provides network-based dental care and reduced fee-for-service plans that provide for 100% of basic preventative dental care costs and discounts for additional procedures. CompDent provides dental coverage to about 2.2 million members through more than 6,000 providers. Operating in 24 states, the company markets its services through a system of over 8,000 independent agents. Subsidiary Dental Health Management offers administrative and management services to individual dental practices. A private investment group is buying CompDent.

Cotton States Life Insurance Company

244 Perimeter Center Pkwy. NE, Atlanta, GA 30346

Telephone: 770-391-8600 **Fax:** 770-391-8986 **Other address:** PO Box 105303, Atlanta, GA 30348 **Metro area:** Atlanta, GA **Web site:** http://www.cottonstatesinsurance.com **Human resources contact:** Wendy M. Chamblee **Sales:** $28.9 million **Number of employees:** 150 **Number of employees for previous year:** 143 **Industry designation:** Insurance—life **Company type:** Public

Cotton States Life Insurance offers individual life insurance products to customers in 10 southern US states. The company's products include individual life and payroll deduction life insurance. Subsidiaries CSI Brokerage Services and CS Marketing Resources broker property, casualty, and accident insurance and group life and health insurance products not offered by the company or its affiliates. Cotton States Life's 265 multiline, exclusive agents work under contract for the company, for affiliate Cotton States Mutual Insurance and its subsidiary, Shield Insurance, and for Cotton States Investment.

Crawford & Company

5620 Glenridge Dr. NE, Atlanta, GA 30342

Telephone: 404-256-0830 **Fax:** 404-433-3532 **Metro area:** Atlanta, GA **Web site:** http://www.crawfordfirstreport.com **Human resources contact:** Nancy Menke **Sales:** $667.3 million **Number of employees:** 7,658 **Number of employees for previous year:** 7,656 **Industry designation:** Medical practice management **Company type:** Public

Crawford & Company is an international insurance services firm providing claims adjustment and risk management services to insurance companies, self-insured corporations, and government entities. Services include its XPressLink initial claims reporting; claims management, evaluation, and resolution; statistical and financial reporting; and medical claims auditing, review, vocational evaluation, and case management. The firm's Risk Sciences Group provides the risk-management and insurance industries with computer-based information systems and analytical forecasting. Crawford & Company serves customers from more than 400 US branches and 300 offices in 50 other countries. SunTrust Banks owns about 60% of the firm.

Cryolife, Inc.

1655 Roberts Blvd. NW, Kennesaw, GA 30144

Telephone: 770-419-3355 **Fax:** 770-590-3741 **Metro area:** Atlanta, GA **Web site:** http://www.cryolife.com **Sales:** $60.7 million **Number of employees:** 330 **Number of employees for previous year:** 315 **Industry designation:** Medical services **Company type:** Public **Top competitors:** Baxter International Inc.; Guidant Corporation; St. Jude Medical, Inc.

CryoLife uses a deep-freeze process called cryopreservation to preserve human tissue for cardiovascular, vascular, and orthopedic transplantation. The cryopreservation process preserves human heart valves, veins, and connective tissues (cartilage, ligaments, and tendons) for use in coronary bypass, vein reconstruction, and knee reconstruction surgeries. The company has relationships with more than 250 tissue banks and organ procurement agencies nationwide. CryoLife also develops implantable biomaterials, such as BioGlue and FibRx, for use as surgical adhesives and sealants. Subsidiary Ideas for Medicine, which Horizon Medical is buying, distributes single-use medical devices.

E3 Corporation

1800 Parkway Place, Ste. 600, Marietta, GA 30067

Telephone: 770-424-0100 **Fax:** 770-424-0050 **Metro area:** Atlanta, GA **Web site:** http://www.e3corp.com **Human resources contact:** Al Shugars **Sales:** $24.9 million (Est.) **Number of employees:** 175 **Industry designation:** Computers—corporate, professional & financial software **Company type:** Private **Top competitors:** Logility, Inc.; i2 Technologies, Inc.; Manugistics Group, Inc.

E3 Corporation makes inventory-management software that helps businesses make purchasing decisions. The company's products are oriented toward four distinct markets—E3TRIM manages warehouse inventories, E3SLIM manages store inventories, E3CRISP manages vendor inventories, and ProfitTrack manages shared inventories. Product prices typically range from $28,000 for E3TRIM to $250,000 for E3SLIM. In addition, E3 offers its customers—distributors, wholesalers, and retail chains—consulting and support services. E3 has installed its systems for more than 600 customers, including Ace Hardware, Best Buy, and CVS Corporation. The company has offices in Australia, Europe, and the US.

Georgia Gulf Corporation

400 Perimeter Center Terrace, Ste. 595, Atlanta, GA 30346

Telephone: 770-395-4500 **Fax:** 770-395-4529 **Metro area:** Atlanta, GA **Human resources contact:** James Worrell **Sales:** $875 million **Number of employees:** 1,041 **Number of employees for previous year:** 1,030 **Industry designation:** Chemicals—diversified **Company type:** Public **Top competitors:** Formosa Plastics Corporation; The Geon Company; The Dow Chemical Company

Georgia Gulf makes electrochemicals, aromatic chemicals, and methanol at plants located primarily in the South. The company's electrochemical products—chlorine, caustic soda, and PVC (polyvinyl chloride)—are used to bleach paper, strengthen textile dyes, and make plastic containers and trim. The acquisition of North American Plastics is expected to enhance the company's PVC market share. Georgia Gulf's aromatic chemical products (cumene, phenol, and acetone) are used by the automotive, cosmetics, and building products industries. The company's principal markets are Asia, Canada, Europe, Latin America, and the US.

Gold Kist Inc.

244 Perimeter Center Pkwy. NE, Atlanta, GA 30346

Telephone: 770-393-5000 **Fax:** 770-393-5262 **Metro area:** Atlanta, GA **Web site:** http://goldkist.com **Human resources contact:** William A. Epperson **Sales:** $1.7 billion **Number of employees:** 18,000 **Number of employees for previous year:** 17,500 **Industry designation:** Agricultural operations **Company type:** Cooperative **Top competitors:** Perdue Farms Incorporated; ConAgra, Inc.; Tyson Foods, Inc.

Gold Kist isn't too chicken to run after Tyson or Perdue. An agricultural cooperative operating in 11 states (mainly in the South), Gold Kist is a top US poultry processor, selling whole chickens and chicken parts to the food service industry and retailers. It also processes pork and breeds catfish and is involved in metal fabrication as well as financing for farmers. The company produces nuts through #1 US pecan processor Young Pecan Company (a partnership with Young Pecan Shelling Company) and Golden Peanut Company (a partnership with Archer-Daniels-Midland and Alimenta). Focusing on food, Gold Kist sold its farm supply assets, including 100 farm stores, to Southern States Cooperative in 1998.

HIE, Inc.

1850 Parkway Place, Ste. 1100, Marietta, GA 30067

Telephone: 770-423-8450 **Fax:** 770-423-8440 **Metro area:** Atlanta, GA **Web site:** http://www.hie.com **Human resources contact:** Debbie Dunn **Sales:** $27.2 million **Number of employees:** 172 **Number of employees for previous year:** 127 **Industry designation:** Computers—corporate, professional & financial software **Company type:** Public **Top competitors:** New Era of Networks, Inc.; DAOU Systems, Inc.; Oacis Healthcare Holdings Corp.

HIE (formerly Healthdyne Information Enterprises) provides information management software mostly for the health care and financial markets. Its integration tools and other software let organizations share, manage, and integrate data, as well as produce reports, from seemingly disparate sources located across LANs and WANs. In addition, HIE offers such consulting services (about 56% of sales) as training, systems analysis and integration, application redesign, maintenance, and support. The company distributes its products through an internal sales force as well as through OEMs, system integrators, and software vendors. About 88% of sales are to customers within the US.

Horizon Medical Products, Inc.

One Horizon Way, Manchester, GA 31816

Telephone: 706-846-3126 **Fax:** 706-846-3146 **Other address:** PO Box 627, Manchester, GA 31816 **Metro area:** Columbus, GA **Web site:** http://www.hmpvascular.com **Human resources contact:** L. Bruce Maloy **Sales:** $39.4 million **Number of employees:** 100 **Industry designation:** Medical products **Company type:** Public **Top competitors:** C. R. Bard, Inc.

Horizon Medical Products makes implantable ports and specialty catheters used in systemic or regional cancer treatments. Vascular access ports include: Triumph-1 (silicone catheter systems), LifePort (titanium and plastic ports), and Infuse-A-Port (implantable ports). Its lines of catheters include Circle C hemodialysis catheters and Pheres-Flow apheresis catheters. Horizon Medical markets its products to vascular surgeons and other physicians and clinicians in the US and 53 other countries through direct sales and a network of distributors. The company has been growing its medical products distribution network through acquisitions, including Cryolife subsidiary Ideas for Medicine and Stepic Corp.

Immucor, Inc.

3130 Gateway Dr., Ste. 600, Norcross, GA 30091

Telephone: 770-441-2051 **Fax:** 770-441-3807 **Other address:** PO Box 5625, Norcross, GA 30091 **Metro area:** Atlanta, GA **Web site:** http://www.immucor.com **Human resources contact:** Tina Sullivan **Sales:** $39.8 million **Number of employees:** 232 **Number of employees for previous year:** 229 **Industry designation:** Medical products **Company type:** Public **Top competitors:** Hemagen Diagnostics, Inc.; TECHNE Corporation; Abaxis, Inc.

Immucor's blood tests answer the classic vampire pickup line: What's your blood type? Used by blood banks, hospitals, and clinical laboratories worldwide, Immucor's products identify human blood properties for blood typing; they also detect foreign antibodies. Immucor has codeveloped an FDA-approved blood analysis device based on its Capture reagent technology; it is marketed as the first fully automated "walk-away" analyzer. Immucor also distributes other companies' products used for monitoring transfusion-therapy patients, transplant typing, and paternity testing. The company markets directly and through distribution agreements in North America and Europe; most of its sales are in the US and Germany.

InfoCure Corporation

1765 The Exchange, Ste. 450, Atlanta, GA 30339

Telephone: 770-221-9990 **Fax:** 770-857-1300 **Metro area:** Atlanta, GA **Web site:** http://www.infocure.com **Human resources contact:** Michael E. Warren **Sales:** $63.7 million **Number of employees:** 832 **Number of employees for previous year:** 390 **Industry designation:** Computers—corporate, professional & financial software **Company type:** Public **Top competitors:** McKesson HBOC, Inc.; National Data Corporation; IDX Systems Corporation

InfoCure treats the dreaded paper pile disease. The company's software, designed to automate the administrative, financial, and clinical operations of a medical practice, is used by medical offices of all sizes, including managed care centers and independent physician alliances. InfoCure offers an electronic data interchange system, which provides electronic transaction processing for billing patients, verifying insurance coverage, filing insurance claims, and collecting payments. Anesthesiology, oral surgery, orthodontics, dentistry, podiatry, and primary care specialties make up the bulk of InfoCure's sales.

Intelligent Systems Corporation

4355 Shackleford Rd., Norcross, GA 30093

Telephone: 770-381-2900 **Fax:** 770-381-2808 **Metro area:** Atlanta, GA **Web site:** http://www.intelsys.com **Human resources contact:** Marcy Powers **Sales:** $21.2 million **Number of employees:** 249 **Number of employees for previous year:** 219 **Industry designation:** Computers—services **Company type:** Public

Intelligent Systems operates through subsidiaries in two industry segments—technology and health care. Subsidiary InterQuad Services provides computer education and training; ChemFree makes a parts washer that cleans and degreases with microbes instead of solvents. Intelligent Enclosures sells mini-environment systems for ultraclean manufacturing; HumanSoft provides patient-information management software for public health agencies. The PsyCare subsidiary develops and administers Christianity-based psychiatric treatment programs in hospitals. Intelligent Systems also operates the Shared Resource Technology Center (a small-business incubator) and invests in developing technology companies.

ISS Group, Inc.

6600 Peachtree-Dunwoody Rd., 300 Embassy Row, Ste. 500, Atlanta, GA 30328

Telephone: 678-443-6000 **Fax:** 678-443-6477 **Metro area:** Atlanta, GA **Web site:** http://iss.net **Human resources contact:** Richard Macchia **Sales:** $35.9 million **Number of employees:** 328 **Number of employees for previous year:** 141 **Industry designation:** Computers—online services **Company type:** Public **Top competitors:** CyberSafe Corporation; Information Resource Engineering, Inc.; Netegrity, Inc.

ISS Group, formerly Internet Security Systems, provides network security monitoring, detection, and response software. Its SAFEsuite line of products protects internal corporate networks, extranets, and the Internet from misuse and security violations. ISS' products are based on its Adaptive Security Management approach, which involves continuous monitoring of network traffic and devices, detection of and response to security risks, and updating security policies. Products are available as individual solutions to particular problems or as a suite of products providing comprehensive network security. Founder and chief technical officer Christopher Klaus owns 26% of ISS.

IVI Checkmate Corp.

1003 Mansell Rd., Roswell, GA 30076

Telephone: 770-594-6000 **Fax:** 770-594-6020 **Metro area:** Atlanta, GA **Web site:** http://www.ivicm.com **Human resources contact:** Carol Falgiano **Sales:** $107.1 million **Number of employees:** 438 **Number of employees for previous year:** 185 **Industry designation:** Optical character recognition **Company type:** Public **Top competitors:** VeriFone, Inc.; Hypercom Corporation; NCR Corporation

Formed from the 1998 merger of Checkmate Electronics and International Verifact, IVI Checkmate is taking a mighty swipe at the electronic payment industry in the US, Canada, and Latin America. The company makes point-of-sale payment scanners used by customers including retailers and financial and health care institutions to reduce fraud and errors by verifying check, debit, and credit payments with magnetic strip and bar code readers and signature-capture technology. The company also makes check readers, thermal receipt printers, smart cards (through a license from French company Ingenico), and credit/debit/electronic benefit transfer (EBT) authorization terminals. Customers include Wal-Mart and J. C. Penney.

iXL Enterprises, Inc.

1888 Emery St., NW, Atlanta, GA 30318

Telephone: 404-267-3800 **Fax:** 404-267-3801 **Metro area:** Atlanta, GA **Web site:** http://www.ixl.com **Human resources contact:** Jodie Littlestone **Sales:** $64.8 million (Est.) **Number of employees:** 1,300 **Industry designation:** Computers—corporate, professional & financial software **Company type:** Private **Top competitors:** USWeb/CKS; Verio Inc.; NETCOM On-Line Communication Services, Inc.

Remember the plant in "Little Shop of Horrors" that kept saying, "Feeeeed me"? That's a bit like iXL Enterprises' appetite over the last few years. Since Bert Ellis founded iXL in 1996, the firm has acquired more than 34 Web, video, and interactive media companies. iXL's Internet services include strategy consulting, e-commerce systems, digital media services, Web site development, and Web publishing technology. It also owns 88% of the Consumer Financial Network (GE Capital owns the rest), which offers loans, life insurance, and other HR benefits to employees of major corporations. New York investment firm Kelso Investment owns about 29% of the firm.

LaRoche Industries Inc.

1100 Johnson Ferry Rd. NE, Atlanta, GA 30342

Telephone: 404-851-0300 **Fax:** 404-851-0421 **Metro area:** Atlanta, GA **Web site:** http://www.larocheind.com **Human resources contact:** Joe Martucci **Sales:** $381 million (Est.) **Number of employees:** 1,120 **Number of employees for previous year:** 800 **Industry designation:** Chemicals—diversified **Company type:** Private **Top competitors:** IMC Global Inc.; Borden Chemicals and Plastics Limited Partnership; Alcoa Inc.

LaRoche by any other name would still smell pretty bad. LaRoche Industries makes nitrogen products (urea, ammonia), chlor-alkali products (chlorine, caustic soda), and specialty chemicals (activated alumina, fluorocarbons). The company markets its nitrogen products for use in fertilizer, explosives, refrigeration, pollution control, and water treatment. LaRoche's chlor-alkali products are used to make plastics and polyvinyl chloride, as well as for water treatment. The company makes or distributes its products in more than 30 US locations, as well as in France and Germany. William LaRoche founded the company (formerly part of U.S. Steel) in 1986.

LHS Group Inc.

6 Concourse Pkwy., Ste. 2700, Atlanta, GA 30328

Telephone: 770-280-3000 **Fax:** 770-280-3099 **Metro area:** Atlanta, GA **Web site:** http://www.lhsgroup.com **Human resources contact:** Vance Schaeffer **Sales:** $163.2 million **Number of employees:** 742 **Number of employees for previous year:** 456 **Industry designation:** Computers—services **Company type:** Public **Top competitors:** ; Convergys Corporation; ALLTEL Corporation

In the global world of telecommunications, someone has to figure out how to pay the bills. LHS Group helps telecommunications service providers in more than 50 countries do just that with its billing and customer care software. Its BSCS (Business Support and Control System) software handles multiple currencies and languages, and helps telecoms manage their daily operations. LHS Group also offers such support services as system design, customization, and installation (about 65% of sales). Chairman and CEO Hartmut Lademacher owns 47% of the firm, which is expanding into the paging, satellite, cable, and Internet markets. About 45% of sales come from European clients.

Logility, Inc.

470 E. Paces Ferry Rd. NE, Atlanta, GA 30305

Telephone: 404-261-9777 **Fax:** 404-238-8450 **Metro area:** Atlanta, GA **Web site:** http://www.logility.com **Human resources contact:** Chad D. Veen **Sales:** $34.7 million **Number of employees:** 214 **Number of employees for previous year:** 185 **Industry designation:** Computers—corporate, professional & financial software **Company type:** Public **Top competitors:** Electronic Data Systems Corporation; TRW Inc.; System Software Associates, Inc.

Getting the goods from point A to point B is what Logility products are all about. The company's Logility Value Chain Solutions software family helps companies maximize their "value chain," which includes everyone from raw materials suppliers to end-product distributors. Manufacturers, distributors, and retailers use Logility software to manage inventory, manufacturing, promotions, transportation, and warehousing. Logility targets consumer goods, food and beverage, and pharmaceutical makers, primarily in the US (90% of sales). Customers include Eastman Chemical, Reynolds Metals, and Sony. Chairman James Edenfield, whose American Software spun off Logility in 1997, owns about 84% of the company.

LogistiCare, Inc.

One Crown Center, Ste. 306, 1895 Phoenix Blvd., College Park, GA 30349

Telephone: 770-907-7596 **Fax:** 770-907-7598 **Metro area:** Atlanta, GA **Web site:** http://www.logisticare.com **Human resources contact:** Cheryl Mallinson **Sales:** $11.5 million (Est.) **Number of employees:** 140 **Industry designation:** Medical services **Company type:** Private

LogistiCare provides nonemergency transportation management services to government health and human service agencies and managed care organizations. The company, which has operations centers in Connecticut, Florida, and Georgia, seeks to be a go-between for third-party payors, transportation carriers, and individuals in need of nonemergency transportation. Its services include processing requests for transportation from eligible individuals and coordinating and purchasing transportation. The company's biggest customer is the Georgia Department of Medical Assistance. After the planned IPO, TGIS Partners (of which chairman William Weksel is a general partner) will own about 40% of LogistiCare.

Magellan Health Services, Inc.

3414 Peachtree Rd. NE, Ste. 1400, Atlanta, GA 30326

Telephone: 404-841-9200 **Fax:** 410-953-5200 **Metro area:** Atlanta, GA **Web site:** http://www.magellanhealth.com **Human resources contact:** Brucie Boggs **Sales:** $1.5 billion **Number of employees:** 11,600 **Number of employees for previous year:** 5,000 **Industry designation:** Medical services **Company type:** Public **Top competitors:** Horizon Health Corporation; Advance Paradigm, Inc.; Behavioral Healthcare Corporation

The US's #1 managed behavioral health care company, Magellan Health Services is navigating a leviathan through some very narrow straits. Cutting costs in the expensive psychiatric industry is a sticky business with slim profit margins, but Magellan has size on its side; it serves more than 60 million people covered by health plans such as Blue Cross and Aetna through three managed behavioral health care companies: Green Spring Health Services, Human Affairs International, and Merit Behavioral Care. Magellan has a 50% stake in Charter Behavioral Health Systems, the US's #1 psychiatric hospital chain. The company also offers nonbehavioral specialty managed care, franchising, and therapeutic foster care.

MAPICS, Inc.

5775-D Glenridge Dr., Atlanta, GA 30328

Telephone: 404-705-3000 **Fax:** 404-705-3445 **Metro area:** Atlanta, GA **Web site:** http://www.mapics.com **Human resources contact:** Eric Blad **Sales:** $129.7 million **Number of employees:** 400 **Number of employees for previous year:** 280 **Industry designation:** Computers—corporate, professional & financial software **Company type:** Public **Top competitors:** Infinium Software, Inc.; SAP AG; System Software Associates, Inc.

MAPICS (formerly Marcam) wants to give companies some direction. It makes enterprise resource planning software for midsized manufacturing companies and divisions of large corporations in industries such as automotive parts, cosmetics, and consumer electronics. The company's MAPICS XA product line integrates customers' production, logistics, maintenance, and financial operations with nearly 50 software applications. Its eWorkPlace lets users access information over intranets and the Internet; COM_Net enables customer transactions over the Internet. MAPICS sells its products through affiliates in more than 70 countries. About 30% of its sales are outside the US.

Mariner Post-Acute Network, Inc.

One Ravinia Dr., Ste. 1500, Atlanta, GA 30346

Telephone: 678-443-7000 **Fax:** 770-393-8054 **Metro area:** Atlanta, GA **Web site:** http://www.marinerhealth.com **Human resources contact:** Ann Weiser **Sales:** $2 billion **Number of employees:** 65,000 **Number of employees for previous year:** 45,000 **Industry designation:** Nursing homes **Company type:** Public **Top competitors:** HCR Manor Care, Inc.; Beverly Enterprises, Inc.; Sun Healthcare Group, Inc.

When the Old Man retired from the sea, he chose Mariner Post-Acute Network. The result of a tangle of mergers among Paragon Health Network, Mariner Health Group, Living Centers of America, and GranCare between 1997 and 1998, the company is a top provider of long-term care in the US (Beverly Enterprises is #1). Mariner Post-Acute Network operates almost 450 inpatient and assisted living centers in some 40 states. Other subsidiaries offer home health, pharmacy, and rehabilitation therapy services. The company also manages medical care and treatment programs in more than 100 acute care hospitals. Leon Black's Apollo Investors owns about one-fourth the company.

Medirisk, Inc.

2 Piedmont Center, Ste. 400, 3565 Piedmont Rd. NE, Atlanta, GA 30305

Telephone: 404-364-6700 **Fax:** 404-364-6710 **Metro area:** Atlanta, GA **Web site:** http://www.medirisk.com **Human resources contact:** Patricia Beaufait **Sales:** $27.2 million **Number of employees:** 276 **Number of employees for previous year:** 209 **Industry designation:** Computers—corporate, professional & financial software **Company type:** Public **Top competitors:** Dow Jones & Company, Inc.; First Data Corporation; National Data Corporation

Medirisk sells access to its health care databases and to the software that analyzes them. The company's products let users (insurers, hospitals, physician practices) compare physician fees, reimbursements, and utilization patterns for all types of treatments across the country. Medirisk's clinical performance products measure the efficiency and effectiveness of care in a variety of medical specialties, and its physician databases offer detailed information about doctors seeking new practice affiliations. Medirisk customers generally purchase single or multiyear licenses to access the database, which continues to grow as Medirisk acquires complementary businesses. Medirisk went public in 1997.

MindSpring Enterprises, Inc.

1430 W. Peachtree St. NW, Ste. 400, Atlanta, GA 30309

Telephone: 404-815-0770 **Fax:** 404-815-8805 **Metro area:** Atlanta, GA **Web site:** http://www.mindspring.net **Human resources contact:** John Bushfield **Sales:** $114.7 million **Number of employees:** 977 **Number of employees for previous year:** 502 **Industry designation:** Computers—online services **Company type:** Public **Top competitors:** MCI WorldCom, Inc.; AT&T Corp.; America Online, Inc.

MindSpring is an Internet access provider that serves about 340,000 subscribers in more than 300 cities nationwide. MindSpring provides its users with Web-friendly amenities such as a graphics viewer, a Web site design package, e-mail, and a Web browser. It also works with businesses as a major provider of Web-hosting services for companies that do not want to operate their own Web sites. The company's growth has been driven primarily by acquisitions, particularly the purchase of some 42,000 individual subscribers from PSINet. Telecommunications firm ITC Holding owns around 30% of MindSpring.

NewCare Health Corporation

6000 Lake Forrest Dr., Ste. 315, Atlanta, GA 30328

Telephone: 404-252-2923 **Fax:** 404-252-2962 **Other address:** PO Box 3318, Tampa, FL 33610 **Metro area:** Atlanta, GA **Human resources contact:** Cathy Parson **Sales:** $33 million **Number of employees:** 1,350 **Number of employees for previous year:** 910 **Industry designation:** Nursing homes **Company type:** Public **Top competitors:** American Retirement Corporation; Summit Care Corporation; Arbor Health Care Company

Specializing in helping the older population, NewCare Health runs senior residential centers located primarily in the southern US. The company owns about 15 long-term-care centers and two assisted-living/independent-living facilities and operates three hospitals in Florida, Georgia, Kansas, Massachusetts, and Texas. The company's skilled-nursing care and ancillary services assist residents needing help with one or more activities of daily living, such as bathing, grooming, cooking, and transportation. NewCare Health subsidiaries include NCS Healthcare of Florida. NewCare's president and chairman face charges relating to alleged criminal violations which occurred at their former company.

Novoste Corporation

4350 International Blvd., Ste. C, Norcross, GA 30093

Telephone: 770-717-0904 **Fax:** 770-717-1283 **Metro area:** Atlanta, GA **Web site:** http://www.novoste.com **Human resources contact:** Susan Smith **Sales:** $100,000 **Number of employees:** 89 **Number of employees for previous year:** 45 **Industry designation:** Medical instruments **Company type:** Public **Top competitors:** Guidant Corporation; Pfizer Inc; United States Surgical Corporation

Novoste is developing a catheter system that uses radiation to help keep arteries open following a coronary angioplasty. Angioplasty increases a patient's blood flow by deploying balloons in arteries to reshape the artery walls. The arteries, however, often narrow again as the body produces excessive cell growth at the site. Novoste's Beta-Cath system is designed to stop such growth by applying localized beta radiation to the inner surface and wall of the artery, targeting only the multiplying cells. A catheter inserted at the arm or leg is guided to the artery, and the radiation is transferred through a handheld device. Novoste expects its system, which is in trials, to reach the market in 2000.

PaySys International, Inc.

One Meca Way, Norcross, GA 30093

Telephone: 770-564-8000 **Fax:** 770-564-8001 **Metro area:** Atlanta, GA **Web site:** http://www.paysys.com **Human resources contact:** Daniel M. DiDomenico **Sales:** $33 million (Est.) **Number of employees:** 400 **Number of employees for previous year:** 345 **Industry designation:** Computers—corporate, professional & financial software **Company type:** Private **Top competitors:** Pegasystems Inc.; ULTRADATA Corporation; Transaction Systems Architects, Inc.

PaySys International makes software that helps bankers and retailers get their due. Founded in 1981, the company makes credit card transaction processing software for banks, financiers, retailers, and third parties. Its customizable VisionPLUS software suite processes bank and retail credit card transactions and performs such tasks as accounts receivable, transaction processing, credit tracking, credit authorization, and fraud prevention. PaySys, which sells its products through a direct sales force, also provides such services as installation, training, maintenance, and support. Customers include American Express and EDS.

Peachtree Software, Inc.

1505 Pavilion Place, Norcross, GA 30093

Telephone: 770-724-4000 **Fax:** 770-806-5166 **Metro area:** Atlanta, GA **Web site:** http://www.peachtree.com **Human resources contact:** Nicola Tidwell **Sales:** $52.5 million **Number of employees:** 410 **Industry designation:** Computers—corporate, professional & financial software **Company type:** Subsidiary **Top competitors:** Platinum Software Corporation; ACCPAC International, Inc.; Intuit Inc.

Would the IRS find your accounts peachy? A subsidiary of UK software company The Sage Group, Peachtree Software provides financial and accounting software applications to small and midsized businesses. Its namesake flagship product helps manage accounts receivable and payable, inventory, payroll, and reporting, and its PeachLink lets users create and host Web pages and perform online sales and purchasing (other e-commerce products perform electronic billing and banking). The company also sells preprinted business forms and tax software updates and offers training and support services. Peachtree products are sold directly and through resellers and distributors.

Physician Health Corporation

One Lakeside Commons, 990 Hammond Dr., Ste. 300, Atlanta, GA 30328

Telephone: 770-673-1964 **Fax:** 770-730-8597 **Metro area:** Atlanta, GA **Human resources contact:** Hazel Wilson **Sales:** $16.6 million (Est.) **Number of employees:** 480 **Number of employees for previous year:** 477 **Industry designation:** Medical practice management **Company type:** Private

Physician Health Corporation provides practice management services to 25 physician networks and 19 physician practices. The company's nonmedical services include billing and payment collection, accounting, payroll services, inventory supply, and managed care contract negotiation. Its also offers ancillary health care services, providing office-based surgery suites, laboratories, and medical equipment. The company operates in Arizona, Florida, Georgia, Illinois, Kentucky, Mississippi, Missouri, Ohio, Tennessee, Texas, and Virginia. Physician Health's planned merger with Medical Industries of America was scrapped in late 1998.

Physicians' Specialty Corp.

1150 Lake Hearn Dr., Ste. 640, Atlanta, GA 30342

Telephone: 404-256-7535 **Fax:** 404-250-0162 **Metro area:** Atlanta, GA **Human resources contact:** Robyn Smith **Sales:** $61.6 million **Number of employees:** 285 **Number of employees for previous year:** 136 **Industry designation:** Medical practice management **Company type:** Public

Physicians' Specialty Corp. provides practice management services to physicians and other health care providers who specialize in the ear, nose, throat, head, and neck (ENT). The company operates through about 60 clinical locations; it is affiliated with about 150 physicians and health care professionals to whom it provides financial and administrative management services, as well as access to ancillary, network development, and payor contracting services. Physicians' Specialty Corp. also holds and administers managed care contracts. Subsidiaries include allergy and facial plastic surgery practices. Dr. Ramie A. Tritt (the firm's chairman and president) and his family own more than one-fourth of the company.

Porex Corporation

500 Bohannon Rd., Fairburn, GA 30213

Telephone: 770-964-1421 **Fax:** 770-969-0954 **Metro area:** Atlanta, GA **Web site:** http://www.porex.com **Human resources contact:** Philip C. White **Sales:** $52.9 million **Number of employees:** 600 **Industry designation:** Chemicals—plastics **Company type:** Subsidiary **Top competitors:** Polymer Group, Inc.; Hoffer Plastics Corporation; AT Plastics, Inc.

Porex, a subsidiary of health care communications company Synetic, makes porous plastic products for health care, consumer, and industrial applications. Its health care products, accounting for more than half of sales, include pipette tips, blood serum filters, surgical implants, and plastic pharmaceutical vials. Its nonmedical plastic components include writing pen tips, automobile battery vents, wastewater treatment filters, and silencers that muffle compressed air noise. Porex sells its products through direct sales and independent distributors and agents, including Allegiance Healthcare and Fisher Scientific. Synetic has put a planned IPO of Porex on hold to pursue growth opportunities through acquisitions.

Radiant Systems, Inc.

1000 Alderman Dr., Alpharetta, GA 30005

Telephone: 770-772-3000 **Fax:** 770-772-3052 **Metro area:** Atlanta, GA **Web site:** http://www.radiantsystems.com **Human resources contact:** Sheree Walker-Stinson **Sales:** $82.9 million **Number of employees:** 581 **Number of employees for previous year:** 265 **Industry designation:** Computers—corporate, professional & financial software **Company type:** Public **Top competitors:** International Business Machines Corporation; Tandem Computers Incorporated; NCR Corporation

Radiant Systems is checking you out. But don't be flattered—it also knows how much popcorn and candy you eat at the movies. Radiant makes touch screen point-of-sale systems for cinema box offices, concession stands, and gasoline stations, and its ReMACS subsidiary provides back office systems that make ordering and inventory tracking easier for retailers. The company's products link point-of-sale data with centralized merchandising functions that ultimately determine how much to order from vendors and suppliers. Radiant also supplies automotive service centers and delivery restaurants, and offers system planning and design services. Customers include Texaco, KFC, and General Cinema Theatres.

Rank America Inc.

5 Concourse Pkwy., Ste. 2400, Atlanta, GA 30328

Telephone: 770-392-9029 **Fax:** 770-392-0585 **Metro area:** Atlanta, GA **Industry designation:** Leisure & recreational services **Company type:** Subsidiary **Parent company:** The Rank Group PLC **Top competitors:** The Walt Disney Company; Planet Hollywood International, Inc.; dick clark productions, inc.

Rank America is a subsidiary that owns and manages the stateside operations of UK-based entertainment company The Rank Group. The company's US holdings include 50% of motion picture theme park and resort Universal Studios Escape in Orlando, Florida (Seagram subsidiary Universal Studios owns the rest). It also owns the Hard Rock brand name, which isn't just reserved for cafes anymore. Hard Rock now encompasses restaurants, recordings, hotels, and merchandise. Rank also owns time-share resort properties, campgrounds, and other real estate holdings in the US through its Resorts USA. Rank America provides its parent with about 40% of its sales.

Ross Systems, Inc.

2 Concourse Pkwy., Ste. 800, Atlanta, GA 30328

Telephone: 770-351-9600 **Fax:** 770-351-0036 **Metro area:** Atlanta, GA **Web site:** http://www.rossinc.com **Human resources contact:** Gary Brown **Sales:** $91.7 million **Number of employees:** 582 **Number of employees for previous year:** 526 **Industry designation:** Computers—corporate, professional & financial software **Company type:** Public **Top competitors:** Oracle Corporation; PeopleSoft, Inc.; Baan Company N.V.

Ross Systems' business software is used by more than 3,000 businesses and other organizations around the world. The company's products include Renaissance CS (available in 16 languages), with financial, decision support, and human resources and payroll packages, as well as extensive enterprise resource planning modules for manufacturers. Ross Systems' software enables organizations to use PC-based client/server computer networks to access data previously stored on centralized computer systems. The company also provides support services, including management consulting, product support, training, and technical consulting. International customers account for about a quarter of sales.

Serologicals Corporation

780 Park North Blvd., Ste. 110, Clarkston, GA 30021

Telephone: 404-296-5595 **Fax:** 404-297-8044 **Metro area:** Atlanta, GA **Web site:** http://www.serologicals.com **Sales:** $123.1 million **Number of employees:** 1,175 **Number of employees for previous year:** 1,100 **Industry designation:** Drugs **Company type:** Public **Top competitors:** NABI; Sera-Tec Biologicals

Serologicals Corporation supplies specialty human antibodies used in therapeutic and diagnostic products made by major health companies. It obtains antibodies through its network of almost 60 donor centers and labs in the US and the UK. Company-supplied immune globulin is used in products to prevent Rh incompatibility in newborns, to treat rabies, and to prevent hepatitis B. Serologicals Corporation also provides over 80 antibodies used to produce blood-typing reagents and biological specimens for use in clinical diagnostic test kit controls. It has two monoclonal manufacturing facilities. Bayer, which accounts for almost 50% of sales, will sell its Pentex Blood Proteins unit to the firm.

Synthetic Industries, Inc.

309 LaFayette Rd., Chickamauga, GA 30707

Telephone: 706-375-3121 **Fax:** 706-375-6953 **Metro area:** Chattanooga, TN **Web site:** http://www.Sind.com **Human resources contact:** Jim Laney Jr. **Sales:** $369 million **Number of employees:** 2,663 **Number of employees for previous year:** 2,015 **Industry designation:** Chemicals—fibers **Company type:** Public **Top competitors:** BP Amoco p.l.c.; W. R. Grace & Co.; Beaulieu Of America, LLC

Synthetic Industries wants you to walk all over it. The maker of polypropylene textiles is the US's #2 maker of carpet backing (almost half of sales), behind BP Amoco. It also makes construction and civil engineering products (concrete-reinforcement fibers) and environmental products (erosion-control textiles and landfill liners). Additionally, Synthetic Industries produces technical textiles including specialty fabrics and industrial yarns and fibers. From its seven plants in Georgia, Illinois, and Tennessee, Synthetic Industries sells more than 2,000 products to 65 markets in North America, Europe, and the Far East. Synthetic Industries, L.P., in which CEO Leonard Chill is a partner, owns 61% of the company.

Theragenics Corporation

5325 Oakbrook Pkwy., Norcross, GA 30093

Telephone: 770-381-8338 **Fax:** 770-931-7998 **Metro area:** Atlanta, GA **Web site:** http://www.theragenics.com **Human resources contact:** Karen Pfeifer **Sales:** $38 million **Number of employees:** 190 **Number of employees for previous year:** 111 **Industry designation:** Medical products **Company type:** Public **Top competitors:** Mentor Corporation; North American Scientific, Inc.

Theragenics develops and manufactures therapeutic radiological devices used to treat cancer. The company's products are used in brachytherapy, in which a physician introduces short-range, short-lived radioactive material directly into cancerous tissues, thereby concentrating the impact of the radiation on the tissue to be destroyed while limiting the effect on surrounding healthy tissues. The company's TheraSeed product is a radioactive implant used to treat localized tumors. Its TheraSphere product is used to treat liver cancer. Theragenics's products are most effective on encapsulated, confined tumors.

WebMD, Inc.

400 The Lenox Bldg., 3399 Peachtree Rd. NE, Atlanta, GA 30326

Telephone: 404-479-7600 **Fax:** 404-479-7651 **Metro area:** Atlanta, GA **Web site:** http://webmd.com **Number of employees:** 146 **Industry designation:** Computers—online services **Company type:** Private **Top competitors:** OnHealth Network Company; Medscape Inc.; MC Informatics, Inc.

WebMD wants to be the cure-all for providing health care information on the Internet. Its subscription-based Web site for medical professionals integrates communications services (e-mail, voice mail, faxing, paging) with continuing medical education courses and medical information and news, and it offers an area for ordering supplies from supply management company McKessonHBOC. WebMD also operates the Health and Wellness Center Web site, which provides free public access to health care information, chat rooms, and message boards. The company's content partners include Thomson Healthcare and InteliHealth. WebMD, which markets itself as the Internet's first health care portal, is growing through acquisitions.

The WMA Corporation

11315 Johns Creek Pkwy., Duluth, GA 30097

Telephone: 770-248-3311 **Fax:** 770-248-3470 **Metro area:** Atlanta, GA **Sales:** $6.8 million (Est.) **Number of employees:** 4 **Industry designation:** Insurance—life **Company type:** Private

The WMA Corporation, through its WMA Life Insurance subsidiary, provides reinsurance for life insurance companies on variable universal life and variable annuity products. All of WMA's business is generated by WMA Agency, which sells life insurance, annuities, and other financial services through a network of independent insurance agents. WMA has reinsurance agreements with three life insurance companies: Western Reserve Life Assurance, Kemper Investors Life Insurance, and American Skandia Life Assurance. The company is expanding current coverages beyond mortality risks.

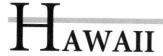

HAWAII

Barnwell Industries, Inc.

1100 Alakea St., Ste. 2900, Honolulu, HI 96813

Telephone: 808-531-8400 **Fax:** 808-531-7181 **Metro area:** Honolulu, HI **Web site:** http://www.brninc.com **Human resources contact:** Mark A. Murashige **Sales:** $11.9 million **Number of employees:** 37 **Number of employees for previous year:** 32 **Industry designation:** Oil & gas—exploration & production **Company type:** Public **Top competitors:** Gulf Canada Resources Limited; Ranger Oil Limited; Canadian Natural Resources Limited

Don't try to keep Barnwell Industries down on the farm—the company ranges far afield with its oil and gas production, water-well drilling, and property development activities. Barnwell Industries explores for and produces oil and gas primarily in Alberta, Canada; it has minor holdings in Saskatchewan. It has proved reserves of about 2.4 million barrels of oil and 40.6 billion cu. ft. of gas. Subsidiary Water Resources International drills water wells and repairs and installs water pumping systems in Hawaii. Barnwell Industries also owns a 50.1% controlling interest in Kaupulehu Developments, a Hawaiian leasehold land company that develops residential, hotel, and golf course properties.

IDAHO

Netivation.com, Inc.

7950 Meadowlark Way, Coeur d'Alene, ID 83815

Telephone: 208-762-2526 **Fax:** 208-762-3525 **Metro area:** Coeur d'Alene, ID **Web site:** http://www.netivation.com **Number of employees:** 36 **Industry designation:** Computers—online services **Company type:** Private **Top competitors:** OnHealth Network Company; America Online, Inc.; WebMD, Inc.

Netivation.com's two Web sites work oddly in tandem: Votenet covers politics (which could make you nauseous) and Medinex covers health care (which could make you better). The development-stage company operates Internet communities that focus on specific topics. Its sites offer e-mail, Web site design and hosting, specialized news, discussion forums, and topic-oriented search engines. Netivation.com plans to generate sales from advertising and sponsorships, e-commerce transactions, and premium membership services, among other sources. Following a planned IPO, brothers Anthony and Gary Paquin (chairman and secretary, respectively) will reduce their stake in the company from about 33% to 23%.

ILLINOIS

Abbott Laboratories

100 Abbott Park Rd., Abbott Park, IL 60064

Telephone: 847-937-6100 **Fax:** 847-937-1511 **Metro area:** Chicago, IL **Web site:** http://www.abbott.com **Human resources contact:** Thomas M. Wascoe **Sales:** $12.5 billion **Number of employees:** 56,236 **Number of employees for previous year:** 54,847 **Industry designation:** Drugs **Company type:** Public **Top competitors:** American Home Products Corporation; Roche Holding Ltd; Merck & Co., Inc.

Abbott Laboratories is a pharmaceuticals company that also produces nutritional supplements and hospital and laboratory equipment. Its pharmaceuticals unit makes antibiotics, antihypertensives, and other drugs such as Norvir, used in treatment of HIV and AIDS. Nutritional products include the infant formula Similac and the adult nutritional supplement Ensure, each a leading product in its field. Abbott's hospital and lab products include medical diagnostic and drug-delivery systems; Abbott is the world's #2 diagnostics company, behind Roche. The company also makes chemical and agricultural products. More than one-third of sales are to foreign markets.

AccuMed International, Inc.

900 N. Franklin St., Ste. 401, Chicago, IL 60610

Telephone: 312-642-9200 **Fax:** 312-642-8684 **Metro area:** Chicago, IL **Web site:** http://www.accumed.com **Human resources contact:** Robert Corbett **Sales:** $19.1 million **Number of employees:** 174 **Number of employees for previous year:** 170 **Industry designation:** Medical products **Company type:** Public **Top competitors:** NeoPath, Inc.; Neuromedical Systems, Inc.; Cytyc Corporation

AccuMed International makes products that use automation to increase the accuracy and productivity of labs that analyze Pap smears, the most widely used screening test for the early detection of cervical cancer. The company's AcCell Cytopathology System includes a computerized microscope and workstation that help pathologists find abnormal tissue samples by electronically recording the location of any abnormalities. AccuMed sold its microbiology line (which accounted for 95% of sales) because of heavy competition and plans to focus on its cytology line.

Aksys, Ltd.

2 Marriott Dr., Lincolnshire, IL 60069

Telephone: 847-229-2020 **Fax:** 847-229-2081 **Metro area:** Chicago, IL **Web site:** http://www.aksys.com **Human resources contact:** Jenny Kavin **Sales:** $100,000 **Number of employees:** 72 **Number of employees for previous year:** 65 **Industry designation:** Medical products **Company type:** Public **Top competitors:** Baxter International Inc.; Gambro AB; Fresenius Medical Care Aktiengesellschaft

Still rotating in the development stage, Aksys is working on hemodialysis products for patients suffering from chronic kidney failure. The company's lead product is the Aksys PHD personal hemodialysis system, which will allow patients to perform hemodialysis daily in their homes or at other non-medical sites. Aksys awaits Food and Drug Administration approval for the system, which will be manufactured by SeaMED Corporation. The company will market its products and related hemodialysis services in the US and Europe; the Japanese sales effort will be aided by plastics colossus Teijin Limited. Aksys is 30%-owned by a partnership that includes Yuval Almog, director Peter McNerney, and Linda Watchmaker.

Alberto-Culver Company

2525 Armitage Ave., Melrose Park, IL 60160

Telephone: 708-450-3000 **Fax:** 708-450-3354 **Metro area:** Chicago, IL **Web site:** http://www.alberto.com **Human resources contact:** Douglas E. Meneely **Sales:** $1.8 billion **Number of employees:** 12,700 **Number of employees for previous year:** 11,000 **Industry designation:** Cosmetics & toiletries **Company type:** Public **Top competitors:** L'Oreal; Unilever; Revlon, Inc.

Whether your problem is bothersome split ends or a bland split chicken, Alberto-Culver makes a product that can help. The firm makes products for hair care (Alberto VO5, Consort), skin care (St. Ives Swiss Formula), and personal care (FDS deodorant); sweeteners and seasonings (Molly McButter, Mrs. Dash, SugarTwin); and household items (Static Guard). Its Sally Beauty subsidiary, the world's #1 professional beauty supply distributor, sells hair care and skin care goods, cosmetics, and styling appliances to professionals and consumers through direct sales and more than 2,000 stores in the US, Canada, and overseas. The Lavin and Bernick families run Alberto-Culver and own about 29% of the company.

AMCOL International Corporation

1500 W. Shure Dr., Ste. 500, Arlington Heights, IL 60004

Telephone: 847-394-8730 **Fax:** 847-577-5582 **Metro area:** Chicago, IL **Web site:** http://www.amcol.com **Human resources contact:** Steve Alexander **Sales:** $521.5 million **Number of employees:** 1,625 **Number of employees for previous year:** 1,546 **Industry designation:** Chemicals—specialty **Company type:** Public **Top competitors:** Oil-Dri Corporation of America

AMCOL International's specialty chemicals are utterly absorbing—its superabsorbent polymers are used in a variety of personal care items (disposable baby diapers and adult incontinence and feminine hygiene products) and account for more than 40% of sales. The company's bentonite clay products are used in clumping cat litter, anticaking agents for agricultural feed, and sand bonding agents for metal castings. Environmental bentonite products include lining products for landfills and treatment equipment for oil and heavy metal wastewater. AMCOL International's products, which also include urethane coatings, are sold worldwide. The company has facilities in Australia, the UK, and the US.

Aon Corporation

123 N. Wacker Dr., Chicago, IL 60606

Telephone: 312-701-3000 **Fax:** 312-701-3100 **Metro area:** Chicago, IL **Web site:** http://www.aon.com **Human resources contact:** Virginia Schooley **Sales:** $6.5 billion **Number of employees:** 33,000 **Number of employees for previous year:** 28,000 **Industry designation:** Insurance—accident & health **Company type:** Public **Top competitors:** Marsh & McLennan Companies, Inc.; Citigroup Inc.; Arthur J. Gallagher & Co.

Aon, whose name means "oneness" in Gaelic, is one of the world's top two insurance brokerage and consulting companies (with Marsh & McLennan). It operates in two major segments: brokerage and consulting services and insurance underwriting. The company's brokerage and consulting operations, which make up the largest part of revenues, include retail and wholesale insurance for groups and businesses, in addition to reinsurance and employee benefits consulting. Aon's older but smaller insurance underwriting segment offers supplementary health, accident, and life insurance and extended warranties for consumer goods.

Applied Systems, Inc.

200 Applied Pkwy., University Park, IL 60466

Telephone: 708-534-5575 **Fax:** 708-534-5943 **Metro area:** Chicago, IL **Web site:** http://www.appliedsystems.com **Human resources contact:** Janet Van Haren **Sales:** $76.1 million (Est.) **Number of employees:** 1,100 **Industry designation:** Computers—corporate, professional & financial software **Company type:** Private **Top competitors:** Delphi Information Systems, Inc.; Policy Management Systems Corporation; INSpire Insurance Solutions, Inc.

Applied Systems' automation software helps insurance agencies get the most out of every policy. The company's main product, The Agency Manager, assists independent agencies with client management, policy pricing, electronic data interchange, policy and claims servicing, and office administration. Its Diamond System is designed to provide insurance carriers with automated billing, real-time processing of policies and claims, and reports. Other software includes PolicyMiner (analyzes policies), Policy-Rollover (identifies blocks of policies to be transferred to a carrier), and FirstRate (compares prices and ratings). Applied Systems, which focuses on property and casualty agencies, also provides support services.

Archer Daniels Midland Company

4666 Faries Pkwy., Decatur, IL 62526

Telephone: 217-424-5200 **Fax:** 217-424-6196 **Other address:** PO Box 1470, Decatur, IL 62525
Metro area: Decatur, IL **Web site:** http://www.admworld.com **Human resources contact:** Sheila
Witts-Mannweiler **Sales:** $16.1 billion **Number of employees:** 23,132 **Number of employees for
previous year:** 17,160 **Industry designation:** Agricultural operations **Company type:** Public **Top
competitors:** ConAgra, Inc.; Cargill, Incorporated; Tate & Lyle PLC

Archer Daniels Midland (ADM)—the self-appointed "supermarket to the world" —is one of the world's largest
processors of corn, wheat, and oilseeds. From corn, it produces syrups, sweeteners, citric acids, and ethanol, among
other items. ADM processes wheat into flour used by bakeries and pasta makers. About two-thirds of the
company's sales come from soybean, peanut, and other oilseed by-products, including vegetable oils, animal feeds,
and pulp. ADM also processes cocoa beans and has a variety of other businesses ranging from fish farming to
banking. It has interests in food processors in Asia, Canada, Europe, and South America. About one-third of
ADM's sales are outside the US.

Archibald Candy Corporation

1137 W. Jackson Blvd., Chicago, IL 60607

Telephone: 312-243-2700 **Fax:** 312-243-5806 **Metro area:** Chicago, IL **Human resources
contact:** Nick Podoba **Sales:** $126.7 million (Est.) **Number of employees:** 2,135 **Number of
employees for previous year:** 2,050 **Industry designation:** Food—confectionery **Company
type:** Private **Parent company:** The Jordan Co. **Top competitors:** Campbell Soup Company; See's
Candies, Inc.; Russell Stover Candies Inc.

Archibald Candy has a sweet story to tell with its boxed candies sold under the Fannie May (since the 1920s) and
Fanny Farmer (since 1994) names. Confections are sold through about 330 company-owned stores and about 6,000
other retailers in 22 midwestern and eastern states. It also sells through catalogs, the Internet, and fundraising
programs. Archibald makes about 75% of its more than 125 products, which include chocolates, mints, and toffee;
it resells some nuts, sweets, and other novelties purchased from outside vendors. To expand its distribution system,
the firm bought Sweet Factory, maker of jelly beans and other non-chocolate candy, in late 1998. Archibald is a
unit of privately held Jordan Industries.

Bally Total Fitness Holding Corporation

8700 W. Bryn Mawr Ave., Chicago, IL 60631

Telephone: 773-380-3000 **Fax:** 773-693-2982 **Metro area:** Chicago, IL **Web site:**
http://www.ballyfitness.com **Human resources contact:** Harold Morgan **Sales:** $742.5 million
Number of employees: 14,800 **Number of employees for previous year:** 13,900 **Industry
designation:** Leisure & recreational services **Company type:** Public **Top competitors:** Kelley
Automotive Group; The Sports Club Company, Inc.; YMCA of the USA

Bally Total Fitness Holding Corporation, through its subsidiaries, operates fitness centers in the US and Canada.
The company operates 320 low-cost fitness centers under the name Bally Total Fitness in 27 states and Canada,
with more than four million members, making it the largest operator in the US. Memberships give clients the use
of its fitness centers, which provide aerobics programs and personal training emphasizing cardiovascular
conditioning, strength development, and improved appearance. Bally targets the 18- to 34-year-old middle-income
segment and offers the option of financing initial membership fees. Most of the company's centers are located in
major metropolitan areas.

Baxter International Inc.

One Baxter Pkwy., Deerfield, IL 60015

Telephone: 847-948-2000 **Fax:** 847-948-3948 **Metro area:** Chicago, IL **Web site:**
http://www.baxter.com **Human resources contact:** Michael J. Tucker **Sales:** $6.6 billion **Number of
employees:** 42,000 **Number of employees for previous year:** 41,000 **Industry designation:**
Medical products **Company type:** Public **Top competitors:** Becton, Dickinson and Company; Fresenius
Medical Care Aktiengesellschaft; Merck & Co., Inc.

Baxter International is the world's leading medical technology manufacturer. The company's products include tissue
heart valves, blood transfusion systems, treatments for hemophilia, home dialysis systems, heart surgery equipment,
and more than 800 intravenous products. Baxter is working on such new products as a human blood substitute,
devices for open- and minimally-invasive-heart surgeries, and a sealant for clotting blood. It's also researching ways
to transplant animal organs into humans. In addition to expanding through new product development, Baxter is
growing its foreign markets, which account for approximately half of its sales.

Bio-logic Systems Corp.

One Bio-logic Plaza, Mundelein, IL 60060

Telephone: 847-949-5200 **Fax:** 847-949-8615 **Metro area:** Chicago, IL **Web site:** http://www.blsc.com **Human resources contact:** Faith Curtis **Sales:** $18 million **Number of employees:** 94 **Number of employees for previous year:** 89 **Industry designation:** Medical instruments **Company type:** Public

Bio-logic Systems designs and sells computer-based electro-diagnostic systems used by hospitals, clinics, universities, and physicians for medical practice and research. Its systems are used to perform medical procedures such as evoked response testing, topographic brain mapping, and other electroencephalographic (EEG) tests conducted by specialists in such fields as neurology, otolaryngology, audiology, anesthesiology, pulmonology, and psychiatry. Bio-logic Systems' products are also used to monitor brain functions in intensive care settings. Subsidiary Neuro Diagnostics makes testing equipment for the human nervous system. The company assembles its products from components made by third parties.

Brookdale Living Communities, Inc.

77 W. Wacker Dr., Ste. 4400, Chicago, IL 60601

Telephone: 312-977-3700 **Fax:** 312-977-3701 **Metro area:** Chicago, IL **Sales:** $77.7 million **Number of employees:** 1,700 **Number of employees for previous year:** 1,060 **Industry designation:** Nursing homes **Company type:** Public **Top competitors:** Sunrise Assisted Living, Inc.; Genesis Health Ventures, Inc.; Advocate Health Care

Brookdale Living Communities makes the old folks feel at home. The operator of assisted-living centers provides residential facilities for middle- and upper-income elderly clients. The company operates more than a dozen facilities in nine states, offering studio, one-bedroom, and two-bedroom units, as well as meal service, 24-hour emergency response, housekeeping, concierge services, transportation, and recreational activities. The company is developing additional facilities in Austin, Texas; New York; Pittsburgh; Raleigh, North Carolina; and Southfield, Michigan; and New York. Chairman Michael Reschke owns nearly 43% of the company.

CCC Information Services Group Inc.

444 Merchandise Mart, World Trade Center, Chicago, IL 60654

Telephone: 312-222-4636 **Fax:** 312-527-2298 **Metro area:** Chicago, IL **Web site:** http://www.cccis.com **Human resources contact:** Kathy Sfikas **Sales:** $188.4 million **Number of employees:** 1,100 **Number of employees for previous year:** 950 **Industry designation:** Computers—corporate, professional & financial software **Company type:** Public **Top competitors:** Automatic Data Processing, Inc.; Applied Systems, Inc.; The Thomson Corporation

CCC Information Services Group thrives on crashes. The firm supplies computer software and services nationwide to the automotive claims industry. Its products, which are typically sold under multiyear contracts to auto insurance agencies and collision repair shops, include TOTAL LOSS, for estimating the worth of totaled vehicles; VINGUARD, for detecting fraudulent claims; EZEST and PATHWAYS, for estimating collision repair costs; and ACCESS, for claims outsourcing. The firm also offers software for capturing digital images of damaged vehicles and a communications service that connects insurers, appraisers, and collision repair shops. Harvard University's endowment fund owns 30% of CCC and has 51% voting rights.

CFC International, Inc.

500 State St., Chicago Heights, IL 60411

Telephone: 708-891-3456 **Fax:** 708-758-5989 **Metro area:** Chicago, IL **Web site:** http://www.cfcintl.com/main.htm **Human resources contact:** Bob Klueppel **Sales:** $51 million **Number of employees:** 266 **Number of employees for previous year:** 252 **Industry designation:** Chemicals—specialty **Company type:** Public **Top competitors:** Bodycote International plc; Lilly Industries, Inc.; General Magnaplate Corporation

You can't fool Mother Nature, but CFC International doesn't intend to—the typical furniture buyer will do just fine. The company applies its proprietary coatings to rolls of plastic film from which its customers transfer the coatings to their products for protective and informative purposes. It produces five primary types of coating products: printed coating such as simulated wood grains for furniture; pigmented coatings used on pharmaceutical products; security products such as magnetic strips used on credit cards; pigmented metal coatings used on beverage cases; and holographic products such as authentication seals. CFC International markets its products worldwide.

CF Industries, Inc.

1 Salem Lake Dr., Long Grove, IL 60047

Telephone: 847-438-9500 **Fax:** 847-438-0211 **Metro area:** Chicago, IL **Web site:** http://www.cfindustries.com **Human resources contact:** William G. Eppel **Sales:** $1.4 billion **Number of employees:** 1,652 **Number of employees for previous year:** 1,609 **Industry designation:** Fertilizers **Company type:** Cooperative **Top competitors:** Potash Corporation of Saskatchewan Inc.; Terra Industries Inc.; IMC Global Inc.

Organized in 1946, CF Industries is an interregional agricultural cooperative that manufactures and markets fertilizers, including nitrogen products (ammonia, granular urea, and UAN solutions), phosphates, and potash products to its members in 48 states and two Canadian provinces. The co-op is owned by 11 regional agricultural co-ops, including Gold Kist, Land O'Lakes, and CENEX. CF Industries operates two nitrogen plants, two phosphate plants, a phosphate mine, and a network of distribution terminals and storage facilities to offer its products worldwide.

Chicago Blackhawk Hockey Team, Inc.

1901 W. Madison St., Chicago, IL 60612

Telephone: 312-455-7000 **Fax:** 312-455-7041 **Metro area:** Chicago, IL **Web site:** http://www.chiblackhawks.com **Sales:** $63.1 million **Number of employees:** 26 **Industry designation:** Leisure & recreational services **Company type:** Subsidiary **Parent company:** Wirtz Corporation **Top competitors:** St. Louis Blues Hockey Club L.L.C.; Detroit Red Wings; Nashville Predators

The Chicago Blackhawks started play in 1926 as one of the six original teams in the National Hockey League (NHL). The franchise belonged to Frederic McLaughlin before Arthur Wirtz and partners James Norris Sr. and James Norris Jr. bought controlling interest in the team in 1952. The Blackhawks enjoy a strong following despite having won only three Stanley Cups in their history (and none since 1961, the NHL's longest drought). The team is also overshadowed by the far more successful Chicago Bulls of the National Basketball Association, with which it shares the United Center arena. The Wirtz Corporation owns the team.

Chicago National League Ball Club, Inc.

1060 W. Addison St., Wrigley Field, Chicago, IL 60613

Telephone: 773-404-2827 **Fax:** 773-404-4111 **Metro area:** Chicago, IL **Web site:** http://www.cubs.com **Human resources contact:** Jenifer Surma **Sales:** $81.5 million **Number of employees:** 1,000 **Industry designation:** Leisure & recreational services **Company type:** Subsidiary **Parent company:** Tribune Company **Top competitors:** St. Louis Cardinals, L.P.; The Cincinnati Reds; Houston Astros Baseball Club

The Chicago National League Ball Club (the Chicago Cubs) first swung into action in 1876. Originally called the White Stockings, its nicknames included Colts, Orphans, and Spuds before it settled on the Cubs in 1907. Media firm Tribune Company (owners of WGN-TV) purchased the Cubs in 1981 from the Wrigley family, and the team is a major source of programming for Tribune's TV and radio stations. The Cubs suffered a loss in 1998 with the death of announcer Harry Caray, but the 1998 season was one for the history books; the team made it to the playoffs for the first time in nine years (but were swept by the Atlanta Braves in the division series) and right fielder Sammy Sosa hit 66 home runs out of the park.

Chicago White Sox Ltd.

Comiskey Park, 333 W. 35th St., Chicago, IL 60616

Telephone: 312-674-1000 **Fax:** 312-674-5116 **Metro area:** Chicago, IL **Web site:** http://www.chisox.com **Human resources contact:** Moira Foy **Sales:** $82.3 million (Est.) **Number of employees:** 200 **Industry designation:** Leisure & recreational services **Company type:** Private **Top competitors:** Kansas City Royals Baseball Corporation; Cleveland Indians Baseball Company, Inc.; Minnesota Twins

The Chicago White Sox want a glimpse of their former glory, which was last sighted around the time of the team's second World Series win in 1917. The so-called Hitless Wonders also won the series in 1906, thanks to some extremely close victories. The team's less-than-glorious moments included the 1919 World Series: the White Sox not only lost, but several team members were also indicted for game fixing. After spending big money on free agents like Albert Belle with minimal results, controlling owner Jerry Reinsdorf (who also owns the Chicago Bulls) is sticking with a young, potentially competitive, and significantly cheaper team. The Chicago White Sox play in Comiskey Park.

Corn Products International, Inc.

6500 S. Archer Rd., Bedford Park, IL 60501

Telephone: 708-563-2400 **Fax:** 708-563-6852 **Other address:** PO Box 345, Argo, IL 60501 **Metro area:** Chicago, IL **Human resources contact:** James Hirchak **Sales:** $1.4 billion **Number of employees:** 5,500 **Number of employees for previous year:** 4,300 **Industry designation:** Food—sugar & refining **Company type:** Public **Top competitors:** Tate & Lyle PLC; Imperial Chemical Industries PLC; Archer Daniels Midland Company

Sweet sodas and diet dishes alike get their base from Bestfoods spinoff Corn Products International. The company makes food ingredients and industrial products from corn and other starch-based raw materials for customers in more than 60 industries, including food and beverages, cosmetics, and paper. More than half of its sales come from corn products, including high-fructose corn syrup used to sweeten soft drinks. Corn Products also produces corn starch (a thickener for diet foods), corn oil, and corn gluten (for animal feed). It sells its products in more than 20 countries (generating about 60% of its sales in North America). Corn Products has 19 plants as well as joint ventures worldwide.

Covenant Ministries of Benevolence

5145 N. California Ave., Chicago, IL 60625

Telephone: 773-989-1610 **Fax:** 773-878-2617 **Metro area:** Chicago, IL **Human resources contact:** Helen J. Clark **Sales:** $258.8 million **Number of employees:** 4,800 **Number of employees for previous year:** 4,720 **Industry designation:** Hospitals **Company type:** Not-for-profit

Covenant Ministries of Benevolence is a not-for-profit organization operating two hospitals, 13 retirement communities, and a health and fitness center. It runs the Emanuel Medical Center in Turlock, California, and the Swedish Covenant Hospital in Chicago. Home to more than 3,500 senior adults, the agency's retirement communities offer assisted living facilities, fitness programs, and adult day care, among other services. Its LifeCenter on the Green, located in Chicago, offers a wide range of fitness services, including women's and senior classes, health screenings and lectures, and cardiac rehabilitation programs. Covenant Ministries traces its roots to the 1886 founding of Home of Mercy in Chicago.

CTI Industries Corporation

22160 N. Pepper Rd., Barrington, IL 60010

Telephone: 847-382-1000 **Fax:** 847-382-1219 **Metro area:** Chicago, IL **Human resources contact:** Carol Slove **Sales:** $20 million **Number of employees:** 186 **Number of employees for previous year:** 161 **Industry designation:** Rubber & plastic products **Company type:** Public **Top competitors:** Amscan Holdings, Inc.; Pioneer Balloon Company; American Greetings Corporation

If CTI Industries' sales balloon, it's because balloons sell. CTI makes and distributes Mylar and latex balloons—decorated with messages and such licensed themes as NASCAR and Precious Moments—sold by retailers and florists in the US and 30 other countries (drugstore chain Eckerd is its top customer). CTI makes its own Mylar balloons and buys latex balloons from a 45%-owned Mexican firm, Pulidos et Terminados Finos. Further inflating the company's sales are toys, novelties, and "message items" such as mugs, banners, inflatable masks, punch balls, and water bombs. In addition, CTI produces laminated and specialty films for commercial uses such as food packaging. Officers and directors own about 43% of CTI.

Cyborg Systems, Inc.

2 N. Riverside Plaza, Chicago, IL 60606

Telephone: 312-454-1865 **Fax:** 312-930-1033 **Metro area:** Chicago, IL **Web site:** http://www.cyborg.com **Human resources contact:** Pat Christensen **Sales:** $68 million (Est.) **Number of employees:** 670 **Number of employees for previous year:** 600 **Industry designation:** Computers—corporate, professional & financial software **Company type:** Private **Top competitors:** Ross Systems, Inc.; PeopleSoft, Inc.; Lawson Software

Resistance is futile. You will be assimilated into the organization. Founded in 1974, Cyborg Systems develops human resource management software for the government, banking, manufacturing, health care, and education markets. It specializes in client/server-based systems (which consist of third-party hardware and the company's proprietary software) that help users assimilate data for such areas as payroll, personnel, pensions administration, timekeeping, and attendance. Cyborg Systems also offers design, consulting, testing, training, and project management services. Customers include Amway, British Airways, and Lockheed Martin. Chairman and CEO Mike Blair owns the company.

Daubert Industries, Inc.

1333 Burr Ridge Pkwy., Ste. 200, Burr Ridge, IL 60521

Telephone: 630-203-6800 **Fax:** 630-203-6907 **Metro area:** Chicago, IL **Web site:** http://www.daubert.com **Human resources contact:** Ginny Winkelmann **Sales:** $136.3 million (Est.) **Number of employees:** 490 **Number of employees for previous year:** 480 **Industry designation:** Chemicals—specialty **Company type:** Private **Top competitors:** Applied Extrusion Technologies, Inc.; Viskase Companies, Inc.; AEP Industries Inc.

When it comes to corrosion, Daubert Industries may be metal's best friend. Its Daubert VCI division makes volatile corrosion inhibitors (protective coatings) for almost every metal—ferrous, nonferrous, or multi-metal. The transparent Daubert protective layer requires no removal because it breaks down immediately upon product unwrapping. The company's Entire Car Protection division offers paints, carpet dyes, detailing products, and under-the-hood cleaners. The company, which began battling metal corrosion in 1935, has sold its release paper (detachable protective sheets) and consumer products (adhesive tapes) divisions to Finnish company UPM-Kymmene.

Dean Foods Company

3600 N. River Rd., Franklin Park, IL 60131

Telephone: 847-678-1680 **Fax:** 847-233-5505 **Metro area:** Chicago, IL **Web site:** http://www.deanfoods.com **Human resources contact:** Daniel M. Dressel **Sales:** $2.7 billion **Number of employees:** 14,500 **Number of employees for previous year:** 11,800 **Industry designation:** Food—dairy products **Company type:** Public **Top competitors:** Groupe Danone; Suiza Foods Corporation; Dairy Farmers of America

Dean Foods has got milk, all right. The diversified dairy and specialty food processor and distributor is the #1 US processor of fluid milk, selling branded and private-label dairy products in the US and Mexico. The dairy division is expanding through acquisitions and brings in about two-thirds of sales. Its pickle division is a leading producer of regional brand and private-label pickles, relishes, and peppers. Its specialty food division is the #1 processor of nondairy creamer for retail and industrial use (including international customers). Dean Foods also operates DFC Trucking, a refrigerated trucking business. The firm sold its vegetable business, which included the Birds Eye brand.

DEKALB Genetics Corporation

3100 Sycamore Rd., DeKalb, IL 60115

Telephone: 815-758-3461 **Fax:** 815-758-3711 **Metro area:** Chicago, IL **Web site:** http://www.dekalb.com **Human resources contact:** John J. McEnery **Sales:** $502.2 million **Number of employees:** 2,058 **Number of employees for previous year:** 2,000 **Industry designation:** Agricultural operations **Company type:** Subsidiary **Top competitors:** Pioneer Hi-Bred International, Inc.; The Dow Chemical Company; Novartis AG

Humans created the corn we eat today through careful selection and tinkering, and DEKALB Genetics carries on the quest for better seed. The company develops crop seed hybrids (corn, sorghum, and sunflower) and varietals (soybean and alfalfa) for sale to farmers worldwide. It is the nation's #2 marketer of hybrid seed corn (behind Pioneer Hi-Bred). The company also develops and markets hybrid swine breeding stock, hogs for slaughter, and related management services for hog producers. DEKALB was bought in 1998 by life sciences company Monsanto; the two companies already shared licensing of biotechnology critical to DEKALB's product line.

Donlar Corporation

6502 S. Archer Ave., Bedford Park, IL 60501

Telephone: 708-563-9200 **Fax:** 708-563-9220 **Metro area:** Chicago, IL **Web site:** http://www.donlar.com **Human resources contact:** Jerilyn Koskan **Sales:** $5 million (Est.) **Number of employees:** 56 **Industry designation:** Chemicals—specialty **Company type:** Private **Top competitors:** Rohm and Haas Company; Uniroyal Chemical Corporation; BASF Aktiengesellschaft

Donlar's specialty polymers are designed to help corn, cotton, and other crops absorb nutrients and fertilizers. They also have industrial and commercial uses, such as inhibiting corrosion and assisting hair and skin to drink in moisturizers. These polymers, thermal polyaspartates (TPAs), are highly charged molecules that attract or repel surfaces and have a high capacity for bonding to water. Such properties make TPAs well suited for tiny jobs such as concentrating herbicides in crops and repelling dirt particles. TPAs are biodegradable, nontoxic, and hypoallergenic. The company's crop nutrition products are sold under the AmiSorb name.

Endorex Corp.

900 N. Shore Dr., Lake Bluff, IL 60044

Telephone: 847-604-7555 **Fax:** 847-604-8570 **Metro area:** Chicago, IL **Web site:** http://www.endorex.com **Sales:** $100,000 **Number of employees:** 17 **Number of employees for previous year:** 13 **Industry designation:** Drugs **Company type:** Public **Top competitors:** American Home Products Corporation; SmithKline Beecham plc; Merck & Co., Inc.

Endorex may be able to help kids stomach their DTP vaccines—literally. The biotechnology company (through subsidiary Orasomal Technologies) is developing oral and mucosal drug-delivery system for vaccines, allergens, and other therapies. It has two joint ventures with Elan focusing on vaccines and drugs that use Elan's Medipad drug delivery system. Endorex also has immunotherapy drugs in trial phases— ImmTher is being tested to treat melanoma and other cancers; Theramide is a cancer vaccine booster. Subsidiary Wisconsin Genetics is developing organic cancer drug perillyl alcohol, in trials for breast, ovarian, and prostate cancers. Elan owns about 14% of Endorex.

Favorite Brands International Inc.

25 Tri-State International, Ste. 222, Lincolnshire, IL 60069

Telephone: 847-374-0900 **Fax:** 847-374-0952 **Metro area:** Chicago, IL **Web site:** http://www.favbrands.com **Human resources contact:** Carrie White **Sales:** $764 million (Est.) **Number of employees:** 4,800 **Number of employees for previous year:** 4,400 **Industry designation:** Food—confectionery **Company type:** Private **Top competitors:** Hershey Foods Corporation; Mars, Inc.; Nestle S.A.

Favorite Brands International has Jet-Puffed itself into the #4 confectioner in the US (behind Hershey, Mars, and Nestle), but the sweets maker is suffering a financial toothache. The company makes brand-name and private-label marshmallow products (Jet-Puffed), fruit snacks (Farley's), gummies (Trolli), caramels, and other candies (Farley's and Sathers). The sweets are sold to US grocery, drug, and convenience stores and major US cereal makers. Favorite Brands was founded in 1995 to acquire Kraft's caramels and marshmallows units; it then bought several other candy makers. Mounting debt forced the company to file for Chapter 11 bankruptcy in 1999. Buyout firm Texas Pacific Group controls the company.

Federal Signal Corporation

1415 W. 22nd St., Oak Brook, IL 60521

Telephone: 630-954-2000 **Fax:** 630-954-2030 **Metro area:** Chicago, IL **Web site:** http://www.federalsignal.com **Sales:** $1 billion **Number of employees:** 6,591 **Number of employees for previous year:** 6,233 **Industry designation:** Protection—safety equipment & services **Company type:** Public

"Better safe than sorry" could easily be the motto of Federal Signal, a maker of safety and rescue equipment. Its Safety Products Group serves government and industry with light, siren, horn, and bell warning signals, as well as weather and power-plant warning and evacuation systems. The Sign Group sells, leases, and repairs customized signs for commercial and industrial clients. Federal Signal's Tool Group supports private industry with die components, precision tooling products, and cutting tools, while the Vehicle Group makes street sweepers, waste-removal vehicles, and fire and rescue trucks. Products are manufactured at nearly 50 plants worldwide and are sold both directly and through distributors.

The Female Health Company

875 N. Michigan Ave., Ste. 3660, Chicago, IL 60611

Telephone: 312-280-1119 **Fax:** 312-280-9360 **Metro area:** Chicago, IL **Web site:** http://www.femalehealth.com **Human resources contact:** Judy Braskamp **Sales:** $5.5 Million **Number of employees:** 76 **Number of employees for previous year:** 66 **Industry designation:** Cosmetics & toiletries **Company type:** Public **Top competitors:** Johnson & Johnson; Pacific Dunlop Investments (USA) Inc.; Carter-Wallace, Inc.

Chicago—home of the Bulls, the Cubs, and The Female Health Company (FHC), maker of condoms for women. FHC seeks to provide more options for women when it comes to preventing pregnancies and sexually transmitted diseases (STDs). The polyurethane female condom is the only product designed for women that is FDA-approved for preventing both pregnancy and STDs. FHC's female condoms are marketed in the US under the Reality name at major drugstores and in other countries mainly under the Femidom name. The company holds patents for the female condom in the US and many countries in Europe and Asia, including Japan and the UK. FHC's London factory can produce more than 60 million female condoms annually.

Ferrara Pan Candy Company

7301 W. Harrison St., Forest Park, IL 60130

Telephone: 708-366-0500 **Fax:** 708-366-5921 **Metro area:** Chicago, IL **Human resources contact:** Joanna Del Real **Sales:** $150 million (Est.) **Number of employees:** 450 **Number of employees for previous year:** 400 **Industry designation:** Food—confectionery **Company type:** Private **Top competitors:** Mars, Inc.; Tootsie Roll Industries, Inc.; Hershey Foods Corporation

Red Hots, Jaw Breakers, Boston Baked Beans, and Lemonheads—these are the candies Baby Boomers blew their allowances on. Ferrara Pan Candy, 90 years old and still operated by descendants of its founders, makes these classic American sweets. Panned candies, made in a rotating drum, are the company's specialty, although it now licenses such products as Gummies, Hanna-Barbera fruit snacks, and seasonal chocolate-covered nuts for holidays. Mouth-puckering Lemonheads, Ferrara Pan's top candy, spawned a line of sweet-and-sour fruit flavors (Applehead, Cherryhead, Grapehead, and Orangehead). Candy makers apprentice a year and a half before stirring up the handmade treats on their own.

First Alert, Inc.

3901 Liberty Street Rd., Aurora, IL 60504

Telephone: 630-851-7330 **Fax:** 630-851-8221 **Metro area:** Chicago, IL **Web site:** http://www.firstalert.com **Human resources contact:** Karolyn Keeley **Sales:** $186.9 million **Number of employees:** 3,142 **Number of employees for previous year:** 2,125 **Industry designation:** Protection—safety equipment & services **Company type:** Subsidiary **Top competitors:** Tyco International Ltd.; Pittway Corporation; Napco Security Systems, Inc.

First Alert can focus on natural fires again. Now that it's no longer catching heat from infamous downsizer "Chainsaw Al" Dunlap, former CEO of parent company Sunbeam, First Alert's remaining employees can return to the business of making the best-selling smoke and carbon monoxide detectors in the US. The company also makes other safety products, including radon detectors, infrared motion detectors, child safety products, fire extinguishers, and escape ladders. First Alert is turning to new markets overseas, including France, Germany, and Japan, where less than 5% of homes have smoke alarms (compared to over 90% in the US). More than 200 employees were extinguished before Dunlap himself was doused.

First Health Group Corp.

3200 Highland Ave., Downers Grove, IL 60515

Telephone: 630-241-7900 **Fax:** 630-719-0076 **Metro area:** Chicago, IL **Web site:** http://www.firsthealth.com **Human resources contact:** Nancy Zambon **Sales:** $503.1 million **Number of employees:** 5,000 **Number of employees for previous year:** 1,500 **Industry designation:** Medical practice management **Company type:** Public **Top competitors:** Foundation Health Systems, Inc.; UnitedHealth Group; Aetna Inc.

First Health Group, formerly HealthCare COMPARE, is a provider of medical cost-management services in the US. The company's First Health Medical Networks manages payor-based PPO networks, including hospitals, physicians, and outpatient care providers, in 49 states, Puerto Rico, and Washington, DC. First Health's medical review programs aid the delivery of medically necessary care and identify cost-effective treatment alternatives to its clients. Its OUCH (Occupational-Urgent Care Health) Systems offers computer-assisted bill reviews and audits, fee schedule reviews, and claims pricing.

Franklin Ophthalmic Instruments Co., Inc.

1265 Naperville Dr., Romeoville, IL 60446

Telephone: 630-759-7666 **Fax:** 630-759-1744 **Metro area:** Chicago, IL **Web site:** http://www.franklin-moi.com **Human resources contact:** James J. Urban **Sales:** $9.6 million **Number of employees:** 32 **Number of employees for previous year:** 29 **Industry designation:** Medical instruments **Company type:** Public **Top competitors:** IRIDEX Corporation; Essilor International SA; Lombart Instrument Company

Vision-care professionals who need new gear can keep their eyes peeled for Franklin Ophthalmic, which sells and services ophthalmic diagnostic instruments and equipment. Through direct mail, trade shows, and a sales force, the firm sells products from high-tech instruments such as slit lamps, retinal cameras, and keratometers (which measure the curvature of the cornea) to basics like examining-room chairs and display projectors. Products come from Nikon, Canon, Marco Ophthalmic, and Reliance Medical Products, among others; the company also sells used and refurbished equipment. Customers are primarily ophthalmologists, optometrists, and medical institutions.

G.D. Searle & Co.

5200 Old Orchard Rd., Skokie, IL 60077

Telephone: 847-982-7000 **Fax:** 847-470-1480 **Metro area:** Chicago, IL **Web site:** http://www.searlehealthnet.com **Human resources contact:** Ann K. M. Gualtieri **Sales:** $2.4 billion **Industry designation:** Drugs **Company type:** Subsidiary **Parent company:** Monsanto Company

Founded in 1888, G.D. Searle has filled apothecary shelves for more than a century. Among its products are such drugs as Calan, a cardiovascular treatment for angina; Aldactone, for edema (swelling); insomnia drug Ambien; and next-generation arthritis treatment Celebrex (which posted near-record sales for a newly released drug). It also has several drugs for women's health, including oral contraceptives, treatments for bacterial infections (Flagyl), and a nasal spray for treatment of endometriosis (Synarel). Searle has a number of drugs in its development pipeline. The company has been a wholly owned subsidiary of biotechnology firm Monsanto since 1985.

Griffith Micro Science International, Inc.

2001 Spring Rd., Ste. 500, Oak Brook, IL 60523

Telephone: 630-571-1280 **Fax:** 630-571-1245 **Metro area:** Chicago, IL **Web site:** http://www.gmsmicro.com **Human resources contact:** Richard Rediehs **Sales:** $75 million (Est.) **Number of employees:** 483 **Industry designation:** Medical services **Company type:** Private **Top competitors:** Environmental Tectonics Corporation; SteriGenics International, Inc.; Isomedix, Inc.

Griffith Micro Science International has an international license to kill ... microbes, that is. The sterilization subsidiary is being spun off from parent Griffith Laboratories. Other manufacturers in North America and Europe use the company's services primarily to sterilize single-use medical products; the plants also sterilize cosmetics, drugs, and foods. Griffith Micro Science operates 11 plants in North America and eight in Europe, and uses both ethylene oxide and gamma radiation sterilization techniques. The company has a joint venture with MDS Nordion to build a gamma radiation sterilization plant in Mexico. After the spinoff, Griffith Laboratories will own more than 65% of the company.

GROWMARK Inc.

1701 Towanda Ave., Bloomington, IL 61701

Telephone: 309-557-6000 **Fax:** 309-829-8532 **Metro area:** Bloomington, IL **Web site:** http://www.growmark.com **Human resources contact:** Stan Nielson **Sales:** $1.3 billion **Number of employees:** 966 **Number of employees for previous year:** 875 **Industry designation:** Agricultural operations **Company type:** Cooperative **Top competitors:** Cenex Harvest States Cooperatives; Agway Inc.; Farmland Industries, Inc.

Fuse farming essentials "growing" and "marketing" and the result is GROWMARK, a retail farm-supply and grain-marketing cooperative. Through its member/owner co-ops—more than 120 in retail and 270-plus in grain marketing—GROWMARK serves more than 250,000 farmers in the midwestern US and Ontario, Canada. Under the FS name, the co-op sells farm supplies such as feed and fuel. Corn and soybeans are among the major crops it markets. GROWMARK's partnerships include ADM/GROWMARK, a grain marketing venture with Archer Daniels Midland; fertilizer maker and distributor CF Industries; pet food producer PRO-PET; seed and feed ventures with Land O'Lakes; and an energy alliance with Countrymark Cooperative and Land O'Lakes.

Halsey Drug Co., Inc.

695 N. Perryville Rd., Crimson Bldg. No. 2, Rockford, IL 61107

Telephone: 815-399-2060 **Fax:** 815-399-9710 **Metro area:** Rockford, IL **Human resources contact:** Beverly Berke **Sales:** $8.8 million **Number of employees:** 160 **Number of employees for previous year:** 142 **Industry designation:** Drugs—generic **Company type:** Public

Halsey Drug Co. makes, sells, and distributes generic drugs. The company's products include analgesics, antibiotics, antituberculars, antihistamines, antihistaminic decongestants, and antitussives. These are sold both under the Halsey label and under private-label arrangements with drugstore chains and drug wholesalers. Halsey's research and development activities consist primarily of developing generic drugs and improving manufacturing processes, as well as developing new chemical products for resale. The company manufactures its products at facilities in New York and Indiana.

HARZA Engineering Company

233 S. Wacker Dr., Chicago, IL 60606

Telephone: 312-831-3000 **Fax:** 312-831-3999 **Metro area:** Chicago, IL **Web site:** http://www.harza.com **Sales:** $109 million (Est.) **Number of employees:** 800 **Number of employees for previous year:** 549 **Industry designation:** Pollution control equipment & services **Company type:** Private

HARZA Engineering specializes in hydroelectricity projects, but it also provides planning, permitting, design, and construction management services for a range of infrastructure work for businesses and government agencies. HARZA's projects have included dams, wastewater treatment facilities, navigation and waterfront projects, and water-supply systems. The firm also offers procurement services, environmental analyses, seismic and geotechnical assessments, and safety analyses. Subsidiary Harza Trade Finance offers project financing, including start-up costs, budgeting, and training. The firm has about 13 US offices and two offices in Brazil and Mexico. Founded in 1920, HARZA is employee-owned.

Health Care Service Corporation

300 E. Randolph, Chicago, IL 60601

Telephone: 312-653-6000 **Fax:** 312-938-8847 **Metro area:** Chicago, IL **Web site:** http://www.bcbsil.com **Human resources contact:** Patrick O'Connor **Sales:** $5.1 billion **Number of employees:** 5,700 **Number of employees for previous year:** 5,650 **Industry designation:** Insurance—accident & health **Company type:** Mutual company **Top competitors:** UnitedHealth Group; The Prudential Insurance Company of America; Humana Inc.

Health Care Service Corporation (HCSC), also known as Blue Cross and Blue Shield of Illinois, is Illinois' oldest health insurer. HCSC provides a wide range of group and individual insurance and medical plans, including indemnity insurance and managed care programs. It has formed an affiliation, which is expected to lead to a merger (now pending regulatory approval), with Blue Cross Blue Shield of Texas. The company also offers life insurance, retirement services, and medical financial services through its FDL, Preferred Financial Corporation, and Nichold Company subsidiaries.

Help at Home, Inc.

223 W. Jackson Blvd., Chicago, IL 60606

Telephone: 312-663-4244 **Fax:** 312-461-0460 **Metro area:** Chicago, IL **Human resources contact:** Gloria Sanchez **Sales:** $23.1 million **Number of employees:** 173 **Number of employees for previous year:** 163 **Industry designation:** Medical services **Company type:** Public **Top competitors:** Sisters of Mercy Health System-St. Louis; Advocate Health Care; Home Health Corporation of America, Inc.

Help at Home provides in-home services such as nutritional planning and assistance, housekeeping, personal care, skilled nursing, rehabilitation, and other medically related social work to disabled and elderly persons. The company has 20 regional contracts with the Illinois Department on Aging, from which it makes about 60% of its sales. Additional referrals come from about 30 contracts with other state and municipal agencies. Because of changes in Medicare reimbursement laws, the company is discontinuing its Medicare home health services. Help At Home has 35 offices in Alabama, Arkansas, Illinois, Indiana, Mississippi, and Missouri. Chairman and CEO Louis Goldstein owns more than 60% of the company.

Hoffer Plastics Corporation

500 N. Collins St., South Elgin, IL 60177

Telephone: 847-741-5740 **Fax:** 847-741-3086 **Metro area:** Chicago, IL **Human resources contact:** Leo Nelson **Sales:** $78.4 million (Est.) **Number of employees:** 715 **Number of employees for previous year:** 675 **Industry designation:** Chemicals—plastics **Company type:** Private **Top competitors:** Berry Plastics Corporation; Cambridge Industries, Inc.; Atlantis Plastics, Inc.

Turning plastic into cash is nothing new at Hoffer Plastics. Founded in 1953 by Robert and Helen Hoffer, the family-owned custom injection-molding company makes custom-designed plastic products for the automotive, construction, electronic, and medical industries. Customers include Briggs & Stratton, Motorola, and Coca-Cola. Hoffer operates a 360,000-sq.-ft. plant in South Elgin, Illinois, which specializes in precision, thin-wall, at-press-color, and insert molding. Other operations include machining, ultrasonic welding, hot stamping, robotic parts handling, subassembly, laser drilling, annealing, and gasketing. Hoffer also offers engineering design (primarily part and tool design) and support services.

Immtech International, Inc.

1890 Maple Ave., Ste. 110, Evanston, IL 60201

Telephone: 847-869-0033 **Fax:** 847-869-0045 **Metro area:** Chicago, IL **Sales:** $19,000 (Est.) **Number of employees:** 3 **Industry designation:** Biomedical & genetic products **Company type:** Private **Top competitors:** Abbott Laboratories; Eli Lilly and Company; Hoffmann-La Roche, Inc.

Like smoking, Immtech International stunts growth. The development-stage biopharmaceutical company uses existing drug technology to develop dications, compounds that inhibit the growth of such unpleasant guests as bacteria, viruses, and parasites. Immtech has compounds in pretrial development for the treatment of cryptosporidiosis and a form of pneumonia common to people with weak immune systems. The company is also synthesizing proteins based on C-reactive protein, which may control the growth of cancerous tumors. Immtech has a number of alliances that give it access to funding and key technology. Medical device firm Criticare Systems will own about 20% of Immtech after the planned IPO.

InstallShield Software Corporation

900 National Pkwy., Ste. 125, Schaumburg, IL 60173

Telephone: 847-240-9111 **Fax:** 847-240-9120 **Metro area:** Chicago, IL **Web site:** http://www.installshield.com **Human resources contact:** John Andrew **Sales:** $22 million (Est.) **Number of employees:** 150 **Industry designation:** Computers—corporate, professional & financial software **Company type:** Private

Computer users no longer have to spend hours installing software on their computers, thanks in part to distribution tools and technologies developed by InstallShield Software. Firms such as Adobe, Microsoft, Netscape (now part of America Online), and Symantec use the InstallShield product family to install and integrate their programs onto the hard drives of Windows-based computers, to distribute their software on the Web, and to create product demos. In fact, nine out of ten leading software vendors use InstallShield, making it the sixth-most owned and used software in the world. InstallShield's products are available in nearly a dozen languages and are sold in more than 40 countries.

It's Just Lunch!, Inc.

432 N. Clark St., Chicago, IL 60610

Telephone: 312-644-9999 **Fax:** 312-644-9474 **Metro area:** Chicago, IL **Human resources contact:** Judy Belzer-Weitzman **Sales:** $9 million (Est.) **Number of employees:** 100 **Industry designation:** Leisure & recreational services **Company type:** Private **Top competitors:** Great Expectations International, Inc.; Together Development Corporation, Inc.; MatchMaker International Development Corp.

It's Just Lunch! gives busy, professional singles an alternative to nightclubs with its lunch-date matchmaking services, marketed from 32 offices nationwide. For between $725 and $1000 (depending on number of dates or duration of membership), singles join the service, interview, and then are set up with potential partners for lunch dates. It's Just Lunch! boasts more than 100,000 dates, 1,400 marriages, 1,100 engagements, and 3,400 seriously dating couples since its inception in 1992. The company was founded by Andrea McGinty after she was jilted six weeks before her wedding. It's Just Lunch! plans to expand into Europe and Asia. Chairman McGinty and her husband, president Daniel Dolan, own the firm.

Landauer, Inc.

Two Science Rd., Glenwood, IL 60425

Telephone: 708-755-7000 **Fax:** 708-755-7016 **Metro area:** Chicago, IL **Web site:** http://www.landauerinc.com **Human resources contact:** Lana Gowen **Sales:** $42.7 million **Number of employees:** 280 **Number of employees for previous year:** 260 **Industry designation:** Protection—safety equipment & services **Company type:** Public **Top competitors:** ICN Pharmaceuticals, Inc.; Pharmacia & Upjohn, Inc.; The Perkin-Elmer Corporation

If your employees are glowing—and not with joy—Landauer can tell you why. A provider of dosimeters (radiation detectors) the company serves corporations, hospitals, and government agencies worldwide. Their badges measure X-ray, gamma ray, and other forms of radiation. Landauer sells its radiation monitors mostly through direct marketing in Canada, the UK, and the US. Subsidiary HomeBuyer's Preferred provides radon monitoring services and related kits to determine possible residential hazards for companies relocating their employees. The company also profits from its 50%-owned joint venture, Nagase-Landauer, in Japan, and its 75% stake in SAPRA-Landauer in Brazil.

Lifeway Foods, Inc.

7625 N. Austin Ave., Skokie, IL 60077

Telephone: 847-967-1010 **Fax:** 847-967-6558 **Metro area:** Chicago, IL **Web site:** http://www.kefir.com **Sales:** $6.8 million **Number of employees:** 43 **Number of employees for previous year:** 35 **Industry designation:** Food—dairy products **Company type:** Public **Top competitors:** General Mills, Inc.; Groupe Danone

It might not go with your kielbasa, but if you're in Chicago you can try a Kefir—Lifeway Foods' yogurt-like dairy beverage. The company also makes Lifeway's Farmer's Cheese (free of animal rennet (calf stomach lining), salt, and sugar); Sweet Kiss (a fruit sugar-flavored dessert spread); and Elita (a cream cheese substitute). Lifeway Foods distributes its products throughout the Chicago area, and in other areas of the US, Canada, and Eastern Europe. The company also operates a Russian theme restaurant in Chicago called Moscow Nites. President and CEO Michael Smolyansky owns about 60% of the company.

McWhorter Technologies, Inc.

400 E. Cottage Place, Carpentersville, IL 60110

Telephone: 847-428-2657 **Fax:** 847-428-9440 **Metro area:** Chicago, IL **Human resources contact:** Mia F. Igyarto **Sales:** $454.9 million **Number of employees:** 1,040 **Number of employees for previous year:** 791 **Industry designation:** Paints & related products **Company type:** Public **Top competitors:** BASF Aktiengesellschaft; E. I. du Pont de Nemours and Company; Rohm and Haas Company

McWhorter Technologies doesn't bother looking beyond surface appearances. Resins and colorants made by McWhorter are used to make a variety of surface coatings, specialty coatings, and reinforced fiberglass. McWhorter's composite polymers, liquid resins, and colorants are used to produce stains, paints, and industrial coatings. Powder-coating products are used in items such as lawn equipment and metal furniture. McWhorter's polyester resins are used to make fiberglass for products such as mega-yachts and hot tubs. McWhorter operates 15 manufacturing plants in China, Europe, and the US.

MedCare Technologies, Inc.

1515 W. 22nd St., Ste. 1210, Oak Brook, IL 60523

Telephone: 630-472-5300 **Fax:** 630-472-5360 **Metro area:** Chicago, IL **Web site:** http://www.medcareonline.com **Human resources contact:** Florence Wagner **Sales:** $100,000 **Number of employees:** 17 **Number of employees for previous year:** 8 **Industry designation:** Medical services **Company type:** Public **Top competitors:** Rochester Medical Corporation; Collagen Aesthetics, Inc.; UroMed Corporation

When the going gets tough or the tough can't stop going, they go to constipation- and incontinence-therapy specialist MedCare Technologies. The company's noninvasive treatments for patients experiencing urinary and fecal incontinence and related problems include biofeedback using electromyography; pelvic-muscle exercises; and bladder and bowel retraining. After a physician prescribes treatment, patients generally begin with weekly hour-long sessions at MedCare Technologies, then progress to less-frequent sessions over three to four months. The company has more than 20 treatment centers in nine states and intends to open more. Chairman and CEO Harmel Rayat owns about 22% of the company.

Medline Industries, Inc.

1 Medline Place, Mundelein, IL 60060

Telephone: 847-949-5500 **Fax:** 847-949-3126 **Metro area:** Chicago, IL **Web site:** http://www.medline.net **Human resources contact:** Dave Anderson **Sales:** $655 million (Est.) **Number of employees:** 2,700 **Number of employees for previous year:** 2,383 **Industry designation:** Medical & dental supplies **Company type:** Private **Top competitors:** Kimberly-Clark Corporation; Allegiance Corporation; Owens & Minor, Inc.

Medline Industries, a private medical equipment distributor and manufacturer, goes toe-to-toe with the bigger guns, selling more than 100,000 products—bandages, liquid-proof surgical gowns, wheelchairs, and more. Medline distributes its products to more than 25,000 customers, including hospitals, extended care facilities, hospital laundries, and home care providers. Medline's five plants make about 70% of its products, which are sold through some 500 sales representatives and 19 distribution centers. Medline is owned by the Mills family, which founded the company in 1910 as a manufacturer of nurses' gowns.

Morton International, Inc.

Morton International Bldg., 100 N. Riverside Plaza, Chicago, IL 60606

Telephone: 312-807-2000 **Fax:** 312-807-2241 **Metro area:** Chicago, IL **Web site:** http://www.mortonintl.com **Human resources contact:** Christopher K. Julsrud **Sales:** $2.5 billion **Number of employees:** 10,600 **Number of employees for previous year:** 10,500 **Industry designation:** Chemicals—specialty **Company type:** Public **Top competitors:** E. I. du Pont de Nemours and Company; Unilever; Cargill, Incorporated

Morton International, the salt processor with the umbrella girl, makes specialty chemicals and is being acquired by specialty chemical and polymer maker Rohm and Haas. Morton's chemical products include adhesives for food packaging, liquid plastic coatings for autos, electronic materials used in printed circuit boards, and dyes used in inks. Specialty chemicals account for nearly 70% of sales. The specialty chemicals are mainly sold in Europe and North America, but also in Asia, and South America. Morton is also a top US salt producer, producing table salt and salt for water conditioning, ice control, and industrial applications. Morton operates production facilities in North America, Europe, and Asia.

Nalco Chemical Company

One Nalco Center, Naperville, IL 60563

Telephone: 630-305-1000 **Fax:** 630-305-2900 **Metro area:** Chicago, IL **Web site:** http://www.nalco.com **Human resources contact:** James F. Lambe **Sales:** $1.6 billion **Number of employees:** 7,000 **Number of employees for previous year:** 6,900 **Industry designation:** Chemicals—specialty **Company type:** Public **Top competitors:** TOTAL SA; LG Group; E. I. du Pont de Nemours and Company

Nalco Chemical—the world's largest maker of water treatment chemicals—aims to provide just the right chemicals for a wide variety of industrial processes, from making paper and steel to mining to generating electricity. Among other functions, Nalco's chemicals clarify water, control corrosion in cooling systems and boilers, help separate liquids and solids, control pollution, and conserve energy. Nalco sells its products through its own representatives in more than 120 countries. Nalco has joint ventures with US Filter and Exxon, and has subsidiaries worldwide. About 40% of the company's sales are outside the US.

NeoPharm, Inc.

100 Corporate North, Ste. 215, Bannockburn, IL 60015

Telephone: 847-295-8678 **Fax:** 847-295-8854 **Metro area:** Chicago, IL **Sales:** $600,000 **Number of employees:** 6 **Number of employees for previous year:** 4 **Industry designation:** Drugs **Company type:** Public **Top competitors:** ALZA Corporation; Zeneca Group PLC; Rhone-Poulenc S.A.

NeoPharm develops drugs used to diagnose and treat various forms of cancer. Broxuridine (BUdR), designed as an indicator of cancer cell proliferation, has completed phase II trials at the National Cancer Institute. BioChem Pharma has secured rights to market BUdR in Canada pending federal approval there. NeoPharm also is working on proprietary liposome products that encapsulate cancer drugs to reduce side effects; Pharmacia & Upjohn has licensed two of these products. In addition, NeoPharm is developing a chimeric protein (IL-13) to be used as an anticancer agent in the treatment of kidney and brain cancer. NeoPharm will produce its drugs through agreements with established pharmaceutical manufacturers.

Northwestern Healthcare

980 N. Michigan Ave., Ste. 1500, Chicago, IL 60601

Telephone: 312-335-6000 **Fax:** 312-335-6020 **Metro area:** Chicago, IL **Web site:** http://www.nhnet.org **Sales:** $1.7 billion **Number of employees:** 16,000 **Number of employees for previous year:** 15,200 **Industry designation:** Hospitals **Company type:** Not-for-profit **Top competitors:** Advocate Health Care; Columbia/HCA Healthcare Corporation

Through its nine member institutions, Northwestern Healthcare provides medical care to some 125,000 people annually. The largest integrated health system in the Chicago area, it boasts a staff of almost 5,000 physicians. The system's managed health care programs cover pediatrics, neonatal care, mental health, cardiac care, and cancer treatment. Other group operations include outpatient and wellness centers, physician practice management units, and hospice and home health care. Like many hospitals around the country, the members of Northwestern Healthcare opted to sacrifice some of their autonomy to join a network whose multitude of services and numerous locations would better attract paying customers.

Oil-Dri Corporation of America

410 N. Michigan Ave., Ste. 400, Chicago, IL 60611

Telephone: 312-321-1515 **Fax:** 312-321-1271 **Metro area:** Chicago, IL **Web site:** http://oildri.com **Human resources contact:** Michael A. Komenda **Sales:** $160.3 million **Number of employees:** 705 **Number of employees for previous year:** 665 **Industry designation:** Chemicals—specialty **Company type:** Public **Top competitors:** Ralston Purina Company; United States Filter Corporation; The Clorox Company

Oil-Dri Corporation of America helps keep cat lovers' homes from stinking to high heaven. The company produces sorbent products for the consumer, industrial, environmental, agricultural, and fluid-purification markets. Cat litter—which Oil-Dri produces for its own Cat's Pride and Lasting Pride brands, Clorox's Fresh Step brand, and retailers' private labels—brings in more than 60% of sales. Some of the company's other products include oil, grease, and water sorbents; filtration, bleaching, and clarification clays; and pet treats. The company operates facilities in Canada, Switzerland, the UK, and the US. The Jaffee family owns 22% of Oil-Dri's stock but controls about two-thirds of its voting power.

Phosphate Resource Partners Limited Partnership

2100 Sanders Rd., Northbrook, IL 60062

Telephone: 847-272-9200 **Fax:** 847-205-4805 **Metro area:** Chicago, IL **Human resources contact:** Russell Lockridge **Sales:** $687.3 million **Number of employees:** 4,284 **Number of employees for previous year:** 3,871 **Industry designation:** Fertilizers **Company type:** Public

Phosphate Resource Partners LP (PLP), formerly Freeport-McMoRan Resource Partners, produces phosphate through its interests in IMC-Agrico, a joint venture between the company and its managing general partner, IMC Global. It mines phosphate rock to make fertilizers and animal feed ingredients in Florida and Louisiana. PLP is involved in legal battles over alleged wrongful transactions involving James Moffett, his Freeport-McMoRan Oil & Gas (which shares oil exploration interests with PLP), and Henry Kissinger, a former director of Freeport-McMoRan, Inc. PLP has also battled declining phosphate demand with temporary mine and plant closings. IMC Global owns more than 50% of PLP.

Provena Health

9223 W. St. Francis Rd., Frankfort, IL 60423

Telephone: 815-469-4888 **Fax:** 815-469-4864 **Metro area:** Chicago, IL **Human resources contact:** John Landstrom **Sales:** $633.8 million **Number of employees:** 11,400 **Number of employees for previous year:** 5,800 **Industry designation:** Hospitals **Company type:** Not-for-profit **Top competitors:** Rush System for Health; Northwestern Healthcare; Advocate Health Care

To stay competitive in the era of managed care, Provena Health was created from the merger of Illinois Catholic hospital groups Franciscan Sisters Health Care (Frankfort), ServantCor (Kankakee), and Mercy Center for Health Care Services (Aurora). One of the largest health systems in Illinois, Provena has seven hospitals, 14 nursing homes, more than 40 clinics, six home health agencies, and its PersonalCare HMO (co-owned with Christie Clinic). The organization, formed in 1997, plans to invite other hospitals and health care plans to join Provena Health, either as affiliates or as full partners. The company has joined MED3000 Group to form Central Health Solutions, a regional physician management group.

Quixote Corporation

One E. Wacker Dr., Chicago, IL 60601

Telephone: 312-467-6755 **Fax:** 312-467-1356 **Metro area:** Chicago, IL **Web site:** http://www.quixotecorp.com **Human resources contact:** Dorothy French **Sales:** $56 million **Number of employees:** 409 **Number of employees for previous year:** 373 **Industry designation:** Rubber & plastic products **Company type:** Public **Top competitors:** Integrated Security Systems, Inc.; Medusa Corporation; Stimsonite Corporation

No crash-test dummy, Quixote is a don in the world of automotive safety products. Operating through its Energy Absorption Systems subsidiary, Quixote is the US's leading maker of such transportation safety products as energy-absorbing highway crash cushions, including the patented Triton Barrier and CushionWall systems. The company also makes accident-avoidance products such as flexible guideposts, portable sign systems, and highway advisory radio systems (HAR) through its TranSafe subsidiary. Other subsidiaries include Spin-Cast Plastics and Safe-Hit. Quixote has shed its compact disc manufacturing and legal stenography operations to focus on road safety products.

Richco, Inc.

5825 N. Tripp Ave., Chicago, IL 60646

Telephone: 773-539-4060 **Fax:** 773-539-6770 **Metro area:** Chicago, IL **Web site:** http://www.richco-inc.com **Human resources contact:** Sandra Varela-Torres **Sales:** $72 million (Est.) **Number of employees:** 544 **Industry designation:** Rubber & plastic products **Company type:** Private **Top competitors:** Deswell Industries, Inc.; Jabil Circuit, Inc.; Illinois Tool Works Inc.

Richco, Inc. (formerly Richco Plastic Company) makes thousands of plastic and metal parts for the electric, electronic, appliance, and fiber-optic industries. The company's products include circuit board hardware, clips and clamps, spacers, rivets, and cable ties. These products hold together and help run almost anything from a Coke machine to a computer. Richco manufactures its products at three facilities in the US, as well as in Malaysia, South Korea, Spain, and the UK. The company also offers services, including custom molding and extrusion, tool building, and design engineering. CEO Craig Richardson and his family own about 80% of Richco.

Sabratek Corporation

5601 W. Howard St., Niles, IL 60714

Telephone: 847-647-2760 **Fax:** 847-647-2582 **Metro area:** Chicago, IL **Web site:** http://www.sabratek.com **Human resources contact:** Joe Guerrero **Sales:** $66.9 million **Number of employees:** 272 **Number of employees for previous year:** 100 **Industry designation:** Medical products **Company type:** Public **Top competitors:** Baxter International Inc.; I-Flow Corporation; Abbott Laboratories

Home is where the pump is. Sabratek markets "Virtual Hospital Room" therapeutic and diagnostic medical products for alternative-site health care. It specializes in multi-therapy infusion pumps and related disposables for home health care providers, long-term-care facilities, clinics, physician's offices, and outpatient centers. Its stationary and mobile infusion therapy systems administer fluid intravenously at a regulated rate and volume. Sabratek's proprietary MediVIEW PC-based software allows real-time programming, monitoring, data capture, and reporting by caregivers at remote sites. Its products are sold directly and through distributors in Africa, Asia, Europe, the Middle East, South America, and the US.

Security Associates International, Inc.

2101 S. Arlington Heights Rd., Ste. 100, Arlington Heights, IL 60005

Telephone: 847-956-8650 **Fax:** 847-956-9360 **Metro area:** Chicago, IL **Web site:** http://www.sai-inc.com **Human resources contact:** Beverly Davis **Sales:** $20.2 million **Number of employees:** 385 **Number of employees for previous year:** 285 **Industry designation:** Protection—safety equipment & services **Company type:** Public **Top competitors:** Protection One, Inc.; Ameritech Corporation; Tyco International Ltd.

Security Associates International is watching. Operating central monitoring stations for independent burglar alarm companies is the company's core business. As a sideline, Security Associates International also protects the interests of its customers as they face large corporate competitors, providing business loans, seminars and information, and marketing tools. The company does not install security systems, but rather it monitors them and reports problems to authorities. It owns four central alarm stations located in Florida, Illinois, Michigan, and Ohio and purchases business and residential accounts from its dealer affiliates. TJS Partners, an investment group led by Thomas J. Salvatore, owns 51% of the company.

SPR Inc.

2015 Spring Rd., Ste. 750, Oak Brook, IL 60523

Telephone: 630-990-2040 **Fax:** 630-575-6262 **Metro area:** Chicago, IL **Web site:** http://www.sprinc.com **Human resources contact:** Patti Paas **Sales:** $85.3 million **Number of employees:** 680 **Number of employees for previous year:** 573 **Industry designation:** Computers—services **Company type:** Public **Top competitors:** Electronic Data Systems Corporation; Andersen Worldwide

SPR puts the SPRing back in old computer systems. As part of its information technology services, SPR analyzes geriatric computer systems and reengineers them to be more manageable and up-to-date. SPR also offers strategic planning, project management and implementation, applications management, and year 2000 remediation. Its information delivery service captures information that is buried within a database, while its proprietary CodeVu software analyzes source code. Clients are large organizations in such industries as health care, manufacturing, transportation, and utilities. Brothers Robert (CEO) and David (EVP) Figliulo each own about 20% of SPR.

SPSS Inc.

444 N. Michigan Ave., Chicago, IL 60611

Telephone: 312-329-2400 **Fax:** 312-329-3558 **Metro area:** Chicago, IL **Web site:** http://www.spss.com **Human resources contact:** Theresa A. Dear **Sales:** $121.4 million **Number of employees:** 781 **Number of employees for previous year:** 535 **Industry designation:** Computers—corporate, professional & financial software **Company type:** Public **Top competitors:** Manugistics Group, Inc.; SAS Institute Inc.

SPSS designs and markets statistical software products to corporations, government agencies, and academic institutions. Marketed under the SPSS, Quantime, In2itive, New View, SigmaPlot, SYSTAT, QI Analyst, Clementine, and allCLEAR brand names, its products are used in a variety of data mining applications including market research, business analysis, scientific research, and quality-improvement analysis. SPSS' desktop products feature point-and-click graphics, report writing, integrated graphics, and data access and management capabilities. SPSS sells its software in more than 50 countries through worldwide telesales, direct-response marketing, and more than 60 distributors.

Stepan Company

Edens and Winnetka Rds., Northfield, IL 60093

Telephone: 847-446-7500 **Fax:** 847-501-2284 **Metro area:** Chicago, IL **Web site:** http://www.stepan.com **Human resources contact:** Craig Gardiner **Sales:** $610.5 million **Number of employees:** 1,372 **Number of employees for previous year:** 1,292 **Industry designation:** Chemicals—specialty **Company type:** Public **Top competitors:** Air Products and Chemicals, Inc.; English China Clays plc; Albright & Wilson plc

Stepan is all bubbly about its business. The company primarily makes surfactants (a key foaming and cleaning agent) for detergent, shampoo, and cosmetic manufacturers. Industrial uses of its foaming agents include latex foams, agricultural herbicides, and oil recovery products. Stepan's other products include polymers, used in urethane foam systems for plastics, building materials, and refrigeration equipment., and specialty products, including flavor intermediates, esters, and synthetic lubricants. Stepan markets its chemicals directly to manufactures in the US and, through joint ventures, to customers in South America and Asia Pacific. The Stepan family owns a controlling stake in the company.

Superior Graphite Co.

120 S. Riverside Plaza, Chicago, IL 60606

Telephone: 312-559-2999 **Fax:** 312-559-9064 **Metro area:** Chicago, IL **Web site:** http://www.graphitesgc.com **Human resources contact:** Alicia Leal **Sales:** $85.4 million (Est.) **Number of employees:** 430 **Number of employees for previous year:** 407 **Industry designation:** Chemicals—fibers **Company type:** Private **Top competitors:** SGL CARBON AG; Hexcel Corporation; Zoltek Companies, Inc.

Superior Graphite wants a slick image and its lubricants are easing but not greasing the way. Products include a dry lubricant made from natural and synthetic graphite. The company adds value to carbons and graphites for a number of industries by creating products such as battery terminals or heavy machinery components. The "SlipPlate" lubricant is used on everything from shovels to forklifts. To manufacture its line of products, the company operates eight plants in the US, Europe, and Mexico. Founded in 1917 by William Carney, the company supplied graphite during World War I. Today the founder's grandson, CEO Peter Carney, runs the family business. Peter's son, Edward Carney, holds the office of President.

TAP Holdings Inc.

Bannockburn Lake Office Plaza, 2355 Waukegan Rd., Deerfield, IL 60015

Telephone: 847-317-5700 **Fax:** 847-940-9801 **Metro area:** Chicago, IL **Web site:** http://www.tapholdings.com **Human resources contact:** Denise Kitchen **Sales:** $1.6 billion **Number of employees:** 1,500 **Industry designation:** Drugs **Company type:** Joint venture

In the competitive field of pharmaceuticals, TAP Holdings is quickly rising to the occasion. The firm's latest development is an erection-inducing drug that makes use of the much-discussed connection between men's brains and their sexual organs. Apomorphine, which is in trials, appears to act more quickly than rival Viagra by directly stimulating nerves in the brain. (On the downside, some test subjects responded with mood-stifling nausea.) The firm is also testing an antitumor drug. Its marketed products include Lupron (for prostate cancer, endometriosis, and anemia) and Prevacid (for ulcers). TAP Holdings is a joint venture between Japan's Takeda Chemical Industries and the US's Abbott Labs.

Technology Solutions Company

205 N. Michigan Ave., Ste. 1500, Chicago, IL 60601

Telephone: 312-228-4500 **Fax:** 312-228-4501 **Metro area:** Chicago, IL **Web site:** http://www.techsol.com **Human resources contact:** Marie Allen **Sales:** $271.9 million **Number of employees:** 1,572 **Number of employees for previous year:** 1,102 **Industry designation:** Computers—services **Company type:** Public **Top competitors:** Computer Sciences Corporation; Andersen Consulting; International Business Machines Corporation

Technology Solutions Company (TSC) wants to take the monkey wrenches out of businesses. The company provides corporate network systems and enterprise resource planning, supply chain, and customer service applications. TSC assesses a company's procedures, then designs and implements systems that streamline them. Its customers are primarily large corporations in the financial services, communications, and manufacturing industries. Among them are Whirlpool, Aetna, and MCI WorldCom. TSC's OrTech Solutions subsidiary sells Oracle products to clients. The company is expanding its business through a series of acquisitions.

Unimed Pharmaceuticals, Inc.

2150 E. Lake Cook Rd., Buffalo Grove, IL 60089

Telephone: 847-541-2525 **Fax:** 847-541-2569 **Metro area:** Chicago, IL **Web site:** http://www.unimed.com **Human resources contact:** Beverly Lascola **Sales:** $15.9 million **Number of employees:** 70 **Number of employees for previous year:** 45 **Industry designation:** Drugs **Company type:** Public

Let's go get stoned? That's not "exactly" the idea behind Unimed Pharmaceutical's appetite-stimulating and nausea-quelling Marinol, but the active ingredient in the drug "is" tetrahydrocannabinol (THC), the primary intoxicant in marijuana. Other drugs sold by Unimed Pharmaceuticals target infections in the lower respiratory and urinary tracts, and treat anemias through use of anabolic androgenic steroids. The company, which targets the HIV/AIDS, endocrinology, infectious disease, and urology markets, is developing two testosterone replacement gels and an antiparasitic drug to combat diarrhea caused by cryptosporidium. Unimed Pharmaceuticals uses third parties to make its products.

Vienna Sausage Manufacturing Company

2501 N. Damen Ave., Chicago, IL 60647

Telephone: 773-278-7800 **Fax:** 773-278-4759 **Metro area:** Chicago, IL **Web site:** http://www.viennabeef.com **Human resources contact:** Jamie Eisenberg **Sales:** $98 million (Est.) **Number of employees:** 600 **Number of employees for previous year:** 540 **Industry designation:** Food—meat products **Company type:** Private **Top competitors:** Kraft Foods, Inc.; Sara Lee Corporation; ConAgra, Inc.

Perhaps Carl Sandburg should have called Chicago "wienie maker for the world" —the city's Vienna Sausage Manufacturing pioneered the processed beef product-cum-cultural icon known as the hot dog. The company first unveiled its frankfurters (made from a secret Viennese recipe) at the 1893 World's Fair in Chicago. The company also makes other sausages, deli meats, desserts, pickles, and soups; it supplies hot dog stands, restaurants, grocery stores, and its own Chicago deli. Domestic and international sales are handled through distribution facilities in Chicago, Los Angeles, Phoenix, and Clearwater, Florida. James Bodman and James Eisenberg own the company and share the titles of chairman and CEO.

Vysis, Inc.

3100 Woodcreek Dr., Downers Grove, IL 60515

Telephone: 630-271-7000 **Fax:** 630-271-7008 **Metro area:** Chicago, IL **Web site:** http://www.vysis.com **Human resources contact:** Susan Zint **Sales:** $23.4 million **Number of employees:** 173 **Number of employees for previous year:** 153 **Industry designation:** Biomedical & genetic products **Company type:** Public **Top competitors:** Applied Imaging Corp.; ONCOR, Inc.

Vysis develops and markets genetic diagnostic products for cancer, prenatal disorders, and other genetic diseases. A subsidiary of oil giant BP Amoco, the company is focusing on diagnostic products for leukemia and breast, bladder, prostate, and cervical cancers. It distributes more than 240 research products in the US and Europe through direct sales and in 28 countries through a worldwide distribution network. Vysis has collaborative agreements with such leading medical research institutions as the Mayo Clinic, St. Jude Children's Research Hospital, and the University of Chicago. BP Amoco owns a 69% stake in Vysis.

Walgreen Co.

200 Wilmot Rd., Deerfield, IL 60015

Telephone: 847-940-2500 **Fax:** 847-914-2804 **Metro area:** Chicago, IL **Web site:** http://www.walgreens.com **Human resources contact:** John A. Rubino **Sales:** $15.3 billion **Number of employees:** 90,000 **Number of employees for previous year:** 85,000 **Industry designation:** Retail—drugstores **Company type:** Public **Top competitors:** Rite Aid Corporation; Eckerd Corporation; CVS Corporation

Walgreen proffers an old-fashioned tonic for fiscal fitness: quality over quantity and homespun growth rather than growth through acquisition. It works. Despite having fewer stores than its top rivals, Walgreen leads the pack in sales and profitability. The company has more than 2,600 Walgreens stores in 36 states and Puerto Rico. Prescription drugs account for about half of sales; the rest come from general merchandise, over-the-counter medications, cosmetics, beverages, and tobacco products. Rather than buy stores, Walgreen builds its own so it can pick prime, high-traffic locations. For shoppers' convenience, nearly half its stores offer drive-thru pharmacies. More than 90% offer one-hour photo processing.

Whittman-Hart, Inc.

311 S. Wacker Dr., Ste. 3500, Chicago, IL 60606

Telephone: 312-922-9200 **Fax:** 312-913-3020 **Metro area:** Chicago, IL **Web site:** http://www.whittman-hart.com **Human resources contact:** Janie Denman **Sales:** $307.6 million **Number of employees:** 2,300 **Number of employees for previous year:** 1,974 **Industry designation:** Computers—services **Company type:** Public **Top competitors:** Andersen Worldwide; International Business Machines Corporation

Whittman-Hart provides information technology consulting and systems integration services, including network design and management, year 2000 compliance, and the development of custom software, electronic commerce capabilities, and Web sites. It also installs Enterprise Resource Planning software developed by other companies. Whittman-Hart has neither a Whittman nor a Hart; founder, chairman, and CEO Robert Bernard took the names from characters in the book "The Paper Chase" to create a sense of heritage. The company focuses on midsize businesses and divisions of "FORTUNE" 1000 companies. It has offices in 15 US cities and a subsidiary in London (World Consulting). Bernard owns about a third of Whittman-Hart.

Wm. Wrigley Jr. Company

410 N. Michigan Ave., Chicago, IL 60611

Telephone: 312-644-2121 **Fax:** 312-644-0097 **Metro area:** Chicago, IL **Web site:** http://www.wrigley.com **Human resources contact:** David E. Boxell **Sales:** $2 billion **Number of employees:** 8,200 **Number of employees for previous year:** 7,800 **Industry designation:** Food—confectionery **Company type:** Public **Top competitors:** Huhtamaki Oyj; Nabisco Holdings Corp.; Warner-Lambert Company

Wm. Wrigley Jr. chews up the competition as the world's #1 maker of chewing gum. Its products include such popular brands as Doublemint, Extra, Freedent, and Juicy Fruit. Its Amurol Confections subsidiary makes novelty gums and candies, including Bubble Tape and Squeezepop. Wrigley commands about 50% of the US chewing-gum market and sells its products in more than 140 countries, with international sales accounting for more than half of the company's revenues. Reflecting its increasing focus overseas, Wrigley closed a plant in California and opened one in Russia. The Wrigley family, now in its fourth generation at the helm, owns more than one-third of the company and controls more than half of the voting shares.

World's Finest Chocolate, Inc.

4801 S. Lawndale Ave., Chicago, IL 60632

Telephone: 773-847-4600 **Fax:** 773-847-7804 **Metro area:** Chicago, IL **Web site:** http://www.wfcusa.com **Human resources contact:** Linda Chatman **Sales:** $160 million (Est.) **Number of employees:** 850 **Number of employees for previous year:** 800 **Industry designation:** Food—confectionery **Company type:** Private **Top competitors:** Hershey Foods Corporation; Archibald Candy Corporation; Mars, Inc.

For every buck you spend on a World's Finest Chocolate (WFC) bar, 50 cents goes to some worthy cause. That's because the confectioner is one of the country's leading producers of candy for fund-raisers. WFC makes chocolate bars, cocoa, and chocolate-covered almonds and raisins at its plants in Chicago, Australia, and Canada. The company has a 238-acre cocoa plantation on the island of St. Lucia and owns Kinney Printing Co., which prints custom wrappers featuring the fund-raising groups' names. For years kids toted cases of candy door-to-door, but WFC now has its Advanced Order Program to take orders first and deliver the goodies later. The Opler family owns the company, which it founded in 1938.

WRP Corporation

500 Park Blvd., Ste. 1260, Itasca, IL 60143

Telephone: 630-285-9191 **Fax:** 630-285-9289 **Metro area:** Chicago, IL **Web site:** http://www.wembleyrubber.com **Human resources contact:** Lisa Romano **Sales:** $65 million **Number of employees:** 64 **Number of employees for previous year:** 57 **Industry designation:** Medical & dental supplies **Company type:** Public **Top competitors:** Safeskin Corporation; London International Group plc; Maxxim Medical, Inc.

WRP Corporation invites you to scrub in and glove up. Through its American Health Products subsidiary, the firm makes latex and vinyl gloves used by the dental, medical, and food service industries. The gloves are made at WRP's 70%-owned plant in Indonesia and then sold under the Glovetex and DermaSafe brands or under third-party private labels. In addition to making gloves, WRP also distributes powdered and powder-free latex examination gloves made by other suppliers. Medical supply giant Owens & Minor and food service supply firm SYSCO account for about 40% and 30% of sales, respectively. Glove supplier Wembley Rubber Products owns about 40% of WRP; the Malaysian firm MBf Holdings indirectly owns about 25%.

YMCA of the USA

101 N. Wacker Dr., Chicago, IL 60606

Telephone: 312-977-0031 **Fax:** 312-977-9063 **Metro area:** Chicago, IL **Web site:** http://www.ymca.net **Human resources contact:** C. L. Parham **Sales:** $2.7 billion **Number of employees:** 27,000 **Number of employees for previous year:** 23,500 **Industry designation:** Leisure & recreational services **Company type:** Not-for-profit

The YMCA of the US is a charitable not-for-profit organization that provides assistance to individual YMCAs in areas such as programming, accounting, finance, insurance, and purchasing. There are about 2,200 YMCAs in the US, located in all 50 states and serving nearly 15 million members, making it the largest not-for-profit community-service organization in the country. Services provided by YMCAs include health and fitness programs, day camps, child care, youth sports, substance abuse prevention, international exchange, and job training. US-based YMCAs belong to the World Alliance of YMCAs, an organization of independent Ys from some 130 countries.

Zebra Technologies Corporation

333 Corporate Woods Pkwy., Vernon Hills, IL 60061

Telephone: 847-634-6700 **Fax:** 847-913-8766 **Metro area:** Chicago, IL **Web site:** http://www.zebra.com **Human resources contact:** Bruce Beebe **Sales:** $336 million **Number of employees:** 745 **Number of employees for previous year:** 627 **Industry designation:** Optical character recognition **Company type:** Public **Top competitors:** Datamax International Corporation; PSC Inc.; Printronix, Inc.

If you see stripes, think Zebra. Zebra Technologies is a leading maker of printers and printing materials (ribbons and ticket stock) used to produce bar codes for automatic identification and data collection systems. Zebra also makes related software for bar coding systems. Its printing systems are used in many applications, including inventory control, just-in-time manufacturing, hospital patient identification, employee time and attendance monitoring, and automated warehousing. International sales in about 80 countries account for almost half of total revenues.

INDIANA

Berry Plastics Corporation

101 Oakley St., Evansville, IN 47706

Telephone: 812-484-0959 **Fax:** 812-424-0128 **Other address:** P.O. Box 959, Evansville, IN 47706 **Metro area:** Evansville, IN **Web site:** http://www.berryplastics.com **Human resources contact:** Brian Norman **Sales:** $227 million (Est.) **Number of employees:** 2,100 **Number of employees for previous year:** 1,040 **Industry designation:** Chemicals—plastics **Company type:** Private **Top competitors:** Kerr Group, Inc.; IPC, Inc.; Sweetheart Cup Company

Practically everybody takes a drink with Berry once in a while. Berry Plastics, a leading manufacturer of injection-molded plastic packaging, makes open-top containers, drink cups and housewares, aerosol overcaps, lawn and garden products, and custom molded products for use in markets such as the food and dairy, personal care, retail, building supplies, and promotion industries. Open-top containers such as those used for dairy products, child-resistant containers, and paint packaging account for almost half of sales. Customers include Coca-Cola, McDonald's, Sherwin-Williams, and Wal-Mart. Berry has sales offices in North America and Europe; it sells its products directly and through local brokers.

Bindley Western Industries, Inc.

10333 N. Meridian St., Ste. 300, Indianapolis, IN 46290

Telephone: 317-298-9900 **Fax:** 317-297-5372 **Metro area:** Indianapolis, IN **Web site:** http://www.bindley.com **Human resources contact:** Thomas J. Weakley **Sales:** $7.6 billion **Number of employees:** 1,283 **Number of employees for previous year:** 909 **Industry designation:** Drugs & sundries—wholesale **Company type:** Public **Top competitors:** McKesson HBOC, Inc.; Bergen Brunswig Corporation; Quality King Distributors Inc.

Bindley Western is the fifth-largest drug wholesaler in the US (McKesson HBOC is #1). The company's customers include Eckerd, CVS, and Rite Aid, which together account for more than a third of the firm's sales. Although sales to drugstore chain warehouses still make up the bulk of earnings, the company's revenues from direct delivery to independent stores, patients, and other direct customers continue to rise. Bindley Western has spun off its subsidiary Priority Healthcare Corp., which serves such higher-margin alternative markets as care providers for patients of kidney disease, cancer, and infectious diseases. Founder and chairman William Bindley owns about 21% of the firm.

Bioanalytical Systems, Inc.

2701 Kent Ave., West Lafayette, IN 47906

Telephone: 765-463-4527 **Fax:** 765-497-1102 **Metro area:** Lafayette, IN **Web site:** http://www.bioanalytical.com **Human resources contact:** Lina L. Reeves-Kerner **Sales:** $18.2 million **Number of employees:** 205 **Number of employees for previous year:** 160 **Industry designation:** Medical services **Company type:** Public **Top competitors:** Covance Inc.; Hewlett-Packard Company; The Perkin-Elmer Corporation

Analyze this! Bioanalytical Systems sells analytical instruments and other products (about 60% of its sales) and provides contract research and development services for the pharmaceutical and biotechnology industries. Its products include bioanalytical separation instrumentation, chemical analyzers, diagnostic kits, and miniaturized in vivo sampling devices. The firm's research services include product purity tests, characterization analysis of compounds, monitoring drug "cocktail" treatment combinations, and testing for drug interactions. Bioanalytical Systems markets its products and services around the world. Chairman and CEO Peter Kissinger and his wife Candice own about 30% of the company.

Biomet, Inc.

Airport Industrial Park, Warsaw, IN 46581

Telephone: 219-267-6639 **Fax:** 219-267-8137 **Other address:** PO Box 587, Warsaw, IN 46581 **Metro area:** South Bend, IN **Web site:** http://www.biomet.com **Human resources contact:** Darlene K. Whaley **Sales:** $651.4 million **Number of employees:** 2,000 **Number of employees for previous year:** 1,800 **Industry designation:** Medical instruments **Company type:** Public **Top competitors:** Bristol-Myers Squibb Company; Sofamor Danek Group, Inc.; DePuy, Inc.

Hail fellow, well Biomet. Biomet makes surgical and nonsurgical medical devices used by orthopedic specialists. Its wares include reconstructive products (hips, knees, and shoulders), fixation devices (bone screws and pins), orthopedic support devices, facial reconstruction products, and operating-room supplies. It also sells electrical bone-growth stimulators and external devices—which are attached to bone and protrude from the skin—through its Electro-Biology (EBI) subsidiary. Reconstructive devices account for about 60% of Biomet's sales, and North America is its biggest market (about 70% of sales). Its subsidiaries include Arthrotek, Biomet Europe, EBI, EBI Medical Systems, and Walter Lorenz Surgical.

Cohesant Technologies Inc.

5845 W. 82nd St., Ste. 102, Indianapolis, IN 46728

Telephone: 317-875-5592 **Fax:** 317-875-5456 **Metro area:** Fort Wayne, IN **Web site:** http://www.COHESANT.COM/ **Human resources contact:** Marcy Bray **Sales:** $11.7 million **Number of employees:** 70 **Number of employees for previous year:** 65 **Industry designation:** Chemicals—specialty **Company type:** Public **Top competitors:** Binks Sames Corporation; Nordson Corporation; Graco Inc.

Loyal customers are adherents of Cohesant Technologies, which through its Glas-Craft and Raven Lining Systems subsidiaries makes spray finishing and coating equipment and epoxy coating and grout products. The construction, transportation, and marine industries use the company's coating and finishing equipment to apply insulation, protective coatings, and sealants. The equipment is also used to make packaging and to fill molds for products such as plumbing fixtures. Cohesant's AquataPoxy and Raven brands of coatings and grouts protect against corrosion in facilities such as water-treatment plants. Chairman and CEO Morton Cohen owns a controlling interest in the firm.

Conseco, Inc.

11825 N. Pennsylvania St., Carmel, IN 46032

Telephone: 317-817-6100 **Fax:** 317-817-2847 **Metro area:** Indianapolis, IN **Web site:** http://www.conseco.com **Human resources contact:** Dennis J. Dunlap **Sales:** $7.7 billion **Number of employees:** 6,800 **Number of employees for previous year:** 3,700 **Industry designation:** Insurance—life **Company type:** Public **Top competitors:** New York Life Insurance Company; The Prudential Insurance Company of America; Metropolitan Life Insurance Company

The consequence of Conseco's actions is consolidation. The company acquires fixer-upper insurance companies and renovates them into sleek moneymakers. The company's portfolio of companies offers life and supplemental health insurance and annuities, primarily targeted at working-class customers through its Bankers Life and Casualty, American Travellers Life Insurance, American Life and Casualty Insurance, and Lincoln American Life Insurance subsidiaries. The company has also moved into finance with the purchase of Green Tree Financial, the #1 mobile home lender in the US. Conseco is facing pressure from insurance firms that have adopted its acquisitive strategy.

DePuy, Inc.

700 Orthopaedic Dr., Warsaw, IN 46580

Telephone: 219-267-8143 **Fax:** 219-267-7196 **Metro area:** South Bend, IN **Web site:** http://www.depuy.com **Human resources contact:** G. Taylor Seward **Sales:** $770.2 million **Number of employees:** 3,220 **Number of employees for previous year:** 2,930 **Industry designation:** Medical products **Company type:** Subsidiary **Top competitors:** Bristol-Myers Squibb Company; Biomet, Inc.; Stryker Corporation

DePuy makes orthopedic devices and supplies used primarily by orthopedic specialists and spinal neurosurgeons to treat patients with bone defects resulting from diseases, deformities, trauma, and sports accidents. A wholly owned subsidiary of Johnson & Johnson, DePuy has a 15% worldwide share of the reconstructive products market and holds the #2 position in the US, behind Bristol-Myers Squibb. Its products include hip replacements; knee, shoulder, and spinal implants; fixative products for bone fractures; and knee braces and other soft goods for sports-related injuries.

Guidant Corporation

111 Monument Circle, 29th Fl., Indianapolis, IN 46204

Telephone: 317-971-2000 **Fax:** 317-971-2040 **Other address:** PO Box 44906, Indianapolis, IN 46244 **Metro area:** Indianapolis, IN **Web site:** http://www.guidant.com **Human resources contact:** Joseph A. Yahner **Sales:** $1.9 billion **Number of employees:** 6,310 **Number of employees for previous year:** 5,100 **Industry designation:** Medical products **Company type:** Public **Top competitors:** Boston Scientific Corporation; Medtronic, Inc.; Johnson & Johnson

Medical device maker Guidant has a healthy heart. The company is a worldwide manufacturer of cardiovascular therapeutic devices and related products. Its cardioverter defibrillators and pacemakers (50% of sales) detect and treat abnormally fast, slow, and irregular heartbeats. The company's vascular products (45% of sales) help open blocked arteries. Guidant also develops minimally invasive surgical devices to reduce procedure times and improve patient recovery. Guidant's products are sold in the US (about 70% of sales) and in more than 70 other countries. Its purchase of Sulzer Medica's pacemaker and defibrillator business made it the world's #2 maker of cardiac rhythm devices after Medtronic.

Holy Cross Health System Corporation

3606 E. Jefferson Blvd., South Bend, IN 46615

Telephone: 219-233-8558 **Fax:** 219-233-8891 **Metro area:** South Bend, IN **Web site:** http://www.hchs.org **Human resources contact:** Brent Miller **Sales:** $1.5 billion **Number of employees:** 19,135 **Number of employees for previous year:** 18,397 **Industry designation:** Hospitals **Company type:** Not-for-profit **Top competitors:** Blue Cross and Blue Shield Association; Columbia/HCA Healthcare Corporation; Tenet Healthcare Corporation

Holy Hoosiers! Holy Cross Health System Corporation (HCHS) is a not-for-profit health care system founded in 1979 and sponsored by the Sisters of the Holy Cross, a Catholic religious order. The order operates seven hospitals in California, Idaho, Indiana, Maryland, and Ohio, as well as a community services organization in Utah. The system also operates an insurance firm, a long-term care organization, and a practice management company. As a part of its network, HCHS runs home health programs, educational programs, health care services for the poor, and a nursing school. HCHS has moved into managed care in recent years, building primary care networks that allow it to pursue the goal of providing for the poor.

Indianapolis Colts

7001 W. 56th St., Indianapolis, IN 46253

Telephone: 317-297-2658 **Fax:** 317-388-0982 **Other address:** PO Box 535000, Indianapolis, IN 46253 **Metro area:** Indianapolis, IN **Web site:** http://www.colts.com **Human resources contact:** Pete Ward **Sales:** $70.9 million (Est.) **Number of employees:** 150 **Industry designation:** Leisure & recreational services **Company type:** Private **Top competitors:** New York Jets Football Club, Inc.; Miami Dolphins Limited; New England Patriots

The story of the NFL's Indianapolis Colts began in 1946 when the bankrupt Miami Seahawks franchise of the old All-American Football Conference was purchased and relocated to Baltimore under the Colts name. In 1984 then-owner Robert Irsay moved the team to Indianapolis. After a league-worst 3-13 record in 1997, the Colts hired a new coaching staff led by Jim Mora, a former New Orleans Saints head coach. However Mora was little help to the ailing team as the Colts scored the exact same record the following season. The team, which is owned by Robert Irsay's son Jim, renegotiated its lease agreement with the City of Indianapolis in 1998, ensuring that the team will stay put until at least 2007.

Lilly Industries, Inc.

733 S. West St., Indianapolis, IN 46225

Telephone: 317-687-6700 **Fax:** 317-687-6710 **Metro area:** Indianapolis, IN **Web site:** http://www.lillyindustries.com **Human resources contact:** A. Barry Melnkovic **Sales:** $619 million **Number of employees:** 2,300 **Number of employees for previous year:** 2,100 **Industry designation:** Chemicals—specialty **Company type:** Public **Top competitors:** Akzo Nobel N.V.; Morton International, Inc.; Ferro Corporation

Lilly Industries helps put the finishing touch on a variety of products with its industrial coatings for wood, metal, and glass. It also makes furniture-care products such as Guardsman Furniture Polish. Lilly's customers typically are manufacturers of furniture, building products, appliances, transportation equipment, and mirrors. Lilly sells directly to its 6,000 clients, often developing finishes to meet specific customers' requirements. In addition, Lilly makes fabric-protection products (Fabri-Coate), as well as private-label automotive chemicals such as fuel injector cleaners. These are sold through retail outlets. The company operates plants and offices in Asia, Australia, Europe, and North America.

Made2Manage Systems, Inc.

9002 Purdue Rd., Indianapolis, IN 46268

Telephone: 317-532-7000 **Fax:** 317-872-6454 **Metro area:** Indianapolis, IN **Web site:** http://www.made2manage.com **Human resources contact:** Lori Roberson **Sales:** $27.2 million **Number of employees:** 239 **Number of employees for previous year:** 149 **Industry designation:** Computers—corporate, professional & financial software **Company type:** Public **Top competitors:** Symix Systems, Inc.; Fourth Shift Corporation; DataWorks Corporation

Some firms are made to manage problems—Made2Manage Systems, with its software for small and midsized manufacturers, wants to be a member of that club. Its Made2Manage for Windows is an integrated, enterprisewide application that covers every aspect of the manufacturing business—sales analysis, inventory, purchasing, scheduling, quality assurance, accounts receivable, and financial reporting. Sales representatives and value-added resellers market the firm's products and services in the US and Canada. Clients are engineer-to-order, make-to-order, make-to-stock, and mixed-mode operations. Underwriter Hambrecht & Quist Group and affiliated entities own 29% of the firm, which went public in 1997.

Pacers Basketball Corporation

300 E. Market St., Indianapolis, IN 46204

Telephone: 317-263-2100 **Fax:** 317-263-2127 **Metro area:** Indianapolis, IN **Web site:** http://www.nba.com/pacers **Human resources contact:** Dale Ratermann **Sales:** $56.4 million (Est.) **Number of employees:** 128 **Industry designation:** Leisure & recreational services **Company type:** Private **Top competitors:** Charlotte Hornets; Chicago Bulls; Atlanta Hawks, Ltd.

Bird is the word for this team. The Indiana Pacers have placed their hopes on coach Larry Bird, an NBA legend and Indiana native, to end a championship drought. After nine years in the American Basketball Association (ABA), the three-time ABA champions joined the NBA in 1976. The team experienced mostly down years until players such as Reggie Miller and Rik Smits led the team to seven straight playoff seasons (1990-96). Bird garnered Coach of the Year honors in 1998 after his Pacers won a franchise record 58 games and took the champion Chicago Bulls to seven games in the conference finals. The Pacers are owned by shopping-center magnates Melvin and Herbert Simon and play in Indianapolis' Market Square Arena.

Standard Management Corporation

9100 Keystone Crossing, Indianapolis, IN 46240

Telephone: 317-574-6200 **Fax:** 317-574-2043 **Metro area:** Indianapolis, IN **Human resources contact:** Pamela Behr **Sales:** $46.9 million **Number of employees:** 141 **Number of employees for previous year:** 139 **Industry designation:** Insurance—life **Company type:** Public **Top competitors:** Financial Industries Corporation; Lincoln Heritage Corporation; Citizens Financial Corporation

Standard Management Corporation (SMC) is a financial services holding company that specializes in life insurance and annuities and grows by acquiring other insurance firms. SMC's main subsidiary, Standard Life, sells life insurance and annuities throughout most of the US; Dixie National Life Insurance offers burial-expense policies. Savers Life Insurance offers retirement products and supplemental Medicare coverage. Other SMC subsidiaries include Standard Marketing (wholesale insurance and annuities), Standard Management International (life insurance in Europe and the Caribbean), and Midwestern National Life Insurance. Chairman and CEO Ronald Hunter owns more than 10% of SMC; Conseco owns about 20%.

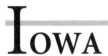

IOWA

Ag Services of America, Inc.

2302 W. First St., Thunder Ridge Ct., Cedar Falls, IA 50613

Telephone: 319-277-0261 **Fax:** 319-277-0144 **Other address:** PO Box 668, Cedar Falls, IA 50613 **Metro area:** Waterloo, IA **Web site:** http://www.agservices.com **Human resources contact:** Robert Boelman **Sales:** $186.1 million **Number of employees:** 119 **Number of employees for previous year:** 107 **Industry designation:** Agricultural operations **Company type:** Public **Top competitors:** Agway Inc.; GROWMARK Inc.; Farmland Industries, Inc.

Ag Services of America is a supplier of agricultural inputs and financing. The company sells seed, fertilizer, and agricultural chemicals and provides multiperil crop insurance and cash advances for rent, fuel, and irrigation to farmers. It buys agricultural supplies from national and regional manufacturers, distributors, and suppliers at volume discounts. Ag Services' strategy is to be a single source for farm supplies and the credit to finance them by taking an interest in the crop itself (customers' farms are visited at least once a year to discuss concerns and strategies). The company's primary market is made up of corn and soybean producers in the central US.

Pioneer Hi-Bred International, Inc.

800 Capital Sq., 400 Locust St., Des Moines, IA 50306

Telephone: 515-248-4800 **Fax:** 515-248-4999 **Metro area:** Des Moines, IA **Web site:** http://www.pioneer.com **Sales:** $1.8 billion **Number of employees:** 5,025 **Number of employees for previous year:** 5,000 **Industry designation:** Agricultural operations **Company type:** Public **Top competitors:** DEKALB Genetics Corporation; Monsanto Company; Novartis AG

Forget T-bills and CDs. Pioneer Hi-Bred International guarantees the best yields around. The nation's largest seller of seed, Pioneer uses genetic research to develop hybrid seeds that produce higher crop yields for farmers, who use the crops primarily as feed for animals. Corn seed accounts for more than 75% of sales; the company also makes seed (hybrid and other varieties) for alfalfa, canola, sorghum, sunflowers, soybeans, and wheat. Pioneer also makes silage (succulent feed) and hay inoculants. About three-quarters of its sales are in the US, but it also sells seed in nearly 100 other countries. The Wallace family owns about 14% of Pioneer. Chemical giant DuPont owns 20% and is buying the entire company.

The Principal Financial Group

711 High St., Des Moines, IA 50392

Telephone: 515-247-5111 **Fax:** 515-246-5475 **Metro area:** Des Moines, IA **Web site:** http://www.principal.com **Human resources contact:** Thomas J. Gaard **Sales:** $8.7 billion **Number of employees:** 17,637 **Number of employees for previous year:** 17,010 **Industry designation:** Insurance—life **Company type:** Mutual company **Top competitors:** Liberty Mutual Insurance Companies; The Hartford Financial Services Group, Inc.

Insurance is a matter of principle for this company. The Principal Financial Group's operating units offer a variety of insurance and financial services. Its flagship company, Principal Mutual Life Insurance (The Principal) offers life and nonmedical health insurance to individuals, groups, and businesses. The company also offers investment services, annuities, mortgage originations and servicing, and mutual funds. Principal Financial has more than 250 locations worldwide including North and South America, Europe, and Asia. A new subsidiary, Principal Bank, offers online banking services. Principal Financial's policyholders have approved its conversion into a mutual holding company.

UroSurge, Inc.

2660 Crosspark Rd., Coralville, IA 52241

Telephone: 319-626-8311 **Fax:** 319-626-8312 **Metro area:** Iowa City, IA **Web site:** http://www.urosurge.com **Sales:** $11,000 (Est.) **Number of employees:** 34 **Industry designation:** Medical products **Company type:** Private **Top competitors:** Biomatrix, Inc.; C. R. Bard, Inc.; Medtronic, Inc.

UroSurge develops medical devices for the management and treatment of genitourinary disorders, primarily urinary incontinence (UI). It markets UroVive (a microballoon around the urethra for treating stress UI) and SANS (electric stimulator to regulate bladder action) in the US, AcuTrainer (electric bladder retrainer) in Europe and the US, and SpiraStent and FilaStent (devices that facilitate urine flow from kidneys and remove kidney stones) internationally. Other products are in the clinical trial stage for US release. UroSurge distributes its products in Australia, Europe, Japan, and South Korea and will market them to urologists and urogynecologists once its direct sales force is in place.

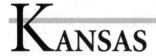

KANSAS

AmVestors Financial Corporation

555 S. Kansas Ave., Topeka, KS 66601

Telephone: 785-232-6945 **Fax:** 785-295-4495 **Metro area:** Topeka, KS **Human resources contact:** Clayton Burklund **Sales:** $216 million **Number of employees:** 148 **Number of employees for previous year:** 100 **Industry designation:** Insurance—life **Company type:** Subsidiary

AmVestors Financial, a wholly owned subsidiary of life insurer AmerUs Life Holdings, sells annuities through its principal subsidiaries, American Investors Life Insurance and Financial Benefit Life Insurance. AmVestors' annuity products include single premium deferred annuities, single premium immediate annuities, and flexible premium deferred annuities. The company markets its products to the growing savings and retirement market and includes features in its policies designed to reduce premature contract terminations and significant withdrawals. AmVestors sells its products through more than 8,000 independent agents in 47 states.

Electronic Processing, Inc.

501 Kansas Ave., Kansas City, KS 66105

Telephone: 913-321-6392 **Fax:** 913-321-1243 **Metro area:** Kansas City, MO-Kansas City, KS **Web site:** http://www.epicorp.com/index.htm **Human resources contact:** Sally D. MacDonald **Sales:** $11.5 million **Number of employees:** 80 **Number of employees for previous year:** 70 **Industry designation:** Computers—corporate, professional & financial software **Company type:** Public **Top competitors:** The Chase Manhattan Corporation; UnionBanCal Corporation

Electronic Processing, Inc. (EPI) develops software and network operations used in bankruptcy management, including legal noticing, claims management, funds distribution, and government reporting. Products include the Trustee Case Management System (for Chapter 7 liquidation filings); and CasePower and the TSI System (both for Chapter 13 individual reorganizations). EPI, which caters to bankruptcy trustees, also provides support services such as consulting, installation, and on-site training. EPI is allied with NationsBank (now BankAmerica) to market an integrated banking services package and bankruptcy management software. Chairman Tom Olofson and his son Christopher (the company's COO) own about 35% of EPI.

Integrated Medical Resources, Inc.

11320 W. 79th St., Lenexa, KS 66214

Telephone: 913-962-7201 **Fax:** 913-962-7063 **Metro area:** Kansas City, MO-Kansas City, KS **Web site:** http://www.for-men.com **Sales:** $21 million **Number of employees:** 161 **Number of employees for previous year:** 151 **Industry designation:** Medical services **Company type:** Public

Integrated Medical Resources operates a national network of nearly 30 medical clinics specializing in the treatment of male sexual dysfunction, particularly impotence. Offering diagnosis, education, and treatment, the company seeks to meet both the medical and emotional needs of patients and their partners. The clinics, operating as The Diagnostic Center for Men (and located mainly in the Southwest, Midwest, and Northeast), place a premium on patient confidentiality by using discreet signs and directly supplying patients with all necessary treatments. About 26% of the company's revenues come from the sale of Rigiscans, in-home monitoring devices that measure naturally occurring erections during sleep.

LabOne, Inc.

10310 W. 84th Terrace, Lenexa, KS 66214

Telephone: 913-888-1770 **Fax:** 913-888-8343 **Metro area:** Kansas City, MO-Kansas City, KS **Web site:** http://www.labone.com **Human resources contact:** Judy Von Feldt **Sales:** $102.2 million **Number of employees:** 895 **Number of employees for previous year:** 665 **Industry designation:** Medical services **Company type:** Public **Top competitors:** Quest Diagnostics Incorporated; SmithKline Beecham plc; Laboratory Corporation of America Holdings

LabOne speedily scrutinizes specimens and samples. Its mainstay is performing lab tests for insurers that wish to prescreen applicants for disease or that want to determine whether a smoker has lied to get lower premiums. LabOne is also certified to perform drug testing for employers. By using express pickup and delivery and a centralized testing lab facility, it has most results available in 24 hours or less. The firm also provides standard clinical lab testing services to health care providers. LabOne serves the US from one centralized operation in Kansas, and its sister company, Lab One Canada, serves its neighbors to the north. Lab Holdings plans to buy the 20% of LabOne that it doesn't already own.

Midwest Grain Products, Inc.

1300 Main St., Atchison, KS 66002

Telephone: 913-367-1480 **Fax:** 913-367-0192 **Other address:** PO Box 130, Atchison, KS 66002 **Metro area:** Kansas City, MO-Kansas City, KS **Human resources contact:** David E. Rindom **Sales:** $223.3 million **Number of employees:** 421 **Number of employees for previous year:** 411 **Industry designation:** Food—flour & grain **Company type:** Public **Top competitors:** Archer Daniels Midland Company; Cargill, Incorporated; High Plains Corporation

Midwest Grain Products puts the proof in the bottle and the texture in most everything else. The company buys wheat and processes it into food ingredients, including vital wheat gluten, wheat proteins, and wheat starch. By-products created during this process are mixed with corn or milo and processed into a variety of alcohol products used in food, beverages, and fuel. To escape the volatile commodities market, Midwest Grain is developing new wheat gluten and starch products, including a material that can be molded like plastic. Members of the founding Cray family, including president and CEO Laidacker "Ladd" Seaberg (son-in-law of chairman Cloud "Bud" Cray Jr.), own about 40% of the company.

National Cooperative Refinery Association

1391 Iron Horse Rd., McPherson, KS 67460

Telephone: 316-241-2340 **Fax:** 316-241-5531 **Web site:** http://www.ncrarefinery.com **Human resources contact:** Ronald Schaumburg **Sales:** $700 million **Number of employees:** 560 **Number of employees for previous year:** 540 **Industry designation:** Oil refining & marketing **Company type:** Cooperative **Top competitors:** Valero Energy Corporation; Tosco Corporation; Farmland Industries, Inc.

Cooperation is a refined art and refining a cooperative art for the National Cooperative Refinery Association (NCRA), which provides three farm supply cooperatives (Cenex Harvest States, GROWMARK, and MFA Oil) with fuel through its oil refinery in Kansas. In 1943, five regional farm supply cooperatives, tired of wartime fuel shortages, created the NCRA to buy the Globe oil refinery in McPherson, Kansas. In 1998 the refinery's production capacity was 75,000 barrels per day. Fuel from the refinery is allocated to member-owners on the basis of ownership percentages. In addition to the refinery, NCRA owns Jayhawk Pipeline, minority interests in two other pipeline companies, and an underground oil storage facility.

Petroglyph Energy, Inc.

6209 N. Hwy. 61, Hutchinson, KS 67502

Telephone: 316-665-8500 **Fax:** 316-665-8577 **Human resources contact:** Susan Bowlby **Sales:** $4.5 million **Number of employees:** 48 **Number of employees for previous year:** 35 **Industry designation:** Oil & gas—exploration & production **Company type:** Public **Top competitors:** Inland Resources Inc.; Snyder Oil Corporation; PetroCorp Incorporated

Petroglyph Energy hopes to see writing on rocks that spells out the location of oil and gas. The exploration and production company's primary activity is its enhanced oil recovery projects in Utah's Lower Green River formation. The company also operates in the Raton Basin in southeast Colorado and northeast New Mexico, where it plans to develop coalbed methane natural gas. In addition, Petroglyph Energy owns a 100% working interest in a South Texas field. The company's proved reserves consist of 18 million barrels of oil equivalent. Petroglyph Energy is laying off 25% of its employees, citing low oil prices.

Seaboard Corporation

9000 W. 67th St., Shawnee Mission, KS 66202

Telephone: 913-676-8800 **Fax:** 913-676-8872 **Metro area:** Kansas City, MO-Kansas City, KS **Web site:** http://www.seaboardcorp.com **Human resources contact:** Douglas W. Schult **Sales:** $1.8 billion **Number of employees:** 12,031 **Number of employees for previous year:** 10,788 **Industry designation:** Food—meat products **Company type:** Public **Top competitors:** ConAgra, Inc.; Dole Food Company, Inc.; Tyson Foods, Inc.

Seaboard is a diversified agribusiness and transportation company with operations in 18 countries in the Americas and Africa. Seaboard sells chicken under the Gold-n-Fresh and Easy Entrees names, mostly in the eastern US and overseas. The company's pork goes to both US and foreign markets, and Seaboard operates a shipping service in the Caribbean. Seaboard also owns the #1 bakery in Puerto Rico. Overseas, it trades grains and seeds, raises and processes shrimp, brokers fruits and vegetables, makes polypropylene bags, operates power plants and feed mills, and grows and refines sugar cane. The descendants of founder Otto Bresky own about three-quarters of the company.

Sisters of Charity of Leavenworth Health Services Corporation

Cantwell Hall, 4200 S. Fourth St., Leavenworth, KS 66048

Telephone: 913-682-1338   **Fax:** 913-682-1052   **Metro area:** Kansas City, MO-Kansas City, KS   **Web site:** http://www.sclhsc.org   **Human resources contact:** Dennis "Mike" Groves   **Sales:** $892.5 million   **Number of employees:** 10,000   **Number of employees for previous year:** 9,000   **Industry designation:** Hospitals   **Company type:** Not-for-profit   **Top competitors:** Health Management Associates, Inc.; Tenet Healthcare Corporation; Province Healthcare Company

In 1857 a group of Catholic sisters arrived in Kansas (then Indian territory) and began teaching and tending the sick; a decade later, they incorporated as the Sisters of Charity of Leavenworth Health Services. The not-for-profit regional health care organization operates more than a dozen hospitals, clinics, and medical centers in California, Colorado, Kansas, and Montana. Its facilities provide health services to lower-income and uninsured people. Along with Boulder-based Lutheran Medical Center, it runs Exempla, a not-for-profit hospital system. The organization has agreed to buy Bethany Medical Center·in Kansas City, Kansas, from Columbia/HCA.

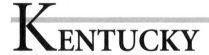

KENTUCKY

Atria Senior Quarters

501 S. Fourth St., Ste. 140, Louisville, KY 40202

Telephone: 502-719-1600   **Fax:** 502-719-1699   **Metro area:** Louisville, KY   **Web site:** http://seniorquarters.com   **Human resources contact:** Maroynn Cohen   **Sales:** $37.2 million (Est.)   **Number of employees:** 1,750   **Number of employees for previous year:** 1,000   **Industry designation:** Nursing homes   **Company type:** Private

In a romance for the aged, Atria Senior Quarters was formed by the merger of Kapson Senior Quarters with its 88%-owned subsidiary, Atria Communities. Both companies focused on independent and assisted living centers for the well (and well-off) but frail elderly, who may need assistance with daily tasks; health monitoring, but not health care. The combined company owns or manages about 100 facilities in more than 25 states. Investment bank Lazard Freres owns the company. The merger was consummated in 1998 over the objections of ARV Assisted Living, an Atria competitor in which Lazard Freres has a significant ownership interest.

Caretenders Health Corp.

100 Mallard Creek Rd., Ste. 400, Louisville, KY 40207

Telephone: 502-899-5355   **Fax:** 502-891-8083   **Metro area:** Louisville, KY   **Human resources contact:** W. Timothy Luckett   **Sales:** $95.2 million   **Number of employees:** 3,400   **Number of employees for previous year:** 2,600   **Industry designation:** Health care—outpatient & home   **Company type:** Public   **Top competitors:** In Home Health, Inc.; American Retirement Corporation; Apria Healthcare Group Inc.

With its home health care and adult day care services, Caretenders Health offers senior citizens an alternative to spending their days in nursing homes. The company's home health care services include in-home infusion therapy, physical therapy, and custodial companion care. Its adult day care centers provide seniors with transportation to and from the centers, meals, and medical attention. Caretenders provides home health care and adult day care programs in nine states, primarily in Kentucky, Ohio, and Maryland. HEALTHSOUTH Rehabilitation owns almost a third of Caretenders.

Churchill Downs Incorporated

700 Central Ave., Louisville, KY 40208

Telephone: 502-636-4400 **Fax:** 502-636-4430 **Metro area:** Louisville, KY **Web site:** http://www.kentuckyderby.com **Human resources contact:** Jeanne A. Keats **Sales:** $147.3 million **Number of employees:** 2,925 **Number of employees for previous year:** 2,600 **Industry designation:** Leisure & recreational services **Company type:** Public **Top competitors:** Players International, Inc.; Aztar Corporation; Argosy Gaming Company

Every year on the first Saturday in May, Churchill Downs hosts the US's most prestigious horse race, the Kentucky Derby. Three-year-old Thoroughbreds have been making the Run for the Roses for more than 120 years. In addition to the Louisville, Kentucky, racetrack, the company operates four off-site betting facilities in Indiana and Kentucky. It also owns Ellis Park racetrack in western Kentucky, and a majority interest in Hoosier Park, a track in Indiana. Churchill Downs conducts races on more than 70 days each year. The company receives half of its sales through gambling, with simulcast revenues comprising the majority of that number.

Dippin' Dots, Incorporated

5101 Charter Oak Dr., Paducah, KY 42001

Telephone: 502-443-8994 **Fax:** 502-443-8997 **Web site:** http://www.dippindots.com **Human resources contact:** Jim Moss **Sales:** $18 million (Est.) **Number of employees:** 100 **Industry designation:** Food—dairy products **Company type:** Private **Top competitors:** Good Humor-Breyers Ice Cream; Eskimo Pie Corporation; TCBY Enterprises, Inc.

State fair staples Dippin' Dots are the product of a scientist with a sweet tooth. Experimenting with cryogenics in 1988, microbiologist Curt Jones flash-froze ice cream into tiny beads, named his creations Dippin' Dots, and opened a store in which to sell them. Today, 20 flavors of Dippin' Dots are sold nationwide at amusement parks, fairs, and the Kennedy Space Center in Florida (where they are called Space Dots). The company sells Dippin' Dots in Europe and Asia, but not in supermarkets: Jones isn't convinced home freezers will keep the pellets (made at 320 below Fahrenheit) cold enough. Dippin' Dots are made in Kentucky and shipped in specialized refrigerated boxes. Jones and his family own the company.

Humana Inc.

The Humana Bldg., 500 W. Main St., Louisville, KY 40202

Telephone: 502-580-1000 **Fax:** 502-580-4188 **Metro area:** Louisville, KY **Web site:** http://www.humana.com **Human resources contact:** Regenold Barefield **Sales:** $9.6 billion **Number of employees:** 19,500 **Number of employees for previous year:** 18,300 **Industry designation:** Health maintenance organization **Company type:** Public **Top competitors:** Kaiser Foundation Health Plan, Inc.; Aetna Inc.; CIGNA Corporation

One of the top health care providers in the US, Humana offers health maintenance organizations (HMOs), preferred provider organizations (PPOs), and Medicare supplement insurance. The company has about 6.2 million members in 16 states and Puerto Rico. Humana tries to cut costs by offering physicians incentives, and by requiring pre-authorization for hospital inpatient services and outpatient surgery. Medicare accounts for almost one-third of sales, but Humana is cutting back its Medicare HMO business. The company markets its HMO and PPO products to employers and other groups, as well as to certain Medicare-eligible individuals.

Jillian's Entertainment Holdings

1387 S. Fourth St., Louisville, KY 40208

Telephone: 502-638-9008 **Fax:** 502-638-0984 **Metro area:** Louisville, KY **Web site:** http://www.jillians.com **Human resources contact:** Barbara Coyne **Sales:** $15 million (Est.) **Number of employees:** 10 **Number of employees for previous year:** 8 **Industry designation:** Leisure & recreational services **Company type:** Private **Top competitors:** Dave & Buster's, Inc.; Hard Rock Cafe International, Inc.; Hooters of America, Inc.

Dave and Buster, meet Jillian. Jillian's Entertainment Holdings operates 30 entertainment centers in 12 states. Similar to Dave & Buster's (D&B), a typical Jillian's offers billiards tables, virtual games, large-screen televisions, and food such as pizza and sandwiches. However, unlike D&B (whose sales are almost 10 times greater than Jillian's), the company focuses on secondary markets such as Columbus, Ohio, and Louisville, Kentucky. Co-founder and CEO Steven Foster took the company private in 1997, buying back all the stock with the help of Boston investment firm J.W. Childs.

Lexmark International Group, Inc.

740 New Circle Rd. NW, Lexington, KY 40550

Telephone: 606-232-2000 **Fax:** 606-232-2403 **Metro area:** Lexington, KY **Web site:** http:// www.lexmark.com **Human resources contact:** Kathleen J. Affeldt **Sales:** $3 billion **Number of employees:** 8,800 **Number of employees for previous year:** 8,000 **Industry designation:** Computers—peripheral equipment **Company type:** Public **Top competitors:** Seiko Corporation; Hewlett-Packard Company; Canon Inc.

Lexmark has good peripheral vision. Lexmark International Group is a leading maker of computer printers and related products, which generate more than 80% of its sales. Its printer line includes laser printers (designed primarily for corporate networks and desktops) and ink-jet printers (for home and business use). Unlike many of its competitors, Lexmark develops and manufactures its own desktop laser printers, which results in fast product cycle times. The company also makes supplies for IBM and other name-brand printers and typewriters. Lexmark's products are sold in more than 15,000 retail outlets in more than 150 countries.

Omnicare, Inc.

50 E. Rivercenter Blvd., Covington, KY 41011

Telephone: 606-291-6800 **Fax:** 606-291-6886 **Metro area:** Cincinnati, OH **Human resources contact:** Janice M. Rice **Sales:** $1.5 billion **Number of employees:** 7,450 **Number of employees for previous year:** 4,699 **Industry designation:** Medical services **Company type:** Public **Top competitors:** Genesis Health Ventures, Inc.; PharMerica Inc.; Cardinal Health, Inc.

Omnicare: it's not everywhere—yet. The top independent provider of pharmacy services to the US nursing home market, the acquisitive company serves almost 6,900 long-term-care facilities in 40 states. It dispenses drugs for nursing homes and provides computerized record keeping and third-party billing for patients in its clients' facilities. Omnicare also offers such consultant pharmacist services as evaluating patient drug-therapy monthly, monitoring drug administration procedures within a nursing facility, and monitoring compliance with government regulations. Related services include infusion therapy and medical supply provision, pharmaceutical research, and wellness maintenance programs.

Pomeroy Select Integration Solutions, Inc.

1020 Petersburg Rd., Hebron, KY 41048

Telephone: 606-586-0600 **Fax:** 606-525-1537 **Metro area:** Cincinnati, OH **Sales:** $45.2 million **Number of employees:** 1,086 **Industry designation:** Computers—services **Company type:** Subsidiary **Top competitors:** TechForce Corporation; Mastech Corporation; CSI Computer Specialists, Inc.

Pomeroy Select Integration Solutions is a data-splattered net-chanic, popping the hoods of corporate computer networks to service their performance. A subsidiary of computer networking equipment specialist Pomeroy Computer Resources (which will retain voting control following the planned IPO), Pomeroy Select offers such services as multi-vendor repair and maintenance, system installation, asset tracking, and computer network design, integration, and management. The company also provides Internet-based training and around-the-clock help desk support. Pomeroy Select primarily targets midsized to large organizations; customers include KN Energy, Lexmark International, and the University of Kentucky.

Res-Care, Inc.

10140 Linn Station Rd., Louisville, KY 40223

Telephone: 502-394-2100 **Fax:** 502-394-2206 **Metro area:** Louisville, KY **Web site:** http://www.rescare.com **Sales:** $522.7 million **Number of employees:** 18,500 **Number of employees for previous year:** 11,900 **Industry designation:** Nursing homes **Company type:** Public **Top competitors:** Magellan Health Services, Inc.; Youth Services International, Inc.; HEALTHSOUTH Corporation

Through its residential, training, and support services, Res-Care offers RESpect and CARE to some 12,000 people with disabilities and mental retardation in 25 states. Specific services include social skills, vocational skills, and functional skills training, as well as counseling and therapy programs. The company also serves more than 9,000 disadvantaged youths at vocational training centers in 17 states and Puerto Rico under the federal Job Corps program. Res-Care has grown by buying up other treatment organizations, including group home providers in Texas and Georgia and a North Carolina provider of services for people with developmental disabilities.

Strategia Corporation

6040 Dutchman's Ln., Louisville, KY 40233

Telephone: 502-426-3434 **Fax:** 502-426-3028 **Other address:** PO Box 37144, Louisville, KY 40233 **Metro area:** Louisville, KY **Web site:** http://www.strategiacorp.com **Human resources contact:** David Workman **Sales:** $11 million **Number of employees:** 118 **Number of employees for previous year:** 62 **Industry designation:** Computers—services **Company type:** Public

Strategia helps businesses and government agencies prepare for and avoid unknown and unplanned data processing interruptions such as natural disasters, fire, and sabotage. As a part of its data processing "insurance," Strategia provides alternate site processing to Bull, IBM, and UNIX-based computer system users at its data centers in Louisville, Kentucky and Paris. Strategia also aids customers in planning for and solving known problems such as the Year 2000 code conversion and the pending European Eurocurrency conversion. Its services are marketed to about 200 medium- to large-sized organizations (including France Telecom) in diverse industries throughout North America and Europe.

Sykes HealthPlan Services, Inc.

11405 Bluegrass Pkwy., Louisville, KY 40299

Telephone: 502-267-4900 **Fax:** 502-263-5680 **Metro area:** Louisville, KY **Human resources contact:** Todd Bartlett **Number of employees:** 975 **Industry designation:** Health care—outpatient & home **Company type:** Joint venture

Sykes HealthPlan Services, a subsidiary of information technology firm Sykes Enterprises, provides outsourced health care management and employee benefits services to corporations and health care providers and payors. The company's services include a 24-hour patient information line, management of prolonged and at-risk patient cases, quality management software (Optimed), COBRA administration, general benefits administration, and retiree benefits services. The company is expanding its customer base (which includes AT&T, Lucent Technologies, and various Blue Cross and Blue Shield companies) through acquisitions and by cross-selling products to existing customers.

Vencor, Inc.

3300 Aegon Center, 400 W. Market St., Louisville, KY 40202

Telephone: 502-596-7300 **Fax:** 502-596-7499 **Metro area:** Louisville, KY **Web site:** http://www.vencor.com **Human resources contact:** Cece Liahagan **Sales:** $3.1 billion **Number of employees:** 76,800 **Industry designation:** Nursing homes **Company type:** Public **Top competitors:** Tenet Healthcare Corporation; Columbia/HCA Healthcare Corporation; Beverly Enterprises, Inc.

Vencor—one of the nation's largest providers of long-term health care—operates more than 60 acute care hospitals and 300 skilled nursing facilities. Vencor split into two separately traded firms in 1998: An operating company (called Vencor) owns the business operations and non-real estate assets; real estate investment trust (REIT) Ventas owns its buildings and other properties. The company sold most of its stake in assisted-living company Atria (now Atria Senior Quarters).

LOUISIANA

Amedisys, Inc.

3029 S. Sherwood Forest Blvd., Ste. 300, Baton Rouge, LA 70816

Telephone: 225-292-2031 **Fax:** 225-295-9685 **Metro area:** Baton Rouge, LA **Web site:** http://www.amedisys.com **Human resources contact:** Cindy Doll **Sales:** $54.5 million **Number of employees:** 665 **Number of employees for previous year:** 456 **Industry designation:** Health care—outpatient & home **Company type:** Public

Because the last thing you want to do when you're sick is drive to a doctor's office, Amedisys has decided to bring health care to you. The company offers home and alternate-site health care to patients, as well as management services to health care providers, primarily in the southern and southeastern US. Sometimes preferred to institutional health care, Amedisys' off-site services include alternate-site infusion therapy for administration of intravenous medications and nutrition, ambulatory surgery centers, home health care nursing, physical and speech therapy, social services, and home health aides. Its management services include staffing and physician support services.

Crystal Oil Company

229 Milam St., Shreveport, LA 71101

Telephone: 318-222-7791 **Fax:** 318-677-5515 **Other address:** PO Box 21101, Shreveport, LA 71120 **Metro area:** Shreveport, LA **Web site:** http://www.crystaloil.com **Human resources contact:** Dom Lanzillotti **Sales:** $22.1 million **Number of employees:** 25 **Number of employees for previous year:** 24 **Industry designation:** Oil & gas—exploration & production **Company type:** Public **Top competitors:** TEPPCO Partners, L.P.; Tejas Energy, LLC; Enterprise Products Company

The means to make money is as clear as crude oil to Crystal Oil. The firm and its subsidiaries own two natural gas storage operations near Hattiesburg, Mississippi, as well as oil and gas interests in Mississippi and Louisiana. Its Hattiesburg and Petal salt caverns have a combined storage capacity of 6.7 billion cu. ft. The firm serves the southeastern and northeastern US through its 33 miles of pipeline, which has links to such major systems as the Transco, Tennessee, Associated, and Koch pipelines. Crystal Oil, which has proved reserves of 113,000 barrels of oil, acquired 29 billion cu. ft. of natural gas through its purchase of properties in DeSoto Parish, Louisiana, where it is drilling additional wells.

ERLY Industries Inc.

8641 United Plaza Blvd., Ste. 300, Baton Rouge, LA 70809

Telephone: 225-922-4658 **Fax:** 225-922-4544 **Metro area:** Baton Rouge, LA **Sales:** $614.3 million **Number of employees:** 1,788 **Number of employees for previous year:** 1,364 **Industry designation:** Food—flour & grain **Company type:** Public **Top competitors:** Mars, Inc.; Riviana Foods Inc.; Riceland Foods, Inc.

Rice processor ERLY Industries is pretty steamed as it tries to reorganize under Chapter 11 bankruptcy protection. Its American Rice subsidiary processes, packages, and markets branded and private-label rice in the US and overseas; domestic brands include Adolphus, Comet, and Wonder. ERLY's smaller Chemonics Industries subsidiary provides consulting services in the fields of agribusiness, natural resources, environmental services, and modernization to emerging-market countries, primarily through contracts with the US government and the World Bank. ERLY has sold off its olive and fire-retardant chemical businesses.

Mcmoran Exploration Co.

1615 Poydras St., New Orleans, LA 70112

Telephone: 504-582-4000 **Fax:** 504-582-4899 **Metro area:** New Orleans, LA **Web site:** http://www.moxy.com **Sales:** $13.6 million **Number of employees:** 331 **Number of employees for previous year:** 16 **Industry designation:** Oil & gas—exploration & production **Company type:** Public

McMoRan Exploration (formerly McMoRan Oil & Gas) explores for, develops, and produces oil and natural gas. A spinoff of former Freeport-McMoRan (bought by IMC Global), the firm operates offshore in the Gulf of Mexico and onshore in the Gulf Coast region. McMoRan Exploration has proved reserves of 40.2 billion cu. ft. of natural gas and 463,000 barrels of oil and condensate. Freeport-McMoRan Services contracted with the firm to handle its management services (administrative, accounting, financial). Through buying Freeport-McMoRan Sulphur, the company began mining and selling sulphur. The new subsidiary has about 54 million long tons of proved sulphur reserves and some five million barrels of proved oil reserves.

Melamine Chemicals, Inc.

Hwy. 18 West, Donaldsonville, LA 70346

Telephone: 225-473-3121 **Fax:** 225-473-0550 **Other address:** PO Box 748, Donaldsville, LA 70346 **Metro area:** Houma-Thibodaux, LA **Web site:** http://www.melamine.com **Human resources contact:** Mike Fowler **Sales:** $60 million **Number of employees:** 153 **Number of employees for previous year:** 93 **Industry designation:** Chemicals—specialty **Company type:** Subsidiary **Top competitors:** Cytec Industries Inc.; H.B. Fuller Company; PPA Technologies, Inc.

Melamine Chemicals, a subsidiary of Borden, Inc., is crystal-clear when it comes to making melamine crystal, a specialty chemical for industrial and commercial use. One of only two melamine producers in the western hemisphere and one of the three largest in the world, the company produces about a million pounds of melamine annually. Most applications involve melamine-formaldehyde resins, which are used in laminates, paper and surface coatings, plastic molding, and textile treatments. Melamine crystals are also used in flame-retardant polyurethane foams and as a concrete plasticizer to make concrete more fluid. Melamine is produced from urea (ammonia and carbon dioxide) supplied mainly by Triad Nitrogen.

New Orleans Saints

5800 Airline Hwy., Metairie, LA 70003

Telephone: 504-733-0255 **Fax:** 504-731-1888 **Metro area:** New Orleans, LA **Web site:** http://www.nfl.com/saints/index.html **Human resources contact:** Charleen Sharpe **Sales:** $80.9 million (Est.) **Number of employees:** 131 **Industry designation:** Leisure & recreational services **Company type:** Private **Top competitors:** San Francisco 49ers; St. Louis Rams Football Company; Atlanta Falcons

The National Football League's New Orleans Saints haven't exactly produced heavenly results over the years. Founded on All Saints' Day in 1966, the team didn't secure its first winning season until 1987. Former Chicago Bears coach Mike Ditka was handed coaching duties in 1997 after the Saints ended the 1996 season with a dismal 3-13 record. The controversial and outspoken Ditka revived fan interest in the franchise, and the team had a fresh start to the 1998 season, winning its first three games (not bad for the only NFL team never to have won a playoff game). However Ditka magic is still a long way off as the team finished the year an improved but still paltry 6-10.

Pan-American Life Insurance Company

601 Poydras St., New Orleans, LA 70130

Telephone: 504-566-1300 **Fax:** 504-566-3950 **Metro area:** New Orleans, LA **Web site:** http://www.palic.com **Human resources contact:** Vicki Cansler **Sales:** $467.9 million **Number of employees:** 1,100 **Industry designation:** Insurance—life **Company type:** Mutual company

Pan-American Life Insurance was founded as a stock company in 1911 to write insurance in the Caribbean basin, but it converted to mutual status in 1952. The company sells life and health insurance and annuities in seven Central and South American countries. Traditional life insurance products have been a declining portion of sales, but Pan-American's strength in the Hispanic market and a new emphasis on pension products provide a base for new growth. Pan-American has exited the US health and life insurance market to focus on sales of retirement products.

PetroQuest Energy, Inc.

625 E. Kaliste Saloom Rd., Ste. 400, Lafayette, LA 70505

Telephone: 318-232-7028 **Fax:** 318-232-0044 **Metro area:** Lafayette, LA **Sales:** $5.3 million **Number of employees:** 26 **Number of employees for previous year:** 9 **Industry designation:** Oil & gas—exploration & production **Company type:** Public

Canada's PetroQuest Energy (formerly Optima Petroleum) and its US subsidiary Optima Energy explore for gas and oil and develop leases primarily in the Gulf Coast of Louisiana. The company seeks projects with oil reserves of five million barrels of oil or 50 billion cu. ft. of natural gas in which it can acquire a 25% to 50% stake. PetroQuest markets its production to third parties, in conjunction with its industry partners. Its share of proved reserves in properties where it has interests total some three trillion cu. ft. of gas and about 875 million barrels of liquid fuels. The company sold off most of its Canadian operations to focus solely on US exploration.

Sterling Sugars, Inc.

PO Box 572, Franklin, LA 70538

Telephone: 318-828-0620 **Fax:** 318-828-1757 **Metro area:** Lafayette, LA **Sales:** $40.7 million **Number of employees:** 207 **Number of employees for previous year:** 102 **Industry designation:** Food—sugar & refining **Company type:** Public **Top competitors:** Tate & Lyle North American Sugars; Imperial Sugar Company

Not quite worth its weight in gold, raw sugar is Sterling Sugars' primary business. The company grows and processes sugar cane, selling raw sugar to refiners and candy makers. Raw sugar accounts for 95% of revenues. The company also sells by-product blackstrap molasses. Sterling Sugars can grind more than 10,000 tons of cane daily at its Louisiana factory. The company owns about 20,000 acres of land in three Louisiana parishes and leases most of it to independent cane farmers. Some land also is used for oil and gas exploration and production. Sterling Sugars' corporate secretary, James Patout Burns Jr., owns about 60% of the company's stock; director Peter Guarisco owns about 20%.

Stone Energy Corporation

625 E. Kaliste Saloom Rd., Lafayette, LA 70508

Telephone: 318-237-0410 **Fax:** 318-232-8061 **Metro area:** Lafayette, LA **Human resources contact:** Flo Ziegler **Sales:** $116.6 million **Number of employees:** 103 **Number of employees for previous year:** 90 **Industry designation:** Oil & gas—exploration & production **Company type:** Public

Stone Energy is an independent oil and gas company that acquires, develops, and exploits oil and natural gas properties in the Gulf Coast basin area. The company operates 14 properties, six onshore Louisiana and eight offshore. Stone Energy focuses on mature properties with established production histories that it believes have significant exploitation and development potential. It has been able to increase its development activities through the expansion of its technical database. The firm has estimated proved reserves of 189.2 billion cu. ft. of natural gas and 17.8 million barrels of oil.

3CI Complete Compliance Corporation

910 Pierremont, #312, Shreveport, LA 71106

Telephone: 318-869-0440 **Fax:** 318-869-4002 **Metro area:** Shreveport, LA **Web site:** http://www.am3ci.com **Human resources contact:** Janice Little **Sales:** $19 million **Number of employees:** 225 **Number of employees for previous year:** 203 **Industry designation:** Pollution control equipment & services **Company type:** Public **Top competitors:** Waste Management, Inc.; Med/Waste, Inc.; Browning-Ferris Industries, Inc.

3CI Complete Compliance treats waste like the plague. Doing business as American 3CI, the firm disposes of medical or biomedical waste (anything that may cause infectious disease) by incineration and other chemical or heat processes. 3CI provides customers with containers, waste transport, and documented tracking of shipping. Its 17,000 customer accounts, mainly in the southern US, include medical centers, clinics, hospitals, dental offices, veterinarians, pharmaceutical companies, laboratories, and retirement homes. The firm also offers safety training and consulting. About half of 3CI is owned by Waste Systems, a subsidiary of #2 medical waste disposer Stericycle.

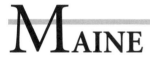

MAINE

Acadia National Health Systems, Inc.

460 Main St., Lewiston, ME 04240

Telephone: 207-777-3423 **Fax:** 207-784-7743 **Metro area:** Lewiston, ME **Web site:** http://www.acadianational.com **Human resources contact:** Richard Hooper **Sales:** $1.1 million **Number of employees:** 34 **Number of employees for previous year:** 16 **Industry designation:** Medical practice management **Company type:** Public **Top competitors:** MedPartners, Inc.; PhyCor, Inc.; FPA Medical Management, Inc.

Acadia National Health Systems knows how to get the bills paid. The company provides practice management products and services, including billing (about 90% of its sales), consulting, software, and administrative services. Clients include health care networks, hospitals, and physician practices. The company also offers billing services for small practices in markets not attractive to major practice management companies. Acquisitive Acadia National Health Systems, which already manages health care practices in four states, plans to establish a division devoted to practice management. Chairman/CEO Paul Chute and vice presidents Jacquelyn Magno and Mark Thatcher each own nearly 20% of the company.

American Skiing Company

Sunday River Rd., Bethel, ME 04217

Telephone: 207-824-8100 **Fax:** 207-824-5158 **Other address:** PO Box 450, Bethel, ME 04217 **Metro area:** Lewiston, ME **Web site:** http://www.peaks.com **Human resources contact:** Judy Klein-Golden **Sales:** $340.4 million **Number of employees:** 7,826 **Number of employees for previous year:** 6,000 **Industry designation:** Leisure & recreational services **Company type:** Public **Top competitors:** Booth Creek Ski Holdings, Inc.; Intrawest Corporation; Vail Resorts, Inc.

American Skiing Company (ASC) has nine resorts nationwide, making it North America's #3 ski resort operator (after Vail Resorts and Intrawest). ASC's resorts include Steamboat in Colorado; Heavenly in California; Sunday River and Sugarloaf in Maine; Attitash Bear Peak in New Hampshire; Sugarbush, Killington, and Mount Snow in Vermont; and the Canyons in Utah. Upgraded facilities and aggressive marketing have boosted ASC's sales. ASC also develops mountainside real estate near its resorts with condos, time-share properties, and other recreation such as golf courses. President and CEO Les Otten owns 54% of ASC.

IDEXX Laboratories, Inc.

One IDEXX Dr., Westbrook, ME 04092

Telephone: 207-856-0300 **Fax:** 207-856-0346 **Metro area:** Portland, ME **Web site:** http://www.idexx.com **Human resources contact:** Sam Fratoni **Sales:** $319.9 million **Number of employees:** 2,100 **Number of employees for previous year:** 1,515 **Industry designation:** Biomedical & genetic products **Company type:** Public **Top competitors:** Diagnostic Products Corporation; EG&G, Inc.; Thermo Electron Corporation

IDEXX Laboratories makes diagnostic test kits and instruments that veterinarians use to detect heartworm, feline leukemia, and other diseases, as well as test systems for food, agricultural, and environmental contaminants. Its products use biotech processes such as DNA and immunoassay testing. The company also provides veterinarians with practice management software and mail-order pharmacy services. IDEXX targets the veterinary and environmental markets, which are less stringently regulated than the human medical market. It sells some 400 products in more than 50 countries.

Nyer Medical Group, Inc.

1292 Hammond St., Bangor, ME 04401

Telephone: 207-942-3630 **Fax:** 207-941-9392 **Human resources contact:** Kurt Kitchen **Sales:** $33.9 million **Number of employees:** 198 **Number of employees for previous year:** 106 **Industry designation:** Medical & dental supplies **Company type:** Public **Top competitors:** CVS Corporation; McKesson HBOC, Inc.; Walgreen Co.

Holding company Nyer Medical Group does business through subsidiaries that cover the medical waterfront. More than half of sales come from D.A.W., which owns Eaton Apothecary, a chain of about 10 Boston-area stores. Three subsidiaries (which together contribute more than 25% of Nyer's sales) provide rescue equipment, fire trucks, and supplies to EMS, fire, and police departments. Several other subsidiaries sell medical equipment and supplies to wholesalers, physicians, health care facilities, and the home health care market throughout New England and in Florida. In 1996 Nyer Medical Group spun off more than 60% of biotech firm Genetic Vectors. Chairman Samuel Nyer owns about two-thirds of the holding company.

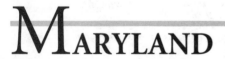

MARYLAND

Appnet Systems, Inc.

6707 Democracy Blvd., Bethesda, MD 20817

Telephone: 301-493-8900 **Fax:** 301-581-2488 **Metro area:** Washington, DC **Web site:** http://www.appnet.net **Human resources contact:** Bob Boehn **Sales:** $17.7 million (Est.) **Number of employees:** 750 **Industry designation:** Computers—services **Company type:** Private **Top competitors:** USWeb/CKS; AGENCY.COM; Harbinger Corporation

When it comes to commerce and communication in the new millennium, AppNet Systems knows there's nothin' but Net. The company helps get its clients moving down the information superhighway by developing e-commerce systems, Web sites, back office Internet applications, and data warehousing and EDI (electronic data interchange) systems. In a bid to expand its services, AppNet has aggressively pursued a string of acquisitions (almost a dozen in one year) to bolster its e-profile. The company counts Ford Motor Company (15% of sales), the US government (13%), America Online, and Arrow Electronics among its clients. Venture capital firm GTCR owns nearly 50% of AppNet.

BioReliance Corporation

9900 Blackwell Rd., Rockville, MD 20850

Telephone: 301-738-1000 **Fax:** 301-738-1036 **Metro area:** Washington, DC **Web site:** http://www.bioreliance.com **Human resources contact:** Connie Robinson **Sales:** $49.8 million **Number of employees:** 414 **Number of employees for previous year:** 371 **Industry designation:** Medical services **Company type:** Public **Top competitors:** SRI International; Covance Inc.; Applied Analytical Industries, Inc.

BioReliance helps biotechnology and pharmaceutical companies suffering from test anxiety. The company provides contract research and manufacturing services at its facilities in Germany, the UK, and the US. BioReliance's BioTesting Services division conducts nonclinical testing of products from preclinical development through licensed production. The BioManufacturing division's BIOMEVA and MAGENTA subsidiaries make microbial and viral products for companies developing gene therapies. Among BioReliance's clients are the US government and the National Institute of Environmental Health Sciences. Chairman Sidney Knafel and his family own about half the company.

BioWhittaker, Inc.

8830 Biggs Ford Rd., Walkersville, MD 21793

Telephone: 301-898-7025 **Fax:** 301-845-7774 **Metro area:** Hagerstown, MD **Web site:** http://www.biowhittaker.com **Human resources contact:** Richard Patchak **Sales:** $56.8 million **Number of employees:** 450 **Number of employees for previous year:** 410 **Industry designation:** Medical products **Company type:** Subsidiary

If someone told you a company's product was made from crab blood, would you guess the company made medical testing products? BioWhittaker, acquired in 1997 as the biotechnology division of specialty chemical firm Cambrex, is a leading supplier of cell cultures (living cells grown in an artificial environment) used for research and detection of viruses and diseases. In addition to ELVIS (a herpes-detection culture), BioWhittaker sells cell-culture media used to sustain artificial cell growth. The company also offers endotoxin-detection products (based on crab blood) that test implantable and injectable medical devices for dangerous contamination. Clients are commercial, government, and university labs.

Bon Secours Health System, Inc.

1505 Marriottsville Rd., Marriottsville, MD 21104

Telephone: 410-442-5511 **Fax:** 410-442-1082 **Metro area:** Baltimore, MD **Web site:** http://www.bshsi.com **Human resources contact:** Virginia Rounsadille **Sales:** $1.2 billion **Number of employees:** 20,000 **Number of employees for previous year:** 19,000 **Industry designation:** Hospitals **Company type:** Not-for-profit **Top competitors:** Carilion Health System; The Johns Hopkins Health System Corporation; Holy Cross Health System Corporation

This company succors its clients. Bon Secours Health System is a not-for-profit organization dedicated to providing health care to all, especially the poor and sick. The company was created in 1983 by the Sisters of Bon Secours, an international Catholic group established in 1824 in Paris. Bon Secours Health System is composed of 14 acute care hospitals, seven long-term care facilities, and a psychiatric hospital. The system also operates clinics, assisted-living facilities, hospices, and home health care services. The organization has facilities in Florida, Maryland, Michigan, Pennsylvania, South Carolina, and Virginia.

Careflow Net, Inc.

15215 Edwards Ferry Rd., Poolesville, MD 20837

Telephone: 301-349-0700 **Fax:** 301-349-0873 **Metro area:** Washington, DC **Web site:** http://www.careflow.com **Human resources contact:** J. Calvin Kaylor **Sales:** $1 million (Est.) **Number of employees:** 11 **Number of employees for previous year:** 9 **Industry designation:** Computers—corporate, professional & financial software **Company type:** Private **Top competitors:** LifeRate Systems, Inc.; MedPlus, Inc.; Comet Software International Ltd.

Founded in 1996, CareFlow⚕t develops information management software. The company's Clinical Document Management system lets medical industry workers electronically access, combine, route, and deliver patient records. Its CareFlow Transcription suite enables secure intranet access for the entire transcription process. Products are sold directly to health care providers and to integrated delivery networks (combinations of hospitals, clinics, and physicians). CareFlow⚕t also offers such services as system development, design, and application customization. Shampa Reddy, the daughter of one of CareFlow's founders, owns about 17%.

Chesapeake Biological Laboratories, Inc.

1111 S. Paca St., Baltimore, MD 21230

Telephone: 410-843-5000 **Fax:** 410-843-4414 **Metro area:** Baltimore, MD **Web site:** http://www.cblinc.com **Human resources contact:** Lauren Kraft **Sales:** $7 million **Number of employees:** 78 **Number of employees for previous year:** 56 **Industry designation:** Medical services **Company type:** Public **Top competitors:** Quintiles Transnational Corp.; Covance Inc.; Kendle International Inc.

Chesapeake Biological Laboratories provides product development and commercial drug production services for pharmaceutical and biotechnology companies. It also produces experimental drugs for use in clinical trials. The company specializes in biopharmaceuticals, which are materials derived from naturally occurring biological substances. Chesapeake Biological provides consulting related to the clinical trial and Food and Drug Administration approval processes. Other services include test-method development and validation, preparation of clinical trial materials, and process design and manufacturing validation.

Condor Technology Solutions, Inc.

170 Jennifer Rd., Ste. 325, Annapolis, MD 21401

Telephone: 410-266-8700 **Fax:** 410-266-8400 **Metro area:** Baltimore, MD **Web site:** http://www.condorweb.com **Sales:** $168.8 million **Number of employees:** 1,075 **Number of employees for previous year:** 530 **Industry designation:** Computers—services **Company type:** Public **Top competitors:** Computer Sciences Corporation; International Business Machines Corporation; Andersen Consulting

Condor Technology Solutions took flight with the acquisition of eight smaller information technology (IT) companies in 1998. Formed to target the needs of midsized organizations, Condor hopes the consolidation will give it an advantage in the highly fragmented IT industry, where midsized companies must often hire multiple firms to handle their needs. Condor helps its clients efficiently adapt to new technologies by offering consulting, systems installation and integration, contract staffing, training, support, and maintenance services through about 25 offices in 11 US states, Germany, and the Netherlands. The company targets insurance, financial, government, technology, and health care markets.

Coventry Health Care Inc.

6705 Rockledge Dr., Ste. 100, Bethesda, MD 20817

Telephone: 615-771-4141 **Fax:** 615-771-4203 **Metro area:** Washington, DC **Human resources contact:** Donald T. Benson **Sales:** $2.1 billion **Number of employees:** 3,050 **Number of employees for previous year:** 2,100 **Industry designation:** Health maintenance organization **Company type:** Public

Coventry Health Care is a managed health care company that provides services to more than one million enrollees in the Midwest and Southeast. The company was formed in 1998 when Coventry Corp. doubled in size by acquiring Principal Financial Group's Principal Health Care unit. Its health care plans cover patients enrolled in health maintenance organizations (HMOs) and preferred provider organizations (PPOs). The company's ASLIC insurance subsidiary underwrites branded flexible provider products, including the company's HMO products. Coventry Health Care also administers self-insured health plans for large employers. Principal Financial Group owns 40% of the firm.

Credit Management Solutions, Inc.

5950 Symphony Woods Rd., Columbia, MD 21044

Telephone: 410-740-1000 **Fax:** 410-884-5298 **Metro area:** Baltimore, MD **Web site:** http://www.cmsinc.com **Human resources contact:** Dave McDonald **Sales:** $16.9 million **Number of employees:** 212 **Number of employees for previous year:** 140 **Industry designation:** Computers—corporate, professional & financial software **Company type:** Public **Top competitors:** The Reynolds and Reynolds Company; International Business Machines Corporation; American Management Systems, Incorporated

Ya can't tell the borrowers without a scorecard. Credit Management Solutions develops software and services for managing volume-intensive credit operations over WANs. Its CreditRevue software analyzes credit applications by considering third-party credit reports and by consulting lenders' internal loan guidelines and loan scorecards. The company's software-based CreditConnection service links credit sources online, thus enabling applications to be sent to multiple lenders and their subsequent decisions to be delivered immediately. The firm also offers credit scoring software produced with Dun & Bradstreet. Chairman and CEO James DeFrancesco owns 39% of the company; EVP Scott Freiman, 20%.

Diehl Graphsoft, Inc.

10270 Old Columbia Rd., Ste. 100, Columbia, MD 21046

Telephone: 410-290-5114 **Fax:** 410-290-8050 **Metro area:** Baltimore, MD **Web site:** http://www.diehlgraphsoft.com **Human resources contact:** Don Webster **Sales:** $7.4 million **Number of employees:** 60 **Number of employees for previous year:** 48 **Industry designation:** Computers—engineering, scientific & CAD-CAM software **Company type:** Public **Top competitors:** Autodesk, Inc.; International Microcomputer Software, Inc.; Intergraph Corporation

Look, but don't touch. Diehl Graphsoft products let designers and engineers do pretty much everything but touch their creations during the design process. Its low-end MiniCAD computer-aided design (CAD) software includes 2-D and 3-D modeling, report generation, a database, programmability, and industry-specific modules for both Mac and PC platforms. The Department of Agriculture and the Fish and Wildlife Service use MiniCAD to design visitor centers, and Air Force engineers design aircraft parts with it. The company also offers training manuals, tutorial software, and technical services for its customers. Founder and CEO Richard Diehl owns about 60% of the company.

Digene Corporation

9000 Virginia Manor Rd., Beltsville, MD 20705

Telephone: 301-470-6500 **Fax:** 301-470-6496 **Metro area:** Washington, DC **Web site:** http://www.digene.com **Sales:** $12 million **Number of employees:** 137 **Number of employees for previous year:** 120 **Industry designation:** Biomedical & genetic products **Company type:** Public **Top competitors:** Meridian Diagnostics, Inc.; Orgenics Ltd.; Abbott Laboratories

For Digene, it's all about women. The company develops and markets DNA and RNA tests that screen for diseases afflicting women. Using its Hybrid Capture technology, Digene has developed the only FDA-approved test for the detection of human papillomavirus (linked to cervical cancer) and currently markets the test to more than 700 customers worldwide—directly in the US and through both subsidiaries and a distribution agreement with Abbott Laboratories internationally (60% of sales). Digene is also developing Hybrid Capture tests for chlamydia, gonorrhea, HIV, and hepatitis. Through a general partnership, Evan Jones (chairman and CEO) and Charles Fleischman (CFO and COO) own almost 40% of the company.

DIGEX, Inc.

One DIGEX Plaza, Beltsville, MD 20705

Telephone: 301-847-5000 **Fax:** 301-847-5215 **Metro area:** Washington, DC **Web site:** http://www.digex.net **Human resources contact:** Peter Daley **Sales:** $15.6 million **Number of employees:** 430 **Number of employees for previous year:** 263 **Industry designation:** Computers—online services **Company type:** Subsidiary

DIGEX calls its Internet services "industrial strength." The company, a subsidiary of telecommunications services provider Intermedia Communications, is one of the US's leading independent Internet carriers. DIGEX works exclusively with business customers and government agencies, including Amtrak, CIGNA, Southwestern Bell, and the World Bank. DIGEX's Internet services include high-speed dedicated connectivity (including telecommute connectivity), corporate Web server hosting and security, and private-label connectivity (for telecommunications providers). The company's high-speed digital backbone and 24-hour network operations center provide high-reliability (99.9%) service from coast to coast.

EntreMed, Inc.

9610 Medical Center Dr., Ste. 200, Rockville, MD 20850

Telephone: 301-217-9858 **Fax:** 301-217-9594 **Metro area:** Washington, DC **Web site:** http://www.entremed.com **Human resources contact:** Susan Cain **Sales:** $5.2 million **Number of employees:** 66 **Number of employees for previous year:** 50 **Industry designation:** Drugs **Company type:** Public

EntreMed develops anti-angiogenic drugs, which inhibit the abnormal growth of new blood vessels. Angiogenesis is associated with cancer, rheumatoid arthritis, and other diseases. EntreMed's anti-angiogenic compounds include Angiostatin and Endostatin, both of which have successfully blocked the growth of blood vessels in cancer tumors; the company receives royalties on the sales on an Endostatin detection kit (ACCUCYTE) it developed with CytImmune Sciences. EntreMed is also working on a blood-cell permeation device that could act as a drug delivery system and has received permission to make the controversial drug thalidomide to treat AIDS-related cancer. Bristol-Myers Squibb owns 7% of the company.

Federal Data Corporation

4800 Hampton Ln., Bethesda, MD 20814

Telephone: 301-986-0800 **Fax:** 301-961-3892 **Metro area:** Washington, DC **Web site:** http://www.feddata.com **Sales:** $336.3 million (Est.) **Number of employees:** 996 **Industry designation:** Computers—services **Company type:** Private

From providing advanced computer systems to conducting biomedical research, Federal Data wants to be the US government's everything—at least in the information technology (IT), engineering, and scientific-contracting arenas. Through its four operating units, Federal Data serves more than 20 government agencies, including NASA and the Department of Defense. Three of the operating groups provide integrated IT systems, computer workstations and servers, and consulting services. The Science and Engineering Group provides IT services, engineering services, and scientific research. An affiliate of The Carlyle Group owns 84% of the company.

FileTek, Inc.

9400 Key West Ave., Rockville, MD 20850

Telephone: 301-251-0600 **Fax:** 301-251-1990 **Metro area:** Washington, DC **Web site:** http://www.filetek.com **Human resources contact:** Debbie Mobley **Sales:** $23.7 million (Est.) **Number of employees:** 98 **Industry designation:** Computers—corporate, professional & financial software **Company type:** Private **Top competitors:** Compaq Computer Corporation; International Business Machines Corporation; Microsoft Corporation

Companies whose data storage systems are about to blow up may be able to defuse the bomb with FileTek's atomic data (information at its most granular level) storage products. The company's StorHouse data warehouse system is designed to manage virtually unlimited amounts of information within files (telephone call records, sales receipt data, and financial transactions). StorHouse, which is easily integrated into current systems, stores data on a variety of media, including inexpensive tapes and optical discs. In 1997 AT&T and U S WEST together accounted for 30% of FileTek's sales. Co-founder and CEO William Thompson owns about 90% of FileTek. The company filed to go public in July 1998.

Gene Logic Inc.

708 Quince Orchard Rd., Gaithersburg, MD 20878

Telephone: 301-987-1700 **Fax:** 301-987-1701 **Metro area:** Washington, DC **Web site:** http://www.genelogic.com **Human resources contact:** Al Lichtenstein **Sales:** $13.2 million **Number of employees:** 157 **Number of employees for previous year:** 97 **Industry designation:** Biomedical & genetic products **Company type:** Public

Gene Logic offers pharmaceutical companies ways to speed up development of new drugs. Its products identify changes in genes associated with a disease and allow drugmakers to gear a drug's development to address those changes. Gene Logic is also developing a Flow-Thru Chip to measure drug efficacy by analyzing gene changes. Its purchase of Oncormed gives it expertise in cancer discovery and treatment using gene technology. The company is developing a database of gene expressions to serve as a reference and a source to predict the effectiveness of test drugs. Gene Logic has strategic alliances with Procter & Gamble, SmithKline Beecham, Japan Tobacco, and Hoechst Schering AgrEvo.

GenVec, Inc.

12111 Parklawn Dr., Rockville, MD 20852

Telephone: 301-816-0396 **Fax:** 301-816-0085 **Metro area:** Washington, DC **Human resources contact:** Marge Meyer **Sales:** $10.2 million (Est.) **Number of employees:** 54 **Industry designation:** Biomedical & genetic products **Company type:** Private

Biotechnology company GenVec has developed a gene therapy designed to induce new blood vessel formation (angiogenesis) in human hearts and other tissue with inadequate blood flow. The therapy, BIOBYPASS, is a harmless respiratory virus that has been engineered to carry the gene that stimulates blood vessel growth. BIOBYPASS is injected into the hearts of patients undergoing coronary artery bypass graft surgery. Still in the clinical testing phase, BIOBYPASS also is intended for treatment of peripheral vascular disease. GenVec has a collaborative agreement with Warner-Lambert to develop and commercialize BIOBYPASS. The company is developing other products for the treatment of cancer and heart disease.

Guilford Pharmaceuticals Inc.

6611 Tributary St., Baltimore, MD 21224

Telephone: 410-631-6300 **Fax:** 410-631-6338 **Metro area:** Baltimore, MD **Web site:** http://www.guilfordpharm.com **Human resources contact:** Lorraine Thomas **Sales:** $12.5 million **Number of employees:** 218 **Number of employees for previous year:** 198 **Industry designation:** Biomedical & genetic products **Company type:** Public **Top competitors:** Cephalon, Inc.; NeoTherapeutics, Inc.; Vertex Pharmaceuticals Incorporated

Guilford Pharmaceuticals is developing drug-delivery systems for treating cancer, and therapeutic and diagnostic products for treating neurological diseases. The company's first approved delivery system, Gliadel, is a medicinal wafer placed in the space left when a brain tumor is removed. Gliadel is being marketed in the US and abroad by Rhone-Poulenc Rorer. In partnership with Amgen, the company's neurological program has developed a series of drugs that can be given orally to regenerate nerve cells in people suffering from spinal injury, Parkinson's, Alzheimer's, and other disorders. Guilford's other neurological products include Dopascan, an intravenous solution used in diagnosing Parkinson's disease.

Hanger Orthopedic Group, Inc.

7700 Old Georgetown Rd., Bethesda, MD 20814

Telephone: 301-986-0701 **Fax:** 301-986-0702 **Metro area:** Washington, DC **Web site:** http://www.hanger.com **Human resources contact:** Ada Brady **Sales:** $187.9 million **Number of employees:** 1,437 **Number of employees for previous year:** 1,213 **Industry designation:** Medical products **Company type:** Public

Hanger Orthopedic Group is a medical practice management company that acquires and operates businesses specializing in orthotic and prosthetic (O&P) rehabilitation. Named for a Civil War amputee, the company has grown from an artificial-limb company into one that operates more than 200 centers in 30 states and the District of Columbia. Hanger still makes orthotics and prosthetics for sale nationwide, but its main business is now the consolidation of the O&P segment: The company has acquired more than 60 businesses since 1986. In addition, Hanger has formed OPNET, a referral network that allows about 280 managed care organizations to contract for O&P services with member practitioners.

Helix/Medlantic

9881 Broken Land Pkwy., Columbia, MD 21046

Telephone: 410-290-6800 **Fax:** 410-290-9958 **Metro area:** Baltimore, MD **Web site:** http://www.medlantic.mhg.edu **Human resources contact:** Linda Hitchcock **Sales:** $1.4 billion **Number of employees:** 21,000 **Number of employees for previous year:** 7,000 **Industry designation:** Hospitals **Company type:** Not-for-profit **Top competitors:** Daughters of Charity National Health System; The Johns Hopkins Health System Corporation; Bon Secours Health System, Inc.

When two not-for-profit health care providers doubled up in 1998, Helix/Medlantic was the result. Formed by the merger of Medlantic Healthcare Group and Helix Health, the company operates seven hospitals, five nursing homes, and other research, outpatient, and home care units in Baltimore and Washington, DC. Its hospitals include Church Hospital, Franklin Square Hospital Center, Good Samaritan Hospital, Harbor Hospital Center, National Rehabilitation Hospital, Union Memorial Hospital, and Washington Hospital Center. The new organization dominates the region. Almost 100,000 patients stay in Helix/Medlantic's hospitals each year, and it treats more than one million more on an outpatient basis.

Howard Hughes Medical Institute

4000 Jones Bridge Rd., Chevy Chase, MD 20815

Telephone: 301-215-8500 **Fax:** 301-215-8937 **Metro area:** Washington, DC **Web site:** http://www.hhmi.org **Human resources contact:** Reed Knight **Sales:** $399.5 million **Number of employees:** 3,000 **Number of employees for previous year:** 2,847 **Industry designation:** Medical services **Company type:** Foundation **Top competitors:** American Cancer Society, Inc.; The Johns Hopkins University; Louisiana State University System

The millions that once belonged to a man afraid of germs and disease are now helping find cures for them. The Howard Hughes Medical Institute (HHMI) is one of the largest private medical research sponsors in the world. Unlike most such organizations, HHMI directly employs the researchers it funds and provides needed equipment and facilities. The institute concentrates primarily on five biomedical areas: cell biology, genetics, immunology, neuroscience, and structural biology. The institute also supports science education through a grant program. Founded in 1953 by Howard Hughes, the institute was the major beneficiary of the sale of Hughes Aircraft to GM and has an endowment of more than $12 billion.

Human Genome Sciences, Inc.

9410 Key West Ave., Rockville, MD 20850

Telephone: 301-309-8504 **Fax:** 301-309-8512 **Metro area:** Washington, DC **Web site:** http://www.hgsi.com **Human resources contact:** Susan B. McKay **Sales:** $29.6 million **Number of employees:** 411 **Number of employees for previous year:** 353 **Industry designation:** Biomedical & genetic products **Company type:** Public **Top competitors:** Genzyme Corporation; Incyte Pharmaceuticals, Inc.; Scios Inc.

Human Genome Sciences (HGS) researches and develops drugs and diagnostic products based on the human gene. The company also researches nonhuman genes, including those of bacteria, fungi, and viruses, which it believes will be useful in creating vaccines and antibiotics. Although HGS has no marketable products, it has several in clinical testing. HGS has formed collaborations with SmithKline Beecham, Takeda Chemical Industries, Schering-Plough, Transgene, Synthelabo, Merck, and The Institute of Genomic Research. These firms pay HGS to develop products useful in treating cancer, heart disease, arthritis, and Lou Gehrig's disease. HGS has 1/3 of a joint venture developing gene therapy for vascular diseases.

The Hunter Group, Inc.

100 E. Pratt St., Ste. 1600, Baltimore, MD 21202

Telephone: 410-576-1515 **Fax:** 410-752-2879 **Metro area:** Baltimore, MD **Web site:** http://www.hunter-group.com **Sales:** $39.2 million **Number of employees:** 426 **Industry designation:** Computers—services **Company type:** Subsidiary **Top competitors:** CACI International Inc; Technology Solutions Company; BrightStar Information Technology Group, Inc.

Data lost in an overwhelming corporate quagmire? Hunt no further. Founded in 1981, The Hunter Group, a subsidiary of information technology consultant Renaissance Worldwide, offers information management consulting services. The company, which provides software training and implementation, has partnerships with enterprise resource planning software vendors such as Lawson Software and PeopleSoft to implement client/server software applications including human resources, finance, and distribution. Consulting services include strategic planning, business process reengineering, and evaluating and selecting vendor products.

ICARUS International, Inc.

1 Central Plaza, 11300 Rockville Pike, Rockville, MD 20852

Telephone: 301-424-4646 **Fax:** 301-424-4647 **Metro area:** Washington, DC **Web site:** http://www.icarus-us.com **Human resources contact:** Lucy Brown **Sales:** $9.1 million (Est.) **Number of employees:** 65 **Number of employees for previous year:** 62 **Industry designation:** Computers—engineering, scientific & CAD-CAM software **Company type:** Private **Top competitors:** Timberline Software Corporation; Aspen Technology, Inc.; Simulation Sciences Inc.

ICARUS International helps engineering become top-flight. Founded in 1969, the company makes automated desktop software (three-fourths of sales) that lets engineers at bulk manufacturing plants in the chemical, food, petroleum refining, and pulp and paper industries simulate, model, and analyze the design, cost, and time requirements of proposed projects. ICARUS, an acronym for Industrial Computer Application Retrieval and Utility Systems, gets most of its revenues from single- and multiyear term license fees. It primarily targets large multinational companies such as Campbell Soup, Mitsubishi Chemical, and Shell Oil. President and CEO Herbert Blecker and his wife, Eunice, own the company.

IGEN International, Inc.

16020 Industrial Dr., Gaithersburg, MD 20877

Telephone: 301-984-8000 **Fax:** 301-947-6998 **Metro area:** Washington, DC **Web site:** http://www.igen.com **Human resources contact:** Cindy Whitman **Sales:** $13.4 million **Number of employees:** 133 **Number of employees for previous year:** 119 **Industry designation:** Medical instruments **Company type:** Public **Top competitors:** Biopool International, Inc.; Diagnostic Products Corporation; Beckman Coulter, Inc.

Electrochemiluminescence, although difficult to spell, is the proprietary technology on which IGEN International bases its medical diagnostic systems. IGEN's systems are used for screening a range of diseases and discovering new drugs. Its patented ORIGEN nucleic acid probe system is used by hospitals, universities, and clinical and life science laboratories for conducting in vitro genetic testing. Companies that pay IGEN licensing and royalty fees for using ORIGEN include Boehringer Mannheim, Organon Teknika, Pfizer, and Eisai. IGEN also collaborates with its customers in research and product development. IGEN is 25%-owned by founder and CEO, Samuel Wohlstadter, who also founded Amgen (blood cell therapy).

Information Systems & Services Inc.

8405 Colesville Rd., Ste. 600, Silver Spring, MD 20910

Telephone: 301-588-3800 **Fax:** 301-588-3986 **Metro area:** Washington, DC **Web site:** http://www.issinet.com **Human resources contact:** Susan Tatterson **Sales:** $6.8 million (Est.) **Number of employees:** 90 **Number of employees for previous year:** 85 **Industry designation:** Computers—services **Company type:** Private

Information Systems & Services Inc. (ISSI) helps government agencies and commercial clients design, install, and manage information systems. The company offers assistance in using the Internet (Web site design, Internet commerce services) and provides training and technical support (including technical writing for training and operation of the system, and graphics production). ISSI also provides Lotus Notes services, helps develop and manage information storage, and assists with system security measures. ISSI's Visual HOMES and World Trade Systems software provide applications specifically designed to work with HUD and the Commerce, Treasury, and State Department regulations, respectively.

Integrated Health Services, Inc.

10065 Red Run Blvd., Owings Mills, MD 21117

Telephone: 410-998-8400 **Fax:** 410-902-2111 **Metro area:** Baltimore, MD **Web site:** http://www.ihs-inc.com **Human resources contact:** Sharon Smith **Sales:** $3 billion **Number of employees:** 86,000 **Number of employees for previous year:** 55,000 **Industry designation:** Medical services **Company type:** Public

Integrated Health Services is one the US's largest post-acute health care companies with more than 2,000 locations in 47 states. It offers rehabilitation, hospice, and diagnostic services. The company operates more than 300 nursing homes. Special services include wound management, cardiac care, and treatment of Alzheimer's. The company also operates institutional pharmacies and a contract therapy business. Integrated Health Services is selling some of its properties, which it will lease back. It is also divesting some underperforming or noncore operations, including its institutional pharmacies.

IT Partners, Inc.

9881 Broken Land Pkwy., Ste. 102, Columbia, MD 21046

Telephone: 410-309-9800 **Fax:** 410-309-9801 **Metro area:** Baltimore, MD **Sales:** $23.8 million (Est.) **Number of employees:** 735 **Industry designation:** Computers—services **Company type:** Private **Top competitors:** Technology Solutions Company; Renaissance Worldwide, Inc.; Perot Systems Corporation

IT Partners wants to win a supporting role in your company's technology picture. Through its wholly owned partner companies, the firm provides information technology (IT) services primarily to midsized corporations with revenues between $25 million and $500 million. Services include consulting, network integration, software and Web site development, and telephony and electronics integration. The company also bundles hardware, software, and services in packages. IT Partners continues to grow by purchasing well-managed local systems integrators, regional business application providers, and national specialty IT services firms.

The Johns Hopkins Health System Corporation

600 N. Wolfe St., Baltimore, MD 21287

Telephone: 410-955-5000 **Fax:** 410-955-6575 **Metro area:** Baltimore, MD **Web site:** http://www.jhu.edu/www/medicine/ **Human resources contact:** Joan Williams **Sales:** $1.8 billion **Number of employees:** 14,000 **Number of employees for previous year:** 13,000 **Industry designation:** Hospitals **Company type:** Not-for-profit **Top competitors:** Mayo Foundation; Columbia/HCA Healthcare Corporation; Bon Secours Health System, Inc.

If you don't eat your apple a day, you may end up in The Johns Hopkins Health System, which operates hospitals and other facilities affiliated with the medical schools of Johns Hopkins University. These include Johns Hopkins Hospital (annually deemed one of the US's best) and Johns Hopkins Bayview Medical Center, both of which are acute-care hospitals. The hospitals, owned by Johns Hopkins Medicine, are staffed by faculty members from the medical school and are the training ground for the medical school. Other divisions include Johns Hopkins Medical Services and Johns Hopkins Employer Health Plans. Johns Hopkins Medicine has contracted with Singapore to build and operate medical and research facilities.

Life Technologies, Inc.

9800 Medical Center Dr., Rockville, MD 20850

Telephone: 301-610-8000 **Fax:** 301-329-8635 **Metro area:** Washington, DC **Web site:** http://www.lifetech.com **Human resources contact:** Janey Flickenger **Sales:** $364.2 million **Number of employees:** 1,759 **Number of employees for previous year:** 1,640 **Industry designation:** Biomedical & genetic products **Company type:** Public

Life Technologies, Inc. (LTI), makes more than 3,000 products used to research life sciences and to make genetically engineered pharmaceuticals and other materials. The company's products include cultures to grow cells in the laboratory and enzymes and biochemicals to identify and manipulate genetic material. It also makes cell culture material and reagents for the production of such genetically engineered pharmaceuticals as interferon and interleuken. LTI sells to more than 20,000 customers, including research labs and pharmaceutical and biotechnology companies. It has operations in Europe, North America, and Asia. Specialty materials maker Dexter Corporation owns more than 70% of the firm.

MedImmune, Inc.

35 W. Watkins Mill Rd., Gaithersburg, MD 20878

Telephone: 301-417-0770 **Fax:** 301-527-4200 **Metro area:** Washington, DC **Web site:** http://www.medimmune.com **Human resources contact:** Robert Obst **Sales:** $200.7 million **Number of employees:** 438 **Number of employees for previous year:** 344 **Industry designation:** Biomedical & genetic products **Company type:** Public **Top competitors:** Merck & Co., Inc.; SmithKline Beecham plc; Glaxo Wellcome plc

MedImmune develops drugs for transplants and infectious diseases. Its product-development strategy emphasizes prevention over treatment. Products include CytoGam, which prevents and treats cytomegalovirus disease in organ transplant patients, and RespiGam (an intravenous treatment), which prevents respiratory syncytial virus (RSV), a leading cause of pneumonia and bronchiolitis in infants. MedImmune has received FDA approval to market Synagis (an injectable treatment for RSV). Products in development include vaccines to prevent genital warts, cervical cancer, Lyme disease, urinary tract infections, and organ transplant rejection.

Meridian Medical Technologies, Inc.

10240 Old Columbia Rd., Columbia, MD 21046

Telephone: 410-309-6830 **Fax:** 410-309-1475 **Metro area:** Baltimore, MD **Web site:** http://www.meridianmeds.com/Home.htm **Human resources contact:** Peter Garbis **Sales:** $44.7 million **Number of employees:** 312 **Number of employees for previous year:** 275 **Industry designation:** Medical products **Company type:** Public **Top competitors:** Glaxo Wellcome plc; Senetek PLC; Medi-Ject Corporation

Severe allergic reactions leave no room for error, so Meridian Medical Technologies makes EpiPen autojectors—spring-loaded, prefilled, pen-like syringes that automatically self-inject precise doses of epinephrine to cut off allergy attacks. The firm had a setback when it had to recall its EpiPen (now reintroduced) and its EpiEZPen (undergoing redesign). It also makes LidoPen for heart attack victims; prefilled syringes for soldiers who need chemical-warfare antidotes; cardiac-analysis systems for heart-attack detection; and devices that measure and transmit a homebound patient's medical condition by telephone. Injectable drug-delivery systems account for 50% of sales; subsidiary STI Military Systems, 47%.

North American Vaccine, Inc.

10150 Old Columbia Rd., Columbia, MD 21046

Telephone: 410-309-7100 **Metro area:** Baltimore, MD **Web site:** http://www.nava.com **Human resources contact:** Arthur Y. Elliot **Sales:** $8.4 million **Number of employees:** 308 **Number of employees for previous year:** 260 **Industry designation:** Drugs **Company type:** Public **Top competitors:** SmithKline Beecham plc; American Home Products Corporation; Merck & Co., Inc.

North American Vaccine (NAV) produces that childhood rite of passage: the shot. NAV's flagship product is Certiva, an acellular whooping cough vaccine that has been combined with diphtheria and tetanus toxoids to form a single vaccine. The company says Certiva causes fewer side effects than current "whole cell" vaccines. It has been approved in Germany, Sweden, Denmark (where an anti-polio component has been added), and the US. NAV is also developing several combination vaccines using Certiva as an anchor component, as well as a new group of conjugate vaccines for a variety of bacterial infections. Abbott Laboratories markets Certiva in the US. BioChem Pharma owns about 40% of NAV.

OAO Technology Solutions, Inc.

7500 Greenway Center Dr., Greenbelt, MD 20770

Telephone: 301-486-0400 **Fax:** 301-486-0415 **Metro area:** Washington, DC **Web site:** http://www.oaot.com **Human resources contact:** Christine M Hazell **Sales:** $113.3 million **Number of employees:** 2,000 **Number of employees for previous year:** 1,600 **Industry designation:** Computers—services **Company type:** Public **Top competitors:** Analysts International Corporation; Computer Task Group, Incorporated; Technisource, Inc.

OAO Technology Solutions is the outsourcer's source. The information technology company provides computer operators, programmers, and system maintenance workers to large outsourcers who contract out portions of their own outsourcing jobs. OAO's megacenter operations management unit brings in about half of the company's sales overseeing the daily operations of large, mostly mainframe computer centers under multi-year contracts. The largest customer in this area is IBM (65% of sales). Its distributed systems management sector administers midsized client/server networks. Digital Equipment, another key client, accounts for about one-fourth of sales. Technology investment firm Safeguard Scientific owns 29% of OAO.

ONCOR, Inc.

209 Perry Pkwy., Gaithersburg, MD 20877

Telephone: 301-963-3500 **Fax:** 301-926-6129 **Metro area:** Washington, DC **Web site:** http://www.oncor.com **Human resources contact:** Stacey Bolton **Sales:** $13.4 million **Number of employees:** 199 **Number of employees for previous year:** 179 **Industry designation:** Biomedical & genetic products **Company type:** Public

Troubled ONCOR has had to surrender its chief technology asset—a test for the recurrence of breast cancer—to satisfy its debts. The test, which the creditor resold to Ventana Medical Systems, had received FDA approval. It allowed doctors to identify patients with a high risk for recurrence and to pinpoint the most effective treatment. ONCOR had also received approval for a leukemia test and has been developing genetic test systems for other cancers, including those of the cervix, prostate, and endometrium. The company continues to try to sell other assets.

Osiris Therapeutics, Inc.

2001 Aliceanna St., Baltimore, MD 21231

Telephone: 410-522-5005 **Fax:** 410-522-6999 **Metro area:** Baltimore, MD **Web site:** http://www.biospace.com/b2/company_profile.cfm?CompanyID=1468 **Human resources contact:** Linda Kosmicki **Sales:** $7.5 million (Est.) **Number of employees:** 105 **Number of employees for previous year:** 70 **Industry designation:** Biomedical & genetic products **Company type:** Private **Top competitors:** American Home Products Corporation; Connetics Corp.; Geron Corporation

Osiris Therapeutics brings connective tissue back to life. The development-stage biomedical company hopes its proprietary technology can be used to regenerate bone marrow, muscle, bone, cartilage, tendons, and other connective tissue by using specialized stem cells taken from the patients themselves. One of Osiris Therapeutics' research projects is focused on regenerating chemotherapy-damaged bone marrow. The firm collaborates with a variety of partners, including the University of Genoa, Italy; the University of Cincinnati (tendon regeneration); Collagenesis (soft-tissue regeneration); and Novartis (treatments for arthritis and osteoporosis).

Peak Technologies Group, Inc.

9200 Berger Rd., Columbia, MD 21046

Telephone: 410-312-6000 **Fax:** 410-312-7381 **Metro area:** Baltimore, MD **Web site:** http://www.peaktech.com **Human resources contact:** Sherry Reed **Sales:** $215.7 million **Number of employees:** 934 **Number of employees for previous year:** 813 **Industry designation:** Optical character recognition **Company type:** Subsidiary **Parent company:** Moore Corporation

Take a peek at Peak Technologies. This distributor of bar-code-based data collection and wireless data transmission systems integrates hardware from a variety of different manufacturers with its own software systems. Peak offers customers complete information-gathering systems for warehousing, inventory management, manufacturing, and distribution. The company also provides technical support and maintenance services for its data capture and printing hardware and software, as well as related supplies and consumables such as bar-code labels, printer ribbons, laser-printer toner cartridges, and spare parts. The company is a subsidiary of Toronto-based business-forms maker Moore Corporation.

Ritz Camera Centers

6711 Ritz Way, Beltsville, MD 20705

Telephone: 301-419-0000 **Fax:** 301-419-2995 **Metro area:** Washington, DC **Web site:** http://www.ritzcamera.com **Human resources contact:** Alan MacDonald **Sales:** $625 million (Est.) **Number of employees:** 7,000 **Industry designation:** Photographic equipment & supplies **Company type:** Private **Top competitors:** Walgreen Co.; Wolf Camera, Inc.; West Marine, Inc.

Picture this: the US's largest photo-specialty chain with more than 800 stores in 47 states and the District of Columbia that provide one-hour photofinishing, digital imaging, and other services. Consider that it sells cameras and accessories, binoculars, wireless phones, video cameras, and more (under such brands as Canon, Epson, Fuji, Minolta, and Nikon), and you can see how Ritz Camera Centers has captured priceless moments since its 1918 inception. Subsidiary Boater's World Marine Centers has about 85 stores nationwide that feature motors, rigging gear, patching fiberglass, lures, rods, reels, and other supplies under such brands as Penn, Shimano, and Shakespeare. President David Ritz owns the firm.

Sherwood Brands, Inc.

6110 Executive Blvd., Ste. 1080, Rockville, MD 20852

Telephone: 301-881-9340 **Fax:** 301-881-0826 **Metro area:** Washington, DC **Human resources contact:** Elana Frydman **Sales:** $18.1 million **Number of employees:** 271 **Number of employees for previous year:** 54 **Industry designation:** Food—confectionery **Company type:** Public **Top competitors:** Mars, Inc.; Keebler Foods Company; Nabisco Holdings Corp.

Sherwood Brands tempts America's sweet tooth with cookies, candies, and chocolates, including Ruger Wafers, demitasse biscuits, COWS butter toffees, Elana Belgian chocolates, School House Candy, and Sour Fruit Burst candies. It also sells Soup du Jour instant soups. A majority of the company's sales come from cookies. Most of Sherwood Brands' products are made according to its recipes and designs by manufacturers in Argentina, Austria, and Belgium. The company sells its sweets to mass merchandisers (including Kmart and several dollar-store chains), vending companies, gourmet distributors, and grocery and drugstore chains, mainly in the US. Founder Uziel Frydman controls 82% of the company's voting power.

Socrates Technologies Corporation

9301 Peppercorn Place, Largo, MD 20774

Telephone: 301-925-2200 **Fax:** 301-925-4150 **Metro area:** Washington, DC **Web site:** http://www.socratespc.com **Human resources contact:** Jean Brown **Sales:** $62 million **Number of employees:** 130 **Number of employees for previous year:** 120 **Industry designation:** Computers—services **Company type:** Public **Top competitors:** Ingram Micro Inc.; Amdahl Corporation; Wang Laboratories, Inc.

Socrates Technologies keeps you from wanting to drink hemlock when you're having computer problems. The company, formerly MVSI, provides information technology services including computer and telecommunications systems integration, Internet connectivity, networking, and training. Subsidiary Technet Computer Services develops custom software for applications such as imaging and multimedia, networking, and year 2000 compliance. Socrates also resells computer products from such industry leaders as 3Com, Oracle, and Texas Instruments. Customers include Unisys and the NBA's Washington Wizards. The company has discontinued its machine vision welding and scanner business.

United Payors & United Providers, Inc.

2275 Research Blvd., 6th Fl., Rockville, MD 20850

Telephone: 301-548-1000 **Fax:** 301-548-8828 **Metro area:** Washington, DC **Web site:** http://www.upup.com **Human resources contact:** Tammy Berman **Sales:** $78.4 million **Number of employees:** 367 **Number of employees for previous year:** 291 **Industry designation:** Medical services **Company type:** Public

United Payors & United Providers (UP&UP) acts as an intermediary between insurance companies and health care providers, enabling claims to be processed more efficiently. For a percentage of health care providers' price concessions, UP&UP saves health insurance companies money and serves a network of about 150,000 physicians and 12,000 hospitals across the US. Subsidiaries include 90%-owned America's Health Card Services, which markets an insurance/credit card, and IM&I-NEWCO, which administers health care benefits for the US Department of Defense. Principal Mutual Life Insurance owns almost 40% of UP&UP.

Usinternetworking, Inc.

One USI Plaza, Annapolis, MD 21401

Telephone: 410-897-4400 **Fax:** 410-573-1906 **Metro area:** Baltimore, MD **Web site:** http://www.usinternetworking.com **Human resources contact:** Brenda Woodsmall **Sales:** $4.1 million (Est.) **Number of employees:** 348 **Industry designation:** Computers—corporate, professional & financial software **Company type:** Private **Top competitors:** PSINet Inc.; DIGEX, Inc.; UUNET WorldCom

A slogan for USinternetworking, Inc. (USI) could be, "Why own when you can rent?" USI's customers sign multiyear contracts for Internet-based access to software from such companies as BroadVision (e-commerce), PeopleSoft (human resources), and Siebel Systems (customer service and sales force automation). The company provides implementation and support services, which helps customers save on both software and support costs. USI also offers hosting services for companies that want to run their own applications over secure Internet-based networks. Customers include Lattice Semiconductor, Lockheed Martin, and NIKE. Investment firm Grotech Capital owns 25% of USI. U S WEST also has a minority stake in the company.

Washington Capitals

One Harry S. Truman Dr., Hyattsville, MD 20785

Telephone: 202-628-3200 **Fax:** 301-386-7012 **Metro area:** Washington, DC **Web site:** http://www.washingtoncaps.com **Human resources contact:** Rosie Beauclair **Sales:** $74.2 million (Est.) **Number of employees:** 100 **Industry designation:** Leisure & recreational services **Company type:** Private **Top competitors:** Carolina Hurricanes Hockey Club; Tampa Bay Lightning; Florida Panthers Holdings, Inc.

Most arenas are built for teams. The Washington Capitals, however, were created to justify a new arena. In 1972 owner Abe Pollin needed a better facility in which to showcase his NBA team, the Baltimore Bullets (now the Washington Wizards). Two tenants in the same stadium would generate more of the support needed to build it. When he heard that the NHL was expanding, Pollin submitted his proposal to own a team. Thus the Washington Capitals were born and began to play in the then-new Capital Centre (now US Airways Arena). After years of struggling, the Capitals finally reached the Stanley Cup Finals in 1998, but were swept out by the Detroit Red Wings. The team now plays in the new MCI Center.

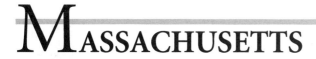

MASSACHUSETTS

ABIOMED, Inc.

33 Cherry Hill Dr., Danvers, MA 01923

Telephone: 978-777-5410 **Fax:** 978-777-8411 **Metro area:** Boston, MA **Web site:** http://www.abiomed.com **Sales:** $22.4 million **Number of employees:** 173 **Number of employees for previous year:** 138 **Industry designation:** Medical instruments **Company type:** Public **Top competitors:** Medtronic, Inc.; St. Jude Medical, Inc.; Baxter International Inc.

ABIOMED develops cardiac-assist technology and dental products. The company makes the BVS-5000 bi-ventricular support system, the first FDA-approved temporary external heart. ABIOMED is developing other cardiac-assist products, including a battery-powered, implantable heart replacement device, the Heart Booster (an implantable device which assists a patient's failing heart), and specialized heart pumps. The company discontinued a dental products subsidiary, which made a periodontal screening system and distributed the Halimeter, used to detect periodontal disease and other sources for halitosis. Research and development contracts make up nearly a quarter of company revenues.

Advanced Magnetics, Inc.

61 Mooney St., Cambridge, MA 02138

Telephone: 617-497-2070 **Fax:** 617-547-2445 **Metro area:** Boston, MA **Web site:** http://www.advancedmagnetics.com **Sales:** $3 million **Number of employees:** 62 **Number of employees for previous year:** 59 **Industry designation:** Medical products **Company type:** Public **Top competitors:** E-Z-EM, Inc.; Schering AG; Nycomed Amersham plc

One thing is clear: Advanced Magnetics makes diagnostic contrast agents. These agents provide clearer images during magnetic resonance imaging (MRI) tests used to detect tumors and other abnormalities. The development-stage company has two products on the market: Feridex I.V. (for the diagnosis of liver lesions) and GastroMARK (used for bowel and abdominal imaging). The company is developing contrast agents for liver and lymph disease detection called Combidex, currently in Phase III trials. In addition to contrast agents, the company makes a line of veterinary blood chemistry tests through its Kalisto Biologicals subsidiary.

Agri-Mark, Inc.

100 Milk St., Methuen, MA 01844

Telephone: 978-689-4442 **Fax:** 978-685-8716 **Other address:** PO Box 5800, Lawrence, MA 01842 **Metro area:** Boston, MA **Web site:** http://www.agrimark.net **Human resources contact:** Robert Porter **Sales:** $575 million **Number of employees:** 500 **Industry designation:** Agricultural operations **Company type:** Cooperative **Top competitors:** Foremost Farms USA; Land O'Lakes, Inc.; Dairy Farmers of America

Milk drinkers who make a habit of Cabot ought to know Agri-Mark, the northeastern dairy cooperative that makes Cabot-brand milk, butter, and cheddar cheese. Formed in 1980, Agri-Mark has about 1,600 members who operate farms throughout New England and New York, producing 2.7 billion pounds of milk a year. It merged with Cabot Creamery in 1992 and now sells Cabot-brand products throughout New England, New York, and the mid-Atlantic states, in parts of Florida and California, and in the UK. Agri-Mark also sells milk to more than 75 fluid bottlers and manufacturers in the eastern US. It owns three processing plants, two in Vermont and one in Massachusetts, which also make cottage cheese, yogurt, and sour cream.

Alkermes, Inc.

64 Sidney St., Cambridge, MA 02139

Telephone: 617-494-0171 **Fax:** 617-494-9263 **Metro area:** Boston, MA **Web site:** http://www.alkermes.com **Human resources contact:** Peter Maguire **Sales:** $25.5 million **Number of employees:** 202 **Number of employees for previous year:** 177 **Industry designation:** Drugs **Company type:** Public **Top competitors:** NPS Pharmaceuticals, Inc.; Vaxcel, Inc.; ALZA Corporation

Alkermes develops drug delivery systems that allow pharmaceuticals to be administered more efficiently. The company's RMP-7 technology, currently in clinical trials, relaxes boundaries between cells and lets drugs in the bloodstream diffuse into the brain, making it potentially helpful in treating brain cancer. Alkermes' proprietary ProLease and Medisorb technologies enable more controlled release of drugs and allow more time between injections. ProLease is being used in the effort to facilitate delivery of human growth hormones. Alkermes has collaborative research agreements with Alza, Genentech, and Johnson & Johnson.

American Biltrite Inc.

57 River St., Wellesley Hills, MA 02181

Telephone: 781-237-6655 **Fax:** 781-237-6880 **Metro area:** Boston, MA **Web site:** http://www.abitape.com **Human resources contact:** Bonnie Posnak **Sales:** $423.9 million **Number of employees:** 3,030 **Number of employees for previous year:** 2,770 **Industry designation:** Chemicals—plastics **Company type:** Public **Top competitors:** Minnesota Mining and Manufacturing Company; O'Sullivan Corporation; Armstrong World Industries, Inc.

American Biltrite Inc. (ABI) sells products that can brighten your neck, your wrists—or your kitchen floor. ABI makes industrial and flooring products and fashion jewelry. Its industrial products include adhesive-coated, pressure-sensitive papers used to protect materials during handling and pressure-sensitive tapes and adhesives used in the footwear, air-conditioning, automotive, and electrical industries. Subsidiary ABI-Canada makes Uni-Turf, a vinyl-based floor covering for indoor sports facilities. ABI has a 49% stake in Congoleum, a producer of floor tile and sheet vinyl flooring. It owns 82% of K&M Associates, which makes and distributes jewelry. The founding Marcus family owns about 55% of ABI.

American Dental Partners, Inc.

301 Edgewater Place, Ste. 320, Wakefield, MA 01880

Telephone: 781-224-0880 **Fax:** 781-224-4216 **Metro area:** Boston, MA **Web site:** http://www.amdpi.com **Sales:** $84.1 million **Number of employees:** 1,155 **Number of employees for previous year:** 910 **Industry designation:** Medical practice management **Company type:** Public

Helping dentists focus on drilling, not billing, American Dental Partners provides management services for dental group practices. The company operates 100 dental facilities in eight states through long-term agreements for its local services, including budgeting, financial reporting, equipment procurement, billing, and hiring support staff. On a national level, the company helps its affiliates with third-party negotiations, new facility leasing, and accounting system implementation. Summit Ventures (of which director Martin Mannion is general partner) owns 35% of the company.

Analogic Corporation

8 Centennial Dr., Peabody, MA 01960

Telephone: 978-977-3000 **Fax:** 978-977-6811 **Metro area:** Boston, MA **Web site:** http://www.analogic.com **Human resources contact:** John W. Kirby **Sales:** $294.5 million **Number of employees:** 1,650 **Number of employees for previous year:** 1,500 **Industry designation:** Instruments—scientific **Company type:** Public **Top competitors:** Analog Devices, Inc.; Semtech Corporation; Mercury Computer Systems, Inc.

Analogic wants to convert you. The company's customizable data acquisition, conversion, and signal processing equipment converts analog signals, such as pressure, temperature, and X-ray intensity, into digital computer language. Its products, including medical image processing equipment (74% of sales), digital signal processors, and industrial test and measurement systems, are used for geophysical exploration, CAT scanners, and automotive test equipment. Analogic, which also owns a hotel adjacent to its headquarters, sells products worldwide through distributors and an independent sales force. Royal Philips Electronics, GE, and Imation account for a third of sales. CEO Bernard Gordon owns 37% of the company.

Anika Therapeutics, Inc.

236 W. Cummings Park, Woburn, MA 01801

Telephone: 781-932-6616 **Fax:** 781-935-4120 **Metro area:** Boston, MA **Web site:** http://www.anikatherapeutics.com **Sales:** $13.9 million **Number of employees:** 61 **Number of employees for previous year:** 48 **Industry designation:** Biomedical & genetic products **Company type:** Public **Top competitors:** Biomatrix, Inc.; Connetics Corp.; OrthoLogic Corp.

Anika Therapeutics is roosterrific. The firm uses hyaluronic acid—a naturally occurring polymer extracted from rooster combs and other sources—to make products which treat and heal bone, cartilage, and soft tissue. An osteoarthritis treatment for racehorses is marketed in the US by Boehringer Ingelheim Vetmedica; a similar product for humans is awaiting FDA approval and will be sold here and in several other countries by a Bristol-Myers Squibb subsidiary. Bausch & Lomb Surgical uses two Anika Therapeutics products to maintain eye shape and protect tissue during eye surgery. Anika Therapeutics is working on a device to prevent post-surgery tissue adhesion, and on a product to speed bone-fracture healing.

ARIAD Pharmaceuticals, Inc.

26 Landsdowne St., Cambridge, MA 02139

Telephone: 617-494-0400 **Fax:** 617-494-8144 **Metro area:** Boston, MA **Web site:** http://www.ariad.com **Human resources contact:** Kathy Lawton **Sales:** $13.1 million **Number of employees:** 120 **Number of employees for previous year:** 89 **Industry designation:** Biomedical & genetic products **Company type:** Public

ARIAD Pharmaceuticals develops proprietary, small-molecule drugs to treat allergies, asthma, immune-related disorders, and osteoporosis by blocking or controlling interactions essential to the disease process. The company is also developing small-molecule drugs for gene and cell therapy. ARIAD Pharmaceuticals has licensing agreements with Harvard University, Massachusetts Institute of Technology, Mount Sinai Hospital, Stanford University, and Yale University, among others; it is also involved in joint ventures with Hoechst Marion Roussel (genomics relating to osteoporosis) and Genovo (gene therapy). All of Ariad's products are in the research or preclinical development stage.

ArQule, Inc.

200 Boston Ave., Medford, MA 02155

Telephone: 781-395-4100 **Fax:** 781-395-1225 **Metro area:** Boston, MA **Web site:** http://www.arqule.com **Human resources contact:** Tony Messina **Sales:** $22.2 million **Number of employees:** 190 **Number of employees for previous year:** 159 **Industry designation:** Drugs **Company type:** Public

ArQule is a development-stage biotechnology company whose Targeted Discovery proprietary technology aids pharmaceutical and agrochemical companies in identifying and quickly developing lead compounds used to create drugs, pesticides, and other products. Through joint discovery programs, ArQule provides partners with Mapping Array compound sets (biological target screening) and Directed Array compound sets (analogs of synthesized lead compounds). The company's partners, including Genzyme, Sepracor, and Cubist Pharmaceuticals, are targeting cancer, HIV, and infectious diseases. ArQule also has collaborative agreements with Abbott Laboratories, Monsanto, and Amersham Pharmacia Biotech.

ASA International Ltd.

10 Speen St., Framingham, MA 01701

Telephone: 508-626-2727 **Fax:** 508-626-0645 **Metro area:** Boston, MA **Web site:** http://www.asaint.com **Human resources contact:** Mary Ann Bishop **Sales:** $35.5 million **Number of employees:** 213 **Number of employees for previous year:** 152 **Industry designation:** Computers—corporate, professional & financial software **Company type:** Public **Top competitors:** Kronos Incorporated; Omega Research, Inc.; ARIS Corporation

ASA International helps businesses operate more efficiently. Its four business software lines include SmartTIME and SmartRULES, which keep track of when employees punch the clock and then process payroll information; Tire Systems, which collects and tracks sales, inventory, work order, and accounting data for tire dealers, retreaders, and wholesalers; Legal Systems, which manages law firms' financial information; and Mozart "commercialware," which handles order management and fulfillment for catalog, direct marketing, and electronic commerce businesses. ASA International's products are sold through a direct sales force. Its customers include more than 900 businesses in Australia, Europe, and the Americas.

Ascent Pediatrics, Inc.

187 Ballardvale St., Ste. B125, Wilmington, MA 01887

Telephone: 978-658-2500 **Fax:** 978-658-3939 **Metro area:** Boston, MA **Web site:** http://www.ascentpediatrics.com **Human resources contact:** Diane Worrick **Sales:** $4.5 million **Number of employees:** 83 **Number of employees for previous year:** 24 **Industry designation:** Drugs **Company type:** Public **Top competitors:** American Home Products Corporation; Johnson & Johnson; Abbott Laboratories

Ascent Pediatrics makes the medicine go down—or up—in the most delightful way. The company develops formulations of already-approved prescription drugs for children that reduce side effects and dosing frequency and are easier to administer. Products include Feverall suppositories (pain and fever); Primsol Trimethoprim solution antibiotic for ear infections that eliminates a compound that can cause allergic reactions; and Pediamist, an over-the-counter nasal saline spray with a metering device. Ascent Pediatrics is also working on treatments for asthma, dermatitis, and cold symptoms. The firm uses proprietary taste-masking technology to make the drugs more palatable for children.

Aspect Medical Systems, Inc.

2 Vision Dr., Natick, MA 01760

Telephone: 508-653-0603 **Fax:** 508-653-6788 **Metro area:** Boston, MA **Web site:** http://www.aspectms.com **Human resources contact:** Margie Ahearn **Sales:** $3.1 million (Est.) **Number of employees:** 77 **Industry designation:** Medical instruments **Company type:** Private

Aspect Medical Systems makes anesthesia-monitoring systems that aid in assessing levels of consciousness during surgery. The company's products are based on its proprietary Bispectral Index (BIS) technology, which directly measures the effects of anesthetics; the systems are designed to help prevent surgical awareness, a phenomenon in which patients become conscious during surgery, even though they appear anesthetized and are unable to communicate. Some victims report post-traumatic stress disorder following the experience. Aspect Medical Systems markets its products in the US through direct sales, and has a distribution agreement with Nihon Kohden to distribute its BIS monitors in Japan.

Aspen Technology, Inc.

10 Canal Park, Cambridge, MA 02141

Telephone: 617-949-1000 **Fax:** 617-949-1030 **Metro area:** Boston, MA **Web site:** http://www.aspentec.com **Human resources contact:** Ernie Valentine **Sales:** $252.6 million **Number of employees:** 1,518 **Number of employees for previous year:** 1,239 **Industry designation:** Computers—engineering, scientific & CAD-CAM software **Company type:** Public **Top competitors:** BTR Siebe plc; MDL Information Systems, Inc.; Honeywell Inc.

Aspen Technology builds computer systems that assist process manufacturers in designing and automating their plants' operations. Companies such as Chevron, Dow Chemical, Procter & Gamble, and Weyerhaeuser use Aspen Technology's software to find more efficient methods of production and management. The company, which has facilities in more than 20 countries, has continued to extend its reach and product line through acquisitions of smaller firms with complementary simulation and modeling technologies. More than 50% of Aspen Technology's sales come from the US.

AutoImmune Inc.

128 Spring St., Lexington, MA 02173

Telephone: 781-860-0710 **Fax:** 781-860-0705 **Metro area:** Boston, MA **Web site:** http://www.autoimmuneinc.com **Human resources contact:** Claudia McNair **Sales:** $100,000 **Number of employees:** 23 **Number of employees for previous year:** 20 **Industry designation:** Drugs **Company type:** Public **Top competitors:** Alteon Inc.; EntreMed, Inc.; Boston Life Sciences, Inc.

Biopharmaceutical company AutoImmune develops orally administered drugs for the treatment of immune system and inflammatory diseases. Colloral, AutoImmune's most advanced product, has been developed to treat rheumatoid arthritis. Other drugs in various stages of development target such disorders as transplant rejection, diabetes, uveitis (an inflammatory eye disease), and multiple sclerosis. The company has agreements with institutions such as Brigham and Women's Hospital, the National Eye Institute, and Eli Lilly to perform research, conduct drug trials, and license technologies in exchange for research funding and potential royalties.

AVANT Immunotherapeutics, Inc.

119 Fourth Ave., Needham, MA 02194

Telephone: 781-433-0771 **Fax:** 781-433-0262 **Metro area:** Boston, MA **Web site:** http://www.tcell.com **Human resources contact:** Paula Freeman **Sales:** $2.2 million **Number of employees:** 53 **Number of employees for previous year:** 36 **Industry designation:** Biomedical & genetic products **Company type:** Public

AVANT Immunotherapeutics, formerly T Cell Sciences, develops treatments for cardiovascular, pulmonary, and autoimmune disorders caused by misregulation of the body's natural defense systems. It also makes vaccine delivery technology. Its leading therapeutic compound, TP10—developed to reduce injury and improve lung function after lung transplant surgery and to inhibit adult respiratory distress syndrome—is undergoing clinical trials. The company is also developing T-cell activation regulators to prevent organ transplant rejection. Also under development is a cholesterol-lowering vaccine against atherosclerosis. The company was formed from the merger of T Cell Sciences and Virus Research Institute in 1998.

Avitar, Inc.

65 Dan Rd., Canton, MA 02021

Telephone: 781-821-2440 **Fax:** 781-821-4458 **Metro area:** Boston, MA **Web site:** http://www.avitarinc.com **Human resources contact:** Roberta Guzman **Sales:** $2.2 million **Number of employees:** 39 **Number of employees for previous year:** 37 **Industry designation:** Medical & dental supplies **Company type:** Public **Top competitors:** Johnson & Johnson; Bristol-Myers Squibb Company; Minnesota Mining and Manufacturing Company

Avitar is avidly advancing medical foam technology. Through its Avitar Technologies subsidiary, the company makes disposable polyurethane foam products for medical, dental, and diagnostic purposes. Avitar's wound dressings (Hydrasorb and Joyce) and custom foam products (including molded dental applicators and disposable ear cushions for hearing devices) account for more than 90% of its sales. The company also makes saliva-sampling devices and drug-abuse test kits, and distributes another manufacturer's urine-based drug abuse and pregnancy test kits. Avitar sells its products through medical and dental distributors who market them around the world.

Aztec Technology Partners, Inc.

50 Braintree Hill Office Park, Ste. 220, Braintree, MA 02184

Telephone: 781-849-1702 **Fax:** 781-849-1802 **Metro area:** Boston, MA **Web site:** http://www.aztecpartners.com **Human resources contact:** Jeanne O'Byrne **Sales:** $208.3 million **Number of employees:** 1,114 **Number of employees for previous year:** 1,067 **Industry designation:** Computers—services **Company type:** Public **Top competitors:** Cambridge Technology Partners (Massachusetts), Inc.; Computer Sciences Corporation; International Business Machines Corporation

Inspired by the 16th century Indians known for "acquiring" their competition and for other technological feats like building cities on top of marsh land, Aztec Technology Partners would make its namesakes proud. Through its numerous regional operating subsidiaries, the company designs, implements, and supports information technology (IT) and telephony systems for companies in a wide range of industries, including communications, health care, financial services, government, and techology. U.S. Office Products Company spun off Aztec Technology Partners in 1998.

Benthos, Inc.

49 Edgerton Dr., North Falmouth, MA 02556

Telephone: 508-563-1000 **Fax:** 508-563-6444 **Metro area:** Boston, MA **Web site:** http://www.benthos.com **Human resources contact:** Kathryn Busa **Sales:** $14 million **Number of employees:** 92 **Number of employees for previous year:** 72 **Industry designation:** Instruments—scientific **Company type:** Public **Top competitors:** Oceaneering International, Inc.; Larson-Davis Incorporated

Benthos' products have gone down with the ship. The company's camera housings enabled the first extravehicular filming of the sunken Titanic. Benthos also makes undersea exploration equipment such as hydrophones to help oil and gas explorers map ocean floor geology. It has adapted its underwater acoustic technology, originally used to find enemy submarines, to detect defects in containers. The company is counting on its TapTone container inspection systems to increase profits. Used by the food, pharmaceutical, and beverage industries, TapTone is popular with big beer makers, since it can electromagnetically "tap" up to 2,000 filled beer bottles a minute and identify bottles that didn't seal properly.

Biogen, Inc.

14 Cambridge Center, Cambridge, MA 02142

Telephone: 617-679-2000 **Fax:** 617-679-2617 **Metro area:** Boston, MA **Web site:** http://www.biogen.com **Human resources contact:** Frank A. Burke Jr. **Sales:** $557.6 million **Number of employees:** 1,114 **Number of employees for previous year:** 797 **Industry designation:** Biomedical & genetic products **Company type:** Public **Top competitors:** Novartis AG; Merck & Co., Inc.; Schering AG

AVONEX calling! Not a peddler of cosmetics, Biogen researches, develops, and markets biopharmaceuticals to treat a variety of ailments; about 55% of total sales are from AVONEX, a drug used to treat relapsing multiple sclerosis. The company is developing a number of drugs to treat inflammation, pulmonary diseases, kidney diseases and disorders, and central nervous system disorders. Biogen also makes money by licensing drugs it has developed to other companies; such products include alpha interferon and a hepatitis B vaccine. Biogen has research agreements with such pharmaceutical firms as Creative BioMolecules, CV Therapeutics, and Merck. The company's products are sold around the world.

BioTransplant Incorporated

Charlestown Navy Yard, Bldg. 75, Third Ave., Charlestown, MA 02129

Telephone: 617-241-5200 **Fax:** 617-241-8780 **Metro area:** Boston, MA **Human resources contact:** Ariane Hodges **Sales:** $8 million **Number of employees:** 63 **Number of employees for previous year:** 57 **Industry designation:** Drugs **Company type:** Public **Top competitors:** Baxter International Inc.; Novartis AG; Roche Holding Ltd

Think you could never have a baboon heart? BioTransplant Incorporated is developing two drug systems to decrease the body's rejection of incompatible organs, both human and animal alike. The development-stage company's AlloMune System attempts to reduce the likelihood of human-to-human organ rejection by creating genetically-mixed bone marrow. Its XenoMune System would create genetically-mixed bone marrow (from miniswine and humans) to enable a human to take an incompatible organ. BioTransplant has teamed with a number of partners to develop its systems, including Novartis, MedImmune, and Stem Cell Sciences. Investment firm HealthCare Ventures owns about one-third of the company.

Boston Biomedica, Inc.

375 West St., West Bridgewater, MA 02379

Telephone: 508-580-1900 **Fax:** 508-580-1110 **Metro area:** Boston, MA **Human resources contact:** Candace Kobyluck **Sales:** $26.1 million **Number of employees:** 282 **Number of employees for previous year:** 191 **Industry designation:** Medical products **Company type:** Public **Top competitors:** SmithKline Beecham plc; Dade Behring; NABI

Boston Biomedica's products evaluate diagnostic tests for such infectious diseases as AIDS, Lyme disease, and hepatitis. Regulatory agencies, test-kit manufacturers, hospitals, care providers, and blood banks use the human-serum based disease-marker kits to ensure the quality of their testing equipment. The company also offers contract research services, clinical trials, and other services. Subsidiary BBI BioSeq develops biomolecular technology products. Subsidiary BBI Biotech researches and develops HIV drugs; it also tests potential HIV vaccines through a contract with the National Institute of Allergy and Infectious Diseases. Chairman and CEO Richard Schumacher owns more than 20% of the company.

Boston Celtics Limited Partnership

151 Merrimac St., Boston, MA 02114

Telephone: 617-523-6050 **Fax:** 617-523-5949 **Metro area:** Boston, MA **Web site:** http://www.nba.com/celtics **Human resources contact:** Barbara Reed **Sales:** $75.7 million **Number of employees:** 55 **Number of employees for previous year:** 43 **Industry designation:** Leisure & recreational services **Company type:** Public **Top competitors:** Miami Heat; New Jersey Nets; New York Knickerbockers

Boston Celtics Limited Partnership owns and operates the Boston Celtics professional basketball team of the National Basketball Association (NBA). The team boasts 16 NBA titles and 24 Hall-of-Famers (including newly inducted Larry Bird). The partnership's revenues come from home-game ticket sales; the licensing of rights to Celtics games for TV, cable, and radio; and merchandising of the Celtics name. After going more than a decade without a championship, the team has tried to resurrect the famous Celtic pride, moving out of historic Boston Garden to the larger FleetCenter and signing a new coach, Rick Pitino, to a whopping $70 million 10-year contract.

Boston Professional Hockey Association Inc.

One FleetCenter, Ste. 250, Boston, MA 02114

Telephone: 617-624-1900 **Fax:** 617-523-7184 **Metro area:** Boston, MA **Web site:** http://www.bostonbruins.com **Human resources contact:** Dale Hamilton **Sales:** $66.1 million (Est.) **Number of employees:** 75 **Industry designation:** Leisure & recreational services **Company type:** Private **Top competitors:** Ottawa Senators; Toronto Maple Leaf Hockey Club; Club de hockey Canadien, Inc.

The Boston Professional Hockey Association, better known as the Boston Bruins, has won the National Hockey League's (NHL) Stanley Cup championship five times. Their last title, however, came in 1972. Head coach Pat Burns brings a lifetime winning record to the Bruins and has won the Jack Adams Trophy (coach of the year) a record three times. Burns imparts his puckish wisdom on one of the NHL's younger teams, featuring such potential stars as Sergei Samsonov (the 1998 NHL Rookie of the Year) and Joe Thornton, a former top draft pick. The team was formed in 1924, making the Bruins the third-oldest surviving team in the NHL. Delaware North chairman Jeremy Jacobs owns the team.

The Boston Red Sox

4 Yawkey Way, Boston, MA 02215

Telephone: 617-267-9440 **Fax:** 617-236-6797 **Metro area:** Boston, MA **Web site:** http://www.redsox.com **Human resources contact:** Michele Julian **Sales:** $92.1 million (Est.) **Number of employees:** 150 **Industry designation:** Leisure & recreational services **Company type:** Private **Top competitors:** New York Yankees; Baltimore Orioles; Toronto Blue Jays Baseball Club

One of the first baseball clubs in the American League, the Boston Red Sox began life in 1901 as the Americans— one of many names it tried before settling on the Red Sox moniker a few years later. The team won its first World Series in 1903 and moved into Fenway Park in 1912. The club would win just four more World Series titles, the last one in 1918. After winning the AL wild card in 1998, the team lost the division series to the Cleveland Indians. Tiring of a park that seats only 33,000, the Boston Red Sox are negotiating to build a new stadium by 2001 that will seat 45,000. Many Bostonians want the team to remain at Fenway Park and are fighting the move. John Harrington is the principal owner of the team.

Boston Scientific Corporation

One Boston Scientific Place, Natick, MA 01760

Telephone: 508-650-8000 **Fax:** 508-647-2200 **Metro area:** Boston, MA **Web site:** http://www.bsci.com **Human resources contact:** Robert G. MacLean **Sales:** $2.2 billion **Number of employees:** 11,000 **Number of employees for previous year:** 9,580 **Industry designation:** Medical instruments **Company type:** Public **Top competitors:** United States Surgical Corporation; Medtronic, Inc.; C. R. Bard, Inc.

Boston Scientific finds a way in. The company makes medical supplies used in surgical procedures. Its products are minimally invasive (inserted into the human body through natural openings or small incisions) and are used to diagnose and treat conditions in a wide variety of medical fields, including cardiology, gastroenterology, pulmonary medicine, radiology, urology, and vascular surgery. Products fashioned by Boston Scientific include catheters, surgical grafts, ureteral stents, polypectomy snares, and lithotripsy devices. Almost one-third of company sales come from international operations.

Cambridge Heart, Inc.

One Oak Park Dr., Bedford, MA 01730

Telephone: 781-271-1200 **Fax:** 781-275-8431 **Metro area:** Boston, MA **Web site:** http://www.cambridgeheart.com **Human resources contact:** Renee Capachoine **Sales:** $2.1 million **Number of employees:** 36 **Number of employees for previous year:** 33 **Industry designation:** Medical products **Company type:** Public

Cambridge Heart conducts research for, develops, manufactures, and sells noninvasive diagnostic products for detecting cardiac disease. Its lead product, the CH 2000 System, performs cardiac stress tests and measures extremely low levels of T-wave alternans, an irregularity in an electrocardiogram indicating the risk of sudden cardiac death. More than 40 manufacturers sell the firm's FDA-approved CH 2000 and accompanying Hi-Resolution electrodes in the US. The CH 2000 System is also sold in Australia, Japan, the Middle East, and Europe through distribution agreements. In addition, Cambridge Heart is researching the use of its cardiac electrical imaging technology to detect ischemic heart disease.

Cambridge Technology Partners (Massachusetts), Inc.

304 Vassar St., Cambridge, MA 02139

Telephone: 617-374-9800 **Fax:** 617-374-8300 **Metro area:** Boston, MA **Web site:** http://www.ctp.com **Human resources contact:** Laura Zak **Sales:** $612 million **Number of employees:** 3,222 **Number of employees for previous year:** 1,926 **Industry designation:** Computers—services **Company type:** Public **Top competitors:** Electronic Data Systems Corporation; Andersen Consulting; International Business Machines Corporation

Software consultant Cambridge Technology Partners (Massachusetts) provides information technology consulting and software development services for companies seeking to shift to client/server networks from older mainframe computers but stymied by the growing complexity of computer technology. It made a name for itself by giving its corporate customers up-front guarantees on how much services would cost and how long a job would take. The company's services include custom and package software deployment, electronic commerce development, information technology strategy, management consulting, network services, and training. Cambridge continues a global expansion, primarily through acquisitions.

CardioTech International, Inc.

11 State St., Woburn, MA 01801

Telephone: 781-933-4772 **Fax:** 781-933-3933 **Metro area:** Boston, MA **Web site:** http://www.technologypark.com/cardiotech **Human resources contact:** John E. Mattern **Sales:** $900,000 **Number of employees:** 10 **Number of employees for previous year:** 9 **Industry designation:** Medical products **Company type:** Public **Top competitors:** W. L. Gore and Associates, Inc.; Thoratec Laboratories Corporation; C. R. Bard, Inc.

If artificial blood becomes a reality, the manufacturers can hook up with CardioTech International, maker of synthetic blood vessels. Formerly a subsidiary of PolyMedica Corporation, the company develops and produces vascular grafts to replace or bypass damaged and diseased arteries and to provide access for dialysis needles in kidney disease patients undergoing hemodialysis. These man-made blood vessels, also called vascular grafts, are made of ChronoFlex, the company's polyurethane-based biomaterial. The company's vascular grafts are in preclinical or clinical trails. CardioTech also makes polyurethane-based biomaterials, including ChronoFlex, for use in a variety of medical devices.

CareGroup, Inc.

375 Longwood Ave., 3rd Fl., Boston, MA 02215

Telephone: 617-975-5000 **Fax:** 617-975-6065 **Metro area:** Boston, MA **Web site:** http://www.caregroup.org **Human resources contact:** Laura Avakian **Sales:** $1.2 billion (Est.) **Number of employees:** 15,000 **Number of employees for previous year:** 13,362 **Industry designation:** Hospitals **Company type:** Private **Top competitors:** Partners HealthCare System, Inc.; Baystate Health Systems, Inc.; Columbia/HCA Healthcare Corporation

Thanks to CareGroup, there's well-being in Beantown. A 1997 agglomeration of Boston-area health care organizations, CareGroup provides care in more than 30 communities in Massachusetts. The system is comprised of six Boston-area hospitals, with Beth Israel Deaconess as its principal institution. CareGroup also includes a variety of specialty clinics, outpatient facilities, and research facilities. Despite the rejection of a proposed merger with Rhode Island's Care New England, CareGroup has not stopped looking for ways to expand. Through an alliance intended to bolster their power with HMOs, CareGroup Provider Service Network and Lahey Clinic serve more than 400,000 managed-care patients.

CareMatrix Corporation

197 First Ave., Needham, MA 02194

Telephone: 781-433-1000 **Fax:** 781-433-1093 **Metro area:** Boston, MA **Web site:** http://www.carematrix.com **Sales:** $147 million **Number of employees:** 2,250 **Number of employees for previous year:** 1,300 **Industry designation:** Nursing homes **Company type:** Public

CareMatrix operates more than 30 assisted-living facilities, primarily along the East Coast. The company provides social and health care services to its residents, including facilities for supportive independent living, skilled nursing/rehabilitation, and Alzheimer's care. CareMatrix focuses on upper-income senior citizens in metropolitan and suburban areas. It also provides management, marketing, development, and other services to other owners of assisted-living communities. CareMatrix is closely related to physician management company PhyMatrix and real estate investment trust Meditrust, which, like CareMatrix, are controlled by Abraham Gosman.

Celerity Solutions, Inc.

270 Bridge St. Ste. 301, Dedham, MA 02026

Telephone: 781-329-1900 **Fax:** 781-461-2421 **Metro area:** Boston, MA **Web site:** http://www.celeritysolutions.com **Sales:** $6 million **Number of employees:** 84 **Number of employees for previous year:** 46 **Industry designation:** Computers—corporate, professional & financial software **Company type:** Public

Celerity Solutions provides software that manages company product supply chains. The company develops, markets, and supports software systems that manage sales and purchase orders, provide inventory control, and help forecast product demand. Other products provide accounts receivable, accounts payable, and general ledger services. Celerity Solutions, which uses a direct sales force to market its products in the US, also sells its products in Europe. Its customers include Honeywell, United Liquors, and Methanex Methanol. The company discontinued its multimedia publishing business.

Chase Corporation

26 Summer St., Bridgewater, MA 02324

Telephone: 508-279-1789 **Fax:** 508-697-6419 **Metro area:** Boston, MA **Web site:** http://www.chasecorp.com/ **Human resources contact:** Theresa Pare **Sales:** $46.2 million **Number of employees:** 222 **Number of employees for previous year:** 215 **Industry designation:** Rubber & plastic products **Company type:** Public **Top competitors:** Ameron International Corporation; Furon Company; Plymouth Rubber Company, Inc.

Duck tape is wonderful stuff, but sometimes the situation calls for a higher-tech solution. Chase Corporation comes to the rescue. The company makes tapes and protective coatings used by the electronic, public utility, and oil industries. Products include insulating and conducting materials for electrical and telephone wire, electrical repair tapes, protective pipe coatings, and thermoelectric insulation for electrical equipment. The company also sells protectants for bridge deck surfaces to municipal transportation clients. Chase has six manufacturing plants in North America. Company co-founder and president emeritus Edward Chase owns 39% of the company. His son Peter, president, CEO, and COO, owns 11%.

Computer People Inc.

125 Jeffrey Ave., Holliston, MA 01746

Telephone: 800-429-1122 **Fax:** 508-429-9595 **Metro area:** Boston, MA **Web site:** http://www.computerpeople.com **Sales:** $140.2 million **Industry designation:** Computers—services **Company type:** Subsidiary **Top competitors:** TSR, Inc.; Analysts International Corporation; OAO Technology Solutions, Inc.

Computer People isn't a 1950s B movie. The firm, a subsidiary of UK-based information technology and human resources specialist Delphi Group, outsources technology personnel to companies needing various services from project development to computer system design and implementation. It also offers international resourcing, executive searches, and an acquisition conversion system program, among other services. Besides dental and 401(k), Computer People's staff get paid vacation and holidays, health insurance and disability benefits. Its customers include AT&T, DaimlerChrysler, IBM, and Microsoft. A division of Computer People, Alpine, performs computer networking and systems design and management consulting.

Concentra Managed Care, Inc.

312 Union Wharf, Boston, MA 02109

Telephone: 617-367-2163 **Fax:** 617-367-8519 **Metro area:** Boston, MA **Web site:** http://www.concentramc.com **Human resources contact:** Darla Walls **Sales:** $616.8 million **Number of employees:** 7,800 **Number of employees for previous year:** 7,270 **Industry designation:** Medical practice management **Company type:** Public

Concentra Managed Care concentrates on providing health care cost containment and case management services to employers and to occupational, auto, and group health payors. The firm's approximately 175 offices in 49 states and Canada offer specialized cost-containment services for occupational and auto injury cases; other services include preferred provider network management, telephonic case management, and medical bill review. At more than 150 locations in 24 states, Concentra also provides occupational health care, including pre-employment screening and injury care. Facing difficulties, the company agreed to be acquired by Welsh, Carson, Anderson & Stowe, which currently holds a 14% stake in Concentra.

Cybex International, Inc.

10 Trotter Dr., Medway, MA 02053

Telephone: 508-533-4300 **Fax:** 508-533-5500 **Metro area:** Boston, MA **Web site:** http://www.cybexintl.com/home/home.html **Human resources contact:** Karen Slein **Sales:** $127.6 million **Number of employees:** 632 **Number of employees for previous year:** 532 **Industry designation:** Medical products **Company type:** Public **Top competitors:** ICON Health & Fitness, Inc.; Soloflex, Inc.; Guthy-Renker Corp.

Cybex International has hearts pounding and pulses racing. The company makes strength training and cardiovascular equipment sold to consumers via independent retailers and to commercial markets including health clubs, hotels, and educational institutions. After merging with Trotter in 1997, Cybex sold its isokinetic testing and rehabilitation line. It now concentrates on cardiovascular products such as treadmills, bikes, and stair climbers as well as strengthening equipment including free-weights and single and multistation units. Investment company UM Holdings Ltd. owns 48% of Cybex and plans to increase its ownership.

Cytyc Corporation

85 Swanson Rd., Boxborough, MA 01719

Telephone: 978-263-8000 **Fax:** 978-635-1033 **Metro area:** Boston, MA **Web site:** http://www.cytyc.com **Human resources contact:** A. Suzanne Meszner-Eltrich **Sales:** $44.3 million **Number of employees:** 209 **Number of employees for previous year:** 124 **Industry designation:** Medical products **Company type:** Public **Top competitors:** Neuromedical Systems, Inc.; NeoPath, Inc.; AutoCyte, Inc.

Cytyc Corporation designs and produces sample-preparation systems used in medical testing. Health care providers use the company's ThinPrep System to diagnose cancer affecting the cervix, lungs, bladder, and gastrointestinal tract. The ThinPrep System stores patients' samples in liquid and incorporates an automated slide-preparation process that results in clearer samples for clinical diagnosis. The company's ThinPrep System has been approved by the Food and Drug Administration to be marketed as a replacement for the conventional Pap smear in the detection of cervical cancer.

Dyax Corp.

One Kendall Sq., Cambridge, MA 02139

Telephone: 617-225-2500 **Fax:** 617-225-2501 **Metro area:** Boston, MA **Web site:** http://www.dyax.com **Human resources contact:** Juanita Jeys **Sales:** $9.8 million (Est.) **Number of employees:** 84 **Industry designation:** Instruments—scientific **Company type:** Private

Dyax's phage display technology is used to develop new therapeutic, diagnostic, and separation products. Dyax has licensed its phage display patents to about 25 companies, including Bristol-Myers Squibb and Merck & Co. Using phage display, Dyax has identified lead compounds with possible applications in treatment of inflammatory diseases and certain cancers. Dyax also develops and produces chromatography separation equipment used to purify therapeutic and diagnostic products during manufacturing. These products are sold worldwide under the Biotage name to more than 50 biotechnology and pharmaceutical companies.

DynaGen, Inc.

99 Erie St., Cambridge, MA 02139

Telephone: 617-491-2527 **Fax:** 617-354-3902 **Metro area:** Boston, MA **Web site:** http://www.dynageninc.com **Human resources contact:** Cynthia Kiley **Sales:** $13.9 million **Number of employees:** 133 **Number of employees for previous year:** 67 **Industry designation:** Medical products **Company type:** Public **Top competitors:** Cardinal Health, Inc.; McKesson HBOC, Inc.

DynaGen, maker of generic medications and medical diagnostic products, is finding a possible NASDAQ delisting a hard pill to swallow. The troubled company's products include more than 500 generic drug compounds (90% of sales); NicCheck, which tests for nicotine in urine; and MycoDot, a tuberculosis diagnostic test distributed primarily in India, China, and Japan. In development are OrthoDyn, a bioactive bone cement; BioLocator, a breast biopsy imaging system; and drug product packaging. Dynagen sells its generic drugs to independent pharmacies (more than 50% of sales), retail pharmacies, pharmaceutical companies, nursing homes, and government agencies.

Dynatech Corporation

3 New England Executive Park, Burlington, MA 01803

Telephone: 781-272-6100 **Fax:** 781-272-2304 **Metro area:** Boston, MA **Web site:** http://www.dynatech.com **Human resources contact:** John A. Mixon **Sales:** $472.9 million **Number of employees:** 2,249 **Number of employees for previous year:** 2,050 **Industry designation:** Instruments—scientific **Company type:** Public **Top competitors:** Tektronix, Inc.; SPX Corporation; Fisher Scientific International Inc.

Although Dynatech primarily makes communications and test equipment, it also tries to put a little color in your life. The firm's test products (about half of sales) analyze and monitor transmission circuits, land-based wireless network equipment, and links between central offices and customers. Its industrial computing and communications unit offers ruggedized computers and other devices (about one-third of sales) suitable for adverse field conditions. Dynatech also sells hardware and software for aircraft cabin video display systems, transferring film to video, and colorizing movies. Investment firm Clayton, Dubilier & Rice, which backed a management-led Dynatech buyout in 1998, owns 92% of the firm.

Elcom International, Inc.

10 Oceana Way, Norwood, MA 02062

Telephone: 781-440-3333 **Fax:** 781-762-1540 **Metro area:** Boston, MA **Web site:** http://www.elcominternational.com **Human resources contact:** Mary Palango **Sales:** $763.6 million **Number of employees:** 996 **Number of employees for previous year:** 258 **Industry designation:** Computers—corporate, professional & financial software **Company type:** Public **Top competitors:** Micro Warehouse, Inc.; Dell Computer Corporation; CDW Computer Centers, Inc.

Elcom International thinks "seeing is believing." The company uses its own Personal Electronic Catalog and Ordering System (PECOS) e-commerce tools to sell PC products and PECOS-brand Internet applications. Subsidiary elcom.com uses PECOS.cm (PECOS commerce manager, interactive browsing and shopping) to sell PCs and PC-related products to business customers, schools, and government agencies. The PECOS line also includes PECOS Procurement Manager (PECOS.pm), an intranet-based procurement system, and PECOS.web Internet ordering and information system. elcom.com licenses PECOS to third parties through Elcom Services Group, an Elcom International subsidiary that provides support for PECOS products as well.

EMC Corporation

35 Parkwood Dr., Hopkinton, MA 01748

Telephone: 508-435-1000 **Fax:** 508-497-6961 **Metro area:** Boston, MA **Web site:** http://www.emc.com **Human resources contact:** Donald W. Amaya **Sales:** $4 billion **Number of employees:** 9,700 **Number of employees for previous year:** 6,400 **Industry designation:** Computers—peripheral equipment **Company type:** Public **Top competitors:** International Business Machines Corporation; Compaq Computer Corporation; Hitachi, Ltd.

EMC can emcee your memory. EMC is the #1 maker (ahead of IBM) of mainframe computer disk memory hardware and software. The company makes RAID (redundant array of independent disks) memory storage and retrieval systems for larger mainframe computers as well as desktop PCs. EMC markets its memory products under the name Symmetrix. Other products let users manage remote data and share information across networks of different computers. EMC continues to broaden its product portfolio, strengthen alliances, and expand its global presence to create more platform-independent systems.

EPIX Medical, Inc.

71 Rogers St., Cambridge, MA 02142

Telephone: 617-499-1400 **Fax:** 617-499-1414 **Metro area:** Boston, MA **Web site:** http://www.epixmed.com **Human resources contact:** Louise Ordman **Sales:** $1.8 million **Number of employees:** 72 **Number of employees for previous year:** 45 **Industry designation:** Medical products **Company type:** Public **Top competitors:** Nycomed Amersham plc; Guerbet SA; Schering AG

EPIX Medical wants to give you that special glow. The development-stage company makes contrast agents which boost the effectiveness of magnetic resonance imaging (MRI) in diagnosing certain conditions by enhancing the visibility of arteries and veins. Its main product, MS-325, is an injectable agent for use in diagnosing vascular diseases, including coronary artery disease and peripheral vascular disease. The company is also testing MS-325 for use in breast cancer detection. EPIX has formed alliances to develop and commercialize its contrast agents with several firms, including Mallinckrodt and Dyax. Other products in development include contrast agents for detecting blood clots and brain function.

Exchange Applications, Inc.

89 South St., Boston, MA 02111

Telephone: 617-737-2244 **Fax:** 617-443-9143 **Metro area:** Boston, MA **Web site:** http://www.exapps.com **Human resources contact:** Kris Zaepfel **Sales:** $24.8 million **Number of employees:** 157 **Number of employees for previous year:** 129 **Industry designation:** Computers—corporate, professional & financial software **Company type:** Public **Top competitors:** Oracle Corporation; SAP AG; Harte-Hanks, Inc.

Exchange Applications' VALEX won't park your car, but it may help you sell your product. The marketing automation software helps marketing professionals analyze the information in their databases and track responses in order to create targeted campaigns. VALEX also works with other business applications to maximize customer management. Exchange Applications supports VALEX with consulting, integration, training, and maintenance services. The company markets VALEX via direct sales and through reselling agreements with companies such as IBM and NCR; customers include FDX, Fleet Financial, and PCS Group. Entities affiliated with Insight Venture Associates own 37% of the company.

Focal, Inc.

4 Maguire Rd., Lexington, MA 02173

Telephone: 781-280-7800 **Fax:** 781-280-7801 **Metro area:** Boston, MA **Web site:** http://www.focalinc.com **Human resources contact:** Jim McEvoy **Sales:** $8.2 million **Number of employees:** 98 **Number of employees for previous year:** 91 **Industry designation:** Medical products **Company type:** Public **Top competitors:** Life Medical Sciences, Inc.; Cohesion Technologies, Inc.; Gliatech, Inc.

For surgeons who don't like leaky patients, Focal is developing sealants to stop leaks during surgery on lungs, brains, hearts, and guts. Focal's liquid sealants, FocalSeal-L and FocalSeal-S, adhere to underlying tissues, withstand air and fluid pressures, expand with tissues, and are absorbed by the body after wounds heal. Having won approval in Europe (for FocalSeal-L), the sealants are undergoing further clinical trials in the US. Focal has a distribution agreement with Ethicon, a division of Johnson & Johnson, for distribution of its sealants outside North America. Focal is also developing other uses for its polymers, including drug delivery systems and tissue coatings that could reduce post-operative scarring.

Galileo Corporation

Galileo Park, Sturbridge, MA 01566

Telephone: 508-347-9191 **Fax:** 508-347-3849 **Other address:** PO Box 550, Sturbridge, MA 01566 **Metro area:** Boston, MA **Web site:** http://www.galileocorp.com **Human resources contact:** Helen Kantor **Sales:** $44.3 million **Number of employees:** 431 **Number of employees for previous year:** 229 **Industry designation:** Fiber optics **Company type:** Public **Top competitors:** SpecTran Corporation; JDS FITEL Inc.; Optical Coating Laboratory, Inc.

Light is firmly at the center of Galileo's universe. Through subsidiary Optical Filter Corporation, Galileo makes fiber-optic and electro-optic components for light and image transmission, identification, and intensification. Its products are used for medical applications, office equipment, telecommunications, and scientific detection and spectroscopy. Subsidiary Leiseganz Medical makes women's health-related medical products, such as ultrasound devices, fetal monitors, and diagnostic instruments. Galileo has sold its medical endoscopic imaging business. The company primarily sells its products to end users and OEMs. Investment firm Andlinger Capital owns 33% of the company.

GelTex Pharmaceuticals, Inc.

9 Fourth Ave., Waltham, MA 02154

Telephone: 781-290-5888 **Fax:** 781-290-5890 **Metro area:** Boston, MA **Web site:** http://www.geltex.com **Human resources contact:** Stephen Burke **Sales:** $32.7 million **Number of employees:** 107 **Number of employees for previous year:** 76 **Industry designation:** Drugs **Company type:** Public **Top competitors:** Bone Care International, Inc.; Merck & Co., Inc.; Bristol-Myers Squibb Company

GelTex Pharmaceuticals develops non-absorbed, polymer-based pharmaceuticals that bind to and eliminate target substances from the intestinal tract. GelTex's pharmaceuticals work in the intestinal tract without being absorbed into the bloodstream, thereby minimizing the potential for adverse side effects. The FDA has approved the company's primary drug RenaGel, which is designed to treat elevated phosphorus levels in patients with chronic kidney failure. The firm is also developing a drug to treat high LDL cholesterol levels, and another to treat obesity by inhibiting the body's absorption of fat. The company has formed a joint venture with a unit of Genzyme to market and distribute RenaGel.

Genzyme Molecular Oncology

One Mountain Rd., Framingham, MA 01701

Telephone: 508-271-2627 **Fax:** 508-271-2604 **Metro area:** Boston, MA **Web site:** http://www.genzyme.com/molecularoncology **Human resources contact:** Susan Lankton-Rivas **Sales:** $782,000 **Industry designation:** Biomedical & genetic products **Company type:** Public **Top competitors:** Genentech, Inc.; Human Genome Sciences, Inc.; Rhone-Poulenc Rorer Inc.

Genzyme Molecular Oncology envisions cancer treatments that won't sicken you. A separately traded division of Genzyme Corporation, the company develops gene-based cancer therapies. Its approaches include tumor targeting (making the cancer more accessible for removal) and immunotherapy, which involves the body in the fight against cancer without weakening it (as chemotherapy does). The firm uses a proprietary technology to identify novel genes to improve diagnosis, and has a program to develop small molecule drugs that will attack cancer targets directly. Genzyme Molecular Oncology has developed a "vaccine" it hopes will breakdown existing tumors and has licensed a protein to cut off blood supply to tumors.

Genzyme Tissue Repair

One Kendall Sq., Cambridge, MA 02139

Telephone: 617-252-7500 **Fax:** 617-252-7600 **Metro area:** Boston, MA **Web site:** http://www.genzyme.com/company/lines/tissue/welcome.htm **Human resources contact:** John V. Heffernan **Sales:** $17.1 million **Number of employees:** 250 **Industry designation:** Biomedical & genetic products **Company type:** Public **Top competitors:** Smith & Nephew plc; Advanced Tissue Sciences, Inc.; Innovative Devices, Inc.

Genzyme Tissue Repair (GTR) burns to treat burns. The company develops products for treating and preventing serious tissue damage. GTR is a separately traded division of Genzyme Corporation. Its main product is Carticel, which is used to aid in the healing of articular knee cartilage. GTR's Epical Service is used to culture skin grafts from a sample the size of a postage stamp of the patient's own skin, growing enough skin to cover a patient's entire body in four weeks. The company is also developing treatments for Parkinson's disease, multiple sclerosis, and Huntington's disease from the company's research on promoting tissue growth.

GE Plastics

One Plastics Ave., Pittsfield, MA 01201

Telephone: 413-448-7110 **Fax:** 413-448-7465 **Metro area:** Pittsfield, MA **Web site:** http://www.ge.com/plastics **Human resources contact:** Robert E. Muir Jr. **Sales:** $6.7 billion **Number of employees:** 14,000 **Industry designation:** Chemicals—plastics **Company type:** Division **Top competitors:** Degussa-Huels AG; BASF Aktiengesellschaft; The Dow Chemical Company

How's this for taking the phrase "pay with plastic" literally? A division of industry giant General Electric, GE Plastics is one of the world's largest suppliers of high-performance polymers for use in automobiles, aircraft, appliances, construction, and other applications. The division designs 11 product families of thermoplastics in three main groups: amorphous (strength and stiffness), semi-crystalline (heat and chemical resistance) and amorphous-crystalline blends (specific applications). GE Plastics' sells mainly to original equipment manufacturers, compounders, and molders in diverse industries. The division, along with other materials operations, accounts for about 7% of General Electric's total sales.

Global Petroleum Corp.

800 South St., Waltham, MA 02254

Telephone: 781-894-8800 **Fax:** 781-398-4160 **Metro area:** Boston, MA **Web site:** http://www.globalp.com **Human resources contact:** Barbara Rosenblum **Sales:** $1.9 billion (Est.) **Number of employees:** 175 **Number of employees for previous year:** 150 **Industry designation:** Oil refining & marketing **Company type:** Private **Top competitors:** Tauber Oil Company; Koch Industries, Inc.; Tosco Corporation

With global ambitions and petroleum sources from around the world, Global Petroleum is an independent wholesaler of gasoline, heating oil, natural gas, and residual fuel oil. From its regional roots, it has grown to annual revenues of more than $2 billion. Global Petroleum sells to retail gas chains, utility power plants, and industrial users. The company makes a proprietary low-sulfur diesel fuel, and Global's Casey Petroleum subsidiary distributes a full line of Mobil lubricants. Founded in 1933 by the father of current president and CEO Alfred Slifka, the company is still owned by the Slifka family.

Haemonetics Corporation

400 Wood Rd., Braintree, MA 02184

Telephone: 781-848-7100 **Fax:** 781-848-5106 **Metro area:** Boston, MA **Web site:** http://www.haemonetics.com **Human resources contact:** Sheila Dryscoll **Sales:** $285.8 million **Number of employees:** 1,687 **Number of employees for previous year:** 1,526 **Industry designation:** Medical products **Company type:** Public **Top competitors:** Sorin Biomedica SpA; Gambro AB; Medtronic, Inc.

Haemonetics Corporation makes a variety of blood-processing systems. Its blood-recovery systems collect and reinfuse a patient's own blood before, during, or after major medical procedures. Haemonetics' automated plasma-collection systems deliver higher-quality plasma twice as fast as manual plasma-collection systems. The company's blood component therapy systems allow donors to donate specific blood components, such as platelets or white blood cells, instead of whole blood, thus increasing donor frequency. The company also makes automated red cell-collection systems, which eliminate the need for secondary separation of red blood cells from whole blood.

Harborside Healthcare Corporation

470 Atlantic Ave., Boston, MA 02210

Telephone: 617-556-1515 **Fax:** 617-556-1565 **Metro area:** Boston, MA **Web site:** http://www.hbrside.com **Human resources contact:** Jan Zdanis **Sales:** $311 million (Est.) **Number of employees:** 9,076 **Number of employees for previous year:** 7,331 **Industry designation:** Medical services **Company type:** Private

Harborside Healthcare provides long-term nursing care, subacute care (for strokes and head injuries, cardiac episodes, and wounds), rehabilitation, and behavioral health services. It also has Alzheimer's disease and hospice programs. The company operates more than 40 facilities in the Mid-Atlantic, the Midwest, the Northeast, and the Southeast. Harborside receives about 40% of its revenues from Medicaid and about 25% from Medicare; the balance comes from private sources. Investors George and Douglas Krupp and Laurence Gerber own about half of Harborside Healthcare, but international buyout firm Investcorp has an agreement to buy 91% of the company.

Harvard Pilgrim Health Care, Inc.

10 Brookline Place West, Brookline, MA 02146

Telephone: 617-745-1000 **Fax:** 617-630-4692 **Metro area:** Boston, MA **Web site:** http://www.harvardpilgrim.org **Human resources contact:** Larry Gibson **Sales:** $2.3 billion **Number of employees:** 5,000 **Industry designation:** Health maintenance organization **Company type:** Not-for-profit **Top competitors:** CIGNA Corporation; UnitedHealth Group; Blue Cross Blue Shield of Massachusetts

Harvard Pilgrim Health Care is Massachusetts' largest provider of managed health care. The company has more than one million members in that state and in Maine, New Hampshire, Rhode Island, and Vermont. Its offerings include health maintenance organizations, point-of-service plans, preferred provider organizations, and plans for Medicare and workers' compensation. Services are offered through a network of more than 22,000 physicians and more than 100 affiliated hospitals. The company was created in 1995 by the merger of Harvard Community Health Plan and Pilgrim Health Care. Affiliate Harvard Pilgrim Health Care Foundation funds teaching, research, and community service programs.

HealthDrive Corporation

25 Needham St., Newton, MA 02161

Telephone: 617-964-6681 **Fax:** 617-630-0141 **Metro area:** Boston, MA **Human resources contact:** Donna Clancy **Sales:** $12.9 million (Est.) **Number of employees:** 206 **Industry designation:** Health care—outpatient & home **Company type:** Private **Top competitors:** Catholic Health East; Integrated Health Services, Inc.; Sun Healthcare Group, Inc.

HealthDrive, through its affiliated medical and dental practices, provides on-site geriatric health care services to residents of about 850 nursing homes, assisted-living facilities, and independent-living senior housing facilities in 11 states. HealthDrive's services include dentistry, optometry, podiatry, and audiology. The company also provides primary care services in Massachusetts. Its operations are concentrated in the northeastern US, but it also serves senior facilities in Florida. HealthDrive filed to go public in April 1998. After the planned IPO, DCC International Holdings will own about 27% of HealthDrive. Chairman, president, and CEO Steven Charlap will own about 20%, and director Alec Jaret will own 10%.

Hemagen Diagnostics, Inc.

34-40 Bear Hill Rd., Waltham, MA 02451

Telephone: 781-890-3766 **Fax:** 781-890-3748 **Metro area:** Boston, MA **Web site:** http://www.hemagen.com **Human resources contact:** Myrna Franzblau **Sales:** $12.3 million **Number of employees:** 114 **Number of employees for previous year:** 108 **Industry designation:** Medical products **Company type:** Public **Top competitors:** IDEXX Laboratories, Inc.; Abbott Laboratories; Sanofi

Hemagen Diagnostics lets no disease go unturned. The company makes more than 125 diagnostic kits to identify infectious and autoimmune diseases such as rheumatoid arthritis, lupus, syphilis, mumps, and toxoplasmosis. Its Reagents Applications division sells medical testing reagents to hospitals and laboratories under the Raichem brand. Subsidiary Cellular Products makes biotech materials and assays for research. Hemagen's majority-owned Brazilian subsidiary markets its products in South America. Most of the company's products are sold to clinical laboratories, but its purchase of Dade Behring's Analyst clinical chemistry system provides it with a line that can be used at the point of care.

Hologic, Inc.

35 Crosby Dr., Bedford, MA 01730

Telephone: 781-999-7300 **Fax:** 781-280-0669 **Metro area:** Boston, MA **Web site:** http://www.hologic.com **Human resources contact:** Dave Brady **Sales:** $115.6 million **Number of employees:** 396 **Number of employees for previous year:** 339 **Industry designation:** Medical instruments **Company type:** Public **Top competitors:** Elscint Limited; Lunar Corporation; Norland Medical Systems, Inc.

Hologic is a hip company. A developer and manufacturer of osteoporosis diagnostic and monitoring products, the company makes X-ray bone densitometers, which measure bone density to diagnose and monitor metabolic bone diseases; Hologic also makes ultrasound devices such as the Sahara Clinical Bone Sonometer, approved by the FDA in 1998, to measure bone density. Together with Ostex International and Serex, Hologic is developing a test to detect biochemical signs of a patient's rate of bone loss. The company also distributes Soredex's Scanora X-ray system for presurgical planning of dental implants and mandibular joint repairs. Customers include pharmaceutical companies Merck and Eli Lilly.

H.P. Hood, Inc.

90 Everett Ave., Chelsea, MA 02150

Telephone: 617-887-3000 **Fax:** 617-887-8990 **Metro area:** Boston, MA **Web site:** http://www.hphood.com **Human resources contact:** Philip Mohan **Sales:** $500 million (Est.) **Number of employees:** 1,200 **Industry designation:** Food—dairy products **Company type:** Private **Top competitors:** Dean Foods Company; Cumberland Farms, Inc.; Suiza Foods Corporation

Founded in 1846 by Harvey P. Hood as a one-man milk-delivery service, H.P. Hood has grown into New England's leading dairy. In addition to being the #1 regional seller of ice cream, low-fat ice cream, and frozen yogurt, the company makes other dairy products, juice, and nondairy creamer. Novelties include the Hoodsie Cup, a single-serving cup of ice cream accompanied by a paddlelike wooden spoon, and FruitStirs (cottage cheese and fruit puree), which are being touted as a power snack. Besides its own brands, H.P. Hood makes private-label, licensed, and franchised products. The company, one of the first to make extended-shelf-life dairy products, has seven plants in six northeastern states.

Implant Sciences Corporation

107 Audubon Rd., #5, Wakefield, MA 01880

Telephone: 781-246-0700 **Fax:** 781-246-1167 **Metro area:** Boston, MA **Web site:** http://www.implantsciences.com **Human resources contact:** Diane Ryan **Sales:** $2.9 million (Est.) **Number of employees:** 33 **Industry designation:** Medical products **Company type:** Private **Top competitors:** International Isotopes Inc.; Theragenics Corporation; Nycomed Amersham plc

Implant Sciences hopes to counter the growth of cancer with the seeds of science. The firm plans to make radioactive seeds (awaiting FDA approval) to treat prostate cancer; it also wants to sell coronary stents, catheters, and other devices with radioactive coatings that make them visible when X-rayed. The company currently uses proprietary ion implantation techniques to alter the surfaces of semiconductors and orthopedic devices (thus minimizing friction and wear). Sales to Biomet and Stryker account for some 48% of sales. Chairman, president, and CEO Anthony Armini will own nearly 27% of the company after it goes public; VP and chief scientist Stephen Bunker will own 14%.

Infinium Software, Inc.

25 Communications Way, Hyannis, MA 02601

Telephone: 508-778-2000 **Fax:** 508-790-6784 **Web site:** http://www.infinium.com **Human resources contact:** Bill Grotezant **Sales:** $114.4 million **Number of employees:** 658 **Number of employees for previous year:** 549 **Industry designation:** Computers—corporate, professional & financial software **Company type:** Public **Top competitors:** PeopleSoft, Inc.; SAP AG; J.D. Edwards & Company

Infinium Software (formerly Software 2000) makes business software for IBM's long-lasting, midrange AS/400 system and also for Windows NT platforms. Products include personnel, accounting, process manufacturing, and materials-management applications. The company targets midsized firms and departments of large companies. About a third of Infinium's sales come from software license fees; the rest is from services. Customers, who buy products directly and through Infinium's global partners, include Mazda, McDonald's, MGM Grand, and Nintendo. Founder and chairman Robert Pemberton owns about 18% of the firm.

Innovasive Devices, Inc.

734 Forest St., Marlborough, MA 01752

Telephone: 508-460-8229   **Fax:** 508-460-6661   **Metro area:** Boston, MA   **Human resources contact:** Charlene Palmer   **Sales:** $11.9 million   **Number of employees:** 131   **Number of employees for previous year:** 125   **Industry designation:** Medical instruments   **Company type:** Public   **Top competitors:** Biomet, Inc.; Smith & Nephew plc; Johnson & Johnson

Innovasive Devices makes sure the leg bone stays connected to the knee bone with its tissue-repair systems. The company's systems are used to repair soft-tissue injuries, primarily for athletes and others needing arthroscopic surgery. Its initial product, the Radial Osteo Compression family of suture fasteners and related arthroscopic instruments, is used to reattach tendons and ligaments to bones and other tissue. Innovasive Devices' products are grouped into four categories: suture fasteners, suture systems, cartilage repair systems, and anterior cruciate ligament repair systems. The company has an agreement with Collagen to develop suture fasteners from collagen-based materials.

Interliant, Inc.

215 First St., Cambridge, MA 02142

Telephone: 617-374-4700   **Fax:** 617-374-4790   **Metro area:** Boston, MA   **Web site:** http://www.interliant.com/sage/index.html   **Human resources contact:** Lori Knowlton   **Sales:** $4.9 million (Est.)   **Number of employees:** 489   **Industry designation:** Computers—online services   **Company type:** Private   **Top competitors:** USinternetworking, Inc.; MindSpring Enterprises, Inc.; AboveNet Communications, Inc.

Interliant, formerly Sage Networks, wants to be the host with the most on the Internet. The company hosts Web sites for more than 37,000 customers, offering virtual, dedicated, and co-located hosting. Interliant also hosts Lotus Notes/Domino-based applications, allowing businesses to rent the use of software. Subscribers can sign on for any or all of a dozen applications hosted by Interliant, including products for messaging, e-commerce, sales, distributed learning, business automation, legal automation, and document sharing. Interliant has grown rapidly, buying 16 Web-hosting and other Internet-related companies in less than two years. Investment firm Charterhouse Group International is a major shareholder.

International Electronics, Inc.

427 Turnpike St., Canton, MA 02021

Telephone: 781-821-5566   **Fax:** 781-821-4443   **Metro area:** Boston, MA   **Web site:** http://www.ieib.com   **Sales:** $9.7 million   **Number of employees:** 69   **Number of employees for previous year:** 64   **Industry designation:** Protection—safety equipment & services   **Company type:** Public   **Top competitors:** Berwind Group; United Security Products, Inc.; Pittway Corporation

The threat of crime pays for International Electronics, manufacturer of electronic security products to deter thieves. The firm makes access control systems, digital keypads, and glass-break detectors (its top-selling products), as well as voice-verification systems through its Ecco Industries unit. Products are marketed under the Door-Gard, Secured Series, Tri-Gard, Glass-Gard, and VoiceKey names. The firm also distributes Weyrad's Viper vibration detector. Customers are security installers and distributors such as Ameritech, Honeywell, and Pittway. More than 85% of International Electronics' sales are in the US.

International Integration Incorporated

101 Main St., Cambridge, MA 02142

Telephone: 617-250-2500   **Fax:** 617-250-2501   **Metro area:** Boston, MA   **Web site:** http://www.i-cube.com   **Human resources contact:** Jane Callanan   **Sales:** $41.2 million   **Number of employees:** 260   **Number of employees for previous year:** 178   **Industry designation:** Computers—services   **Company type:** Public   **Top competitors:** Intelligroup, Inc.; Cambridge Technology Partners (Massachusetts), Inc.; Computer Management Sciences, Inc.

International Integration Incorporated, known as i-Cube, provides custom software development and computer application migration services to large global companies such as Boeing, DaimlerChrysler, Hewlett-Packard, and IBM. Its services, which also include information systems consulting and customer support, target companies making the shift from inflexible legacy systems to specially tailored client/server networks. Joint marketing agreements with companies such as Hewlett-Packard have helped i-Cube expand its customer base and increase name recognition. The company has offices in Cambridge, Massachusetts, Los Angeles, and Mannheim, Germany.

Jeepers! Inc.

60 Hickory Dr., Waltham, MA 02154

Telephone: 781-890-1800 **Fax:** 781-890-1810 **Metro area:** Boston, MA **Web Site:** http://www.jeepers.com **Sales:** $16.4 million (Est.) **Number of employees:** 1,250 **Industry designation:** Leisure & recreational services **Company type:** Private **Top competitors:** CEC Entertainment, Inc.; Discovery Zone, Inc.

Jeepers! positions itself as the indoor theme park company that offers food, fun, and a monkey; the company owns 15 jungle-themed parks (12 Jeepers! Parks and three Jungle Jim's Playlands). The facilities target both the birthday party crowd and the "I'm bored" market segment (families with children under 12). Each location offers amusement park rides (indoor roller coasters, bumper cars), skill games (Skee Ball), simulator games, and family dining. The company is licensed to sell Pizza Hut products at all its Jeepers! Parks. Jeepers! has indoor parks in Arizona, Illinois, Kansas, Maryland, Michigan, New York, Texas, and Utah; it plans to open about 35 more by the end of 1999.

Keane, Inc.

10 City Sq., Boston, MA 02129

Telephone: 617-241-9200 **Fax:** 617-241-9507 **Metro area:** Boston, MA **Web Site:** http://www.keane.com **Human resources contact:** Renee Southard **Sales:** $1.1 billion **Number of employees:** 8,008 **Number of employees for previous year:** 6,018 **Industry designation:** Computers—services **Company type:** Public **Top competitors:** Electronic Data Systems Corporation; Andersen Consulting; International Business Machines Corporation

Software services firm Keane has two business units: Its Information Services Division (95% of sales) provides software design, development, integration, and management services to corporations and government agencies, while its Healthcare Services Division develops financial, patient care, and clinical applications for hospitals and long-term care facilities. Clients include IBM (12% of sales), General Electric, the US Department of Justice, Johns Hopkins Hospital, Microsoft, and the US Customs Service. Keane, an early entrant into the year 2000 compliance market, has become a major provider of services dealing with the millennium bug. The Keane family owns about 20% of the company.

LeukoSite, Inc.

215 First St., Cambridge, MA 02142

Telephone: 671-621-9350 **Fax:** 671-621-9349 **Metro area:** Boston, MA **Web Site:** http://www.leukosite.com **Sales:** $12.1 million **Number of employees:** 67 **Number of employees for previous year:** 54 **Industry designation:** Drugs **Company type:** Public

LeukoSite develops treatments for cancer and inflammatory, autoimmune, and viral diseases associated with malfunctioning leukocytes (white blood cells). The company has a monoclonal antibody that has completed Phase I and II FDA clinical trials (LDP-03, also known as CAMPATH), and two other drugs are undergoing clinical trials in the UK. Leukosite also has seven small-molecule drug research programs. The company is developing drugs to fight transplant rejection and to aid in the treatment of leukemia, asthma, stroke, inflammatory bowel disease, arthritis, arteriosclerosis, and HIV. the company's partners include Warner-Lambert, Roche, and Kyowa Hakko .

Lifeline Systems, Inc.

640 Memorial Dr., Cambridge, MA 02139

Telephone: 617-679-1000 **Fax:** 617-923-1384 **Metro area:** Boston, MA **Web Site:** http://www.lifelinesys.com **Human resources contact:** Heather E. Edelman **Sales:** $64.4 million **Number of employees:** 635 **Number of employees for previous year:** 535 **Industry designation:** Medical products **Company type:** Public

Personal monitoring systems and response services by Lifeline Systems are designed to help elderly or physically disadvantaged individuals get emergency help. Its Lifeline product includes a help button worn or carried by a subscriber and a communicator connected to a phone line in the subscriber's home. When pressed, the button sends a radio signal to the communicator. An automatic phone call to a response center allows emergency help to be dispatched. Its other products include CarePartner Telephone with special features for those with visual or hearing limitations. Lifeline Systems, which Protection One has agreed to buy, markets its services to hospitals and other health care providers in the US and Canada.

LoJack Corporation

333 Elm St., Dedham, MA 02026

Telephone: 781-326-4700 **Fax:** 781-326-7255 **Metro area:** Boston, MA **Web site:** http://www.lojack.com **Human resources contact:** Mark Bornemann **Sales:** $74.5 million **Number of employees:** 414 **Number of employees for previous year:** 377 **Industry designation:** Protection—safety equipment & services **Company type:** Public **Top competitors:** Directed Electronics, Inc.; OnStar; GSE, Inc.

LoJack's signature product—a chilling thought for those driving hot cars—helps police recover stolen vehicles. When a car with a LoJack transponder is stolen, police track the car by its radio signal. LoJack contracts with law enforcement agencies to furnish tracking computers, then markets transponders to car dealers, fleet operators, and consumers. The tracking system has been implemented in 17 US states and the District of Columbia. Lojack also sells conventional vehicle security devices, including LoJack Prevent, a passive starter disabler, and LoJack Alert, a remote alarm. Internationally, private security companies and law enforcement agencies in 18 countries are licensed to use LoJack technology.

Lycos, Inc.

400-2 Totten Pond Rd., Waltham, MA 02154

Telephone: 781-370-2700 **Fax:** 781-370-2600 **Metro area:** Boston, MA **Web site:** http://www.lycos.com **Human resources contact:** Gretchen McAuliffe **Sales:** $56.1 million **Number of employees:** 456 **Number of employees for previous year:** 137 **Industry designation:** Computers—online services **Company type:** Public **Parent company:** CMG Information Services, Inc. **Top competitors:** Excite, Inc.; Yahoo! Inc.; Infoseek Corporation

One of the fastest-growing Internet companies barreling down the information superhighway, Lycos has finally joined the Internet consolidation flurry. The company has agreed to merge with USA Networks' 61%-owned Ticketmaster Online-CitySearch to create an e-commerce powerhouse, USA/Lycos Interactive Networks. The Lycos Network (a family of Web sites including Lycos, Tripod, and Angelfire) is visited by more than 28 million people each month and offers Web searching, chat rooms, e-mail, news, and free personal homepages. About 75% of Lycos' revenue comes from advertising, but it also receives revenue through e-commerce agreements and through licensing agreements with partners such as Bertelsmann and Microsoft.

MacroChem Corporation

110 Hartwell Ave., Lexington, MA 02173

Telephone: 781-862-4003 **Fax:** 781-862-4338 **Metro area:** Boston, MA **Web site:** http://www.macrochem.com **Sales:** $100,000 **Number of employees:** 29 **Number of employees for previous year:** 22 **Industry designation:** Medical products **Company type:** Public **Top competitors:** Novartis AG; Cygnus, Inc.; Elan Corporation, plc

MacroChem is developing transdermal drug-delivery systems, which allow drugs to be absorbed through the skin via creams, gels, patches, and the like. MacroChem is trying to attract business partners by applying its SEPA (Soft Enhancer of Percutaneous Absorption) system to FDA-approved drugs. The company is testing its system's use with drugs used to treat impotence (Topiglan), testosterone deficiency, arthritis pain, and skin conditions. MacroChem has also developed a delivery with potential applications in cosmetics and other topical products (moisturizers, sunscreens, insect repellents). Ascent Pediatrics has licensed SEPA for possible use in treating allergies and respiratory disorders.

The Manufacturers Life Insurance Company of North America

116 Huntington Ave., Boston, MA 02116

Telephone: 617-266-6004 **Fax:** 617-375-0297 **Metro area:** Boston, MA **Sales:** $274.2 million **Number of employees:** 233 **Number of employees for previous year:** 200 **Industry designation:** Insurance—life **Company type:** Subsidiary **Parent company:** The Manufacturers Life Insurance Company **Top competitors:** Pacific Mutual Holding Company; The Minnesota Mutual Life Insurance Company; Life USA Holding, Inc.

At The Manufacturers Life Insurance Company of North America (Manulife North America), coverage requires no assembly. Manulife North America, a subsidiary of The Manufacturers Life Insurance Company, Canada's largest mutual life insurer, primarily sells variable and fixed annuities through its Venture program. The company also offers Venture Life, a single premium variable life insurance policy for estate planning. Manulife North America, through partner Wood Logan Associates, markets its products in all states except New Hampshire and New York: subsidiary Manulife New York covers New York. Although the company itself is a stock company, its parent company is demutualizing.

Massachusetts Mutual Life Insurance Company

1295 State St., Springfield, MA 01111

Telephone: 413-788-8411 **Fax:** 413-744-8889 **Metro area:** Springfield, MA **Web site:** http://www.massmutual.com **Human resources contact:** Susan A. Alfano **Sales:** $10.7 billion **Number of employees:** 5,000 **Industry designation:** Insurance—life **Company type:** Mutual company **Top competitors:** The Northwestern Mutual Life Insurance Company; The Prudential Insurance Company of America; New York Life Insurance Company

Massachusetts Mutual Life Insurance needs structure in its life; a different one, that is. While mulling a shift from its mutual ownership structure, MassMutual offers its client base of upper-income individuals and small businesses a variety of life insurance and pension products. Its Investment Group offers investment management products (securities and real estate) and includes subsidiaries OppenheimerFunds (mutual fund management), David L. Babson & Company (individual and institutional investor services), and Cornerstone Real Estate (real estate equities management). In recent years Massachusetts Mutual Life has begun moving into new markets overseas, including Argentina and Chile.

MathSoft, Inc.

101 Main St., Cambridge, MA 02142

Telephone: 617-577-1017 **Fax:** 617-577-8829 **Metro area:** Boston, MA **Web site:** http://www.mathsoft.com **Human resources contact:** Mary Gruol **Sales:** $24.4 million **Number of employees:** 174 **Number of employees for previous year:** 160 **Industry designation:** Computers—engineering, scientific & CAD-CAM software **Company type:** Public **Top competitors:** Visual Numerics, Inc.; SAS Institute Inc.; Franklin Electronic Publishers, Incorporated

MathSoft designs technical calculation and data analysis software (about 85% of sales) for technical personnel, academicians, and students. The software, which is used for mathematical calculations and creating publications, also lets users access the company's digital publications to alter formulas and work problems. Products include the flagship Mathcad and Electronic Books mathematical calculation software; the StudyWorks math and science line for high school and college students and educators; Axum, for preparing charts; and S-PLUS for statistical analysis. MathSoft also distributes digital versions of publishers' reference works, and licenses its own technology to third parties.

Matritech, Inc.

330 Nevada St., Newton, MA 02160

Telephone: 617-928-0820 **Fax:** 617-928-0821 **Metro area:** Boston, MA **Web site:** http://www.matritech.com **Human resources contact:** Paula Roycroft **Sales:** $1.4 million **Number of employees:** 51 **Number of employees for previous year:** 46 **Industry designation:** Biomedical & genetic products **Company type:** Public

Matritech is a biomedical company that develops diagnostic tests for various cancers. Using its proprietary nuclear matrix protein (NMP) technology (pioneered by MIT and the Johns Hopkins University School of Medicine), the company is developing cell-based, serum-based, and urine-based NMP diagnostics to help doctors detect and monitor breast, cervical, colorectal, and prostate cancers. Using such fluids analysis methods provides cancer patients with an alternative to the often painful instrument-based exams. Matritech is co-marketing its first product, its NMP-22 Test Kit for bladder cancer, with Laboratory Corporation of America Holdings.

Millennium Pharmaceuticals, Inc.

640 Memorial Dr., Cambridge, MA 02139

Telephone: 617-679-7000 **Fax:** 617-225-0884 **Metro area:** Boston, MA **Web site:** http://www.mlnm.com **Human resources contact:** Linda K. Pine **Sales:** $133.7 million **Number of employees:** 730 **Number of employees for previous year:** 520 **Industry designation:** Biomedical & genetic products **Company type:** Public **Top competitors:** Genentech, Inc.; Chiron Corporation; Amgen Inc.

Millennium Pharmaceuticals develops treatments and diagnostics for such conditions as obesity, type II diabetes, asthma, cancer, and central nervous system disorders. Its approach is to look for the genetic basis of a disease and stop it at its roots. The company has forged research and development alliances with leading pharmaceutical companies, including Hoffmann-La Roche; Becton, Dickinson and Company; Eli Lilly; and Bayer, with whom Millennium has signed a $465 million deal. The company has discovered genes responsible for obesity, appetite control, and predispositions to type II diabetes and manic depression. Millennium licenses its technology to Monsanto for use in plant agriculture and human health care.

New England Patriots

60 Washington St., Foxboro, MA 02035

Telephone: 508-543-8200 **Fax:** 508-543-0285 **Metro area:** Boston, MA **Web site:** http://www.patriots.com **Human resources contact:** Joanne Nichols **Sales:** $84 million (Est.) **Number of employees:** 133 **Industry designation:** Leisure & recreational services **Company type:** Private **Top competitors:** New York Jets Football Club, Inc.; Miami Dolphins Limited; Buffalo Bills, Inc.

The Boston Patriots hit the hashmarks in 1959 as part of the American Football League (AFL). In 1971 the team changed its name to the New England Patriots and moved to Foxboro, Massachusetts, after the AFL merged with the NFL. The Patriots made it to the Super Bowl in 1985 but were pounded by the dominating Chicago Bears. The team fared little better in its second Super Bowl appearance in 1997 against the Green Bay Packers. That Super Bowl was the fourth-most-watched program in TV history. New England has fielded such football greats as Hall of Fame tackle John Hannah and now features talented quarterback Drew Bledsoe. Boston businessman Robert Kraft owns the team, which is moving to Hartford, Connecticut.

NewsEdge Corporation

80 Blanchard Rd., Burlington, MA 01803

Telephone: 781-229-3000 **Fax:** 781-229-3030 **Metro area:** Boston, MA **Web site:** http://www.newsedge.com **Human resources contact:** Al Zink **Sales:** $79.5 million **Number of employees:** 412 **Number of employees for previous year:** 202 **Industry designation:** Computers—online services **Company type:** Public **Top competitors:** WavePhore, Inc.; The Dialog Corporation plc; OneSource Information Services, Inc.

Formed when online information provider Desktop Data bought rival Individual, NewsEdge supplies information to more than 1.2 million users in North America, Europe, and Asia; it delivers more than 50,000 news stories a day. Its products and services include NewsEdge Insight (value-added industry and company news delivered via intranets and the Internet), NewsEdge Live (real-time news delivered over LANs, WANs, and intranets), NewsEdge NewsPage (customized news offered over the Internet), and NewsEdge NewsTools (software, including NewsObjects, for integrating news into other applications). In 1998 the company spun off its ClariNet Communications (now NaviLinks) unit to focus on its core business.

Nextera Enterprises, Inc.

One Cranberry Hill, Lexington, MA 02421

Telephone: 781-778-4400 **Fax:** 781-778-4500 **Metro area:** Boston, MA **Web site:** http://www.nextera.com **Human resources contact:** Dave Fritts **Sales:** $67.6 million (Est.) **Number of employees:** 600 **Number of employees for previous year:** 496 **Industry designation:** Computers—services **Company type:** Private **Top competitors:** Towers Perrin; Bain & Company; Keane, Inc.

The junk bond king and the king of junking Bill Gates are ready to tell you how to run your business. Nextera Enterprises, an independent consulting arm of education software specialist Knowledge Universe—formed by famed financier Michael Milken and Oracle chairman Lawrence Ellison—offers corporate strategy planning, personnel development, and other information technology consulting services to multinational firms. Customers include IBM, Levi Strauss & Co., and SmithKline Beecham. Nextera Enterprises is using acquisitions to build its services base, which like Knowledge Universe emphasizes education and training. Following the planned IPO, Knowledge Universe will own nearly 90% of the company.

Nitinol Medical Technologies, Inc.

27 Wormwood St., Boston, MA 02210

Telephone: 617-737-0930 **Fax:** 617-737-0924 **Metro area:** Boston, MA **Web site:** http://www.nitinolmed.com **Human resources contact:** Henne Johnson **Sales:** $32.2 million **Number of employees:** 50 **Number of employees for previous year:** 39 **Industry designation:** Medical instruments **Company type:** Public **Top competitors:** Arterial Vascular Engineering, Inc.; Boston Scientific Corporation; Guidant Corporation

Nitinol Medical Technologies develops medical devices—stents and filters—that are implanted via minimally invasive surgery to treat vascular or other conditions. One device treats holes in the heart, a condition suffered primarily by children. A Nitinol Medical Technologies filter is used to prevent pulmonary embolisms. A self-expanding stent holds open arteries, veins, and other body passages that have closed or become obstructed due to aging, disease, or trauma. The products are designed to reduce patient trauma, recovery time, and cost compared with more invasive treatments. Nitinol has bought almost 25% of Image Technologies, developers of an imaging system used for minimally invasive surgeries.

Nutramax Products, Inc.

51 Blackburn Dr., Gloucester, MA 01930

Telephone: 978-283-1800 **Fax:** 978-281-7824 **Metro area:** Boston, MA **Web site:** http://www.nutramax.com **Human resources contact:** Carol Woloss **Sales:** $128.4 million **Number of employees:** 1,200 **Number of employees for previous year:** 1,000 **Industry designation:** Cosmetics & toiletries **Company type:** Public **Top competitors:** Perrigo Company; SmithKline Beecham plc; Johnson & Johnson

NutraMax Products helps smooth out the rough spots, wherever they might be. The company is the #1 maker of private-label cough drops and throat lozenges, electrolyte oral maintenance solutions for children, disposable baby bottles, disposable douches, and ready-to-use enemas. The company also markets contact lens care products, over-the-counter and generic prescription ophthalmics, toothbrushes, dental floss, first-aid products, and liquid adult nutrition products. NutraMax sells its products through drugstores, mass merchandisers, and supermarkets, as well as institutional customers such as hospitals and nursing homes. Founder, president, and CEO Donald Lepone owns nearly 8% of NutraMax.

Occupational Health + Rehabilitation Inc

175 Derby St., Ste. 36, Hingham, MA 02043

Telephone: 781-741-5175 **Fax:** 781-741-5499 **Metro area:** Boston, MA **Sales:** $23.1 million **Number of employees:** 393 **Number of employees for previous year:** 301 **Industry designation:** Medical practice management **Company type:** Public **Top competitors:** NovaCare, Inc.; Concentra Managed Care, Inc.; HEALTHSOUTH Corporation

Occupational Health + Rehabilitation (formerly Telor Ophthalmic Pharmaceuticals) has its eye on success in the workers' accident field. After failing to develop a treatment for eye diseases, Telor acquired Occupational Health + Rehabilitation and its physician practice management business. The company specializes in treating work-related injuries through 16 health care centers in the Northeast; it also provides workplace patient care at some locations. The company's programs emphasize injury prevention strategies such as physical exams, drug testing, and safety programs. Occupational Health + Rehabilitation is building up its business through joint ventures with hospitals, acquisitions, and strategic startups.

Organogenesis Inc.

150 Dan Rd., Canton, MA 02021

Telephone: 781-575-0775 **Fax:** 781-575-1570 **Metro area:** Boston, MA **Web site:** http://www.organogenesis.com **Human resources contact:** Caryle Connelly **Sales:** $9 million **Number of employees:** 142 **Number of employees for previous year:** 125 **Industry designation:** Biomedical & genetic products **Company type:** Public **Top competitors:** Advanced Tissue Sciences, Inc.; Ortec International, Inc.; Genzyme Corporation

Organogenesis has the skinny on replacement tissue. The company's primary product is Apligraf, a human skin substitute that has received FDA approval for use in treating certain skin ulcers; the product is already available in Canada. Apligraf also has applications in burn and wound treatment. The product is cultured from foreskins obtained in infant circumcision and is rejection-resistant. The company's GRAFTPATCH, used to reinforce soft tissue, is also FDA-approved. Products under development include a liver-assist device and cell and gene therapies. Novartis has worldwide marketing rights to Apligraf.

Parametric Technology Corporation

128 Technology Dr., Waltham, MA 02154

Telephone: 781-398-5000 **Fax:** 781-398-6000 **Metro area:** Boston, MA **Web site:** http://www.ptc.com **Human resources contact:** Carl Ockerbloom **Sales:** $1 billion **Number of employees:** 4,911 **Number of employees for previous year:** 3,432 **Industry designation:** Computers—engineering, scientific & CAD-CAM software **Company type:** Public **Top competitors:** Autodesk, Inc.; Dassault Systemes S.A.; Structural Dynamics Research Corporation

Parametric Technology appreciates model behavior. The company is a leading maker of mechanical computer-aided design, manufacturing, and engineering software. Its flagship product, Pro/ENGINEER, has a slew of add-on modules that let users create models for products ranging from cellular phones to car bodies. Almost half of Parametric's sales come from training, consulting, and other services. Customers include Airbus Industrie, Rolls-Royce, General Electric, and Lockheed Martin. Parametric continues to expand through acquisitions, focusing on product information software companies.

PAREXEL International Corporation

195 West St., Waltham, MA 02154

Telephone: 781-487-9900 **Fax:** 781-487-0525 **Metro area:** Boston, MA **Web site:** http://www.parexel.com **Human resources contact:** Michael Brandt **Sales:** $285.4 million **Number of employees:** 3,700 **Number of employees for previous year:** 2,400 **Industry designation:** Medical services **Company type:** Public **Top competitors:** Covance Inc.; Pharmaceutical Product Development, Inc.; Quintiles Transnational Corp.

PAREXEL International's M.O. is contract R&D. The company's services include clinical trial and data management, biostatistical analysis, medical and regulatory consulting, performance improvement, and clinical pharmacology. The company provides its services to some of the largest pharmaceutical and biotechnology firms and works on about 2,000 projects a year. The firm's Pediatric Drug Development Services conducts trials on pediatric drugs. Unlike many of its competitors, PAREXEL has significant business overseas, where it derives about 40% of its sales. Recent strategic acquisitions have moved the company beyond pharmaceutical R&D into medical marketing.

Pegasystems Inc.

101 Main St., Cambridge, MA 02142

Telephone: 617-374-9600 **Fax:** 617-374-9620 **Metro area:** Boston, MA **Web site:** http://www.pegasystems.com **Human resources contact:** Ira Vishner **Sales:** $44.4 million **Number of employees:** 400 **Number of employees for previous year:** 220 **Industry designation:** Computers—corporate, professional & financial software **Company type:** Public **Top competitors:** Oracle Corporation; Mosaix, Inc.; CFI ProServices, Inc.

Pegasystems makes software designed to allow transaction-intensive service enterprises to automate and better manage their business operations. Its software helps integrate a broad range of customer interactions, including account set-up, record retrieval, correspondence, investigations, and sales. Products such as PegaREACH and PegaCONNECT are used by the financial services, insurance, health care management, telecommunications, and utilities industries, with clients ranging from Sears to the Bank of Ireland. The company also licenses its software to First Data Resources, a credit card processor. Founder and CEO Alan Trefler owns about 75% of the company.

Photoelectron Corporation

5 Forbes Rd., Lexington, MA 02173

Telephone: 781-861-2069 **Fax:** 781-259-0482 **Metro area:** Boston, MA **Web site:** http://www.photoelectron.com **Human resources contact:** Monica Hall **Sales:** $700,000 **Number of employees:** 48 **Number of employees for previous year:** 41 **Industry designation:** Medical instruments **Company type:** Public **Top competitors:** Matrix Pharmaceutical, Inc.; QLT PhotoTherapeutics Inc.; Theragenics Corporation

Like a menacing creature from outer space, Photoelectron wants to irradiate you from the inside out. The development-stage company makes the Photon Radiosurgery System (PRS), a device for eliminating cancerous tumors. The PRS delivers a high dose of radiation through a minimally invasive, needle-like probe that emits precisely controlled, low-energy X-rays from its tip, irradiating a tumor from the inside out. Compared to other radiation therapies, the PRS allows higher dosages of radiation to be delivered in a shorter time. Photoelectron plans to use the PRS to treat breast, kidney, liver, skin, and other tumors. Founder, chairman, and CEO Peter Nomikos owns nearly half of the company.

Physicians Quality Care, Inc.

950 Winter St., Ste. 2410, Waltham, MA 02154

Telephone: 978-439-0300 **Fax:** 978-667-3353 **Metro area:** Boston, MA **Sales:** $30.4 million (Est.) **Number of employees:** 43 **Number of employees for previous year:** 34 **Industry designation:** Medical practice management **Company type:** Private **Top competitors:** Medaphis Corporation; PhyCor, Inc.; FPA Medical Management, Inc.

The doctor's stitchin' might not be straight, but you'll get a good billin' thanks to Physicians Quality Care (PQC). The physician practice management company handles staffing, billing, and other administrative tasks for multispecialty medical practice groups. PQC forms professional corporations or associations with clients, who either sell their assets to or merge with these affiliated groups and become shareholders in PQC. Focusing on northern Connecticut, western Massachusetts, and Maryland, the company has long-term service agreements with more than 200 doctors. PQC also has 50% interest in two management companies in Atlanta covering 350 physicians. Bain Capital Funds owns about one-third of the company.

Physiometrix, Inc.

5 Billerica Park, 101 Billerica Ave., North Billerica, MA 01862

Telephone: 978-670-2422 **Fax:** 978-670-2817 **Metro area:** Boston, MA **Web site:** http://www.physiometrix.com **Human resources contact:** Marie McCahon **Sales:** $600,000 **Number of employees:** 48 **Number of employees for previous year:** 31 **Industry designation:** Medical instruments **Company type:** Public **Top competitors:** Nihon Kohden Corp.; Bio-logic Systems Corp.; ThermoSpectra Corporation

Physiometrix had a brain wave. Its medical devices monitor brain activity; they include the HydroDot NeuroMonitoring System, which is used for performing clinical electroencephalograph (EEG) procedures. The Equinox EEG System incorporates the HydroDot device in a complete package. The Neurolink product is a multichannel data device that processes the digital signal coming from the patient. Physiometrix also makes several models of EEG headpieces under the e-net name for different needs. Products under development include the Patient State Analyzer, which is designed for monitoring brain activity in the operating room; it will be distributed by General Electric's Marquette division.

PolyMedica Corporation

11 State St., Woburn, MA 01801

Telephone: 781-933-2020 **Fax:** 781-938-6950 **Metro area:** Boston, MA **Web site:** http://www.polymedica.com **Human resources contact:** Diane Gately **Sales:** $73.8 million **Number of employees:** 349 **Number of employees for previous year:** 196 **Industry designation:** Medical & dental supplies **Company type:** Public **Top competitors:** Abbott Laboratories; American Home Products Corporation; Bristol-Myers Squibb Company

PolyMedica Corporation is no parrot savant. The company distributes home test kits, insulin, syringes, and other supplies (made by Bayer, Roche, and Johnson & Johnson's LifeScan, among others) to diabetes patients through its Liberty Medical Supply mail-order business. The company also sells digital thermometers and its AZO urinary discomfort product line over the counter in supermarkets and drugstores. In addition, PolyMedica sells prescription urological products. PolyMedica's diabetes supply business sells directly to individuals, primarily senior citizens eligible for Medicare, and through contracts with managed-care organizations. PolyMedica operates facilities in Colorado, Florida, and Massachusetts.

PRAECIS PHARMACEUTICALS INCORPORATED

One Hampshire St., Cambridge, MA 02139

Telephone: 617-494-8400 **Fax:** 617-494-8414 **Metro area:** Boston, MA **Human resources contact:** Mary O'Malley **Sales:** $20.7 million (Est.) **Number of employees:** 71 **Industry designation:** Drugs **Company type:** Private **Top competitors:** Pfizer Inc; Warner-Lambert Company; Zeneca Group PLC

PRAECIS PHARMACEUTICALS hopes its peptide-based drug therapies will be the precise answer to diseases aggravated by testosterone or estrogen. Its abarelix is intended to halt prostate cancer growth by dropping patients' testosterone to the castration level. The drug, which is in clinical trials, may also be used to treat such conditions as benign prostatic hyperplasia, breast cancer, and endometriosis. Abarelix development allies include Amgen and Synthelabo (which has distribution rights in Europe, the Middle East, South America, and some African countries). Praecis withdrew its 1998 planned IPO, citing a poor market for biotech stocks.

Psychemedics Corporation

1280 Massachusetts Ave., Cambridge, MA 02138

Telephone: 617-868-7455 **Fax:** 617-864-1639 **Metro area:** Boston, MA **Web site:** http://www.psychemedics.com **Sales:** $17.7 million **Number of employees:** 127 **Number of employees for previous year:** 125 **Industry designation:** Medical products **Company type:** Public **Top competitors:** SmithKline Beecham plc; LabOne, Inc.; Laboratory Corporation of America Holdings

Don't give anyone a lock of hair as a keepsake—it could end up at Psychemedics Corporation, which provides testing services to detect substance abuse through the analysis of hair samples. Tests not only reveal that a substance has been consumed, but also provide historical data that can show drug use over a period of time. The company markets its services to employers, law enforcement, insurance agencies, physicians, and parents for detection of cocaine, marijuana, opiates, methamphetamine, and PCP. It also has a test for methadone for use in the treatment industry. Psychemedics' largest customer is GM.

Repligen Corporation

117 Fourth Ave., Needham, MA 02194

Telephone: 781-449-9560 **Fax:** 781-453-0048 **Metro area:** Boston, MA **Web site:** http://www.repligen.com **Human resources contact:** Barbara Burnim Day **Sales:** $2.4 million **Number of employees:** 24 **Number of employees for previous year:** 20 **Industry designation:** Biomedical & genetic products **Company type:** Public **Top competitors:** Abbott Laboratories; OXIS International, Inc.; IJL BioSystems, Inc.

Repligen speeds up drug research. The biopharmaceutical firm's processes help researchers rapidly synthesize libraries of up to one million chemicals; the processes are used to identify specific compounds that will interact with biological targets implicated in a disease. A successful match may help inhibit the disease. Repligen holds the rights to Secretin (a possible treatment for autism) and to a recombinant form of Protein A, which the firm uses to make mass-produced antibodies that may aid in disease treatment. Repligen, which has received grants from the National Institutes of Health, has agreements to collaborate with drugmakers Glaxo Wellcome, Pfizer, and Cambridge NeuroScience.

Restrac, Inc.

91 Hartwell Ave., Lexington, MA 02421

Telephone: 781-869-5000 **Fax:** 781-869-5050 **Metro area:** Boston, MA **Web site:** http://www.restrac.com **Human resources contact:** Robert J. Lederman Jr. **Sales:** $30.9 million **Number of employees:** 177 **Number of employees for previous year:** 159 **Industry designation:** Computers—corporate, professional & financial software **Company type:** Public **Top competitors:** SAP AG; Geac Computer Corporation Limited; PeopleSoft, Inc.

Ever wonder what prospective employers do with your resume? Some use Restrac's software to identify potential employees. Its software enables human resource departments to create and manage electronic resume pools, scan resumes for specific qualifications, and track interview schedules. Restrac's products, which include Restrac Resume Reader (developed with PeopleSoft and marketed with that company's software) and Restrac Hire, use Verity's text search software. The company also offers Restrac WebHire, an Internet-based candidate sourcing and management service, on a subscription basis. Restrac markets its products directly. Its more than 375 customers include AT&T, Merrill Lynch, Pfizer, and RJR Nabisco.

SafeScience, Inc.

Park Square Bldg., 31 St. James Ave., Ste. 520, Boston, MA 02116

Telephone: 617-621-3133 **Fax:** 617-621-0902 **Metro area:** Boston, MA **Web site:** http://www.safesci.com **Number of employees:** 16 **Number of employees for previous year:** 6 **Industry designation:** Biomedical & genetic products **Company type:** Public

Using nature's blessings to fight nature's pests and diseases, SafeScience (formerly IGG International) derives drugs and fungicides from naturally occurring substances. A development-stage biotechnology company, SafeScience operates through two subsidiaries. Its International Gene Group has developed GBC 590, a complex-carbohydrate glycoprotein being tested for treatment of cancer. Subsidiary Agricultural Glycosystems develops fertilizers, fungicides, insecticides, and transgenic plants; its products include the fungicide Greenleaf Plant Defense Booster. SafeScience conducts research at independent labs.

Safety 1st, Inc.

210 Boylston St., Chestnut Hill, MA 02167

Telephone: 617-964-7744 **Fax:** 617-332-0125 **Metro area:** Boston, MA **Human resources contact:** Stephanie Sestito **Sales:** $121.3 million **Number of employees:** 315 **Number of employees for previous year:** 235 **Industry designation:** Protection—safety equipment & services **Company type:** Public **Top competitors:** Playtex Products, Inc.; The First Years Inc.

Safety 1st puts children first with its child safety and child care products. Its well-known yellow and black diamond-shaped "Baby on Board" automobile signs secured the national attention needed to expand its distribution and product line. Its safety products include outlet plugs, cabinet locks, and balcony guards; its child care line (70% of sales) features items such as baby monitors, potty trainers, and activity gyms. Safety 1st's home security items include door and window locks, bolts, and latches. Its 375 products are sold to about 2,500 customers in the US and more than 60 other countries; Wal-Mart, Toys "R" Us, and Kmart account for about 50% of sales. CEO Michael Lerner owns almost 40% of the company.

Sapient Corporation

One Memorial Dr., Cambridge, MA 02142

Telephone: 617-621-0200 **Fax:** 617-621-1300 **Metro area:** Boston, MA **Web site:** http://www.sapient.com **Human resources contact:** Mike Millet **Sales:** $160.4 million **Number of employees:** 1,450 **Number of employees for previous year:** 817 **Industry designation:** Computers—engineering, scientific & CAD-CAM software **Company type:** Public **Top competitors:** International Business Machines Corporation; Andersen Consulting; Computer Sciences Corporation

Sapient serves its clients with client/servers and Web-based technology and integrated software systems. The company's QUADD (Quality Design and Delivery) program is a rapid-development, workshop-based system that designs, installs, and tests interactive client/server computer systems. The company offers its customers a fixed price and guaranteed delivery date for its software systems. The firm specializes in designing software systems for financial services, telecommunications, manufacturing, energy, and health and social services organizations. The company was founded in 1991 by co-CEOs Jerry Greenberg and Stuart Moore, who each own about 25% of Sapient.

SAZTEC International, Inc.

43 Manning Rd., Billerica, MA 01821

Telephone: 978-901-9600 **Fax:** 978-901-9601 **Metro area:** Boston, MA **Web site:** http://www.saztec1.com/800/htm/home.htm **Human resources contact:** Kent L. Meyer **Sales:** $8.3 million **Number of employees:** 268 **Number of employees for previous year:** 242 **Industry designation:** Computers—services **Company type:** Public **Top competitors:** Docucon, Incorporated; Innodata Corporation; COGNICASE Inc.

SAZTEC switches sources. SAZTEC International provides information conversion services. The company helps convert information (data, graphics, text) from several sources, including microfilm and paper, to such computer-usable formats as HTML and SGML languages. After a client approves a test database, SAZTEC begins the formal conversion, tracking documents throughout the process. The company also provides consulting, data entry, database maintenance, and project management services both on- and off-site. It primarily services the electronic publishing industry, including libraries, market research companies, online information vendors, and publishers. Amsterdam-based Tallard BV owns 45% of SAZTEC.

Segue Software, Inc.

1320 Centre St., 4th Fl., Newton Center, MA 02159

Telephone: 617-796-1000 **Fax:** 617-796-1610 **Metro area:** Boston, MA **Web site:** http://www.segue.com **Human resources contact:** Betsy R. Rudnick **Sales:** $42 million **Number of employees:** 167 **Number of employees for previous year:** 125 **Industry designation:** Computers—services **Company type:** Public **Top competitors:** Rational Software Corporation; Mercury Interactive Corporation; Compuware Corporation

Cashing in on e-commerce, Segue Software supplies software testing tools for businesses engaging in high-volume online transactions. Customers ranging from Dow Jones to AT&T use product suites from Segue, such as LiveQuality and Silk, to test the reliability of databases, Web links, Web-enabled software, Java code, load capacity, and client/server functions. The company offers training, consulting, and technical support for its products, plus year 2000 compliance services. Segue distributes and licenses its products through a direct sales force, system integrators, and value-added resellers in Australia, Canada, Europe, Japan, and the US.

Selfcare, Inc.

200 Prospect St., Waltham, MA 02154

Telephone: 781-647-3900 **Fax:** 781-647-3939 **Metro area:** Boston, MA **Web site:** http://selfcareinc.com **Sales:** $52.3 million **Number of employees:** 419 **Number of employees for previous year:** 325 **Industry designation:** Medical products **Company type:** Public

Selfcare makes home medical test kits, including pregnancy and fertility tests that are sold under both the Selfcare name and private labels at most US pharmacies. Other Selfcare tests detect the presence of HIV, hepatitis, Lyme disease, and chlamydia. The company also makes a glucose-monitoring system for diabetics. Selfcare's FastTake glucose test is distributed worldwide by the Johnson & Johnson unit LifeScan. In addition, Selfcare has US marketing rights for several women's nutritional supplements, including Stresstabs, Ferro-Sequels, and Posture. It has sold the infectious disease diagnostics business of its Cambridge Diagnostics Ireland subsidiary to Trinity Biotech.

Sepracor Inc.

111 Locke Dr., Marlborough, MA 01752

Telephone: 508-481-6700 **Fax:** 508-357-7499 **Metro area:** Boston, MA **Web site:** http://www.sepracor.com **Human resources contact:** Shizuko Yamaji **Sales:** $17.4 million **Number of employees:** 300 **Number of employees for previous year:** 149 **Industry designation:** Drugs **Company type:** Public **Top competitors:** Glaxo Wellcome plc; Bayer AG; Johnson & Johnson

Sepracor develops and commercializes improved chemical entities that are new, patented forms of existing pharmaceuticals. These products can offer reduced side effects, improved safety, new uses, and improved dosage forms over traditional compounds. Sepracor is developing pharmaceuticals to address asthma, allergies, pain, urological disorders, sleep disorders, periodontal disease, and depression. It developed Allegra as an alternative to Seldane (the FDA withdrew its approval of Seldane in 1997). The company is also developing antihistamines similar to Claritin and Hismanal. Sepracor has licensed to Johnson & Johnson the rights to an improved version of that company's own Propulsid heartburn medication.

Sight Resource Corporation

100 Jeffrey Ave., Holliston, MA 01746

Telephone: 508-429-6916 **Fax:** 508-429-6023 **Metro area:** Boston, MA **Web site:** http://www.sightresource.com **Number of employees:** 596 **Number of employees for previous year:** 488 **Industry designation:** Medical services **Company type:** Public **Top competitors:** Vision Twenty-One, Inc.; LensCrafters, Inc.; Cole National Corporation

Sight Resource provides eyewear products and services through almost 90 eye care centers in the Midwest and New England. Its stores—Cambridge Eye Doctors, E.B. Brown Opticians, Vision Plaza, Vision World—offer prescription eyewear and contacts; most have an in-house optometrist. Some centers also provide hearing aids and audiology services. The firm's regional laboratories and distribution centers provide the stores with lab services and supplies. Sight Resource, in conjunction with affiliated ophthalmological surgeons, operates four laser vision correction centers. The firm also offers a managed primary eye care program under the SightCare name.

Simplex Time Recorder Co.

1 Simplex Plaza, Gardner, MA 01441

Telephone: 978-632-2500 **Fax:** 978-630-7867 **Metro area:** Fitchburg, MA **Web site:** http://www.simplexnet.com **Human resources contact:** Russ Smith **Sales:** $695 million (Est.) **Number of employees:** 6,300 **Number of employees for previous year:** 5,800 **Industry designation:** Protection—safety equipment & services **Company type:** Private

The common phrase "punch the clock" might have an entirely different meaning if it were not for Simplex Time Recorder, inventor of the practical time clock and modern marketer of security, fire-alarm, communications, and time-management systems. The company's products, including WinSTAR, a Windows-based attendance system, are sold from some 140 offices in North America. It also has operations in 46 countries, with manufacturing subsidiaries in Asia, Australia, Europe, Latin America, and Canada. Founder Edward Watkins invented the first functional time clock in 1894—existing models could track only one worker's time. The Watkins family still owns Simplex.

SpecTran Corporation

50 Hall Rd., Sturbridge, MA 01566

Telephone: 508-347-2261 **Fax:** 508-347-2747 **Metro area:** Boston, MA **Web site:** http://www.spectran.com **Human resources contact:** Sue Jowett **Sales:** $70.9 million **Number of employees:** 531 **Number of employees for previous year:** 504 **Industry designation:** Fiber optics **Company type:** Public **Top competitors:** Corning Incorporated; Ortel Corporation; Lucent Technologies Inc.

If you were wondering what ever happened to those thousand points of light, SpecTran uses them in its optical fibers and specialty fibers and cables. Optical fibers are flexible, hair-thin strands of glass that transmit information in the form of light pulses from one point to another much more efficiently than copper wire. SpecTran's Specialty unit makes custom fibers and cables for use in short-haul datacom, geophysical exploration, military data and voice communications, industrial automation, and laser delivery. It also makes fibers through its communications division for telephony and computer networks. Through a joint venture with General Cable, SpecTran also makes fiber-optic cables and accessories.

Stream International Inc.

275 Dan Rd., Canton, MA 02021

Telephone: 781-575-6800 **Fax:** 781-575-6999 **Metro area:** Boston, MA **Web site:** http://www.stream.com **Human resources contact:** Lewis Legon **Sales:** $186 million (Est.) **Number of employees:** 5,000 **Number of employees for previous year:** 4,764 **Industry designation:** Computers—services **Company type:** Private **Top competitors:** TeleTech Holdings, Inc.; Sykes Enterprises, Inc.; SITEL Corporation

Stream International provides outsourced technical support and help desks for big computer industry players, including Microsoft and Hewlett-Packard. The company is one of three independent businesses formed from the restructuring of Stream International Holdings; the others are Corporate Software & Technology (software resale) and Modus Media International (media-related manufacturing and fulfillment); the outsourcing business kept the Stream International name. The company was formed by a merger between Corporate Software Inc. and commercial printer R. R. Donnelley & Sons' Global Software Services. R. R. Donnelley owns 87% of Stream International, and Bain Capital and other investors control the rest.

Suburban Ostomy Supply Co., Inc.

75 October Hill Rd., Holliston, MA 01746

Telephone: 508-429-1000 **Fax:** 508-429-7921 **Metro area:** Boston, MA **Human resources contact:** Stephanie Carr **Sales:** $94.4 million **Number of employees:** 289 **Number of employees for previous year:** 173 **Industry designation:** Medical & dental supplies **Company type:** Subsidiary

Suburban Ostomy Supply sells wholesale medical supplies and home health care products, primarily for use by ostomy, incontinent, and diabetic patients or those with difficult-to-heal wounds. The company's 7,800 products include ostomy appliances, adult diapers, blood-glucose meters, and wound dressings. Suburban Ostomy Supply has more than 23,000 customers. Independent suppliers account for about 80% of sales; national home health care chains and managed care organizations make up the remainder. The company has distribution centers in California, Georgia, Illinois, Indiana, Massachusetts, and Texas. In 1998 wheelchair maker Invacare bought 95% of the company.

Thermedics Detection Inc.

220 Mill Rd., Chelmsford, MA 01824

Telephone: 781-622-1000 **Fax:** 781-622-1123 **Metro area:** Boston, MA **Web site:** http://www.tdxinc.com/ **Human resources contact:** Fred Florio **Sales:** $91.6 million **Number of employees:** 520 **Number of employees for previous year:** 218 **Industry designation:** Instruments—scientific **Company type:** Public **Top competitors:** Barringer Technologies Inc.

Thermedics Detection makes high-speed detection and measurement devices for manufacturers, and explosives-detection equipment for airports and border crossings. Its Alexus systems detect trace elements in plastic bottles used by beverage producers, including Coca-Cola (which accounts for one-fourth of the company's revenues) and Perrier. The InScan system helps manufacturers fill containers with consistent amounts. The Quadra Beam measures product moisture, fats, adhesives, and coatings. EGIS systems detect trace amounts of explosives and are used by federal agencies. Thermedics Detection sells products in more than 30 countries. Thermedics Inc., a Thermo Electron subsidiary, owns more than 75% of the company.

Thermo Cardiosystems Inc.

470 Wildwood St., Woburn, MA 01888

Telephone: 781-932-8668 **Fax:** 781-933-4476 **Other address:** PO Box 2697, Woburn, MA 01888 **Metro area:** Boston, MA **Web site:** http://www.thermo.com/subsid/tca.html **Human resources contact:** Anne Pol **Sales:** $66.8 million **Number of employees:** 471 **Number of employees for previous year:** 420 **Industry designation:** Medical products **Company type:** Public **Top competitors:** Baxter International Inc.; Arrow International, Inc.; Medtronic, Inc.

Thermo Cardiosystems manufactures HeartMate, an implantable, pneumatic left- ventricular assist system (LVAS) that takes over the function of the heart's left ventricle (its primary pumping chamber) in patients awaiting a heart transplant. The HeartMate is one of only two LVAS devices approved for commercial sale by the FDA (Baxter unveiled the other in 1998). The company also makes an electric HeartMate device, but this product is available only in Europe and Canada. The company's International Technidyne subsidiary makes blood coagulation testing equipment and related disposables. Thermo Cardiosystems is a member of the Thermo Electron family of technology companies (its parent owns 55%).

Thermo Optek Corporation

8-E Forge Pkwy., Franklin, MA 02038

Telephone: 781-622-1000 **Fax:** 781-622-1123 **Metro area:** Boston, MA **Web site:** http://www.thermo.com/subsid/toc.html **Human resources contact:** Fred Florio **Sales:** $447.3 million **Number of employees:** 2,437 **Number of employees for previous year:** 2,341 **Industry designation:** Instruments—scientific **Company type:** Public **Top competitors:** Varian Associates, Inc.; Bio-Rad Laboratories, Inc.; The Perkin-Elmer Corporation

Thermo Optek's light-based instruments analyze the elemental and molecular composition of solids, liquids, and gases. Because light is nondestructive, Thermo Optek's equipment is used in a variety of applications such as crime analysis, semiconductor manufacturing, and quality assurance. Airlines rely on its instruments to assess when internal engine maintenance must be performed; the beverage industry uses its systems to identify mineral and vitamin content for nutrition labels; and municipalities use it to monitor water and air quality. Thermo Optek's own sales force, dealers, and distributors market its products worldwide. Thermo Electron owns 92% of Thermo Optek.

ThermoRetec Corporation

9 Pond Ln., Ste. 5A, Concord, MA 01742

Telephone: 978-371-3200 **Fax:** 978-371-9124 **Metro area:** Boston, MA **Web site:** http://www.thermo.com/subsid/thn.html **Human resources contact:** Fred Florio **Sales:** $128.4 million **Number of employees:** 952 **Number of employees for previous year:** 720 **Industry designation:** Pollution control equipment & services **Company type:** Public **Top competitors:** Tetra Tech, Inc.; Radian International LLC; Omega Environmental, Inc.

Dirt-rich ThermoRetec has made its money by cleaning soil. Formerly known as Thermo Remediation, ThermoRetec provides environmental-liability management services, including industrial, nuclear, and soil remediation, as well as waste-fluids recycling. ThermoRetec also offers environmental management consulting and develops computer systems designed to collect environmental data. Contracts with the US government account for 10% of revenues. Thermo TerraTech, a publicly traded environmental services subsidiary of Thermo Electron, owns 71% of the rapidly growing company.

ThermoSpectra Corporation

8 E. Forge Pkwy., Franklin, MA 02038

Telephone: 508-541-0401 **Fax:** 508-520-4881 **Metro area:** Boston, MA **Web site:** http://www.thermo.com/subsid/ths.html **Human resources contact:** Anne Pol **Sales:** $191 million **Number of employees:** 1,400 **Number of employees for previous year:** 790 **Industry designation:** Instruments—scientific **Company type:** Public **Top competitors:** Oxford Instruments PLC; Hewlett-Packard Company; Seiko Corporation

ThermoSpectra can see through problems. The company makes precision-imaging, inspection, temperature-control, and measurement instruments. Its digital storage oscilloscopes are used to record and analyze crash-test data and to test airbags, its X-ray microanalyzers help find and analyze imperfections in semiconductors, and its X-ray inspection systems are used to inspect finished products such as printed circuit boards and automotive electronics. More than 20% of sales are outside the US. Thermo Instrument Systems, a publicly traded subsidiary of Thermo Electron, owns 77% of ThermoSpectra. As part of a major restructuring, Thermo Electron plans to take ThermoSpectra private as a Thermo Instrument Systems unit.

Thermo TerraTech Inc.

81 Wyman St., Waltham, MA 02254

Telephone: 781-622-1000 **Fax:** 781-622-1207 **Other address:** PO Box 9046, Waltham, MA 02254 **Metro area:** Boston, MA **Web site:** http://www.thermo.com/subsid/ttt.html **Human resources contact:** Anne Pol **Sales:** $298.8 million **Number of employees:** 2,736 **Number of employees for previous year:** 2,407 **Industry designation:** Pollution control equipment & services **Company type:** Public **Parent company:** Thermo Electron Corp. **Top competitors:** Bechtel Group, Inc.; Radian International LLC; The IT Group, Inc.

Thermo TerraTech offers housecleaning services for the great outdoors, including environmental-liability management, laboratory-based testing, bioremediation (using naturally occurring microbes to decontaminate soil and water), and recycling. The company's major customers include oil companies, public utilities, large industrial plants, and federal and local governments. Thermo TerraTech also offers engineering, design, and construction management services. Formerly named Thermo Process, Thermo TerraTech is an 84%-owned subsidiary of Thermo Electron.

Transcend Therapeutics, Inc.

640 Memorial Dr., Cambridge, MA 02139

Telephone: 617-374-1200 **Fax:** 617-374-1201 **Metro area:** Boston, MA **Web site:** http://www.tsnd.com **Human resources contact:** Elizabeth McBride **Sales:** $5 million **Number of employees:** 23 **Number of employees for previous year:** 13 **Industry designation:** Drugs **Company type:** Public

Transcend Therapeutics is developing drugs for the treatment of diseases associated with oxidative stress, such as acute respiratory distress syndrome (ARDS) and multiple organ dysfunction (MOD). Procysteine, the company's lead product candidate, has been tested in two Phase II clinical trials involving ARDS patients, but a Phase III study has been canceled, leaving the future of the drug in question. The drug is intended to alleviate these diseases without causing the tissue damage in the body's major organs that sometimes occurs with mechanical ventilation. There are currently no commercially available drug treatments for ARDS or MOD. KeraVision is buying Transcend Therapeutics.

Transkaryotic Therapies, Inc.

195 Albany St., Cambridge, MA 02139

Telephone: 617-349-0200 **Fax:** 617-349-0599 **Metro area:** Boston, MA **Web site:** http://www.biospace.com/b2/company_profile.cfm?CompanyID=1548 **Human resources contact:** Andrea Jeffrey **Sales:** $5.8 million **Number of employees:** 149 **Number of employees for previous year:** 130 **Industry designation:** Biomedical & genetic products **Company type:** Public **Top competitors:** Aastrom Biosciences, Inc.; ARIAD Pharmaceuticals, Inc.; Vical Incorporated

Transkaryotic Therapies operates at the cellular level. The development-stage biopharmaceutical company specializes in researching gene therapies that activate malfunctioning genes, causing them to produce proteins that are necessary for proper operation. A prime example is the failure of cells to produce blood clotting factors that result in hemophilia A. Unlike many companies in the field, Transkaryotic Therapies does not rely on using cloned genes, instead it is developing a way to graft activating DNA sequences directly to the genes, which will then reproduce correctly. The company has research collaborations with Hoechst Marion Roussel and the National Institutes of Health.

Tufts Health Plans

333 Wyman St., Waltham, MA 02254

Telephone: 781-466-9400 **Fax:** 781-466-8590 **Metro area:** Boston, MA **Web site:** http://www.tufts-healthplan.com **Human resources contact:** Paula LaPalme **Sales:** $1.2 billion **Number of employees:** 2,341 **Number of employees for previous year:** 1,200 **Industry designation:** Health maintenance organization **Company type:** Not-for-profit **Top competitors:** Harvard Pilgrim Health Care, Inc.; Oxford Health Plans, Inc.; CIGNA Corporation

Tufts Health Plans, formerly Tufts Associated Health Plans, provides management, administrative, and marketing services for its affiliates and subsidiaries, including Tufts Associated Health Maintenance Organization (TAHMO), Total Health Plan (THP), and TAHP Brokerage. Its provider network includes about 16,000 physicians and has more than 950,000 members. TAHMO offers HMO and point-of-service plans through its Tufts Health Plan of New England subsidiary. It also offers third-party administration services through its Tufts Benefits Administrators subsidiary. THP provides support to participants in insured and self-insured point-of-service arrangements.

Vertex Pharmaceuticals Incorporated

130 Waverly St., Cambridge, MA 02139

Telephone: 617-577-6000 **Fax:** 617-577-6680 **Metro area:** Boston, MA **Web site:** http://www.vpharm.com **Human resources contact:** Michael S. Walsh **Sales:** $44.4 million **Number of employees:** 223 **Number of employees for previous year:** 178 **Industry designation:** Drugs **Company type:** Public **Top competitors:** Abbott Laboratories; Amgen Inc.; Merck & Co., Inc.

Vertex Pharmaceuticals develops drugs that combat autoimmune, inflammatory, neurodegenerative, and viral diseases. Vertex drugs in various stages of development include Agenerase (amprenavir, for treatment of the HIV virus and AIDS), two compounds for treament of cancer multidrug resistance, and a compound for the treatment of autoimmune diseases. Vertex is developing experimental nerve drugs to combat symptoms of illnesses such as Parkinson's disease. The company has collaborative agreements with Biochem Therapeutics, Eli Lilly, Glaxo Wellcome, Hoechst Marion Roussel, Kissei Pharmaceuticals, and Schering AG.

Viant Corporation

89 South St., Boston, MA 02111

Telephone: 617-531-3700 **Fax:** 617-531-3803 **Metro area:** Boston, MA **Web site:** http://www.viant.com **Human resources contact:** Diane Hall **Sales:** $8.8 million (Est.) **Number of employees:** 119 **Number of employees for previous year:** 20 **Industry designation:** Computers—online services **Company type:** Private **Top competitors:** iXL Enterprises, Inc.; USWeb/CKS; Proxicom, Inc.

Viant (formerly Silicon Valley Internet Partners) wants to be a giant in the world of Internet consulting. Building on its expertise in business consulting, systems integration, and Internet technology, Viant offers everything from intranet development to the creation of online catalog and customer service systems. The company has entered into a joint venture with Carat Freeman (high-tech media planning and buying) to offer clients a broad package of Internet and media services. It was founded in 1996 by Eric Greenberg, who later went on to found Viant rival Scient. Kleiner Perkins, General Motors, and several other venture capital firms own the company.

Vivid Technologies, Inc.

10E Commerce Way, Woburn, MA 01801

Telephone: 781-938-7800 **Fax:** 781-939-3996 **Metro area:** Boston, MA **Web site:** http://www.vividusa.com **Sales:** $38.7 million **Number of employees:** 125 **Number of employees for previous year:** 109 **Industry designation:** Protection—safety equipment & services **Company type:** Public **Top competitors:** L-3 Communications Holdings, Inc.; Barringer Technologies Inc.; InVision Technologies, Inc.

Vivid Technologies would like to wish you a pleasant—and bomb-free—flight. The company makes automated inspection systems that detect explosives and other contraband in checked and carry-on baggage. Deployed in several of the world's largest airports, Vivid's systems use dual-energy X-rays. Its checked-baggage systems were developed with BAA (formerly the British Airport Authority) after the 1988 bombing of Pan Am Flight 103 over Lockerbie, Scotland, essentially created the industry. The company works with Italian X-ray maker Gilardoni to make its carry-on-baggage inspection system. Vivid gets research money from the US government to design detection systems that meet FAA requirements.

Wang Laboratories, Inc.

600 Technology Park Dr., Billerica, MA 01821

Telephone: 978-967-5000 **Fax:** 978-625-5055 **Metro area:** Boston, MA **Web site:** http://www.wang.com **Human resources contact:** Albert A. Notini **Sales:** $1.9 billion **Number of employees:** 21,000 **Number of employees for previous year:** 9,300 **Industry designation:** Computers—services **Company type:** Public **Top competitors:** Hewlett-Packard Company; International Business Machines Corporation; Electronic Data Systems Corporation

Companies that need to combine a variety of computers, operating systems, and software applications turn to Wang Laboratories. The company is shedding its image as an old computer hardware manufacturer by focusing on system and telecommunications network integration and by providing IT services worldwide. Clients include multinational companies, institutions, and defense and civilian government agencies; the US government accounts for 20% of sales. To spread its network services skills, Wang has continued an acquisition strategy. Olivetti has a 16% stake in the company, and Microsoft owns 8%. To reflect its geographic growth, the company is operating as Wang Global and plans to make that moniker its legal name.

Waters Corporation

34 Maple St., Milford, MA 01757

Telephone: 508-478-2000 **Fax:** 508-482-3361 **Metro area:** Boston, MA **Web site:** http://www.waters.com **Human resources contact:** Brian K. Mazar **Sales:** $618.8 million **Number of employees:** 2,640 **Number of employees for previous year:** 1,865 **Industry designation:** Instruments—scientific **Company type:** Public **Top competitors:** The Perkin-Elmer Corporation; Thermo Electron Corporation

As a leading maker of high-performance liquid chromatography and thermal analysis instruments, Waters Corporation sells researchers, scientists, and engineers the tools to separate and identify 80% of all known chemicals and materials. Liquid chromatography instruments are used to develop new drugs, identify the nutritional content of food, and test air and water quality. Thermal analysis identifies physical characteristics of polymers. Waters' Micromass subsidiary makes mass spectrometers for use with liquid chromatography technologies. Pharmaceutical companies, universities, government agencies, and a wide range of industrial companies worldwide use Waters' products.

Wave Systems Corp.

480 Pleasant St., Lee, MA 01238

Telephone: 413-243-1600 **Fax:** 413-243-0045 **Metro area:** Pittsfield, MA **Web site:** http://www.wavesys.com **Human resources contact:** Lisa Dorris **Sales:** $1.5 million **Number of employees:** 80 **Number of employees for previous year:** 41 **Industry designation:** Computers—peripheral equipment **Company type:** Public **Top competitors:** America Online, Inc.; Rainbow Technologies, Inc.; Open Market, Inc.

Wave Systems surfs the Net for profit. The company's WaveMeter system monitors Internet hits, then uses that collected data to track credit and fees, manage decryption keys, and calculate royalties. Its customers include electronic content providers GT Interactive and Psygnosis. WaveMeter technology also enables secure online publishing and purchasing, and the company operates the Great Stuff Network, an online mall featuring books, games, graphics, and other digital products from suppliers like Monotype. Joint venture GlobalWave distributes Wave products in Europe and the Middle East. Peter Sprague, National Semiconductor's chairman for 30 years, is Wave's chairman and CEO.

ZipLink, Inc.

900 Chelmsford St., Tower One, 5th Fl., Lowell, MA 01851

Telephone: 978-551-8100 **Fax:** 978-551-2777 **Metro area:** Boston, MA **Web site:** http://www.ziplink.net **Human resources contact:** Joyce Moriarty **Sales:** $7.1 million (Est.) **Number of employees:** 54 **Industry designation:** Computers—online services **Company type:** Private **Top competitors:** Concentric Network Corporation; UUNET WorldCom; PSINet Inc.

The missing ZipLink of Internet access services for Internet appliances and Internet service providers (ISPs) has been found. ZipLink has 19 SuperPOPs (points of presence that allow unlimited local access numbers, expanding the network) in 16 large cities; traffic is routed over a 45-megabits-per-second backbone network. Offering wholesale dial-up services, ZipLink essentially acts as an ISP for ISPs that serve retail customers. ZipLink also provides service for Internet appliances (such as set-top boxes that provide Internet functions through a TV screen instead of a PC), including WebTV. The Zachs family and Northern Telecom own significant stakes in the company.

ZOLL Medical Corporation

32 Second Ave., Burlington, MA 01803

Telephone: 781-229-0020 **Fax:** 781-272-5578 **Metro area:** Boston, MA **Web site:** http://www.zoll.com/ **Human resources contact:** Maureen Callahan **Sales:** $55.1 million **Number of employees:** 375 **Number of employees for previous year:** 348 **Industry designation:** Medical instruments **Company type:** Public **Top competitors:** Laerdal Medical Corporation; Medtronic Physio-Control Inc.; Hewlett-Packard Company

ZOLL Medical makes noninvasive cardiac defibrillators and pacemakers for emergency resuscitation and heartbeat regulation. The devices are used by hospital staff and emergency personnel in the field. The company also makes disposable electrodes that permit defibrillation, pacing, and other uses through a single set of electrodes. Through subsidiary Westech Mobile Solutions, ZOLL also makes hardware and software for electronic data collection and billing by ambulance companies. While maintaining its domestic sales to hospitals, ZOLL has increased its sales to the international and first responder markets.

MICHIGAN

Aastrom Biosciences, Inc.

24 Frank Lloyd Wright Dr., Lobby L, Ann Arbor, MI 48105

Telephone: 734-930-5777 **Fax:** 734-665-0485 **Other address:** PO Box 376, Ann Arbor, MI 48106 **Metro area:** Detroit, MI **Web site:** http://www.aastrom.com **Human resources contact:** Emilie Stawiarski **Sales:** $200,000 **Number of employees:** 87 **Number of employees for previous year:** 72 **Industry designation:** Biomedical & genetic products **Company type:** Public **Top competitors:** Amgen Inc.; Novartis AG

Development-stage Aastrom Biosciences' automated cell therapy systems are designed to replace human cells damaged by cancer chemotherapy. Its AastromReplicell, a cell production system being tested for approval in the US and Europe, grows cells in laboratory conditions; these can be used to replace blood cells, bone marrow cells, and immune cells. The system is designed to be less costly, faster, and less invasive than such traditional cell-replacement methods as blood transfusions and bone marrow transplants. The company is also developing the Aastrom Gene Loader, through which therapeutic genes can be transferred into target cells. Cobe Laboratories, which owns 20% of Aastrom, will market the CPS worldwide.

American Dental Technologies, Inc.

28411 Northwestern Hwy., Ste. 1100, Southfield, MI 48034

Telephone: 248-395-3900 **Fax:** 248-395-3901 **Metro area:** Detroit, MI **Human resources contact:** Nancy Barron **Sales:** $28.3 million **Number of employees:** 118 **Number of employees for previous year:** 92 **Industry designation:** Medical products **Company type:** Public **Top competitors:** BioLase Technology, Inc.; Premier Laser Systems, Inc.

American Dental Technologies takes dentistry into high-tech. The company's PulseMaster dental laser performs surgery and other procedures on gums and teeth using pulses of laser energy delivered through flexible fiber-optics that can reach into difficult recesses. Other products include KPC (kinetic cavity preparation) systems—tools that remove tooth decay and surrounding structure with a narrow stream of alpha alumina particles propelled by compressed air. American Dental Technologies sells to general dental practitioners and specialists through independent dealers. The firm also makes precision air abrasive jet machining systems for industry.

Blue Cross Blue Shield of Michigan

600 E. Lafayette Blvd., Detroit, MI 48226

Telephone: 313-225-9000 **Fax:** 313-225-5629 **Metro area:** Detroit, MI **Web site:** http://www.bcbsm.com **Human resources contact:** George F. Francis III **Sales:** $7.7 billion **Number of employees:** 8,827 **Number of employees for previous year:** 7,980 **Industry designation:** Insurance—accident & health **Company type:** Not-for-profit **Top competitors:** PHP Healthcare Corporation; Aetna Inc.; Omnicare, Inc.

Blue Cross Blue Shield of Michigan (BCBSM) is one of the nation's top Blue Cross Blue Shield health insurance associations, serving more than 4.5 million members, including autoworkers for GM and Ford. BCBSM insurance plans include traditional indemnity, Blue Preferred (PPO), Blue Care Network (HMO), and Blue MedSave (medical savings plans). The company also offers workers compensation insurance, health assessment, and health care management services. BCBSM is pursuing additional revenue without having to alter its not-for-profit status. The purchase of Preferred Provider Organization of Michigan, a private health care manager operating in four states, is a part of this drive.

Cambridge Industries, Inc.

555 Horace Brown Dr., Madison Heights, MI 48071

Telephone: 248-616-0500 **Metro area:** Detroit, MI **Web site:** http://www.cambrinc.com **Human resources contact:** Alan M. Swiech **Sales:** $426.1 million (Est.) **Number of employees:** 4,207 **Industry designation:** Chemicals—plastics **Company type:** Private **Top competitors:** Magna International Inc.; United Technologies Corporation

Cambridge Industries manufactures plastic components for cars, pickups, and heavy trucks. The largest supplier of sheet-molding components in the US, it makes automotive products in three categories: exterior (fenders, spoilers, and hoods); structural/functional/powertrain (structural beams, fuel tank shields, and firewalls); and interior (liftgate and door trim panels, shift knobs, and glove compartment doors and assemblies). Its customers include Ford, Honda, Volkswagen, Kenworth, and Volvo Heavy Truck. The company has about 20 manufacturing facilities in Brazil, Canada, and the US. It has a joint venture with Mexican Industries of Michigan to make injection-molded interior systems and subsystems.

Caraco Pharmaceutical Laboratories, Ltd.

1150 Elijah McCoy Dr., Detroit, MI 48202

Telephone: 313-871-8400 **Fax:** 313-871-8314 **Metro area:** Detroit, MI **Web site:** http://www.caraco.com **Sales:** $871,000 **Number of employees:** 43 **Number of employees for previous year:** 32 **Industry designation:** Drugs—generic **Company type:** Public **Top competitors:** Halsey Drug Co., Inc.; Global Pharmaceutical Corporation; Xechem International, Inc.

Caraco Pharmaceutical Laboratories develops generic drugs for the prescription and over-the-counter markets. Caraco currently markets nine products primarily to drug wholesalers through agreements with other pharmaceutical companies. These products include nifedipine (made by R.P. Scherer for Caraco), metroprolol tartrate and paromomycin (originally made by Hexal-Pharma), and selegeline (developed by Caraco for Apotex). The company also has a development and marketing agreement with Clonmel Chemicals for a product awaiting FDA approval. Sun Pharmaceutical Industries, which has agreed to sell development and marketing rights for 25 products to Caraco, owns almost 40% of the company.

Championship Auto Racing Teams, Inc.

755 W. Big Beaver Rd., Ste. 800, Troy, MI 48084

Telephone: 248-362-8800 **Fax:** 248-362-8810 **Metro area:** Detroit, MI **Web site:** http://www.cart.com **Sales:** $62.5 million **Number of employees:** 79 **Number of employees for previous year:** 48 **Industry designation:** Leisure & recreational services **Company type:** Public **Top competitors:** Indy Racing League; National Association for Stock Car Auto Racing; Formula One

Championship Auto Racing Teams (CART) organizes, regulates, and sanctions 19 races for Indy Cars (high-performance, single-seat, open-wheeled race cars that can reach speeds of 240 mph). Sanction fees, paid by race promoters, account for more than half of CART's sales. CART team owners (who pick up expenses) include David Letterman, Paul Newman, and Walter Payton; drivers include Michael Andretti and Al Unser Jr. Most CART races are held in the US, but teams also race in Australia, Brazil, Canada, and Japan. In 1996 CART initiated the U.S. 500 to compete with the Indianapolis 500. A group of about 25 race team owners owns 68% of the company.

Chelsea Milling Company

201 W. North St., Chelsea, MI 48118

Telephone: 734-475-1361 **Fax:** 734-475-7577 **Other address:** PO Box 460, Chelsea, MI 48118 **Metro area:** Detroit, MI **Web site:** http://www.jiffymix.com **Human resources contact:** Patricia McGraw **Sales:** $100 million (Est.) **Number of employees:** 350 **Industry designation:** Food—flour & grain **Company type:** Private **Top competitors:** Aurora Foods Inc.; The Pillsbury Company; General Mills, Inc.

Chelsea Milling Company (CMC) gets you out of the kitchen in a "Jiffy." The family-owned and -run business makes 19 Jiffy-brand mixes for fruit, buttermilk, and cornbread muffins and biscuits; brownies; pizza and pie crusts; and frosting. The Holmes family runs a self-contained company: CMC stores wheat in its silos, mills flour and blends it with other ingredients, dispenses its products into 1.4 million boxes each day, and even does some of the transporting to the supermarkets around the US that sell its mixes. Shunning advertising, the company keeps prices at less than 50 cents a single-batch box. The family purchased the Chelsea mill in 1887; Mabel White Holmes created the first Jiffy mix in 1930.

Complete Business Solutions, Inc.

32605 W. Twelve Mile Rd., Ste. 250, Farmington Hills, MI 48334

Telephone: 248-488-2088 **Fax:** 248-488-2089 **Metro area:** Detroit, MI **Web site:** http://www.cbsinc.com **Human resources contact:** Nanjappa S. Venugopal **Sales:** $376.6 million **Number of employees:** 2,067 **Number of employees for previous year:** 1,632 **Industry designation:** Computers—services **Company type:** Public **Top competitors:** Andersen Consulting; Cap Gemini S.A.; International Business Machines Corporation

Complete Business Solutions, Inc. (CBSI) likes to finish what it starts. The company provides a variety of information technology services, including software development, year 2000 compliance, and contract programming, to customers such as Citibank, Ford, IBM, Southern California Edison, and the State of Michigan. Subsidiary CBS India provides low-cost support at two software development centers and a training center in India, and a branch in Singapore. President and CEO Rajendra Vattikuti owns about 35% of CBSI. The company is using acquisitions to strengthen its presence in the eastern and western US.

Country Fresh Inc.

2555 Buchanan Ave. SW, Grand Rapids, MI 49548

Telephone: 616-243-0173 **Fax:** 616-243-5926 **Metro area:** Grand Rapids, MI **Human resources contact:** Bill Reynolds **Sales:** $353 million **Number of employees:** 500 **Industry designation:** Food—dairy products **Company type:** Cooperative

Founded in 1946, Country Fresh processes and distributes dairy and juice products. Under regional brands such as Embest, McDonald Dairy, Frostbite Brands, and Southeastern Juice, the company sells dairy staples, fresh juices, and frozen desserts. In addition, Country Fresh has a licensing agreement with Smilk Inc. to produce and distribute Smilk (a fruit-flavored, nonfat milk for children). Country Fresh operates processing plants in Indiana, Michigan, Ohio, and Tennessee; it distributes its products throughout the Midwest and in Virginia. In 1997 the cooperative sold its operations for shares in dairy industry consolidator Suiza Foods.

Detrex Corporation

24901 Northwestern Hwy., Ste. 500, Southfield, MI 48075

Telephone: 248-358-5800 **Fax:** 248-358-5803 **Other address:** PO Box 5111, Southfield, MI 48086 **Metro area:** Detroit, MI **Web site:** http://www.detrex.com **Human resources contact:** Margie Limpert **Sales:** $86 million **Number of employees:** 366 **Number of employees for previous year:** 353 **Industry designation:** Chemicals—specialty **Company type:** Public

A specialty chemical company, Detrex produces cleaning solvents, lubricants, paints, and related products and services for the manufacturing and service industries. Its subsidiaries include Elco (lubricants), Siebert-Oxidermo (paints), and Harvel Plastics (PVC pipe). The company's chemical products and services account for more than 80% of sales; sales of chemical equipment make up the remainder. Detrex also recycles cleaning solvents and industrial wastes and designs and sells materials-handling equipment. About 12% of the company's sales are to customers outside the US.

Detroit Lions

1200 Featherstone Rd., Pontiac, MI 48342

Telephone: 248-335-4131 **Fax:** 248-335-1403 **Metro area:** Detroit, MI **Web site:** http://detroitlions.com **Human resources contact:** Cheryl Carrier **Sales:** $74.2 million (Est.) **Number of employees:** 142 **Industry designation:** Leisure & recreational services **Company type:** Private **Top competitors:** Tampa Bay Buccaneers; The Green Bay Packers, Inc.; Minnesota Vikings Football Club

As befits the Motor City, the Detroit Lions have a speedster in the backfield—Barry Sanders, winner of three National Football League (NFL) rushing titles. Despite Sanders' skills, the Lions haven't won an NFL title since 1957, and the team's last division title came in 1993. Team owner William Ford, grandson of automobile pioneer Henry Ford, overhauled his coaching staff in 1997 and brought in Bobby Ross to replace Wayne Fontes. Ross will have to work fast—Ford has announced he wants to win the Super Bowl. The team, founded in 1934, is getting a new domed stadium in downtown Detroit.

The Detroit Medical Center

Orchestra Place, 3663 Woodward Ave., Detroit, MI 48201

Telephone: 313-578-2000 **Fax:** 313-578-3990 **Metro area:** Detroit, MI **Web site:** http://www.dmc.org **Human resources contact:** Dan Zuhlke **Sales:** $1.4 billion **Number of employees:** 16,288 **Number of employees for previous year:** 13,879 **Industry designation:** Hospitals **Company type:** Not-for-profit **Top competitors:** Mercy Health Services; Henry Ford Health System; William Beaumont Hospital

The seeds for the Detroit Medical Center were planted in 1955, when four Detroit hospitals joined efforts to provide coordination between the hospitals and Wayne State University's medical school. Today the medical center (which became a nonprofit corporation in 1985) serves patients throughout southeast Michigan with about 3,000 health care facility beds and 3,300 physicians. The center is made up of eight hospitals, more than 100 outpatient facilities, and two nursing centers. The Detroit Medical Center is the teaching and clinical research site for Wayne State University; it is also allied with the Barbara Ann Karmanos Cancer Institute.

The Detroit Pistons Basketball Company

The Palace of Auburn Hills, Two Championship Dr., Auburn Hills, MI 48326

Telephone: 248-377-0100 **Fax:** 248-377-4262 **Metro area:** Detroit, MI **Web site:** http://www.nba.com/pistons **Human resources contact:** Bill Newton **Sales:** $85.9 million (Est.) **Number of employees:** 300 **Number of employees for previous year:** 250 **Industry designation:** Leisure & recreational services **Company type:** Private **Top competitors:** Charlotte Hornets; Pacers Basketball Corporation; Chicago Bulls

The Detroit Pistons is one of the oldest teams in the National Basketball Association (NBA). Founded in 1941 as the Fort Wayne (Indiana) Zollner Pistons by auto piston maker Fred Zollner, the team went on to become one of the perennial also-rans of its league. The team's move to Detroit in 1957 failed to improve its standing. After a brief flowering in the late 1980s, the team returned to its lackluster ways, despite the stalwart efforts of forward Grant Hill. The Pistons, one of the most valuable teams in the NBA, is owned by an investment group led by William Davidson, billionaire CEO of Guardian Industries. The group also owns the team's playing venue, the Palace Sports and Entertainment arena.

Detroit Red Wings

Joe Louis Arena, 600 Civic Center Dr., Detroit, MI 48226

Telephone: 313-396-7544 **Fax:** 313-567-0296 **Metro area:** Detroit, MI **Web site:** http://www.detroitredwings.com/wings.html **Human resources contact:** Linda Vivian **Sales:** $80.1 million (Est.) **Number of employees:** 120 **Industry designation:** Leisure & recreational services **Company type:** Private **Top competitors:** Chicago Blackhawk Hockey Team, Inc.; St. Louis Blues Hockey Club L.L.C.; Nashville Predators

Founded in 1926 as the Cougars, the Detroit Red Wings are one of the oldest teams still playing in the NHL. The team boasts such greats as Gordie Howe (who played until he was 52) and current captain Steve Yzerman, the team's leader for more than a decade. Fans in Detroit are known for throwing the occasional octopus onto the ice; the custom started in the 1950s, when teams needed only eight wins in two playoff rounds to win the championship (thus the octopus, with eight legs). The Red Wings have won nine Stanley Cup titles, including 1997 and 1998. Mike Ilitch, who also owns the Detroit Tigers baseball team and Little Caesar Enterprises, bought the team in 1982.

Detroit Tigers, Inc.

2121 Trumbull Ave., Detroit, MI 48216

Telephone: 313-962-4000 **Fax:** 313-965-2138 **Metro area:** Detroit, MI **Web site:** http://www.detroittigers.com **Human resources contact:** Lara Baremor **Sales:** $50.6 million (Est.) **Number of employees:** 82 **Industry designation:** Leisure & recreational services **Company type:** Private **Top competitors:** Kansas City Royals Baseball Corporation; Chicago White Sox Ltd.; Cleveland Indians Baseball Company, Inc.

One of the American League's (AL) original baseball clubs, the Detroit Tigers first hit the field in 1901. In the decades since, it has become the AL's second-winningest team (behind the New York Yankees) and been home to baseball luminaries such as Ty Cobb and Hughie Jennings. Detroit's Tiger Stadium, which opened in 1912 as Navin Field, is also one of the oldest major league ballparks. The stadium will be replaced by Comercia Park, scheduled for completion in 2000. The new stadium will increase overall attendance and give the team new income from the sale of luxury suits. The club is owned by Michael Ilitch, who also owns the Detroit Red Wings hockey team and Little Caesar Enterprises.

Eltrax Systems, Inc.

2000 Town Center., Ste. 690, Southfield, MI 48075

Telephone: 248-358-1699 **Fax:** 248-358-2743 **Metro area:** Detroit, MI **Web site:** http://www.eltrax.com **Human resources contact:** John Lamirande **Sales:** $50.7 million **Number of employees:** 300 **Number of employees for previous year:** 155 **Industry designation:** Computers—services **Company type:** Public

Eltrax Systems designs, installs, and monitors computer network systems for corporate and government customers. The company buys the modems, routers, switches, and other network products it installs from manufacturers such as ADTRAN, Motorola, and 3Com. Sales efforts by Eltrax Systems include hosting technical seminars, attending trade shows, publishing newsletters, and conducting direct mailings. The company started as an X-ray imaging and electronic information card business, but it has jettisoned those pursuits to enter the network systems market. Customers include businesses and government agencies with employees who telecommute. Eltrax's 1999 purchase of Sulcus Hospitality Technologies doubles its size.

Guardian Industries Corp.

2300 Harmon Rd., Auburn Hills, MI 48326

Telephone: 248-340-1800 **Fax:** 248-340-9988 **Metro area:** Detroit, MI **Web site:** http://www.guardian.com **Human resources contact:** Bruce Cummings **Sales:** $2 billion (Est.)
Number of employees: 14,000 **Number of employees for previous year:** 13,000 **Industry designation:** Glass products **Company type:** Private **Top competitors:** Owens Corning; Asahi Glass Company, Limited; PPG Industries, Inc.

Giving its customers a break never would occur to Guardian Industries, the world's fourth-largest glassmaker. With facilities in 15 countries on five continents, Guardian primarily produces float glass and fabricated glass products for the automobile and construction markets. It also makes architectural glass and fiberglass insulation. President and CEO William Davidson owns the Detroit Pistons basketball team and, like the Pistons, has a reputation for playing rough—using such tactics as hiring top people away from rivals and aggressively copying the glassmaking technology of competitors. Davidson's family founded the company in 1932. He took it public in 1968 and in 1985 bought it back for himself.

HDS Services

33469 Fourteen Mile Rd., Farmington Hills, MI 48331

Telephone: 248-324-9500 **Fax:** 248-324-1825 **Metro area:** Detroit, MI **Web site:** http://www.hdsservices.com **Human resources contact:** Judith Simmons **Sales:** $171 million (Est.)
Number of employees: 600 **Industry designation:** Leisure & recreational services **Company type:** Private **Top competitors:** ARAMARK Corporation; Sodexho Marriott Services, Inc.; Compass Group PLC

Whether you live to eat or eat to live, HDS Services prides itself on serving up a pleasant dining experience. Founded in 1965 by owner William Triplett, HDS originally provided food service management to hospitals. It has since expanded its customer base to include long-term health facilities, retirement centers, schools, corporations, and clubs and resorts throughout the US. Its food management services include customized dining room and cafeteria management, special event catering, a line of prewrapped foods, and fresh-baked goods. In addition, the company's McVety & Associates division provides consulting services to other food service operators.

Key Plastics, Inc.

21333 Haggerty Rd., Ste. 200, Novi, MI 48375

Telephone: 248-449-6100 **Fax:** 248-449-6199 **Metro area:** Detroit, MI **Web site:** http://www.keyplastics.com **Human resources contact:** Richard J. Blough **Sales:** $371.5 million (Est.)
Number of employees: 5,000 **Number of employees for previous year:** 3,730 **Industry designation:** Chemicals—plastics **Company type:** Private **Top competitors:** Lear Corporation; Donnelly Corporation; United Technologies Corporation

If you unlock Key Plastics, you'll find a company that designs and manufactures plastic parts for cars and trucks around the world. The company operates 14 manufacturing plants and two paint facilities in North America; it also has three dual-purpose facilities in Europe. Key Plastics' products include door handles, radio bezels, and speaker grilles. The company's major customers are Ford, General Motors, DaimlerChrysler, and suppliers to these carmakers; together they make up about 80% of sales. Company founders David Benoit, George Mars, and Joel Tauber own more than half of Key Plastics. (Benoit is CEO; the other two are directors.) Other employees own the rest of the 30-year-old company.

McClain Industries, Inc.

6200 Elmridge Rd., Sterling Heights, MI 48310

Telephone: 810-264-3611 **Fax:** 810-264-7191 **Metro area:** Detroit, MI **Human resources contact:** Carl Jaworski **Sales:** $116.6 million **Number of employees:** 810 **Number of employees for previous year:** 740 **Industry designation:** Pollution control equipment & services **Company type:** Public **Top competitors:** Standard Automotive Corporation; Waste Technology Corp.; Dover Corporation

McClain Industries helps to haul it away with dump-truck bodies and solid-waste-handling equipment that it makes at plants in Alabama, Georgia, Michigan, Ohio, and Oklahoma. Through subsidiaries including Galion and E-Z Pack, it produces baling equipment, transfer trailers, sludge and detachable roll-off containers, compactors, and bodies for garbage and recycling trucks. It sells to distributors and solid-waste-handling companies such as Waste Management. The company also operates a steel-tube mill and processes and warehouses steel products. McClain Industries sells through its own sales subsidiary and independent dealers. CEO Kenneth McClain and SVP Robert McClain own about 31% and 24% of the company, respectively.

Mechanical Dynamics, Inc.

2301 Commonwealth Blvd., Ann Arbor, MI 48105

Telephone: 734-994-3800 **Fax:** 734-994-6418 **Metro area:** Detroit, MI **Web site:** http://www.adams.com **Human resources contact:** Linda Moore **Sales:** $36.6 million **Number of employees:** 283 **Number of employees for previous year:** 234 **Industry designation:** Computers—engineering, scientific & CAD-CAM software **Company type:** Public **Top competitors:** Engineering Animation, Inc.; The MacNeal-Schwendler Corporation; 3D Systems Corporation

Mechanical Dynamics, Inc. (MDI) is an integrated manufacturer of virtual prototyping software. Its products allow engineers and designers to visually and mathematically simulate prototypes—a measure that reduces the need for building test models and the time it takes to get products to market. MDI markets primarily to automobile manufacturers and their suppliers; Ford accounts for about 10% of its revenues. MDI's products include ADAMS/Solver (to solve equations of motion), ADAMS/View (interactive graphics software), and ADAMS/Vehicle (for simulating full vehicle dynamics). The company, which operates in Asia, Europe, and North America, also provides consulting, training, and technical support services.

Michigan Milk Producers Association

41310 Bridge St., Novi, MI 48376

Telephone: 248-474-6672 **Fax:** 248-474-0924 **Other address:** PO Box 8002, Novi, MI 48376 **Metro area:** Detroit, MI **Web site:** http://www.mimilk.com **Human resources contact:** Cindy Tilden **Sales:** $444 million **Number of employees:** 190 **Industry designation:** Food—dairy products **Company type:** Cooperative **Top competitors:** Land O'Lakes, Inc.; Dean Foods Company; Dairy Farmers of America

Ice cream and other dairy products might lack a key ingredient without Michigan Milk Producers Association (MMPA). The dairy cooperative serves nearly 3,000 farmers in Michigan, Ohio, Indiana, and Wisconsin, producing a variety of milks (standardized, skim, sweet condensed, instant nonfat, dried whole), dried sweet and standardized cream, and ice-cream mixes. MMPA sells its products as ingredients to food manufacturers across the US, mainly in the Midwest, who make baby formulas, candy, ice cream, and yogurt. It does not sell directly to consumers. The co-op, founded in 1916, operates two Michigan plants and provides its farmer-members with product quality incentives and training as well as customized blending.

Miller Exploration Company

3104 Logan Valley Rd., Traverse City, MI 49685

Telephone: 616-941-0004 **Fax:** 616-941-8312 **Web site:** http://www.mexp.com **Human resources contact:** Vicki Schuch **Sales:** $7.4 million **Number of employees:** 32 **Number of employees for previous year:** 18 **Industry designation:** Oil & gas—exploration & production **Company type:** Public **Top competitors:** Denbury Resources Inc.; National Energy Group, Inc.; Clayton Williams Energy, Inc.

Producing oil and gas from salt domes is thirsty work, but it's always Miller time in the Mississippi Salt Basin, where Miller Exploration owns 22 prospects. The company, which has estimated proved reserves of 51 billion cu. ft. of natural gas and one million barrels of oil, uses 3D seismic data analysis and imaging in its exploration efforts. Miller also operates in the onshore Gulf Coast regions of Texas and Louisiana (on 7 prospects), and in the Michigan Basin (where it has interests in 300 producing wells). The company's Michigan Basin operations consist primarily of long-lived, lower-volume Antrim Shale production.

National TechTeam, Inc.

835 Mason St., Ste. 200, Dearborn, MI 48124

Telephone: 313-277-2277 **Fax:** 313-277-6409 **Metro area:** Detroit, MI **Web site:** http://www.techteam.com **Human resources contact:** Victoria Neville **Sales:** $117.5 million **Number of employees:** 1,904 **Number of employees for previous year:** 1,294 **Industry designation:** Computers—services **Company type:** Public **Top competitors:** The Capita Group Plc; Unisys Corporation; Metro Information Services, Inc.

National TechTeam provides a variety of computer support services to international corporate clientele. Its call center services (about 45% of sales) primarily involve technical support and product information. The company's corporate computer services include technical staffing (about 30% of sales), software training, application development, contract programming, networking, design, and systems integration (about 15%). National TechTeam also leases and finances high-tech equipment in the US and Canada. Hewlett-Packard and Ford each account for about 20% of sales.

Neogen Corporation

620 Lesher Place, Lansing, MI 48912

Telephone: 517-372-9200 **Fax:** 517-372-0108 **Metro area:** Lansing, MI **Web site:** http://www.neogen.com **Human resources contact:** Lon M. Bohannon **Sales:** $18.5 million **Number of employees:** 210 **Number of employees for previous year:** 186 **Industry designation:** Medical products **Company type:** Public **Top competitors:** Meridian Diagnostics, Inc.; The Perkin-Elmer Corporation; IDEXX Laboratories, Inc.

Bacteriophobes have a friend in Neogen, a maker and distributor of more than 140 diagnostic test kits for the food safety, animal health, pharmacology, and agricultural markets. Its single-use kits are used by the food industry to detect such food-borne bacteria as "E. coli," listeria, and salmonella; Neogen tests also check for pesticide residue and naturally occurring toxins. Other kits ferret out hormones, steroid residues, plant diseases, and sexually transmitted diseases. Diagnostic products account for about 80% of sales. Subsidiary Ideal Instruments sells a line of more than 250 veterinary instruments and drug delivery systems for animals. Neogen has more than 2,000 customers in more than 75 countries.

Newstar Resources Inc.

104 W. Front St., Monroe, MI 48161

Telephone: 734-243-0719 **Fax:** 734-243-5503 **Other address:** PO Box 1306, Monroe, MI 48161 **Metro area:** Detroit, MI **Web site:** http://www.newstarresources.com **Sales:** $5.8 million **Number of employees:** 25 **Industry designation:** Oil & gas—exploration & production **Company type:** Public

Newstar Resources acquires, explores for, and develops oil and gas reserves. Its subsidiary, Newstar Energy USA, has wells in Ohio and Michigan that produce more than 5,000 barrels of oil equivalent daily. The northern locale of those fields allows the company to sell directly to local markets, where it enjoys slightly higher market prices. Newstar Energy also explores for oil and gas reserves in Texas, Michigan, and Louisiana. The company plans to tap oil deposits beneath Lake Michigan from drilling operations on the shoreline—a controversial project that was recently approved by Michigan's Department of Environmental Quality.

Penske Motorsports, Inc.

13400 Outer Dr. West, Detroit, MI 48239

Telephone: 313-592-5000 **Fax:** 313-592-7332 **Metro area:** Detroit, MI **Web site:** http://www.penskemotorsports.com **Sales:** $116.9 million **Number of employees:** 175 **Number of employees for previous year:** 163 **Industry designation:** Leisure & recreational services **Company type:** Public **Top competitors:** Dover Downs Entertainment, Inc.; Speedway Motorsports, Inc.; International Speedway Corporation

A leading US promoter and marketer of professional motorsports, Penske Motorsports owns and operates four motor speedways: the Michigan Speedway, the North Carolina Speedway, the Nazareth Speedway (Pennsylvania), and the California Speedway, which conduct NASCAR and Indy car races. The company also owns 45% of the Homestead-Miami Speedway in Florida. Penske Motorsports makes and markets motor sports-related apparel, souvenirs, and collectibles through subsidiary Motorsports International, and distributes Goodyear racing tires through Competition Tire subsidiaries. Race car legend and chairman Roger Penske owns about 55% of the company.

Perrigo Company

515 Eastern Ave., Allegan, MI 49010

Telephone: 616-673-8451 **Fax:** 616-673-9328 **Metro area:** Kalamazoo, MI **Web site:** http://www.perrigo.com **Human resources contact:** Mike Stewart **Sales:** $902.6 million **Number of employees:** 4,868 **Number of employees for previous year:** 4,122 **Industry designation:** Drugs **Company type:** Public **Top competitors:** The Procter & Gamble Company; Bristol-Myers Squibb Company; Johnson & Johnson

If you're buying a private-label personal care product at Wal-Mart or Kroger, chances are you're buying something made by Perrigo. The nation's largest manufacturer of over-the-counter pharmaceuticals and personal care products for the store-brand market, Perrigo makes products that use knockoff packaging and discount pricing to compete with leading national brands. It makes some 1,300 products—including pain relievers, cough and cold remedies, dental care, deodorant, hair care, baby care products, nutritional supplements, and vitamins—for retailers such as Wal-Mart (24% of sales), CVS, Target, and Kmart and for wholesalers such as Topco and McKesson HBOC.

Rockwell Medical Technologies, Inc.

28025 Oakland Oaks Dr., Wixom, MI 48393

Telephone: 248-449-3353 **Fax:** 248-449-3363 **Metro area:** Detroit, MI **Sales:** $5.3 million **Number of employees:** 50 **Number of employees for previous year:** 41 **Industry designation:** Medical products **Company type:** Public **Top competitors:** Minntech Corporation; Fresenius Medical Care Aktiengesellschaft; Gambro AB

Rockwell Medical Technologies rocks on. The company makes hemodialysis concentrates, dialysis kits, and other hemodialysis products. Subsidiary Rockwell Transportation delivers supplies to customers via a fleet of nine trucks. The company directly markets and distributes its products to hemodialysis providers in the US and Venezuela, as well as through sales representatives and independent distributors. Rockwell Medical plans to become a one-stop source for hemodialysis providers by offering more than 120 concentrates, chemicals, and hemodialysis supplies. The company was formed to acquire the assets of the heavily indebted Rockwell Medical Supplies and its delivery operation Rockwell Transportation.

R.P. Scherer Corporation

2301 W. Big Beaver Rd., Troy, MI 48084

Telephone: 248-649-0900 **Fax:** 248-649-2079 **Metro area:** Detroit, MI **Web site:** http://www.rpscherer.com **Human resources contact:** Sherryl Shewach **Sales:** $620.7 million **Number of employees:** 3,600 **Number of employees for previous year:** 3,500 **Industry designation:** Medical products **Company type:** Public **Top competitors:** Elan Corporation, plc; ALZA Corporation; Abbott Laboratories

Cardinal Health subsidiary R.P. Scherer is the world's top maker of softgels used to encase drugs and vitamins. The company also develops and markets other drug delivery systems, including hard-shell capsules and freeze-dried wafers that dissolve on the tongue. Softgel products account for about 90% of sales. R.P. Scherer's business is not all drugs—the company also uses its softgel process for paint balls, skin care products, and bath beads. The firm has operations in the US and 11 other countries (international sales are about 70% of total). The Food and Drug Administration has approved the Zydis form of Schering-Plough's Claritin (allergy medicine).

Sisters of St. Joseph Health System

455 E. Eisenhower Pkwy., Ste. 300, Ann Arbor, MI 48108

Telephone: 734-741-1700 **Fax:** 734-741-5796 **Metro area:** Detroit, MI **Web site:** http://www.ssjhs.org/ssjhs.html **Human resources contact:** Elizabeth Veenhuis **Sales:** $1.5 billion **Number of employees:** 22,000 **Number of employees for previous year:** 18,700 **Industry designation:** Hospitals **Company type:** Not-for-profit **Top competitors:** Mercy Health Services; Henry Ford Health System; The Detroit Medical Center

Sisters of St. Joseph Health System, owned by Sisters of St. Joseph of Nazareth (established in 1889), is the largest health care corporation in Michigan. It has four regional health divisions: Detroit's St. John Health System, Flint's Genesys Health System, Kalamazoo's Borgess Health Alliance, and Tawas City's St. Joseph Health Services of Northeastern Michigan. In addition, the Catholic health provider distributes medical equipment and supplies (St. Joseph Health Enterprises) and provides medical treatment at its various home health centers, nursing homes, outpatient surgery centers, mental health hospitals, and substance-abuse facilities.

SofTech, Inc.

4695 44th St. SE, Ste. B-130, Grand Rapids, MI 49512

Telephone: 616-957-2330 **Fax:** 616-956-0077 **Metro area:** Grand Rapids, MI **Web site:** http:// www.softech.com **Human resources contact:** Randy Rand **Sales:** $20 million **Number of employees:** 214 **Number of employees for previous year:** 102 **Industry designation:** Computers—services **Company type:** Public **Top competitors:** Unigraphics Solutions Inc.; Parametric Technology Corporation; Autodesk, Inc.

SofTech adds a gentle touch to CAD design. The company, which previously sold and supported Parametric Technology products, has used acquisitions to grow into a provider of 2-D computer aided design (CAD) and manufacturing (CAM) products and related services. Its Advanced Manufacturing Technology (AMT) division makes the Prospector (mold making) and ToolMaker (tool design) software lines. Subsidiary Adra Systems offers the Cadra family of software, which automates CAD and CAM functions from the design stage through manufacturing. SofTech's services include consulting, engineering, integration, staff placement, and training.

Somanetics Corporation

1653 E. Maple Rd., Troy, MI 48083

Telephone: 248-689-3050 **Fax:** 248-689-4272 **Metro area:** Detroit, MI **Web site:** http://www.somanetics.com **Human resources contact:** Mary Ann Victor **Sales:** $2.5 million **Number of employees:** 46 **Number of employees for previous year:** 41 **Industry designation:** Medical instruments **Company type:** Public **Top competitors:** Protocol Systems, Inc.; Invivo Corporation; Respironics, Inc.

Somanetics sells a window to the brain known as the INVOS Cerebral Oximeter. The device offers a noninvasive method of monitoring blood-oxygen levels in the brain. Based on its in vivo optical spectroscopy (INVOS) technology, the Cerebral Oximeter's SomaSensors attach to each side of the patient's forehead, and the company's proprietary software displays oxygen levels on a computer screen. Somanetics markets to surgeons, anesthesiologists, and other health care providers through a direct sales force and independent distributors in the US and in more than 50 foreign countries. The company is developing a version of the Cerebral Oximeter for children and plans to license its technology to other manufacturers.

Stryker Corporation

2725 Fairfield Rd., Kalamazoo, MI 49002

Telephone: 616-385-2600 **Fax:** 616-385-1062 **Other address:** PO Box 4085, Kalamazoo, MI 49003 **Metro area:** Kalamazoo, MI **Web site:** http://www.strykercorp.com **Human resources contact:** David Huisjen **Sales:** $1.1 billion **Number of employees:** 10,974 **Number of employees for previous year:** 5,691 **Industry designation:** Medical instruments **Company type:** Public **Top competitors:** Pfizer Inc; Bristol-Myers Squibb Company; DePuy, Inc.

Is this an operating room or Dad's workshop? Stryker's line of surgical equipment includes power instruments like drills, saws, drill bits, rasps, and even cement mixers sold under the Stryker, Dimso, and Osteonics names. Surgical products, including endoscopy diagnostic and surgical instruments and joint implants, account for about 75% of sales. The company also makes stretchers and hospital beds and provides rehabilitation services (Physiotherapy Associates). Stryker subsidiaries include Howmedica (it bought the #3 maker of reconstructive instruments from Pfizer) and 75%-owned Matsumoto Medical Instruments, which distributes products by Stryker and other makers in Japan.

Versus Technology, Inc.

2600 Miller Creek Rd., Traverse City, MI 49684

Telephone: 616-946-5868 **Fax:** 616-946-6775 **Web site:** http://www.versustech.com **Human resources contact:** Andrea Beadle **Sales:** $3.2 million **Number of employees:** 36 **Number of employees for previous year:** 33 **Industry designation:** Computers—engineering, scientific & CAD-CAM software **Company type:** Public **Top competitors:** EXECUTONE Information Systems, Inc.

You're bound to lose a game of hide-and-seek versus Versus Technology. The company sells infrared location tracking systems and cellular products, mainly to the health care sector. The systems enable remote monitoring of patients and equipment, restrict access to secured sites, and allow two-way cellular communication. Potential markets for its infrared tracking systems include prisons, schools, and government buildings. Through its Olmsted Engineering subsidiary, Versus makes the ACUCARV suite of CAD/CAM software for controlling industrial machines that make molds, dies, and patterns.

William Beaumont Hospital

3601 W. 13 Mile Rd., Royal Oak, MI 48073

Telephone: 248-551-5000 **Fax:** 248-551-1555 **Metro area:** Detroit, MI **Web site:** http://www.beaumont.edu **Human resources contact:** Wesley Kokko **Sales:** $794.1 million (Est.) **Number of employees:** 10,700 **Number of employees for previous year:** 7,680 **Industry designation:** Hospitals **Company type:** Private **Top competitors:** The Detroit Medical Center; Henry Ford Health System; Mercy Health Services

William Beaumont Hospital consists of two teaching hospitals, both ranked among the busiest in the US for inpatient admissions. It also includes medical buildings, a rehabilitation center, a primary health care clinic, five nursing homes, a research institute, and a comprehensive home care service, all serving the Detroit area. A number of special programs are available, including the Preventative and Nutritional Medicine Clinic for treatment of obesity and related illnesses, an eating-disorders treatment facility, and InterHealth, a health service for international travelers. The Michigan hospitals, one in Royal Oak and the other in Troy, are affiliated with Wayne State University.

Wolverine Packing Company

1340 Winder, Detroit, MI 48207

Telephone: 313-259-7500 **Fax:** 313-568-1909 **Metro area:** Detroit, MI **Web site:** http://www.wolverinepacking.com **Human resources contact:** Denise Goodrich **Sales:** $300 Million (Est.) **Number of employees:** 150 **Industry designation:** Food—meat products **Company type:** Private **Top competitors:** IBP, inc.; Rosen's Diversified, Inc.; ConAgra, Inc.

If Mary lost her little lamb anywhere near Detroit, it probably ended up at Wolverine Packing. The wholesale meat packer and distributor slaughters, processes, trims, and packs veal and lamb. Wolverine Packing also sells frozen beef, pork, lamb, veal, and poultry to retailers and to the food service industry, including schools. The company's distribution division offers next-day delivery of frozen, fresh, and processed meats. Wolverine markets its veal as Bonnie Maid Premium Veal. The company was founded in 1937 and has operations in Detroit's Eastern Market district. CEO Jim Bonahoom owns the company.

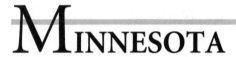

MINNESOTA

Allina Health System

5601 Smetana Dr., Minnetonka, MN 55343

Telephone: 612-992-2000 **Fax:** 612-992-2126 **Other address:** PO Box 9310, Minneapolis, MN 55440 **Metro area:** Minneapolis-St. Paul, MN **Web site:** http://www.allina.com **Human resources contact:** Mike Howe **Sales:** $2.5 billion **Number of employees:** 21,200 **Number of employees for previous year:** 20,800 **Industry designation:** Hospitals **Company type:** Not-for-profit **Top competitors:** Columbia/HCA Healthcare Corporation; Mayo Foundation; SSM Health Care System Inc.

Allina Health System is a not-for-profit health care system that focuses on prevention and community programs as an alternative means of keeping its members healthy. Allina's health plans, doctors, and hospitals cover Minnesota, North and South Dakota, and Wisconsin. The system's Medica Health Plans, which serves more than one million members, offers HMO, PPO, and senior health plans through a network of more than 12,000 health care providers. The Allina Medical Group includes more than 50 clinics. Allina also owns or manages nearly 20 hospitals, seven nursing homes, and a senior housing complex.

American Crystal Sugar Company

101 N. Third St., Moorhead, MN 56560

Telephone: 218-236-4400 **Fax:** 218-236-4422 **Metro area:** Fargo-Moorhead, ND **Web site:** http://www.crystalsugar.com **Human resources contact:** David A. Berg **Sales:** $676.6 million **Number of employees:** 1,263 **Number of employees for previous year:** 1,202 **Industry designation:** Food—sugar & refining **Company type:** Cooperative **Top competitors:** United States Sugar Corp.; Imperial Sugar Company; Tate & Lyle PLC

Call it saccharine, but for American Crystal Sugar, business is all about sharing. A cooperative, the sugar-beet giant is owned by about 2,800 growers in the Red River Valley of North Dakota and Minnesota. American Crystal, formed in 1899 and converted into a co-op in 1973, divides the 35-mile-wide valley into five districts, each served by a processing plant. During an annual eight-month "campaign," the plants operate continuously, turning beets into sugar, molasses, and beet pulp. The products (under the Crystal brand name and the licensed Pillsbury Best label) are sold through marketing co-ops United Sugars and Midwest Agri-Commodities. The cooperative owns 46% of ProGold, a corn-sweeteners joint venture.

Analysts International Corporation

7615 Metro Blvd., Minneapolis, MN 55439

Telephone: 612-835-5900 **Fax:** 612-897-4555 **Metro area:** Minneapolis-St. Paul, MN **Web site:** http://www.analysts.com **Human resources contact:** Lori Buegler **Sales:** $587.4 million **Number of employees:** 5,300 **Number of employees for previous year:** 4,650 **Industry designation:** Computers—services **Company type:** Public **Top competitors:** Computer Task Group, Incorporated; Keane, Inc.; Andersen Consulting

Feeling outsmarted by your computer network? Analysts International Corporation (AiC) provides a wide variety of programming and software. The company offers custom programming, project management, systems analysis and design, software-related consulting, year 2000 software remediation, and specialized training. AiC's TechWest division, which has grown rapidly since its inception, provides technical outsourcing (both staff and software) to corporations such as U S WEST (20% of sales), IBM (more than 15%), and Motorola. AiC has about 45 branch and field offices located throughout the US and in Canada and the UK.

Angeion Corporation

7601 Northland Dr., Brooklyn Park, MN 55428

Telephone: 612-315-2000 **Fax:** 612-315-2099 **Metro area:** Minneapolis-St. Paul, MN **Web site:** http://www.angeion.com **Human resources contact:** Robert S. Garin **Sales:** $4.6 million **Number of employees:** 238 **Number of employees for previous year:** 199 **Industry designation:** Medical products **Company type:** Public

Angeion's medical products treat irregular heartbeats. The products—implantable cardioverter defibrillators (ICDs) and radio-frequency catheter ablation systems (RFCAs)—have premarket approval in the US. ICDs treat rapid beating in the lower chambers of the heart, delivering a shock when an aberrant rhythm is detected. When rapid beating occurs in the heart's upper chambers, RFCAs may be an alternative to invasive surgery. The catheter is guided into the heart, where energy zaps the affected tissue. French pharmaceutical firm Synthelabo (which owns about 20% of Angeion) markets Angeion's products in Europe and Japan; joint venture ELA*Angeion markets ICDs in the US.

Apogee Enterprises, Inc.

7900 Xerxes Ave. South, Ste. 1800, Minneapolis, MN 55431

Telephone: 612-835-1874 **Fax:** 612-835-3196 **Metro area:** Minneapolis-St. Paul, MN **Human resources contact:** Warren Planitzer **Sales:** $912.8 million **Number of employees:** 6,672 **Number of employees for previous year:** 6,553 **Industry designation:** Glass products **Company type:** Public **Top competitors:** Safelite AutoGlass Corp.; PPG Industries, Inc.; Corning Incorporated

Getting cracked up over the glass business, Apogee Enterprises makes glass products for the commercial, automotive, and construction markets. The company's auto glass segment encompasses about 340 Harmon AutoGlass service centers in 43 states, more than 70 wholesale Glass Depot centers, and windshield maker Curvlite. Its glass technologies segment makes specialized coated glass for items including antiglare computer monitors and energy efficient windows for high-rise structures. The building products and services segment makes specialized coated glass and metal building exteriors, called curtainwall. The family of longtime Apogee leader Russell Baumgardner owns about 8% of the company.

Appliance Recycling Centers of America, Inc.

7400 Excelsior Blvd., Minneapolis, MN 55426

Telephone: 612-930-9000 **Fax:** 612-930-1800 **Metro area:** Minneapolis-St. Paul, MN **Human resources contact:** Cindy Janzig **Sales:** $12 million **Number of employees:** 158 **Number of employees for previous year:** 157 **Industry designation:** Pollution control equipment & services **Company type:** Public

Wanna make that old refrigerator disappear? Appliance Recycling Centers of America will retrieve it, recycle it, and maybe even recondition it to sell to someone else. The company offers environmentally sound recycling of household appliances for appliance retailers, waste and property management companies, and utilities (although electric utility deregulation has put a damper on that segment). The company sells reconditioned appliances at its Encore Recycled Appliances stores in California, Minnesota, Missouri, and Ohio. It has reclamation contracts with utility Southern California Edison (which accounts for about 40% of sales) and Whirlpool. Chairman and CEO Edward Cameron owns 26% of the company.

ATS Medical, Inc.

3905 Annapolis Ln., Minneapolis, MN 55447

Telephone: 612-553-7736 **Fax:** 612-553-1492 **Metro area:** Minneapolis-St. Paul, MN **Web site:** http://www.atsmedical.com **Human resources contact:** Marge McCardle **Sales:** $18 million **Number of employees:** 74 **Number of employees for previous year:** 62 **Industry designation:** Medical instruments **Company type:** Public **Top competitors:** Medtronic, Inc.; St. Jude Medical, Inc.; Baxter International Inc.

ATS Medical makes mechanical heart valves sold outside the US. It touts its ATS Open Pivot valve as an improvement over other pyrolytic carbon valves in several measures, including lower noise levels, improved implantability, increased X-ray visibility, improved blood flow, and reduced risk of blood clots. ATS Medical sells to about 30 independent distributors in more than 40 countries, including Japan and the European Union nations. The company is conducting clinical trials required for FDA approval in the US. It is also seeking authorization to sell the valve in Australia and Canada.

Bio-Vascular, Inc.

2575 University Ave., St. Paul, MN 55114

Telephone: 651-603-3700 **Fax:** 651-642-9018 **Metro area:** Minneapolis-St. Paul, MN **Web site:** http://www.biovascular.com **Human resources contact:** Gail Kaleta **Sales:** $12 million **Number of employees:** 175 **Number of employees for previous year:** 94 **Industry designation:** Medical products **Company type:** Public **Top competitors:** Baxter International Inc.; W. L. Gore and Associates, Inc.; Medtronic, Inc.

The next time you have open heart surgery, don't be surprised if you feel the need to moo. Using collagen derived from the lining of cows' hearts, Bio-Vascular makes Tissue-Guard products for use in cardiac, neurological, ophthalmic, thoracic, and vascular surgery. These products help reconstruct, reinforce, and repair tissue and prevent blood, other bodily fluids, and air from leaking following surgery. In addition to its patches and stapling buttresses, Bio-Vascular makes a line of blood occluders and stents, as well as arterial blockage probes. Through its Jer-Neen Manufacturing subsidiary, the company makes wire components for medical devices and procedures. Bio-Vascular's products are sold around the world.

Canterbury Park Holding Corporation

1100 Canterbury Rd., Shakopee, MN 55379

Telephone: 612-445-7223 **Fax:** 612-496-6400 **Other address:** PO Box 508, Shakopee, MN 55379 **Metro area:** Minneapolis-St. Paul, MN **Web site:** http://www.canterburypark.com **Human resources contact:** Mary Fleming **Sales:** $19.2 million **Number of employees:** 205 **Number of employees for previous year:** 195 **Industry designation:** Leisure & recreational services **Company type:** Public **Top competitors:** Minnesota Vikings Football Club; Lakes Gaming, Inc.; Minnesota Twins

Pilgrimages to this Canterbury involve tales of big scores and lost glory at the track. Canterbury Park Holding owns Canterbury Park in Shakopee, Minnesota (near Minneapolis-St. Paul), which features live Thoroughbred and quarter horse racing and televised pari-mutuel wagering on races from other tracks year-round. Pari-mutuel betting on live and simulcast races at Canterbury Park allows bettors to wager against each other and for the park to keep a percentage of the betting pool. The park also features special events such as motorcycle and snowmobile racing, arts and crafts shows, and concerts (including the Lilith Fair). Curtis Sampson, father of president Randy Sampson, owns more than 40% of the company.

Cenex Harvest States Cooperatives

5500 Cenex Dr., Inver Grove Heights, MN 55077

Telephone: 651-451-5151 **Fax:** 651-451-5568 **Other address:** PO Box 64089, St. Paul, MN 55164 **Metro area:** Minneapolis-St. Paul, MN **Web site:** http://www.cenexharveststates.com **Human resources contact:** Allen J. Anderson **Sales:** $5.6 billion **Number of employees:** 2,404 **Number of employees for previous year:** 2,178 **Industry designation:** Agricultural operations **Company type:** Cooperative **Top competitors:** Cargill, Incorporated; ConAgra, Inc.; Archer Daniels Midland Company

Cenex Harvest States Cooperatives likes to go with the grain, not against it. Formed by Harvest States' 1998 merger with CENEX, the co-op represents some 300,000 farmers in 17 central and western states; it's the US's #2 agricultural co-op, behind Farmland Industries. Grain trading is the co-op's primary business; it purchases, sells, and arranges for the transfer of its members' crops. The co-op processes soybeans into products such as mayonnaise, margarine, salad dressing, and animal feed. Its wheat-milling operations grind durum and semolina wheat into flour used mainly for pastas. The co-op also offers crop-protection products, plant food, fuel, and insurance. It also runs about 160 farm supply stores.

CIMA LABS INC.

10000 Valley View Rd., Eden Prairie, MN 55344

Telephone: 612-947-8700   **Fax:** 612-947-8770   **Metro area:** Minneapolis-St. Paul, MN   **Human resources contact:** Ronald Gay   **Sales:** $7.2 million   **Number of employees:** 74   **Number of employees for previous year:** 63   **Industry designation:** Medical products   **Company type:** Public   **Top competitors:** Fuisz Technologies Ltd.; R.P. Scherer Corporation

CIMA LABS makes pills that can be ingested without water or chewing. Through its patented technology, OraSolv, CIMA LABS uses coating to microencapsulate a drug into a tablet that dissolves quickly in the mouth. In addition, the coating effectively masks the medication's taste. The pills will be primarily marketed to children and elderly patients. The firm is also developing DuraSolv, which works the same as OraSolv, but which is a more durable pill that can be packaged more efficiently and at a lower cost than OraSolv. The company has partnerships with brand name drug manufacturers such as Bristol-Myers Squibb, SmithKline Beecham, and Novartis.

CNS, Inc.

4400 W. 78th St., Minneapolis, MN 55435

Telephone: 612-820-6696   **Fax:** 612-835-5229   **Other address:** PO Box 39082, Minneapolis, MN 55439   **Metro area:** Minneapolis-St. Paul, MN   **Web site:** http://www.cnxs.com   **Human resources contact:** Michelle Belining   **Sales:** $53.6 million   **Number of employees:** 52   **Number of employees for previous year:** 42   **Industry designation:** Medical products   **Company type:** Public   **Top competitors:** The Procter & Gamble Company; Respironics, Inc.; American Home Products Corporation

Snore no more! CNS markets the Breathe Right nasal strip, a nonprescription disposable device that improves breathing by lifting the side walls of the nose outward to open the nasal passages. The company targets the product to allergy sufferers, snorers, and athletes. CNS also markets Breathe Right nasal spray and pillow covers to keep pillow-born dust mites out of the air a sleeper breathes. CNS also makes the BANISH personal smoke deodorizing mist. Other products under development include a chewable, dietary fiber tablet. The company contracts out all its manufacturing operations. CNS has product distribution in more than 40 countries. About 10% of its sales are generated outside the US.

Datakey, Inc.

407 W. Travelers Trail, Burnsville, MN 55337

Telephone: 612-890-6850   **Fax:** 612-890-2726   **Metro area:** Minneapolis-St. Paul, MN   **Web site:** http://www.datakey.com   **Human resources contact:** Tami Nelson   **Sales:** $5.9 million   **Number of employees:** 60   **Number of employees for previous year:** 55   **Industry designation:** Protection—safety equipment & services   **Company type:** Public   **Top competitors:** The National Registry, Inc.; Visa International; Information Resource Engineering, Inc.

Think of Datakey as a high-tech doorkeeper. Datakey makes durable and portable memory keys, badges, magnetic stripe cards, and cryptographic tokens for businesses that rely on information security. Such devices can store more than a million bits of data to be used in communications, computer, and building security, as well as in vending and process control applications. The company also makes the access and interface devices into which the cards and tokens are inserted. Datakey offers hardware and software that protects computer-aided drawings and other electronic documents with encryption and digital signatures to prevent theft of information and intellectual property.

Datalink Corporation

7423 Washington Ave. South, Minneapolis, MN 55439

Telephone: 612-944-3462   **Fax:** 612-944-7869   **Metro area:** Minneapolis-St. Paul, MN   **Web site:** http://www.datalink.com   **Human resources contact:** Amy Zapolski   **Sales:** $90 million (Est.)   **Number of employees:** 130   **Number of employees for previous year:** 77   **Industry designation:** Computers—services   **Company type:** Private   **Top competitors:** International Business Machines Corporation; Computer Sciences Corporation; Unisys Corporation

Datalink Corporation creates high-end, custom-designed data storage systems for big companies and organizations such as American Express, Allstate, NASA, and UAL's United Airlines. The company also sells to original equipment manufacturers and value-added resellers. Datalink's storage systems include data capture equipment such as scanners, data management software, and storage devices using CD-ROM, optical, RAID (redundant array of independent disks), and tape technologies. Datalink uses an open system standard, combining products made by several manufacturers to create its highly customized systems. Following its IPO, CEO Greg Meland will own about one-third of Datalink, which has offices nationwide.

Digital Biometrics, Inc.

5600 Rowland Rd., Minnetonka, MN 55343

Telephone: 612-932-0888 **Fax:** 612-932-7181 **Metro area:** Minneapolis-St. Paul, MN **Web site:** http://www.digitalbiometrics.com **Human resources contact:** Karen Stennes **Sales:** $11.3 million **Number of employees:** 89 **Number of employees for previous year:** 81 **Industry designation:** Optical character recognition **Company type:** Public **Top competitors:** Printrak International Inc.; Identix Incorporated; Rheinmetall Berlin AG

Digital Biometrics lets your fingerprints do the walking. The company's TENPRINTER product enables law enforcement personnel and others to capture, digitize, and print fingerprints and transmit the images over telephone lines. Another Digital Biometrics product, Squad Car Identification, is a portable fingerprint capture system used in police patrol cars for on-the-spot identification of suspects. The company's products are used with computer-based automatic fingerprint indentification systems. Digital Biometrics also makes TRAK-21, a system used by casinos to track players' wagers. Government agencies account for 70% of the company's sales.

Digital River, Inc.

9625 W. 76th St., Ste. 150, Eden Prairie, MN 55344

Telephone: 612-253-1234 **Fax:** 612-253-8497 **Metro area:** Minneapolis-St. Paul, MN **Web site:** http://www.digitalriver.com **Human resources contact:** Nancy Brown **Sales:** $20.9 million **Number of employees:** 148 **Number of employees for previous year:** 75 **Industry designation:** Computers—online services **Company type:** Public **Top competitors:** Preview Systems, Inc.; Beyond.com; TechWave Inc.

The opportunity to spend money is only a point and click away for cyber-consumers on the Digital River. The company provides electronic commerce services to software publishers and online retail clients, including the creation of Web stores, data mining (used in market research), and merchandising services. Digital River maintains a database of more than 100,000 software products sold and delivered on its electronic software delivery system. The company also has services for fraud prevention, export control, and online registration. The more than 2,000 clients currently riding the Digital River include Corel, Cyberian Outpost, and Lotus Development. President and CEO Joel Ronning owns about 20% of the company.

Eagle Pacific Industries, Inc.

2430 Metropolitan Center, 333 S. Seventh St., Minneapolis, MN 55402

Telephone: 612-305-0339 **Fax:** 612-371-9651 **Metro area:** Minneapolis-St. Paul, MN **Web site:** http://www.eaglepacific.com **Human resources contact:** Larry Zabloudil **Sales:** $74 million **Number of employees:** 337 **Number of employees for previous year:** 331 **Industry designation:** Rubber & plastic products **Company type:** Public

Eagle Pacific Industries isn't afraid of a little pressure, considering it's an extruder of polyvinyl chloride (PVC) pipe and polyethylene tubing products gauged to withstand different pressures. The firm makes small- and medium-diameter plastic pipe and tubing products, including the Pure Core and Eagle-Tough Turf brands. Eagle Pacific Industries' products are sold primarily in the Midwest and Northwest and are used in construction, commercial and residential plumbing, turf irrigation, municipal water and sewage, natural gas distribution, and telecommunications. As Eagle Pacific grows its PVC operations through acquisitions, a US subsidiary of Germany-based manufacturer RWE-DEA is buying control of the firm.

Endocardial Solutions, Inc.

1350 Energy Ln., Ste. 110, St. Paul, MN 55108

Telephone: 651-644-7890 **Fax:** 651-644-7897 **Metro area:** Minneapolis-St. Paul, MN **Web site:** http://www.endocardial.com **Sales:** $100,000 **Number of employees:** 62 **Number of employees for previous year:** 50 **Industry designation:** Medical instruments **Company type:** Public

Endocardial Solutions, Inc. (ESI) designs and manufactures a minimally invasive system for diagnosing tachycardia, a potentially fatal arrhythmia. The company's EnSite catheters and clinical workstations (which are now in clinical trials in the US and Europe) together produce a high-resolution, real-time, three-dimensional color display of electrical activity in the heart chamber, thus allowing doctors to locate and diagnose tachycardia and to determine the best course of treatment. In 1997 Medtronic, Inc., signed an agreement regarding overseas distribution of ESI's products, and Medtronic Asset Management owns nearly 25% of the company.

Everest Medical Corporation

13755 First Ave. North, Minneapolis, MN 55441

Telephone: 612-473-6262 **Fax:** 612-473-6465 **Metro area:** Minneapolis-St. Paul, MN **Web site:** http://www.everestmedical.com **Human resources contact:** Julie Seurer **Sales:** $10.8 million **Number of employees:** 105 **Number of employees for previous year:** 79 **Industry designation:** Medical instruments **Company type:** Public **Top competitors:** Johnson & Johnson; Boston Scientific Corporation; Imagyn Medical Technologies, Inc.

Everest Medical's tallest order is laparoscopic equipment. The company makes laparoscopic surgical instruments ranging from specialized forceps and scissors to surgical electrodes which cut tissue and coagulate blood using a tiny electrical arc. The devices are used in minimally-invasive surgeries in such areas as gynecology, gastroenterology, and cardiology. Everest Medical's electrical cutting products are bipolar, which means the all electrodes are contained within the device, as opposed to less contained monopolar devices, which require the patient to be in contact with a return electrode to cause a single electrode in the instrument to arc.

GalaGen Inc.

4001 Lexington Ave. North, Arden Hills, MN 55126

Telephone: 651-481-2105 **Fax:** 651-481-2380 **Metro area:** Minneapolis-St. Paul, MN **Web site:** http://www.galagen.com **Human resources contact:** Sue Rehberger **Sales:** $100,000 **Number of employees:** 19 **Number of employees for previous year:** 17 **Industry designation:** Drugs **Company type:** Public **Top competitors:** AMBI Inc.; OraVax, Inc.; IgX Corp.

Holy cow! Development-stage GalaGen makes nutritional products and pharmaceuticals from bovine colostrum, the antibody-rich milk produced just after birthing. GalaGen collects colostrum from 400,000 cows owned by Land O'Lakes (which also owns 16% of GalaGen). The company is developing clinical treatments for antibiotic-associated diarrhea, oral fungal infections, and stomach ulcers. It already sells nutritional products to more than 500 hospitals and health care providers. It also sells consumer nutritional beverages through an agreement with manufacturing and marketing partner Lifeway Foods. GalaGen licenses research technology from Chiron, which owns another 30% of the company.

GFI America, Inc

2815 Blaisdell Ave. South, Minneapolis, MN 55408

Telephone: 612-872-6262 **Fax:** 612-870-4955 **Metro area:** Minneapolis-St. Paul, MN **Web site:** http://www.gfiamerica.com **Human resources contact:** Clark Peterson **Sales:** $510 million (Est.) **Number of employees:** 1,200 **Number of employees for previous year:** 1,125 **Industry designation:** Food—meat products **Company type:** Private **Top competitors:** Rosen's Diversified, Inc.; IBP, inc.; Packerland Packing Company

Sure, protein is brain food, but that's not where GFI America's SmartMeat gets its name. Trimmed of fat and prepared without chemical preservatives or artificial flavoring, SmartMeat is part of the beef processor's lineup of portion-cut and value-added meats sold to restaurants, supermarkets, and food processors in the US and internationally. Selected cattle are fed to the company's specifications, then processed at its four midwestern plants. They emerge as bulk ground beef, steaks, taco meat, fajitas, meatloaf, sausage, and other products under labels including SmartMeat and ReelTender. President and CEO Robert Goldberger and his brother Howard founded the company in 1974; their family still owns GFI America.

Hawkins Chemical, Inc.

3100 E. Hennepin Ave., Minneapolis, MN 55413

Telephone: 612-331-6910 **Fax:** 612-331-5304 **Metro area:** Minneapolis-St. Paul, MN **Web site:** http://www.hawkinschemical.com/ **Human resources contact:** Teresa Moran **Sales:** $94.7 million **Number of employees:** 156 **Number of employees for previous year:** 151 **Industry designation:** Chemicals—specialty **Company type:** Public **Top competitors:** Jones Chemicals, Inc.; Corporate Express, Inc.; Albemarle Corporation

Hawkins Chemical and its subsidiaries process and distribute bulk specialty chemicals. The Hawkins Water Treatment Group provides water- and wastewater-treatment equipment and chemicals for testing water samples; it is also a regional distributor of laundry, dry cleaning, and janitorial supplies. The Hawkins Terminal Division stores and distributes bulk chemicals (primarily liquid caustic soda, phosphoric acid, and aqua ammonia); makes bleach; and repackages liquid chlorine. The company has a patented form of liquid sodium phosphate for use in the processed-food industry. Hawkins Chemical operates in nine midwestern states. Employees own 22% of the company through a trust.

Health Fitness Corporation

3500 W. 80th St., Ste. 130, Bloomington, MN 55431

Telephone: 612-831-6830 **Fax:** 612-831-7264 **Metro area:** Minneapolis-St. Paul, MN **Human resources contact:** Tina Oskey **Sales:** $33.7 million **Number of employees:** 1,600 **Number of employees for previous year:** 1,510 **Industry designation:** Health care—outpatient & home **Company type:** Public

Health Fitness Corporation operates corporate and hospital-based fitness centers and freestanding physical therapy clinics. The company provides staffing and consulting services, management systems, and wellness products for its center clients. It provides a full range of rehabilitative and chronic pain relief services. Health Fitness Corporation is under contract to manage about 140 corporate and hospital fitness centers for clients including Hewlett Packard/ Palo Alto and Tishman of California. The company plans to sell its freestanding physical therapy clinics to reduce its debt.

Hormel Foods Corporation

One Hormel Place, Austin, MN 55912

Telephone: 507-437-5611 **Fax:** 507-437-5489 **Metro area:** Rochester, MN **Web site:** http:// www.hormel.com **Human resources contact:** James A. Jorgenson **Sales:** $3.3 billion **Number of employees:** 11,200 **Number of employees for previous year:** 11,000 **Industry designation:** Food—meat products **Company type:** Public **Top competitors:** ConAgra, Inc.; IBP, inc.; Smithfield Foods, Inc.

Hormel Foods estimates Americans consume 3.6 cans of SPAM per second, and that's just one of many facts at the fingertips of the company responsible for the well-known brand of canned ham. Hormel is the nation's #1 turkey processor and #3 pork processor (behind Smithfield Foods and IBP), making Jennie-O turkey products, Cure 81 hams, Always Tender fresh pork, and Dinty Moore beef stew. The company has expanded into value-added food products such as Chi-Chi's Mexican foods and House of Tsang sauces. Hormel has joint ventures in Australia, China (the biggest market for pork in the world), Mexico, and the Philippines. The Hormel Foundation, a charitable trust, owns 43% of the company's stock.

Hutchinson Technology Incorporated

40 W. Highland Park, Hutchinson, MN 55350

Telephone: 320-587-3797 **Fax:** 320-587-1810 **Metro area:** Minneapolis-St. Paul, MN **Web site:** http://www.htch.com **Human resources contact:** Rebecca A. Albrecht **Sales:** $407.6 million **Number of employees:** 7,764 **Number of employees for previous year:** 7,181 **Industry designation:** Computers—peripheral equipment **Company type:** Public **Top competitors:** K.R. Precision Co.; Nippon Hatsujo Kogyo Co.; Magnecomp International Limited

Disk drive makers know the way across Hutchinson's suspension bridge. Hutchinson Technology makes 70% of the world's disk drive suspension assemblies, the component that supports the read-write head above the spinning magnetic disk in a hard drive. The company supplies many of the major disk drive makers, including TDK and IBM (the two account for nearly half of sales between them). Hutchinson is focused on developing suspension assembly technologies that accommodate smaller read-write heads. Smaller heads can read and write more data tracks, increasing a disk drive's memory and performance. Hutchinson is also using its technical expertise to expand into the medical device market.

Image Systems Corporation

6103 Blue Circle Dr., Minnetonka, MN 55343

Telephone: 612-935-1171 **Fax:** 612-935-1386 **Metro area:** Minneapolis-St. Paul, MN **Web site:** http://www.imagesystemscorp.com **Human resources contact:** Laura S. Sorensen **Sales:** $8.2 million **Number of employees:** 41 **Number of employees for previous year:** 40 **Industry designation:** Medical instruments **Company type:** Public **Top competitors:** Siemens AG; BARCO N.V.

Bright ideas come from Image Systems Corporation in the form of the high-brightness, high-resolution video monitors. The company's gray scale and color monitors, which have three to ten times the resolution and twice the brightness of a typical monitor, are marketed primarily to the original equipment manufacturers (OEMs) and the medical field and are used particularly in radiology, where image quality is critical. The monitors are also used for air traffic control, scientific analysis, image processing, and electronic and mechanical design. Image Systems provides monitors to the Defense Department under an OEM contract with IBM. The family of president Dean Scheff owns more than 60% of Image Systems.

Imation Corp.

One Imation Place, Oakdale, MN 55128

Telephone: 651-704-4000 **Fax:** 651-704-3444 **Metro area:** Minneapolis-St. Paul, MN **Web site:** http://www.imation.com **Human resources contact:** Jacqueline Chase **Sales:** $2 billion **Number of employees:** 9,800 **Number of employees for previous year:** 9,400 **Industry designation:** Computers—peripheral equipment **Company type:** Public **Top competitors:** E. I. du Pont de Nemours and Company; Sony Corporation; Eastman Kodak Company

Image and information storage specialist Imation is one of the world's top makers of removable magnetic and optical technology media (diskettes, storage tapes, and other products) used to capture, process, store, reproduce, and distribute information and images via computers. Imation's more than 10,000 products include digital color proofing systems, photographic films (it's a top world supplier of private-label brands), printing plates, single-use cameras, and medical imaging systems. Exports account for about half of its sales. Formed when 3M spun off some of its less-lucrative business lines, Imation has sold its CD-ROM operations and most of its medical imaging business.

ITI Technologies, Inc.

2266 N. Second St., North St. Paul, MN 55109

Telephone: 651-777-2690 **Fax:** 651-779-4890 **Metro area:** Minneapolis-St. Paul, MN **Web site:** http://www.securitypro.com/index.html **Human resources contact:** Martha Carlson **Sales:** $109 million **Number of employees:** 645 **Number of employees for previous year:** 641 **Industry designation:** Protection—safety equipment & services **Company type:** Public

ITI Technologies keeps an eye on things with its burglar alarms, fire detectors, and access-control systems. The company makes wireless, hard-wire, and hybrid security systems for sale through its dealer network and to large security companies, private-label customers such as Westar, and electric and gas utilities. Other ITI products include building-access systems; LifeGard, a personal emergency-response system for the elderly; and Meter Minder, a security system add-on that monitors utility usage. ITI manufactures its products in the US and Mexico and sells them worldwide. Foreign sales, mostly through subsidiary CADDX Controls, account for about 15% of revenues.

LecTec Corporation

10701 Red Circle Dr., Minnetonka, MN 55343

Telephone: 612-933-2291 **Fax:** 612-933-4808 **Metro area:** Minneapolis-St. Paul, MN **Web site:** http://www.lectec.com **Human resources contact:** Alice Ong **Sales:** $12.9 million **Number of employees:** 85 **Number of employees for previous year:** 72 **Industry designation:** Medical instruments **Company type:** Public **Top competitors:** Hewlett-Packard Company; ALZA Corporation; Medtronic Physio-Control Inc.

LecTec licks some sticky problems with its sticky products. The company makes diagnostic electrodes and adhesive gels, medical tapes, and transdermal drug delivery patches based on its patented hydrogel membrane technology. Products include its TheraPatch, over-the-counter cold remedies, and pain relief patches. It also is developing a non-nicotine smoking cessation remedy. The company's conductive products (hydrogels, electrodes) are its biggest seller, bringing in more than 60% of total sales. LecTec sells its products in Asia, Europe, and North and South America.

Lifecore Biomedical, Inc.

3515 Lyman Blvd., Chaska, MN 55318

Telephone: 612-368-4300 **Fax:** 612-368-3411 **Metro area:** Minneapolis-St. Paul, MN **Web site:** http://www.lifecore.com **Human resources contact:** Julia Jensen **Sales:** $25.6 million **Number of employees:** 159 **Number of employees for previous year:** 157 **Industry designation:** Biomedical & genetic products **Company type:** Public **Top competitors:** Anika Therapeutics, Inc.; Life Medical Sciences, Inc.; SULZER Corporation

Lifecore Biomedical hopes you like most of your biomedical products "al dente." Its Oral Restorative division accounts for a majority of revenues. The division makes dental implants made from titanium to replace lost or extracted teeth; it also makes tissue-regeneration products for treatment of periodontal disease and tooth loss. Lifecore also produces hyaluronate, a lubricating carbohydrate which prevent organs from growing together after surgery. The material is used primarily in cataract surgery and is under development for use in general surgery and drug delivery. Hyaluronate was originally extracted from rooster combs (the company now makes the product with its own fermentation process).

Life USA Holding, Inc.

300 S. Hwy. 169, Ste. 95, Interchange North Bldg., Minneapolis, MN 55426

Telephone: 612-546-7386 **Fax:** 612-525-6000 **Metro area:** Minneapolis-St. Paul, MN **Human resources contact:** Jeanelle Arch **Sales:** $362.6 million **Number of employees:** 461 **Number of employees for previous year:** 434 **Industry designation:** Insurance—life **Company type:** Public **Top competitors:** New York Life Insurance Company; The Prudential Insurance Company of America; Metropolitan Life Insurance Company

Through subsidiary LifeUSA Insurance, Life USA Holding sells fixed-rate annuities and life insurance. The company's Accumulator, IDEAL, and Universal Annuity Life policies are structured to encourage holders to choose annuity payments over lump sums upon maturity. Life USA also markets policies for the US subsidiary of German-insurer Allianz Life. Subsidiary LifeUSA Securities offers its own family of mutual funds and markets 22 others. LifeUSA Marketing, working through field marketing organizations, markets the company's products via some 67,000 agents operating in every state except New York.

Malt-O-Meal Company

80 S. Eighth St., Ste. 2600, Minneapolis, MN 55402

Telephone: 612-338-8551 **Fax:** 612-339-5710 **Metro area:** Minneapolis-St. Paul, MN **Web site:** http://www.malt-o-meal.com **Human resources contact:** Jeff Zibley **Sales:** $300 million (Est.) **Number of employees:** 900 **Industry designation:** Food—flour & grain **Company type:** Private **Top competitors:** Kellogg Company; The Quaker Oats Company; General Mills, Inc.

Cheerios or Toasty O's? Malt-O-Meal Company wants breakfast eaters to follow "its" O's. Malt-O-Meal is a leading manufacturer of discount bagged and store-brand hot and cold cereals that resemble major national cereal brands. Under such product names as Malt-O-Meal hot cereal (in several flavors), Toasty O's, Crispy Rice, Tootie Fruities, Coco-Roos, and Golden Puffs, the company's 39 cereal brands are distributed nationwide and include store brands such as IGA, Cub Foods, Janet Lee, Kroger, and Safeway. John Campbell founded the family-owned company in 1919.

Mayo Foundation

200 First St. SW, Rochester, MN 55905

Telephone: 507-284-2511 **Fax:** 507-284-8713 **Metro area:** Rochester, MN **Web site:** http://www.mayo.edu **Human resources contact:** Gregory Warner **Sales:** $2.6 billion **Number of employees:** 30,497 **Number of employees for previous year:** 28,671 **Industry designation:** Hospitals **Company type:** Not-for-profit **Top competitors:** Columbia/HCA Healthcare Corporation; Tenet Healthcare Corporation; Daughters of Charity National Health System

This Mayo—100% corporate-fat-free—is good for you. The not-for-profit Mayo Foundation provides health care, most notably for difficult medical conditions, through its renowned Mayo Clinic in Rochester, Minnesota. The foundation also operates major facilities in Jacksonville, Florida, and Phoenix and Scottsdale, Arizona, as well as a network of 11 affiliated community-based hospitals and clinics in Iowa, Minnesota, and Wisconsin. Each year about 400,000 patients check into Mayo's facilities. The foundation also conducts research and trains physicians, nurses, and other health professionals. It dates back to a frontier practice launched by William Mayo in 1863.

MedAmicus, Inc.

15301 Hwy. 55 West, Plymouth, MN 55447

Telephone: 612-559-2613 **Fax:** 612-559-7548 **Metro area:** Minneapolis-St. Paul, MN **Human resources contact:** Donna Richardson **Sales:** $8 million **Number of employees:** 80 **Number of employees for previous year:** 75 **Industry designation:** Medical products **Company type:** Public **Top competitors:** C. R. Bard, Inc.; Baxter International Inc.; St. Jude Medical, Inc.

With products aimed at two major medical markets—cardiovascular ailments and urinary incontinence—MedAmicus is a friend indeed. The company makes percutaneous venous vessel introducers, used by physicians to insert infusion catheters, implantable ports, and pacemaker leads into veins. MedAmicus' LuMax Cystometry System uses fiber optics to help physicians diagnose and treat male and female incontinence, as well cardiovascular, respiratory, and neurological diseases. The company has marketing agreements for its vessel introducers with C.R. Bard and with Medtronic, which accounts for 55% of sales. MedAmicus also has a distribution pact to sell Schick Technologies' bone-density measurement device.

Medi-Ject Corporation

161 Cheshire Ln., Minneapolis, MN 55441

Telephone: 612-475-7700 **Fax:** 612-476-1009 **Metro area:** Minneapolis-St. Paul, MN **Web site:** http://www.mediject.com **Human resources contact:** Ellen Hendricksen **Sales:** $2.8 million **Number of employees:** 43 **Number of employees for previous year:** 36 **Industry designation:** Medical instruments **Company type:** Public **Top competitors:** IOMED, Inc.; Bioject Medical Technologies Inc.; Aradigm Corporation

Medi-Ject develops needle-free injection systems for a wide array of drugs that patients can use on their own. The company's principal product, the Medi-Jector system, is a handheld, spring-powered device that injects drugs using a very thin, high-pressure stream of liquid, eliminating the need to pierce the skin with a hypodermic needle. Its systems, used primarily for insulin delivery, are suitable for a variety of treatments, including multiple sclerosis and hepatitis. Medi-Ject has marketing and development agreements with several pharmaceutical companies, including Becton, Dickinson, which owns about a third of Medi-Ject's stock. The company is also developing a pen-sized injection system powered by a gas spring.

Mercury Waste Solutions, Inc.

302 N. Riverfront Dr., Ste. 100A, Mankato, MN 56001

Telephone: 507-345-0522 **Fax:** 507-345-1483 **Web site:** http://www.mwsi.com **Human resources contact:** Mark Stennes **Sales:** $6.3 million **Number of employees:** 51 **Number of employees for previous year:** 36 **Industry designation:** Pollution control equipment & services **Company type:** Public

Mercury Waste Solutions is a waste-disposal firm that serves utilities and other companies that use mercury to make batteries, switches, fluorescent lamps, and measurement equipment. Half of the company's sales come from fees charged for retorting mercury waste (distilling it from other wastes) with its own proprietary processes. The firm also stores mercury waste and recycles fluorescent and other mercury-containing lamps and ballasts. The company is growing through acquisitions and has operations in Georgia, Indiana, Minnesota, New York, and Wisconsin. Chairman and CEO Brad Buscher owns 35% of the firm; president and COO Mark Edlund owns 20%.

MGI PHARMA, Inc.

9900 Bren Rd. East, Ste. 300E, Opus Center, Minnetonka, MN 55343

Telephone: 612-935-7335 **Fax:** 612-935-0468 **Metro area:** Minneapolis-St. Paul, MN **Human resources contact:** Shirley Anderson **Sales:** $17.6 million **Number of employees:** 78 **Number of employees for previous year:** 65 **Industry designation:** Drugs **Company type:** Public **Top competitors:** SciClone Pharmaceuticals, Inc.; Connetics Corp.; Roberts Pharmaceutical Corporation

MGI PHARMA finds homes for orphan drugs. The company acquires and develops drugs that probably won't be best-sellers but fit small medical niches, primarily in the oncology market. Products currently being marketed include Salagen Tablets for the treatment of radiation-induced chronic dry mouth in head and neck cancer patients and for patients with Sjogren's Syndrome and Didronel IV Infusion, used to treat hypercalcemia of malignancy, a life-threatening disorder. Other products include an iron deficiency treatment marketed for Schein Pharmaceutical and a family of anticancer drugs. MGI attempts to reduce the risk of product failure by acquiring promising products that are past the initial discovery stage.

The Minnesota Mutual Life Insurance Company

400 Robert St. North, St. Paul, MN 55101

Telephone: 651-665-3500 **Fax:** 651-665-4488 **Metro area:** Minneapolis-St. Paul, MN **Web site:** http://www.minnesotamutual.com **Human resources contact:** Keith M. Campbell **Sales:** $1.7 billion **Number of employees:** 2,187 **Number of employees for previous year:** 1,950 **Industry designation:** Insurance—life **Company type:** Mutual company **Top competitors:** New York Life Insurance Company; The Prudential Insurance Company of America; The Northwestern Mutual Life Insurance Company

With 10,000 lakes in their state, Minnesotans have learned to be careful. Minnesota Mutual Life helps them take that caution a step further. The company's nationwide agency network sells individual and group life and disability insurance, annuities, and investment and pension products. The company also provides mortgage life insurance, homeowners and auto insurance, and provides investment and pension management services, including the Advantus family of mutual funds. Subsidiary Ministers Life Resources provides financial services for church members and religious professionals. Minnesota Mutual Life is examining the possibility of converting to mutual holding company status.

Minnesota Timberwolves

600 First Ave. North, Minneapolis, MN 55403

Telephone: 612-337-3865 **Fax:** 612-673-1699 **Metro area:** Minneapolis-St. Paul, MN **Web site:** http://www.nba.com/timberwolves **Sales:** $51.8 million (Est.) **Number of employees:** 65 **Number of employees for previous year:** 60 **Industry designation:** Leisure & recreational services **Company type:** Private **Top competitors:** Houston Rockets; San Antonio Spurs, Ltd.; Utah Jazz

Can Randy Moss play hoops, too? The Minnesota Timberwolves joined the National Basketball Association (NBA) as an expansion club in 1989. The team proceeded to struggle through its first seven NBA campaigns, never mustering more than 29 wins in a season. However, with the talents of youthful forward Kevin Garnett, the team has made the playoffs the past two years, although it has yet to win a series. Former Minnesota Senator Glen Taylor, whose Taylor Corporation is the largest printer of wedding invitations in the US (with about 90% of the market), owns a controlling interest in the team. There are 14 minority owners.

Minnesota Twins

34 Kirby Puckett Place, Minneapolis, MN 55415

Telephone: 612-375-1366 **Fax:** 612-375-7480 **Metro area:** Minneapolis-St. Paul, MN **Web site:** http://www.mntwins.com **Human resources contact:** Rachel Dorn **Sales:** $46.8 million (Est.) **Number of employees:** 109 **Industry designation:** Leisure & recreational services **Company type:** Private **Top competitors:** Chicago White Sox Ltd.; Kansas City Royals Baseball Corporation; Cleveland Indians Baseball Company, Inc.

The Minnesota Twins competed as Major League Baseball's Washington Senators until 1960, when the club moved to the frozen sister cities of St. Paul-Minneapolis (hence the name Twins). The team won World Series championships in 1987 and 1991 and has fielded such players as Tony Oliva, Kirby Puckett, and Rod Carew. Billionaire owner Carl Pohlad has threatened to sell the Twins to North Carolina businessman Don Beaver if Minnesota continues its refusal to build the team a new stadium (the Twins share the Hubert Humphrey Metrodome with the Minnesota Vikings). The deal must be approved by a majority of American and National League owners, who are reluctant to have the team move to North Carolina.

Minnesota Vikings Football Club

9520 Viking Dr., Eden Prairie, MN 55344

Telephone: 612-828-6500 **Fax:** 612-828-6540 **Metro area:** Minneapolis-St. Paul, MN **Web site:** http://www.nfl.com/vikings/index.html **Sales:** $77.7 million (Est.) **Number of employees:** 130 **Industry designation:** Leisure & recreational services **Company type:** Private **Top competitors:** The Green Bay Packers, Inc.; Detroit Lions; Tampa Bay Buccaneers

Founded in 1960, a decade later the Vikings became the first modern expansion team to win an NFL championship game and play in the Super Bowl. Recent years have seen fan apathy and infighting between head coach Denny Green and the former owners. However, relief from the squabbling came in the unlikely form of Texas billionaire Red McCombs, the new owner. Since paying about $250 million for the team in 1998, the former owner of the San Antonio Spurs and Denver Nuggets has shown faith in Green's coaching abilities and promised the Twin Cities a Super Bowl victory. McCombs and the Vikes almost delivered on that promise during the 1998-99 season but the team lost to the Atlanta Falcons in the NFC championship game.

Minntech Corporation

14605 28th Ave. North, Minneapolis, MN 55447

Telephone: 612-553-3300 **Fax:** 612-553-3387 **Metro area:** Minneapolis-St. Paul, MN **Web site:** http://www.minntech.com **Human resources contact:** Robert Lysaght **Sales:** $69.4 million **Number of employees:** 386 **Number of employees for previous year:** 377 **Industry designation:** Medical products **Company type:** Public **Top competitors:** Baxter International Inc.; Gambro AB; Fresenius Medical Care Aktiengesellschaft

Minntech helps patients stay bloody clean. The company produces medical devices, sterilants, and water purification products under the names Renal Systems, Minntech, and Fibercor for use in kidney dialysis, open-heart surgery (its biggest sectors), endoscopy, and the separation and disinfecting of pure water for medical use. Minntech develops all its core technologies in-house. The firm has subsidiaries in the Netherlands and in Japan. Customers include pharmaceutical, hospital, and biotechnology companies. Its five largest customers account for one-fourth of company sales.

National Computer Systems, Inc.

11000 Prairie Lakes Dr., Eden Prairie, MN 55344

Telephone: 612-829-3000 **Fax:** 612-829-3167 **Metro area:** Minneapolis-St. Paul, MN **Web site:** http://www.ncs.com **Human resources contact:** Gary Martini **Sales:** $505.4 million **Number of employees:** 3,500 **Number of employees for previous year:** 2,700 **Industry designation:** Optical character recognition **Company type:** Public **Top competitors:** Bell & Howell Company; John H. Harland Company; Houghton Mifflin Company

Form follows function. National Computer Systems (NCS) makes the forms and processing equipment used in automated testing and document processing applications. Using either electronic or paper forms (the latter incorporating the company's optical recognition technology), the company creates, scores, and sorts tests, applications, and profiles. Major customers include school districts, government agencies, and health care organizations. NCS also offers database management services for telecommunications providers. Its Virtual University Enterprises unit offers online software certification.

NetRadio Corporation

43 Main St. SE, Ste. 149, Minneapolis, MN 55414

Telephone: 612-378-2211 **Fax:** 612-378-9540 **Metro area:** Minneapolis-St. Paul, MN **Web site:** http://www.netradio.com **Sales:** $255,000 (Est.) **Number of employees:** 43 **Industry designation:** Computers—online services **Company type:** Private **Top competitors:** CDnow, Inc.; broadcast.com inc.; Best Buy Co., Inc.

With NetRadio, you can listen to "Itsy Bitsy Spider" while surfing the Web. The company's NetRadio.com Web site allows customers to download audio files from more than 120 music, news, sports, and entertainment channels. The channels are grouped into such categories as Cafe Jazz, Classical, Electronica, New Age, Vintage Rock, and World Music. For those who like what they hear, NetRadio operates CDPoint, an online music store where listeners can purchase tunes. Computer software and music distributor Navarre Corporation owns about 77% of the company; NetRadio chairman Eric Paulson and director Charles Cheney are officers of and own interests in Navarre. ValueVision International owns about 22% of NetRadio.

ONTRACK Data International, Inc.

6321 Bury Dr., Stes. 13-21, Eden Prairie, MN 55346

Telephone: 612-937-1107 **Fax:** 612-937-5815 **Metro area:** Minneapolis-St. Paul, MN **Web site:** http://www.ontrack.com **Human resources contact:** Cindy Mustful **Sales:** $35.8 million **Number of employees:** 303 **Number of employees for previous year:** 291 **Industry designation:** Computers—services **Company type:** Public **Top competitors:** Comdisco, Inc.; DriveSavers; Network Associates, Inc.

Beset by virus problems? Forget laughter—ONTRACK Data International has the best medicine. The company is the world's #1 data recovery services provider; it rescues lost or corrupted electronic data from hard disk drives and other storage devices. ONTRACK provides data recovery services (about 75% of sales) through labs in California; Minnesota; New Jersey; Washington, DC; Germany; Japan; London; and Paris. On-site and after-hours emergency services are available. ONTRACK also offers computer data evidence services for legal proceedings and sells software for hard drive installations, virus monitoring and removal, data protection, and data recovery.

Orphan Medical, Inc.

13911 Ridgedale Dr., Ste. 475, Minnetonka, MN 55305

Telephone: 612-513-6900 **Fax:** 612-541-9209 **Metro area:** Minneapolis-St. Paul, MN **Web site:** http://www.orphan.com/index.dbm **Sales:** $600,000 **Number of employees:** 44 **Number of employees for previous year:** 33 **Industry designation:** Drugs **Company type:** Public **Top competitors:** Glaxo Wellcome plc; MGI PHARMA, Inc.; Hoechst AG

Orphan Medical sells drugs for inadequately treated or uncommon diseases. Taking advantage of incentives offered under the Orphan Drug Act of 1983, the company develops and markets drugs for rare diseases and conditions affecting small patient populations, a market often neglected by large pharmaceutical companies. Orphan Medical keeps costs low by licensing promising drugs from others, then conducting clinical trials to obtain FDA marketing approval. The company currently markets only a few drugs, including drugs to treat the rare genetic disorder homocystinuria (Cystadane) and meningeal leukemia or lymphocytic lymphoma (Elliotts B Solution).

Patterson Dental Company

1031 Mendota Heights Rd., St. Paul, MN 55120

Telephone: 651-686-1600 **Fax:** 651-686-9331 **Metro area:** Minneapolis-St. Paul, MN **Web site:** http://www.pattersondental.com **Human resources contact:** Mary H. Baglien **Sales:** $778.2 million **Number of employees:** 3,214 **Number of employees for previous year:** 2,913 **Industry designation:** Medical & dental supplies **Company type:** Public **Top competitors:** Zila, Inc.; Sybron International Corporation; Henry Schein, Inc.

Patterson Dental has a mouthful of the dental products industry. The company is the #2 distributor of dental products (Henry Schein is #1). The company supplies a full line of over 80,000 products (including a line of some 2,000 private-label items) to dentists, dental laboratories, and institutions. Its products include X-ray film and solutions, impression and restorative materials, hand instruments, sterilization products, dental chairs and lights, compressors, and diagnostic equipment. Dental supplies account for over 60% of sales, while equipment makes up nearly 30%. Patterson Dental markets its products via a sales force of about 900 operating in the US and Canada.

Photran Corporation

21875 Grenada Ave., Lakeville, MN 55044

Telephone: 612-469-4880 **Fax:** 612-469-4886 **Metro area:** Minneapolis-St. Paul, MN **Human resources contact:** James Waters **Sales:** $4.4 million **Number of employees:** 120 **Number of employees for previous year:** 109 **Industry designation:** Glass products **Company type:** Public **Top competitors:** Donnelly Corporation; Galileo Corporation; Optical Coating Laboratory, Inc.

Photran manufactures optically and electrically conductive thin-film-coated products. Its manufacturing process applies microscopically thin layers of materials—including metal, metal oxide, nitride, carbide, and flouride—to improve the durability, optical properties, and electrical properties of glass, metal, or plastic. Photran's products are used in flat-panel displays, laptop computer monitors, electronic games, photocopiers, bar code scanners, projection televisions, and other consumer goods. The company has plans to produce specialty glass for picture framing. Most of Photran's sales are to Asian customers, one of which contributes more than half of Photran's total sales.

Possis Medical, Inc.

9055 Evergreen Blvd. NW, Minneapolis, MN 55433

Telephone: 612-780-4555 **Fax:** 612-780-2227 **Metro area:** Minneapolis-St. Paul, MN **Human resources contact:** Irving R. Colacci **Sales:** $6.1 million **Number of employees:** 188 **Number of employees for previous year:** 168 **Industry designation:** Medical products **Company type:** Public **Top competitors:** American BioMed, Inc.; CardioTech International, Inc.; Sulzer Medica Ltd.

Possis Medical makes catheter systems used to remove blood clots, and blood-vessel grafts designed to treat patients with cardiovascular or vascular disease. Its AngioJet Thrombectomy System, a minimally invasive catheter system, removes blood clots without surgery. Its Perma-Flow Coronary Bypass Graft helps bypass surgery patients with inadequate veins. The Perma-Seal Graft is used as a vascular graft for dialysis patients. Some products are still in clinical trials in the US, but the Perma-Seal Graft and the AngioJet System are approved for certain uses in the US and abroad; products are marketed to physicians directly and by third-party distributors.

Rehabilicare Inc.

1811 Old Hwy. 8, New Brighton, MN 55112

Telephone: 651-631-0590 **Fax:** 651-638-0476 **Metro area:** Minneapolis-St. Paul, MN **Web site:** http://www.rehabilicare.com **Human resources contact:** Alla Byrne **Sales:** $33.8 million **Number of employees:** 252 **Number of employees for previous year:** 92 **Industry designation:** Medical products **Company type:** Public **Top competitors:** Dynatronics Corporation; Empi, Inc.; Henley Healthcare, Inc.

Rehabilicare takes pains to take pain away. The company makes electrotherapy devices for rehabilitation and pain management that work through electrical pulse generators connected by electrodes to the patient's skin. Its neuromuscular stimulation devices are designed to activate muscles and increase strength and mobility. It also makes RehabiliCaine, an analgesic patch. The company makes its own products and sells to health care providers in the US and UK. Rehabilicare more than doubled in size with its purchase of Staodyn, a maker of electrotherapeutic devices. It further bolstered its position by buying the Homecare division of Henley Healthcare, a distributor of home electrotherapy products.

Rochester Medical Corporation

One Rochester Medical Dr., Stewartville, MN 55976

Telephone: 507-533-9600 **Fax:** 507-533-4232 **Metro area:** Rochester, MN **Human resources contact:** Brian J. Wierzbinski **Sales:** $9.5 million **Number of employees:** 180 **Number of employees for previous year:** 117 **Industry designation:** Medical products **Company type:** Public **Top competitors:** C. R. Bard, Inc.; Tyco International Ltd.; Hollister Incorporated

It's all about quality of life. Rochester Medical focuses on products and devices used in the management of urinary dysfunction. The company's products, which are designed to help with urinary incontinence and urinary retention, include male external catheters and urethral inserts for women. Proprietary products include catheters with antibacterial properties. Rochester Medical markets directly to distributors, institutions, and home care providers; the manufacturing company also sells through private-label and marketing arrangements with such firms as Mentor and ConvaTec, a division of Bristol-Myers Squibb.

St. Jude Medical, Inc.

One Lillehei Plaza, St. Paul, MN 55117

Telephone: 651-483-2000 **Fax:** 651-482-8318 **Metro area:** Minneapolis-St. Paul, MN **Web site:** http://www.sjm.com **Human resources contact:** Jan M. Webster **Sales:** $1 billion **Number of employees:** 3,984 **Number of employees for previous year:** 3,772 **Industry designation:** Medical instruments **Company type:** Public **Top competitors:** Guidant Corporation; Medtronic, Inc.; Baxter International Inc.

Does your heart go pitter-patter? St. Jude Medical develops and markets devices for cardiovascular applications and is the world's leading manufacturer of mechanical heart valves. The company's Heart Valve Disease Management division makes mechanical and tissue heart valves as well as annuloplasty rings. The Cardiac Rhythm Management division makes pacemakers (for fast, slow, and irregular heartbeats) and implantable defibrillators. The Daig division makes angiography catheters, guidewires, guiding sheaths, and catheters used for diagnostic heart mapping. St. Jude's products are sold in more than 100 countries through a combination of direct-sales personnel and independent manufacturers' representatives.

SpectraScience, Inc.

3650 Annapolis Ln. Ste. 101, Minneapolis, MN 55447

Telephone: 612-509-9999 **Fax:** 612-509-9805 **Metro area:** Minneapolis-St. Paul, MN **Web site:** http://www.spectrascience.com **Sales:** $100,000 **Number of employees:** 11 **Number of employees for previous year:** 9 **Industry designation:** Medical services **Company type:** Public **Top competitors:** C. R. Bard, Inc.; EndoSonics Corporation; Boston Scientific Corporation

Development-stage SpectraScience is scoping out the diagnostic possibilities. The company makes spectroscopic devices which use light to help detect and differentiate between cancerous and healthy tissue and to detect cardiovascular disease. The company's Optical Biopsy System looks for cancer in the gastrointestinal tract using minimally invasive endoscopic surgery. It may also be useful for detection of cancer in the lungs, urinary tract, cervix, prostate, and bladder. SpectraScience's other product, the Spectroscopic Guidewire System, is used to detect coronary blockages (blood clots, fatty deposits in the arteries). Both products are awaiting approval in the US and Europe.

SurModics, Inc.

9924 W. 74th St., Eden Prairie, MN 55344

Telephone: 612-829-2700 **Fax:** 612-829-2743 **Metro area:** Minneapolis-St. Paul, MN **Web site:** http://www.surmodics.com **Human resources contact:** Joan Blum **Sales:** $9.8 million **Number of employees:** 97 **Number of employees for previous year:** 85 **Industry designation:** Medical products **Company type:** Public **Top competitors:** Landec Corporation; Spire Corporation; Norsk Hydro ASA

SurModics doesn't just want to scratch the surface of the medical devices market—it also wants to coat it with its own special agent. The company's PhotoLink product is a light-activated coating that makes a covalent bond between medical device surfaces and a variety of chemicals, improving such attributes as infection resistance, drug-delivery diffusion, and lubricity. PhotoLink is used on such devices as catheters, shunts, pacemakers, and urological and gynecological devices. SurModics has licensing agreements with companies including Abbott Laboratories. In addition to PhotoLink, the company makes stabilization products for immunoassay diagnostic tests and a format for in vitro diagnostic tests.

Urologix, Inc.

14405 21st Ave. North, Minneapolis, MN 55447

Telephone: 612-475-1400 **Fax:** 612-475-1443 **Metro area:** Minneapolis-St. Paul, MN **Web site:** http://www.urologix.com **Human resources contact:** Bridgette Kamais **Sales:** $11.2 million **Number of employees:** 139 **Number of employees for previous year:** 87 **Industry designation:** Medical instruments **Company type:** Public **Top competitors:** Boston Scientific Corporation; VidaMed, Inc.; EDAP TMS S.A.

For men whose prostate has them prostrate, Urologix has the answer. The company's Targis System is designed to treat benign prostate hyperplasia, or enlargement of the prostate. Targis uses a noninvasive catheter-based therapy that applies microwave heat to the diseased areas of the prostate, while cooling and protecting urethral tissue. The treatment, an alternative to drug therapy, does not require anesthesia or surgery and can be administered on an outpatient basis. The Targis System is sold in the US, the European Union, and Japan. The company has international marketing and distribution agreements with Boston Scientific and Japanese medical devices firm Nihon Kohdon.

Uroplasty, Inc.

2718 Summer St. NE, Minneapolis, MN 55413

Telephone: 612-378-1180 **Fax:** 612-378-2027 **Metro area:** Minneapolis-St. Paul, MN **Web site:** http://www.uroplasty.com **Sales:** $4.3 million **Number of employees:** 38 **Industry designation:** Medical products **Company type:** Public **Top competitors:** Advanced UroScience, Inc.; Mentor Corporation; C. R. Bard, Inc.

Uroplasty makes and sell products for the treatment of urinary incontinence. The company's primary product is Macroplastique, an injectable bulking agent used to treat stress urinary incontinence, the most common form of incontinence, which occurs as a result of intra-abdominal pressure caused by coughing, laughing, or exercise. Macroplastique is also used to treat incontinence that can occur after prostate surgery, and vesicoureteral reflux (the backward flow of urine from the bladder into the kidney), which occurs mostly in children. The company has received approval to sell the product throughout the European Union and is seeking FDA approval for the US.

The Valspar Corporation

1101 Third St. South, Minneapolis, MN 55415

Telephone: 612-332-7371 **Fax:** 612-375-7723 **Metro area:** Minneapolis-St. Paul, MN **Web site:** http://www.valspar.com **Human resources contact:** Gary E. Gardner **Sales:** $1.2 billion **Number of employees:** 3,800 **Number of employees for previous year:** 3,200 **Industry designation:** Paints & related products **Company type:** Public **Top competitors:** PPG Industries, Inc.; The Sherwin-Williams Company; Akzo Nobel N.V.

In 1866 Valspar's progenitor hired American artist Winslow Homer's chemist brother to make varnishes. Today the company still makes varnishes, along with other consumer, packaging, and industrial coatings. Its special products group also makes resins and emulsions used in coatings and colorants. The company sells a number of brands, including Valspar, Laura Ashley, Magicolor, and Masury. Customers include home centers, farm store chains, and specialty paint stores. Lowes Corporation accounts for more than 10% of company sales. To manufacture its products, Valspar operates plants throughout North America, the Asia/Pacific region, and Europe as well as in South Africa.

Verdant Brands Inc.

9555 James Ave. South, Ste. 200, Bloomington, MN 55431

Telephone: 612-703-3300 **Fax:** 612-887-1300 **Metro area:** Minneapolis-St. Paul, MN **Web site:** http://www.verdantbrands.com/ **Human resources contact:** Lisa Stasek **Sales:** $48.2 million **Number of employees:** 231 **Number of employees for previous year:** 57 **Industry designation:** Chemicals—specialty **Company type:** Public **Top competitors:** The Scotts Company; Virbac Corporation; Novartis AG

Verdant Brands (formerly Ringer Corporation) develops and sells lawn, garden, and turf products. The company makes environment-minded alternative pesticides under the Safer brand and traditional pesticides under the Dexol brand. Verdant's granular fertilizer products control the release of nutrients for extended uniform plant feeding and are marketed under the Restore, Supreme Garden Fertilizer, and Safer Lawn Fertilizer brand names. The company's Oxygen Plus and Safer brand water-soluble products enhance root growth. Subsidiary Dexol makes most of its traditional pesticides, with subcontractors making the rest. The company doubled its size in 1998 by acquiring rival pesticide maker Consep.

VirtualFund.com, Inc.

7090 Shady Oak Rd., Eden Prairie, MN 55344

Telephone: 612-941-8687 **Fax:** 612-941-8652 **Metro area:** Minneapolis-St. Paul, MN **Web site:** http://www.virtualfund.com **Human resources contact:** Mary Paige **Sales:** $80.7 million **Number of employees:** 404 **Number of employees for previous year:** 350 **Industry designation:** Computers—peripheral equipment **Company type:** Public **Top competitors:** ENCAD, Inc.; Raster Graphics, Inc.; Hewlett-Packard Company

VirtualFund.com (formerly LaserMaster Technologies) wants to conquer the worlds of printers and cyberspace. A maker of printers and supplies for the professional graphics industry, the company is branching into Web hosting, e-commerce software, and related IT consulting services. Specializing in wide-format, color ink jet printers; filmsetters; and related supplies, VirtualFund.com's customers range from commercial printers to photo labs. The company generates all of its revenue through sales of its printers and consumables. Subsidiary RSPnetwork has its sights set on creating a string of service providers to help clients become active in e-commerce.

Mississippi

Delta and Pine Land Company

One Cotton Row, Scott, MS 38772

Telephone: 601-742-4500 **Fax:** 601-742-4196 **Human resources contact:** George Williams **Sales:** $192.3 million **Number of employees:** 581 **Number of employees for previous year:** 580 **Industry designation:** Agricultural operations **Company type:** Public **Top competitors:** Pioneer Hi-Bred International, Inc.; The Dow Chemical Company

Cotton-pickin' Delta and Pine Land (D&PL) leads the US in cottonseed production. It also breeds, produces, and sells soybean seed. D&PL uses breeding programs and advanced biotechnology to develop cottonseed with improved crop yield and fiber characteristics. Together with Monsanto, which is buying D&PL, it has developed herbicide-tolerant (Roundup Ready) cotton and soybeans, as well as pest-resistant (Bollgard) cottonseed. D&PL is researching the controversial "terminator" gene, which germinates once and would necessitate annual seed purchases. D&PL's cotton varieties are grown mainly in Arizona and east of Texas. The company has facilities in the US as well as in Africa, Asia, Australia, and Latin America.

Sanderson Farms, Inc.

225 N. 13th Ave., Laurel, MS 39440

Telephone: 601-649-4030 **Fax:** 601-426-1461 **Other address:** PO Box 988, Laurel, MS 39441 **Web site:** http://www.sandersonfarms.com **Human resources contact:** Robin Robinson **Sales:** $521.4 million **Number of employees:** 6,358 **Number of employees for previous year:** 6,155 **Industry designation:** Food—meat products **Company type:** Public **Top competitors:** Pilgrim's Pride Corporation; Gold Kist Inc.; Tyson Foods, Inc.

Sanderson Farms is making (chicken) scratches on the surface of the poultry processing field. The company sells ice-pack, chill-pack, and frozen chicken in whole, cut-up, and boneless forms. The company markets to retailers, distributors, and fast-food operators, principally in the southeastern, southwestern, and western US. Its chicken processing operations encompass five hatcheries, four feed mills, and six processing plants. Through its foods division (about 15% of sales) the firm sells more than 200 processed and prepared food items, including frozen entrees such as chicken and dumplings, lasagna, and seafood gumbo, under the Sanderson Farms label. The founding Sanderson family owns 47% of the company.

Staple Cotton Cooperative Association

214 W. Market St., Greenwood, MS 38935

Telephone: 601-453-6231 **Fax:** 601-453-6274 **Other address:** PO Box 547, Greenwood, MS 38935 **Web site:** http://www.staplcotn.com **Human resources contact:** Eugene A. Stansel Jr. **Sales:** $704.5 million **Number of employees:** 197 **Number of employees for previous year:** 156 **Industry designation:** Agricultural operations **Company type:** Cooperative **Top competitors:** Plains Cotton Cooperative Association; Dunavant Enterprises Inc.; Calcot, Ltd.

Wear underwear? Chances are Staplcotn had a hand in it. Staple Cotton Cooperative Association, the US's oldest cotton-marketing co-op, provides marketing and warehousing services to its nearly 7,500 members in 36 states. Founded in 1921 by Mississippi cotton producer Oscar Bledsoe and 10 Delta growers, the co-op's Staplcotn business now sells almost two million bales of cotton annually, produced by more than 6,000 growers. Most of the yield is sold to the US textile industry to make men's knit underwear, T-shirts, sheets, towels, and denim. Customers include Fruit of the Loom and Levi's. The co-op's Staplchiscount subsidiary offers low-interest loans for equipment, buildings, and land to members and non-members alike.

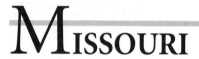

Missouri

Agribrands International, Inc.

9811 South Forty Dr., St. Louis, MO 63124

Telephone: 314-812-0500 **Fax:** 314-812-0400 **Metro area:** St. Louis, MO **Web site:** http://www.agribrands.com/ **Human resources contact:** Cheryl Howery **Sales:** $1.4 billion **Number of employees:** 5,736 **Number of employees for previous year:** 5,550 **Industry designation:** Agricultural operations **Company type:** Public **Top competitors:** Archer Daniels Midland Company; Ag Processing Inc; Cargill, Incorporated

Agribrands International really knows what it's like to "pig out" or be "hungry as a horse." In markets outside the US, Agribrands produces feed and other nutritional products for hogs, dairy cows, cattle, poultry, rabbits, horses, shrimp, and fish. Spun off by pet-food giant Ralston Purina in 1998, Agribrands has nearly 75 plants in 16 countries. The company generates nearly 45% of its sales from the Americas (excluding the US); sales to Europe and the Asia/Pacific region make up the balance. The company's customers are primarily wholesalers and farmers who buy in bulk. Agribrands sells its feed under the Purina and Chow brand names, among others.

All Star Gas Corporation

119 W. Commercial St., Lebanon, MO 65536

Telephone: 417-532-3103 **Fax:** 417-532-8529 **Other address:** PO Box 303, Lebanon, MO 65536 **Human resources contact:** Debi Neugebauer **Sales:** $86.5 million **Number of employees:** 625 **Number of employees for previous year:** 600 **Industry designation:** Oil refining & marketing **Company type:** Public **Top competitors:** AmeriGas Partners, L.P.; Ferrellgas Partners, L.P.; Suburban Propane Partners, L.P.

The prospect of selling 100 million gallons of propane each year puts a twinkle in the eye of All Star Gas. All Star Gas serves some 112,000 residential, agricultural, and commercial customers in 19 states from Washington to Florida with about 130 retail service centers and a fleet of more than 300 delivery trucks. The company buys propane from refineries, gas processing plants, underground storage facilities, and pipeline terminals. All Star Gas also markets a variety of propane appliances, supplies, and related equipment and rents steel propane storage tanks with capacities of up to 30,000 gallons. CEO Paul Lindsey and his wife Kristin, also an executive at All Star Gas, own more than 65% of the company.

Americo Life, Inc.

1055 Broadway, Kansas City, MO 64105

Telephone: 816-391-2700 **Fax:** 816-391-2083 **Metro area:** Kansas City, MO-Kansas City, KS
Human resources contact: Bill Marden **Sales:** $438.3 million (Est.) **Number of employees:** 623
Number of employees for previous year: 420 **Industry designation:** Insurance—life **Company
type:** Private

Americo Life is a holding company for subsidiaries that primarily sell life insurance. The company owns seven life
insurance companies, including Great Southern Life of Dallas, Texas, and National Farmers Union of Kansas City,
Missouri. It also owns a half interest in Financial Assurance Life of Kansas City, Missouri, and Annuity Service of
Austin, Texas. Other business interests include real estate partnerships and a half interest in Argus Health Systems,
a prescription-drug claim-processing company. Chairman Michael Merriman owns about a 30% interest in the
company, which is a subsidiary of Financial Holding.

AVAX Technologies, Inc.

4520 Main St., Ste. 930, Kansas City, MO 64111

Telephone: 816-960-1333 **Fax:** 816-960-1334 **Metro area:** Kansas City, MO-Kansas City, KS **Web
site:** http://www.avax-tech.com **Human resources contact:** Erika Rich **Sales:** $100,000 **Number of
employees:** 13 **Number of employees for previous year:** 6 **Industry designation:** Biomedical
& genetic products **Company type:** Public **Top competitors:** Bristol-Myers Squibb Company; Chiron
Corporation; Schering-Plough Corporation

AVAX Technologies is a development-stage biopharmaceutical company that concentrates on cancer treatments. Its
leading technology is a method to produce vaccines against cancer recurrence using a patient's own modified cancer
cells. The company's first product using this technology is M-Vax, a treatment for melanoma (skin cancer); it is
also developing O-Vax to treat ovarian cancer. AVAX does not engage in pure research, instead licensing the
underlying technology for its products from Rutgers University, the University of Medicine and Dentistry of New
Jersey, and The Texas A&M University System.

Bartlett and Company

4800 Main St., Ste. 600, Kansas City, MO 64112

Telephone: 816-753-6300 **Fax:** 816-753-0062 **Metro area:** Kansas City, MO-Kansas City, KS
Human resources contact: Bill Webster **Sales:** $750 million (Est.) **Number of employees:** 575
Number of employees for previous year: 560 **Industry designation:** Food—flour & grain
Company type: Private **Top competitors:** Archer Daniels Midland Company; Cactus Feeders, Inc.;
Cargill, Incorporated

When the cows come home, Bartlett and Company will be ready. The company's primary business is grain
merchandising, but it also runs cattle feedlots and mills flour. Bartlett operates grain storage facilities in Kansas
City, Kansas; St. Joseph and Waverly, Missouri; and Nebraska City, Nebraska. It has terminal elevators in Council
Bluffs, Iowa; Kansas City and Wichita, Kansas; and St. Joseph, Missouri, as well as more than 10 country elevators.
Bartlett's cattle operations are based in Texas; its flour mills are in Kansas, North Carolina, and South Carolina.
Founded in 1907 as Bartlett Agri Enterprises, the company is still owned by its founding family and has been run
by Paul Bartlett Jr. since 1961.

BHA Group Holdings, Inc.

8800 E. 63rd St., Kansas City, MO 64133

Telephone: 816-356-8400 **Fax:** 816-353-1873 **Metro area:** Kansas City, MO-Kansas City, KS **Web
site:** http://www.bha.com **Human resources contact:** Stephen Kelly **Sales:** $142.4 million **Number
of employees:** 1,025 **Number of employees for previous year:** 860 **Industry designation:**
Pollution control equipment & services **Company type:** Public **Top competitors:** MFRI, Inc.; Donaldson
Company, Inc.; ITEQ, Inc.

If smoke gets in your eyes, then maybe you should call BHA Group Holdings, a leading maker of replacement parts
and accessories for industrial air pollution control equipment. The company's products include fabric filters,
electrically charged collector plates, and high-efficiency expanded polytetrafluoroethylene (ePTFE) membrane
products. The company also provides rehabilitation and conversion services for pollution control equipment. BHA
serves customers operating in nearly all areas of the industrial marketplace in Asia, Europe, and the Americas.

BJC Health System

4444 Forest Park Ave., St. Louis, MO 63108

Telephone: 314-286-2000 **Fax:** 314-286-2060 **Metro area:** St. Louis, MO **Web site:** http://www.bjc.org **Human resources contact:** William M. Behrendt **Sales:** $1.6 billion **Number of employees:** 25,500 **Number of employees for previous year:** 23,696 **Industry designation:** Hospitals **Company type:** Not-for-profit **Top competitors:** Sisters of Mercy Health System-St. Louis; SSM Health Care System Inc.; Tenet Healthcare Corporation

BJC Health System is the largest health care provider in the St. Louis area. It operates a network of more than 100 health care facilities in mid-Missouri (including greater St. Louis) and southern Illinois. Affiliated with Washington University School of Medicine through two of its member teaching hospitals, Barnes-Jewish Hospital and St. Louis Children's Hospital, BJC operates 14 hospitals, six nursing homes, its own health plan, and numerous outpatient care centers. With a group of some 2,000 doctors, BJC jointly owns Joint Contracting, a company set up to bargain with managed care plans.

Blue Cross and Blue Shield of Missouri

1831 Chesnut St., St. Louis, MO 63103

Telephone: 314-923-4444 **Fax:** 314-923-5002 **Metro area:** St. Louis, MO **Web site:** http://www.abcbs.com **Human resources contact:** Morris Burger **Sales:** $719.4 million **Number of employees:** 1,700 **Number of employees for previous year:** 1,600 **Industry designation:** Insurance—accident & health **Company type:** Not-for-profit **Top competitors:** Humana Inc.; Aetna Inc.; UnitedHealth Group

Blue Cross and Blue Shield of Missouri provides HMO, PPO, point-of-service, and medical indemnity coverage to St. Louis and 84 Missouri counties. As a not-for-profit insurer of last resort, the company receives state tax breaks, but it is also vulnerable to competition from for-profit care providers. In response, in 1994 it set up for-profit managed care company RightCHOICE, which serves more than two million people. As part of the process of converting to for-profit status, Blue Cross and Blue Shield of Missouri wants to transfer its 80% stake in RightCHOICE into a charitable foundation; RightCHOICE would then absorb the rest of the company and operate as a Blue Cross Blue Shield licensee.

Carondelet Health System

13801 Riverport Dr., Ste. 300, St. Louis, MO 63043

Telephone: 314-770-0333 **Fax:** 314-770-0444 **Metro area:** St. Louis, MO **Web site:** http://www.chs-stl.com **Human resources contact:** Nancy Heet **Sales:** $961 million **Number of employees:** 15,800 **Number of employees for previous year:** 15,500 **Industry designation:** Hospitals **Company type:** Not-for-profit **Top competitors:** Catholic Health Initiatives; Tenet Healthcare Corporation; Columbia/HCA Healthcare Corporation

Through a network of over 20 health care facilities, Carondelet Health System carries on its healing mission in some 10 US states, including Arizona, Missouri, and California. Besides hospitals such as St. Joseph Health System in Kansas City, Missouri, the system also operates skilled nursing care facilities, behavioral treatment centers, hospice care facilities, and home health service provider organizations. The Sisters of St. Joseph Carondelet, a Catholic entity whose members emigrated from France in 1836 and founded St. Mary's Hospital in Arizona in 1880, still sponsors the Carondelet Health System.

C.D. Smith Drug Company

3907 S. 48th Terrace, St. Joseph, MO 64503

Telephone: 816-232-5471 **Fax:** 816-279-1682 **Other address:** PO Box 789, St. Joseph, MO 64503 **Metro area:** St. Joseph, MO **Web site:** http://www.cdsdrug.com **Human resources contact:** Laura Peppers **Sales:** $544.1 million (Est.) **Number of employees:** 318 **Industry designation:** Drugs & sundries—wholesale **Company type:** Private **Top competitors:** Cardinal Health, Inc.; Bergen Brunswig Corporation; McKesson HBOC, Inc.

C.D. Smith Drug Company distributes wholesale pharmaceuticals to more than 3,000 customers in the midwestern US and New England. The company sells branded and generic drugs, over-the-counter health care products, and health and beauty aids. C.D. Smith Drug operates OptiSource, a generic buying program through which the company and 16 other regional distributors combine to purchase drugs at prices comparable to those paid by larger competitors. The company's SBS Pharmaceuticals (acquired during C.D. Smith Drug's purchase of another wholesale pharmaceutical distributor) repackages and distributes branded and generic drugs. After the planned IPO, the employee stock ownership plan will own nearly half of the company.

Cerner Corporation

2800 Rockcreek Pkwy., Ste. 601, Kansas City, MO 64117

Telephone: 816-221-1024 **Fax:** 816-474-1742 **Metro area:** Kansas City, MO-Kansas City, KS **Web site:** http://www.cerner.com **Human resources contact:** Julie Wilson **Sales:** $330.9 million **Number of employees:** 837 **Number of employees for previous year:** 663 **Industry designation:** Computers—corporate, professional & financial software **Company type:** Public **Top competitors:** Shared Medical Systems Corporation; IDX Systems Corporation

Cerner designs information systems for the health care industry. Its clinical and administrative information systems connect large health care providers' multisite departments, from emergency rooms to nurses' stations to pharmacies. Extensive patient records, as a result, are always available to physicians. The company's products run on Digital Equipment Corporation (absorbed by Compaq) and IBM servers. Customers include hospitals, health maintenance organizations, clinics, physicians, and integrated health organizations. Co-founders Neal Patterson (chairman and CEO) and Clifford Illig (president) each own 11% of Cerner.

Clark USA, Inc.

8182 Maryland Ave., St. Louis, MO 63105

Telephone: 314-854-9696 **Fax:** 314-854-1580 **Metro area:** St. Louis, MO **Web site:** http://www.clarkusa.com **Human resources contact:** Juli Sherman **Sales:** $4.3 billion (Est.) **Number of employees:** 7,500 **Number of employees for previous year:** 7,400 **Industry designation:** Oil refining & marketing **Company type:** Private **Top competitors:** Exxon Corporation; USX-Marathon Group; BP Amoco p.l.c.

High costs associated with upgrading its Texas refinery have made Clark USA a financial clunker in the last few years. One of the largest independent oil refiners in the US, Clark USA's main operating unit, Clark Refining & Marketing, produces petroleum products, including crude oil, liquid petroleum gas, and automotive and aviation fuel. Besides the refinery in Texas, it owns two more in Illinois, and has more than 15 distribution terminals and about 700 gasoline/convenience stores, primarily in the Midwest. The Blackstone Group, an investment company, owns 68% of Clark, and Occidental Petroleum owns a 31% stake.

Dairy Farmers of America

10220 N. Executive Hills Blvd., Kansas City, MO 64190

Telephone: 816-801-6455 **Fax:** 816-801-6456 **Metro area:** Kansas City, MO-Kansas City, KS **Web Site:** http://www.dfamilk.com **Human resources contact:** Ray Silver **Sales:** $3.8 billion **Number of employees:** 5,300 **Number of employees for previous year:** 3,200 **Industry designation:** Food—dairy products **Company type:** Cooperative **Top competitors:** Groupe Danone; Dean Foods Company; Land O'Lakes, Inc.

They're partners in cream: Mid-America Dairymen (previously the #1 milk co-op), the Southern Region of Associated Milk Producers, Milk Marketing, and Western Dairymen Cooperative. The four groups have formed the Dairy Farmers of America (DFA), the largest US dairy cooperative, with 24,000 members in 43 states. The co-op controls about a quarter of the US milk supply. Under such brand names as Borden, DFA sells milk, cheese, butter, and other products to wholesale and retail customers worldwide; it also produces Frito-Lay's cheese dips, Baskin-Robbins Ice Cream, and Starbucks' Frappuccino coffee drink. DFA provides marketing, research and development, and legislative lobbying for its members.

D & K Healthcare Resources, Inc.

8000 Maryland Ave., Ste. 920, St. Louis, MO 63105

Telephone: 314-727-3485 **Fax:** 314-727-5759 **Metro area:** St. Louis, MO **Web site:** http://www.dkwd.com **Human resources contact:** Lisa White **Sales:** $612.4 million **Number of employees:** 261 **Number of employees for previous year:** 234 **Industry designation:** Drugs & sundries—wholesale **Company type:** Public **Top competitors:** Cardinal Health, Inc.; AmeriSource Health Corporation; Bergen Brunswig Corporation

Need drugs? D & K Healthcare Resources can get 'em to you PDQ. Operating in about 20 midwestern and southern states, the regional wholesale drug distributor supplies pharmaceuticals (about 90% of sales) and over-the-counter health and beauty aids to some 700 independent and franchise pharmacies, regional drugstore chains, hospitals, alternative care facilities, and managed care organizations. About half of its sales are to independent pharmacies, while health care facilities and organizations account for another 30%. Its products are distributed from warehouses in Kentucky, Minnesota, and Missouri. D & K Healthcare Resources owns 50% of Pharmaceutical Buyers, a group purchasing organization.

Data Research Associates, Inc.

1276 N. Warson Rd., St. Louis, MO 63132

Telephone: 314-432-1100 **Fax:** 314-993-8927 **Other address:** PO Box 8495, St. Louis, MO 63132 **Metro area:** St. Louis, MO **Web site:** http://www.dra.com **Human resources contact:** Maggie Bell **Sales:** $32.5 million **Number of employees:** 215 **Number of employees for previous year:** 204 **Industry designation:** Computers—services **Company type:** Public **Top competitors:** Dawson Holdings PLC; Geac Computer Corporation Limited; Follett Corporation

Products by Data Research Associates (DRA) allow librarians the luxury of filing the card catalog system under "Extinct." DRA is a systems integrator for libraries and other information providers. The company's systems enable users to search a local library catalog and remote databases, allowing access to full text and graphics. DRA systems also manage library circulation and generate collection, usage, and borrower reports for the library staff. Designed for all sizes and classes of libraries (including academic, business, and public libraries), DRA systems are used by more than 2,400 libraries on four continents.

Daughters of Charity National Health System

4600 Edmundson Rd., St. Louis, MO 63134

Telephone: 314-253-6700 **Fax:** 314-253-6491 **Other address:** PO Box 45998, St. Louis, MO 63145 **Metro area:** St. Louis, MO **Web site:** http://www.dcnhs.org **Human resources contact:** David A. Smith **Sales:** $6.2 billion **Number of employees:** 65,000 **Number of employees for previous year:** 60,000 **Industry designation:** Hospitals **Company type:** Not-for-profit **Top competitors:** Catholic Health Initiatives; Columbia/HCA Healthcare Corporation; Tenet Healthcare Corporation

Ah, sweet charity! The Daughters of Charity National Health System (DCNHS) is a network of about 80 Catholic hospitals, nursing homes, community clinics, rehabilitation centers, and psychiatric wards in 15 states and the District of Columbia. It is the #1 Catholic hospital system in the US (ahead of Catholic Health Initiatives). The network is sponsored by four US provinces of the Daughters of Charity religious order and governed by a board made up primarily of sisters of the order that is led, however, by a non-clergy CEO. Although its traditional mission is caring for children and the poor, DCNHS has displayed a financial acumen that has earned it some $2 billion in investments and the nickname "Daughters of Currency."

DST Systems, Inc.

333 W. 11th St., Kansas City, MO 64105

Telephone: 816-435-1000 **Fax:** 816-435-8618 **Metro area:** Kansas City, MO-Kansas City, KS **Web site:** http://www.dstsystems.com **Human resources contact:** Joan Horan **Sales:** $1.1 billion **Number of employees:** 6,000 **Number of employees for previous year:** 5,600 **Industry designation:** Computers—corporate, professional & financial software **Company type:** Public **Top competitors:** First Data Corporation; SunGard Data Systems Inc.; Fiserv, Inc.

DST Systems provides information processing services and computer software products and services to mutual funds (it has about 30% of the market), insurance providers, and banks. Its clients include Janus Capital and T. Rowe Price Corp. DST's Emerging Business unit consists of 50%-owned Argus Health Systems (prescription claims processing) and DBS Systems Corp. (cable television subscriber-management software). In 1998 DST, Boston EquiServe, and First Chicago Trust teamed up to form EquiServe, the largest provider of corporate stock transfers in the US. The company has operations worldwide; about 16% of its sales are outside the US. Former railroad firm Kansas City Southern Industries owns about 41% of DST.

Express Scripts, Inc.

14000 Riverport Dr., Maryland Heights, MO 63043

Telephone: 314-770-1666 **Fax:** 314-291-3669 **Metro area:** St. Louis, MO **Web site:** http:// www.express-scripts.com **Human resources contact:** Karen Matteuzzi **Sales:** $2.8 billion **Number of employees:** 1,570 **Number of employees for previous year:** 1,513 **Industry designation:** Insurance—accident & health **Company type:** Public **Top competitors:** Walgreen Co.; SmithKline Beecham plc; Merck & Co., Inc.

Express Scripts is one of the largest pharmacy benefits management companies in the US. The company's 12 million members have access to a network of 50,000 pharmacies, in addition to mail-order prescription services and a planned online pharmacy. Express Script's customers are primarily HMOs, with other clients including self-insured businesses and insurance companies. Unlike other large pharmacy benefits companies, Express Scripts is not owned by a drug company, assuring wider purchase options for the company. Express Scripts also offers eye care, infusion therapy, and a 24-hour help line. New York Life owns 45% of the company.

Farmland Industries, Inc.

3315 N. Oak Trafficway, Kansas City, MO 64116

Telephone: 816-459-6000 **Fax:** 816-459-6979 **Other address:** P.O. Box 7305, Kansas City, MO 64116 **Metro area:** Kansas City, MO-Kansas City, KS **Web site:** http://www.farmland.com **Human resources contact:** Holly D. McCoy **Sales:** $8.8 billion **Number of employees:** 16,100 **Number of employees for previous year:** 14,600 **Industry designation:** Agricultural operations **Company type:** Cooperative **Top competitors:** IBP, inc.; Cenex Harvest States Cooperatives; Cargill, Incorporated

At the end of the workday for Farmland Industries' members, it's time for a hoedown. Farmland Industries is the #1 agricultural cooperative in the US and is a competitor in agribusiness worldwide, exporting products (primarily grain) to about 90 countries. It is a major beef packer in the US and also a top producer of pork products. Farmland Industries is owned by 1,500 local co-ops, which are made up of about 600,000 farmers in the US, Canada, and Mexico. The co-op's operations, many accomplished through joint ventures, include crop processing, fertilizer plants, a petroleum refinery, grain elevators, feed mills, beef and pork processing plants, and a fleet of trucks, railcars, and barges.

HealthCore Medical Solutions, Inc.

11904 Blue Ridge Blvd., Grandview, MO 64030

Telephone: 816-763-4900 **Fax:** 816-765-6573 **Metro area:** Kansas City, MO-Kansas City, KS **Web site:** http://www.solutionscard.com **Human resources contact:** Sharon Polk **Sales:** $100,000 **Number of employees:** 16 **Number of employees for previous year:** 13 **Industry designation:** Medical services **Company type:** Public **Top competitors:** MedicalControl, Inc.; Anthem Insurance Companies, Inc.; SafeGuard Health Enterprises, Inc.

It's no platinum card, but for an annual fee of $55-100 individuals without insurance can get discounts on health care with cards from HealthCore Medical Solutions. The firm provides a noninsurance alternative to health care with its HealthCare Solutions Card, which entitles members to discounts (from 5% to 60% off) at participating networks of health care providers, including eye care, dental, hearing, pharmacy, and chiropractic providers. Customers can also use their cards for such health care services as occupational therapy, medical equipment, and vitamins. HealthCore offers the Savings Solutions Card for customers in the New York City area and the Medical Solutions Card for hospital and physician services.

Health Midwest

2304 E. Meyer Blvd., Kansas City, MO 64132

Telephone: 816-276-9297 **Fax:** 816-276-9222 **Metro area:** Kansas City, MO-Kansas City, KS **Web site:** http://www.healthmidwest.org **Human resources contact:** Sue Heiman **Sales:** $669.1 million **Number of employees:** 13,200 **Number of employees for previous year:** 11,000 **Industry designation:** Hospitals **Company type:** Not-for-profit **Top competitors:** Columbia/HCA Healthcare Corporation; Saint Luke's Shawnee Mission Health System; Catholic Health Initiatives

Health Midwest operates about 15 hospitals in metropolitan Kansas City, and serves people within a 150-mile radius of the city. With more than 2,000 physicians and about 100 service locations, Health Midwest is not only the largest health care provider in the area, but is also a major employer. Services include primary care, rehabilitation, and home health care. Specialized programs and community outreach services include childbirth classes, health screenings, a program for older adults, physician referral, and a family practice residency program. Despite expansion efforts by health care giant Columbia/HCA, Health Midwest and other local hospitals retain top market shares in the area.

Hoechst Marion Roussel, Inc.

10236 Marion Park Dr., Kansas City, MO 64137

Telephone: 816-966-5000 **Fax:** 816-966-3803 **Metro area:** Kansas City, MO-Kansas City, KS **Web site:** http://www.hmri.com **Human resources contact:** Tommy White **Sales:** $7.8 billion **Number of employees:** 40,670 **Number of employees for previous year:** 39,595 **Industry designation:** Drugs **Company type:** Subsidiary **Parent company:** Hoechst Group

Hoechst Marion Roussel's mission is to develop new drug therapies and bring them quickly to global markets. Through partnerships with health care providers, it offers value-added programs addressing health economics, information management, patient involvement, and professional education. Hoechst Marion Roussel's drug treatments target illnesses such as cardiovascular disease, respiratory disorders, infections, cancer, arthritis and rheumatism, and central nervous system disorders. The company, formed by the 1995 merger of the pharmaceutical operations of Hoechst, Marion Merrel Dow, and Roussel Uclaf, became a wholly owned subsidiary of Hoechst in 1997.

Intensiva HealthCare Corporation

7733 Forsyth Blvd., 8th Fl., St. Louis, MO 63105

Telephone: 314-725-0112 **Fax:** 314-725-0443 **Metro area:** St. Louis, MO **Human resources contact:** Cordia Young-Brown **Sales:** $69.6 million **Number of employees:** 1,475 **Number of employees for previous year:** 572 **Industry designation:** Medical services **Company type:** Subsidiary **Top competitors:** Olsten Corporation; Harborside Healthcare Corporation

Intensiva Healthcare provides specialized, acute long-term medical care for patients who require intensive monitoring and treatment. The company leases underused hospital space to serve patients who have multiple problems and unstable conditions and must be hospitalized for more than 25 days. By leasing space and purchasing certain services (such as laboratory work and housekeeping) from a host hospital, Intensiva Healthcare offers patients immediate access to a general hospital and doctors without the inconvenience of being moved to a specialty location. The company operates in more than 21 hospitals in nine states. Intensiva is a subsidiary of Select Medical Corporation.

Jack Henry & Associates, Inc.

663 Hwy. 60, Monett, MO 65708

Telephone: 417-235-6652 **Fax:** 417-235-8406 **Other address:** PO Box 807, Monett, MO 65708 **Metro area:** Springfield, MO **Web site:** http://www.jackhenry.com **Human resources contact:** Michelle Hunter **Sales:** $113.4 million **Number of employees:** 605 **Number of employees for previous year:** 447 **Industry designation:** Computers—services **Company type:** Public **Top competitors:** CFI ProServices, Inc.; BancTec, Inc.; The BISYS Group, Inc.

Jack Henry & Associates (JHA) helps your hometown bank operate like a national financial powerhouse. The firm provides integrated hardware and software systems for small banks and other institutions that automate transaction and data processing functions. Its growing line also includes ATM networking tools, digital check imaging software, and Internet banking products. Maintenance and other services account for about 30% of sales. The company continues to expand by acquiring smaller, similar firms. Co-founder and VC Jack Henry and his son, chairman Michael Henry, own 23% of JHA. EVP Jerry Hall, also a founder, owns 9%.

Jones Pharma Inc.

1945 Craig Rd., St. Louis, MO 63146

Telephone: 314-576-6100 **Fax:** 314-469-5749 **Metro area:** St. Louis, MO **Web site:** http://www.jmedpharma.com **Sales:** $103.4 million **Number of employees:** 562 **Number of employees for previous year:** 508 **Industry designation:** Drugs **Company type:** Public **Top competitors:** American Home Products Corporation; Johnson & Johnson; BASF Aktiengesellschaft

Jones Pharma (formerly Jones Medical Industries) makes and distributes specialty pharmaceutical products. About half of the company's sales are generated by the thyroid-disorder drugs Tapazole, Levoxyl, Triostat, and Cytomel. Its other products include Thrombin-JMI for controlling blood loss during surgery (more than 20% of sales); anesthetic Brevital Sodium (about 10%); and veterinary pharmaceuticals Soloxine, Tussigon, and Pancrezyme (about 9%). Jones Pharma makes more than half of its products and contracts out the manufacturing of the remainder. The company sold its branded nutritional products division to Twinlab.

Kansas City Chiefs

One Arrowhead Dr., Kansas City, MO 64129

Telephone: 816-920-9300 **Fax:** 816-923-4719 **Metro area:** Kansas City, MO-Kansas City, KS **Web site:** http://www.kcchiefs.com **Human resources contact:** Dennis Watley **Sales:** $85.6 million (Est.) **Number of employees:** 100 **Industry designation:** Leisure & recreational services **Company type:** Private **Top competitors:** Oakland Raiders; The Denver Broncos Football Club; Seattle Seahawks

The Kansas City Chiefs originally kicked off as the American Football League's Dallas Texans in 1959 but moved to Kansas City, Missouri, in 1963 (the AFL and NFL merged in the late 1960s). In one of the NFL's smallest markets, the Chiefs consistently sell out 79,000-seat Arrowhead Stadium, which is rented from the Jackson County Sports Complex Authority for a nominal fee. In 1999 coach Marty Schottenheimer resigned after his first losing season in 10 years with the team; he was replaced by Gunther Cunningham, the team's defensive coordinator. The Chiefs are owned by founder Lamar Hunt and his family. Hunt is credited with naming the Super Bowl, which the Chiefs won only once—Super Bowl IV in 1970.

Kansas City Life Insurance Company

3520 Broadway, Kansas City, MO 64111

Telephone: 816-753-7000 **Fax:** 816-753-4902 **Metro area:** Kansas City, MO-Kansas City, KS **Web site:** http://www.kclife.com **Human resources contact:** Kathryn Church **Sales:** $483.8 million **Number of employees:** 697 **Number of employees for previous year:** 689 **Industry designation:** Insurance—life **Company type:** Public

There's life in Kansas City? You betcha! Kansas City Life Insurance. It sells individual life and annuity products through general agents in nearly every state in the US. The company also offers variable annuity and universal life insurance. It has two life insurance subsidiaries: Sunset Life, based in Olympia, Washington, offers the same types of policies as Kansas City Life, primarily west of the Mississippi; and Old American Insurance (OAIC), which shares offices with its parent company in Kansas City, Missouri, and focuses mainly on burial and other final-needs insurance. Chairman Joseph Bixby and members of his family own about half of the company.

Kansas City Royals Baseball Corporation

One Royal Way, Kansas City, MO 64129

Telephone: 816-921-8000 **Fax:** 816-921-1366 **Other address:** PO Box 419969, Kansas City, MO 64141 **Metro area:** Kansas City, MO-Kansas City, KS **Web site:** http://www.kcroyals.com **Human resources contact:** Lynne Elder **Sales:** $51.2 million (Est.) **Number of employees:** 131 **Number of employees for previous year:** 130 **Industry designation:** Leisure & recreational services **Company type:** Private **Top competitors:** Chicago White Sox Ltd.; Minnesota Twins; Cleveland Indians Baseball Company, Inc.

Bankrolled by patent-medicine millionaire Ewing Kauffman in 1969, the Kansas City Royals quickly became a baseball success story. Led by All-Star George Brett, the club finished first or second in its American League division 14 times in its first 20 years and won the World Series in 1985. When Kauffman died in 1993, he left the team to the city in a charitable trust that was given six years to find a buyer who would keep it in Kansas City. Although a buyer has been found (the $75 million purchase by New York lawyer Miles Prentice and a group of about 25 largely local investors is awaiting approval), the long period of limbo has chased away some of the team's players.

KV Pharmaceutical Company

2503 S. Hanley Rd., St. Louis, MO 63144

Telephone: 314-645-6600 **Fax:** 314-645-6732 **Metro area:** St. Louis, MO **Human resources contact:** Georgia Tsopeis **Sales:** $98.5 million **Number of employees:** 353 **Number of employees for previous year:** 333 **Industry designation:** Drugs **Company type:** Public **Top competitors:** Mylan Laboratories Inc.; McKesson General Medical Corporation; Owen Healthcare, Inc.

Just a spoonful of KV Pharmaceutical helps the medicine go down. The company makes generic drugs and advanced drug-delivery processes. Its ETHEX subsidiary sells generic drugs to wholesalers, distributors, independent pharmacies, and drugstore chains; it accounts for 80% of KV Pharmaceutical's sales. The firm's time-release processes are used in pills, lotions, and creams; other drug-delivery products include taste-masking products for unpalatable drugs. The company also markets pharmaceutical compounds used to make vitamins in tablet and capsule form. The Hermelin family, which includes KV Pharmaceutical's chairman and vice chairman, owns about one-third of the company.

Laser Vision Centers, Inc.

540 Maryville Centre Dr., Ste. 200, St. Louis, MO 63141

Telephone: 314-434-6900 **Fax:** 314-434-2424 **Metro area:** St. Louis, MO **Web site:** http://www.laservision.com **Human resources contact:** Tammi Johns **Sales:** $23.5 million **Number of employees:** 83 **Number of employees for previous year:** 56 **Industry designation:** Medical products **Company type:** Public **Top competitors:** Sterling Vision, Inc.; LCA-Vision; TLC The Laser Center Inc.

Through both fixed-site and mobile operations, Laser Vision Centers provides ophthalmologists with access to its 40 excimer lasers for treatment of refractive vision disorders such as nearsightedness and astigmatism. The company operates fixed-site centers, independently or through joint operating agreements, in the US, Canada, and Europe; mobile centers operate in the US, Canada, and the UK. Laser Vision has an agreement with Columbia/HCA Healthcare to provide excimer laser equipment to about 20 of that company's ambulatory surgery centers across the US. Laser Vision Centers also provides technical support and training. Big British bank Schroders plc owns almost one-fifth of the company.

Mallinckrodt Inc.

675 McDonnell Blvd., St. Louis, MO 63134

Telephone: 314-654-2000 **Fax:** 314-654-5380 **Other address:** PO Box 5840, St. Louis, MO 63134 **Metro area:** St. Louis, MO **Web site:** http://www.mallinckrodt.com **Human resources contact:** Bruce K. Crockett **Sales:** $2.4 billion **Number of employees:** 12,800 **Number of employees for previous year:** 7,871 **Industry designation:** Medical products **Company type:** Public **Top competitors:** Abbott Laboratories; Syncor International Corporation; Pharmacia & Upjohn, Inc.

Mallinckrodt manufactures and distributes health care products, including imaging agents for radiological, cardiological, urological, and nuclear medicine applications. Its critical-care segment makes products for anesthesiology, respiratory care, and blood analysis. Mallinckrodt also makes various specialty pharmaceuticals such as acetaminophen, codeine salts, and morphine. The company has sold its catalyst businesses and plans to sell its specialty chemicals segment (chemical additives, polymer stearates, and other chemicals) to focus on health care products. Mallinckrodt maintains manufacturing facilities in Europe and North America.

Milnot Company

100 S. Fourth St., Ste. 1010, St. Louis, MO 63102

Telephone: 314-436-7667 **Fax:** 314-436-7679 **Metro area:** St. Louis, MO **Human resources contact:** Scott Meader **Sales:** $92 million (Est.) **Number of employees:** 185 **Industry designation:** Food—canned **Company type:** Private **Top competitors:** Dairy Farmers of America; Hormel Foods Corporation; Nestle S.A.

Milnot really knows how to milk a cow for all its worth. Founded in 1912 as the Litchfield Creamery in Litchfield, Illinois, Milnot makes canned milk products and other foodstuffs under names such as Milnot, Dairy Sweet, Chilli Man, La Famous, and Bravos. Products include sweetened and condensed milk, regular and skim evaporated milk, chili, chip dips, salsa, and various canned meat products. With its purchase of Beech-Nut from Ralcorp, the company became the nation's #2 maker of baby food (behind Gerber). Milnot, owned by Madison Dearborn Partners of Chicago, also makes private-label products at its plants in Colorado, Illinois, and Missouri.

PANACO, Inc.

1050 W. Blue Ridge Blvd., PANACO Bldg., Kansas City, MO 64145

Telephone: 816-942-6300 **Fax:** 816-942-6305 **Metro area:** Kansas City, MO-Kansas City, KS **Web site:** http://www.panaco.com **Human resources contact:** Larry M. Wright **Sales:** $37.8 million **Number of employees:** 71 **Number of employees for previous year:** 46 **Industry designation:** Oil & gas—exploration & production **Company type:** Public

PANACO acquires, develops, and operates oil and gas properties. The company owns or has interests in about 255 oil wells and about 355 natural gas wells in the Gulf of Mexico and onshore in the Gulf Coast region. PANACO's strategy is to acquire producing properties, particularly from larger integrated oil companies, and develop them by completing existing wells and drilling developmental and exploratory wells. The firm markets its oil and gas to companies such as BP Amoco, Citgo, Conoco, Texaco, Unocal, and Vastar. Noted investor Carl Icahn owns about 19% of the company.

Premium Standard Farms, Inc.

423 W. Eighth St., Ste. 200, Kansas City, MO 64105

Telephone: 816-472-7675 **Fax:** 816-843-1450 **Metro area:** Kansas City, MO-Kansas City, KS **Web site:** http://www.psfarms.com **Human resources contact:** Tom Irish **Sales:** $295 million **Number of employees:** 2,200 **Industry designation:** Food—meat products **Company type:** Subsidiary **Top competitors:** Cargill, Incorporated; Murphy Family Farms; Carroll's Foods, Inc.

Premium Standard Farms is the third-largest hog producer in the US (after Murphy Family Farms and Carroll's Foods). The company controls production from birth to slaughter, making feed and selling live hogs, fresh pork, and processed products. It has facilities in rural northern Missouri and in Texas. Not everyone is hog wild about Premium Standard Farms: The company has faced protests (including one headlined by singer Willie Nelson) and paid fines over the economic and environmental impact of its large-scale hog operations. Premium Standard Farms reorganized under Chapter 11 bankruptcy protection in 1996. Continental Grain, one of the world's largest grain companies, owns 51% of Premium Standard Farms.

RehabCare Group, Inc.

7733 Forsyth Blvd., Ste. 1700, St. Louis, MO 63105

Telephone: 314-863-7422 **Fax:** 314-863-0769 **Metro area:** St. Louis, MO **Web site:** http://www.rehabcare.com **Human resources contact:** Stephen J. Toth **Sales:** $207.4 million **Number of employees:** 7,500 **Number of employees for previous year:** 2,366 **Industry designation:** Medical services **Company type:** Public **Top competitors:** HEALTHSOUTH Corporation; NovaCare, Inc.; Mariner Post-Acute Network, Inc.

RehabCare Group is a major US provider of contract rehabilitation services, serving more than 150 hospitals, long-term-care units, and outpatient facilities in all 50 states. The company manages and provides staff for medical rehabilitation, skilled nursing, and therapy operations primarily at acute-care hospitals (more than 50% of sales), but also at outpatient clinics and even schools. Subsidiary Healthcare Staffing Solutions offers temporary and permanent therapist staffing services to hospitals, nursing homes, and contract therapy companies throughout the US. The company is growing through acquisitions and has acquired StarMed Staffing, the temporary staffing service of Medical Resources, Inc.

Reliv International, Inc.

136 Chesterfield Industrial Blvd., Chesterfield, MO 63006

Telephone: 314-537-9715 **Fax:** 314-537-9753 **Metro area:** St. Louis, MO **Web site:** http://www.reliv.com **Human resources contact:** Lynne Kopp **Sales:** $51.9 million **Number of employees:** 228 **Number of employees for previous year:** 162 **Industry designation:** Vitamins & nutritional products **Company type:** Public **Top competitors:** Slim-Fast Foods Company; Avon Products, Inc.; The Quaker Oats Company

Reliv International, which grew out of founder Robert Montgomery's belief that nutritional supplements enabled his quick recovery from brain surgery, wants people all over the world to live healthier lives with its products. Reliv develops, manufactures, and sells nutritional supplements, weight-management and dietary fiber products, skin care products, granola bars, sports drink mixes, and a line of soy-based entrees. These products are sold by subsidiaries to independent distributors in Australia, Canada, Mexico, New Zealand, the UK, and the US. The company's products are manufactured both at Reliv's facility in Missouri and by contract manufacturers.

RightCHOICE Managed Care, Inc.

1831 Chestnut St., St. Louis, MO 63103

Telephone: 314-923-4444 **Fax:** 314-923-5002 **Metro area:** St. Louis, MO **Web site:** http://www.abcbs.com **Human resources contact:** Morris Berger **Sales:** $767.5 million **Number of employees:** 1,800 **Number of employees for previous year:** 1,700 **Industry designation:** Health maintenance organization **Company type:** Public **Top competitors:** BJC Health System; Sisters of Mercy Health System-St. Louis; Deaconess Health Systems

As Alliance Blue Cross Blue Shield, RightCHOICE Managed Care provides health care benefits to more than two million members, most of whom live in the St. Louis area. The company's services include preferred provider organization (PPO), point-of-service, health maintenance organization (HMO), Medicare supplement, and specialty managed care plans, as well as managed indemnity benefit plans. The not-for-profit Blue Cross and Blue Shield of Missouri parked most of its assets in RightCHOICE in 1994 and owns 80% of the company. It hopes to transfer its stake, however, into a charitable foundation, after which it would be absorbed or liquidated by RightCHOICE. The reorganization has not been approved by regulators.

Russell Stover Candies Inc.

1000 Walnut St., Kansas City, MO 64106

Telephone: 816-842-9240 **Fax:** 816-842-5593 **Metro area:** Kansas City, MO-Kansas City, KS **Human resources contact:** Robinn S. Weber **Sales:** $510 million (Est.) **Number of employees:** 6,000 **Number of employees for previous year:** 5,900 **Industry designation:** Food—confectionery **Company type:** Private **Top competitors:** Favorite Brands International Inc.; Nestle S.A.; Mars, Inc.

For Russell Stover Candies, life is like a ... chocolate Elvis? The largest US producer of boxed chocolates is protecting its sweet position with an army of icons. Facing growing competition as candy bar makers such as Hershey and Mars enter the boxed-chocolate arena, it has licensed the use of images of Superman, Snoopy, Bugs Bunny, Elvis (a big hit on Valentine's Day), and Barbie. Boxed chocolates make up 85% of sales, but the firm is breaking out of the box with plans to introduce bagged Halloween candy. Founded by Russell Stover in 1923, the company is owned by brothers Tom and Scott Ward, whose father, Louis, acquired it in 1960. Stover sells candies under the Russell Stover and Whitman's brand names.

St. Louis Blues Hockey Club L.L.C.

Kiel Center, 1401 Clark Ave., St. Louis, MO 63103

Telephone: 314-622-2500 **Fax:** 314-622-2588 **Metro area:** St. Louis, MO **Web site:** http://www.stlouisblues.com **Human resources contact:** Dave Coverstone **Sales:** $70 million (Est.) **Number of employees:** 150 **Industry designation:** Leisure & recreational services **Company type:** Private **Top competitors:** Chicago Blackhawk Hockey Team, Inc.; Detroit Red Wings

The St. Louis Blues Hockey Club is named after a song by W. C. Handy, who has often been called the father of the blues. True to the club's name, the team has been pretty low-down since joining the National Hockey League in 1967. St. Louis made three appearances in the Stanley Cup finals in its first three years as a team, only to be swept 4-0 each time. The St. Louis Blues, owned by Sid Salomon, are in the Central Division of the Western Conference; the team plays home games in the 19,200-seat Kiel Center. The club's main logo is the Bluenote—a stylized musical note with wings.

St. Louis Cardinals, L.P.

Busch Stadium, 250 Stadium Plaza, St. Louis, MO 63102

Telephone: 314-421-3060 **Fax:** 314-425-0640 **Metro area:** St. Louis, MO **Web site:** http://www.stlcardinals.com **Human resources contact:** Marian Rhodes **Sales:** $82.9 million (Est.) **Industry designation:** Leisure & recreational services **Company type:** Private **Top competitors:** Chicago National League Ball Club, Inc.; The Cincinnati Reds; Houston Astros Baseball Club

They take their beer and baseball seriously in St. Louis: beer-garden owner Chris Von der Ahe created the St. Louis Brown Stockings in 1882 in order to sell more brew. The team moved from the American Association to the National League in 1892 and was renamed the Cardinals in 1900. Since then the team has played in 15 league championships and won the World Series nine times—the last in 1982. The Cardinals became one of 1998's hottest tickets as fans watched Cardinal first baseman Mark McGwire destroy Roger Maris' single-season home-run record of 61 slams. (McGwire hit an astounding 70 dingers out of the park.) An investment group led by St. Louis banker Andrew Baur and William DeWitt Jr. owns the team.

St. Louis Rams Football Company

One Rams Way, St. Louis, MO 63045

Telephone: 314-982-7267 **Fax:** 314-770-9261 **Metro area:** St. Louis, MO **Web site:** http://www.stlouisrams.com **Sales:** $91.9 million (Est.) **Industry designation:** Leisure & recreational services **Company type:** Private **Top competitors:** Atlanta Falcons; San Francisco 49ers; New Orleans Saints

After the St. Louis Cardinals professional football team left for Arizona in 1988, the city went without a team for seven years. That changed in 1995 when owner and chairperson Georgia Frontiere, one of the few female owners in professional sports, moved the Los Angeles Rams (founded in Cleveland in 1936) to the city of the Gateway Arch. Playing in the Trans World Dome, the St. Louis Rams field a young team—with wide receiver Isaac Bruce and quarterback Tony Banks, both age 25, among them—that have yet to make the most of their talent. The Rams have not won their division since 1985, when they were still in Los Angeles.

Sheffield Pharmaceuticals, Inc.

425 Woodsmill Rd., Ste. 270, St. Louis, MO 63017

Telephone: 314-579-9899 **Fax:** 314-579-9799 **Metro area:** St. Louis, MO **Human resources contact:** Judy Roeske Bullock **Sales:** $400,000 **Number of employees:** 12 **Number of employees for previous year:** 9 **Industry designation:** Drugs **Company type:** Public

Sheffield Pharmaceuticals is a development-stage company seeking to develop and commercialize its proprietary drug delivery system, the Premaire Metered Solution Inhaler (the Premaire MSI System) and four respiratory drugs. The reusable, handheld, metered solution inhaler can deliver up to two months' supply of drugs to treat asthma and chronic obstructive pulmonary disease. Sheffield acquired the exclusive worldwide rights to the Premaire MSI System from Siemens AG, and through an option agreement with Zambon Group SpA of Milan seeks to develop and market respiratory drugs delivered by its inhaler. It is also looking to out-license its portfolio of early-stage biomedical technologies.

Siegel-Robert Inc.

12837 Flushing Meadows Dr., St. Louis, MO 63131

Telephone: 314-965-2444 **Fax:** 314-544-8472 **Metro area:** St. Louis, MO **Human resources contact:** John Maxwell **Sales:** $485 million (Est.) **Number of employees:** 3,100 **Industry designation:** Rubber & plastic products **Company type:** Private **Top competitors:** Plastronics Plus; Triple S Plastics, Inc.; International Smart Sourcing, Inc.

Siegel-Robert doesn't mind molding away or getting yanked around. Injection-molded plastic products by the firm include car door handles and other parts for the automotive, appliance, and electronic industries. It also makes car emblems, radiator grilles, exterior mirror housings, and side moldings. Developer of the auto industry's first all-plastic exterior mirror housings, the company supplies companies such as General Motors. Its mirrors appear on the Chevrolet Venture, Oldsmobile Silhouette, and Pontiac Trans Sport minivans. To reduce costs and increase part consistency, Siegel-Robert has switched from conventional molding to co-injection molding. CEO Halvor Anderson partially owns the company.

Sigma-Aldrich Corporation

3050 Spruce St., St. Louis, MO 63103

Telephone: 314-771-5765 **Fax:** 314-286-7874 **Metro area:** St. Louis, MO **Web site:** https://www.sigma-aldrich.com **Human resources contact:** Terry R. Colvin **Sales:** $1.2 billion **Number of employees:** 6,666 **Number of employees for previous year:** 5,110 **Industry designation:** Chemicals—specialty **Company type:** Public **Top competitors:** Laporte plc; Holliday Chemical Holdings PLC; ICN Pharmaceuticals, Inc.

Sigma-Aldrich sells chemicals used in research and development, usually to labs with orders averaging $225. It has lots of customers—approximately 145,000 of them, 55% of which are foreign. The company distributes more than 83,000 chemicals (it makes about 46% and buys the rest) used in biochemistry, synthetic chemistry, and pharmacology. Sigma-Adrich's diagnostic kits detect heart, liver, and kidney diseases. Catalog sales account for most orders. Subsidiary B-Line sells metal products, such as strut and pipe supports, cable trays to hold telephone cables, electrical fasteners, and fuse boxes, to electrical, mechanical, and telecommunications wholesalers. Founder Alfred Bader owns about 5% of Sigma-Aldrich.

Sisters of Mercy Health System-St. Louis

2039 N. Geyer Rd., St. Louis, MO 63131

Telephone: 314-965-6100 **Fax:** 314-957-0466 **Metro area:** St. Louis, MO **Web site:** http://www.smhs.com **Human resources contact:** Stephen Isenhower **Sales:** $2.2 billion **Number of employees:** 26,000 **Number of employees for previous year:** 25,300 **Industry designation:** Hospitals **Company type:** Not-for-profit **Top competitors:** Columbia/HCA Healthcare Corporation; BJC Health System; Tenet Healthcare Corporation

It's a sister act. Sponsored by the Sisters of Mercy of the St. Louis Regional Community, Sisters of Mercy Health System provides a range of health care and social services through its network of facilities in Arkansas, Illinois, Kansas, Louisiana, Mississippi, Missouri, Oklahoma, and Texas. Through nine regional units, the system runs about 25 hospitals, home health programs, a psychiatric hospital, long-term care facilities, physician practices, and outpatient facilities. Sisters of Mercy also runs several charitable foundations and provides charity care to patients unable to pay for services. For-profit subsidiary Mercy Health Plans offers managed care health plans in Arkansas, Kansas, Missouri, and Texas.

Spartech Corporation

7733 Forsyth Blvd., Ste. 1450, Clayton, MO 63105

Telephone: 314-721-4242 **Fax:** 314-721-1447 **Metro area:** St. Louis, MO **Web site:** http://www.spartech.com **Human resources contact:** Matthew T. Sweeney **Sales:** $653.9 million **Number of employees:** 2,700 **Number of employees for previous year:** 2,125 **Industry designation:** Chemicals—plastics **Company type:** Public **Top competitors:** Tenneco Inc.; Cabot Corporation; M. A. Hanna Company

Spartech goes through more plastic sheets than a chronically thirsty bedwetter. A leading North American plastic-sheet extruder, the company processes more than one billion pounds of material annually. Its rigid sheet and rollstock division makes plastics used in products including industrial signage, showers, spas, and burial-vault liners. Spartech's fast-growing color and specialty compounds unit makes plastic for footwear, lawn and garden equipment, and loose-leaf binders. Its molded products division makes food packaging, thermoplastic wheels and tires, and housewares. Spartech has 38 plants in North America and Europe. The US accounts for 87% of the firm's sales. Vita International owns 44% of the company.

SSM Health Care System Inc.

477 N. Lindbergh Blvd., St. Louis, MO 63141

Telephone: 314-994-7800 **Fax:** 314-994-7900 **Metro area:** St. Louis, MO **Web site:** http://www.ssmhc.com/inet.nsf **Human resources contact:** Steven Barney **Sales:** $2.1 billion **Number of employees:** 19,439 **Number of employees for previous year:** 19,200 **Industry designation:** Hospitals **Company type:** Not-for-profit **Top competitors:** Columbia/HCA Healthcare Corporation; Tenet Healthcare Corporation; BJC Health System

Founded in 1872 by the Sisters of St. Mary, the not-for-profit SSM Health Care System is one of the largest Catholic health systems in the country. SSM owns, operates, and manages nearly 30 hospitals, rehabilitation clinics, and nursing homes, with a total of almost 5,500 licensed beds. Its health care facilities are located in Illinois, Missouri, Oklahoma, and Wisconsin (SSM divested ventures in South Carolina to focus on its other operations). Its health-related businesses include information systems, home care management, and clinical engineering and other support services.

Tripos, Inc.

1699 S. Hanley Rd., St. Louis, MO 63144

Telephone: 314-647-1099 **Fax:** 314-647-9241 **Metro area:** St. Louis, MO **Web site:** http://www.tripos.com **Human resources contact:** David Summers **Sales:** $25.6 million **Number of employees:** 187 **Number of employees for previous year:** 147 **Industry designation:** Computers—corporate, professional & financial software **Company type:** Public **Top competitors:** Pharmacopeia, Inc.

Research company Tripos provides software, software consulting, chemical compound libraries, and contract and collaborative research services to the biotechnology, pharmaceutical, and other life science industries. Tripos' chemical library business uses computer-assisted design to help researchers find molecular structures that aid in the development of new drugs. The company also sells third-party hardware that is used to operate its software products. Tripos sells its products and services in North America, Europe, and Pacific Rim countries. Foreign customers account for more than 40% of the company's sales. Tripos' customers include Genelabs and Cell Pathways.

Unigraphics Solutions Inc.

13736 Riverport Dr., Maryland Heights, MO 63043

Telephone: 314-344-5900 **Fax:** 314-344-4180 **Metro area:** St. Louis, MO **Web site:** http://www.ugsolutions.com **Human resources contact:** Mike Desmond **Sales:** $403.6 million **Number of employees:** 2,200 **Number of employees for previous year:** 2,000 **Industry designation:** Computers—engineering, scientific & CAD-CAM software **Company type:** Public

Unigraphics Solutions, a computer-aided design (CAD) software provider, offers such software products as the high-end Unigraphics program and a Windows-driven version called Solid Edge, both of which are based on Unigraphics' Parasolid core software. The programs allow designers to kick the virtual tires—and also open doors, trunks, and hoods—of a CAD car model before it is constructed. It also makes a software product called IMAN that organizes and manages design data. Customers include General Motors, Boeing, and other makers of automobiles, aircraft, machinery, and electronics. Unigraphics also provides program customization, training, and technical support. Electronic Data Systems owns about 86% of the company.

Young Innovations, Inc.

13705 Shoreline Ct. East, Earth City, MO 63045

Telephone: 314-344-0010 **Fax:** 314-344-0021 **Metro area:** St. Louis, MO **Human resources contact:** Vicki Giaimo **Sales:** $36.6 million **Number of employees:** 200 **Number of employees for previous year:** 173 **Industry designation:** Medical & dental supplies **Company type:** Public **Top competitors:** DENTSPLY International Inc.; Allegheny Teledyne Incorporated; The Gillette Company

Young Innovations makes and markets single-use dental instruments and supplies. Used primarily in preventive dentistry and infection control, the products include disposable and metal prophy angles, cups, brushes, pastes, fluorides, and fluoride applicators sold under the Young and Denticator brand names. The company's Panoramic PC 1000 X-ray machine produces images of a patient's dental arch and its Laser 1000 cephalometric X-ray produces images of a patient's anterior skull. Young Innovations also makes private-label products for third parties. Its products are sold worldwide through medical and dental distributors. The trust of George E. Richmond, president and CEO, owns almost 50% of the company's stock.

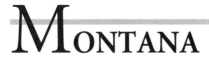

MONTANA

Kampgrounds of America, Inc.

860 N. 31st St., Billings, MT 59101

Telephone: 406-248-7444 **Fax:** 406-248-7414 **Web site:** http://www.koakampgrounds.com **Sales:** $25 million (Est.) **Number of employees:** 357 **Number of employees for previous year:** 300 **Industry designation:** Leisure & recreational services **Company type:** Private **Top competitors:** International Leisure Hosts, Ltd.; Rank America Inc.; Thousand Trails, Inc.

Kampgrounds of America (KOA) provides kamping in komfort to anyone wanting to spend some time in the great outdoors. KOA is North America's largest system of open-to-the-public campgrounds, with more than 75,000 sites at about 600 campgrounds throughout Canada, Japan, Mexico, and the US. The campgrounds offer cabins, on-site convenience stores, restrooms, laundry facilities, utility hookups, and swimming pools and other forms of entertainment. The company generates sales through camping registration fees and franchise fees (only 10 of the campground sites are company-owned). Founded in 1962 by real estate developer Dave Drum, KOA is owned by the family of investor Oscar Tang.

Ribi ImmunoChem Research, Inc.

553 Old Corvallis Rd., Hamilton, MT 59840

Telephone: 406-363-6214 **Fax:** 406-363-6129 **Metro area:** Missoula, MT **Web site:** http://www.ribi.com **Human resources contact:** Sue Kerner **Sales:** $6.1 million **Number of employees:** 112 **Number of employees for previous year:** 103 **Industry designation:** Biomedical & genetic products **Company type:** Public **Top competitors:** Rhone-Poulenc S.A.; BioChem Pharma, Inc.; Chiron Corporation

This Ribi will stimulate, but not for your pleasure. Ribi ImmunoChem Research develops biopharmaceuticals that stimulate the immune system to generate natural agents and signals to treat and prevent human diseases. It is also developing immunostimulants that direct the immune system to respond to a particular cancer or infectious disease. With partners SmithKline Beecham and Wyeth-Lederle Vaccines and Pediatrics, the company is developing vaccines for such diseases as hepatitis A, B, and C and Lyme disease. With partners Schering-Plough, Biomira, and the National Cancer Institute, Ribi ImmunoChem is also developing a number of vaccines to treat such cancers as breast, lung, ovarian, skin, and prostate cancer.

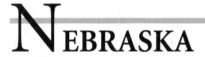

NEBRASKA

George Risk Industries, Inc.

GRI Plaza, 802 S. Elm St., Kimball, NE 69145

Telephone: 308-235-4645 **Fax:** 308-235-2609 **Web site:** http://www.grisk.com **Human resources contact:** Penny Stull **Sales:** $11.5 million **Number of employees:** 250 **Number of employees for previous year:** 230 **Industry designation:** Computers—peripheral equipment **Company type:** Public **Top competitors:** Pittway Corporation; Key Tronic Corporation; Tyco International Ltd.

Butch and Sundance might have gotten honest jobs if George Risk Industries (GRI) had been around in the late 1800s. GRI makes burglar alarm systems and components, including holdup switches used by banks and home-installed panic buttons for direct access to alarm monitoring centers. While security products make up about 90% of its sales, GRI also manufactures computer keyboards and keypads, a passel of switches, and control boards used by the FAA's air traffic controllers. The company serves the commercial, aerospace, industrial, and medical fields. GRI's goods have traveled to outer space and have gone to war in the Persian Gulf. Chairman and president Ken Risk, the founder's son, owns 48% of the company.

IBP, inc.

IBP Ave., Dakota City, NE 68731

Telephone: 402-494-2061 **Fax:** 402-241-2068 **Other address:** PO Box 515, Dakota City, NE 68731 **Metro area:** Sioux City, IA **Web site:** http://www.ibpinc.com **Human resources contact:** Kenneth J. Kimbro **Sales:** $12.8 billion **Number of employees:** 38,000 **Number of employees for previous year:** 34,000 **Industry designation:** Food—meat products **Company type:** Public **Top competitors:** Smithfield Foods, Inc.; Cargill, Incorporated; ConAgra, Inc.

The world's largest producer of fresh beef and the #2 US pork processor (behind Smithfield Foods), IBP processes more than nine billion pounds of meat per year—almost 15% of the US total. Products include fresh, boxed beef and pork and processed meat products. IBP sells to grocery retailers, distributors, the food service industry, and other meat processors. It sells the less-edible leftovers to manufacturers of animal feed, cosmetics, gelatin, leather, and pharmaceuticals. To buffer itself against commodity price swings, the company is diversifying into higher-margin, value-added products such as deli meats, pizza toppings, smoked hams, and taco meat.

Isco, Inc.

4700 Superior St., Lincoln, NE 68504

Telephone: 402-464-0231 **Fax:** 402-458-5502 **Other address:** PO Box 5347, Lincoln, NE 68505 **Metro area:** Lincoln, NE **Web site:** http://www.isco.com **Human resources contact:** Sheryl Wright **Sales:** $47.9 million **Number of employees:** 488 **Number of employees for previous year:** 423 **Industry designation:** Instruments—scientific **Company type:** Public **Top competitors:** Milltronics Ltd.; Dionex Corporation; Hach Company

Isco makes water quality testing instruments for government agencies, laboratories, and industrial customers. Products include Flowlink software for pinpointing repairs; flow meters; water and wastewater samplers (36% of sales) for determining pollution levels; and parameter monitoring devices that measure characteristics such as conductivity, pH, and temperature. Isco also makes high-pressure pumps, fluid extraction devices for sample preparation, and liquid chromatography equipment that separates molecule mixtures into components. Subsidiary Geomation makes measurement and control systems for geotechnical and environmental applications. Founder and CEO Robert Allington owns 48% of the company.

Transaction Systems Architects, Inc.

224 S. 108th Ave., Ste. 7, Omaha, NE 68154

Telephone: 402-334-5101 **Fax:** 402-390-8077 **Metro area:** Omaha, NE **Web site:** http://www.tsainc.com **Human resources contact:** Ann Toth **Sales:** $289.8 million **Number of employees:** 2,054 **Number of employees for previous year:** 1,372 **Industry designation:** Computers—corporate, professional & financial software **Company type:** Public **Top competitors:** Harbinger Corporation; Sterling Commerce, Inc.; Deluxe Corporation

Transaction Systems Architects (TSA) moves money. The firm makes electronic funds transfer software used to process transactions involving ATMs, home banking, credit and debit cards, point-of-sale terminals, and wire transfers. TSA's customers include banks, retailers, and third-party transaction processors. The bulk of the company's sales stem from its BASE24 software for high-reliability Compaq computers. TSA also makes network integration and systems migration tools and interactive voice response software. Software license fees contribute more than half of sales; another 43% comes from technical services and maintenance fees. TSA continues to expand its product and geographic breadth through acquisitions.

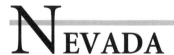

NEVADA

A-55, Inc.

5270 Neil Rd., Reno, NV 89502

Telephone: 775-826-8300 **Fax:** 775-826-8383 **Metro area:** Reno, NV **Web site:** http://www.a-55.com **Human resources contact:** Kristina Gunnerman **Number of employees:** 53 **Number of employees for previous year:** 50 **Industry designation:** Chemicals—specialty **Company type:** Private **Top competitors:** Cinergy Corp.; American Electric Power Company, Inc.; Consolidated Natural Gas Company

A-55 helps electricity generators and petroleum refiners scrape the bottom of the barrel. Its A-55 Additive is combined with a blend of water and heavy residual oils (A-55 Clean Fuels) to produce fuel that burns cleaner than traditional fuels. A-55 Clean Fuels are suitable for open-flame applications that include electricity generation boilers and internal combustion engines. The company has sold enough additives to Commonwealth Edison of Illinois for it to burn almost three million gallons of A-55 Clean Fuels at one of its generating plants. A-55 also sells to mass transit providers, the trucking industry, and industrial customers. Founder and CEO Rudolf Gunnerman owns nearly 80% of the firm.

AgriBioTech, Inc.

120 Corporate Park Dr., Henderson, NV 89014

Telephone: 702-566-2440 **Fax:** 702-566-2450 **Metro area:** Las Vegas, NV **Web site:** http://www.agribiotech.com **Human resources contact:** Ruth Lytle **Sales:** $205.1 million **Number of employees:** 1,079 **Number of employees for previous year:** 325 **Industry designation:** Agricultural operations **Company type:** Public **Top competitors:** DEKALB Genetics Corporation; Pioneer Hi-Bred International, Inc.

Grass seed company AgriBioTech has grown like a weed—too quickly. Formed in 1987 to consolidate smaller companies, AgriBioTech has acquired more than 30 seed operations since 1995 to become one of the world's largest forage (grown to feed animals) and cool-season turf grass (for golf courses and lawns) seed companies. The company researches and processes seed (contracting farmers to do the growing) and distributes seed in all 50 states and to more than 50 countries worldwide. AgriBioTech also sells soybean, corn, vegetable, and grain seeds. Facing heavy debt and a diminished stock price, the acquisitive company has considered finding a buyer for itself.

American Pacific Corporation

3770 Howard Hughes Pkwy., Ste. 300, Las Vegas, NV 89109

Telephone: 702-735-2200 **Fax:** 702-735-4876 **Metro area:** Las Vegas, NV **Human resources contact:** Linda G. Ferguson **Sales:** $52.3 million **Number of employees:** 218 **Number of employees for previous year:** 200 **Industry designation:** Chemicals—specialty **Company type:** Public **Top competitors:** E. I. du Pont de Nemours and Company; Arch Chemicals, Inc.; Nippon Kayaku Co., Ltd.

American Pacific knows how to have a blast. The company's products launch rockets, propel missiles, deploy airbags, and suppress fires. The specialty chemicals firm makes ammonium perchlorate (AP; rocket fuel oxidizer), Halotron (ozone-friendly fire suppressant), sodium azide (airbag deployment chemical), and environmental protection equipment such as its OdorMaster system for use at sewage treatment plants. American Pacific, with operations in Utah and Nevada, is the only US producer of AP. The company also has real estate interests near Las Vegas. Customers include commercial satellite launchers, Cordant Technologies (39% of sales), NASA, and the US military. Specialty chemicals make up 91% of sales.

DBT Online, Inc.

5550 W. Flamingo Rd., Ste. B-5, Las Vegas, NV 89103

Telephone: 702-257-1112 **Fax:** 702-257-1109 **Metro area:** Las Vegas, NV **Web site:** http://www.dbtonline.com **Human resources contact:** Kevin A. Barr **Sales:** $46.9 million **Number of employees:** 247 **Number of employees for previous year:** 215 **Industry designation:** Computers—services **Company type:** Public **Top competitors:** OneSource Information Services, Inc.; West Group; LEXIS-NEXIS

DBT Online is a holding company for Patlex, Database Technology, and Information Connectivity Group. The latter two subsidiaries form DBT's Electronic Information Group, which provides online access and cross-referencing of public records from governmental and commercial sources. The company's most notable product is its AutoTrack Plus, which searches for basic information (addresses, date of birth) as well as drivers license information, vehicle registration numbers, and bankruptcy information. Patlex Corporation receives royalties from licenses on laser patents and protects them from infringement. Director Hank Asher controls 25% of the company.

Equinox International

10190 Covington Cross Dr., Las Vegas, NV 89134

Telephone: 702-877-2287 **Fax:** 702-228-0288 **Metro area:** Las Vegas, NV **Web site:** http://www.equinoxinternational.com **Human resources contact:** Susan Archangel **Sales:** $250 million (Est.) **Number of employees:** 300 **Number of employees for previous year:** 250 **Industry designation:** Cosmetics & toiletries **Company type:** Private

Equinox International sells all-natural personal care products, long-distance service, and hopes of financial success to its distributors. The direct-sales company offers its body-, home-, and car-care items; homeopathic medicines; and dietary supplements through about 80,000 independent sales reps in the US and Mexico under a system of cooperative (multilevel) marketing. Equinox, despite claims of being a "marketing opportunity to anyone with a dream for a better life," has itself been the subject of numerous complaints by consumers, ex-distributors, and states' attorneys general. Oft-investigated founder and CEO Bill Gouldd added the second "d" to his name on the recommendation of a spiritual adviser.

On Stage Entertainment, Inc.

4625 W. Nevso Dr., Las Vegas, NV 89103

Telephone: 702-253-1333 **Fax:** 702-253-1122 **Metro area:** Las Vegas, NV **Human resources contact:** Christopher R. Grobl **Sales:** $15.7 million **Number of employees:** 269 **Number of employees for previous year:** 151 **Industry designation:** Leisure & recreational services **Company type:** Public **Top competitors:** Feld Entertainment, Inc.

On Stage Entertainment is a live theatrical production company whose flagship production, "Legends in Concert," features impersonators who pay tribute to such notables as Elvis Presley, the Beatles, Madonna, and Dolly Parton. The company has resident productions at resort hotels, casinos, and theaters throughout the US, as well as traveling productions and cruise ship shows in the US and abroad. On Stage also produces musical reviews, magic shows, ice shows, and corporate entertainment events. In addition, the company sells "Legends in Concert" souvenir merchandise, which includes clothing and video and audio tapes. CEO and chairman John Stuart owns about 55% of On Stage.

Sierra Health Services, Inc.

2724 N. Tenaya Way, Las Vegas, NV 89128

Telephone: 702-242-7000 **Fax:** 702-242-9711 **Other address:** PO Box 15645, Las Vegas, NV 89114 **Metro area:** Las Vegas, NV **Web site:** http://www.sierrahealth.com **Human resources contact:** Ross Lagatutta **Sales:** $1 billion **Number of employees:** 4,700 **Number of employees for previous year:** 2,800 **Industry designation:** Health maintenance organization **Company type:** Public **Top competitors:** PacifiCare Health Systems, Inc.; Foundation Health Systems, Inc.; Aetna Inc.

Nevada's #1 managed care company, Sierra Health Services operates an HMO and offers home and hospice care, standard insurance, and health care administrative services. Subsidiaries include Behavioral Healthcare Options (mental health and substance abuse insurance), Family Health Care Services (home health care), Family Home Hospice (terminal care), Health Plan of Nevada (HMO), Sierra Health and Life Insurance Company, Sierra Insurance Group (workers' compensation), and Southwest Realty. Sierra also owns Nevada's largest multispecialty medical group, Southwest Medical Associates.

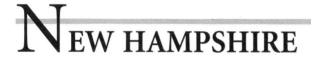

NEW HAMPSHIRE

Bottomline Technologies (de), Inc.

155 Fleet St., Portsmouth, NH 03801

Telephone: 603-436-0700 **Fax:** 603-436-0300 **Metro area:** Boston, MA **Web site:** http://www.bottomline.com **Human resources contact:** Lisa Kolosey **Sales:** $29 million **Number of employees:** 235 **Number of employees for previous year:** 198 **Industry designation:** Computers—corporate, professional & financial software **Company type:** Public **Top competitors:** CheckFree Holdings Corporation; CyberCash, Inc.; Sterling Commerce, Inc.

No more riding the paper trail: Bottomline Technologies' electronic data interchange (EDI) software enables companies to move the money cow electronically. Its PayBase software helps users make, receive, and manage payments (payroll, commissions, bills) and notifies payees via e-mail or fax. The Windows NT-based suite works with a company's existing software and has the optional LaserCheck printing system and a tax payment module. The Federal Reserve Bank offers members Bottomline-developed software (FEDI) for receiving payments electronically. Customers include Charles Schwab, Dow Jones, and Harvard University. Co-founders Daniel McGurl (CEO) and James Loomis (a director) each own about 16% of the company.

Chemfab Corporation

701 Daniel Webster Hwy., Merrimack, NH 03054

Telephone: 603-424-9000 **Fax:** 603-424-9028 **Other address:** PO Box 1137, Merrimack, NH 03054 **Metro area:** Boston, MA **Web site:** http://www.chemfab.com **Sales:** $104.5 million **Number of employees:** 641 **Number of employees for previous year:** 584 **Industry designation:** Chemicals—fibers **Company type:** Public **Top competitors:** Bayer AG; E. I. du Pont de Nemours and Company; BASF Aktiengesellschaft

Chemfab's advanced polymer fiber products cover the Georgia Dome, line the space shuttles' cargo bays, and protect US Navy personnel against shipboard fire. Why? Its fabrics (polymeric composite materials) are extremely strong and flexible and are resistant to heat, water, and chemicals. The company's products are also used in food processing (for example, to make conveyor belts) and in laboratory packaging, as well as to cover satellite dishes and microwave antennae. Chemfab is building a 1-million-sq.-ft. membrane to cover the huge Millennium Dome being built outside London. The company has operations in Brazil, China, Ireland, Japan, Spain, the UK, and the US. About 32% of its sales are outside the US.

Diatide, Inc.

9 Delta Dr., Londonderry, NH 03053

Telephone: 603-437-8970 **Fax:** 603-437-8977 **Metro area:** Boston, MA **Web site:** http://www.diatide.com **Human resources contact:** Mary Wallace **Sales:** $6.4 million **Number of employees:** 88 **Number of employees for previous year:** 73 **Industry designation:** Drugs **Company type:** Public

Diatide discovers and develops proprietary radiopharmaceuticals for use in nuclear medicine imaging procedures. The company is developing Techtides, synthetic peptides that can be used as medical imaging agents to detect chronic and life-threatening diseases by giving physicians information on cells, tissues, and organs, in addition to traditional anatomical information. The FDA has given marketing approval to Diatide's AcuTect, used to detect blood clots that can cause pulmonary embolism. Nycomed Amersham, a producer of medical imaging agents, has an agreement with Diatide to co-promote Techtides in the US and distribute them abroad.

Fisher Scientific International Inc.

One Liberty Ln., Hampton, NH 03842

Telephone: 603-926-5911 **Fax:** 603-926-0222 **Metro area:** Boston, MA **Web site:** http://www.Fisher1.com **Human resources contact:** Tom Rea **Sales:** $2.3 billion **Number of employees:** 6,800 **Number of employees for previous year:** 6,600 **Industry designation:** Instruments—scientific **Company type:** Public **Top competitors:** VWR Scientific Products Corporation; Sybron International Corporation; E. I. du Pont de Nemours and Company

Fisher Scientific International is the world's #1 seller of science equipment and supplies to laboratories, hospitals, schools, researchers, and government agencies. Using catalogs and its Web site, Fisher Scientific sells some 245,000 products in 145 countries. Its wares include science instruments (microscopes, centrifuges, and balances), chemicals, lab supplies, workstations, Internet software, and a chemical inventory tracking system (ChemTrace). The company offers products from 3,200 independent suppliers, as well as products bearing the Fisher name. After a 1998 recapitalization, Thomas H. Lee Company and Donaldson, Lufkin & Jenrette's DLJ Merchant Banking unit own about 80% of the company.

The General Chemical Group Inc.

Liberty Ln., Hampton, NH 03842

Telephone: 603-929-2606 **Fax:** 603-929-2404 **Metro area:** Boston, MA **Web site:** http://www.genchem.com **Human resources contact:** A. Christiaan Muns **Sales:** $700.1 million **Number of employees:** 2,799 **Number of employees for previous year:** 2,402 **Industry designation:** Chemicals—diversified **Company type:** Public **Top competitors:** GAF Corporation; PPG Industries, Inc.; The Dow Chemical Company

The General Chemical Group doesn't split atoms, but it is splitting its businesses. A leading maker of soda ash and calcium chloride, the company is spinning off to the public its specialty chemicals and manufacturing units (two-thirds of sales). To be named GenTek Inc., the split-off company will produce chemicals for printing plates, drugs and agricultural and personal-care goods and provide refinery and chemical regeneration services. The new company's manufacturing unit will make precision metal products, primarily car engine parts. The manufacturing division includes subsidiary Defiance, Inc., a maker of precision automotive parts. Chairman Paul Montrone owns 44% of General Chemical Group.

Silknet Software, Inc.

50 Phillippe Cote St., Manchester, NH 03101

Telephone: 603-625-0070 **Fax:** 603-625-0428 **Metro area:** Manchester, NH **Web site:** http://www.silknet.com **Human resources contact:** Karen Hume **Sales:** $3.6 million (Est.) **Number of employees:** 121 **Industry designation:** Computers—corporate, professional & financial software **Company type:** Private **Top competitors:** BroadVision, Inc.; The Vantive Corporation; Siebel Systems, Inc.

When you make software that Microsoft wants to use, you must be doing something right. That's the enviable position in which Silknet Software, a maker of customer service software, finds itself. The company's eBusiness System, eService, and eCommerce brand products enable businesses to leap into cyberspace and perform marketing, sales, e-commerce, and customer service functions via the Web. The Windows-based software can also be tailored to users' specific needs. In addition to Microsoft, Silknet's customer list includes 3Com and Compaq. Chairman, president, and CEO James Wood, who founded Silknet in 1995, owns about 20% of the company. Internet investment powerhouse CMGI owns 24%.

Storage Computer Corporation

11 Riverside St., Nashua, NH 03062

Telephone: 603-880-3005 **Fax:** 603-889-7232 **Metro area:** Boston, MA **Web site:** http://www.storage.com **Human resources contact:** Jeamme McCreaby **Sales:** $17.1 million **Number of employees:** 138 **Number of employees for previous year:** 113 **Industry designation:** Computers—peripheral equipment **Company type:** Public **Top competitors:** Hewlett-Packard Company; Sun Microsystems, Inc.

Storage Computer makes software-driven storage systems that can store more than four terabytes of data. Its RAID 7 technology combines industry standard disk drives into a single "mega" drive and is used by its Virtual Storage Architecture. Virtual Storage Architecture, the basis of its StorageSuite products, treats the storage area as a complete and coherent space that can be used simultaneously by multiple users. It also offers disaster recovery and management products to protect, monitor, and control stored data. Its products are sold worldwide through direct sales, resellers, distributors, affiliates, and minority-owned entities. CEO Theodore Goodlander and family own almost 65% of the company.

NEW JERSEY

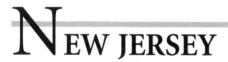

Able Energy, Inc.

344 Rte. 46, Rockaway, NJ 07866

Telephone: 973-625-1012 **Fax:** 973-625-8097 **Metro area:** Allentown, PA **Web site:** http://www.ableenergy.com **Human resources contact:** Colleen Harrington **Sales:** $16.4 million (Est.) **Number of employees:** 63 **Industry designation:** Oil refining & marketing **Company type:** Private

Operating in Florida, New Jersey, and Pennsylvania, Able Energy provides retail distribution of heating oil and other fuels to residential and commercial customers through subsidiaries Able Oil, Able Melbourne, and Able Montgomery. The company also installs and repairs home heating equipment and markets diesel fuel, gasoline, and lubricants. Able Propane distributes liquid propane gas and propane equipment in New Jersey. Subsidiary A & O provides environmental consulting and engineering services, including fuel-tank testing and remediation. After the company's planned IPO, CEO Timothy Harrington will own about 52% of Able Energy.

ADM Tronics Unlimited, Inc.

224 -S Pegasus Ave., Northvale, NJ 07647

Telephone: 201-767-6040 **Fax:** 201-784-0620 **Metro area:** New York, NY **Web site:** http://www.admtronics.com **Sales:** $1.5 million **Number of employees:** 19 **Number of employees for previous year:** 11 **Industry designation:** Chemicals—specialty **Company type:** Public **Top competitors:** Biomet, Inc.; Orthofix International N.V.; OrthoLogic Corp.

ADM Tronics Unlimited makes chemical products, primarily for use in the printing and packaging industries. Its water-based primers, cosmetic and medical adhesives, coatings, resins, and chemical additives account for about 65% of sales. ADM Tronics also develops medical devices: Using a beam generated by audio and radio waves, its Sonotron Device treats osteoarthritis and inflammatory joint conditions in humans. Legal and regulatory issues have hampered its distribution. FDA-approved electronic therapy devices include Aurex-3, to treat ringing in the ears, and SofPulse, to relieve pain and swelling after cosmetic surgery. CEO Alfonso Di Mino and his family own about 50% of the company.

Advanced Nutraceuticals, Inc.

500 Metuchen Rd., South Plainfield, NJ 07080

Telephone: 908-668-0088 **Fax:** 908-561-9682 **Metro area:** New York, NY **Human resources contact:** Linda Attridge **Sales:** $50.8 million (Est.) **Number of employees:** 196 **Industry designation:** Vitamins & nutritional products **Company type:** Private **Top competitors:** Rexall Sundown, Inc.; Weider Nutrition International, Inc.; Twinlab Corporation

Depressed because you missed your St. John's-wort? Cheer up, Advanced Nutraceuticals will help you get your daily dose. The company sources and processes herbal and other compounds and makes, packages, and distributes private-label and brand-name herbal remedies and nutritional supplements. The company was formed by a merger of ACTA Products, Bactolac Pharmaceuticals, Northridge Laboratories, and Quality Botanical Ingredients, which engage in processing and contract manufacturing activities. Clients include specialty and mass-market retailers and network marketers. Founding officers Gregory Pusey and Barry Loder are veterans of Nutrition for Life International, which sells nutritional supplements.

Algos Pharmaceutical Corporation

Collingwood Plaza, 4900 Rte. 33, Neptune, NJ 07753

Telephone: 732-938-5959 **Fax:** 732-938-2825 **Metro area:** New York, NY **Human resources contact:** Karen Lyle **Sales:** $100,000 **Number of employees:** 21 **Number of employees for previous year:** 12 **Industry designation:** Drugs **Company type:** Public **Top competitors:** Chiroscience Group plc; Allelix Biopharmaceuticals Inc.; Bayer Corporation

When ordinary aspirin won't cure a killer headache, Algos Pharmaceutical just might have the pill for you. The development stage company researches alternative pain relievers for migraines, cancer pain, and postoperative pain. MorphiDex (its lead product), HydrocoDex, and OxycoDex combine narcotic and non-narcotic analgesics to relieve cancer pain, while LidoDex (developed with partner Interneuron Pharmaceuticals) treats migraines. Algos is working with the National Institute on Drug Abuse to develop a treatment for opiate and cocaine addiction. The firm is also developing an anticonvulsant to treat chronic pain in patients with spinal cord injuries, as well as a treatment for urge urinary incontinence.

Alpharma Inc.

One Executive Dr., Fort Lee, NJ 07024

Telephone: 201-947-7774 **Fax:** 201-947-5541 **Other address:** PO Box 1399, Fort Lee, NJ 07024 **Metro area:** New York, NY **Web site:** http://www.alpharma.com **Human resources contact:** Loraine Catarcio **Sales:** $604.6 million **Number of employees:** 3,000 **Number of employees for previous year:** 2,600 **Industry designation:** Drugs **Company type:** Public

Alpharma produces generic and proprietary drugs and animal health products at facilities in Europe, Indonesia, and the US. The company sells its generic drugs, over-the-counter cough and cold remedies, and creams and lotions to drug wholesalers, mass merchandisers, hospitals, and managed care providers. Alpharma's international division sells primarily in Western Europe, Indonesia, and the Middle East. The company's fine chemicals division supplies bulk antibiotics for use in the firm's own drugs and in third-party drugs. Alpharma's animal antibiotics and feed additives are sold to livestock producers and feed makers. A.L. Industrier, a Norwegian firm, owns almost 40% of the company's stock.

American Home Products Corporation

5 Giralda Farms, Madison, NJ 07940

Telephone: 973-660-5000 **Fax:** 973-660-7026 **Metro area:** New York, NY **Web site:** http://www.ahp.com **Human resources contact:** Rene R. Lewin **Sales:** $13.5 billion **Number of employees:** 60,523 **Number of employees for previous year:** 59,747 **Industry designation:** Drugs **Company type:** Public **Top competitors:** Novartis AG; Merck & Co., Inc.; Rhone-Poulenc S.A.

American Home Products (AHP) makes health care and agricultural products. The company generates more than 60% of its sales from pharmaceuticals. AHP makes estrogen-replacement drug Premarin (one of the top-selling prescription drugs in the US) and consumer products (Advil, Robitussin). AHP's subsidiaries include Cyanamid (herbicides and insecticides), Fort Dodge (animal health care products), Whitehall-Robins Healthcare (consumer health products), Wyeth-Ayerst Laboratories (prescription drugs), and Genetics Institute (biotechnology). It also owns a majority stake in biotech firm Immunex Corp.

Anthra Pharmaceuticals, Inc.

103 Carnegie Center, Ste. 102, Princeton, NJ 08540

Telephone: 609-514-1060 **Fax:** 609-514-0534 **Metro area:** Philadelphia, PA **Web site:** http://www.anthra.com **Human resources contact:** Rose Lucia **Number of employees:** 33 **Number of employees for previous year:** 30 **Industry designation:** Drugs **Company type:** Private **Top competitors:** U.S. Bioscience, Inc.; SuperGen, Inc.; Corixa Corporation

Anthra Pharmaceuticals has found a new pharmaceutical star in its Valstar bladder cancer treatment. The development-stage company acquires and develops late-stage drug candidates that treat bladder, ovarian, and prostate cancer, as well as complications from metastatic cancer. Anthra has licensed Valstar—which was approved by the Food and Drug Administration in 1998—to Medeva for sale in the US. In addition, Anthra has acquired the US development and marketing rights to Bonefos, a treatment for hypercalcemia and lytic bone disease, from Schering AG. Anthra Pharmaceuticals has facilities in Europe and the US.

Barringer Technologies Inc.

219 South St., Murray Hill, NJ 07974

Telephone: 908-665-8200 **Fax:** 908-665-8298 **Metro area:** New York, NY **Web site:** http://www.barringer.com **Sales:** $20.5 million **Number of employees:** 135 **Number of employees for previous year:** 119 **Industry designation:** Protection—safety equipment & services **Company type:** Public **Top competitors:** Vivid Technologies, Inc.; Thermedics Detection Inc.; InVision Technologies, Inc.

Barringer Technologies makes bomb and drug detectors for security and law enforcement agencies worldwide. Its flagship product, the IONSCAN, is a portable desktop unit that detects trace amounts of a substance smaller than one-billionth of a gram in about six seconds. Used in prisons and by forensics departments and the military, IONSCAN's buyers include the Eurotunnel, the Federal Aviation Administration (FAA), the US Coast Guard, and more than 40 airports around the world. The company is developing two new products with the aid of FAA grants: a document scanner to detect trace amounts of explosives on passenger documents, and an automated baggage scanner. About 39% of the company's sales are overseas.

Becton, Dickinson and Company

One Becton Dr., Franklin Lakes, NJ 07417

Telephone: 201-847-6800 **Fax:** 201-847-6475 **Metro area:** New York, NY **Web site:** http://www.bd.com **Human resources contact:** James V. Jerbasi **Sales:** $3.1 billion **Number of employees:** 21,700 **Number of employees for previous year:** 18,900 **Industry designation:** Medical & dental supplies **Company type:** Public **Top competitors:** Bristol-Myers Squibb Company; Johnson & Johnson; Abbott Laboratories

Becton, Dickinson is sanguine about injection and infusion equipment. The company is the leading maker of syringes in the US and one of the top manufacturers in the world. Its Medical Supplies and Devices segment makes diabetes care, infusion therapy, and drug injection products, and its Diagnostic Systems segment makes flow cytometry (cell analysis) systems, immunodiagnostic test kits, sample-collection devices, and tissue culture labware. Becton, Dickinson's best-sellers include Hypak prefillable syringes and Vacutainer blood-collection products. The company has operations in more than 40 countries and has established manufacturing plants in China and India.

Beechwood

100 Walnut Ave., Clark, NJ 07066

Telephone: 732-382-5400 **Fax:** 732-382-5575 **Metro area:** New York, NY **Web site:** http://www.bdsi.com **Human resources contact:** Nima Kelly **Sales:** $47 million (Est.) **Number of employees:** 400 **Industry designation:** Computers—services **Company type:** Private **Top competitors:** American Management Systems, Incorporated; Andersen Consulting; Architel Systems Corporation

Beechwood (formerly Beechwood Data Systems) makes OSS (operations support systems) software for the telecommunications industry. Its products automate business functions such as billing and order processing and integrate incompatible computer systems so they can communicate with each other. The company focuses on new local telephone companies, creating computer interfaces for carriers that work together and for companies that are merging and need to integrate their systems. Chairman Don Rankin and VC Paul Hummel own Beechwood, which they founded in 1987.

Benjamin Moore & Co.

51 Chestnut Ridge Rd., Montvale, NJ 07645

Telephone: 201-573-9600 **Fax:** 201-573-0046 **Metro area:** New York, NY **Web site:** http://www.benjaminmoore.com **Human resources contact:** Charles C. Vail **Sales:** $666.3 million **Number of employees:** 2,050 **Number of employees for previous year:** 2,000 **Industry designation:** Paints & related products **Company type:** Public **Top competitors:** The Sherwin-Williams Company; PPG Industries, Inc.; Imperial Chemical Industries PLC

Coatings manufacturer Benjamin Moore is well known for its paints, stains, and clear finishes, which are sold through independently owned distributors. In addition to ready-mixed colors, sold under such brands as Benjamin Moore Paints, Wall Satin, and Benwood, the company can match almost any color with its Computer Color Matching and Moor-O-Matic III Color Systems. Benjamin Moore also makes production finish coatings for manufacturers of flexible packaging, beverage and food containers, furniture, and roof decking. It has more than 20 manufacturing facilities in Australia, New Zealand, Canada, and the US. Descendants of brothers Benjamin and Robert Moore, who founded the company in 1883, control the company.

Bio-Imaging Technologies, Inc.

830 Bear Tavern Rd., West Trenton, NJ 08628

Telephone: 609-883-2000 **Fax:** 609-883-7719 **Metro area:** Philadelphia, PA **Web site:** http://www.bioimaging.com **Human resources contact:** Maria Kraus **Sales:** $3.6 million **Number of employees:** 35 **Number of employees for previous year:** 34 **Industry designation:** Medical services **Company type:** Public **Top competitors:** Quintiles Transnational Corp.; ClinTrials Research Inc.; Collaborative Clinical Research, Inc.

When a medical breakthrough is made, Bio-Imaging Technologies wants to be the first to see it. The contract research organization (CRO) processes and analyzes medical images for clients conducting clinical trials on drugs or medical devices. Its software system Bio/ImageBase lets clients and FDA medical reviewers review the images and related data electronically. Bio-Imaging also offers technical consulting, training, and end-user support. It markets services directly in the US and Europe, primarily to developers of cancer, central nervous system, and cardiovascular disease treatments, as well as diagnostic imaging and anti-inflammatory agents. Covance, a leading CRO, owns nearly 30% of the company.

Biomatrix, Inc.

65 Railroad Ave., Ridgefield, NJ 07657

Telephone: 201-945-9550 **Fax:** 201-945-0363 **Metro area:** New York, NY **Web site:** http://www.biomatrix.com/index.htm **Human resources contact:** Nina Esaki **Sales:** $47.6 million **Number of employees:** 223 **Number of employees for previous year:** 105 **Industry designation:** Biomedical & genetic products **Company type:** Public **Top competitors:** Lifecore Biomedical, Inc.; Fidia S.P.A.; Genzyme Corporation

Biomatrix is combing for biomedical success. The firm makes proprietary biological polymers called hylans (a purified form of hyaluronic acid, which is found in rooster combs) for therapeutic uses. The company's Synvisc is a lubricant injected into arthritic joints to reduce pain and increase mobility; its skin care line includes Hylaform (which still awaits FDA approval), an injectable substance used to fix wrinkles and scars. Synvisc and the company's other products (Hylashield eye drops and Gelvisc Vet for animal arthritis) are marketed by several distributors in the US and abroad, including Wyeth-Ayerst and Bayer AG, among others. Co-founders Endre Balazs and his wife Janet Denlinger own 30% of Biomatrix.

Bio-Reference Laboratories, Inc.

481 Edward H. Ross Dr., Elmwood Park, NJ 07407

Telephone: 201-791-2600 **Fax:** 201-791-1941 **Metro area:** New York, NY **Web site:** http://www.bio-referencelabs.com **Human resources contact:** Carol Rusert **Sales:** $46.6 million **Number of employees:** 672 **Number of employees for previous year:** 430 **Industry designation:** Medical services **Company type:** Public **Top competitors:** Quest Diagnostics Incorporated; SmithKline Beecham plc; Laboratory Corporation of America Holdings

Bio-Reference Laboratories operates clinical laboratories in northern New Jersey and New York. The company offers a wide range of chemical diagnostic tests, including blood and urine analysis, hematology services, and serology. Other tests include Pap smears, radioimmunoassay, toxicology, and tissue pathology. The lab picks up test specimens from physicians' offices and generally has the results back to the physician within 24 hours. The company markets its services to physicians, hospitals, and clinics in the greater New York area. Bio-Reference intends to expand its laboratory operations through acquisitions, particularly in the area of specialty testing, such as certain cancer tests.

Bio-Technology General Corp.

70 Wood Ave. South, Iselin, NJ 08830

Telephone: 732-632-8800 **Fax:** 732-632-8844 **Metro area:** New York, NY **Web site:** http://www.oxandrin.com/aboutbtg.html **Human resources contact:** Leah Berkozits **Sales:** $70.9 million **Number of employees:** 271 **Number of employees for previous year:** 247 **Industry designation:** Biomedical & genetic products **Company type:** Public

Bio-Technology General researches, develops, manufactures, and markets genetically engineered and other products for health care. The company focuses primarily on developing therapeutic products targeted toward conditions such as endocrine disorders, cardiopulmonary diseases, and ophthalmic and skin disorders. Its key products include Bio-Tropin (human growth hormone) for the treatment of short stature; Oxandrin (oxandrolone), for treatment of weight loss due to chronic infection, extensive surgery, and severe trauma; Androtest-SL (sublingual testosterone) for hypogonadism; and Bio-Hep-B, a third-generation vaccine against hepatitis B virus. The company is also developing a treatment for gout.

BiznessOnline.com, Inc.

1720 Rte. 34, Wall, NJ 07719

Telephone: 732-280-6408 **Fax:** 732-280-6409 **Metro area:** New York, NY **Web site:** http://www.biznessonline.com **Human resources contact:** Mark E. Munro **Sales:** $6.2 million (Est.) **Number of employees:** 60 **Industry designation:** Computers—online services **Company type:** Private **Top competitors:** MindSpring Enterprises, Inc.; EarthLink Network, Inc.; Verio Inc.

Internet service provider BiznessOnline.com is looking for both "bizness" and residential customers in secondary markets in the northeastern US. The company's Global 2000 Communications unit provides Internet services to 4,000 residential and small to medium-sized business customers in the Albany, New York area. BiznessOnline.com has agreed to purchase four more ISPs with a total of 16,000 subscribers in New York and Connecticut. The company offers dial-up and dedicated Internet access, Web site design and hosting, and e-commerce services. President and CEO Mark Munro owns nearly 65% of the company; after the planned IPO, his ownership will drop to 43%.

Bush Boake Allen Inc.

7 Mercedes Dr., Montvale, NJ 07645

Telephone: 201-391-9870 **Fax:** 201-391-0860 **Metro area:** New York, NY **Web site:** http://www.bushboakeallen.com **Human resources contact:** Ronald A. Landis **Sales:** $485.4 million **Number of employees:** 1,977 **Number of employees for previous year:** 1,964 **Industry designation:** Chemicals—specialty **Company type:** Public **Top competitors:** Roche Holding Ltd; International Flavors & Fragrances Inc.; Universal Foods Corporation

Flavor and fragrance maker Bush Boake Allen (BBA) knows the nose. Its business consists of two operating segments: flavors and fragrance (which account for more than three-quarters of sales) and aroma chemicals. Its flavor products are used in soft drinks, snack foods, dairy products, and alcoholic drinks. The fragrance segment makes chemicals used in soaps, detergents, and toiletries. The company's aroma chemicals are used as raw materials in fragrance compounds. BBA has operations in 39 countries and sells to food and consumer products makers in Africa, Asia, Australia, Europe, and North and South America. Union Camp, a chemical and paper producer, owns about 70% of the company.

Cantel Industries, Inc.

1135 Broad St., Clifton, NJ 07013

Telephone: 973-470-8700 **Fax:** 973-471-0054 **Metro area:** New York, NY **Sales:** $40 million **Number of employees:** 171 **Number of employees for previous year:** 150 **Industry designation:** Medical instruments **Company type:** Public **Top competitors:** Allegiance Corporation; McKesson General Medical Corporation; Owens & Minor, Inc.

Cantel Industries markets and services optics equipment for medical, consumer, and industrial use in North and South America. US subsidiary MediVators makes disinfection and disposal equipment for endoscopes and medical sharps at its facility in Minnesota. Canadian subsidiary Carsen Group distributes endoscopes, related surgical accessories, and scientific products, including microscopes and micromanipulators. Industrial products include borescopes, fiberscopes, and video-image scopes. Cantel Industries also distributes consumer goods (primarily from Japanese maker Olympus Optical) such as binoculars, handheld dictation equipment, and 35 mm and digital cameras.

CareInsite, Inc.

669 River Dr., River Drive Center II, Elmwood Park, NJ 07407

Telephone: 201-703-3400 **Fax:** 201-703-3401 **Metro area:** New York, NY **Human resources contact:** Bob Seifert **Number of employees:** 100 **Industry designation:** Medical practice management **Company type:** Private **Top competitors:** Quintiles Transnational Corp.; Misys plc; Medical Manager Corporation

CareInsite is scaring up scratch to develop a Web-based network for use by health care providers and their patients. The company's product will offer e-commerce, information, and messaging services to doctors, suppliers, laboratories, and administrators. The network is being developed using software by health care information systems provider Cerner Corporation. CareInsite currently provides services to and owns 20% of The Health Information Connection LLC (or THINC), a venture that offers health care information to managed care providers in the New York area. CareInsite is 80%-owned by plastics and health care communications firm Synetic and 20%-owned by Cerner.

CCA Industries, Inc.

200 Murray Hill Pkwy., East Rutherford, NJ 07073

Telephone: 201-330-1400 **Fax:** 201-935-0675 **Metro area:** New York, NY **Human resources contact:** Kelly Merritt **Sales:** $41.1 million **Number of employees:** 139 **Number of employees for previous year:** 132 **Industry designation:** Cosmetics & toiletries **Company type:** Public **Top competitors:** Revlon, Inc.; Colgate-Palmolive Company; L'Oreal

CCA Industries sells health and beauty aids that wash, whiten, and wax. The company's products include Nutra Nail fingernail treatments, Pro Perm and Wash 'n Curl hair treatments, Hair Off depilatories, Sudden Change skin care products, Plus+White oral hygiene products, Eat 'n Lose and Hungrex Plus dietary products, and a line of fragrances sold through its Fragrance Corp. subsidiary. The company hires third parties to make everything except its hot-wax depilatory. CCA Industries sells its products to major food and drug retailers, mass merchandisers, and beauty aid wholesalers in the US (Wal-Mart accounts for about 30% of sales; Walgreen, about 10%).

Celgene Corporation

7 Powder Horn Dr., Warren, NJ 07059

Telephone: 732-271-1001 **Fax:** 732-271-4184 **Metro area:** New York, NY **Web site:** http://www.celgene.com **Human resources contact:** Lisa Desnoyers **Sales:** $1.1 million **Number of employees:** 94 **Number of employees for previous year:** 79 **Industry designation:** Drugs **Company type:** Public **Top competitors:** Immunex Corporation; Medeva PLC; EntreMed, Inc.

Celgene is a drug company specializing in immunotherapy medications. The company's immunotherapy products are small-molecule compounds that suppress the body's production of proteins that cause inflammatory and immunological diseases. The drugs include a form of thalidomide (blamed for thousands of birth defects when prescribed as a sedative in Europe), which the FDA approved in 1998 to treat leprosy. The company is also exploring the use of thalidomide to treat brain tumors. Celgene is working on a treatment for chronic pain and its own version of Ritalin (used to treat children with attention deficit disorder), which Biovail will market in Canada.

Checkpoint Systems, Inc.

101 Wolf Dr., Thorofare, NJ 08086

Telephone: 609-848-1800 **Fax:** 609-848-0937 **Other address:** PO Box 188, Thorofare, NJ 08086 **Metro area:** Philadelphia, PA **Web site:** http://www.checkpointsystems.com **Human resources contact:** Teresa McHale **Sales:** $362.4 million **Number of employees:** 3,605 **Number of employees for previous year:** 2,628 **Industry designation:** Protection—safety equipment & services **Company type:** Public **Top competitors:** Sensormatic Electronics Corporation; Sentry Technology Corporation; Diebold, Incorporated

Checkpoint Systems makes and markets electronic article surveillance (EAS) systems and closed-circuit television systems used to monitor activity in locations such as retail stores and libraries. It also makes electronic tags (such as paper-thin radio-frequency labels) that are attached to merchandise and trigger an alarm when moved beyond a specified area without being deactivated or removed. Checkpoint holds about one-third of the US's EAS market (behind Sensormatic's 55% share). The company has manufacturing operations in the Dominican Republic and Puerto Rico.

Chem International, Inc.

201 Rte. 22, Hillside, NJ 07205

Telephone: 973-926-0816 **Fax:** 973-926-1735 **Metro area:** New York, NY **Web site:** http://www.cheminternational.com **Human resources contact:** Christina M. Kay **Sales:** $16 million **Number of employees:** 96 **Number of employees for previous year:** 77 **Industry designation:** Vitamins & nutritional products **Company type:** Public **Top competitors:** Twinlab Corporation; Weider Nutrition International, Inc.; IVC Industries, Inc.

Keeping its customers healthy and happy is the mission of Chem International, a manufacturer of vitamins, nutritional supplements, and herbal products. The company manufactures products under its private label, Vitamin Factory, for sale at its retail store in Hillside, New Jersey, and through the mail. Subsidiary Manhattan Drug manufactures vitamins and nutritional supplements for sale to distributors, multilevel marketers, and specialized health care providers. Rexall Sundown accounts for about 45% of Chem International's sales. The company also supplies nutritional supplements to Herbalife and dietary supplements to Pilon International.

Church & Dwight Co., Inc.

469 N. Harrison St., Princeton, NJ 08543

Telephone: 609-683-5900 **Fax:** 609-497-7269 **Metro area:** Philadelphia, PA **Human resources contact:** George Dombroski **Sales:** $684.4 million **Number of employees:** 1,137 **Number of employees for previous year:** 937 **Industry designation:** Soap & cleaning preparations **Company type:** Public **Top competitors:** Colgate-Palmolive Company; Unilever; The Procter & Gamble Company

Church & Dwight is the world's leading producer of sodium bicarbonate, popularly known as baking soda. The company's ARM & HAMMER baking soda is used as leavening, deodorizer, scratchless cleaner for kitchen surfaces and cooking appliances, and swimming-pool pH stabilizer. The company makes other consumer products (which together account for 80% of sales) including cat litter, laundry detergent, carpet deodorizer, air fresheners, dishwashing powder, toothpaste, and antiperspirants. Church & Dwight also owns the Brillo scouring-pad brand and has interests in industrial sodium bicarbonate and specialty products.

Computer Horizons Corp.

49 Old Bloomfield Ave., Mountain Lakes, NJ 07046

Telephone: 973-299-4000 **Fax:** 973-402-7988 **Metro area:** New York, NY **Web site:** http://www.computerhorizons.com **Human resources contact:** Michelle Friedery **Sales:** $514.9 million **Number of employees:** 4,834 **Number of employees for previous year:** 3,630 **Industry designation:** Computers—services **Company type:** Public **Top competitors:** Andersen Worldwide; Computer Sciences Corporation; Hewlett-Packard Company

Computer Horizons provides a range of information technology services to major corporations. Through offices in Canada, India, the UK, and the US, the company offers staffing services (more than 50% of sales), computer network development and integration, document management, year 2000 compliance software (about a fourth of sales), consulting, and outsourcing, among other services and products. Clients include AT&T (which accounts for 12% of sales), Prudential, and other "FORTUNE" 500 companies with large information technology budgets and recurring software or staffing needs.

Computron Software, Inc.

301 Rte. 17 North, Rutherford, NJ 07070

Telephone: 201-935-3400 **Fax:** 201-935-7678 **Metro area:** New York, NY **Web site:** http://www.computronsoftware.com **Human resources contact:** Michelle May **Sales:** $63.5 million **Number of employees:** 504 **Number of employees for previous year:** 454 **Industry designation:** Computers—corporate, professional & financial software **Company type:** Public **Top competitors:** Computer Associates International, Inc.; FileNET Corporation

Software developed and marketed by Computron Software enables businesses to manage financial information, access archived data, and automate business cycle information such as budget, expense, and procurement data. Its Computron Financials suite of accounting software supports international currencies, languages, and tax formulas, and can be customized according to an industry's information needs. The Computron COOL software provides online access, retrieval, and warehousing of archival data. The company's software supports most database systems and is compatible with UNIX and Windows NT.

Comtrex Systems Corporation

102 Executive Dr., Ste. 1, Moorestown, NJ 08057

Telephone: 609-778-0090 **Fax:** 609-778-9322 **Metro area:** Philadelphia, PA **Web site:** http://www.comtrex.com **Human resources contact:** Lisa J. Mudrick **Sales:** $6.4 million **Number of employees:** 60 **Number of employees for previous year:** 35 **Industry designation:** Computers—peripheral equipment **Company type:** Public **Top competitors:** PAR Technology Corporation; JDA Software Group, Inc.; MicroTouch Systems, Inc.

Comtrex Systems makes point-of-sale terminals and software for the retail dining industry. The company's systems combine traditional fast food and sit-down restaurant cash register functions with computer control and data collecting capabilities. Its open-architecture PCS-5000 system uses terminals with keyboards or touch-screen monitors linked to the client's computer network; upgradable software is sold separately. Accounting for about two-thirds of sales, PCS-5000 systems are replacing the company's Sprint and SuperSprint terminals. Comtrex Systems sells its products through authorized dealers in the US, Canada, Europe, and Australia. More than 60% of sales are outside the US.

The Connell Company

45 Cardinal Dr., Westfield, NJ 07090

Telephone: 908-233-0700 **Fax:** 908-233-1070 **Metro area:** New York, NY **Web site:** http://www.connellco.com/index.html **Human resources contact:** Rosalie Fleming **Sales:** $1.3 billion (Est.) **Number of employees:** 225 **Number of employees for previous year:** 220 **Industry designation:** Food—flour & grain **Company type:** Private **Top competitors:** Continental Grain Company; Riceland Foods, Inc.; Cargill, Incorporated

Business is sweet at The Connell Company, a leading international distributor of sugar and rice. Connell's core business is rice distribution, which is accomplished through subsidiary Connell Rice & Sugar. The Connell Company has branched out into equipment leasing; Connell Finance handles everything from locomotives to large passenger aircraft. Other Connell subsidiaries distribute canned foods and heavy equipment; provide investment, brokerage, and financial services; export equipment and supplies; and develop commercial properties. The Connell Company has offices in Malaysia, Senegal, Taiwan, Thailand, and the US. Owner Grover Connell (a well-connected Democrat) heads the company, which was founded in 1912.

Covance Inc.

210 Carnegie Center, Princeton, NJ 08540

Telephone: 609-452-4440 **Fax:** 609-452-9375 **Metro area:** Philadelphia, PA **Web site:** http://www.covance.com **Human resources contact:** Kathleen A. Weslock **Sales:** $731.6 million **Number of employees:** 7,200 **Number of employees for previous year:** 6,000 **Industry designation:** Medical services **Company type:** Public **Top competitors:** Pharmaceutical Product Development, Inc.; Quintiles Transnational Corp.; PAREXEL International Corporation

Covance, formerly Corning Pharmaceutical Services, is the #2 contract research organization in the US (Quintiles Transnational is #1). The company develops and carries out preclinical and clinical trials of potential commercial drugs. Covance also offers health economics and outcomes and laboratory testing and will assist a company in moving a drug through the regulatory approval process. Other services include packaging, manufacturing, and economic analysis. Customers include pharmaceutical companies, hospitals, managed care organizations, and laboratory testing services in the chemical, agrochemical, and food industries. Covance has operations in 17 countries around the world.

Cover-All Technologies Inc.

18-01 Pollitt Dr., Fair Lawn, NJ 07410

Telephone: 201-794-4800 **Fax:** 201-794-6527 **Metro area:** New York, NY **Web site:** http://www.cover-all.com **Human resources contact:** Raul F. Calvo **Sales:** $7.9 million **Number of employees:** 45 **Number of employees for previous year:** 40 **Industry designation:** Computers—corporate, professional & financial software **Company type:** Public **Top competitors:** CCC Information Services Group Inc.; Delphi Information Systems, Inc.; Policy Management Systems Corporation

It's got insurance companies covered. Cover-All Technologies (formerly Warner Insurance Services) develops management software for casualty insurance firms through its COVER-ALL Systems subsidiary. Used by more than 50 companies, its Classic product line is a self-contained, LAN-based, PC software package that automates insurance issuance, ratings, renewals, and other transactions. To meet the needs of larger customers, its TAS 2000 products offer the same features as the Classic line, but over client/server WANs. COVER-ALL markets its products directly and through distributors and outside consultants. Customers include Inspire Insurance Solutions, Secura, and Millers Insurance Group.

Cytec Industries Inc.

5 Garret Mountain Plaza, West Paterson, NJ 07424

Telephone: 973-357-3100 **Fax:** 973-357-3060 **Metro area:** New York, NY **Web site:** http://www.cytec.com **Human resources contact:** James W. Hirsch **Sales:** $1.4 billion **Number of employees:** 5,200 **Number of employees for previous year:** 4,700 **Industry designation:** Chemicals—specialty **Company type:** Public **Top competitors:** E. I. du Pont de Nemours and Company; Hexcel Corporation; H.B. Fuller Company

Cytec Industries produces specialty chemicals (56% of sales), specialty materials, and building-block chemicals for numerous industrial uses. The firm's specialty chemicals are used in water treatment, papermaking, mining, and other processes. Cytec's specialty materials include aerospace composites and adhesives, as well as catalysts used in oil refining. Cytec also makes building-block chemicals such as methanol, melamine, and acrylamide. The firm has 28 facilities in the US and seven other countries. Non-US operations account for nearly 30% of sales, and US exports add another 11%. In 1997 the firm bought composite maker Fiberite (since renamed Cytec Fiberite).

Dataram Corporation

PO Box 7528, Princeton, NJ 08543

Telephone: 609-799-0071 **Fax:** 609-799-6734 **Metro area:** Philadelphia, PA **Web site:** http://www.dataram.com **Human resources contact:** Pat Demers **Sales:** $77.3 million **Number of employees:** 88 **Number of employees for previous year:** 60 **Industry designation:** Computers—peripheral equipment **Company type:** Public **Top competitors:** Kingston Technology Company; SMART Modular Technologies, Inc.; PNY Technologies, Inc.

Dataram hopes that its memory is the first to go—where sales are concerned, that is. The company makes gigabyte add-in memory boards and modules that expand the capacity of UNIX and Windows-based network servers and workstations. Its products, which use dynamic random-access memory (DRAM), are compatible with industry leaders such as Compaq, Hewlett-Packard, IBM, Silicon Graphics, and Sun Microsystems. Dataram sells its products directly and through value-added resellers and distributors such as Ingram Micro. The compan targets customers primarily in the US (71% of sales), Canada, Western Europe, and Asia.

Datascope Corp.

14 Philips Pkwy., Montvale, NJ 07645

Telephone: 201-391-8100 **Fax:** 201-307-5400 **Metro area:** New York, NY **Human resources contact:** James Cooper **Sales:** $242.4 million **Number of employees:** 1,300 **Number of employees for previous year:** 1,200 **Industry designation:** Medical instruments **Company type:** Public **Top competitors:** Baxter International Inc.; United States Surgical Corporation; St. Jude Medical, Inc.

Datascope helps keep body and soul together. The company makes medical instruments for the health care industry, including the VasoSeal, a hemostatic device that rapidly seals arterial punctures, and knitted and woven polyester vascular grafts and patches for reconstructive blood vessel surgeries. The company also makes intra-aortic balloon pump systems that increase the heart's output and reduce its workload, and Passport multifunction patient monitoring devices. Datascope markets its products worldwide to medical segments including cardiology, anesthesiology, cardiovascular and vascular surgery, emergency departments, and intensive care units.

Datatec Systems, Inc.

20-C Commerce Way, Totowa, NJ 07512

Telephone: 973-890-4800 **Fax:** 973-890-2888 **Metro area:** New York, NY **Web site:** http://www.datatec.com **Human resources contact:** Mary Simon **Sales:** $76.8 million **Number of employees:** 750 **Number of employees for previous year:** 560 **Industry designation:** Computers—services **Company type:** Public **Top competitors:** Computer Management Sciences, Inc.; Technology Solutions Company; Computer Horizons Corp.

Datatec Systems will design your computer network and move your furniture. The company (formerly Glasgal Communications) provides configuration, integration, and installation services for complex computer networks. Its Integrator's Workbench software organizes design and configuration information, which expedites Datatec's services (it completes about 4,500 jobs each month) and helps keep project costs down. Installation services include equipment set-up, reorganizing and adding fixtures (such as cabinets, desks, and partitions), and a complete test of the network. Datatec provides information technology services in North America for clients such as Blockbuster, Cisco Systems, and Pizza Hut.

Dendrite International, Inc.

1200 Mount Kemble Ave., Morristown, NJ 07960

Telephone: 973-425-1200 **Fax:** 973-425-1919 **Metro area:** New York, NY **Web site:** http://www.drte.com **Human resources contact:** Martha Kerr **Sales:** $112.5 million **Number of employees:** 771 **Number of employees for previous year:** 679 **Industry designation:** Computers—corporate, professional & financial software **Company type:** Public **Top competitors:** Comshare, Incorporated; IMS HEALTH Incorporated

Dendrite International has just the thing to cure communication ills in pharmaceutical sales units. Series 6, its core software product, promotes information exchange between field reps and the office. It aids in bid and contract development, record keeping, planning, and activity analysis. Dendrite also offers stand-alone products for specific functions, such as delivering customer, prescription, or industry information to traveling sales reps via modems. The systems, which can be customized, include a file server, laptop or handheld computers, and software. Its ForceOne product is geared to the over-the-counter pharmaceutical market. Dendrite conducts most of its business in France, the UK, and the US.

Derma Sciences, Inc.

214 Carnegie Center, Ste. 100, Princeton, NJ 08540

Telephone: 609-514-4744 **Fax:** 609-514-0502 **Metro area:** Philadelphia, PA **Web site:** http://www.dermasciences.com **Sales:** $4 million **Number of employees:** 74 **Number of employees for previous year:** 20 **Industry designation:** Drugs **Company type:** Public **Top competitors:** Bristol-Myers Squibb Company; Johnson & Johnson; ProCyte Corporation

Time alone won't heal some wounds, so Derma Sciences makes sprays, ointments, dressings, and irrigation products for chronic wounds (bedsores, venous ulcers, and diabetic leg ulcers), incisions, and burns. The company's treatments protect wounds from infection, and a proprietary zinc-nutrient technology stimulates healing. Because chronic wounds afflict the elderly more than any other segment of the population, Derma Sciences sells to nursing homes, hospitals, and home health care agencies throughout the US. The company also has distribution agreements in Canada, Egypt, Indonesia, Israel, the Philippines, and South Africa. Derma Sciences outsources its manufacturing to plants in Canada, the UK, and the US.

DynamicWeb Enterprises, Inc.

271 Route 46 West, Fairfield Commons, Bldg. F, Ste. 209, Fairfield, NJ 07004

Telephone: 973-276-3100 **Fax:** 973-575-9830 **Metro area:** New York, NY **Web site:** http://www.dynamicweb.com **Human resources contact:** Pat Baker **Sales:** $1.2 million **Number of employees:** 42 **Number of employees for previous year:** 24 **Industry designation:** Computers—corporate, professional & financial software **Company type:** Public **Top competitors:** Open Market, Inc.; Sterling Commerce, Inc.; Harbinger Corporation

DynamicWeb Enterprises is into swapping. The company makes software and provides services that enable businesses to trade online. Its EDIxchange Enterprise Suite of e-commerce software helps users create product catalogs, view and edit purchase orders, send electronic invoices, and generate shipping notices. DynamicWeb also offers on-site and remote consulting services such as systems analysis, integration, and corporate e-commerce strategy planning. It targets the manufacturing, pharmaceutical, retail, telecommunications, and transportation industries. Customers include Church & Dwight, Rite Aid, and RJR Nabisco. Chairman Steven Vanechanos Jr. and his father, Steven Sr. (SVP), together own 22% of the company.

ECCS, Inc.

One Sheila Dr., Tinton Falls, NJ 07724

Telephone: 732-747-6995 **Fax:** 732-747-6542 **Metro area:** New York, NY **Web site:** http://www.eccs.com **Human resources contact:** Sharon Wallace **Sales:** $28.5 million **Number of employees:** 125 **Number of employees for previous year:** 96 **Industry designation:** Computers—peripheral equipment **Company type:** Public **Top competitors:** EMC Corporation; Mylex Corporation

ECCS produces high-performance computer data storage products intended to provide a less-costly alternative to traditional mainframe storage systems. Its primary product, Synchronix, employs redundant array of independent disks technology to protect against data loss as a result of software or hardware failure. Other products by ECCS include external disks, optical and tape systems, and internal disk and tape storage devices. The company sells to businesses and the federal government and to original equipment manufacturers such as Unisys and Tandem.

EchoCath, Inc.

4326 US Rte. 1, Monmouth Junction, NJ 08852

Telephone: 609-987-8400 **Fax:** 609-987-1019 **Other address:** PO Box 7224, Princeton, NJ 08543 **Metro area:** New York, NY **Sales:** $1.1 million **Number of employees:** 18 **Number of employees for previous year:** 15 **Industry designation:** Medical instruments **Company type:** Public **Top competitors:** C. R. Bard, Inc.; EndoSonics Corporation

Development-stage EchoCath designs and makes minimally invasive surgery products that use ultrasound technology in new ways. Among its products are ones that are designed to monitor internal blood flow; mark and display catheters and other objects within the body; and view tissues and internal organs in three-dimensional real time. Although some of EchoCath's products are cleared for market in the US, others are awaiting FDA and European approval. Companies which have had collaborative agreements with EchoCath include C.R. Bard, EP MedSystems, and Medtronic.

Elite Pharmaceuticals, Inc.

165 Ludlow Ave., Northvale, NJ 07647

Telephone: 201-750-2646 **Fax:** 201-750-2755 **Metro area:** New York, NY **Human resources contact:** Robert Deline **Sales:** $51,958 **Number of employees:** 9 **Number of employees for previous year:** 8 **Industry designation:** Drugs **Company type:** Public **Top competitors:** Andrx Corporation; ALZA Corporation; Elan Corporation, plc

Elite Pharmaceuticals is the holding company for Elite Laboratories, a development-stage company working on controlled-release pharmaceutical products. The company intends to develop less-expensive, generic versions of existing controlled-release drugs that are nearing the end of their exclusivity period. The company's six products, all of which are in various stages of testing, include angina and hypertension therapies, a nonsteroidal analgesic drug, and a drug to lower blood glucose by stimulating insulin production in the pancreas. Elite Laboratories also provides contract R&D sponsored by other drug companies including Novo Nordisk and SmithKline Beecham.

Engelhard Corporation

101 Wood Ave., Iselin, NJ 08830

Telephone: 732-205-5000 **Fax:** 732-321-1161 **Metro area:** New York, NY **Web site:** http://www.engelhard.com **Human resources contact:** John C. Hess **Sales:** $4.2 billion **Number of employees:** 6,425 **Number of employees for previous year:** 6,400 **Industry designation:** Chemicals—specialty **Company type:** Public **Top competitors:** BASF Aktiengesellschaft; Akzo Nobel N.V.; Imperial Chemical Industries PLC

Specialty chemical maker Engelhard has operations in three segments. Its engineered materials and industrial commodities management unit gathers minerals and uses them to make such industrial products as conductive pastes and electroplating materials. Engelhard's catalysts and chemicals unit produces catalysts used in the automotive, petroleum, chemical, food-processing, and pharmaceutical industries. The company's pigments and additives group makes products used in paper, plastics, ink, packaging, and paints and other coatings. Minorco, a Luxembourg-based company affiliated with Anglo American Corporation of South Africa, is selling its 32% stake.

EPITAXX, Inc.

7 Graphics Dr., West Trenton, NJ 08628

Telephone: 609-538-1800 **Fax:** 609-538-1684 **Metro area:** Philadelphia, PA **Web site:** http://www.epitaxx.com **Human resources contact:** Connie McGee **Sales:** $25.3 million (Est.) **Number of employees:** 210 **Number of employees for previous year:** 208 **Industry designation:** Fiber optics **Company type:** Private **Top competitors:** Siemens AG; Mitsubishi Electric Corporation; Fujitsu Limited

EPITAXX makes semiconductor optical detectors and receivers for the fiber-optic communications industry. Its InGaAs (indium gallium arsenide) detectors and receivers are used in high-capacity terrestrial and undersea fiber-optic systems, multichannel cable television distribution, digital local-loop and access networks, and computer networking. The company also makes testing and measurement equipment used by defense and industry markets. It offers customization services to its customers (which include Lucent and Hewlett-Packard). Flat-glass maker Nippon Sheet Glass owns 70% of EPITAXX.

EP MedSystems, Inc.

100 Stierli Ct., Mount Arlington, NJ 07856

Telephone: 973-398-2800 **Fax:** 973-398-8636 **Metro area:** Allentown, PA **Sales:** $7.5 million **Number of employees:** 75 **Number of employees for previous year:** 60 **Industry designation:** Medical products **Company type:** Public **Top competitors:** Angeion Corporation; Cardiac Control Systems, Inc.; Cambridge Heart, Inc.

EP MedSystems skips no beats, designing products that diagnose, monitor, and treat cardiac arrhythmias. The company is developing the ALERT system, which treats arrhythmia by delivering low levels of electricity to the heart via catheter. Already marketed in Europe, the system is undergoing clinical trials in the US. Other products include the EP-3 Stimulator, the only computerized electrophysiology clinical stimulator in the US, and the EP WorkMate, which monitors heart activity and stores arrhythmia data. Through subsidiary ProCath, the company also manufactures diagnostic catheters. EP MedSystems is building its own sales staff to market its products in the US; it markets abroad through other distributors.

Faulding Oral Pharmaceuticals

200 Elmora Ave., Elizabeth, NJ 07207

Telephone: 908-527-9100 **Fax:** 908-527-0649 **Metro area:** New York, NY **Human resources contact:** Lisa Zimmer **Sales:** $112.7 million **Number of employees:** 500 **Number of employees for previous year:** 479 **Industry designation:** Drugs—generic **Company type:** Subsidiary **Top competitors:** Hoechst AG; Glaxo Wellcome plc; IVAX Corporation

Open up and say, "Faahh-lding." Faulding Oral Pharmaceuticals develops and manufactures generic drug products. The oral pharmaceuticals arm of Australian drug firm F.H. Faulding, the group includes Purepac Pharmaceutical, Faulding Laboratories, and CMAX, an Australian drug testing firm. Among the generic drugs the division makes are clonazepam, diclofenac, and pentoxifylline. Faulding's customers include drug wholesalers, national and regional retail drugstores, and drug distributors. Parent F. H. Faulding & Co. acquired full ownership of the firm in 1998 as part of a restructuring to better compete against pharmaceutical giants.

Flemington Pharmaceutical Corporation

43 Emery Ave., Flemington, NJ 08822

Telephone: 908-782-3431 **Fax:** 908-782-2445 **Metro area:** New York, NY **Web site:** http://www.flemington-pharma.com **Human resources contact:** Harry A. Dugger III **Sales:** $871,000 **Number of employees:** 9 **Number of employees for previous year:** 4 **Industry designation:** Drugs **Company type:** Public **Top competitors:** Fuisz Technologies Ltd.; R.P. Scherer Corporation; Anesta Corp.

Flemington Pharmaceutical's provides drug development consulting to European companies. To reduce its reliance on a few major customers (three of which account for about two-thirds of revenues), Flemington Pharmaceuticals is branching out—developing new ways to deliver popular over-the-counter and prescription drugs. The company's patent-pending delivery systems include lingual sprays and soft-bite gelatin capsules, which allow fast absorption. Proposed products include osteoporosis treatments, hormone therapy, sleep inducers, and cardiovascular drugs. Founder/CEO/President Harry Dugger and Chairman John Moroney respectively own about 40% and 20% of the company, which went public in 1997.

HealthCare Imaging Services, Inc.

200 Schulz Dr., Red Bank, NJ 07701

Telephone: 732-224-9292 **Fax:** 732-224-9329 **Metro area:** New York, NY **Human resources contact:** Dolores Lessone **Sales:** $16.5 million **Number of employees:** 136 **Number of employees for previous year:** 71 **Industry designation:** Medical services **Company type:** Public **Top competitors:** Medical Resources, Inc.; InSight Health Services Corp.; Universal Health Services, Inc.

HealthCare Imaging Services has expanded from MRIs to PPMs. The company operates 12 medical imaging centers throughout New York and New Jersey and is moving into physician practice management (PPM). The company's move into practice management includes a contract to manage a 60-physician practice in New Jersey. The company's centers generally offer MRI services, but also offer CAT, mammography, X-ray, ultrasound, and bone densitrometry imaging at some locations. It leases the services to health care providers including health care plans and individual physician practices.

Hoffmann-La Roche, Inc.

340 Kingsland St., Nutley, NJ 07110

Telephone: 973-235-5000 **Fax:** 973-562-2208 **Metro area:** New York, NY **Human resources contact:** Bradley Smith **Sales:** $800 million **Number of employees:** 1,100 **Industry designation:** Drugs **Company type:** Subsidiary **Parent company:** Roche Holding AG **Top competitors:** Abbott Laboratories; Glaxo Wellcome plc; Rhone-Poulenc S.A.

Druggernaut Hoffmann-La Roche is the inexorable force behind Roche Holding Ltd, with businesses ranging from pharmaceuticals to fragrances. The Roche subsidiary develops and makes drugs to treat AIDS, cancer, heart disease, and obesity, among other conditions. Not all of Hoffmann-La Roche's products, however, address the grim side of life: The firm also makes vitamins, animal feed additives, fragrances for consumer products, and flavorings for drinks, foods, tobacco products, and pharmaceuticals. Hoffmann-La Roche has an agreement to co-market its Parkinson's drug Tasmar along with Du Pont's Sinemet. The company takes its name from its Swiss founder, Fritz Hoffmann-La Roche.

Hooper Holmes, Inc.

170 Mount Airy Rd., Basking Ridge, NJ 07920

Telephone: 908-766-5000 **Fax:** 908-953-6304 **Metro area:** New York, NY **Web site:** http://www.hooperholmes.com **Human resources contact:** Frank Stiner **Sales:** $185.2 million **Number of employees:** 1,735 **Number of employees for previous year:** 1,700 **Industry designation:** Medical services **Company type:** Public **Top competitors:** ChoicePoint Inc.

Talk about a high-pressure exam. Hooper Holmes, the largest health information services firm in the US, collects data on life and health insurance prospects for the insurance industry. The company performs more than two million medical exams a year through its network of about 200 offices nationwide. More than 90% of the company's revenues come from its Portamedic business, which offers exams in an applicant's home or office. Clients include Prudential, Northwestern Mutual, First Colony, and State Farm. Its Infolink service provides inspection reports and doctors' statements to insurance companies. Hooper Holmes also is seeking to use its mobile testing capabilities in the clinical research market.

HumaScan Inc.

125 Moen Ave., Cranford, NJ 07016

Telephone: 908-709-3434 **Fax:** 908-709-4646 **Metro area:** New York, NY **Web site:** http://www.humascan.com **Human resources contact:** Kenneth S. Hollander **Sales:** $100,000 **Number of employees:** 46 **Number of employees for previous year:** 12 **Industry designation:** Medical instruments **Company type:** Public **Top competitors:** Siemens Corporation; ThermoTrex Corporation; Fischer Imaging Corporation

Breast cancer is red hot, and HumaScan can feel the heat. The company has licensed from Scantek Medical the rights to make and sell its BreastAlert Differential Temperature Sensor in the US and Canada. The BreastAlert consists of two disposable sensor pads that are worn next to each breast for about 15 minutes. Because the increased metabolic activity associated with early-stage breast cancer produces excess heat, the sensors detect temperature variations. The sensors change color if increased heat is detected, alerting doctors to a potential tumor. HumaScan sells its pads for about $25 per set to gynecologists and general practitioners. The Travelers Group owns about 25% of the company.

IBS Interactive, Inc.

2 Ridgedale Ave., Ste. 350, Cedar Knolls, NJ 07927

Telephone: 973-285-2600 **Fax:** 973-285-4777 **Metro area:** New York, NY **Web site:** http://www.interactive.net **Human resources contact:** Jeffrey E. Brenner **Sales:** $9.8 million **Number of employees:** 128 **Number of employees for previous year:** 46 **Industry designation:** Computers—services **Company type:** Public

IBS Interactive provides outsourced computer networking, programming, applications development, and Internet services to businesses, government agencies, and not-for-profit organizations. Its systems integration services include design, implementation, and maintenance. Internet services include dedicated leased line and frame relay connections, Web hosting, dial-up access, and e-mail services. Customers have included Aetna, Bell Atlantic, Unilever, and the US Department of Defense. President Nicholas Loglisci, chief technical officer Clark Frederick, and chief information officer Frank Altieri each own about 12% of IBS, which is growing through acquisitions.

IDM Environmental Corp.

396 Whitehead Ave., South River, NJ 08882

Telephone: 732-390-9550 **Fax:** 732-390-9545 **Other address:** PO Box 388, South River, NJ 08882 **Metro area:** New York, NY **Web site:** http://www.idm-corp.com **Human resources contact:** George Pasalano **Sales:** $17.9 million **Number of employees:** 237 **Number of employees for previous year:** 191 **Industry designation:** Pollution control equipment & services **Company type:** Public **Top competitors:** Enron Global Power & Pipelines L.L.C.; Allied Waste Industries, Inc.; Waste Management, Inc.

IDM Environmental cleans up on environmental cleanups. It offers plant decommissioning, dismantling, and relocation (primarily for chemical companies) as well as asbestos abatement and hazardous waste and radiological remediation. The company offers design, construction, and engineering services, with a concentration in hands-on remediation for specialized environmental and hazardous projects. IDM also has joined the energy services arena, with agreements to design, build, own, and operate waste-to-energy facilities in El Salvador and the former Soviet state of Georgia. The company's clients include industrial plants, utilities, and government agencies in the US and overseas.

IgX Corp.

One Springfield Ave., Summit, NJ 07960

Telephone: 908-598-4663 **Fax:** 908-598-4673 **Metro area:** New York, NY **Web site:** http://www.igxcorporation.com **Human resources contact:** Leslie Jones **Number of employees:** 31 **Industry designation:** Drugs **Company type:** Private **Top competitors:** Ophidian Pharmaceuticals, Inc.; Merck & Co., Inc.; Astra AB

Is there a chicken in the house? The bird best known for its breakfast delectables is now working for IgX Corp. in the fight against cryptosporidiosis. The company is developing treatments for gastrointestinal infections using avian technology, a process in which hens injected with pathogens produce antibodies that concentrate in the yolks of their eggs. IgX then processes the antibodies for oral delivery in humans. The company thinks this type of treatment, called passive immunity, is an effective way to combat pathogens' resistance to antibiotics. Subsidiary IgX Oxford is working on a hepatitis B treatment using Monsanto's proprietary compound N-nonyl-DNJ. CEO Albert Henry will own 52% of IgX after the IPO.

Immunomedics, Inc.

300 American Rd., Morris Plains, NJ 07950

Telephone: 973-605-8200 **Fax:** 973-605-8282 **Metro area:** New York, NY **Web site:** http://www.immunomedics.com **Human resources contact:** Donna Bobb Ransom **Sales:** $7.6 million **Number of employees:** 115 **Number of employees for previous year:** 91 **Industry designation:** Biomedical & genetic products **Company type:** Public **Top competitors:** NeoRx Corporation; Palatin Technologies, Inc.; Chiron Corporation

Immunomedics offers oncologists a sneak preview of that worst of horror shows—cancer—and hopes to provide a way to a happy ending. The biopharmaceutical firm operates in two areas: diagnostics and therapeutics. It has nine in vivo imaging products for several forms of cancer, soft-tissue infections, appendicitis, inflammatory lesions, and non-Hodgkin's lymphoma; most products are still in trials. CEA-Scan (colorectal cancer imaging) has been approved in the US and the European Union; LeukoScan (infection imaging) is marketed in Europe and awaiting the FDA's OK. Immunomedics is also developing monoclonal antibodies that deliver radiation, chemotherapy, or other treatments directly to disease sites.

Infu-Tech, Inc.

910 Sylvan Ave., Englewood Cliffs, NJ 07632

Telephone: 201-567-4600 **Fax:** 201-567-1072 **Metro area:** New York, NY **Sales:** $26.5 million **Number of employees:** 128 **Number of employees for previous year:** 112 **Industry designation:** Medical services **Company type:** Public **Top competitors:** Pediatric Services of America, Inc.; Apria Healthcare Group Inc.; Coram Healthcare Corporation

Infu-Tech provides infusion therapy to patients in their own homes, in nursing homes and subacute care facilities, and at the company's ambulatory IV suites. Its Intravenous Infusion unit provides such therapy services as chemotherapy, enteral and parenteral nutrition, chronic pain management, and hydration therapy. The Contract Services unit provides infusion therapy products, as well as urology and wound care products to residents of long-term-care facilities. Infu-Tech's Disease Management unit develops preventative programs for patients suffering from such conditions as asthma, diabetes, and congestive heart failure. Kuala Healthcare owns about 60% of the company.

Integra LifeSciences Corporation

105 Morgan Ln., Plainsboro, NJ 08536

Telephone: 609-275-0500 **Fax:** 609-799-3297 **Metro area:** Philadelphia, PA **Web site:** http://www.integra-ls.com **Human resources contact:** Linda Nathan **Sales:** $17.5 million **Number of employees:** 178 **Number of employees for previous year:** 166 **Industry designation:** Biomedical & genetic products **Company type:** Public

Integra LifeSciences' products literally get under your skin. The firm develops, makes, and sells implants and biomaterials for regenerating human tissues damaged by surgery, disease, or accident. Its flagship Integra Artificial Skin line (which accounts for about 45% of sales) replaces skin and reduces the need for conventional autografts. The remainder of the firm's sales come from absorbable medical products, which are used for delivering drugs, controlling bleeding and infection, aiding in dental surgery, and wound care. Integra LifeSciences has marketing relationships with such firms as Johnson & Johnson and Sulzer Medica. Chairman Richard Caruso owns 48% of Integra.

Intelligroup, Inc.

499 Thornall St., Edison, NJ 08837

Telephone: 732-590-1600 **Fax:** 732-362-2100 **Metro area:** New York, NY **Web site:** http://www.intelligroup.com **Human resources contact:** Jeffrey Weiner **Sales:** $144.9 million **Number of employees:** 772 **Number of employees for previous year:** 369 **Industry designation:** Computers—services **Company type:** Public **Top competitors:** Andersen Worldwide; International Business Machines Corporation; Cap Gemini S.A.

Intelligroup's expertise is the deployment of complex business software systems from top providers such as SAP, Baan, Oracle, and PeopleSoft. The company also provides systems integration and Internet/intranet application services and develops custom software. Its own 4Sight software products provide tools for implementing and managing projects based on third-party software. Intelligroup operates a programming center in India, and sells its services to large companies worldwide, including PricewaterhouseCoopers and Bristol-Myers Squibb. About 40% of sales come from consulting on teams formed by other IT firms. Co-chairmen Ashok Pandey, Rajkumar Koneru, and Nagarjun Valluripalli each own about 18% of the company.

Interferon Sciences, Inc.

783 Jersey Ave., New Brunswick, NJ 08901

Telephone: 732-249-3250 **Fax:** 732-249-6895 **Metro area:** New York, NY **Web site:** http://www.interferonsciences.com **Human resources contact:** Jeanne Howarth **Sales:** $3 million **Number of employees:** 100 **Number of employees for previous year:** 77 **Industry designation:** Drugs **Company type:** Public **Top competitors:** Merck & Co., Inc.; Minnesota Mining and Manufacturing Company; Schering-Plough Corporation

Interferon Sciences makes products based on natural alpha interferons, which are proteins made from human white blood cells that aid the body's natural defenses against diseases. The company's ALFERON N Injection is an FDA-approved injectible form of natural alpha interferon used in the treatment of genital warts. Interferon Sciences is developing that product for the treatment of viral and immune systems diseases (such as HIV), hepatitis C, and multiple sclerosis, although the FDA has yet to approve ALFERON N's use as a treatment for HIV. The company has also developed a topical gel, which is being tested as a treatment for cervical dysplasia, intravaginal warts, and genital herpes.

Isomedix, Inc.

11 Apollo Dr., Whippany, NJ 07981

Telephone: 973-887-4700 **Fax:** 973-887-1476 **Metro area:** New York, NY **Web site:** http://www.isomedix.com **Human resources contact:** Suzan Chang-Johnson **Sales:** $45.2 million **Number of employees:** 346 **Number of employees for previous year:** 336 **Industry designation:** Medical services **Company type:** Subsidiary **Top competitors:** Griffith Micro Science International, Inc.; SteriGenics International, Inc.; Medical Sterilization, Inc.

Isomedix asks, "where's the beef?" The wholly owned subsidiary of sterilization equipment maker STERIS provides contract gamma radiation and ethylene oxide sterilization services to manufacturers of prepackaged products. The FDA has approved its petition to use irradiation to kill bacteria in meat. Isomedix operates a network of contract sterilization facilities throughout the US. It processes syringes, needles, scalpels, surgeons' gloves, and intravenous tubes. Consumer products include cotton balls, food packaging materials, baby bottle nipples, cosmetic brushes and applicators, and talc. The company markets its sterilization services to manufacturers of single-use medical devices and consumer products.

i-STAT Corporation

303 College Rd. East, Princeton, NJ 08540

Telephone: 609-243-9300 **Fax:** 609-243-9311 **Metro area:** Philadelphia, PA **Web site:** http://www.i-stat.com **Human resources contact:** Bill Beattie **Sales:** $39.1 million **Number of employees:** 531 **Number of employees for previous year:** 499 **Industry designation:** Medical instruments **Company type:** Public

i-STAT Corporation makes blood analysis products that provide health care professionals with diagnostic information at the point of patient care. i-STAT offers handheld, automated blood analyzers that can perform several common, critical tests using two or three drops of blood in a couple of minutes while the patient waits. Each i-STAT system consists of a microprocessor-based analyzer and disposable test cartridges containing biosensor-laden silicon chips. The company produces the i-STAT systems for the critical care departments of hospitals throughout the world. Hewlett-Packard owns 14% of i-STAT; Abbott Laboratories owns about 12%.

Johnson & Johnson

One Johnson & Johnson Plaza, New Brunswick, NJ 08933

Telephone: 732-524-0400 **Fax:** 732-524-3300 **Metro area:** New York, NY **Web site:** http://www.jnj.com **Human resources contact:** Russell C. Deyo **Sales:** $23.7 billion **Number of employees:** 90,500 **Number of employees for previous year:** 89,300 **Industry designation:** Medical products **Company type:** Public **Top competitors:** The Procter & Gamble Company; Merck & Co., Inc.; Bristol-Myers Squibb Company

Johnson & Johnson is one of the world's largest and most diversified health care product makers. The company operates in three sectors: consumer products (with brands like Tylenol and Motrin analgesics, Reach toothbrushes, Band-Aid bandages), professional products (AcuVue contact lenses, surgical instruments, joint replacements), and pharmaceuticals (including Ergamisol cancer treatment, Hismanal antihistamine, and Ortho-Novum oral contraceptives). Johnson & Johnson expands its product line through acquisitions (it has made more than 30 this decade) and partnerships with smaller firms (they provide the technology; Johnson & Johnson provides the marketing muscle).

KCS Energy, Inc.

379 Thornall St., Edison, NJ 08837

Telephone: 732-632-1770 **Fax:** 732-603-8960 **Metro area:** New York, NY **Web site:** http://www.kcsenergy.com **Human resources contact:** Kathryn M. Kinnamon **Sales:** $129.5 million **Number of employees:** 229 **Number of employees for previous year:** 209 **Industry designation:** Oil & gas—exploration & production **Company type:** Public **Top competitors:** Mitchell Energy & Development Corp.; Barrett Resources Corporation; BP Amoco p.l.c.

After kissing its pipeline operations goodbye, KCS Energy is focusing on oil and gas exploration and production in the Gulf Coast, Rocky Mountain, Midcontinent, and West Texas regions. The company also has interests in the Gulf of Mexico and Michigan's Niagaran Reef Trend. Natural gas makes up about three-fourths of the company's oil and gas reserves. KCS Energy's 1996 purchase of the InterCoast Oil and Gas (now Medallion Resources) doubled its energy production and reserves. Among other factors, markedly lower oil and gas prices in 1997 played a role in KCS Energy's $92 million loss for the year. Chairman Stewart Kean owns about 9% of the company.

KTI, Inc.

7000 Boulevard East, Guttenberg, NJ 07093

Telephone: 201-854-7777 **Fax:** 201-854-1771 **Metro area:** New York, NY **Web site:** http://www.hawkassociates.com/kti **Human resources contact:** Kelly Stllakis **Sales:** $96.2 million **Number of employees:** 493 **Number of employees for previous year:** 188 **Industry designation:** Pollution control equipment & services **Company type:** Public

KTI turns trash into power. The company converts commercial and municipal waste into electricity through incineration and then recycles the remaining ash to obtain scrap metals and materials used in commercial construction, asphalt, concrete, and roadbed applications. KTI disposes of 60% of Maine's garbage in this manner. Other KTI facilities turn wood waste into electricity, recycle paper and plastics, and dispose of commercial and industrial specialty wastes. The company operates processing facilities and marketing offices in the eastern US and Oregon and is expanding its reach through frequent acquisitions.

Kuala Healthcare Inc.

910 Sylvan Ave., Englewood Cliffs, NJ 07632

Telephone: 201-567-4600 **Fax:** 201-567-8536 **Metro area:** New York, NY **Human resources contact:** Gerry Kelly **Sales:** $63.9 million **Number of employees:** 950 **Number of employees for previous year:** 926 **Industry designation:** Nursing homes **Company type:** Public **Top competitors:** Beverly Enterprises, Inc.; Genesis Health Ventures, Inc.; Apria Healthcare Group Inc.

Kuala means "quality" according to Kuala Healthcare, but we won't blame you for thinking of the Qantas bear or luau menu items. Kuala operates nursing homes and provides medical services to nonhospitalized patients. The company's five nursing homes in New Jersey and Philadelphia provide provide meals, lodging, and care services. Publicly traded subsidiary Infu-Tech, of which Kuala owns about 60%, provides infusion therapy to patients in long-term care facilities and at home. Another subsidiary distributes Eli Lilly pharmaceuticals in Russia. The company is developing new assisted-care sites. A joint venture agreement with Care One will give that company a 49% stake in Kuala's nursing homes and all of its entire institutional pharmacy operations.

The Liposome Company, Inc.

One Research Way, Princeton Forrestal Center, Princeton, NJ 08540

Telephone: 609-452-7060 **Fax:** 609-452-1890 **Metro area:** Philadelphia, PA **Web site:** http://www.lipo.com **Human resources contact:** George G. Renton **Sales:** $77.9 million **Number of employees:** 301 **Number of employees for previous year:** 280 **Industry designation:** Biomedical & genetic products **Company type:** Public **Top competitors:** ALZA Corporation; NeXstar Pharmaceuticals, Inc.; NeoPharm, Inc.

The Liposome Company develops and markets lipid- and liposome-based drugs for treating cancer and other illnesses. (Liposomes are man-made cells that can be used to deliver drugs, often with fewer side effects than with ordinary drug-delivery systems.) The company sells ABELCET for treating systemic fungal infections; in addition, it is developing Evacet, TLC ELL-12, and Bromotaxol (all of which may help treat cancer) and is working on a gene-based drug-delivery system. Liposome markets its products directly in the US, the UK, and Canada and has marketing agreements abroad with other firms. Through his Ross Financial Corp., Kenneth Dart (expatriate emperor of Dart Container Corp.) owns 25% of the company.

Lucille Farms, Inc.

150 River Rd., Montville, NJ 07045

Telephone: 973-334-6030 **Fax:** 973-402-6361 **Other address:** PO Box 517, Montville, NJ 07045 **Metro area:** New York, NY **Web site:** http://www.lucille-farms.com **Sales:** $36.2 million **Number of employees:** 72 **Number of employees for previous year:** 64 **Industry designation:** Food—dairy products **Company type:** Public **Top competitors:** Land O'Lakes, Inc.; Southern Foods Group Incorporated; Kraft Foods, Inc.

What's pizza without the mozzarella? Lucille Farms makes mozzarella, provolone, and feta cheese for sale to pizza chains, independent pizzerias, restaurants, hospitals, schools, and other businesses and institutions. Conventional mozzarella cheese accounts for about 90% of the firm's sales. Using a proprietary formula that it intends to apply to other types of cheese, Lucille Farms also produces a line of fat-free, cholesterol-free, and low-fat mozzarella substitutes sold under the Mozzi-RITE and Tasty-Lite Cheese brand names. Lucille Farms produces about 500,000 pounds of cheese weekly at its plant in Swanton, Vermont. Co-founders Philip, Gennaro, and Alfonso Falivene together own nearly 35% of Lucille Farms.

New Jersey

MDY Advanced Technologies, Inc.

21-00 Rte. 208 South, Fair Lawn, NJ 07410

Telephone: 201-797-6676 **Fax:** 201-797-6852 **Metro area:** New York, NY **Web site:** http://www.mdyadvtech.com **Human resources contact:** David Stott **Sales:** $8 million (Est.) **Number of employees:** 43 **Number of employees for previous year:** 37 **Industry designation:** Computers—services **Company type:** Private

Within hours of the World Trade Center bombing, three major law firms in the complex called MDY Advanced Technologies, a disaster-recovery and computer consulting company, to restore their data-processing and billing operations. Founded in 1988, MDY also provides records management and file-conversion software and network integration through its TransferXpress, CompareRite, Related Documents, and RMS products. As part of its disaster planning and recovery services, MDY maintains a "hot site" equipped with desks, phones, and computers where clients can resume business following a disaster. Founders Galina Datskovsky and husband Mark Moerdler own MDY, which has offices in Florida, New Jersey, and Washington, DC.

Medarex, Inc.

1545 Rte. 22 East, Annandale, NJ 08801

Telephone: 908-713-6001 **Fax:** 908-713-6002 **Other address:** PO Box 953, Annandale, NJ 08801 **Metro area:** New York, NY **Web site:** http://www.medarex.com **Human resources contact:** Nancy Dawley **Sales:** $6.8 million **Number of employees:** 89 **Number of employees for previous year:** 64 **Industry designation:** Biomedical & genetic products **Company type:** Public **Top competitors:** Chiron Corporation; ImClone Systems Incorporated; Genentech, Inc.

Medarex and its subsidiaries use monoclonal antibody and immunology technologies to discover and develop treatments for cancer, autoimmune diseases, and other life-threatening disorders. Its products are designed either to block "bad" or to trigger and enhance "good" immune system responses. Many in late-stage clinical testing for FDA approval, some products target cancers (prostate, colon, kidney) and tumors (head, neck, kidney); others are designed to treat glaucoma, secondary cataracts, and a type of acute leukemia. Medarex also clones human monoclonal antibodies for itself and its partners, including Merck and Novartis. Subsidiary GenPharm develops antibodies from bioengineered animals.

MEDIQ Incorporated

One MEDIQ Plaza, Pennsauken, NJ 08110

Telephone: 609-662-3200 **Fax:** 609-665-2391 **Metro area:** Philadelphia, PA **Human resources contact:** Dina Lichtman **Sales:** $180.9 million (Est.) **Number of employees:** 1,271 **Number of employees for previous year:** 927 **Industry designation:** Medical products **Company type:** Private **Top competitors:** Universal Hospital Services, Inc.; Home Health Corporation of America, Inc.; Kinetic Concepts, Inc.

MEDIQ owns MEDIQ/PRN Life Support Services, which rents some 650 types of medical machines such as monitors and ventilators to health care facilities nationwide. It also rents specialized surface products (such as mattress covers that help prevent bedsores) and sells replacement parts, accessories, and disposable products relating to its equipment. The company's Comprehensive Asset Management Program offers consulting to health care equipment clients. To cut inventory costs, MEDIQ has arranged to share rental profits with some equipment makers rather than buy the machines. Investment firm Bruckman, Rosser, Sherrill & Co. owns more than 40% of the company.

MedQuist Inc.

5 Greentree Centre, Ste. 311, Marlton, NJ 08053

Telephone: 609-596-8877 **Fax:** 609-596-3351 **Metro area:** Philadelphia, PA **Web site:** http://www.medquist.com **Human resources contact:** Tami Martin **Sales:** $84.6 million **Number of employees:** 2,400 **Number of employees for previous year:** 857 **Industry designation:** Medical practice management **Company type:** Public **Top competitors:** Transcend Services, Inc.; EquiMed, Inc.; Digital Dictation, Inc.

MedQuist takes doctors' chicken-scratching and makes it legible. It provides transcription and information management services to more than 1,400 hospitals, physician groups, and other health care organizations nationwide. With a nationwide network of service centers, the company provides systems and software to replace or supplement clients' in-house medical transcription departments. In addition to providing its services to medical records departments, the acquisitive company (which swallowed up its primary rival, MRC Group, in 1998) plans to provide transcription for specific departments, including cardiology and oncology. MedQuist is the transcriptionist for online physicians' resource WebMD.

Merck & Co., Inc.

One Merck Dr., Whitehouse Station, NJ 08889

Telephone: 908-423-1000 **Fax:** 908-423-2592 **Other address:** PO Box 100, Whitehouse Station, NJ 08889 **Metro area:** New York, NY **Web site:** http://www.merck.com **Human resources contact:** Deborah K. Smith **Sales:** $26.9 billion **Number of employees:** 57,300 **Number of employees for previous year:** 53,800 **Industry designation:** Drugs **Company type:** Public **Top competitors:** Glaxo Wellcome plc; Novartis AG; Pfizer Inc

Merck is the #1 drugmaker in the US and is tied for first in the world with Glaxo Wellcome in prescription drugs. The company develops products for both humans and animals; almost two-fifths of its sales come from treating ailments associated with American eating habits—high cholesterol, hypertension, and heart failure. Leading this battle against too many greasy burgers are Merck's Zocor and Mevacor, two prominent cholesterol drugs. In addition, Merck has the top-selling US drugs for hypertension (Vasotec, Prinivil), as well as newer, promising drugs such as Crixivan (AIDS treatment), Propecia (for male baldness), and Maxalt (for migraine headaches). Also under development is a new arthritis drug, Vioxx.

Metalogics, Inc.

Riverview Historical Plaza, 33-41 Newark St., Ste. 4-C, Hoboken, NJ 07030

Telephone: 201-656-0906 **Fax:** 201-656-0901 **Metro area:** New York, NY **Web site:** http://www.meta4inc.com **Human resources contact:** Deborah Stein **Sales:** $1.6 million (Est.) **Number of employees:** 18 **Industry designation:** Computers—services **Company type:** Private **Top competitors:** Computer Associates International, Inc.; Deloitte Touche Tohmatsu International; Ernst & Young International

Metalogics software keeps hospital computer networks from needing emergency care. The company's Java-based Intelligent Configuration Management (ICM) software monitors large, integrated networks of computers, medical equipment, and building systems (security, elevators), and handles current or impending problems. ICM, which is installed in about 60 facilities, includes real-time monitoring functions, a year 2000 compliance program and a help desk that logs and tracks reported problems. Metalogics also does facilities engineering, consulting, and IT training. After the planned IPO, CEO and co-founder William Doyle will reduce his stake from 60% to 37%, and co-founder James Urbaniak's will drop from 40% to 25%.

Metrologic Instruments, Inc.

90 Coles Rd., Blackwood, NJ 08012

Telephone: 609-228-8100 **Fax:** 609-228-6673 **Metro area:** Philadelphia, PA **Web site:** http://www.metrologic.com **Human resources contact:** John L. Patton **Sales:** $65.6 million **Number of employees:** 400 **Number of employees for previous year:** 378 **Industry designation:** Optical character recognition **Company type:** Public **Top competitors:** PSC Inc.; Symbol Technologies, Inc.; Scan-Optics, Inc.

Your library book, cereal box, and the package you got today all have the "mark." Bar code, that is. Bar code scanner systems, such as those made by Metrologic Instruments, let libraries, supermarkets, and package handlers track, price, and code diverse items. Metrologic makes handheld, fixed-position, and in-counter scanners. Laser-based models make up the bulk of sales (90%), although a new holographic system is making inroads in the area of high-volume, unattended package handling. The company makes all its own components and offers proprietary software (ScanSet, ScanSelect) for the systems. Metrologic makes private-label products for Matsushita Inter-Techno, Rockwell Automation, and Symbol Technologies.

Milestone Scientific Inc.

220 S. Orange Ave., Livingston Corporate Park, Livingston, NJ 07039

Telephone: 973-716-0087 **Fax:** 973-535-2829 **Metro area:** New York, NY **Human resources contact:** Thomas M. Stuckey **Sales:** $2.9 million **Number of employees:** 38 **Number of employees for previous year:** 15 **Industry designation:** Medical products **Company type:** Public

Say ah-h-h-h. Milestone Scientific develops and manufactures health care equipment and disposable products, mainly for use by dental practitioners. The company's primary product is the Wand, a computer-controlled device (the size of a pen) that allows dentists to administer local anesthesia with more precision and much less pain—significantly reducing patient anxiety and waiting time. Other products include accessories for dental drill tips, clinical flosses, and the Sharps Disposal System, a heat sterilizer that safely disposes of used needles and other sharp instruments. The company also owns the US distribution arm of UK-based Wisdom, an oral hygiene company that sells toothbrushes and related products.

Millennium Sports Management, Inc.

Ross' Corner, U.S. Hwy. 206 and County Rte. 565, Augusta, NJ 07822

Telephone: 973-383-7644 **Fax:** 973-383-7522 **Other address:** PO Box 117, Augusta, NJ 07822 **Metro area:** Allentown, PA **Sales:** $656,554 **Number of employees:** 9 **Industry designation:** Leisure & recreational services **Company type:** Public **Top competitors:** The Sports Authority, Inc.; New York Yankees; Metropolitan Baseball Club Inc.

Millennium Sports Management is a baseball lover's dream. Its New Jersey-based Skylands Park Sports and Recreation Center provides fans the opportunity to watch baseball games in a 4,300-seat stadium, hone their skills in an indoor recreation facility, and purchase equipment and apparel through the Skylands Sporting Goods store. Millennium Sports owns a minority stake in the New Jersey Cardinals, a minor league baseball team that plays its home games in Skylands Parks. In addition to Cardinals games, the stadium hosts more than 90 college, high school, and other amateur events. The company is also involved in a joint venture with Golf Stadiums to develop a Stadium Golf resort in Naples, Florida.

New Brunswick Scientific Co., Inc.

44 Talmadge Rd., Edison, NJ 08818

Telephone: 732-287-1200 **Fax:** 732-287-4222 **Other address:** PO Box 4005, Edison, NJ 08818 **Metro area:** New York, NY **Web site:** http://www.nbsc.com **Sales:** $46.5 million **Number of employees:** 433 **Number of employees for previous year:** 412 **Industry designation:** Instruments—scientific **Company type:** Public **Top competitors:** B. Braun-Melsungen AG; CELLEX BIOSCIENCES, Inc.

If you're in the mood to shake your beaker, New Brunswick Scientific (NBS) could help. NBS makes equipment used in biotechnology to create, measure, and control conditions needed to grow and detect microorganisms. Although known for its durable New Brunswick Shaker, NBS makes other products, including fermentors, bioreactors, sterilizers, tissue culture rotators, and centrifuges. Its equipment is used in medical, biological, chemical, and environmental research and development facilities. NBS owns 80 percent of DGI BioTechnologies, which specializes in assay systems that aid in the discovery of new drugs. Brothers David and Sigmund Freedman, both NBS directors, together own nearly 30 percent of the company.

New Jersey Devils

50 Rte. 120 North, East Rutherford, NJ 07073

Telephone: 201-935-6050 **Fax:** 201-935-2127 **Other address:** PO Box 504, East Rutherford, NJ 07073 **Metro area:** New York, NY **Web site:** http://www.newjerseydevils.com **Human resources contact:** Peter McMullen **Sales:** $54.4 million (Est.) **Number of employees:** 150 **Industry designation:** Leisure & recreational services **Company type:** Private **Top competitors:** New York Rangers; Philadelphia Flyers; Pittsburgh Penguins

During the past two decades, the New Jersey Devils have gone from being a National Hockey League embarrassment to a Stanley Cup winner. The team was founded as the 1974 expansion Kansas City Scouts, then moved to Denver in 1976 to become the Colorado Rockies. It was bought in 1982 by a group led by principal owner John McMullen and moved to the East Coast. Renamed the Devils, hockey great Wayne Gretzky called the team a "Mickey Mouse organization" that was ruining the league. Twelve years later, the Devils had their revenge when they shut out the Detroit Red Wings in the 1995 Stanley Cup Finals. The Devils play in the Continental Airlines Arena in East Rutherford, New Jersey.

New Jersey Nets

390 Murray Hill Pkwy., East Rutherford, NJ 07073

Telephone: 201-935-8888 **Fax:** 201-939-7812 **Metro area:** New York, NY **Web site:** http://www.nba.com/nets **Sales:** $65.5 million (Est.) **Number of employees:** 100 **Industry designation:** Leisure & recreational services **Company type:** Private **Top competitors:** Washington Wizards; New York Knickerbockers; Miami Heat

It's been a long, strange trip for the New Jersey Nets. The team was formed in 1967 as the New Jersey Americans and was a member of the American Basketball Association (ABA). After its first season, the club moved across the river and became the New York Nets. With Julius "Dr. J" Erving, the Nets won two ABA championships before joining the NBA (and losing Erving) in 1976. (The team moved back to the Garden State that year.) A group that includes comedian Bill Cosby and Community Youth Organization, a trust to benefit urban-area youth in New Jersey, owns the team. The Nets plans to merge its business operations with Major League Baseball's New York Yankees into a new comany called YankeeNets.

New York Giants

Giants Stadium, East Rutherford, NJ 07073

Telephone: 201-935-8111 **Fax:** 201-935-8493 **Metro area:** New York, NY **Web site:** http://www.nfl.com/giants **Human resources contact:** Nicole Kelly **Sales:** $82.3 million (Est.) **Number of employees:** 135 **Industry designation:** Leisure & recreational services **Company type:** Private **Top competitors:** Dallas Cowboys Football Club, Ltd.; Arizona Cardinals; Philadelphia Eagles

One of the oldest teams in the NFL, the New York Giants date back to 1925 when Tim Mara bought a football franchise for the nation's biggest city for $500. Over the course of its more than 70-year history, the Big Blue Machine has won four NFL championships (1927, 1934, 1938, 1956) and two Super Bowls (1987 and 1991). Notable Giants have included head coaches Steve Owen and Bill Parcels, quarterback Phil Simms, and linebacker Lawrence Taylor. The team is co-owned by Wellington Mara (Tim's son) and billionaire Robert Tisch (a former Postmaster General and co-chairman of Loews Corporation). New York plays its home games at Giants Stadium in East Rutherford, New Jersey.

ObjectSoft Corporation

Continental Plaza III, 433 Hackensack Ave., Hackensack, NJ 07601

Telephone: 201-343-9100 **Fax:** 201-343-0056 **Metro area:** New York, NY **Web site:** http://www.objectsoftcorp.com **Human resources contact:** Janis Barsuk **Sales:** $600,000 **Number of employees:** 19 **Number of employees for previous year:** 18 **Industry designation:** Computers—services **Company type:** Public **Top competitors:** International Business Machines Corporation; True North Communications Inc.

If you ever find yourself renewing your driver's license or paying a parking fine through a computerized kiosk, you may have ObjectSoft to thank. The firm offers interactive services via the Internet and public kiosks. Sales come from kiosk sales or (on ObjectSoft-owned units) advertising sales. The City of New York (84% of sales) has ObjectSoft kiosks that provide access to certain city records, as well as birth certificates or other documents for a fee, while SmartSign kiosks provide information about city events and places of interest. ObjectSoft's FastTake units allow video store customers to search for titles. Chairman David Sarna and president George Febish together own about one-third of the company.

Osteotech, Inc.

51 James Way, Eatontown, NJ 07724

Telephone: 732-542-2800 **Fax:** 732-542-9312 **Metro area:** New York, NY **Human resources contact:** Charles Jannetti **Sales:** $59.2 million **Number of employees:** 231 **Number of employees for previous year:** 210 **Industry designation:** Medical services **Company type:** Public **Top competitors:** Orthofix International N.V.; OrthoLogic Corp.; Collagen Aesthetics, Inc.

Osteotech makes no bones about its business—well, yes, it does. It uses tissue from deceased human donors to make bone and tissue products for the orthopedic, neurological, oral/maxillofacial, dental, and general surgery markets in the US and Europe. Its Grafton product line offers surgeons a variety of processed bone for grafting procedures. Osteotech processes bone, ligaments, and tendons for transplantation, and provides ceramic and titanium plasma spray coating services to the orthopedic, dental, ear, nose, and throat implant markets. The American Red Cross and the Musculoskeletal Transplant Foundation account for nearly all of Osteotech's sales.

PacificHealth Laboratories, Inc.

1460 Rte. 9 North, Woodbridge, NJ 07095

Telephone: 732-636-6141 **Fax:** 732-636-7410 **Metro area:** New York, NY **Sales:** $1 million **Number of employees:** 10 **Number of employees for previous year:** 7 **Industry designation:** Vitamins & nutritional products **Company type:** Public **Top competitors:** SmithKline Beecham plc; Herbalife International, Inc.; Nature's Sunshine Products, Inc.

PacificHealth Laboratories' dietary supplements might have what it takes to get Mark McGwire's attention—especially since they're pitched by former grid star Joe Montana. Its ENDUROX supplements, which are based on the Chinese herb ciwujia, are touted as sports performance and recovery products. It is also developing an antidepressant based on St. John's wort; natural analgesics (licensed from Dermagenics); and a weight loss product. The firm sells through mass merchandisers; nutritional supplement and independent health food retailers; and health clubs. The Chinese Academy of Preventive Medicine contributes to product development. CEO Robert Portman owns about 25% of the company, which went public in 1997.

Palatin Technologies, Inc.

214 Carnegie Center, Ste. 100, Princeton, NJ 08540

Telephone: 609-520-1911 **Fax:** 609-452-0880 **Metro area:** Philadelphia, PA **Web site:** http://www.palatin.com **Sales:** $100,000 **Number of employees:** 23 **Number of employees for previous year:** 16 **Industry designation:** Medical products **Company type:** Public **Top competitors:** Syncor International Corporation; Nycomed Amersham plc; Mallinckrodt Inc.

Palatin Technologies fights the dragons of cancer. The development-stage company produces biopharmaceutical technologies for diagnostic imaging, cancer therapy, and drug development. Products include LeuTech, which is designed to provide quicker diagnoses of infections and occult abscesses in the body. PT-14 is under development as a treatment for sexual dysfunction. MIDAS technology prohibits peptides from changing shape, reducing their side effects when used as drugs. Palatin has an alliance with Japanese firm Nihon Medi-Physics to use MIDAS to develop radiopharmaceuticals.

PaperClip Software, Inc.

611 Route 46, Hasbrouck Heights, NJ 07604

Telephone: 201-329-6300 **Fax:** 201-329-6321 **Metro area:** New York, NY **Web site:** http://www.paperclip.com **Human resources contact:** Dennis Marchand **Sales:** $2 million **Number of employees:** 43 **Industry designation:** Computers—corporate, professional & financial software **Company type:** Public **Top competitors:** Documentum, Inc.; Universal Document Management Systems, Inc.; FileNET Corporation

Ever wish you could combine parts of your computer programs into one accessible database? Paperclip Software lets you do just that. Its document- and workflow-management software eases the clutter of paper by locating and extracting networked computer applications, documents, and images from a user's application screen to be clipped together in a database. Clients have the option of buying different software licenses—production, desktop, and viewer—that vary in price and offer access to certain product features. The company also offers integration services to its authorized resellers and corporate customers.

Papetti's Hygrade Egg Products, Inc.

One Papetti Plaza, Elizabeth, NJ 07206

Telephone: 908-354-4844 **Fax:** 908-354-8660 **Metro area:** New York, NY **Human resources contact:** Jack Novak **Number of employees:** 950 **Industry designation:** Food—meat products **Company type:** Subsidiary **Top competitors:** Cal-Maine Foods, Inc.; Cargill, Incorporated

Papetti's Hygrade Egg Products receives "hymarks" from parent company Michael Foods for being the part of the operation that brings in nearly two-thirds of the diversified food processor's sales. (Papetti's sister company in the egg division is M.G. Waldbaum.) Papetti's makes processed egg products: extended shelf-life eggs, dried eggs, and egg substitutes (Better'n Eggs, Table Ready, Chef's Eggs). Papetti's Hygrade Egg sells to food service, industrial, and retail markets. Michael Foods' 1997 acquisition of Papetti's (which breaks more than 16 million eggs per day) made it the US's largest egg producer and the world's largest egg processor. Stock-wielding Papetti family members still hold a 14% "stake in eggs."

Pharmaceutical Formulations, Inc.

460 Plainfield Ave., Edison, NJ 08818

Telephone: 732-985-7100 **Fax:** 732-819-3330 **Metro area:** New York, NY **Human resources contact:** Rick Perles **Sales:** $80.8 million **Number of employees:** 378 **Number of employees for previous year:** 348 **Industry designation:** Drugs—generic **Company type:** Public **Top competitors:** Pharmaceutical Resources, Inc.; Copley Pharmaceutical, Inc.; Duramed Pharmaceuticals, Inc.

Pharmaceutical Formulations probably has a few formulations in your medicine cabinet. The company makes more than 120 types of over-the-counter generic drugs: pain relievers, cold and allergy medications, and antacids. The majority of its products are packaged under customers' brand names, with less than 1% sold under the company's Health+Cross and Health Pharm trade names. The firm sells to more than 50 retailers, most of which are drugstores, supermarkets, and mass merchandisers. Its largest customers include Costco Wholesale (20% of sales) and Walgreens (17% of sales). Pharmaceutical Formulations is approximately two-thirds owned by ICC Industries, a chemical, plastics, and pharmaceutical products firm.

Pharmacopeia, Inc.

101 College Rd. East, Princeton, NJ 08540

Telephone: 609-452-3600 **Fax:** 609-452-3671 **Metro area:** Philadelphia, PA **Web site:** http://www.pcop.com **Human resources contact:** Kenneth McCarthy **Sales:** $92.2 million **Number of employees:** 546 **Number of employees for previous year:** 197 **Industry designation:** Medical services **Company type:** Public

Pharmacopeia uses small-molecule combinatorial chemistry to develop drug discovery programs. The company has used its proprietary tagging technology, Encoded Combinatorial Libraries on Polymeric Support (ECLiPS), to generate large libraries of more than 3.9 million diverse small molecules for pharmaceutical research. Its Molecular Simulations subsidiary makes molecular modeling and simulation software. The company's ability to produce diverse and targeted compound libraries accelerates the drug discovery process and increases drug production. Pharmacopeia has a number of collaborative agreements with such firms as Bayer, Novartis, Daiichi, Zeneca, Regeneron, and Schering-Plough.

Philipp Brothers Chemicals

One Parker Plaza, Ste. 1400, Fort Lee, NJ 07024

Telephone: 201-944-6020 **Fax:** 201-944-7916 **Metro area:** New York, NY **Web site:** http://www.philipp-brothers.com **Human resources contact:** Maria Engel **Sales:** $250 million (Est.) **Number of employees:** 500 **Industry designation:** Chemicals—specialty **Company type:** Private **Top competitors:** Elf Atochem; Novartis AG; E. I. du Pont de Nemours and Company

Philipp Brothers Chemicals and its subsidiaries are one big happy chemically dependent family. Among the companies' products are metals used for electroplating, povidone iodine for mouthwash, and fine chemicals potassium nitrate and sodium fluoride. Unit Phibro-Tech recycles copper, nickel, iron, ammonia, and other waste materials and is the US's largest hydrometallurgical waste recycler. Mineral Resource Technologies offers ash and mineral by-product managing services, and Agtrol International makes fungicides and plant growth regulators. Serving the agricultural, metalworking, and personal care products industries, about 38% of the companies' sales are outside the US. President Jack Bendheim owns the company.

Physician Computer Network, Inc.

1200 The American Rd., Morris Plains, NJ 07950

Telephone: 973-490-3100 **Fax:** 973-490-3103 **Metro area:** New York, NY **Web site:** http://www.pcn.com **Human resources contact:** Hank Halat **Sales:** $95.8 million **Number of employees:** 725 **Number of employees for previous year:** 640 **Industry designation:** Computers—corporate, professional & financial software **Company type:** Public **Top competitors:** InfoCure Corporation; McKesson HBOC, Inc.; IDX Systems Corporation

In the medical world, paperwork grows like a virus. Physician Computer Network makes software that battles that bug. PCN Health Network, and its add-on modules, automates routine tasks such as billing, scheduling, and documentation in doctors' offices. HealthPoint ACS, developed with pharmaceutical maker Glaxo Wellcome, is a clinical system that stores patient information, provides drug interaction alerts, and authorizes prescription refills. Physician Computer Network, a leading supplier of practice management systems, is facing a number of shareholder lawsuits for allegedly issuing false financial statements. Chairman Jeffry Picower owns 43% of the company.

Phytotech, Inc.

One Deer Park Dr., Ste. 1, Monmouth Junction, NJ 08852

Telephone: 732-438-0900 **Fax:** 732-438-1209 **Metro area:** New York, NY **Web site:** http://www.phytotech.com **Sales:** $461,000 (Est.) **Number of employees:** 18 **Industry designation:** Pollution control equipment & services **Company type:** Private **Top competitors:** E. I. du Pont de Nemours and Company; Monsanto Company; The Dow Chemical Company

As a development-stage biotechnology company, Phytotech really gets to the root of waste removal. Phytotech cultivates plants specially selected and engineered to absorb and store large amounts of heavy metals, such as lead and uranium, from water and soil at toxic waste sites. The company's plant-based remediation technology is intended to cost less than traditional technology and to be performed on-site to minimize environmental disturbance. The company has agreements for its initial commercial projects and is targeting its technology to metal smelters, paint makers, and owners of contaminated sites. Grants account for more than 80% of the firm's revenues.

Pure World, Inc.

376 Main St., Bedminster, NJ 07921

Telephone: 908-234-9220 **Fax:** 908-234-9355 **Other address:** PO Box 74, Bedminster, NJ 07921
Metro area: New York, NY **Web site:** http://www.pureworld.com **Human resources contact:** John
W. Galuchie Jr. **Sales:** $24 million **Number of employees:** 67 **Number of employees for
previous year:** 53 **Industry designation:** Vitamins & nutritional products **Company type:** Public

Pure World has its business down to an extract science. Through subsidiary Madis Botanicals, Pure World extracts
natural ingredients from plants, develops them, and sells them to the cosmetic, food and flavor, nutraceutical
(dietary supplement), and pharmaceutical industries. From more than 15,000 pounds of raw material each day,
Pure World makes solid, liquid, and powdered botanical extracts—including St. John's Wort, aloe, and coal tar
(used in anti-dandruff shampoo)—that customers use to create finished products for sale to consumers. Paul and
Natalie Koether own 65% of the company. Pure World also owns 35% of Gaia Herbs, a privately held maker of
natural products sold by retailers.

PVC Container Corporation

401 Industrial Way West, Eatontown, NJ 07724

Telephone: 732-542-0060 **Fax:** 732-542-7706 **Metro area:** New York, NY **Human resources
contact:** Diane Murphy **Sales:** $69.7 million **Number of employees:** 769 **Number of employees
for previous year:** 361 **Industry designation:** Chemicals—plastics **Company type:** Public **Top
competitors:** Silgan Holdings, Inc.; The Geon Company

If you are having trouble containing yourself, PVC Container would like to help out. The company makes plastic
bottles and containers from polyvinyl chloride (PVC) compounds, high-density polyethylene (HDPE), and
polyethylene terephthalate (PET) resins. The bottles are used to package foods, toiletries, cosmetics, and chemicals
for the home, garden, and lawn. In an effort to diversify, PVC has produced a line of plastic furniture, as well as
plastic moldings and electrical and electronic housings. The company also sells its PVC resins to competitors.
Kirtland Capital Partners II owns 59% of the company.

Response USA, Inc.

11-H Princess Rd., Lawrenceville, NJ 08648

Telephone: 609-896-4500 **Fax:** 609-896-3535 **Metro area:** Philadelphia, PA **Web site:** http://
www.responseusa.com **Human resources contact:** Brenda Brown **Sales:** $16.5 million **Number of
employees:** 332 **Number of employees for previous year:** 137 **Industry designation:**
Protection—safety equipment & services **Company type:** Public **Top competitors:** Protection One, Inc.;
Tyco International Ltd.; Lifeline Systems, Inc.

Response USA is waiting for your call. The company sells, installs, monitors, and maintains electronic security
systems, including access controls, burglar alarms, fire alarms, and sprinkler systems, for residences and businesses,
primarily in the northeastern US. Response USA also markets two types of personal emergency-response systems.
One, used mainly by elderly people and people with disabilities, allows them to send distress signals via portable
transmitters. The other, designed primarily for Alzheimer's patients, emits a continuous signal to alert monitors
when an individual leaves a safe area. Response USA serves about 77,000 subscribers.

R.F. Management Corp.

95 Madison Ave., Ste. 301, Morristown, NJ 07960

Telephone: 973-292-2833 **Fax:** 973-267-2412 **Metro area:** New York, NY **Human resources
contact:** Connie Boscia **Sales:** $10.7 million **Number of employees:** 6 **Number of employees
for previous year:** 5 **Industry designation:** Medical practice management **Company type:** Public
Top competitors: Medical Resources, Inc.; Primedex Health Systems, Inc.; UtiliMED, Inc.

R.F. Management gets a charge out of its business. The company manages freestanding diagnostic imaging centers,
offering such services as contract negotiation, patient billing, and equipment procurement. Its clients include centers
in New Jersey (through its subsidiaries Northern New Jersey Medical Management and Atrium Radiology) and
Pennsylvania. In addition to managing imaging centers, the company operates two mobile MRI units for health
care providers with which it signs daily, weekly, or monthly rental agreements. Through its Hamilton McGregor
International subsidiary, the company also constructs outpatient medical suites (more than 50% of sales).

Rheometric Scientific, Inc.

One Possumtown Rd., Piscataway, NJ 08854

Telephone: 732-560-8550 **Fax:** 732-560-7451 **Metro area:** New York, NY **Web site:** http://www.rheosci.com **Human resources contact:** Matthew Bilt **Sales:** $37.5 million **Number of employees:** 241 **Number of employees for previous year:** 230 **Industry designation:** Instruments—scientific **Company type:** Public **Top competitors:** NUMAR Corporation; Instron Corporation

Rheometric Scientific makes testing and analysis instruments and related software. Its rheometers, viscometers, thermal analyzers, and process-control monitors measure physical properties such as elasticity, thermal behavior, and viscosity in a variety of materials, including plastics, petrochemicals, cosmetics, and foods. The test systems (which control motion to within two-millionths of an inch) contain actuators that manipulate samples, controlled furnaces to heat the samples, sensors that measure these results, and microprocessors to analyze findings. Rheometric primarily targets manufacturers, research laboratories, and schools. Materials technology company Axess owns 77% of the company.

R-Tec Technologies, Inc.

61 Mallard Dr., PO Box 282, Allamuchy, NJ 07820

Telephone: 908-850-8593 **Fax:** 908-850-4670 **Metro area:** Allentown, PA **Number of employees:** 12 **Industry designation:** Chemicals—specialty **Company type:** Private **Top competitors:** USTMAN Technologies, Inc.; Arizona Instrument Corporation; Team, Inc.

R-Tec Technologies plans to raise the red flag on gas leaks. The firm's reactive paint changes from blue to fluorescent yellow when leaking gas passes through it. The paint is for application to caps, valves, and joints in pipe systems and in refrigeration and air-conditioning systems. R-Tec has three products ready for production: R-Tect 22 (Freon leaks), R-Tect CO2, and R-Tect Natural Gas. R-Tec has contracts with other businesses to manufacture its paints and market them to the chemical, natural gas, air-conditioning, and aviation industries. After the planned IPO, president Philip Lacqua and VPs Nancy Vitolo and Marc Scola each will reduce their share of the firm from one-third to about one-fourth.

Schering-Plough Corporation

One Giralda Farms, Madison, NJ 07940

Telephone: 973-822-7000 **Fax:** 973-822-7048 **Metro area:** New York, NY **Web site:** http://www.sch-plough.com **Human resources contact:** John Ryan **Sales:** $8.1 billion **Number of employees:** 25,100 **Number of employees for previous year:** 22,700 **Industry designation:** Drugs **Company type:** Public **Top competitors:** Rhone-Poulenc Rorer Inc.; Glaxo Wellcome plc; Amgen Inc.

Schering-Plough develops and markets prescription drugs, animal health products, over-the-counter (OTC) drugs, and foot care and sun care products. Its pharmaceuticals include Claritin (antihistamine), its top-selling product and the #1 antihistamine in the world, and genetically engineered products like Intron A, an antiviral/anticancer agent. Schering-Plough's well-known OTC brand names include Afrin (nasal sprays), Coppertone (sun care), and Dr. Scholl's (foot care). The company's animal care operations include a line of anti-infective drugs. Schering-Plough also makes Paas Easter-egg decorating kits.

Sigma Plastics Group

Page & Schuyler Ave., Bldg. #8, Lyndhurst, NJ 07071

Telephone: 201-933-6000 **Metro area:** New York, NY **Sales:** $765 million (Est.) **Number of employees:** 3,000 **Number of employees for previous year:** 2,500 **Industry designation:** Chemicals—plastics **Company type:** Private **Top competitors:** E. I. du Pont de Nemours and Company; Bemis Company, Inc.; Sealed Air Corporation

Although plastic film and sheet products by Sigma Plastics both shrink and stretch, the company itself prefers only to expand. Having grown through acquisitions, Sigma Plastics produces shrink and stretch film, converter-grade packaging, and merchandise, garment, grocery, and trash bags. The company manufactures its diverse range of plastic products at its plants in Canada, the UK, and the US. Sigma also owns Delta Plastics and Polystar Films. It holds a majority interest in Essex Plastics and 50% interest in Aargus Plastics. It has a joint venture with the UK's IPEL to sell shrink film in Europe.

Sybron Chemicals Inc.

Birmingham Rd., Birmingham, NJ 08011

Telephone: 609-893-1100 **Fax:** 609-894-8641 **Other address:** PO Box 66, Birmingham, NJ 08011 **Metro area:** Philadelphia, PA **Web site:** http://www.sybronchemicals.com **Human resources contact:** Stephen R. Adler **Sales:** $222.8 million **Number of employees:** 738 **Number of employees for previous year:** 722 **Industry designation:** Chemicals—specialty **Company type:** Public **Top competitors:** Henkel of America, Inc.; AMCOL International Corporation; Ciba Specialty Chemicals Corporation

Stone-washed denim, drain build-up removers, fabric dyes, microbes to clean up chemical spillls—they are all products made by Sybron Chemicals, an international chemical manufacturer. Its more than 1,600 chemical products encompass two key areas: textiles and environmental products. The largest segment (which accounts for about 70% of sales) provides wet-process chemical products for the textile industry, including the major textile centers of Europe. These products scour, bleach, print, dye and finish fabrics. The company's environmental products include chemicals for home and industrial water treatment; biochemicals for waste, contaminated soil, and groundwater treatment; and specialty polymers.

Synaptic Pharmaceuticals Corporation

215 College Rd., Paramus, NJ 07652

Telephone: 201-261-1331 **Fax:** 201-261-0623 **Metro area:** New York, NY **Sales:** $9.4 million **Number of employees:** 127 **Number of employees for previous year:** 125 **Industry designation:** Biomedical & genetic products **Company type:** Public **Top competitors:** Neurogen Corporation; Elan Corporation, plc; Interneuron Pharmaceuticals, Inc.

Synaptic Pharmaceuticals wants to make sure its signals cross just right. The biotech firm is developing a process to discover and clone human receptor genes associated with specific disorders. By developing drugs designed to work with certain receptors (which receive cell-to-cell signals within the human body), the company hopes to create treatments that are more effective and have fewer side effects than traditional drugs. It focuses on several disorders, including Alzheimer's, migraine headaches, anxiety, depression, enlargement of the prostate, and obesity. Synaptic is collaborating with several pharmaceutical firms, including Merck and Novartis.

Synetic, Inc.

669 River Dr., Elmwood Park, NJ 07407

Telephone: 201-703-3400 **Fax:** 201-703-3401 **Metro area:** New York, NY **Human resources contact:** Merla Horst **Sales:** $64.9 million **Number of employees:** 745 **Number of employees for previous year:** 711 **Industry designation:** Rubber & plastic products **Company type:** Public **Top competitors:** Medex, Inc.; Furon Company; Baxter International Inc.

When Cher needs bodywork done in the future she won't have to go to her plastic surgeon, she can go online. Synetic, a healthcare plastics and communications group, makes surgical plastics and provides medical information services. Its plastics division, Porex Technologies, makes plastics used mostly in medicine, including blood filters, pipette tips, and plastic surgery implant parts. The goal of the communications branch, Avicenna, is to use the Internet to provide a fast, secure, data delivery network for health care professionals in order to cut costs and improve patient care. Synetic has made key alliances with other medical networks to further its aim. Chairman Martin Wygood owns almost 30% of the company.

Triarco Industries, Inc.

400 Hamburg Tpke., Wayne, NJ 07470

Telephone: 973-942-5100 **Fax:** 973-942-8873 **Metro area:** New York, NY **Web site:** http://www.triarco.com **Human resources contact:** Tony Zagarino **Sales:** $42 million (Est.) **Number of employees:** 144 **Industry designation:** Vitamins & nutritional products **Company type:** Private **Top competitors:** Pure World, Inc.

The booming nutrition market is a natural for Triarco Industries. The company processes ingredients for nutritional supplements, selling more than 700 products, including herbs (more than half of sales), minerals, enzymes, and teas. Triarco sells these ingredients to nutritional supplement manufacturers that distribute their products through marketers such as Amway, mass-market stores, and specialty retailers such as General Nutrition Companies (its products use Triarco's first branded ingredients, Fingerprint Botanicals). The company also researches growing methods for raw materials. After Triarco's planned IPO, the family of CEO and founder Roger Rohde Sr. will own about 70% of the company.

Tutogen Medical Inc.

1719 Rte. 10, Parsippany, NJ 07054

Telephone: 973-359-8444 **Fax:** 973-359-8410 **Metro area:** New York, NY **Web site:** http://www.tutogen.com **Sales:** $8.9 million **Number of employees:** 92 **Number of employees for previous year:** 70 **Industry designation:** Biomedical & genetic products **Company type:** Public **Top competitors:** Baxter International Inc.; Johnson & Johnson; CryoLife, Inc.

Tutogen Medical brings recycling into a whole other realm. The company, formerly Biodynamics International, processes human donor tissue, or allografts, for neurological, ophthalmological, orthopedic, and plastic surgery, as well as animal tissue (xenografts) for several other procedures. The company's patented Tutoplast procedure is used to dehydrate and sterilize the tissue so it cannot transmit diseases such as AIDs or Creuzfeldt-Jakob Disease. A German subsidiary provides specialty surgical products and services in more than 40 countries. About two-thirds of Tutogen's sales are from outside the US. Renaissance Capital Partners owns more than 60% of the company.

Unigene Laboratories, Inc.

110 Little Falls Rd., Fairfield, NJ 07004

Telephone: 973-882-0860 **Fax:** 973-227-6088 **Metro area:** New York, NY **Web site:** http://www.unigene.com **Human resources contact:** William Steinhauer **Sales:** $3 million **Number of employees:** 72 **Number of employees for previous year:** 69 **Industry designation:** Biomedical & genetic products **Company type:** Public **Top competitors:** Novo Nordisk A/S; Sanofi; Eli Lilly and Company

Unigene Laboratories is a development-stage pharmaceutical company that focuses on the manufacture and delivery of products based on the hormone calcitonin as a treatment for osteoporosis. The company is seeking US and European approval for its FORTICAL injectable calcitonin. Parke-Davis holds the license for the firm's oral calcitonin technology. Unigene Laboratories has a joint venture with Qingdao General Pharmaceutical for the production and marketing of injectable and nasal calcitonin in China. The firm also has collaborative research programs with Rutgers and Yale universities.

Vestcom International, Inc.

1100 Valley Brook Ave., Lyndhurst, NJ 07071

Telephone: 201-935-7666 **Fax:** 201-935-9987 **Metro area:** New York, NY **Web site:** http://www.vestcomintl.com **Sales:** $108.7 million **Number of employees:** 1,070 **Number of employees for previous year:** 1,015 **Industry designation:** Computers—peripheral equipment **Company type:** Public

Vestcom International provides computer output and document management services to about 1,400 customers from 23 facilities in 14 US states and in Quebec and Ontario. The company, which produces and distributes time-sensitive documents (invoices, bills, and statements) on paper, compact disc, microfiche, and microfilm, plans to offer document distribution through the Internet. Vestcom also provides computer-generated labels for retail stores and demand publishing of frequently revised publications (user manuals, technical materials). Vestcom ships materials on daily, weekly, monthly, or quarterly bases. Customers include financial, telecommunications, pharmaceutical, publishing, and manufacturing companies.

Vikonics, Inc.

370 North St., Teterboro, NJ 07608

Telephone: 201-641-8077 **Fax:** 201-641-7728 **Metro area:** New York, NY **Sales:** $1.6 million **Number of employees:** 14 **Industry designation:** Protection—safety equipment & services **Company type:** Public **Top competitors:** STRATESEC, Inc.; Delta Protection SA

Ever wonder: While the army is guarding us, who's guarding the army? Vikonics sells computer-based security systems to the US Army, the Air Force, and even the Marines. Fort Meade accounts for 33% of the company's sales, the US Capitol for 20%. Vikonics' customizable systems combine modular software and hardware components, including intrusion-detection systems, entry- and access-control devices, and alarm sensor interfaces. The systems can be monitored remotely or locally. In addition to government agencies, Vikonics sells to commercial customers such as American Express, defense contractors such as Raytheon, and dealers. About 10% of its sales are to international customers.

Vital Signs, Inc.

20 Campus Rd., Totowa, NJ 07512

Telephone: 973-790-1330 **Fax:** 973-790-3307 **Metro area:** New York, NY **Web site:** http://www.vital-signs.com **Human resources contact:** Elizabeth Greenberg **Sales:** $126.4 million **Number of employees:** 1,052 **Number of employees for previous year:** 1,037 **Industry designation:** Medical & dental supplies **Company type:** Public **Top competitors:** Ballard Medical Products; Smiths Industries plc; Baxter International Inc.

Vital Signs makes disposable medical products for in during anesthesia (nearly half of sales), critical care, and respiratory care functions. Disposable medical products have gained popularity because of their cost-effectiveness and reduced risk of infection. Vital Signs' anesthesia products include face masks, laryngoscopes, and breathing circuits. Respiratory products from the company include blood-pressure cuffs, humidifiers, and suction devices; Vital Signs also makes CPR mannequins for emergency training. About 12% of the company's sales are to foreign customers. Founder and CEO Terence Wall and his family own more than 50% of Vital Signs.

Warner-Lambert Company

201 Tabor Rd., Morris Plains, NJ 07950

Telephone: 973-540-2000 **Fax:** 973-540-3761 **Metro area:** New York, NY **Web site:** http://www.warner-lambert.com **Human resources contact:** Raymond M. Fino **Sales:** $10.2 billion **Number of employees:** 41,000 **Number of employees for previous year:** 40,000 **Industry designation:** Drugs **Company type:** Public **Top competitors:** Merck & Co., Inc.; The Gillette Company; Bristol-Myers Squibb Company

Warner-Lambert brings a breath of fresh air: Listerine, Clorets, and Certs are three of its best-known products. Other consumer products include the Zantac 75 heartburn remedy, topical antibiotic Neosporin, Sudafed cold remedies, and Efferdent denture-cleaning products. It also makes Schick razors and Trident, Dentyne, and Chiclets chewing gum. Warner-Lambert's Parke-Davis and Goedecke pharmaceuticals divisions make analgesics, anesthetics, and hemostatic agents as well as diabetes (Rezulin) and cholesterol treatments (including best-seller Lipitor). The company, which gets almost half of sales from outside the US, has operations in 34 countries. It is looking to build its pipeline with the planned purchase of Agouron.

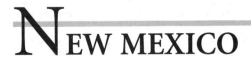

NEW MEXICO

Presbyterian Healthcare Services

5901 Harper Dr. NE, Albuquerque, NM 87109

Telephone: 505-923-5678 **Fax:** 505-923-5277 **Metro area:** Albuquerque, NM **Web site:** http://www.phs.org/ **Human resources contact:** Rita Arthur **Sales:** $402.4 million **Number of employees:** 7,400 **Industry designation:** Hospitals **Company type:** Not-for-profit **Top competitors:** Blue Cross and Blue Shield of Texas Inc.; Foundation Health Systems, Inc.; Catholic Health Initiatives

Presbyterian Healthcare Services (PHS) cares for more than 400,000 New Mexicans. It operates the largest HMO in New Mexico, with over 160,000 enrolled. Its individual health plans for individuals, spouses, and dependents cover everything from preventive to emergency care. PHS hospitals offer small group plans for companies under 50 employees and group health plans with HMO and point-of-service options. Enrollees include the State of New Mexico, University of New Mexico, and Intel. Its network of 13 hospitals, six community health centers, and four clinics stretches from Cimarron to Socorro.

Sun Healthcare Group, Inc.

101 Sun Ave. NE, Albuquerque, NM 87109

Telephone: 505-821-3355 **Fax:** 505-858-4735 **Metro area:** Albuquerque, NM **Web site:** http://www.sunh.com **Human resources contact:** Maureen Frank **Sales:** $2 billion **Number of employees:** 68,900 **Number of employees for previous year:** 35,900 **Industry designation:** Nursing homes **Company type:** Public **Top competitors:** Vencor, Inc.; Beverly Enterprises, Inc.; NovaCare, Inc.

Retirees don't have to move to the coast to find a place in the sun. Sun Healthcare Group provides long-term, subacute, and related health care services through about 580 facilities in Australia, Germany, Spain, the UK, and the US. The company's Sundance Rehabilitation provides physical, occupational, and speech therapies, and its SunCare unit offers respiratory therapy. CareerStaff Unlimited provides temporary therapy staffing. Sun Healthcare owns pharmacies serving company-operated and nonaffiliated facilities in the US and the UK and distributes disposable medical products. About 55% of the acquisitive company's revenues come from Medicare and Medicaid reimbursements.

Thermo BioAnalysis Corporation

504 Airport Rd., Santa Fe, NM 87504

Telephone: 508-528-0551 **Fax:** 505-473-9221 **Metro area:** Santa Fe, NM **Web site:** http://www.thermo.com/subsid/tba.html **Human resources contact:** Mary Wanda **Sales:** $227.1 million **Number of employees:** 1,700 **Number of employees for previous year:** 979 **Industry designation:** Medical instruments **Company type:** Public **Parent company:** Thermo Instrument Systems Inc. **Top competitors:** The Perkin-Elmer Corporation; Hewlett-Packard Company; Waters Instruments, Inc.

Thermo BioAnalysis makes scientific testing instruments and supplies as well as software that helps organize and analyze testing data, particularly chromatography data. The company's instruments include mass spectrometers, which are used to identify unknown substances; DNA amplifiers and hybridization ovens, used to identify DNA sequences; and capillary electrophoresis equipment, used in DNA fingerprinting. In addition, the company makes equipment that detects and measures radiation levels and lab equipment such as pipettes and titer plates. The company sells directly and through distributors throughout the world. High-tech hothouse Thermo Electron owns about 85% of the company.

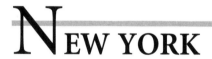

NEW YORK

Albany Molecular Research, Inc.

21 Corporate Circle, Albany, NY 12203

Telephone: 518-464-0279 **Fax:** 518-464-0289 **Metro area:** Albany, NY **Web site:** http://www.albmolecular.com **Human resources contact:** James J. Grates **Sales:** $8.8 million **Number of employees:** 122 **Industry designation:** Drugs **Company type:** Public

Albany Molecular Research provides contract chemistry research and development services to pharmaceutical firms. Its services (including medicinal chemistry, chemical development, analytical chemistry, and small-scale manufacturing) have traditionally been provided by in-house chemistry divisions at pharmaceutical companies, but Albany Molecular Research believes drugmakers and biotechnology firms will be eager to use outsourcing to reduce the time and cost involved in drug development. The company also conducts some proprietary research (it receives royalties from Hoechst Marion Roussel for the antihistamine Allegra). CEO Thomas D'Ambra owns about 35% of the company.

Alloy Online, Inc.

115 W. 30th St., #201, New York, NY 10001

Telephone: 212-244-4307 **Fax:** 212-244-4311 **Metro area:** New York, NY **Web site:** http://www.alloyonline.com **Sales:** $10.2 million (Est.) **Number of employees:** 25 **Industry designation:** Computers—online services **Company type:** Private **Top competitors:** iTurf Inc.; America Online, Inc.; GeoCities

Ready to cash in on the baggy pants generation, Alloy Online targets Generation Y Web surfers with content and e-commerce. The company's Web site is the hip destination for some 400,000 registered users who participate in its online community, which offers such features as free e-mail, homepages, chat rooms, and instant messaging. The site also provides content aimed at the under-25 set, including music news, video Webcasts, celebrity interviews, and even homework assistance. Alloy's online store sells clothing, beauty products, music, and magazine subscriptions. Although most of its revenue comes from merchandise sales, the company plans to increase its advertising and sponsorship income.

AMBI Inc.

4 Manhattanville Rd., Purchase, NY 10577

Telephone: 914-701-4500 **Fax:** 914-696-0860 **Metro area:** New York, NY **Web site:** http://www.ambiinc.com **Human resources contact:** Nancy Hutter **Sales:** $20.8 million **Number of employees:** 40 **Number of employees for previous year:** 36 **Industry designation:** Vitamins & nutritional products **Company type:** Public **Top competitors:** Mannatech, Incorporated; Balchem Corporation; PowerBar, Inc.

AMBI wants to wipe out fat and germs. Its Nutrition 21 subsidiary sells bulk form dietary products, including weight-loss supplement Chromax (chromium picolinate), Selenomax (selenium), Zinmax (zinc picolinate), and Magnemax (manganese picolinate). Customers include Leiner Health Products, TwinLabs, and General Nutrition Centers. AMBI sells salt alternative Cardia in the US through an alliance with American Home Products. AMBI retail products include Lite Bites nutrition bars, sold through a catalog, QVC home-shopping programs, and an Internet site. AMBI is also developing two drugs that treat various infections. Burns Philp & Company, an Australian food manufacturer and marketer, owns 30% of AMBI.

American Biogenetic Sciences, Inc.

1375 Akron St., Copiague, NY 11726

Telephone: 516-789-2600 **Fax:** 516-789-1661 **Metro area:** New York, NY **Web site:** http://www.mabxa.com **Sales:** $200,000 **Number of employees:** 43 **Number of employees for previous year:** 35 **Industry designation:** Biomedical & genetic products **Company type:** Public

American Biogenetic Sciences engages in research and development related to cardiovascular and neurobiology products. The company conducts research in China, Israel, the US, and Europe at its own facilities and through collaborations with institutions such as the Russian Academy of Medical Sciences. American Biogenetic Sciences develops in vivo and in vitro diagnostic tests that use monoclonal antibodies generated through an antigen-free mouse colony. The company is also developing a blood test for detecting Alzheimer's disease and chemical compounds to stop the progression of strokes, Alzheimer's, Parkinson's disease, amyotrophic lateral sclerosis, and other conditions.

American Bio Medica Corporation

300 Fairview Ave., Hudson, NY 12534

Telephone: 518-822-8882 **Fax:** 518-822-0391 **Metro area:** Poughkeepsie, NY **Web site:** http://www.americanbiomedica.com **Human resources contact:** Terri Drobner **Sales:** $2.2 million **Number of employees:** 50 **Number of employees for previous year:** 24 **Industry designation:** Medical products **Company type:** Public **Top competitors:** Biosite Diagnostics Incorporated; Roche Holding Ltd; MEDTOX Scientific, Inc.

Thanks to American Bio Medica's drug-testing kits, the difference between one line or two could mean no job for you. The company's Rapid Drug Screen products indicate the presence of such illegal substances as PCP, marijuana, cocaine, amphetamines, and opiates in a urine sample within minutes. Used by company drug-testing programs, law enforcement agencies, hospitals, and other institutions, the tests offer two, five, and eight panel options (each panel tests for different substances). The company's Rapid One is a line of drug-specific tests that detect one substance only. Manufactured at the company's facilities in New York, the tests are sold worldwide primarily to distributors, including Abbott Laboratories.

American International Petroleum Corporation

444 Madison Ave., New York, NY 10022

Telephone: 212-688-3333 **Fax:** 212-688-6657 **Metro area:** New York, NY **Web site:** http://www.aipcorp.com **Human resources contact:** Michael Dodge **Sales:** $800,000 **Number of employees:** 76 **Number of employees for previous year:** 73 **Industry designation:** Oil & gas—exploration & production **Company type:** Public

American International Petroleum is an independent oil and gas exploration and production company. Subsidiary American International Refinery, based in Lake Charles, Louisiana, refines crude extracted from Mexico and Venezuela to produce asphalt, which it sells to the truck-rack paving market in Louisiana, Mississippi, and Texas. Other products include vacuum-gas oil, naphtha, and jet, diesel, and industrial fuel, which it is preparing to sell in Alabama, Florida, and Georgia. Another subsidiary, American International Petroleum Kazakhstan, explores for oil and gas in a 20,000-square-kilometer region in Kazakhstan.

American Medical Alert Corp.

3265 Lawson Blvd., Oceanside, NY 11572

Telephone: 516-536-5850 **Fax:** 516-536-5276 **Metro area:** New York, NY **Web site:** http://www.amacalert.com **Human resources contact:** Corey M. Aronin **Sales:** $8.3 million **Number of employees:** 103 **Number of employees for previous year:** 82 **Industry designation:** Computers—services **Company type:** Public **Top competitors:** Lifeline Systems, Inc.; Humana Inc.; Response USA, Inc.

It's kind of like having a guardian angel hovering around, but without the wings. With personal emergency response systems from American Medical Alert, elderly people and people with disabilities, or those ill or in distress can speak to an emergency medical dispatcher at a specially equipped 24-hour monitoring center, who will then send help or contact relatives. The company's Voice of Help System comes in wall-mounted or stand-alone models and is activated by the push of a button on the unit or on a portable device. It can also monitor fire and burglar alarms. The company sells the systems to individuals, hospitals, and retirement communities. Monitoring, the bulk of sales, is provided on a monthly fee basis.

Ampacet Corporation

660 White Plains Rd., Tarrytown, NY 10591

Telephone: 914-631-6600 **Fax:** 914-631-7197 **Metro area:** New York, NY **Web site:** http://www.ampacet.com **Human resources contact:** Bob Oakes **Sales:** $415 million (Est.) **Number of employees:** 830 **Number of employees for previous year:** 750 **Industry designation:** Chemicals—specialty **Company type:** Private **Top competitors:** NL Industries, Inc.; Hitox Corporation of America; E. I. du Pont de Nemours and Company

Ampacet helps manufacturers of plastic products show their true hues with its custom color and additive concentrates. Using polyethylene, polypropylene, polystyrene, polyamide, and polyester resins, Ampacet makes compounds and concentrates that allow plastics manufacturers to produce consistent colors and chemical characteristics for their extruded and molded products. The company's additives are used in trash bags, food packaging, diaper liners, and other plastic products. Founded in 1937, Ampacet operates manufacturing plants in Belgium, Canada, Italy, and the US and maintains warehouses in Belgium, Canada, Denmark, France, Germany, Italy, Singapore, and the UK. CEO Norman E. Alexander owns the firm.

AppliedTheory Corporation

40 Cutter Mill Rd., Ste. 405, Great Neck, NY 11021

Telephone: 516-466-8422 **Fax:** 516-466-8650 **Metro area:** New York, NY **Web site:** http://www.appliedtheory.com **Human resources contact:** Debbie Newman **Sales:** $22.6 million (Est.) **Number of employees:** 151 **Industry designation:** Computers—online services **Company type:** Private **Top competitors:** UUNET WorldCom; PSINet Inc.; Concentric Network Corporation

Internet service provider (ISP) AppliedTheory has long brought theory into practice. The ISP provides Internet connectivity, including high-speed dedicated Internet access and virtual private networks; Web-enabled database integration, including site design; and Web hosting. Established in 1985 as NYSERNet to bring New York universities onto the Net, AppliedTheory has about 650 customers, mainly New York public institutions and midsized businesses (and midsized departments of large corporations). Long-distance carrier IXC owns 34% of AppliedTheory, and Grumman Hill Investments another 17%. IXC is building a coast-to-coast network, over which AppliedTheory will reach Internet customers outside New York.

ATC Group Services Inc.

104 E. 25th St., 10th Fl., New York, NY 10010

Telephone: 212-353-8280 **Fax:** 212-353-8306 **Metro area:** New York, NY **Web site:** http://www.atc-enviro.com **Sales:** $119.4 million (Est.) **Number of employees:** 2,043 **Number of employees for previous year:** 1,630 **Industry designation:** Pollution control equipment & services **Company type:** Private **Top competitors:** GZA GeoEnvironmental Technologies, Inc.; Ecology and Environment, Inc.; Radian International LLC

ATC Group Services clears the air. The firm provides environmental consulting, testing, and remediation services to industrial, municipal, and government clients. With offices in 35 states, the firm provides environmental management services such as asbestos testing, soil and groundwater assessment, and risk assessment. The firm offers environmental management software that tracks environmental maintenance schedules and makes risk management assessments. Subsidiary Environmental Warranty sells environmental insurance products. In 1998 ATC Group Services founder Morry Rubin was bought out and ATC was taken private by managers and investment firm Weiss, Peck & Green, which holds more than two-thirds of the stock.

Balchem Corporation

2007 Rte. 284, Slate Hill, NY 10973

Telephone: 914-355-5300 **Fax:** 914-355-6314 **Other address:** PO Box 175, Slate Hill, NY 10973 **Metro area:** New York, NY **Web site:** http://www.balchem.net **Human resources contact:** Lucy Klaus **Sales:** $28.7 million **Number of employees:** 131 **Number of employees for previous year:** 116 **Industry designation:** Chemicals—specialty **Company type:** Public **Top competitors:** Clariant Ltd.; Monsanto Company; Praxair, Inc.

Balchem manufactures high-performance encapsulated ingredients in the food, feed, and aquaculture markets and repackages specialty gases for use in medical sterilization. The company's CAP-SHURE product line includes food encapsulates such as vitamin C, leavening agents, fermentation aids, iron, and salt. Balchem's encapsulate technology prevents food products from reacting prematurely with their environments or from degrading during processing and storage. The company also makes blowing and nucleating agents for the foamed-plastic industry under the Safoam brand name. Balchem's manufacturing facilities are located in Slate Hill, New York, and Green Pond, South Carolina.

Barr Laboratories, Inc.

2 Quaker Rd., Pomona, NY 10970

Telephone: 914-362-1100 **Fax:** 914-362-2774 **Other address:** PO Box 2900, Pomona, NY 10970 **Metro area:** New York, NY **Web site:** http://www.barrlabs.com **Human resources contact:** Catherine F. Higgins **Sales:** $377.3 million **Number of employees:** 557 **Number of employees for previous year:** 467 **Industry designation:** Drugs—generic **Company type:** Public **Top competitors:** Glaxo Wellcome plc; Merck & Co., Inc.; Novartis AG

Barr Laboratories thinks brands are for cattle. The company makes and distributes generic prescription drugs. Products include more than 70 drugs for cancer, hypertension, heart disease, and infections, as well as anxiety, depression, and similar disorders. Barr distributes sodium warfarin, the generic equivalent of DuPont's Coumadin anticoagulant, and a generic version of the patented breast cancer drug Nolvadex (tamoxifen citrate; both the branded and generic versions are made by Zeneca Pharmaceuticals). It also produces generic equivalents of such drugs as Pediazole, Percocet, and Valium. Former chairman Bernard Sherman owns about 42% of the company.

Bausch & Lomb Incorporated

One Bausch & Lomb Place, Rochester, NY 14604

Telephone: 716-338-6000 **Fax:** 716-338-6007 **Metro area:** Rochester, NY **Web site:** http://www.bausch.com **Human resources contact:** Daryl M. Dickson **Sales:** $2.4 billion **Number of employees:** 15,000 **Number of employees for previous year:** 13,000 **Industry designation:** Medical products **Company type:** Public **Top competitors:** Luxottica Group S.p.A.; Johnson & Johnson; Allergan, Inc.

Bausch & Lomb is a leading maker of contact lenses, lens care solutions (ReNu and Sensitive Eyes brands), and eyedrops. It also makes sunglasses, including Ray-Ban, Killer Loop, and Liz Claiborne, and Miracle-Ear hearing aids. The company's pharmaceuticals unit makes ophthalmic products and other prescription and over-the-counter medications, including Minoxidil hair-regrowth solutions. The Charles River Laboratories unit breeds genetically unique strains of animals used in drug research and provides biomedical products and services. Bausch & Lomb is moving out of diversified health care markets and the sunglasses business to focus on its core eye care products.

Biospecifics Technologies Corp.

35 Wilbur St., Lynbrook, NY 11563

Telephone: 516-593-7000 **Fax:** 516-593-7039 **Metro area:** New York, NY **Sales:** $5.8 million **Number of employees:** 38 **Number of employees for previous year:** 35 **Industry designation:** Drugs **Company type:** Public **Top competitors:** Warner-Lambert Company; Genzyme Corporation; Knoll AG

Biospecifics Technologies develops pharmaceutical products and licenses them to other companies for sale. Its main product, Collagenase ABC, is an enzyme that dissolves connective tissue, and treats second- and third-degree burns and skin ulcers. Biospecifics is also testing the product to treat glaucoma and skin deformities. Most sales stem from a distribution pact with BASF subsidiary Knoll Pharmaceutical, which sells collagenase products in the US and Canada (90% of all sales); products are also marketed in South America and Europe. Nucleolysin, a collagenase product used to treat herniated spinal disks, is sold in the Netherlands Antilles. Chairman and president Edwin Wegman owns half of the company.

Box Hill Systems Corp.

161 Avenue of the Americas, New York, NY 10013

Telephone: 212-989-4455 **Fax:** 212-989-6817 **Metro area:** New York, NY **Web site:** http://www.boxhill.com **Human resources contact:** Sheryl Brinker **Sales:** $72.5 million **Number of employees:** 162 **Number of employees for previous year:** 155 **Industry designation:** Computers—peripheral equipment **Company type:** Public **Top competitors:** MTI Technology Corporation; Network Appliance, Inc.; Datalink Corporation

Box Hill Systems is watching your back. The company makes data storage and backup products primarily for UNIX systems and offers related services. Its storage products include disk arrays (for numerous disk drives), RAID (redundant array of independent disks), and Fibre Box storage systems. Backup products include tape drives, enterprise-wide backup software, and media changers, such as the Magna Box and the Echo Box. Box Hill targets data-intensive industries; financial and telecommunications firms account for about 40% of sales. Products are distributed in Europe, the Pacific Rim, South America, and the US. Chairman and CTO Benjamin Monderer, EVP Carol Turchin, and VP Mark Mays own 55% of Box Hill.

Bridge Information Systems, Inc.

3 World Financial Center, 27th Fl., New York, NY 10285

Telephone: 212-372-7100 **Fax:** 212-372-7148 **Metro area:** New York, NY **Web site:** http://www.bridge.com **Human resources contact:** Julie Brown **Sales:** $1.3 billion (Est.) **Number of employees:** 4,500 **Number of employees for previous year:** 1,200 **Industry designation:** Computers—online services **Company type:** Private **Top competitors:** The Thomson Corporation; Bloomberg L.P.; Reuters Group PLC

Bridge Information Systems is the #2 provider (behind Reuters) of financial information to the global financial services community. Bridge's owner, Welsh, Carson, Anderson & Stowe, has spent over $1 billion to assemble a new financial information company. Bridge's 1998 acquisition of rival Dow Jones' real-time service, which is now Bridge's Telerate division, nearly tripled its size. Bridge also acquired ADP's installed base of 80,000 terminals in a deal that gave ADP a minority stake in Bridge. The company's use of standard PCs, rather than proprietary systems, translates to lower costs, which allow Bridge to compete on price and expand beyond the traditional financial services markets.

Bristol-Myers Squibb Company

345 Park Ave., New York, NY 10154

Telephone: 212-546-4000 **Fax:** 212-546-4020 **Metro area:** New York, NY **Web site:** http://www.bms.com **Human resources contact:** Charles G. Tharp **Sales:** $18.3 billion **Number of employees:** 53,600 **Number of employees for previous year:** 51,200 **Industry designation:** Drugs **Company type:** Public **Top competitors:** Rhone-Poulenc Rorer Inc.; Glaxo Wellcome plc; Merck & Co., Inc.

Bristol-Myers Squibb is perhaps best known to the public as a stalwart of the personal care industry. Among its market-leading products are Clairol and Excedrin, but more than half its sales come from pharmaceuticals. The company focuses its efforts on cardiovascular treatments and related products such as cholesterol-reduction drugs and anticancer and anti-infective drugs. Its efforts in this field are increasingly based on technologies developed through cooperative research agreements. Bristol-Myers Squibb also makes baby formula, wound-treatment, and orthopedic products.

Buffalo Bills, Inc.

One Bills Dr., Orchard Park, NY 14127

Telephone: 716-648-1800 **Fax:** 716-649-6446 **Metro area:** Buffalo, NY **Web site:** http://www.nfl.com/bills **Sales:** $78.7 million (Est.) **Number of employees:** 125 **Number of employees for previous year:** 100 **Industry designation:** Leisure & recreational services **Company type:** Private **Top competitors:** New York Jets Football Club, Inc.; New England Patriots; Miami Dolphins Limited

The Buffalo Bills have a notorious NFL tradition: a good team that always finds a way to lose. The Bills appeared in the Super Bowl a record four consecutive seasons (1991 through 1994) and lost every time. It first hit the gridiron in 1960 as part of the American Football League (the AFL merged with the NFL in the late 1960s). The Bills are pinning their future Super Bowl hopes on new head coach Wade Phillips (the team's former defensive coordinator) and quarterback Doug Flutie (a Heisman Trophy winner and six-time Canadian Football League Most Outstanding Player). Buffalo plays in Orchard Park, New York at Ralph Wilson Stadium, named for the Detroit businessman who has owned the team since its inception.

Cadus Pharmaceutical Corporation

777 Old Saw Mill River Rd., Tarrytown, NY 10591

Telephone: 914-467-6200 **Fax:** 914-345-3565 **Metro area:** New York, NY **Web site:** http://www.cadus.com **Human resources contact:** Suzanne Wakamoto **Sales:** $12.6 million **Number of employees:** 108 **Number of employees for previous year:** 103 **Industry designation:** Drugs **Company type:** Public

Cadus Pharmaceutical develops drugs to treat diseases caused by signal malfunctions between and within human cells. The firm uses genetically engineered yeast cells similar to human genes to study gene functions and search for applicable drugs. It is developing small-molecule drugs for asthma and a type of lung cancer and is also collaborating with SmithKline Beecham, Bristol-Myers Squibb, and Solvay Pharmaceuticals to find drugs to treat cardiovascular disease, central nervous system disorders, gastrointestinal problems, and other ailments. With the Massachusetts Institute of Technology, the firm is developing the Living Chip, a research-results database. Investor Carl Icahn owns 27% of the firm.

Carlisle Companies Incorporated

250 S. Clinton St., Ste. 201, Syracuse, NY 13202

Telephone: 315-474-2500 **Fax:** 315-474-2008 **Metro area:** Syracuse, NY **Web site:** http://www.carlisle.com **Human resources contact:** John Barsanti Jr. **Sales:** $1.5 billion **Number of employees:** 9,500 **Number of employees for previous year:** 8,500 **Industry designation:** Rubber & plastic products **Company type:** Public **Top competitors:** Wabash National Corporation; Pirelli S.p.A.; Meritor Automotive, Inc.

Carlisle Companies grows its diversified manufacturing businesses the old fashioned way—cash flow. The firm focuses on construction materials (rubber, plastic, and FleeceBack sheeting), industrial components (small tires and wheels), automotive components (rubber and plastic components), and plastic foodservice equipment (dishes and tableware), and it holds each operation to one key measure—the ability to generate cash. Carlisle uses the cash to fund new products and acquisitions. The company sells to manufacturers and suppliers, with the aftermarket accounting for 40% of company sales. Carlisle has operations in the US, Canada, and Europe. The US accounts for 90% of sales.

Catholic Healthcare Network

155 E. 56th St., 2nd Fl., New York, NY 10022

Telephone: 212-752-7300 **Fax:** 212-752-7547 **Metro area:** New York, NY **Web site:** http://www.chcn.org **Human resources contact:** Exzera Hope **Sales:** $2 billion **Industry designation:** Hospitals **Company type:** Not-for-profit **Top competitors:** Eastern Mercy Health System; North Shore-Long Island Jewish Health System; New York City Health and Hospitals Corporation

While it may not have the high profile of the late Mother Teresa, New York's Catholic Healthcare Network is nonetheless dedicated to providing high-quality health care (rooted in the values of the Catholic Church) to people who need it, regardless of their income or status. The network includes more than 45 hospitals, nursing homes, and affiliated health care providers (such as children's homes and medical centers). Catholic Healthcare Network is co-sponsored by the Archdiocese of New York and the Sisters of Charity of Saint Vincent de Paul of New York.

Cognizant Technology Solutions Corporation

1700 Broadway, 26th Fl., New York, NY 10019

Telephone: 212-887-2385 **Fax:** 212-887-2450 **Metro area:** New York, NY **Web site:** http://www.dbss.com **Human resources contact:** Mansoor Ahmed **Sales:** $58.6 million **Number of employees:** 1,560 **Number of employees for previous year:** 240 **Industry designation:** Computers—services **Company type:** Public **Top competitors:** Mastech Corporation; Complete Business Solutions, Inc.

Cognizant Technology Solutions (CTS) is mindful of your technology systems. The company provides services primarily to large companies that include software development, application management, computer date corrections (which together generate about 90% of sales), and currency conversion. CTS has recruited and trained about 1,000 programmers who work at six software development centers in India. The company also has offices in Boston, Chicago, London, Toronto, and Washington, DC. Nearly 60% of its sales come from Dun & Bradstreet's current or former divisions, a percentage Cognizant is working to reduce. Cognizant Corporation controls 95% of the voting power of CTS.

Command Security Corporation

Lexington Park, Lagrangeville, NY 12540

Telephone: 914-454-3703 **Fax:** 914-454-0075 **Other address:** PO Box 340, Lagrangeville, NY 12540 **Metro area:** Poughkeepsie, NY **Web site:** http://www.cscny.com **Human resources contact:** Debra M. Miller **Sales:** $53.2 million **Number of employees:** 3,833 **Number of employees for previous year:** 3,734 **Industry designation:** Protection—safety equipment & services **Company type:** Public **Top competitors:** Borg-Warner Security Corporation; Pinkerton's, Inc.; Wackenhut Corporation

Command Security's watchdogs wear uniforms and walk on two legs. The firm's more than 3,700 hourly guards perform security tasks for commercial, industrial, aviation, and governmental clients. With 18 offices in California, Connecticut, Florida, Georgia, Illinois, New Jersey, New York, and Pennsylvania, the company provides armed and unarmed personal protection, surveillance, airport security, and crowd control (Command Security kept rock fans in line at Woodstock '94). Other services include private investigating, vehicular and foot patrolling, airline passenger screening, and plant security. Command Security provides contract billing, collection, and payroll services for other security companies.

Commodore Applied Technologies, Inc.

150 E. 58th St., Ste. 3400, New York, NY 10155

Telephone: 212-308-5800 **Fax:** 212-753-0731 **Metro area:** New York, NY **Web site:** http://www.commodore.com **Human resources contact:** Melissa Berkowitz **Sales:** $19.5 million **Number of employees:** 169 **Number of employees for previous year:** 140 **Industry designation:** Pollution control equipment & services **Company type:** Public **Top competitors:** Browning-Ferris Industries, Inc.; Raytheon Company; Lockheed Martin Corporation

Commodore Applied Technologies uses technology to clean up the mess the modern world has made of the environment. The firm markets a patented solvated electron technology (SET) that cleans soils and other materials by destroying toxic contaminants. Through a joint venture with an Allegheny Teledyne subsidiary, the company is adapting this technology for the safe destruction of chemical weapon materials. Commodore Applied Technologies has also developed a process for separating metals and biochemicals from wastewater (through subsidiary Commodore Separation Technologies). Director Bentley Blum controls more than 40% of the stock of the company, which markets primarily to government and industry in the US.

Community Care Services, Inc.

18 Sargent Place, Mount Vernon, NY 10550

Telephone: 914-665-9050 **Fax:** 914-665-9063 **Metro area:** New York, NY **Human resources contact:** Colleen Gaglio **Sales:** $19.1 million **Number of employees:** 128 **Number of employees for previous year:** 65 **Industry designation:** Medical products **Company type:** Public

Community Care Services sells and rents medical equipment in New York and New Jersey. The company works with health care providers to meet patients' home health care needs by providing and servicing needed equipment. Community Care provides durable medical equipment including hospital beds, wheelchairs, and respiratory machinery and such disposables as dressings and bandages. The company and its former CEO and CFO are under investigation by the Justice Department for Medicare fraud. Former chairman Alan Sheinwald owns about 33% of the company's stock; current chairman Dean Sloane owns about 26%.

Complete Management, Inc.

254 W. 31st St., New York, NY 10001

Telephone: 212-273-0600 **Fax:** 212-594-1645 **Metro area:** New York, NY **Human resources contact:** Carri Ellen Angel **Sales:** $72.4 million **Number of employees:** 920 **Number of employees for previous year:** 772 **Industry designation:** Medical practice management **Company type:** Public **Top competitors:** Medaphis Corporation; MedPartners, Inc.; PhyCor, Inc.

Complete Management answers the cry for help from hospitals swamped in red tape. The company offers administrative and other services to health care providers primarily in the New York City area. In addition to its administrative services, the management firm leases office space and equipment, hires and trains nonmedical personnel, advises on regulatory compliance, and provides other services to help clients cut costs. The company also helps its clients establish diagnostic imaging services and operates its own imaging centers in two New York City hospitals and has a mobile MRI unit serving two New York counties. Greater Metropolitan Medical Services accounts for almost 30% of its sales.

Computer Associates International, Inc.

One Computer Associates Plaza, Islandia, NY 11788

Telephone: 516-342-5224 **Fax:** 516-342-5329 **Metro area:** New York, NY **Web site:** http://www.cai.com **Human resources contact:** Deborah J. Coughlin **Sales:** $4.7 billion **Number of employees:** 11,400 **Number of employees for previous year:** 9,850 **Industry designation:** Computers—corporate, professional & financial software **Company type:** Public **Top competitors:** International Business Machines Corporation; Microsoft Corporation; Oracle Corporation

Computer Associates International (CA) CEO Charles Wang likens his company's software to plumbing under a sink—not the fancy faucet on top. The world's #3 independent software company (after Microsoft and Oracle; Microsoft and IBM are #1 and #2 overall), CA offers more than 500 software products, from data access to network management tools. Its flagship Unicenter program gives customers centralized control over their software, hardware, and networks. Other products include Jasmine (multimedia), CA-Fix/2000 (year 2000 remediation), and Remotely Possible (remote control networking). CA, which has a history of gobbling up smaller software firms, is turning an acquisitive eye toward computer services providers.

Computer Concepts Corp.

80 Orville Dr., Bohemia, NY 11716

Telephone: 516-244-1500 **Fax:** 516-563-8085 **Metro area:** New York, NY **Web site:** http://www.computerconcepts.com **Human resources contact:** Cathy Athans **Sales:** $29.7 million **Number of employees:** 252 **Number of employees for previous year:** 186 **Industry designation:** Computers—corporate, professional & financial software **Company type:** Public

Computer Concepts develops and sells data-access software for PCs and client/server environments as well as systems management software for corporate data centers. Its d.b.Express software allows users to access and analyze information in more than 85% of the relational databases used worldwide, to use information obtained from spreadsheets, and to analyze data on the Internet without first downloading. Through subsidiary SOFTWORKS, which it is spinning off, the company markets 19 software products that address applications and systems performance, data and storage management, and year 2000 conversions. Customers include telecommunications and financial concerns, government agencies, and equipment manufacturers.

Computer Generated Solutions, Inc.

1675 Broadway, New York, NY 10019

Telephone: 212-408-3800 **Fax:** 212-977-7474 **Metro area:** New York, NY **Web site:** http://www.cgsinc.com **Human resources contact:** Dan Dird **Sales:** $80 million (Est.) **Number of employees:** 1,000 **Number of employees for previous year:** 890 **Industry designation:** Computers—services **Company type:** Private **Top competitors:** Hewlett-Packard Company; International Business Machines Corporation; Electronic Data Systems Corporation

Computer Generated Solutions (CGS) is a computer servicing firm that provides an array of technology services such as help desk support, network services, call center management, technical training, and new systems development. CGS is also active in systems integration, and offers its clients expertise in both computer software and hardware (the company is partnered with IBM and specializes in providing IBM hardware). CGS' ACS Optima modular software package is used by more than 500 firms in the apparel industry, and the company offers a number of software tools to assist in year 2000 conversions. CEO Philip Friedman founded CGS in 1984; he and his brother Victor own the company.

CONMED Corporation

310 Broad St., Utica, NY 13501

Telephone: 315-797-8375 **Fax:** 315-797-0321 **Web site:** http://www.conmed.com **Human resources contact:** Elizabeth Bowers **Sales:** $336.4 million **Number of employees:** 2,161 **Number of employees for previous year:** 957 **Industry designation:** Medical instruments **Company type:** Public **Top competitors:** Minnesota Mining and Manufacturing Company; United States Surgical Corporation; Stryker Corporation

Doctors and their patients get a charge out of CONMED's surgical equipment. The company makes a wide range of instruments used in surgical and medical procedures, including electrosurgical systems, powered surgical instruments, suction equipment, arthroscopic devices, and imaging systems. Electrosurgery instruments such as pencils, ground pads, and generators use an electrical current to cut and cauterize tissue. Almost half of the company's sales are electrosurgery products, while arthroscopic devices account for another 33%. Brand names include Apex, BioScrew, MicroChoice, and TroGARD. About one-quarter of total sales are overseas. The company has expanded its product offerings through acquisitions.

Coty Inc.

237 Park Ave., New York, NY 10017

Telephone: 212-850-2300 **Fax:** 212-850-2544 **Metro area:** New York, NY **Web site:** http://www.cotyusinc.com **Sales:** $1.6 billion **Industry designation:** Cosmetics & toiletries **Company type:** Subsidiary **Top competitors:** Revlon, Inc.; The Procter & Gamble Company; Unilever

Coty scents have turned heads since Francois Coty founded the company in 1904 with his first perfume, La Rose Jacqueminot. Coty is the world's leading maker of fragrances for men and women. Its boudoir includes moderately priced scents sold by mass retailers. Brands include Vanilla Fields (the #1 women's fragrance in the US), Stetson, Aspen, !ex'cla.ma'tion, and Jovan. Rather than launching new brands, Coty is introducing variations of existing products (Stetson County, Dark Vanilla). The company also sells cosmetics, lotions, aromatherapy and foot care items, Calgon bath and body products, and other skin treatments. Coty is a wholly owned subsidiary of Joh. A Benckiser GmbH, a maker of consumer goods.

CPAC, Inc.

2364 Leicester Rd., Leicester, NY 14481

Telephone: 716-382-3223 **Fax:** 716-382-3031 **Metro area:** Rochester, NY **Web site:** http://www.cpac-fuller.com **Human resources contact:** Maryann Merle **Sales:** $106.1 million **Number of employees:** 662 **Number of employees for previous year:** 567 **Industry designation:** Chemicals—specialty **Company type:** Public **Top competitors:** Eastman Kodak Company; Amway Corporation; Avon Products, Inc.

Holding company CPAC sells specialty chemicals and other products worldwide through subsidiaries such as Fuller Brush and Stanley Home Products. Bought by CPAC in 1994, Fuller Brush makes more than 2,000 industrial and consumer products, including cleaning chemicals, brooms, and personal care products. Stanley Home Products sells its more than 250 personal care and cleaning products through a network of distributors via the hostess or party plan. Trebla Chemical develops photography chemicals designed to minimize pollution and increase recycling. Allied Diagnostic Imaging Resources provides X-ray chemicals, and CPAC's equipment Division makes silver-recovery equipment.

Curative Health Services, Inc.

150 Motor Pkwy., Hauppauge, NY 11788

Telephone: 516-232-7000 **Fax:** 516-232-9322 **Other address:** PO Box 9052, East Setauket, NY 11733 **Metro area:** New York, NY **Web site:** http://www.curative.com **Sales:** $104 million **Number of employees:** 731 **Number of employees for previous year:** 671 **Industry designation:** Health care—outpatient & home **Company type:** Public

Curative Health Services, Inc., formerly known as Curative Technologies, Inc., is a disease management company specializing in chronic wound care. The company's Wound Care Center network consists of 61 operating clinics utilizing its Procuren product, a topical therapeutic (produced from a patient's own blood) containing growth factors that promote wound healing. Chronic nonhealing wounds are often associated with insufficient blood circulation (common in patients with diabetes and venous stasis disease) and can lead to infection, gangrene, and amputation.

Czarnikow-Rionda Inc.

1 William St., New York, NY 10004

Telephone: 212-806-0700 **Fax:** 212-968-0825 **Metro area:** New York, NY **Human resources contact:** Donna White **Sales:** $800 million (Est.) **Number of employees:** 48 **Number of employees for previous year:** 33 **Industry designation:** Food—sugar & refining **Company type:** Private **Top competitors:** Cargill, Incorporated; The Connell Company; United Sugars Corp.

Sugar brokerage Czarnikow-Rionda had its beginnings in the 1870s when founder Manuel Rionda and his siblings left Cuba. Rionda became involved in the sugar trade in New York and in 1909 took over a trading firm, renaming it Czarnikow-Rionda. For decades the firm was a dominant seller of sugar exported from Cuba; it also owned six plantations in Cuba (through Cuban Trading Company) and was involved in all levels of production, from cane growing to refining. When Fidel Castro seized power in 1959, the firm lost its Cuban holdings; Rionda's relatives fled to the US to build new sugar operations, one of which became the Fanjul family's powerful Flo-Sun. CEO Daniel Gutman is Czarnikow-Rionda's majority owner.

Dairylea Cooperative Inc.

5001 Brittonfield Pkwy., East Syracuse, NY 13057

Telephone: 315-433-0100 **Fax:** 315-433-2345 **Other address:** PO Box 4844, Syracuse, NY 13221 **Metro area:** Syracuse, NY **Sales:** $750 million **Number of employees:** 200 **Number of employees for previous year:** 150 **Industry designation:** Food—dairy products **Company type:** Cooperative **Top competitors:** Dairy Farmers of America; North Central AMPI, Inc.; Foremost Farms USA

Dairylea Cooperative is a major milk marketing and agricultural service organization owned by a herd of more than 2,800 dairy farmers in the northeastern US. In addition to marketing efforts, the cooperative invests in dairy companies, provides members with financial and farm-management services, and markets livestock. Dairylea subsidiary Agri-Service Agencies, Inc., provides life, health, dental, and workers' compensation insurance for workers in agriculture-related businesses nationwide. In hopes of lowering its members' operational costs, Dairylea is also leading a pilot program for the deregulation of New York State's energy services.

Daxor Corporation

350 Fifth Ave., Ste. 7120, New York, NY 10118

Telephone: 212-244-0555 **Fax:** 212-244-0806 **Metro area:** New York, NY **Human resources contact:** Octavia Atanasiu **Sales:** $2.6 million **Number of employees:** 31 **Number of employees for previous year:** 30 **Industry designation:** Medical services **Company type:** Public **Top competitors:** The American Red Cross; North Shore-Long Island Jewish Health System; New York City Health and Hospitals Corporation

A decade of legal wrangling almost put Daxor on ice, but the company's sperm and blood banks are again open to attract new, uh, deposits. The sperm banks, operated through subsidiary Idant Laboratory, target men undergoing procedures that may impair fertility (cancer treatment, vasectomies). The company also offers anonymous third-party semen from donors recruited from some 130 colleges in the New York and New Jersey area. Blood services include autologous blood banking services, in which donors deposit their own blood for possible later use during surgery or emergency situations. Daxor also produces a device that measures the amount of blood in one's body.

Deja News, Inc.

437 Fifth Ave., 6th Fl., New York, NY 10016

Telephone: 212-481-4920 **Fax:** 212-481-4909 **Metro area:** New York, NY **Web site:** http://www.dejanews.com **Human resources contact:** Julie Rachui **Sales:** $5 million (Est.) **Number of employees:** 80 **Number of employees for previous year:** 56 **Industry designation:** Computers—online services **Company type:** Private **Top competitors:** Yahoo! Inc.; America Online, Inc.; GeoCities

Founded in 1995, Deja News provides free access to some 80,000 online discussion forums, including Usenet news groups (Web interfaces that enable interaction among others with similar interests) and its own user groups. Registered users can post messages to the forums and search messages posted within the past three years. Users can also create their own online communities to discuss topics of interest. Deja News also provides discussion-forum search services and content for several third-party sites, including Yahoo! and America Online. The company generates revenues from advertising and sponsorships on its Web site. Austin Ventures and publisher Ziff-Davis are main backers of the company.

Del Laboratories, Inc.

178 EAB Plaza, Uniondale, NY 11556

Telephone: 516-844-2020 **Fax:** 516-844-1515 **Metro area:** New York, NY **Web site:** http://www.dellabs.com **Human resources contact:** Charlie Schneck **Sales:** $274.9 million **Number of employees:** 1,560 **Number of employees for previous year:** 1,480 **Industry designation:** Cosmetics & toiletries **Company type:** Public **Top competitors:** The Procter & Gamble Company; Unilever; Revlon, Inc.

Del Laboratories makes and markets cosmetics and over-the-counter pharmaceuticals. The company's beauty products include nail care products, color cosmetics, beauty implements, bleaches, and hair removers under the Sally Hansen name. Cosmetics include the #1 nail care brand (leading Unilever's Cutex), a leading nail polish brand, and the Naturistics line of bath products. Del's pharmaceutical segment features #1 oral analgesic Orajel, cold sore medication Tanac, acne treatment Propa pH, Arthricare arthritis medication, and Pronto lice treatment. President and CEO Dan Wassong owns about 33% of the company.

Detection Systems, Inc.

130 Perinton Pkwy., Fairport, NY 14450

Telephone: 716-223-4060 **Fax:** 716-223-9180 **Metro area:** Rochester, NY **Web site:** http://detectionsys.com **Human resources contact:** Chris Kather **Sales:** $126.3 million **Number of employees:** 1,100 **Number of employees for previous year:** 744 **Industry designation:** Protection—safety equipment & services **Company type:** Public **Top competitors:** Napco Security Systems, Inc.; Checkpoint Systems, Inc.; Pittway Corporation

Detection Systems has a sixth sense for finding business. The electronic detection, control, and communications equipment made by the company is used worldwide by firms that provide commercial and residential fire protection and security services. Products include smoke detectors, motion detectors, handheld alarm transmitters, and closed-circuit TV equipment. Brands include Detection Systems, Radionics, Security Escort, and DS Vision. Detection Systems offers products that can transmit or receive alarm signals over telephone lines, cellular networks, or secure radio networks. Its manufacturing facilities are in Australia, China, the UK, and the US. Video monitoring firm Ultrak owns a 20% stake in the firm.

DHB Capital Group Inc.

11 Old Westbury Rd., Old Westbury, NY 11568

Telephone: 516-997-1155 **Fax:** 516-997-1144 **Metro area:** New York, NY **Human resources contact:** Dawn Schlegel **Sales:** $33.3 million **Number of employees:** 357 **Number of employees for previous year:** 290 **Industry designation:** Protection—safety equipment & services **Company type:** Public **Top competitors:** DePuy, Inc.; Riddell Sports Inc.; Armor Holdings, Inc.

Feeling vulnerable? DHB Capital Group can help. The company manufactures and sells bulletproof vests, protective athletic equipment, and orthopedic devices. DHB's Armor Group makes both concealable and tactical body armor from Kevlar and other materials, selling its products to law enforcement agencies and armed forces in the US, Europe, and the Middle East. Its Sports Group specializes in protective padding and braces for the injury-prone athlete; it also markets orthopedic equipment and medical supplies to doctors and hospitals. Chairman and CEO David Brooks owns 57% of the company.

Discovery Laboratories, Inc.

509 Madison Ave., 14th Fl., New York, NY 10022

Telephone: 212-223-9504 **Fax:** 212-688-7978 **Metro area:** New York, NY **Web site:** http://www.discoverylabs.com **Sales:** $700,000 **Number of employees:** 13 **Number of employees for previous year:** 9 **Industry designation:** Drugs **Company type:** Public **Top competitors:** Genentech, Inc.; Forest Laboratories, Inc.; Glaxo Wellcome plc

Discovery Laboratories is a development-stage pharmaceutical company that acquires, develops, and commercializes critical-care drugs. By focusing on drugs that have been previously tested on humans or animals, the company reduces risk and speeds development. It has three licensed investigational drug candidates under development: SuperVent, for treating airway diseases such as cystic fibrosis and chronic bronchitis; Surfaxin, for treating infant and adult respiratory distress and meconium aspiration syndrome; and ST-630 for postmenopausal osteoporosis. It also has licensed drugs for pancreatitis and chemotherapy-induced hair loss, both acquired in its merger with Ansan Pharmaceuticals.

DoubleClick Inc.

41 Madison Ave., 32nd Fl., New York, NY 10010

Telephone: 212-683-0001 **Fax:** 212-655-4635 **Metro area:** New York, NY **Web site:** http://www.doubleclick.net **Human resources contact:** Laura Ianuly **Sales:** $80.2 million **Number of employees:** 482 **Number of employees for previous year:** 185 **Industry designation:** Computers—online services **Company type:** Public **Top competitors:** America Online, Inc.; Flycast Communications Corporation; 24/7 Media, Inc.

DoubleClick works to turn double takes into click throughs. The online advertising firm offers highly targeted ad delivery through its DART technology, a dynamic analysis tool that collects information on audience behavior and response, and uses that information to target ad placement. DoubleClick delivers ads to more than 450 sites in its DoubleClick Network, including the AltaVista search engine (about 45% of sales), "Billboard" Online, and "U.S. News and World Report." DoubleClick serves advertisers including Microsoft (about 7% of sales), AT&T, and IBM. The company has operations in Australia, Canada, Europe, and the US.

EarthWeb Inc.

3 Park Ave., New York, NY 10016

Telephone: 212-725-6550 **Fax:** 212-725-6559 **Metro area:** New York, NY **Web site:** http://www.earthweb.com **Human resources contact:** Rebecca Haralabatos **Sales:** $3.3 million **Number of employees:** 121 **Number of employees for previous year:** 53 **Industry designation:** Computers—online services **Company type:** Public **Top competitors:** CMP Media Inc.; Ziff-Davis Inc.; CNET, Inc.

EarthWeb provides online information and services to information technology (IT) professionals worldwide. The company's collection of Web sites, including developer.com and datamation.com, offers access to some 150,000 technical resources as well as more than 500 technical books and proprietary tutorials. In addition, the company offers bulletin boards and question-and-answer sessions in which IT professionals can share information and help each other. EarthWeb's online shopping service features more than 700 products from more than 100 vendors, including Microsoft and Lotus. The company, which attracts more than one million users a month, generates virtually all of its sales from advertising.

Ecology and Environment, Inc.

368 Pleasant View Dr., Lancaster, NY 14086

Telephone: 716-684-8060 **Fax:** 716-684-0844 **Metro area:** Buffalo, NY **Web site:** http://www.ecolen.com **Human resources contact:** Laird Robertson **Sales:** $61.5 million **Number of employees:** 800 **Number of employees for previous year:** 700 **Industry designation:** Pollution control equipment & services **Company type:** Public **Top competitors:** Waste Management, Inc.; The IT Group, Inc.; Bechtel Group, Inc.

Every day is Earth Day at environmental consulting and testing company Ecology and Environment—almost half its revenues come from cleaning up Superfund sites for the US government. Ecology and Environment's services include environmental-impact assessments, air pollution control, wastewater analyses, and other site-planning and laboratory services. The company maintains 23 US offices and operates in 36 other countries. Founders and senior executives own 65% of the company, and an investment group headed by First Carolina Investors owns 32%.

Emisphere Technologies, Inc.

765 Old Saw Mill River Rd., Tarrytown, NY 10591

Telephone: 914-347-2220 **Fax:** 914-347-2498 **Metro area:** New York, NY **Web site:** http://www.emisphere.com **Human resources contact:** Barbara Mohl **Sales:** $15.9 million **Number of employees:** 72 **Number of employees for previous year:** 64 **Industry designation:** Drugs **Company type:** Public **Top competitors:** Endorex Corp.; Anesta Corp.; TheraTech, Inc.

Development-stage Emisphere Technologies is creating drug-delivery systems for people who literally can't stomach the treatments they need for diabetes, clotting disorders, asthma, and other health problems. The company's delivery compounds are intended to allow oral ingestion of drugs that normally are blocked by enzymes in the gastrointestinal system. Emisphere Technologies is also developing vaccines that can be administered orally. The company has alliances with Eli Lilly and Novartis. It is also involved in a 50/50 joint venture with Elan to develop and sell oral carriers for the anticoagulant heparin.

Empire Beef Co., Inc.

171 Weidner Rd., Rochester, NY 14624

Telephone: 716-235-7350 **Fax:** 716-235-1776 **Metro area:** Rochester, NY **Human resources contact:** Michael Prebost **Sales:** $548 million (Est.) **Number of employees:** 240 **Number of employees for previous year:** 170 **Industry designation:** Food—meat products **Company type:** Private **Top competitors:** ConAgra, Inc.; Smithfield Foods, Inc.; IBP, inc.

Protein has given Empire Beef its bulk. The wholesale meat processor and distributor ships more than five million pounds of meat each week. Empire Beef's products include beef, pork, lamb, veal, seafood, poultry, cheese, and processed meats. The firm also offers food service and retail products. Empire Beef serves customers in the US (in the Northeast and Southeast) and internationally (including the Caribbean and the Far East). Operations include a fleet of more than 80 tractor trailers. Harry Levine started the firm as a small slaughtering plant in 1937; slaughter operations later stopped. The Levine family (Harry's grandson Steve is CEO) owns Empire Beef.

Enamelon, Inc.

15 Kimball Ave., Yonkers, NY 10704

Telephone: 914-237-1308 **Fax:** 914-237-4024 **Metro area:** New York, NY **Web site:** http://www.enamelon.com **Sales:** $14.3 million **Number of employees:** 49 **Number of employees for previous year:** 32 **Industry designation:** Cosmetics & toiletries **Company type:** Public **Top competitors:** The Procter & Gamble Company; SmithKline Beecham plc; Colgate-Palmolive Company

Even toothpaste isn't simple anymore. Enamelon wants to take a bite out of the world's toothpaste market with dental care products designed to enhance "remineralization" —strengthening of tooth enamel and prevention of cavities. Founded in 1992 by Chairman and CEO Steven Fox, the company has introduced its first product, Enamelon all-family toothpaste, to the US's $1.8 billion toothpaste market. The toothpaste containing sodium fluoride, calcium, and phosphate ions dispenses two streams of paste that mix to create a form of salted calcium, said to add minerals to the tooth surface. The company has additional patents pending and is expanding into Canada. Fox owns 28% of Enamelon.

Enzo Biochem, Inc.

60 Executive Blvd., Farmingdale, NY 11735

Telephone: 516-755-5500 **Fax:** 516-755-5561 **Metro area:** New York, NY **Web site:** http://www.enzo.com **Human resources contact:** Debbie Sohmer **Sales:** $40.4 million **Number of employees:** 230 **Number of employees for previous year:** 210 **Industry designation:** Biomedical & genetic products **Company type:** Public **Top competitors:** Chiron Corporation; Quest Diagnostics Incorporated; Laboratory Corporation of America Holdings

Enzo Biochem has three subsidiaries through which it develops and sells molecular biology- and genetic engineering-based health care products and provides contract laboratory services to health care providers. The company operates clinical reference laboratories and provides diagnostic testing in the New York City area through its Enzo Clinical Labs subsidiary, which account for some 70% of Enzo's sales. The company's Enzo Therapeutics unit develops antisense technology, which blocks disease-causing genes within cells to treat cancer and other diseases. Subsidiary Enzo Diagnostics makes DNA probe tests, which are used to detect diseases at the genetic level.

The Estee Lauder Companies Inc.

767 Fifth Ave., New York, NY 10153

Telephone: 212-572-4200 **Fax:** 212-572-6633 **Metro area:** New York, NY **Web site:** http://www.elcompanies.com **Human resources contact:** Andrew J. Cavanaugh **Sales:** $3.6 billion **Number of employees:** 15,300 **Number of employees for previous year:** 14,700 **Industry designation:** Cosmetics & toiletries **Company type:** Public **Top competitors:** Revlon, Inc.; Shiseido Company, Limited; L'Oreal

Estee, Jane, and Bobbi are close friends to women around the world. With brands including Estee Lauder, professional-style Bobbi Brown "essentials," and trendy, teen-oriented "jane," —not to mention Clinique—Estee Lauder sells skin care, cosmetic, and fragrance products in more than 100 countries. The company's upscale lines (available in department stores, through specialty retailers, and in company stores) account for nearly half of all US prestige cosmetic sales. Estee Lauder has increased its botanical beauty product offerings (Origins) with the purchase of Aveda, which also expanded its distribution into 30,000 beauty salons. The founding Lauder family owns 70% of the company.

Family Golf Centers, Inc.

225 Broadhollow Rd., Melville, NY 11747

Telephone: 516-694-1666 **Fax:** 516-694-0918 **Metro area:** New York, NY **Web site:** http://familygolf.com **Human resources contact:** Rose Johnson **Sales:** $122.2 million **Number of employees:** 3,719 **Number of employees for previous year:** 1,496 **Industry designation:** Leisure & recreational services **Company type:** Public **Top competitors:** The Arnold Palmer Golf Company; Proformance Research Organization, Inc.; Golden Bear Golf, Inc.

Family Golf Centers is the largest golf range operator in North America, with about 120 facilities, including seven Golden Bear Golf Centers in the US and Canada. The company offers golf lessons and facilities for driving, putting, chipping, and sand play. Some of the centers are located adjacent to golf courses; most include a coaching studio and a clubhouse with a full-line pro shop where the company sells both its own and third-party golf equipment and apparel. The golf centers also have miniature golf courses, cafes or snack bars, and video games. To offset seasonal business Family Golf also operates about 30 ice skating and family-entertainment facilities and has plans to build and acquire more.

FeatureCast, Inc.

1650 Broadway, Ste. 408, New York, NY 10019

Telephone: 212-315-1275 **Fax:** 212-765-8159 **Metro area:** New York, NY **Number of employees:** 25 **Industry designation:** Computers—online services **Company type:** Private **Top competitors:** InfoSpace.com, Inc.; The Walt Disney Company; NaviLinks Inc.

FeatureCast is the result of the merger of E-Ticket (an idealab! company) and RealTime Syndication Network (RTSN). FeatureCast produces and distributes online content using the expertise of its founding companies. Through E-Ticket, FeatureCast owns exclusive rights to popular online properties (including "America's Most Wanted Online" and "National ENQUIRER Online") and profits from the traffic generated by these popular sites. FeatureCast also distributes ready-made online content through RTSN, which provides Web-ready content, such as real-time sports information and multiplayer games, to hundreds of third-party Web sites.

Firecom, Inc.

39-27 59th St., Woodside, NY 11377

Telephone: 718-899-6100 **Fax:** 718-899-1932 **Metro area:** New York, NY **Sales:** $14.1 million **Number of employees:** 123 **Industry designation:** Protection—safety equipment & services **Company type:** Public **Top competitors:** Firetector Inc.; American Protective Services, Inc.; Detection Systems, Inc.

Firecom sparks feelings of security in its customers. It designs, makes, tests, distributes, and services customizable fire safety and security systems, which it sells under the Firecom brand. Its products, including fire detection equipment, audio-visual systems, and controls, protect buildings by sensing and reporting fires, sounding alarms, notifying the fire department, controlling building functions, and enabling building-wide communications. In addition the firm distributes third-party electronic building systems (such as the Life Safety brand). Although Firecom sells its products nationwide, it primarily serves the greater New York City area. Chairman and CEO Paul Mendez owns 74% of the firm.

FONAR Corporation

110 Marcus Dr., Melville, NY 11747

Telephone: 516-694-2929 **Fax:** 516-249-3734 **Metro area:** New York, NY **Web site:** http://www.fonar.com **Human resources contact:** Fred Peipman **Sales:** $27.6 million **Number of employees:** 444 **Number of employees for previous year:** 346 **Industry designation:** Medical instruments **Company type:** Public **Top competitors:** General Electric Company; Siemens AG; Hitachi, Ltd.

FONAR is the very image of magnetic resonance imaging. A pioneer in the MRI field, FONAR today makes "and" manages scanning equipment. Its U.S. Health Management subsidiary (about 75% of FONAR's sales) provides management services to nearly 40 diagnostic imaging centers and other health care providers. FONAR's products include the QUAD series of "open" MRIs with high field strength; the units, priced between $780,000 and $980,000, are marketed by distributors and at trade shows. FONAR is developing a breast MRI scanner and an operating-room scanner. The company sells to hospitals and other health care providers in the US and several other nations. Chairman Raymond Damadian owns about 20% of FONAR.

foreignTV.com, Inc.

162 Fifth Ave., Ste. 1005A, New York, NY 10010

Telephone: 212-206-1121 **Metro area:** New York, NY **Web site:** http://www.foreigntv.com **Number of employees:** 7 **Industry designation:** Computers—online services **Company type:** Private **Top competitors:** broadcast.com inc.; America Online, Inc.; Yahoo! Inc.

foreignTV.com wants to show you the world. The development-stage company plans to broadcast foreign news, human interest stories, interviews, cultural events, and other content in English through Web sites such as parisTV.com and london-TV.com. It will receive proprietary content from company-owned bureaus established in major cities throughout the world. foreignTV.com will utilize streaming video technology to transmit its broadcasts. The general public will be allowed access to the company's sites for free; foreigntv.com will generate sales through advertising and e-commerce. After a planned IPO, CEO Jonathan Braun and chairman William Lane will reduce their stakes in the company to 31% and 27%, respectively.

Forest Laboratories, Inc.

909 Third Ave., New York, NY 10022

Telephone: 212-421-7850 **Fax:** 212-750-9152 **Metro area:** New York, NY **Human resources contact:** Bernard E. McGovern **Sales:** $455.2 million **Number of employees:** 1,854 **Number of employees for previous year:** 1,663 **Industry designation:** Drugs **Company type:** Public **Top competitors:** IVAX Corporation; Schering-Plough Corporation; Eli Lilly and Company

Forest Laboratories develops and manufactures name-brand and generic prescription and nonprescription pharmaceutical products. The company's pharmaceutical line ranges from Cervidil (used to help speed the birthing process) to citalopram, an approval-pending antidepressant that would compete with Prozac. Aerosol asthma drug Aerobid makes up more than 20% of the company's sales; Lorcet, a strong analgesic, contributes the second-largest chunk of revenue at about 10%. Forest Laboratories, which has subsidiaries in the UK and Ireland, markets directly to doctors, drugstore chains, wholesalers, and distributors.

Frisby Technologies, Inc.

77 E. Main St., Ste. 2000, Bay Shore, NY 11706

Telephone: 516-969-8570 **Fax:** 516-969-8579 **Metro area:** New York, NY **Web site:** http://www.frisby.com **Human resources contact:** Stephen P. Villa **Sales:** $2.9 million **Number of employees:** 30 **Number of employees for previous year:** 13 **Industry designation:** Chemicals—specialty **Company type:** Public **Top competitors:** R. G. Barry Corporation; Aavid Thermal Technologies, Inc.; Outlast Technologies, Inc.

Frisby Technologies puts a spin on thermal additives and foams used in consumer and industrial products. Its Thermasorb heat-absorbing powders can be added to materials such as foams and coolants, among others. ComforTemp breathable polyurethane foams are embedded with Thermasorb. Both use phase-change materials that absorb and reject heat according to preset temperature ranges. Frisby Technologies' products are used in gloves, boots, and helmets through partnerships with such companies as LaCrosse Footwear and Bell Sports. The products can also be used in protective clothing, packaging materials, electronics, and avionics cooling systems. Chairman Gregory Frisby owns 58% of the company.

Frontline Communications Corporation

One Blue Hill Plaza, 6th Fl., Pearl River, NY 10965

Telephone: 914-623-8553 **Fax:** 914-623-8669 **Other address:** PO Box 1548, Pearl River, NY 10965 **Metro area:** New York, NY **Web site:** http://www.fcc.net/default2.html **Human resources contact:** Michael Olbermann **Sales:** $300,000 **Number of employees:** 46 **Number of employees for previous year:** 5 **Industry designation:** Computers—online services **Company type:** Public **Top competitors:** Microsoft Corporation; CompuServe Interactive Services, Inc.; America Online, Inc.

Frontline Communications provides Internet services primarily for individual and small-business subscribers in suburban New York and New Jersey. The company's dial-up Internet access services, which include e-mail and access to the World Wide Web, are provided through a telecommunications network of leased high-speed data lines and 10 points-of-presence (POPs). Frontline has more than 1,700 subscribers on monthly or quarterly payment plans with unlimited access. The company also provides technical support for Web site design and maintenance as well as dedicated leased lines for business users. Frontline plans to expand its services to the New York City metropolitan area, including New Jersey and Connecticut.

Fuji Photo Film U.S.A., Inc.

555 Taxter Rd., Elmsford, NY 10523

Telephone: 914-789-8100 **Fax:** 914-789-8295 **Metro area:** New York, NY **Web site:** http://www.fujifilm.com/home/corp/corp.htm **Human resources contact:** Joe Convery **Industry designation:** Photographic equipment & supplies **Company type:** Subsidiary **Parent company:** Fuji Photo Film Co., Ltd. **Top competitors:** Bayer AG; Eastman Kodak Company; Canon Inc.

Smile, you're on film produced by Fuji Photo Film U.S.A (Fujifilm). A subsidiary of Tokyo-based Fuji Photo Film, Fujifilm primarily makes film and cameras and processes film. It also makes computer disks, graphic arts materials, microfilm, motion picture film, and printers. The company has operations in 23 states, with its largest manufacturing facility in Greenwood, South Carolina. Fujifilm has been engaged in a price war with Eastman Kodak in a successful bid for market share. The US film market is dominated by Kodak, but Fujifilm's share is creeping upward and is expected to hit 20%. Worldwide, Fuji and Kodak are tied.

Getty Petroleum Marketing Inc.

125 Jericho Tpke., Jericho, NY 11753

Telephone: 516-338-6000 **Fax:** 516-338-1582 **Metro area:** New York, NY **Human resources contact:** Carolann Gaites **Sales:** $892.8 million **Number of employees:** 624 **Number of employees for previous year:** 521 **Industry designation:** Oil refining & marketing **Company type:** Public

Getty Petroleum Marketing is a major independent distributor of motor and heating fuels. The company operates in 12 northeastern and mid-Atlantic states through more than 1,300 service stations, some of which maintain convenience stores, automotive repair centers, or car washes. It also runs 10 distribution terminals and bulk plants, which are used for storing and distributing petroleum products purchased from regional suppliers. Spun off from Getty Petroleum (now Getty Realty) to handle its parent's petroleum-marketing and heating-oil businesses, it leases about 75% of its retail stores from Getty Realty.

Globix Corporation

295 Lafayette St., 3rd Fl., New York, NY 10012

Telephone: 212-334-8500 **Fax:** 212-334-8552 **Metro area:** New York, NY **Web site:** http://www.globix.com **Human resources contact:** Dennis Nelson **Sales:** $20.6 million **Number of employees:** 204 **Number of employees for previous year:** 91 **Industry designation:** Computers—online services **Company type:** Public **Top competitors:** PSINet Inc.; UUNET WorldCom; Concentric Network Corporation

When businesses in New York City get tired of crashing on the information superhighway, they can turn to Globix (formerly Bell Technology Group) for Internet-related third-party hardware and software and systems integration. Globix also operates as an Internet service provider (ISP), offering dedicated access, Web site design and hosting, e-commerce support, and training programs. Customers include the American Red Cross, Dow Jones, General Media International (Penthouse), Microsoft, the NHL, and Standard & Poors. Globix is expanding its New York operations and building facilities in London and the San Francisco Bay area. Founder and CEO Marc Bell owns 25% of the company and controls 50% of the voting rights.

Graham-Field Health Products, Inc.

400 Rabro Dr. East, Hauppauge, NY 11788

Telephone: 516-582-5900 **Fax:** 516-582-2775 **Metro area:** New York, NY **Human resources contact:** Peggy Brunn **Sales:** $262 million **Number of employees:** 2,236 **Number of employees for previous year:** 1,421 **Industry designation:** Medical products **Company type:** Public **Top competitors:** Sunrise Medical Inc.; Medline Industries, Inc.; Invacare Corporation

Graham-Field Health Products comes in third in the wheelchair race behind Invacare and Sunrise Medical. Rather than concentrate on sleek racing models, the firm specializes in chairs in the power, pediatric, and geriatric fields. It also distributes more than 45,000 different types of medical supplies, including sphygmomanometers (blood-pressure measurement devices), stethoscopes, EKG instruments, durable medical equipment, antiseptics, and sterile, disposable medical products. Its Fuqua Enterprises subsidiary makes and supplies such medical furnishings as beds and seating and bathroom safety products. The company has been growing rapidly through acquisitions and distributes to customers in the US and abroad.

Greka Energy Corporation

575 Madison Ave., Ste. 1006, New York, NY 10022

Telephone: 212-605-0470 **Fax:** 212-605-0454 **Metro area:** New York, NY **Sales:** $200,000 **Number of employees:** 15 **Number of employees for previous year:** 5 **Industry designation:** Oil & gas—exploration & production **Company type:** Public

Greka Energy, formerly Horizontal Ventures, is an oil and gas producer that drills sideways to capture reserves from declining wells. The company acquires fields with proved reserves and production infrastructure in place (primarily in California and Illinois) and then uses a low-cost, horizontal drilling technology to recover oil remaining after more conventional drilling. Greka Energy has drilled more than 40 wells for clients such as Chevron, Texaco, Exxon, and OXY. Aside from exploitation and development, the company is moving into exploration drilling.

Griffin Land & Nurseries, Inc.

1 Rockefeller Plaza, New York, NY 10020

Telephone: 212-218-7910 **Fax:** 212-218-7917 **Metro area:** New York, NY **Human resources contact:** Tammy Pollack **Sales:** $51.2 million **Number of employees:** 332 **Number of employees for previous year:** 259 **Industry designation:** Agricultural operations **Company type:** Public **Parent company:** Culbro Corporation **Top competitors:** Hines Horticulture, Inc.; HomeBase, Inc.; The Home Depot, Inc.

Plant and plot yourself in Griffin Land & Nurseries and what do you get ... plant containers and real estate. Subsidiary Imperial Nurseries grows and distributes container-grown plants such as azaleas and rhododendrons. The nursery has seven wholesale centers in five states (another is being planned for New Jersey) and sells primarily to landscapers. Among Griffin's primary real estate activities is the development of its 600 acres near Bradley International Airport in Connecticut. The company also owns 33% of the UK's Centaur Communications, a private publisher of business magazines such as "Marketing Week" and "New Media Age." The Cullman family owns over 45% of the company.

Halstead Energy Corporation

33 Hubbells Dr., Mount Kisco, NY 10549

Telephone: 914-666-3200 **Fax:** 914-666-6743 **Other address:** P.O. Box 660, Mount Kisco, NY 10549 **Metro area:** New York, NY **Sales:** $13.3 million **Number of employees:** 31 **Number of employees for previous year:** 28 **Industry designation:** Oil refining & marketing **Company type:** Public **Top competitors:** Gulf Oil, L.P.; National Propane Partners, L.P.; Petroleum Heat and Power Co., Inc.

Halstead Energy is the suburban New York City HQ for fuel. Through its HQ Propane subsidiary, the company retails liquid propane gas and related equipment and services to 7,000 homes and businesses in the affluent suburban counties surrounding NYC. HQ Propane has three separate divisions. HQ Terminal wholesales fuel oil to third parties and provides gasoline, fuel oil, and diesel storage services for petroleum companies. HQ Gasoline supplies and operates 25 gas stations and convenience stores under the ATI, Gulf, and Getty names, while its Dino Oil division distributes gasoline throughout the Big Apple and the surrounding metropolitan area. The Tarricone family controls the company and serves as its officers.

Health Management Systems, Inc.

401 Park Ave. South, New York, NY 10016

Telephone: 212-685-4545 **Fax:** 212-889-8776 **Metro area:** New York, NY **Web site:** http://www.hmsy.com **Human resources contact:** Lewis D. Levetown **Sales:** $105.3 million **Number of employees:** 860 **Number of employees for previous year:** 837 **Industry designation:** Medical practice management **Company type:** Public **Top competitors:** IDX Systems Corporation; Shared Medical Systems Corporation; McKesson HBOC, Inc.

Health Management Systems supplies information management services, data processing services, and software to hospitals and health care providers, government health agencies, and other health care companies. The company, which has more than 1,000 clients, develops systems for retroactive insurance claims reprocessing and third-party liability recovery. In response to managed care's emphasis on up-front cost savings, Health Management Systems has moved into electronic data interchange services such as electronic billing and managed care decision-support systems. The company's biggest client, Columbia/HCA, accounts for 10% of the company's revenues.

Healthplex, Inc.

60 Charles Lindbergh Blvd., Uniondale, NY 11553

Telephone: 516-542-2200 **Fax:** 516-794-3186 **Metro area:** New York, NY **Web site:** http://www.healthplex.com **Sales:** $13.7 million **Number of employees:** 82 **Number of employees for previous year:** 63 **Industry designation:** Medical practice management **Company type:** Public **Top competitors:** Oxford Health Plans, Inc.; Metropolitan Life Insurance Company; The Prudential Insurance Company of America

Healthplex's services are duplex—the company supports and offers dental plans in New York and New Jersey; it also offers document-imaging technology. On the dental front, its major client is a dental care plan provider controlled by Healthplex officers and directors; Healthplex provides the client company with such services as claims processing, marketing, and data processing. Through subsidiaries, Healthplex also offers its own dental plan and markets dental plans. Subsidiary O.A.SYS develops document-imaging software and hardware, which it markets to hospitals. President Martin Kane and his brother, VP George Kane, own a combined 28% of Healthplex; Chairman Stephen Cuchel owns another 14%.

Henry Schein, Inc.

135 Duryea Rd., Melville, NY 11747

Telephone: 516-843-5500 **Fax:** 516-843-5658 **Metro area:** New York, NY **Web site:** http://www.henryschein.com **Human resources contact:** Leonard A. David **Sales:** $1.9 billion **Number of employees:** 6,000 **Number of employees for previous year:** 5,000 **Industry designation:** Medical & dental supplies **Company type:** Public **Top competitors:** Owens & Minor, Inc.; Patterson Dental Company; Allegiance Corporation

Henry Schein is the largest dental equipment supplier in the US and Europe. The dental market accounts for nearly 70% of its sales. The company is also expanding into the medical and veterinary equipment supply businesses. Henry Schein sells about 50,000 products to 230,000 customers worldwide. Its dental products include anesthetics, infection control items, impression materials, and X-ray equipment. Medical and veterinary items include branded and generic pharmaceuticals and surgical supplies. The company's direct marketing approach boosts sales through lower prices. Henry Schein is buying companies to expand its core lines. Chairman and CEO Stanley Bergman and his family own almost 36% of the company.

ICC Industries Inc.

460 Park Ave., New York, NY 10022

Telephone: 212-521-1700 **Fax:** 212-521-1794 **Metro area:** New York, NY **Web site:** http://www.iccchem.com **Human resources contact:** Frances Foti **Sales:** $1 billion (Est.) **Number of employees:** 2,729 **Number of employees for previous year:** 2,550 **Industry designation:** Chemicals—diversified **Company type:** Private **Top competitors:** Formosa Plastics Corporation; IVAX Corporation; International Flavors & Fragrances Inc.

ICC Industries keeps US pharmaceutical companies supplied with the raw materials used in manufacturing drugs. An international maker and marketer of chemicals, plastics, and pharmaceutical products, ICC also trades and distributes nutritional supplements and food ingredients. Its operates through its main subsidiary, ICC Chemical Corporation, which maintains trading and marketing offices in Asia, Europe, South America, and the US. The company's Prior Energy Corporation has natural gas distribution interests in Alabama, Florida, Mississippi, and Tennessee. ICC Industries also owns 67% of Pharmaceutical Formulations, a manufacturer and distributor of generic over-the-counter drugs.

IFS International, Inc.

Rensselaer Technology Park, 185 Jordan Rd., Troy, NY 12180

Telephone: 518-283-7900 **Fax:** 518-283-7336 **Metro area:** Albany, NY **Web site:** http://WWW.IFSINTL.COM **Human resources contact:** Len DeForge **Sales:** $5.2 million **Number of employees:** 95 **Number of employees for previous year:** 52 **Industry designation:** Computers—corporate, professional & financial software **Company type:** Public **Top competitors:** Transaction Systems Architects, Inc.

Presto! IFS International makes money appear from a box. The company's electronic funds transfer software allows credit and debit card transaction processing from ATMs and point-of-sale terminals. Its TPII software family is used primarily by financial institutions in emerging countries, including parts of Eastern Europe. Through an agreement with VISA, IFS is testing a system in Europe that allows cardholders to load a fixed amount of purchasing power onto a smart card at an ATM, then debit purchases from the card. Digital Equipment, which accounts for 20% of sales, licenses IFS software for use in some of its electronic funds transfer systems. The company has subsidiaries in Germany and the UK.

ImClone Systems Incorporated

180 Varick St., 7th Fl., New York, NY 10014

Telephone: 212-645-1405 **Fax:** 212-645-2054 **Metro area:** New York, NY **Web site:** http://www.imclone.com **Human resources contact:** Marilyn Ramirez **Sales:** $4.2 million **Number of employees:** 138 **Number of employees for previous year:** 110 **Industry designation:** Biomedical & genetic products **Company type:** Public **Top competitors:** Chiron Corporation; Corixa Corporation; Genentech, Inc.

ImClone Systems's drug candidates are of mice and men. The biopharmaceutical firm develops chimerized (made from mouse and human antibodies) treatments and vaccines for cancer. The company's main product under development (with druggernaut Merck) is C225, a cancer cell inhibitor known to boost the effectiveness of chemotherapy agents. ImClone Systems is also developing cancer-related angiogenesis inhibitors, cancer vaccines for small-cell lung carcinoma and melanoma, and endothelial stem cells to deliver gene therapies. The company conducts much of its research with partners, including CombiChem and Memorial Sloan-Kettering Cancer Center. ImClone Systems has facilities in New York and New Jersey.

IMPATH Inc.

521 W. 57th St., New York, NY 10019

Telephone: 212-698-0300 **Fax:** 212-258-2137 **Metro area:** New York, NY **Web site:** http://www.impath.com **Human resources contact:** Anne Druck **Sales:** $56.3 million **Number of employees:** 509 **Number of employees for previous year:** 288 **Industry designation:** Medical services **Company type:** Public **Top competitors:** APACHE Medical Systems, Inc.; UroCor, Inc.; DIANON Systems, Inc.

IMPATH slices, dices, and juliennes (cancer data, that is). The company contracts with health care providers to analyze tumor specimens, then uses its database of cancer treatments and outcomes to diagnose the cancer, recommend treatment, and predict its outcome. Focusing on breast cancer, leukemias, lymphomas, and difficult-to-diagnose tumors, the company expands its database by adding case information illustrating diagnosis and treatment options. IMPATH targets hospitals and doctors that can't afford to maintain the specialized equipment and staff needed for cancer analysis, as well as managed care organizations seeking cost-effective cancer care. IMPATH is expanding via acquisitions.

IntegraMed America, Inc.

One Manhattanville Rd., Purchase, NY 10577

Telephone: 914-253-8000 **Fax:** 914-253-8008 **Metro area:** New York, NY **Human resources contact:** Rita Gruber **Sales:** $38.6 million **Number of employees:** 414 **Number of employees for previous year:** 372 **Industry designation:** Medical services **Company type:** Public

IntegraMed America (formerly IVF America) provides physician practice management to medical providers specializing in women's reproductive health care, particularly infertility and assisted reproductive technology. The firm's operations consist of 12 network sites with 21 locations in 9 states and the District of Columbia. Approximately 60 physicians use the company's management services, which include access to capital, technology, administrative services, marketing and practice development, and information-systems assistance in the development of clinical strategies. One of the company's sites specializes in menopause-related health issues. IntegraMed America continues to grow through acquisitions.

International Flavors & Fragrances Inc.

521 W. 57th St., New York, NY 10019

Telephone: 212-765-5500 **Fax:** 212-708-7132 **Metro area:** New York, NY **Human resources contact:** Eric Campbell **Sales:** $1.4 billion **Number of employees:** 4,670 **Number of employees for previous year:** 4,640 **Industry designation:** Chemicals—specialty **Company type:** Public **Top competitors:** Unilever; Roche Holding Ltd; Bush Boake Allen Inc.

International Flavors & Fragrances (IFF) has a nose for business—it's one of the world's leading originators and manufacturers of artificial flavors and aromas. Flavors are sold principally to producers of prepared foods, dairy foods, beverages, confections, and pharmaceuticals. IFF's fragrances (about 60% of sales) are used in the manufacture of perfumes, cosmetics, soaps, and other household and personal care products. Foreign sales account for more than two-thirds of revenues, due in part to growing demand in such emerging markets as Eastern Europe. IFF operates manufacturing facilities, sales offices, and laboratories in Africa, Asia, Australia, Europe, and North and South America.

International Smart Sourcing, Inc.

320 Broad Hollow Rd., Farmingdale, NY 11735

Telephone: 516-752-1950 **Fax:** 516-752-1971 **Metro area:** New York, NY **Human resources contact:** Steven Sgammato **Sales:** $6.1 million (Est.) **Number of employees:** 105 **Industry designation:** Rubber & plastic products **Company type:** Private

International Smart Sourcing (formerly International Plastic Technologies) makes injection-molded plastic components and assemblies for consumer, industrial, and military use. Its Electronic Hardware subsidiary produces knobs, handles, and dials for electronics equipment and instrumentation switches. Subsidiary Compact Disc Packaging has a license to make and sell the Pull Pack CD packaging system, which uses a drawer design instead of the standard hinge jewel boxes. The firm also has a license to make the Ultratherm handheld massager through its Duralogic Technologies subsidiary. Chairman David Kassel will reduce his ownership in the company from 36% to 22% after the IPO.

i-traffic, Inc.

375 W. Broadway, 5th Fl., New York, NY 10012

Telephone: 212-219-0050 **Fax:** 212-219-3434 **Metro area:** New York, NY **Web site:** http://www.itraffic.com **Human resources contact:** Joanne Kivlahan **Sales:** $5 million (Est.) **Number of employees:** 70 **Industry designation:** Computers—online services **Company type:** Private **Top competitors:** Leo Burnett Company, Inc.; iXL Enterprises, Inc.; Organic Online, Inc.

A variety of online merchants—including Bertelsmann Online, CDNow, CNN/SI Store, Internet Shopping Network, and NetGrocer—rely on i-traffic to manage their Internet advertising. The employee-owned company provides media buying services and placement of online ads such as banners, buttons, and remote storefronts. It also helps establish strategic alliances and affiliations, and provides ad testing, analysis, and support. i-traffic has developed a service for NetGrocer that allows online users to make purchases through a banner ad without leaving the host Web site. As the industry trend toward consolidation continues, the company is reportedly seeking to be acquired, but wants to retain its name and independence.

iTurf Inc.

435 Hudson St., New York, NY 10014

Telephone: 212-741-7785 **Fax:** 212-807-9069 **Metro area:** New York, NY **Web site:** http://www.iturf.com **Human resources contact:** Tracy Koenig **Sales:** $134,000 **Number of employees:** 25 **Industry designation:** Computers—online services **Company type:** Subsidiary **Top competitors:** GeoCities; The Gap, Inc.; Alloy Online, Inc.

Reality bites for Generation Y. So that they won't feel less than zero, online company iTurf targets consumers between 10 and 24 with its network of community, content, and e-commerce Web sites. Its gURL.com sites offer an online magazine, an e-mail service, free homepages, and third-party content targeting teen girls and young women. Among iTurf's retail sites are dELiAs.cOm (young women's apparel), TSISoccer.com (athletic wear), contentsonline.com (furnishings), and droog.com (apparel for young men). The company generates most of its revenue from retail sales, advertising fees, and licensing fees. iTurf plans to spin off from its parent, apparel retailer dELiA*s, in an IPO.

iVillage Inc.

170 Fifth Ave., 4th Fl., New York, NY 10010

Telephone: 212-604-0963 **Fax:** 212-604-9133 **Metro area:** New York, NY **Web site:** http://www.ivillage.com **Human resources contact:** Donna Introcaso **Sales:** $15 million **Number of employees:** 200 **Number of employees for previous year:** 193 **Industry designation:** Computers—online services **Company type:** Public **Top competitors:** Lifetime Television; Oxygen Media, Inc.; Women.com Networks, Inc.

It takes an iVillage to publish Web sites for women. Promoting itself as one of the leading providers of interactive programming for women, iVillage's sites provide information and advice on careers, investing, nutrition, and health. Its nearly 750,000 members have access to e-mail, message boards, and other proprietary content. Information channels include Parent Soup, Better Health, and Work at Home. The company generates revenue from advertising and e-commerce fees. CEO Candice Carpenter has been successful at raising cash, most recently garnering $32.5 million from a variety of investors, including the Bank of Kuwait. America Online owns about 10% of the company and NBC owns 7%.

Juniper Group, Inc.

111 Great Neck Rd., Ste. 604, Great Neck, NY 11021

Telephone: 516-829-4670 **Fax:** 516-829-4691 **Metro area:** New York, NY **Sales:** $1.4 million **Number of employees:** 12 **Number of employees for previous year:** 11 **Industry designation:** Medical practice management **Company type:** Public **Top competitors:** PhyCor, Inc.; Medaphis Corporation; First Health Group Corp.

This juniper hopes its approach to the medical business will keep the company evergreen. Through its PartnerCare and Juniper Healthcare Containment Systems subsidiaries, Juniper Group offers physician practice management, liability assessment programs, cost containment, and other health care management services. PartnerCare provides a managed-care revenue enhancement program that reduces hospitals' operating costs. Juniper Group has also formed Nuclear Cardiac Imaging to provide nuclear diagnostic services to physicians in their offices for a per-test fee. Juniper Group has been scaling back its motion picture distribution activities. Marc Harris' offshore Harris Organization owns about 25% of the company.

Juno Online Services, Inc.

1540 Broadway, New York, NY 10036

Telephone: 212-597-9000 **Fax:** 212-597-9100 **Metro area:** New York, NY **Web site:** http://www.juno.com **Sales:** $21.7 million (Est.) **Number of employees:** 147 **Industry designation:** Computers—online services **Company type:** Private **Top competitors:** Microsoft Corporation; USA Networks, Inc.; America Online, Inc.

Scared of the Internet? Don't worry, Juno Online Services will hold your hand. The Internet service provider (ISP) offers a gradual path to the Internet for mainstream users, beginning with free basic e-mail (some 6.6 million accounts created) supported by advertising that users download with their mail. Billable services include enhanced e-mail (76,000 subscribers), which allows users to send attachments, and Web access (115,000 subscribers) provided through the Lycos Internet portal. Juno, which leases its network capacity from telecommunications providers, offers local dial-up access to most of the US population through more than 1,600 points of presence (POPs). Chairman David Shaw owns 62% of the company.

Kinray, Inc.

152-35 10th Ave., Whitestone, NY 11357

Telephone: 718-767-1234 **Fax:** 718-767-4388 **Metro area:** New York, NY **Web site:** http://mall6.register.com/kinray **Human resources contact:** Howard Hershberg **Sales:** $900 million (Est.) **Number of employees:** 275 **Number of employees for previous year:** 250 **Industry designation:** Drugs & sundries—wholesale **Company type:** Private **Top competitors:** Neuman Distributors, Inc.; McKesson HBOC, Inc.; Quality King Distributors Inc.

Kinray, the US's #3 privately held wholesale drug distributor (behind Neuman and Quality King), is nothing if not independent. It provides drugs, health and beauty products, medical equipment, small electronics, and school supplies and has a 500-item private label program. The company serves nearly 1,500 pharmacies in Connecticut, New Jersey, New York, and Pennsylvania. Kinray spearheaded creation of the Wholesale Alliance Cooperative, a group of about 20 independent regional drug distributors that hopes to aid independent pharmacies in their dealings with such third-party payors as HMOs and PPOs. The company was founded in 1936 by Joseph Rahr. His son, CEO and president Stewart Rahr, owns the company.

Lakeland Industries, Inc.

711-2 Koehler Ave., Ronkonkoma, NY 11779

Telephone: 516-981-9700 **Fax:** 516-981-9751 **Metro area:** New York, NY **Web site:** http://www.lakeland.com **Sales:** $47.3 million **Number of employees:** 766 **Number of employees for previous year:** 416 **Industry designation:** Protection—safety equipment & services **Company type:** Public **Top competitors:** Vallen Corporation; Worksafe Industries Inc.; Mine Safety Appliances Company

Lakeland Industries provides protection for on-the-job hazards more harmful than spilled coffee. Through several divisions, the company makes suits for toxic-waste cleanup (Chemland), fire- and heat-resistant apparel (Fireland), industrial work gloves (Highland), and industrial and medical woven-cloth garments (Uniland). Lakeland Industries is licensed to use DuPont specialty fabrics, including Kevlar and Tyvek. It has plants in Alabama, Missouri, and Mexico. Using about 20 independent sales representatives, Lakeland Industries markets its protective gear to the steel, aluminum, nuclear, automotive, and chemical industries; fire departments; utilities; and refineries. Chairman Raymond Smith owns 23% of the firm.

Mail.com, Inc.

11 Broadway, 6th Fl., New York, NY 10004

Telephone: 212-425-4200 **Fax:** 212-425-3487 **Metro area:** New York, NY **Web site:** http://www.mail.com **Human resources contact:** Keith Nagle **Sales:** $1.5 million (Est.) **Number of employees:** 92 **Number of employees for previous year:** 29 **Industry designation:** Computers—online services **Company type:** Private **Top competitors:** USA.NET, Inc.; Critical Path, Inc.; America Online, Inc.

Mail.com, bienvenue, welcome. Mail.com greets its clients with a cabaret of e-mail services. More than five million registered users have signed up for the company's Internet messaging, which Mail.com provides in collaboration with about 50 of the Web's most popular entertainment, news, sports, and search sites (including CNET, CNN, IDG, Prodigy, and Snap), as well as Internet service providers. The company's services include fax and voice-messaging and free lifetime e-mail accounts. Mail.com generates revenues from advertising, direct response, and e-commerce activities and from member subscriptions. Mail.com was launched in 1996 as iName, Inc. Founder and CEO Gerald Gorman owns about 35% of the company.

Malcolm Pirnie, Inc.

104 Corporate Park Dr., White Plains, NY 10602

Telephone: 914-694-2100 **Fax:** 914-694-2986 **Metro area:** New York, NY **Web site:** http://www.pirnie.com **Human resources contact:** Daniel R. Shevchik **Sales:** $149.6 million (Est.) **Number of employees:** 1,112 **Industry designation:** Pollution control equipment & services **Company type:** Private **Top competitors:** Montgomery Watson; ICF Kaiser International, Inc.; CH2M Hill Companies, Ltd.

Founded by two Boston sanitary engineers in 1895, Malcom Pirnie has been helping clean up water and wastewater for more than 100 years. Engineers working in 40 offices in the US consult on environmental management and restoration projects, including air and water pollution control and solid- and hazardous-waste management. Services include planning and feasibility studies, pollution control designs, construction observation, and facility management. Clients include the US Environmental Protection Agency and the Army Corps of Engineers; agencies in 17 states and hundred of cities; and the World Bank. The company is owned by senior management.

Manchester Equipment Co., Inc.

160 Oser Ave., Hauppauge, NY 11788

Telephone: 516-435-1199 **Fax:** 516-435-2113 **Metro area:** New York, NY **Web site:** http://www.manchesterequipment.com **Human resources contact:** Brian Milack **Sales:** $202.5 million **Number of employees:** 322 **Number of employees for previous year:** 263 **Industry designation:** Computers—services **Company type:** Public **Top competitors:** PC Warehouse Investment, Inc.; InaCom Corp.; Software Spectrum, Inc.

It may sound like the British are coming, but Manchester Equipment generates about 71% of its sales from integrating and reselling computer hardware, software, and networking products in the New York metropolitan area. The company also offers computer maintenance and repair, network management, and systems design services. Manchester's subsidiaries include Coastal Office Products, a provider and reseller of microcomputer servers; Electrograph Systems, a distributor of microcomputer peripherals; computer technology consultant ManTech Computer; and Manchester International, which sells computer products to resellers in the US and abroad. CEO Barry Steinberg owns 58% of the company.

MatchMaker International Development Corp.

331 Alberta Dr., Amherst, NY 14226

Telephone: 716-835-4046 **Fax:** 913-642-1702 **Metro area:** Buffalo, NY **Web site:** http://www.matchmakerintl.com **Sales:** $2 million (Est.) **Number of employees:** 225 **Industry designation:** Leisure & recreational services **Company type:** Private **Top competitors:** It's Just Lunch!, Inc.; Great Expectations International, Inc.

Among the larger dating services in the country, Matchmaker International Development has 30 offices, mostly in the eastern and midwestern US. Potential customers pay membership fees, are given interviews with company representatives, and asked to complete a compatibility questionnaire. Then Matchmaker representatives analyze the questionnaires and introduce members to others who have similar values, interests, and goals. Matchmaker leaves the date arrangements, and any ensuing sparks, up to the two parties. The company has about 1,500 active members at any one time.

MEDE America Corporation

90 Merrick Ave., Ste. 501, East Meadow, NY 11554

Telephone: 516-542-4500 **Fax:** 516-542-4508 **Metro area:** New York, NY **Web site:** http://www.mede.com **Human resources contact:** J. C. Gibson **Sales:** $42.3 million **Number of employees:** 367 **Number of employees for previous year:** 356 **Industry designation:** Computers—corporate, professional & financial software **Company type:** Public **Top competitors:** QuadraMed Corp.; Medic Computer Systems, Inc.; Shared Medical Systems Corporation

MEDE makes managing medical claims mindless. MEDE America offers computer software and services that let dentists, hospitals, pharmacies, and other health care providers across the US process and track insurance claims. The company's software, including MEDE Claim and MEDE Eligibility, electronically process and track provider enrollment and eligibility data and patient insurance claims. MEDE maintains almost 550 connections with major insurance companies, Medicare systems, and Blue Cross systems. Former chairman Thomas McInerney and director Anthony de Nicola, through investment firm Welsh, Carson, Anderson & Stowe, own 45% of the company, which processes more than 900,000 claims per day for about 65,000 clients.

Medical Action Industries Inc.

150 Motor Pkwy., Ste. 205, Hauppauge, NY 11788

Telephone: 516-231-4600 **Fax:** 516-231-3075 **Metro area:** New York, NY **Human resources contact:** Richard Satin **Sales:** $54.6 million **Number of employees:** 200 **Number of employees for previous year:** 189 **Industry designation:** Medical & dental supplies **Company type:** Public **Top competitors:** Medline Industries, Inc.; Rexam PLC; Johnson & Johnson

Medical Action Industries is soaking up success. Its main products are laparotomy sponges and operating-room towels, which together account for about 70% of sales. Medical Action Industries also makes gauze sponges, fluffs, and dressings, which are used in medical, dental, and veterinary centers. The 1999 purchase of Acme United Corporation's medical products unit (hospital kits and trays, disposable instruments) expanded Medical Action Industries' product line. Major clients include Allegiance, Owens & Minor, and McKesson General Medical. Chairman, CEO, and president Paul Meringola owns 11% of the company; his brother Joseph owns nearly 15%.

Medical Sterilization, Inc.

225 Underhill Blvd., Syosset, NY 11791

Telephone: 516-496-8822 **Fax:** 516-496-8328 **Metro area:** New York, NY **Web site:** http://www.medst.com **Human resources contact:** Ann Parasco **Sales:** $9.9 million **Number of employees:** 120 **Number of employees for previous year:** 96 **Industry designation:** Medical services **Company type:** Public **Top competitors:** Kimberly-Clark Corporation; Angelica Corporation; Sterile Recoveries, Inc.

Medical Sterilization helps hospitals and surgical centers in the Northeast keep clean by providing off-site sterilization and reprocessing of reusable surgical instruments and related items. The company returns items prepackaged in sterile containers for specific surgical procedures, including newborn delivery, tonsillectomy, and open-heart surgery. Medical Sterilization has about 85 specialized sets, including such items as utensils, surgical gowns, and basins. Medical Sterilization also provides contract sterilization. The firm and TFX Equities formed joint venture SSI Surgical Services to market sterilization and reprocessing services across North America. TFX Equities owns about 48% of Medical Sterilization.

Mediware Information Systems, Inc.

1121 Old Walt Whitman Rd., Melville, NY 11747

Telephone: 516-423-7800 **Fax:** 516-423-0161 **Metro area:** New York, NY **Web site:** http://www.mediware.com **Human resources contact:** Lori Craag **Sales:** $20.5 million **Number of employees:** 145 **Number of employees for previous year:** 133 **Industry designation:** Computers—corporate, professional & financial software **Company type:** Public **Top competitors:** Medaphis Corporation; Cerner Corporation; Medical Technology Systems, Inc.

Mediware Information Systems sells data management systems (not ready-to-wear scrubs) for pharmacies, blood banks, and surgical centers. Its systems combine third-party hardware and software with proprietary software to help manage department activities. Mediware's Hemocare system performs such blood bank functions as managing blood inventory, tracking records, and billing; and its Web-based IntraMed.net application monitors plan coverages, referrals, and benefits, among other items. Digimedics and WORx help hospitals keep tabs on their pharmacies, while StarPath manages pathology departments and Surgiware manages people, operating rooms, and equipment. Products are sold directly and through resellers.

Memorial Sloan-Kettering Cancer Center

1275 York Ave., New York, NY 10021

Telephone: 212-639-3573 **Fax:** 212-639-3576 **Metro area:** New York, NY **Web site:** http://www.mskcc.org **Human resources contact:** Michael Browne **Sales:** $693.5 million **Number of employees:** 6,142 **Number of employees for previous year:** 5,799 **Industry designation:** Hospitals **Company type:** Not-for-profit **Top competitors:** New York City Health and Hospitals Corporation; Columbia University in the City of New York; Partners HealthCare System, Inc.

Ranked as one of the nation's top cancer centers, Memorial Sloan-Kettering Cancer Center includes Memorial Hospital for pediatric and adult cancer care and the Sloan-Kettering Institute for cancer research activities. The center specializes in bone-marrow transplants and chemotherapy and offers programs in cancer prevention, treatment, research, and education. More than 500 scientists and physicians staff Memorial Sloan-Kettering, which annually admits almost 20,000 patients and logs nearly 250,000 outpatient visits. Other services include oncology nursing, pain management, and rehabilitation. The center's budget includes close to $60 million in federal and corporate research grants.

Metropolitan Baseball Club Inc.

Shea Stadium, 12301 Roosevelt Ave., Flushing, NY 11368

Telephone: 718-507-6387 **Fax:** 718-507-6395 **Metro area:** New York, NY **Web site:** http://www.mets.com **Human resources contact:** Ray A. Scott **Sales:** $80.5 million (Est.) **Number of employees:** 200 **Number of employees for previous year:** 180 **Industry designation:** Leisure & recreational services **Company type:** Private **Top competitors:** The Atlanta Braves; The Philadelphia Phillies; Montreal Baseball Club Inc.

The Metropolitan Baseball Club, better known as the New York Mets, played its first game on April 13, 1962, against Pittsburgh and lost. Losing soon became a habit, and that season the team set a 20th-century record for losses—120. All that changed in 1969 when the "Miracle Mets" won the World Series, capping a worst-to-first comeback from the previous year. Nelson Doubleday and Fred Wilpon bought the team in 1980, and six years later the Mets reclaimed the World Series crown. The Mets have struggled since then, but don't blame frugality on the part of owners anymore: the team signed catcher Mike Piazza to a seven-year, $91 million contract, paying him the equivalent of more than $80,000 per game.

Metropolitan Life Insurance Company

1 Madison Ave., New York, NY 10010

Telephone: 212-578-2211 **Fax:** 212-578-3320 **Metro area:** New York, NY **Web site:** http://www.metlife.com **Human resources contact:** Anne E. Hayden **Sales:** $24.4 billion **Number of employees:** 44,979 **Number of employees for previous year:** 43,500 **Industry designation:** Insurance—life **Company type:** Mutual company **Top competitors:** The Prudential Insurance Company of America; American International Group, Inc.; State Farm Mutual Automobile Insurance Company

Metropolitan Life Insurance (MetLife) is the US's second-largest life insurance company (behind Prudential). The company offers a variety of life insurance products and personal property/casualty insurance (homeowners and auto coverage), as well as savings, retirement, and other financial services for groups and individuals. Its insurance affiliates include Metropolitan Property and Casualty, Metropolitan Tower, and Texas Life. MetLife is the product of a merger between Metropolitan Life Insurance and New England Mutual, which expanded MetLife's traditional middle-income customer base to include upper-income clientele. MetLife plans to convert from mutual to stock ownership in 1999.

Micros-to-Mainframes, Inc.

614 Corporate Way, Valley Cottage, NY 10989

Telephone: 914-268-5000 **Fax:** 914-268-9695 **Metro area:** New York, NY **Web site:** http://www.mtm.com **Human resources contact:** Dottie Sloaman **Sales:** $69.6 million **Number of employees:** 155 **Number of employees for previous year:** 125 **Industry designation:** Computers—services **Company type:** Public **Top competitors:** Tech Data Corporation; MicroAge, Inc.; InaCom Corp.

Systems integrator Micros-to-Mainframes sells computer hardware and software, including microcomputers, printers, displays, videoconferencing equipment, and other peripherals. The company, which sells such products from companies like Dell (23% of sales), Compaq (16%), 3Com, and Novell, also provides support services (22% of sales) including system design, installation, maintenance, and network integration. Micros-to-Mainframes has two e-commerce Web sites (www.orderpc.com and www.orderpcsupplies.com) to sell its products to home shoppers. Chairman Howard Pavony and president and CEO Steven Rothman each own 25% of the company, which serves about 500 customers in the tri-state area surrounding New York City.

MIM Corporation

100 Clearbrook Rd., Elmsford, NY 10523

Telephone: 914-460-1600 **Fax:** 914-460-1660 **Metro area:** New York, NY **Web site:** http://www.mimcorp.net **Human resources contact:** Joseph DeMarte **Sales:** $451.1 million **Number of employees:** 275 **Number of employees for previous year:** 163 **Industry designation:** Medical practice management **Company type:** Public **Top competitors:** Advance Paradigm, Inc.; Express Scripts, Inc.; National Prescription Administrators Inc.

MIM is a pharmacy management organization that targets nursing homes, HMOs, and other managed care organizations with a promise to help them control their pharmacy benefit costs. MIM works with its client companies and with retail pharmacies and drug manufacturers to develop formularies, establish financial risk-sharing arrangements, and encourage the substitution of lower-cost generic drugs for brand-name drugs. Almost 70% of the company's revenues come from health services related to TennCare, a Medicaid waiver program for formerly Medicaid-eligible and certain uninsured Tennessee residents.

Minerals Technologies Inc.

The Chrysler Bldg., 405 Lexington Ave., New York, NY 10174

Telephone: 212-878-1800 **Fax:** 212-878-1801 **Metro area:** New York, NY **Web site:** http://www.shareholder.com/minerals **Human resources contact:** Howard R. Crabtree **Sales:** $609.2 million **Number of employees:** 2,260 **Number of employees for previous year:** 2,250 **Industry designation:** Chemicals—specialty **Company type:** Public

Minerals Technologies develops and produces performance-enhancing mineral, mineral-based, and synthetic mineral products for the paper, steel, food, pharmaceutical, paint, and polymer manufacturing industries. The company supplies precipitated calcium carbonate (PCC) to the North American paper industry; it also sells mineral-based monolithic refractory materials, which enable industrial furnaces to withstand high temperatures. Minerals Technologies operates six mining and processing plants and 15 refractory facilities worldwide, as well as more than 50 satellite PCC plants at customer paper plants.

MiningCo.com, Inc.

220 E. 42nd St., 24th Fl., New York, NY 10017

Telephone: 212-849-2000 **Metro area:** New York, NY **Web site:** http://www.miningco.com **Sales:** $3.7 million **Number of employees:** 113 **Number of employees for previous year:** 104 **Industry designation:** Computers—online services **Company type:** Public **Top competitors:** Yahoo! Inc.; Infoseek Corporation; America Online, Inc.

MiningCo.com won't leave you in the dark when it comes to quality Web content. The company is a Web directory with 600 GuideSites, each dedicated to a single topic and managed by an expert human guide. GuideSites are broken down into 13 channels and nearly 70 sections covering topics such as arts and entertainment, business, and news and issues. The company's guides, who go through a rigorous 16-week training, maintain their Web sites from more than 40 states and 18 countries. Its editorial staff monitors guides' sites in order to ensure that they provide quality, up-to-date information. CEO Scott Kurnit and COO William Day founded MiningCo.com in 1996. Kurnit owns about 13% of the firm.

Misonix, Inc.

1938 New Hwy., Farmingdale, NY 11735

Telephone: 516-694-9555 **Fax:** 516-694-9412 **Metro area:** New York, NY **Web site:** http://www.misonix.com **Sales:** $26.8 million **Number of employees:** 143 **Number of employees for previous year:** 108 **Industry designation:** Instruments—scientific **Company type:** Public **Top competitors:** Met-Pro Corporation; United States Filter Corporation; Emerson Electric Co.

Misonix makes ultrasonic and filtration equipment for medical and industrial markets. Its Sonicator product is a liquid processor and cell disruptor used (among other things) to extract protein from cells and to remove gas from solvents. The Sonimist is an ultrasonic spray nozzle used to remove radioactive particles, rust, blood, and oil from laboratory equipment. Filtration products from Misonix include an activated charcoal filter for use in containment hoods in laboratory settings. The company licenses its ultrasonic soft-tissue aspiration technology to Medical Device Alliance and is developing ultrasonic cutting technology with United States Surgical. Misonix owns about 87% of UK-based Labcaire Systems.

Mobius Management Systems, Inc.

120 Old Post Rd., Rye, NY 10580

Telephone: 914-921-7200 **Fax:** 914-921-1360 **Metro area:** New York, NY **Web site:** http://www.mobius-inc.com **Human resources contact:** Deborah Gross **Sales:** $56.5 million **Number of employees:** 335 **Number of employees for previous year:** 282 **Industry designation:** Computers—corporate, professional & financial software **Company type:** Public **Top competitors:** Computron Software, Inc.; New Dimension Software, Ltd.; FileNET Corporation

Mobius Management Systems makes managing data mo' better. The company makes data management software (about two-thirds of sales) for the financial, health care, manufacturing, and retail markets. Its Electronic Data Warehouse (EDW) suite accesses, stores, manages, retrieves, and distributes massive amounts of transactional data, including credit card transactions and check statements. EDW also lets users access files, including audio and video data, over the Web and corporate intranets, and provides industry-specific templates for viewing. Other products include software for enhancing tape-storage devices and the cross-application transfer of numerical data. CEO Mitchell Gross owns about 30% of the company.

Montefiore Medical Center

111 E. 210th St., Bronx, NY 10467

Telephone: 718-920-4321 **Fax:** 718-920-6321 **Metro area:** New York, NY **Human resources contact:** George Dugan **Sales:** $958.4 million **Number of employees:** 7,935 **Number of employees for previous year:** 7,570 **Industry designation:** Hospitals **Company type:** Not-for-profit **Top competitors:** Catholic Healthcare Network; New York City Health and Hospitals Corporation; Franciscan Health Partnership, Inc.

As the university hospital for the Albert Einstein College of Medicine, Montefiore Medical Center is a leading teaching and research center. More than a century old, the hospital serves residents of New York City (particularly the Bronx, where it is located) and suburban Westchester county. Specialties include vascular and infectious diseases, asthma and allergies, infertility, and pain management. It also has a geriatric program and a children's medical center. The hospital has a partnership with Bentley Health Care, created by renowned oncologist Bernard Salick, to open three cancer clinics, an AIDS center, and a network of AIDS/HIV facilities in the Bronx, Manhattan, and Westchester County.

The MONY Group Inc.

1740 Broadway, New York, NY 10019

Telephone: 212-708-2000 **Fax:** 212-708-2056 **Metro area:** New York, NY **Web site:** http://www.mony.com **Human resources contact:** Thomas J. Conklin **Sales:** $2 billion **Number of employees:** 2,324 **Industry designation:** Insurance—life **Company type:** Public **Top competitors:** New York Life Insurance Company; The Prudential Insurance Company of America; Metropolitan Life Insurance Company

Claiming to have sold the nation's first mutual life insurance policy in 1843, The MONY Group sells traditional life insurance and annuity products worldwide. In recent years it has moved into financial services, developing subsidiaries that offer investment-oriented products. These include Enterprise Capital Management (mutual funds), MONY Brokerage (retail brokerage services), and MONY Securities (securities brokerage). Other subsidiaries offer insurance and financial services overseas. Ending its more than 150-year run as a mutual insurer, The Mutual Life Insurance Company of New York demutualized and went public, becoming a subsidiary of holding company The MONY Group.

Multex.com, Inc.

33 Maiden Ln., 5th Fl., New York, NY 10038

Telephone: 212-859-9800 **Fax:** 212-859-9810 **Metro area:** New York, NY **Web site:** http://www.multex.com **Human resources contact:** Olympia Romero **Sales:** $13.2 million **Number of employees:** 149 **Number of employees for previous year:** 120 **Industry designation:** Computers—online services **Company type:** Public **Top competitors:** Primark Corporation; The Thomson Corporation; Market Guide Inc.

Multex.com (formerly Multex Systems) offers information and research services to institutional and individual investors worldwide. Its subscription Web site, MultexNET, offers a database of more than 900,000 research reports from about 400 contributors, including brokerage firms, investment banks, and independent researchers. In addition, the company offers an Internet community for individual investors (Multex Investor Network), an electronic document distribution service (MultexEXPRESS), and a research-on-demand service that provides reports that clients can download to their computers. Multex.com's services are also available through alliances with companies such as Bloomberg, Reuters, and America Online.

Nastech Pharmaceutical Company Inc.

45 Davids Dr., Hauppauge, NY 11788

Telephone: 516-273-0101 **Fax:** 516-273-0252 **Metro area:** New York, NY **Human resources contact:** Carol Wenig **Sales:** $9.6 million **Number of employees:** 46 **Number of employees for previous year:** 32 **Industry designation:** Drugs **Company type:** Public **Top competitors:** Novartis AG; Merck & Co., Inc.; Glaxo Wellcome plc

Nastech Pharmaceutical Company gets paid through the nose. The company targets its drugmaking efforts on making nasally administered drugs used to treat everything from migraines to stomach ulcers to chronic vitamin deficiencies. Most of the company's products are nasally administered versions of drugs already extant in oral or injectable forms. Commercially available Nastech products include Stadol, a narcotic analgesic marketed through Bristol-Myers Squibb, and Nascobal, a vitamin B-12 product marketed in the US through Schwarz Pharma. The company has eight nasally administered products under development.

National Basketball Association

Olympic Tower, 645 Fifth Ave., New York, NY 10022

Telephone: 212-407-8000 **Fax:** 212-754-6414 **Metro area:** New York, NY **Web site:** http://www.nba.com **Human resources contact:** Loretta Hackett **Sales:** $1.9 billion **Number of employees:** 1,000 **Number of employees for previous year:** 850 **Industry designation:** Leisure & recreational services **Company type:** Association **Top competitors:** National Football League; National Hockey League; Major League Baseball

The NBA is the #3 US sports league, behind the NFL and Major League Baseball. The 29-team league, divided into the Eastern and Western Conference, includes two Canadian teams, the Vancouver Grizzlies and the Toronto Raptors. The NBA also operates the Women's NBA (WNBA). A six month lockout by the owners stalled the opening of the 1998-99 NBA season while the owners and players argued furiously over salary issues. Now that the labor dispute has been settled, the league plans to play a 50-game season (a normal season has 82 games). When operational, the NBA is a multifaceted business with activities in consumer products, network television, and new media projects. NBA games are broadcast to 190 countries.

National Football League

280 Park Ave., New York, NY 10017

Telephone: 212-450-2000 **Fax:** 212-681-7573 **Metro area:** New York, NY **Web site:** http://www.nfl.com **Human resources contact:** John Buzzeo **Sales:** $2.4 billion **Number of employees:** 400 **Industry designation:** Leisure & recreational services **Company type:** Not-for-profit **Top competitors:** National Basketball Association; National Hockey League; Major League Baseball

Are you ready for some football? The National Football League (NFL) has been the nation's most popular sports league since football surpassed baseball in the 1970s as America's favorite spectator sport. The organization has 30 franchised teams organized into the American and National Football Conferences. The teams are run as separate businesses, but share about three-quarters of their revenues with each other. The NFL acts as a trade association for the teams' owners to promote the game, license team names and logos, collect dues, and develop new programs. The NFL has sealed the most expensive sports TV rights negotiations ever, awarding television contracts to ABC, ESPN, CBS, and Fox for nearly $18 billion.

National Hockey League

1251 Avenue of the Americas, 47th Fl., New York, NY 10020

Telephone: 212-789-2000 **Fax:** 212-789-2020 **Metro area:** New York, NY **Web site:** http://www.nhl.com **Human resources contact:** Janet A. Meyers **Sales:** $1.3 billion **Number of employees:** 289 **Number of employees for previous year:** 257 **Industry designation:** Leisure & recreational services **Company type:** Association **Top competitors:** National Football League; National Basketball Association; Major League Baseball

Billed as the league of the coolest game on earth, the National Hockey League (NHL) consists of 27 hockey teams in the US and Canada. The league, founded in 1917, is divided into the Eastern Conference (which consists of the Atlantic, Northeast, and Southeast Divisions) and the Western Conference (Central, Northwest, and Pacific Divisions). After years of flagging fan interest, the NHL has gone on the marketing offensive, jettisoning the sport's old ice-belt, thugs-on-blades image to appeal to a new generation of fans. The league's hopes for positive exposure in the 1998 Olympics were dashed due to poor coverage, a poor showing by the Americans, and their poor sportsmanship in trashing their dorms.

National Home Health Care Corp.

700 White Plains Rd., Scarsdale, NY 10583

Telephone: 914-722-9000 **Fax:** 914-722-9239 **Metro area:** New York, NY **Sales:** $34.3 million **Number of employees:** 1,800 **Number of employees for previous year:** 1,700 **Industry designation:** Health care—outpatient & home **Company type:** Public **Top competitors:** Apria Healthcare Group Inc.; New York Health Care, Inc.; Home Health Corporation of America, Inc.

National Home Health Care, through subsidiaries, provides health care services in metropolitan New York. Health Acquisition (which operates as Allen Health Care Services) offers round-the-clock home health services through RNs and personal care aides. New England Home Care serves Connecticut's Fairfield, Hartford, Litchfield, Middlesex, and New Haven counties with mental health, high-risk pregnancy, and pediatrics services in addition to standard home health services. Accredited Health provides home health services in New Jersey. Chairman/CEO Frederick Fialkow and son Steven (president, COO) own more than one-third of the acquisitive company, which has an approximately 30% stake in Florida's SunStar Healthcare.

National Medical Health Card Systems, Inc.

26 Harbor Park Dr., Port Washington, NY 11050

Telephone: 516-626-0007 **Fax:** 516-484-0679 **Metro area:** New York, NY **Web site:** http://www.nmhcs.com **Sales:** $100 million (Est.) **Number of employees:** 75 **Industry designation:** Health maintenance organization **Company type:** Private **Top competitors:** Express Scripts, Inc.; Merck & Co., Inc.; ProVantage Health Services, Inc.

National Medical Health Card Systems hopes to play its cards right. The company manages pharmacy benefits programs for other health care providers. Via the plans of sponsor companies, National Medical Health Card covers more than 430,000 individuals. The company monitors costs, provides in-depth customer and drug information, and offers consulting services to its clients, which generally include HMOs, unions, corporations, and local governments. The company offers its services through a network of 42,000 participating pharmacies. Vytra Health Plans Long Island accounts for more than 40% of the company's sales. Chairman and CEO Bert Brodsky will own about 60% of the company after the planned IPO.

NBTY, Inc.

90 Orville Dr., Bohemia, NY 11716

Telephone: 516-567-9500 **Fax:** 516-563-1180 **Metro area:** New York, NY **Web site:** http://www.nbty.com/ **Human resources contact:** Pamela Antros **Sales:** $572.1 million **Number of employees:** 3,000 **Number of employees for previous year:** 1,460 **Industry designation:** Vitamins & nutritional products **Company type:** Public **Top competitors:** Twinlab Corporation; Nature's Sunshine Products, Inc.; Rexall Sundown, Inc.

Got wort? Cashing in on the market for preventive health care, homeopathic remedies such as St. John's wort, and nutraceuticals, NBTY makes over 900 kinds of nutritional supplements, including vitamins, minerals, amino acids, and herbs. The company sells its products under the Nature's Bounty, Natural Wealth, Nutrition Headquarters, American Health, and Good 'N Natural brand names, among others. NBTY sells through independent and chain pharmacies, wholesalers, supermarkets, and health foods stores, as well as by direct mail. It operates more than 230 Vitamin World stores in 40 states and Guam and more than 400 stores in the UK under the Holland & Barrett name.

Neuromedical Systems, Inc.

2 Executive Blvd., Ste. 306, Suffern, NY 10901

Telephone: 914-368-3600 **Fax:** 914-368-3896 **Metro area:** New York, NY **Web site:** http://www.nsix.com **Human resources contact:** Patrick O'Reilly **Sales:** $9.4 million **Number of employees:** 241 **Number of employees for previous year:** 231 **Industry designation:** Medical products **Company type:** Public **Top competitors:** NeoPath, Inc.; AutoCyte, Inc.; Cytyc Corporation

The same technology for blowing Commie nuclear missiles out of the sky is now being used to detect cancerous cervical cells on Pap smears. Neuromedical Systems makes the PAPNET Testing System, a computerized image-gathering and processing service used by laboratories to reexamine Pap smears to prevent false negatives. Neuromedical Systems once rescreened most of the slides at its own labs in Hong Kong, the Netherlands, and the US, then returned the slides to clients to be analyzed with its PAPNET Review Station. However, the company is now selling both the imaging and analyzing components directly to independent laboratories under the brand PAPNET-on-Cyte. Goldman Sachs owns about one-fourth of the company.

New York Health Care, Inc.

1850 McDonald Ave., Brooklyn, NY 11223

Telephone: 718-375-6700 **Fax:** 718-375-1555 **Metro area:** New York, NY **Web site:** http://www.nyhc.com **Human resources contact:** Jerry Braun **Sales:** $13.2 million **Number of employees:** 1,200 **Number of employees for previous year:** 623 **Industry designation:** Health care—outpatient & home **Company type:** Public

New York Health Care makes house calls—the licensed home health care agency provides paraprofessional services to patients in the greater New York City area. The company has contracts with social services agencies and hospitals, including Mt. Sinai Medical Center and New York Methodist Hospital. Special services and features include a maternity/neonatal home health care service (Special Deliveries), staff members who are experienced in keeping a Kosher home, and others who are fluent in Spanish, Yiddish, and Russian. New York Health Care has purchased several home health firms since 1988. Jerry Braun, the firm's president, CEO, and COO, holds 25% of the company.

New York Islanders

Nassau Coliseum, 1255 Hempstead Tpke., Uniondale, NY 11553

Telephone: 516-794-4100 **Fax:** 516-542-9348 **Metro area:** New York, NY **Web site:** http://www.xice.com **Human resources contact:** Margret Barrett **Sales:** $46.2 million (Est.) **Number of employees:** 160 **Industry designation:** Leisure & recreational services **Company type:** Private **Top competitors:** Philadelphia Flyers; Pittsburgh Penguins; New York Rangers

The National Hockey League's (NHL) New York Islanders first skated onto the ice as an expansion team in 1972. The team had its share of disappointment in its first few years, but then dominated the NHL in the early 1980s, winning four Stanley Cup championships from 1980 to 1983. Notable Islanders include such Hall of Fame players as Denis Potvin and Mike Bossy. Howard Milstein and Steven Gluckstern each own 45% of the team, although Milstein would be forced to divest his ownership in the Islanders if his group's $800 million offer to buy the NFL's Washington Redskins is accepted (NFL rules prevent cross-ownership of teams in most cases).

New York Jets Football Club, Inc.

1000 Fulton Ave., Hempstead, NY 11550

Telephone: 516-560-8100 **Fax:** 516-560-8198 **Metro area:** New York, NY **Web site:** http://www.newyorkjets.com **Human resources contact:** Michael Gerstle **Sales:** $76.2 million (Est.) **Number of employees:** 100 **Industry designation:** Leisure & recreational services **Company type:** Private **Top competitors:** Miami Dolphins Limited; Buffalo Bills, Inc.; New England Patriots

It's easy to remember the successes of the New York Jets Football Club—you can count them on one finger. In 1969 "Broadway" Joe Namath managed to confound gamblers everywhere and lead the Jets to an upset victory over the Baltimore Colts in Super Bowl III. Otherwise, there has been little for the franchise to cheer about since the then New York Titans joined the American Football League in 1963. These days the Jets are relying on veteran coach Bill Parcels (aka "Tuna") to get the team off the ground and flying right. In 1998 he led the team to its first ever division title since joining the National Football League in 1970. Oil baron Leon Hess has owned the team since 1984.

New York Knickerbockers

Madison Square Garden, 2 Penn Plaza, New York, NY 10121

Telephone: 212-465-6471 **Fax:** 212-465-6026 **Metro area:** New York, NY **Web site:** http://www.nba.com/knicks **Human resources contact:** Aimee Kaye **Sales:** $86.2 million **Number of employees:** 34 **Number of employees for previous year:** 30 **Industry designation:** Leisure & recreational services **Company type:** Subsidiary **Parent company:** ITT Corporation **Top competitors:** New Jersey Nets; Miami Heat; Washington Wizards

The New York Knickerbockers have been among the league's best in three nonconsecutive decades. Founded in 1946 the Knicks are one of only two NBA teams still playing in its original home city (Boston is the other). New York played for the NBA title three times in the 1950s. In the early 1970s the team won two NBA titles with future Hall of Famers Willis Reed, Walt Frazier, and future senator Bill Bradley. The Knicks were ascendant again in the 1990s behind center Patrick Ewing. Although New York advanced to the NBA Finals in 1994 under coach Pat Riley, it lost to the Houston Rockets. What's a knickerbocker? The style of pants worn by New York's Dutch settlers in the 1600s. Cablevision owns the franchise.

New York Life Insurance Company

51 Madison Ave., New York, NY 10010

Telephone: 212-576-7000 **Fax:** 212-576-8145 **Metro area:** New York, NY **Web site:** http://www.newyorklife.com **Human resources contact:** Richard A. Hansen **Sales:** $17.3 billion **Number of employees:** 12,570 **Number of employees for previous year:** 12,190 **Industry designation:** Insurance—life **Company type:** Mutual company **Top competitors:** John Hancock Mutual Life Insurance Company; Metropolitan Life Insurance Company; The Prudential Insurance Company of America

Though not the only New York life insurance company, "the" New York Life Insurance Company is one of the US's top five providers of life and disability insurance policies, annuities, mutual funds, and other investments. It also provides third-party asset management services to institutions and has an agreement with the AARP to provide insurance to its members. Girding its loins to face the increased competition in its consolidating field, the company has sold its health care operations. Outside the US, New York Life has operations in Argentina, Bermuda, Hong Kong, Indonesia, Mexico, South Korea, Taiwan, and the UK.

New York Rangers

Madison Square Garden, 2 Penn Plaza, New York, NY 10121

Telephone: 212-465-6000 **Fax:** 212-465-6026 **Metro area:** New York, NY **Web site:** http://www.newyorkrangers.com **Human resources contact:** Pamela Marquis **Sales:** $74.9 million **Number of employees:** 48 **Number of employees for previous year:** 40 **Industry designation:** Leisure & recreational services **Company type:** Subsidiary **Parent company:** ITT Corporation **Top competitors:** New Jersey Devils; Philadelphia Flyers; Pittsburgh Penguins

For the 1926-27 season the National Hockey League granted Madison Square Garden a franchise for its own team, the New York Rangers; with that, the league launched one of the stalwarts of pro hockey. The Rangers made 15 playoff appearances in its first 16 seasons in the league and won four Stanley Cups over its history. The latest of these championships came in 1994 under the leadership of All Star center Mark Messier. Other notable Rangers include Hall of Famers Eddie Giacomin and all-time Ranger scoring leader Rod Gilbert (both players' jerseys hang in the Garden's rafters). The team is a subsidiary of cable TV giant Cablevision Systems, which owns the Rangers.

New York Yankees

Yankee Stadium, Bronx, NY 10451

Telephone: 718-293-4300 **Fax:** 718-293-8431 **Metro area:** New York, NY **Web site:** http://www.yankees.com **Human resources contact:** Harvey Winston **Sales:** $144.7 million (Est.) **Industry designation:** Leisure & recreational services **Company type:** Private **Top competitors:** The Boston Red Sox; Toronto Blue Jays Baseball Club; Baltimore Orioles

Those "Damn Yankees" are at it again. Formed in 1903, the New York Yankees have won 24 World Series titles and a record 35 American League pennants with the help of such icons as Babe Ruth, Lou Gehrig, and Joe DiMaggio. With an all-star lineup in the 1990s (at $63 million in 1998, the second most expensive roster in baseball behind the Baltimore Orioles), the Yankees won a World Series title in 1996 and set an AL record in 1998 for most regular season wins (114) before winning the World Series by sweeping the San Diego Padres in four games. Owner George Steinbrenner, who led a partnership that bought the team in 1973 from CBS, plans to merge the Yankees' business operations with the NBA's New Jersey Nets.

Niagara Frontier Hockey Limited Partnership

One Seymour H. Knox III Plaza, Buffalo, NY 14203

Telephone: 716-855-4100 **Fax:** 716-855-4110 **Metro area:** Buffalo, NY **Web site:** http://www.sabres.com **Human resources contact:** Vanessa Barrons **Sales:** $41.5 million (Est.) **Number of employees:** 100 **Industry designation:** Leisure & recreational services **Company type:** Private **Top competitors:** Ottawa Senators; Toronto Maple Leaf Hockey Club; Club de hockey Canadien, Inc.

With the 1998 NHL Most Valuable Player as goalie, it takes a lot to rattle the Buffalo Sabres. Led by star goalie Dominik "The Dominator" Hasek, the Sabres play in the Northeast division of NHL's Eastern Conference. First skating onto the ice in 1970, the team won its first and only Stanley Cup in the 1974-75 season. Still, the dearth of titles has not stopped fans from coming to see the Sabres' home games at Marine Midland Arena. Niagara Frontier Hockey Limited Partnership chairman John Rigas and his family own the team. Co-founder of Adelphia Communications (a Pennsylvania cable-company), Rigas was a former minority owner of the Sabres.

Norland Medical Systems, Inc.

106 Corporate Park Dr., Ste. 106, White Plains, NY 10604

Telephone: 914-694-2285 **Fax:** 920-563-8626 **Metro area:** New York, NY **Web site:** http://www2.norland.com **Sales:** $20.5 million **Number of employees:** 106 **Number of employees for previous year:** 40 **Industry designation:** Medical instruments **Company type:** Public **Top competitors:** CompuMed, Inc.; Lunar Corporation; Hologic, Inc.

Norland Medical Systems makes and markets bone densitometry systems used to help diagnose and monitor osteoporosis and other bone disorders. The desktop to full-sized equipment uses various technologies—X-ray, ultrasound, and peripheral scans—to analyze human, animal (research), and in vitro bone mass. In addition, the FDA has approved the firm's Body Composition Option, which measures soft-tissue and fat mass and can be used in treatments for AIDS, cystic fibrosis, renal failure, and weight disorders. The company sells in 40 countries and has distribution rights for medical diagnostic products manufactured by Norland Corporation, Schick, Stratec Medizintechnik, and Vitel.

North Shore-Long Island Jewish Health System

145 Community Dr., Great Neck, NY 11021

Telephone: 516-465-8000 **Fax:** 516-465-8396 **Metro area:** New York, NY **Web site:** http://warp.interstat.net/nshs/ **Human resources contact:** Ronald Stone **Sales:** $2.1 billion **Number of employees:** 27,000 **Industry designation:** Hospitals **Company type:** Not-for-profit **Top competitors:** New York City Health and Hospitals Corporation; Catholic Healthcare Network; Franciscan Health Partnership, Inc.

The result of a merger of two top-tier medical systems, North Shore-Long Island Jewish Health System operates a health care network serving New York City boroughs Brooklyn, Queens, and Staten Island, plus Nassau and Suffolk Counties. Its two anchor hospitals, North Shore University Hospital and Long Island Jewish Hospital, are affiliated with prestigious medical schools (NYU and Albert Einstein College of Medicine, respectively). The outfit, one of the largest hospital groups in the Northeast, has more than 4,000 beds in 10 hospitals, including a rehab center, a biomedical research center, a children's hospital, and an ambulatory surgery center. The company has a tie-up with PhyMatrix to develop care centers.

OCG Technology, Inc.

450 W. 31st St., New York, NY 10001

Telephone: 212-967-3079 **Fax:** 212-967-3217 **Metro area:** New York, NY **Web site:** http://www.ocgt.com **Sales:** $815,213 **Number of employees:** 7 **Number of employees for previous year:** 4 **Industry designation:** Medical instruments **Company type:** Public **Top competitors:** Medaphis Corporation; MC Informatics, Inc.; United American Healthcare Corporation

The computer will see you now. OCG Technology's PrimeCare Patient Management System gives doctors fast access to medical records that patients fill out via computer questionnaire. (OCG recommends patients access it in the waiting room, presumably instead of reading year-old "People" magazines.) Made by subsidiary PrimeCare Systems and marketed by OCG to health care providers, the PrimeCare System is sold on a pay-per-use basis. OCG also makes CodeCompiler, which keeps up with Medicare codes, and the Cardioentegraph for detecting heart disease. Subsidiary Mooney-Edwards Enterprises offers computer and consulting services to health care providers. In 1998 OCG fell below Nasdaq listing criteria and was delisted.

OmniCorder Technologies, Inc.

25 E. Loop Rd., Stony Brook, NY 11790

Telephone: 516-444-6499 **Fax:** 516-444-8825 **Metro area:** New York, NY **Web site:** http://www.omnicorder.com **Human resources contact:** Tamara Hoen **Number of employees:** 8 **Industry designation:** Medical instruments **Company type:** Private **Top competitors:** Caprius, Inc.; Biofield Corp.; Biomira Inc.

Milton Friedman probably didn't have this in mind when he spoke of "trickle-down," but Star Wars spending is now making its way to the public. OmniCorder Technologies wants to develop a device for early detection of breast cancer using Dynamic Area Telethermometry (DAT) technology developed for the Department of Defense's Missile Defense Initiative. DAT, which OmniCorder licenses from Lockheed Martin and the California Technology Institute, operates by way of hypersensitive infrared detectors. The company plans to license the DAT System to HMOs and PPOs. OmniCorder's screening device has not yet received FDA approval. CEO Mark Fauci owns more than 70% of the company.

OneMain.com, Inc.

50 Hawthorne Rd., Southampton, NY 11968

Telephone: 516-287-4084 **Fax:** 516-287-4767 **Web site:** http://www.onemain.com **Human resources contact:** Dewey K. Shay **Sales:** $56.7 million **Number of employees:** 696 **Number of employees for previous year:** 600 **Industry designation:** Computers—online services **Company type:** Public **Top competitors:** MCI WorldCom, Inc.; America Online, Inc.; AT&T Corp.

OneMain.com wants to be the one main Internet service provider (ISP) for Main Street, USA. Focusing on the underserved small town, suburban, and rural markets, OneMain.com is acquiring 17 existing ISPs in Arkansas, California, Florida, Illinois, Indiana, Kansas, Missouri, Ohio, Pennsylvania, and Tennessee, which it plans to organize into seven operating groups. The combined ISPs serve 273,000 subscribers. OneMain.com will promote dial-up and high-speed Internet access, Web hosting, e-mail, and Internet relay chat as a "Hometown Internet" service, allowing customers to use local phone numbers to connect (instead of pricier long-distance numbers).

Ortec International, Inc.

3960 Broadway, 2nd Fl., New York, NY 10032

Telephone: 212-740-6999 **Fax:** 212-740-6963 **Metro area:** New York, NY **Sales:** $300,000 **Number of employees:** 22 **Number of employees for previous year:** 16 **Industry designation:** Medical products **Company type:** Public **Top competitors:** Integra LifeSciences Corporation; LifeCell Corporation; Advanced Tissue Sciences, Inc.

Yo, Ortec! Slip me some skin! The development-stage company has developed Composite Cultured Skin (CCS), a wound dressing made of a bovine collagen matrix seeded with epidermal and dermal cells. The matrix not only covers a wound but also stimulates the body to regenerate new skin. Ortec International has received FDA approval to use CCS to treat epidermolysis bullosa, a congenital skin disease that causes severe blisters to form and upper layers of skin to slough. CCS may also have uses in cosmetic or reconstructive surgeries and in treating burns, diabetic and venous skin ulcers, and other skin diseases.

OSI Pharmaceuticals, Inc.

106 Charles Lindbergh Blvd., Uniondale, NY 11553

Telephone: 516-222-0023 **Fax:** 516-222-0114 **Metro area:** New York, NY **Human resources contact:** Edmund L. Henault **Sales:** $19.5 million **Number of employees:** 164 **Number of employees for previous year:** 156 **Industry designation:** Biomedical & genetic products **Company type:** Public **Top competitors:** AXYS Pharmaceuticals, Inc.; GeneMedicine, Inc.; Cell Genesys, Inc.

Development-stage OSI Pharmaceuticals (formerly Oncogene Science) uses proprietary technology to discover drug candidates to treat cancer, chronic anemia, muscular dystrophy, HIV, neurological disorders, and diabetes. The company's drug screens use genetically engineered human cells to identify effective drug compounds. OSI Pharmaceuticals also develops robotic high-throughput screening for more efficient generation of lead drug compounds. The company has established collaborative agreements with such companies as Bayer, Pfizer, Sankyo, and Hoechst Marion Roussel. OSI is working with the EPA to develop ways of using the company's technology to test the safety of chemicals used in everyday products.

Oxygen Media, Inc.

1370 Avenue of the Americas, 22nd Fl., New York, NY 10019

Telephone: 212-833-4400 **Fax:** 212-833-4455 **Metro area:** New York, NY **Web site:** http://www.oxygen.com **Human resources contact:** Kate Moody **Number of employees:** 100 **Industry designation:** Computers—online services **Company type:** Private **Top competitors:** Women.com Networks, Inc.; iVillage Inc.; Lifetime Television

Oxygen Media wants to bring a breath of fresh air to the male-oriented worlds of the Internet and cable TV. Founded in 1998 by former Disney and Nickelodeon executive Geraldine Laybourne, Oxygen develops branded content for women, including its three Internet sites (Thrive, MomsOnline, Electra) that focus on health and family issues. Oxygen also plans to launch a cable network in 2000 that will offer original programming and reruns from partners Harpo (producer of "The Oprah Winfrey Show") and Carsey-Werner ("Roseanne," "The Cosby Show"). The company plans to introduce more Web sites that will support and feed off of the Oxygen cable network. Other investors in the startup include America Online and Disney/ABC.

Paracelsian, Inc.

Cornell Technology Park, 266 Langmuir Laboratories, 95 Brown Rd., #1005, Ithaca, NY 14850

Telephone: 607-257-4224 **Fax:** 607-257-2734 **Metro area:** Elmira, NY **Web site:** http://www.paracelsian.com **Sales:** $55,700 **Number of employees:** 12 **Number of employees for previous year:** 7 **Industry designation:** Biomedical & genetic products **Company type:** Public **Top competitors:** SmithKline Beecham plc; Laboratory Corporation of America Holdings; Quest Diagnostics Incorporated

Paracelsus studied the curative properties of mineral water; development-stage namesake Paracelsian studies the healing power of herbs and develops drugs based on traditional Chinese herbal medicine. Its BioFIT quality-assurance assay system (distributed by a Cardinal Health subsidiary) and its drug-screening assay system work to verify the consistency of herbal extracts and to derive drugs from them. Its AH-Immunoassay toxicological-screening assay system quickly tests for dioxin pollution in the environment. Paracelsian is also working on herbal treatments for breast and prostate cancer. Directors Colin Campbell and Nelson Campbell (father and son) together own more than one-third of Paracelsian.

PAR Technology Corporation

PAR Technology Park, 8383 Seneca Tpke., New Hartford, NY 13413

Telephone: 315-738-0600 **Fax:** 315-738-0411 **Metro area:** Utica, NY **Web site:** http://www.partech.com **Human resources contact:** Ken Giffune **Sales:** $122.3 million **Number of employees:** 930 **Number of employees for previous year:** 880 **Industry designation:** Computers—peripheral equipment **Company type:** Public **Top competitors:** MICROS Systems, Inc.; Key Technology, Inc.; Point of Sale Limited

Thousands of people, eating behind the wheel, got their food fast in part because of PAR Technology. PAR makes touch pad point-of-sale equipment that inputs and displays orders at fast-food restaurants. It also makes middleware (software that lets different computers communicate) that monitors inventory, scheduling, and quality control in manufacturing and warehousing. Customers include McDonald's, Diageo's Burger King, and TRICON Global's KFC, Pizza Hut, and Taco Bell. PAR's Qscan system inspects packaged foods for objects like seed pits or glass, and its government segment makes systems for testing weapons and detecting, tracking, and targeting ground vehicles. Founder and president John Sammon owns about 45%.

Patient Infosystems, Inc.

46 Prince St., Rochester, NY 14607

Telephone: 716-242-7200 **Fax:** 716-244-1367 **Metro area:** Rochester, NY **Human resources contact:** Aneli Rivera **Sales:** $2.3 million **Number of employees:** 67 **Number of employees for previous year:** 46 **Industry designation:** Medical services **Company type:** Public

Take two tablets and Patient Infosystems will call you in the morning. The company designs, develops, and operates data management programs that contact medical patients to determine their condition and compliance with treatment protocols. The firm gathers data via a semi-automated telephone system and then processes it and generates reports for health care providers, pharmaceutical companies, and others. The firm receives payment based on the number of patients enrolled in its programs (a figure that remains low). Patient Infosystems has contracts with Bristol-Myers and other companies to provide data management for patients with asthma, diabetes, congestive heart failure, and other coronary conditions.

PennCorp Financial Group, Inc.

590 Madison Ave., New York, NY 10022

Telephone: 212-896-2700 **Fax:** 919-786-8344 **Metro area:** New York, NY **Human resources contact:** Pam Hutton **Sales:** $663.8 million **Number of employees:** 1,500 **Number of employees for previous year:** 1,371 **Industry designation:** Insurance—accident & health **Company type:** Public

PennCorp Financial Group is a holding company for about a dozen life and health insurance companies that offer low-cost life insurance, fixed-benefit accident and sickness insurance, and annuity products throughout Canada and the US. The company's products, which are targeted to middle-income individuals in rural and suburban areas, are sold through a variety of distribution channels, including exclusive agents, general agents, and payroll deduction programs. Troubled PennCorp has sold some of its units (career sales, professional insurance) to reduce debt.

Penwest Pharmaceuticals Co.

2981 Rte. 22, Patterson, NY 12563

Telephone: 914-878-3414 **Fax:** 914-878-3484 **Metro area:** Poughkeepsie, NY **Web site:** http://www.penw.com **Human resources contact:** Camille Roca **Sales:** $29 million **Number of employees:** 120 **Number of employees for previous year:** 118 **Industry designation:** Drugs **Company type:** Public **Top competitors:** Biovail Corporation International; ALZA Corporation; Elan Corporation, plc

Timing is everything to Penwest Pharmaceuticals, a developer of time-release drug delivery systems. The company's focus is developing its proprietary TIMERx drug release technology. TIMERx can be used in a variety of oral drugs to precisely control the release of active ingredients. Penwest is collaborating with pharmaceutical companies to develop drugs that utilize the TIMERx system. The company also makes and distributes excipients, the inactive ingredients in tablets and capsules that control binding, lubrication, and disintegration. Penwest was spun off from Penford Corporation in 1998.

Polymer Research Corp. of America

2186 Mill Ave., Brooklyn, NY 11234

Telephone: 718-444-4300 **Fax:** 718-241-3930 **Metro area:** New York, NY **Web site:** http://www.polymer-rd.com **Human resources contact:** Betty Friedman **Sales:** $5.4 million **Number of employees:** 53 **Number of employees for previous year:** 52 **Industry designation:** Chemicals—specialty **Company type:** Public **Top competitors:** Aceto Corporation; Sybron Chemicals Inc.; Ciba Specialty Chemicals Corporation

Transformation is a daily occurrence at Polymer Research Corp. of America (PRCA)—the company chemically "grafts" organic and inorganic substances to modify polymers and produce products such as plastics and resins. Modified polymers can resist scratching or add strength to an end product, such as tires. Rather than producing polymer products for sale, PRCA conducts contract research and development for other companies. Customers include pharmaceutical, packaging, tire, and plastics companies. The company does manufacture textile printing inks, but product sales account for only 23% of company revenues. Chairman and CEO Carl Horowitz and his wife, Irene, own 28% of PRCA.

Prodigy Communications Corporation

44 S. Broadway, White Plains, NY 10601

Telephone: 914-448-8000 **Fax:** 914-448-8083 **Metro area:** New York, NY **Web site:** http://www.prodigy.com **Human resources contact:** Nicholas Lapko **Sales:** $134.2 million **Number of employees:** 304 **Industry designation:** Computers—online services **Company type:** Public **Top competitors:** UUNET WorldCom; AT&T Corp.; CompuServe Interactive Services, Inc.

Prodigy Communications (formerly Prodigy, Inc.), the first graphical online service in the US, has morphed into a national Internet service provider (ISP). Its Prodigy Internet subscribers can get Internet access, Web hosting, and e-commerce services. Prodigy still offers its original online services, including e-mail and chat groups, as Prodigy Classic. The company, which has a total of 638,000 subscribers, is both expanding its Internet business products and targeting the US Spanish-speaking population. Mexican telecom holding company Carso Global Telecom is Prodigy's principal stockholder, with a nearly 50% stake, and Mexico's largest phone company, Telmex, owns about 20%.

Pro-Fac Cooperative, Inc.

90 Linden Place, Rochester, NY 14625

Telephone: 716-383-1850 **Fax:** 716-383-1281 **Other address:** PO Box 682, Rochester, NY 14603 **Metro area:** Rochester, NY **Human resources contact:** Lois J. Warlick-Jarvie **Sales:** $719.7 million **Number of employees:** 3,727 **Number of employees for previous year:** 3,684 **Industry designation:** Food—canned **Company type:** Cooperative **Top competitors:** Tri Valley Growers; Del Monte Foods Company; Dole Food Company, Inc.

Pro-Fac proves that fruits and veggies really do make you big and strong. The co-op's Agrilink Foods subsidiary provides marketing and processing services to more than 600 fruit- and vegetable-growing member/owners nationwide. Agrilink doubled its size when it purchased Birds Eye, Freshlike, and VegAll vegetable operations in 1998 and the Agripac frozen-vegetable business in 1999. Agrilink's Curtice Burns unit makes fruit fillings, vegetables, canned and frozen fruits, and popcorn. Agrilink also includes Nalley Fine Foods (chili, stew, pickles, dressings, syrup, salsa) and a unit that makes potato chips and salty snacks. Formed in 1960, Pro-Fac produces private-label and brand-name foods.

Progenics Pharmaceuticals, Inc.

777 Old Saw Mill River Rd., Tarrytown, NY 10591

Telephone: 914-789-2800 **Fax:** 914-789-2817 **Metro area:** New York, NY **Web site:** http://www.progenics.com **Human resources contact:** Robert A. McKinney **Sales:** $14 million **Number of employees:** 40 **Number of employees for previous year:** 32 **Industry designation:** Drugs **Company type:** Public **Top competitors:** IDEC Pharmaceuticals Corporation; Vertex Pharmaceuticals Incorporated; Agouron Pharmaceuticals, Inc.

Progenics Pharmaceuticals runs the gamut from A to C: it is developing drugs to combat AIDS precursor HIV and cancer. Primary products under development are GMK and MGV vaccines for melanoma and other cancers. Bristol-Myers Squibb is collaborating on these products. Also in the pipeline are PRO 542, designed to prevent HIV from infecting healthy cells by bonding with the virus before it strikes the cells, and PRO 367, designed to kill HIV-infected cells. Partners in its HIV research include Genzyme Transgenics, Roche Holding, and Pharmacopeia. In the meantime, the company has begun selling diagnostic reagents and assays developed during its research. Paul Tudor Jones's Tudor Investment owns 31% of the company.

PRT Group Inc.

342 Madison Ave., 11th Fl., New York, NY 10173

Telephone: 212-922-0800 **Fax:** 212-922-0806 **Metro area:** New York, NY **Web site:** http://www.prt.com **Human resources contact:** Carol Anderson **Sales:** $85.6 million **Number of employees:** 867 **Number of employees for previous year:** 700 **Industry designation:** Computers—services **Company type:** Public **Top competitors:** Cambridge Technology Partners (Massachusetts), Inc.; Renaissance Worldwide, Inc.; Perot Systems Corporation

PRT Group's service station keeps a company's computer network rolling down the data highway. The firm provides information technology (IT) services to global companies in the financial services, consumer products, communications, and health care industries. Its services include group and individual staffing for long- and short-term IT projects, which account for more than 50% of its sales. Other support includes consulting, IT planning, software development, maintenance outsourcing, and year 2000 date changes. Customers J.P. Morgan, Philip Morris, and Prudential Insurance each account for more than 10% of sales. Brothers Douglas (chairman and CEO), Gregory (COO), and Paul Mellinger own 32% of the company.

PSC Inc.

675 Basket Rd., Webster, NY 14580

Telephone: 716-265-1600 **Fax:** 716-265-6400 **Metro area:** Rochester, NY **Web site:** http://www.pscnet.com **Human resources contact:** Dennis T. Hopwood **Sales:** $217.2 million **Number of employees:** 1,200 **Number of employees for previous year:** 1,150 **Industry designation:** Optical character recognition **Company type:** Public **Top competitors:** NCR Corporation; Symbol Technologies, Inc.; Metrologic Instruments, Inc.

The steady beeping of bar code scanners—such as those made by PSC—has replaced the "cha-ching" of cash registers in stores. In addition to retail checkout, bar code scanners are used for inventory management, shipping, automated luggage and parcel sorting, and other functions. PSC makes handheld and fixed-position scanners, as well as automated machines used in retail, commercial, and industrial segments. The company's U-Scan Express self-checkout system lets customers scan and pay for purchases without a salesperson or checker. PSC also sells accessories (antennae, printers, power supplies) for use with its systems. PSC is looking for growth in foreign markets, where almost half of its sales occur.

Razorfish, Inc.

107 Grand St., 3rd Fl., New York, NY 10013

Telephone: 212-966-5960 **Fax:** 212-966-6915 **Metro area:** New York, NY **Web site:** http://www.razorfish.com **Human resources contact:** Elizabeth Semple **Sales:** $13.8 million (Est.) **Number of employees:** 380 **Number of employees for previous year:** 350 **Industry designation:** Computers—services **Company type:** Private **Top competitors:** Proxicom, Inc.; Modem Media.Poppe Tyson, Inc.; Icon Medialab International AB

Razorfish is sucking up the tank's other inhabitants in its efforts to dominate the Internet-design aquarium. The company specializes in high-end Internet development and the all-encompassing services that go with it—consultation, implementation, management, and enhancement. Razorfish's clients include Microsoft, eBay, Time Warner, the Smithsonian Institution, Charles Schwab, and Ericsson. Razorfish continues a strategy of buying up other high-end Internet development firms (including Sweden's Spray, whose shareholders own a 38% stake in Razorfish) to grow geographically and expand its client base. Advertising firm Omnicom Group also owns 38% of the company.

Regeneron Pharmaceuticals, Inc.

777 Old Saw Mill River Rd., Tarrytown, NY 10591

Telephone: 914-347-7000 **Fax:** 914-347-2113 **Metro area:** New York, NY **Web site:** http://www.regeneron.com **Human resources contact:** Vicki Gaddy **Sales:** $38.2 million **Number of employees:** 371 **Number of employees for previous year:** 270 **Industry designation:** Biomedical & genetic products **Company type:** Public **Top competitors:** Genentech, Inc.; Amgen Inc.; Rhone-Poulenc Rorer Inc.

Regeneron Pharmaceuticals seeks to develop and commercialize protein-based and small-molecule drugs to treat neurological, inflammatory, and muscle diseases, as well as cancer and other serious conditions. One of the company's principal interests is the discovery and development of neurotrophic factors (naturally occurring proteins that are required for nerve cells, or neurons, to grow and sustain themselves). Regeneron has signed a long-term agreement with Procter & Gamble to jointly develop and market AXOKINE, a neurotrophic drug for the treatment of diabetes-related obesity. The company also has partnership agreements with Amgen, Glaxo-Wellcome, Medtronic, Sumitomo, and other companies.

REXX Environmental Corporation

350 Park Ave., New York, NY 10022

Telephone: 212-750-7755 **Fax:** 212-789-8924 **Metro area:** New York, NY **Sales:** $2.3 million **Number of employees:** 159 **Number of employees for previous year:** 150 **Industry designation:** Pollution control equipment & services **Company type:** Public

REXX Environmental Corporation helps business and governmental clients get clean. Through subsidiary Watkins Contracting, the company provides environmental services such as asbestos removal, soil remediation, hazardous materials clean-up, and demolition, primarily within California. REXX Environmental once operated as Oak Hill Sportswear Corporation, a designer, importer, manufacturer, and marketer of moderately priced women's clothing and accessories, but in 1995 management performed a corporate demolition, selling off the underperforming sportswear operations. REXX Environmental adopted its current form and name in 1998 following the acquisition of Watkins, a privately held environmental services contractor.

RMS Titanic, Inc.

17 Battery Place, Ste. 203, New York, NY 10004

Telephone: 212-558-6300 **Fax:** 212-482-1912 **Metro area:** New York, NY **Web site:** http://www.titanic-online.com **Sales:** $4.7 million **Number of employees:** 4 **Number of employees for previous year:** 3 **Industry designation:** Leisure & recreational services **Company type:** Public

Riding the wave of interest created by the popular movie, RMS Titanic is capitalizing on its controversial but exclusive salvage rights to the legendary ship that sank in 1912. The company has recovered 5,000 artifacts from the wreck during five expeditions and preserves and displays the items in worldwide public exhibitions. The company also sells photos, replicas, and souvenir coal, among other merchandise. In addition, it makes money through licensing agreements for books and video products, furniture replication, and exploratory expeditions. Though unrelated to the movie, RMS Titanic has benefited from increased merchandise sales since its release (1998 first half earnings jumped a whopping 380%).

Ronnybrook Farm Dairy, Inc.

Prospect Hill Rd., Ancramdale, NY 12503

Telephone: 518-398-6455 **Fax:** 518-398-6464 **Metro area:** Poughkeepsie, NY **Sales:** $842,000 (Est.) **Number of employees:** 11 **Industry designation:** Food—dairy products **Company type:** Private

Ronnybrook Creamline brand milk and other dairy products by Ronnybrook Farm Dairy are sold in New York and northern New Jersey. The dairy's products go to more than 150 supermarkets and delis, about 50 food service clients, the Culinary Institute of America, and directly to the public through outdoor green markets and the company's distribution center. All of the company's raw milk comes from Ronnybrook Farms, a local dairy farm owned and operated by the Osofsky family. The dairy also produces milk and cream (in glass bottles), butter, ice cream, yogurt, and assorted cheeses. Following the company's planned IPO, brothers Richard, Sidney, and Ronald Osofsky will each own about 17% of Ronnybrook Farm Dairy's stock.

Schick Technologies, Inc.

31-00 47th Ave., Long Island City, NY 11101

Telephone: 718-937-5765 **Fax:** 718-937-5962 **Metro area:** New York, NY **Web site:** http://www.schicktech.com **Human resources contact:** Arthur King **Sales:** $38.5 million **Number of employees:** 392 **Number of employees for previous year:** 173 **Industry designation:** Medical instruments **Company type:** Public **Top competitors:** Trex Medical Corporation; DENTSPLY International Inc.; Siemens AG

Smile pretty for the camera! Schick Technologies makes medical and dental digital imaging equipment. Its main product is CDR (computed dental radiography), an X-ray system that uses less radiation than conventional equipment, fits inside the mouth, incorporates an oral camera, and produces the images on a computer instead of film. The company also makes the accuDEXA, a bone densitometer. Schick is developing a digital mammography device capable of producing low-cost computer images of a wide surface area. Schick's products are based on technology developed at the California Institute of Technology's Jet Propulsion Laboratory. The company has facilities in New Jersey and New York.

Seneca Foods Corporation

1162 Pittsford-Victor Rd., Pittsford, NY 14534

Telephone: 716-385-9500 **Fax:** 716-385-4249 **Metro area:** Rochester, NY **Web site:** http://www.senecafoods.com **Human resources contact:** Cindy Ford **Sales:** $703.2 million **Number of employees:** 3,062 **Number of employees for previous year:** 2,572 **Industry designation:** Food—canned **Company type:** Public **Top competitors:** Chiquita Brands International, Inc.; Pro-Fac Cooperative, Inc.; Del Monte Foods Company

Seneca Foods has a "can-do" attitude. As a major produce processor, Seneca cans and freezes fruits and vegetables for sale to the retail and food service industries under its own brands, including Seneca, Libby's, and Aunt Nellie's, and for private-label brands. It is the primary packer of Pillsbury's Green Giant brand of vegetables. Once the producer of the nation's top-selling frozen apple juice concentrate, the company sold nearly all of its juice operations to Northland Cranberries in 1998. Seneca's only nonfood division, Seneca Flight Operations, is an air charter in upstate New York. Chairman Arthur Wolcott and president and CEO Kraig Kayser and their families control 40% voting power in the company.

SFX Entertainment, Inc.

650 Madison Ave., 16th Fl., New York, NY 10022

Telephone: 212-838-3100 **Fax:** 212-702-0126 **Metro area:** New York, NY **Sales:** $884.3 million **Number of employees:** 1,300 **Number of employees for previous year:** 950 **Industry designation:** Leisure & recreational services **Company type:** Public **Top competitors:** Feld Entertainment, Inc.; TBA Entertainment Corporation; Ticketmaster Group, Inc.

Concert promoter SFX Entertainment is a spinoff of SFX Broadcasting (which is now part of Capstar Broadcasting). SFX Entertainment owns, leases, or manages about 82 venues in 31 of the top 50 markets in the US. The company promotes such events as concerts, touring Broadway shows, and motorsports. SFX has acquired promoters Delsener/Slater Enterprises (metropolitan New York City), Bill Graham Presents (San Francisco Bay area), and PACE Entertainment (nationwide), among others. The company expanded into the sports arena with its purchase of Falk Associates Management Enterprises (FAME), an agency that represents primarily NBA players including Patrick Ewing.

Shiseido Cosmetics (America) Ltd.

900 Third Ave., 15th Fl., New York, NY 10022

Telephone: 212-805-2300 **Fax:** 212-688-0109 **Metro area:** New York, NY **Human resources contact:** Barbara Aubin **Industry designation:** Cosmetics & toiletries **Company type:** Subsidiary **Parent company:** Shiseido Company, Limited **Top competitors:** Revlon, Inc.; L'Oreal; The Procter & Gamble Company

If you want to kiss and makeup, Shiseido can help. Shiseido Cosmetics (America) is a subsidiary of Shiseido Company, Japan's largest cosmetics firm. The parent company produces makeup and skin care products (accounting for about three-fourths of sales), toiletries, and professional beauty salon products. Shiseido Cosmetics (America) manufactures makeup and skin care products sold worldwide. Shiseido Company sells its products in about 50 countries but gets only about 15% of sales outside Japan. To aid its goal of increasing international sales to 25% of the total, it has bought various North American operations from Helene Curtis and Lamaur Corp.

SIGA Pharmaceuticals, Inc.

420 Lexington Ave., Ste. 620, New York, NY 10170

Telephone: 212-672-9100 **Fax:** 212-697-3130 **Metro area:** New York, NY **Web site:** http://www.siga.com **Sales:** $700,000 **Number of employees:** 19 **Number of employees for previous year:** 10 **Industry designation:** Drugs **Company type:** Public

SIGA Pharmaceuticals is a development stage company that produces vaccines, antibiotics, and novel anti-infectives for infectious diseases. The company is working on developing a vaccine for strep throat that can be given directly through the mucus-lined surfaces (mouth, nose, lungs, and gastrointestinal and urogenital tracts) that are the usual entry points for most infectious agents. Other vaccines are being developed to prevent sexually transmitted diseases. SIGA Pharmaceuticals is also working on anti-infective drugs that keep bacteria from attaching to human tissue, and has an alliance with the Ludwig Institute for Cancer Research to develop cancer vaccines.

StarMedia Network, Inc.

29 West 36th Street, 5th Fl., New York, NY 10018

Telephone: 212-548-9600 **Fax:** 212-631-9100 **Metro area:** New York, NY **Web site:** http://www.starmedia.com **Human resources contact:** Tyrone Fripp **Sales:** $5.3 million (Est.) **Number of employees:** 247 **Industry designation:** Computers—online services **Company type:** Private **Top competitors:** Cisneros Group of Companies; Yahoo! Inc.; quepasa.com, inc.

StarMedia Network offers Spanish- and Portuguese-speaking Web surfers the chance to plug in to cyberspace. The company's starmedia.com Web portal is the world's largest Spanish-language Web site and features local content from Latin American and US newspapers as well as e-mail, chat rooms, bulletin boards, and home pages. The company is hoping to foster a sense of community among Hispanic Web surfers and is beefing up its efforts to draw US visitors. StarMedia generates revenue through e-commerce and advertising. Chase Venture Capital Associates owns about 27% of the company. Chairman and CEO Fernando Espuelas and president Jack Chen, who co-founded StarMedia Network in 1996, each own about 14% of the company.

Sunnydale Farms, Inc.

400 Stanley Ave., Brooklyn, NY 11207

Telephone: 718-257-7600 **Fax:** 718-257-7466 **Metro area:** New York, NY **Human resources contact:** Susan Prager **Sales:** $145 million **Industry designation:** Food—dairy products **Company type:** Subsidiary **Top competitors:** Nestle S.A.; Dean Foods Company; Suiza Foods Corporation

Sunnydale Farms nurses New York City's appetite for milk. The company is a major processor of milk and other dairy products in the Big Apple, nearby Long Island and Westchester County, and Connecticut and New Jersey. As part of recent consolidation in the dairy industry, Sunnydale was bought in 1998 by Parmalat USA, a subsidiary of Italy's Parmalat Finanziaria, the world's leading fluid (not powdered) milk producer. Parmalat hopes to provide technological and marketing assistance to Sunnydale and to introduce Parmalat products that have proved successful at its other US dairy operations.

Superior Supplements, Inc.

270 Oser Ave., Hauppauge, NY 11788

Telephone: 516-231-0783 **Fax:** 516-231-3515 **Metro area:** New York, NY **Sales:** $10.3 million **Number of employees:** 61 **Number of employees for previous year:** 19 **Industry designation:** Vitamins & nutritional products **Company type:** Public **Top competitors:** NBTY, Inc.; Perrigo Company; IVC Industries, Inc.

Superior Supplements knows that eating right is just part of staying healthy. The dietary supplement maker's health-centric product line includes vitamins, minerals, herbs, and specialty nutritional supplements. Products are available in capsule, powder, and tablet form and are sold to third-party drug retailers who market them in convenience, drug, health food, and discount stores under their own brands. The company has agreements with PDK Labs to supply and package specially manufactured vitamins and dietary supplements; sales to PDK account for almost 90% of revenues. Barry Gersten owns more than half of the company he founded.

Swissray International, Inc.

200 E. 32nd St., Ste. 34-B, New York, NY 10016

Telephone: 212-545-0095 **Fax:** 212-545-7912 **Metro area:** New York, NY **Web site:** http://www.swissray.com **Sales:** $22.9 million **Number of employees:** 116 **Number of employees for previous year:** 110 **Industry designation:** Medical instruments **Company type:** Public **Top competitors:** Toshiba Corporation; Siemens AG; General Electric Company

Giving Superman's X-ray eyes a run for the money, Swissray International sells X-ray and imaging equipment to the health care industry. Its products include imaging equipment used in radiology, such as mobile X-ray and remote control examination systems. The company's AddOn-Multi-System generates instant digital X-ray images. The SwissVision workstation allows sectioning and enlargement of X-rays and transfers of images through networks and telecommunications systems. Swissray has contracts to build X-ray systems for Philips Medical Systems. Its products are sold by medical equipment suppliers in the US and Europe.

Symbol Technologies, Inc.

One Symbol Plaza, Holtsville, NY 11742

Telephone: 516-738-2400 **Fax:** 516-738-5990 **Metro area:** New York, NY **Web site:** http://www.symbol.com **Human resources contact:** Robert Blonk **Sales:** $977.9 million **Number of employees:** 3,700 **Number of employees for previous year:** 3,200 **Industry designation:** Optical character recognition **Company type:** Public **Top competitors:** Telxon Corporation; Fujitsu Limited; NCR Corporation

Symbol Technologies is the world leader in bar code scanners and portable data terminals, with customers including General Motors and the US Postal Service. Its products use laser technology and wireless LANs to retrieve data, such as product and price information, everywhere from the grocery store to the stock market. The company makes bar code scanners (handheld laser scanners, fixed-station card-reading devices), portable data-collection devices (handheld computers, radio modems), and software and programming tools (DOS-based programs, application-development kits). Symbol serves customers in such industries as warehousing and distribution, parcel delivery and postal service, retail, and health care.

Taro Pharmaceutical Industries Ltd.

5 Skyline Dr., Hawthorne, NY 10532

Telephone: 914-345-9001 **Fax:** 914-345-8728 **Metro area:** New York, NY **Web site:** http://www.taropharma.com **Human resources contact:** Nitza Lifshitz **Sales:** $66.7 million **Industry designation:** Drugs—generic **Company type:** Public **Top competitors:** Warner-Lambert Company; Novartis AG; Medicis Pharmaceutical Corporation

Generic drugs are Taro's future. Taro Pharmaceutical Industries makes generic and proprietary drugs to treat dermatologic conditions, epilepsy, and other diseases. The company specializes in topical corticosteroids with such products as hydrocortisone valerate cream and ointment and clobetasol proprionate solution, among other products. It also makes teril carbamazepine tablets that are equivalent to Tegretol, Novartis' epilepsy treatment. Other drugs include clomipramine hydrochloride, an antidepressant, and acetazolamide, a diuretic. Taro sells its products through HMOs, drugstore chains, drug distributors, and grocery stores.

Tate & Lyle North American Sugars

1114 Avenue of the Americas, New York, NY 10036

Telephone: 212-789-9700 **Fax:** 212-789-9746 **Metro area:** New York, NY **Web site:** http://www.tlna.com **Industry designation:** Food—sugar & refining **Company type:** Subsidiary **Parent company:** Tate & Lyle PLC **Top competitors:** Imperial Sugar Company; Sterling Sugars, Inc.; American Crystal Sugar Company

Tate & Lyle North American Sugars sweetens the pot for its UK-based parent company, Tate & Lyle PLC. The company accounts for more than 20% of the US sugar market with its Domino Sugar brand and also sells sugar in Canada under the Redpath name. Both brands include white, brown, dark brown, and confectioners sugars. Tate & Lyle North American Sugars also operates Western Sugar, which processes beet sugar in six plants in the western US. Domino Sugar traces its roots back to two brothers who founded a New York refinery in 1807. Tate & Lyle is a global producer of sugar, cereal sweeteners, and starches that also has popular brands in Europe, Africa, and Australia.

theglobe.com, inc.

31 W. 21st St., New York, NY 10010

Telephone: 212-886-0800 **Fax:** 212-367-8588 **Metro area:** New York, NY **Web site:** http://www.theglobe.com **Human resources contact:** David Tonkin **Sales:** $5.5 million **Number of employees:** 80 **Industry designation:** Computers—online services **Company type:** Public **Top competitors:** GeoCities; Microsoft Corporation; Lycos, Inc.

theglobe.com provides free Internet services, including Web site building, chat rooms, e-mail, and a marketplace for various products. Seeking to be a portal for mouse potatoes, it also offers movie reviews, horoscopes, games, and personal ads for its 2.3 million members. Founded in 1995 by Cornell grads Todd Krizelman and Stephan Paternot, theglobe.com derives most of its sales from advertising. The company also sells subscriptions for clients who need enhanced services. Major ad clients include Lee Jeans and Coca Cola. The firm also has a number of corporate partnerships, including one with ad industry rag "Advertising Age." Chairman Michael Egan owns about 50% of the firm.

TheStreet.com, Inc.

2 Rector St., 14th Fl., New York, NY 10006

Telephone: 212-271-4004 **Fax:** 212-271-4005 **Metro area:** New York, NY **Web site:** http://www.thestreet.com **Human resources contact:** Simon Clark **Sales:** $4.6 million (Est.) **Number of employees:** 122 **Number of employees for previous year:** 45 **Industry designation:** Computers—online services **Company type:** Private **Top competitors:** Microsoft Corporation; The Motley Fool, Inc.; Morningstar, Inc.

TheStreet.com delivers in-your-face Wall Street news and analysis to about 37,000 subscribers via its Web site. It covers equities and mutual funds and offers news and opinion columns from its own staff and guest analysts. Tough-talking co-founder Jim Cramer predicts the site will overtake Dow Jones and Reuters in financial coverage. TheStreet.com has deals in place with Yahoo! and America Online to drive traffic to its site. Cramer, a hedge-fund manager, and "The New Republic" editor in chief Martin Peretz launched the venture in 1996. Cramer, Peretz, SOFTBANK, and The New York Times Company own interests in TheStreet.com.

Town Sports International, Inc.

888 Seventh Ave., New York, NY 10106

Telephone: 212-246-6700 **Fax:** 212-246-8422 **Metro area:** New York, NY **Web site:** http://www.nysc.com **Human resources contact:** Anthony Imcona **Sales:** $82.4 million (Est.) **Number of employees:** 2,600 **Industry designation:** Leisure & recreational services **Company type:** Private **Top competitors:** Bally Total Fitness Holding Corporation; Kelley Automotive Group

Town Sports International owns or operates 64 fitness clubs serving some 175,000 members in the Northeast and Mid-Atlantic. About 80% of the clubs are located in or around New York (including 18 clubs in New Jersey and Connecticut) under the New York Sports Club name. Other locations include Washington, DC; Boston; and Philadelphia. The company establishes club clusters, groupings which allow it to sell higher-priced memberships offering multiple-club access. Its clubs offer cardio-aerobic and strength-training equipment as well as aerobic classes, private training, and physical therapy, among other services. In addition, each region's flagship club offers swimming pools and racquetball and basketball courts.

Transworld HealthCare, Inc.

555 Madison Ave., New York, NY 10022

Telephone: 212-750-0064 **Fax:** 212-750-7221 **Metro area:** New York, NY **Web site:** http://www.twhh.com **Human resources contact:** Fatin Biner **Sales:** $155.3 million **Number of employees:** 680 **Number of employees for previous year:** 440 **Industry designation:** Health care—outpatient & home **Company type:** Public **Top competitors:** Lincare Holdings Inc.; Salick Health Care, Inc.; Star Multi Care Services, Inc.

Transworld HealthCare delivers. The company provides medical products and services to US and UK patients in their homes. US operations (which account for about 45% of sales) include infusion therapy and home medical equipment sales. The company's primary US service areas are New Jersey and New York; it also sells specialty mail-order pharmaceutical and medical supplies nationwide and in Puerto Rico. Transworld Healthcare's UK subsidiary provides medical supplies, respiratory therapy, and nursing services from some 70 locations. Investment group Hyperion Partners II owns more than 67% of Transworld HealthCare.

TSR, Inc.

400 Oser Ave., Hauppauge, NY 11788

Telephone: 516-231-0333 **Fax:** 516-435-1428 **Metro area:** New York, NY **Web site:** http://www.tsrconsulting.com **Sales:** $70.4 million **Number of employees:** 387 **Number of employees for previous year:** 347 **Industry designation:** Computers—services **Company type:** Public **Top competitors:** Analysts International Corporation; Metamor Worldwide, Inc.; Computer Horizons Corp.

TSR has the IT girl, but she ain't Clara Bow. TSR provides contract computer programmers to "FORTUNE" 1000 companies to augment their in-house information technology staffs. The company can call on a pool of about 35,000 technical personnel to provide services, including mainframe computer operations, voice and data communications, and network computing support in metropolitan New York, New England, and the Mid-Atlantic. TSR also offers companies a way to check their computer codes for year 2000 compliance using its proprietary Catch/21 software. Catch/21 automates a large part of the conversion process. Chairman and CEO Joseph Hughes owns 35% of the company.

24/7 Media, Inc.

1250 Broadway, New York, NY 10001

Telephone: 212-231-7100 **Fax:** 212-760-1774 **Metro area:** New York, NY **Web site:** http://www.247media.com **Human resources contact:** Audrey Blauner **Sales:** $19.9 million **Number of employees:** 200 **Number of employees for previous year:** 100 **Industry designation:** Computers—online services **Company type:** Public **Top competitors:** DoubleClick Inc.; NetGravity, Inc.; CMGI, Inc.

24/7 Media is an Internet advertising and marketing firm that makes money by selling ads and promotions to its Web site affiliates. The company offers advertisers a broad base of online content by operating the 24/7 Network (a group of more than 80 Web sites) and the ContentZone, a network of more than 2,000 small to medium-sized Web sites. Customers can buy ad space on a specific Web site, within a particular content channel, or across an entire network. In addition, 24/7 Media licenses its Adfinity and dbCommerce software products, which use demographics to deliver ads to specific audiences and help track the effectiveness of ads.

Twinlab Corporation

2120 Smithtown Ave., Ronkonkoma, NY 11779

Telephone: 516-467-3140 **Fax:** 516-630-3490 **Metro area:** New York, NY **Web site:** http://www.twinlab.com **Human resources contact:** Nestor Navarri **Sales:** $333.4 million **Number of employees:** 974 **Number of employees for previous year:** 634 **Industry designation:** Vitamins & nutritional products **Company type:** Public **Top competitors:** Herbalife International, Inc.; Celestial Seasonings, Inc.

Twinlab makes vitamins, sports drinks, and herbal supplements sold primarily in health foods stores. Most of its nearly 1,000 products are marketed under the Twinlab name; its herbal supplements are marketed under the name Nature's Herbs. The company also sells Alvita brand tea. The company sells its products internationally primarily through specialty stores, such as GNC, and a growing cadre of independent distributors. Twinlab is developing its direct-mail operations, through which it will sell its existing nutritional supplements, as well as new products under development. It also publishes the monthly magazine "All Natural Muscular Development," which focuses on steroid-free bodybuilding.

UniHolding Corporation

96 Spring St., New York, NY 10012

Telephone: 212-219-9496 **Fax:** 212-925-2184 **Metro area:** New York, NY **Human resources contact:** Andrea Kay **Sales:** $83.5 million **Number of employees:** 700 **Number of employees for previous year:** 680 **Industry designation:** Medical services **Company type:** Public **Top competitors:** Covance Inc.; SmithKline Beecham plc; Laboratory Corporation of America Holdings

If you come down with something between the Eiffel Tower and the Vatican and you're not sure what it is, try visiting one of UniHolding's testing facilities. Through a minority stake in subsidiaries in Italy, Spain, Switzerland, Turkey, and the UK, the company operates a network of about 20 clinical laboratory testing facilities that serve general practitioners, hospitals, health care providers, and specialists. The company's labs and specimen-collection centers offer a broad range of tests to diagnose, monitor, and treat medical conditions. Chairman Edgard Zwirn controls the network's operations through his majority ownership in UniHolding's main subsidiary.

Universal American Financial Corp.

6 International Dr., Ste. 190, Rye Brook, NY 10573

Telephone: 914-934-5200 **Fax:** 914-934-0700 **Metro area:** New York, NY **Human resources contact:** Joan M. Ferrarone **Sales:** $51.3 million **Number of employees:** 265 **Number of employees for previous year:** 231 **Industry designation:** Insurance—life **Company type:** Public

Universal American Financial is a life, accident, and health insurance holding company for American Pioneer Life, American Progressive Life and Health, and American Exchange Life. Universal targets the senior market by offering Medicare supplement, home health care and nursing home, and hospital indemnity insurance. Universal uses independent marketing groups to sell its products throughout the US. WorldNet, a subsidiary, provides communication, managed care, and claims adjudication to the company and third parties. Chairman and CEO Richard Barasch and his family own about half of Universal American.

Vasomedical, Inc.

180 Linden Ave., Westbury, NY 11590

Telephone: 516-997-4600 **Fax:** 516-997-2299 **Metro area:** New York, NY **Web site:** http://www.vasomedical.com **Human resources contact:** Joseph A. Giacalone **Sales:** $5.2 million **Number of employees:** 32 **Number of employees for previous year:** 26 **Industry designation:** Medical instruments **Company type:** Public **Top competitors:** Hoechst AG; St. Jude Medical, Inc.; Astra AB

Vasomedical's noninvasive treatment device for coronary heart disease, EECP, has some angina patients' blood pumping. During the company's Medicare-covered treatments for angina and coronary heart disease, cuffs are applied to a patient's calves, thighs, and buttocks; the cuffs are inflated and deflated in sync with the patient's heart beat, which increases and decreases aortic blood pressure. After about 35 one-hour treatments, patients may experience years of symptomatic relief. Vasomedical's EECP device consists of a control unit, air compressor, compression cuffs, and electrocardiogram and pulse-monitoring unit. The EECP is marketed to hospitals, clinics, and cardiac health care professionals worldwide.

V.I. Technologies, Inc.

155 Duryea Rd., Melville, NY 11747

Telephone: 516-752-7314 **Fax:** 516-752-8768 **Metro area:** New York, NY **Human resources contact:** Jacqueline Roberts **Sales:** $33.8 million **Number of employees:** 265 **Number of employees for previous year:** 235 **Industry designation:** Medical products **Company type:** Public

V.I. Technologies (VITEX) uses its proprietary viral inactivation technologies to eliminate dangerous viruses from its blood products, including plasma, red blood cells, and platelets. The company's transfusion plasma, created and distributed in conjunction with the American Red Cross under the name PLAS+SD, uses solvent/detergent viral inactivation technology to eliminate viruses such as hepatitis A, B, and C and HIV. VITEX has other strategic agreements with Bayer, United States Surgical Corporation, and Pall Corporation. The New York Blood Center (of which VITEX chairman David Tendler is a member of the board of trustees) owns about 29% of VITEX's stock.

NORTH CAROLINA

Applied Analytical Industries, Inc.

5051 New Centre Dr., Wilmington, NC 28403

Telephone: 910-392-1606 **Fax:** 910-791-4711 **Metro area:** Wilmington, NC **Human resources contact:** Eugene T. Haley **Sales:** $80.4 million **Number of employees:** 850 **Number of employees for previous year:** 750 **Industry designation:** Medical services **Company type:** Public

Applied Analytical Industries provides drug development and support services to pharmaceutical and biotechnology companies worldwide. The company's services range from drug formulation and development to regulatory and compliance consulting, providing US and European companies an alternative to internal development programs. In addition to its fee-for-service business, Applied Analytical Industries licenses internally developed drugs and drug technologies, focusing on generic products, patented technologies, and line extensions. Its products include hormone pharmaceuticals developed by 40%-owned Endeavor Pharmaceuticals. Frederick Sancilio owns almost 30% of the firm.

AutoCyte, Inc.

780 Plantation Dr., Burlington, NC 27215

Telephone: 336-222-9707 **Fax:** 336-222-8819 **Metro area:** Greensboro, NC **Web site:** http://www.rias.com **Sales:** $4.8 million **Number of employees:** 83 **Number of employees for previous year:** 78 **Industry designation:** Medical instruments **Company type:** Public **Top competitors:** Cytyc Corporation; NeoPath, Inc.; Neuromedical Systems, Inc.

AutoCyte wants gynecologists to move from Pap to PREP with its cytology equipment, designed to make cervical cancer screenings more efficient and accurate. AutoCyte believe its automated PREP system is better than standard Pap smears because it can not only preserve more cells but can do so for several months, allowing follow-up testing from the original sample. After slides are prepared with PREP, AutoCyte's SCREEN system uses automated microscopes, digital color cameras, and monitors to diagnose samples. The company's products, which are sold overseas, are awaiting clearance from the FDA. Former parent Roche Image Analysis Systems owns nearly 25% of the company.

The Body Shop Incorporated

5036 One World Way, Wake Forest, NC 27587

Telephone: 919-554-4900 **Fax:** 919-554-4361 **Metro area:** Raleigh-Durham, NC **Human resources contact:** Kathy Schwartz **Industry designation:** Cosmetics & toiletries **Company type:** Subsidiary **Parent company:** The Body Shop International PLC **Top competitors:** Intimate Brands, Inc.; Garden Botanika, Inc.; The Estee Lauder Companies Inc.

Hoping to stimulate Americans in body and soul, The Body Shop (US subsidiary of UK-based The Body Shop International) sells natural skin and hair care products through about 290 owned and franchised shops in the US. Known for activism as much as aromatherapy, the company uses minimal packaging, encourages recycling, and campaigns for social causes. The Body Shop appears worn out from body blows such as declining sales, unhappy franchise owners, and heavy competition (from stores with similar product lines, such as Intimate Brands' Bath & Body Works and chains such as the Gap adding personal care lines). The company has aimed to get in shape with new management through a joint venture with Bellamy Retail Group.

Broadway & Seymour, Inc.

128 S. Tryon St., Charlotte, NC 28202

Telephone: 704-372-4281 **Fax:** 704-344-3015 **Metro area:** Charlotte, NC **Web site:** http://www.bsis.com **Human resources contact:** Mary Stokes **Sales:** $69 million **Number of employees:** 465 **Number of employees for previous year:** 450 **Industry designation:** Computers—corporate, professional & financial software **Company type:** Public

Broadway & Seymour is an information technology company that provides software and services to financial institutions, law firms, and professional service companies. Products include TouchPoint, a software system that retrieves customer data for use in offices, branches, and call centers; Elite Billing System, an online accounting and billing software; and Elite Case Management System, a software for tracking legal cases. Broadway & Seymour offers systems maintenance and support services to customers on a renewable-contract basis. Chase Manhattan Bank accounts for about 13% of the company's business. Sales to customers in Europe make up about 10% of the company's revenue.

Carolina Hurricanes Hockey Club

5000 Aerial Center Pkwy., Ste. 100, Morrisville, NC 27560

Telephone: 919-467-7825 **Fax:** 919-462-7030 **Metro area:** Raleigh-Durham, NC **Web site:** http://www.caneshockey.com **Human resources contact:** Mike Amendola **Sales:** $25.1 million (Est.) **Number of employees:** 105 **Number of employees for previous year:** 90 **Industry designation:** Leisure & recreational services **Company type:** Private **Top competitors:** Florida Panthers Holdings, Inc.; Tampa Bay Lightning; Washington Capitals

The National Hockey League's Carolina Hurricanes met with an icy reception upon moving to North Carolina in 1997 (the former Hartford Whalers spent about 20 years in Connecticut). Its average attendance of about 7,500 is last in the NHL, and majority owner Peter Karmanos, who bought the team in 1994, lost $30 million in the Canes' first year in North Carolina. The club was lured from Connecticut by the promise of a new arena (the $152 million Entertainment and Sports Arena is scheduled for completion by the 1999-2000 season) and the chance to earn a percentage of concessions, parking, and box seats. Owners hope that the team's move to Raleigh from its temporary location in Greensboro will help it find more fans.

Carolina Panthers

800 S. Mint St., Charlotte, NC 28202

Telephone: 704-358-7000 **Fax:** 704-358-7618 **Metro area:** Charlotte, NC **Web site:** http://www.cpanthers.com **Sales:** $83 million (Est.) **Industry designation:** Leisure & recreational services **Company type:** Private **Top competitors:** Atlanta Falcons; San Francisco 49ers; New Orleans Saints

In 1959 Jerry Richardson (now owner of the Carolina Panthers) earned $4,864 for catching a Johnny Unitas touchdown pass to win the championship game between the Baltimore Colts and the New York Giants. Richardson used the money to buy a restaurant. In 1993 (many business deals later) Richardson scored again with his $140 million purchase of the NFL expansion team. The Panthers hit the grid in 1995, earning a respectable 7-9 season. In 1996 respectable became awesome as the Panthers beat Super Bowl champs Dallas in first-round playoffs. The Panther's new home, $184 million Ericsson Stadium, also opened that year. Even without a winning season, the team secures a spot near the top of the list for franchise value.

Carroll's Foods, Inc.

2822 W. Hwy. 24, Warsaw, NC 28398

Telephone: 910-293-3434 **Fax:** 910-293-3199 **Metro area:** Fayetteville, NC **Web site:** http://www.carrollsfoods.com **Human resources contact:** Dick Reece **Sales:** $500 million (Est.) **Number of employees:** 2,500 **Industry designation:** Food—meat products **Company type:** Private **Top competitors:** ConAgra, Inc.; Murphy Family Farms; Premium Standard Farms, Inc.

Carroll's Foods is hog-wild about pork and poultry. The US's #2 hog producer (after Murphy Family Farms), the company has farms in Iowa, North and South Carolina, Utah, Virginia, Brazil, and Mexico. Carroll's is being acquired by top pork processor Smithfield Foods in a deal that will make the resulting company #1 in both US hog production and processing (the two are exclusive representatives of the extra-lean NPD line of pigs in the US and Mexico). Smithfield will then acquire Carroll's share of the Circle Four Farms hog operation in southwestern Utah. Carroll's also is one of the largest turkey producers in the US. President F. J. "Sonny" Faison Jr. owns Carroll's.

CEM Corporation

3100 Smith Farm Rd., Matthews, NC 28105

Telephone: 704-821-7015 **Fax:** 704-821-7894 **Other address:** PO Box 200, Matthews, NC 28106 **Metro area:** Charlotte, NC **Web site:** http://www.cemx.com **Human resources contact:** Stephen V. Spradling **Sales:** $32.4 million **Number of employees:** 177 **Number of employees for previous year:** 176 **Industry designation:** Instruments—scientific **Company type:** Public **Top competitors:** Arizona Instrument Corporation; Thermo Electron Corporation; J.M. Voith AG

CEM breaks the beakers and cools the burners. CEM—short for chemistry, electronics, and mechanics—claims a 70% share of the market for microwave-based instruments that perform testing, analysis, and process control in laboratory and industrial markets. Its MARS and MDS heating systems, which analyze samples by dissolving them in acid, account for one-third of sales. The company sells its products direct in the US and through independent dealers worldwide to the food, chemicals, tobacco, textiles, pulp and paper, and other industries. President and CEO Michael Collins owns 16% of the company.

Charlotte Hornets

100 Hive Dr., Charlotte, NC 28217

Telephone: 704-357-0252 **Fax:** 704-357-0289 **Metro area:** Charlotte, NC **Web site:** http://www.nba.com/hornets **Human resources contact:** Debby Benson **Sales:** $56.4 million (Est.) **Number of employees:** 65 **Number of employees for previous year:** 50 **Industry designation:** Leisure & recreational services **Company type:** Private **Top competitors:** Pacers Basketball Corporation; Chicago Bulls; Atlanta Hawks, Ltd.

In Charlotte, North Carolina, basketball don't mean a thing if it ain't got that sting. Although the Charlotte Hornets play in one of the National Basketball Association's (NBA) smallest markets, the team racks up attendance figures and merchandise sales that rank among the league's best. Admitted to the NBA as an expansion club in 1987, the Hornets began play during the 1988-89 season. A playoff contender during most of the late 1990s, the Hornets have had more problems off the court than on, as team owner George Shinn and power forward Anthony Mason have been accused of sexual misconduct. Both Mason and Shinn have civil suits pending.

Closure Medical Corporation

5250 Greens Dairy Rd., Raleigh, NC 27616

Telephone: 919-876-7800 **Fax:** 919-790-1041 **Metro area:** Raleigh-Durham, NC **Human resources contact:** Diane Lewis **Sales:** $9.6 million **Number of employees:** 96 **Number of employees for previous year:** 61 **Industry designation:** Medical products **Company type:** Public **Top competitors:** Anika Therapeutics, Inc.; Cohesion Technologies, Inc.; Fusion Medical Technologies, Inc.

Closure Medical Corporation may not be able to heal your unresolved childhood psychological traumas, but it can seal the lacerations that accompanied them. Closure's primary product, Dermabond, is a tissue glue designed to close cuts and wounds. Dermabond forms a flexible, waterproof coating over the wound that keeps it clean, making sutures and bandages superfluous. The company's products are based on cyanoacrylate, an adhesive material compatible with living tissue. Closure also produces adhesives for periodontal and veterinary treatments. The company has marketing agreements with Johnson & Johnson's Ethicon and Innocoll of Germany. Co-founders Rolf and William Schmidt each own about a fourth of Closure.

C3, Inc.

3800 Gateway Blvd., Ste. 310, Morrisville, NC 27560

Telephone: 919-468-0399 **Fax:** 919-468-0486 **Metro area:** Raleigh-Durham, NC **Human resources contact:** Linda Hahn **Sales:** $4 million **Number of employees:** 49 **Number of employees for previous year:** 35 **Industry designation:** Chemicals—diversified **Company type:** Public **Top competitors:** Anglo American Corporation of South Africa Limited; Dia Met Minerals Ltd.; Comcast Corporation

Diamonds are C3's best friends. The company markets its patented, lab-created moissantie gemstones to the jewelry industry as a substitute for diamonds. Composed of silicon and carbon, the mineral moissanite (aka silicon carbide or SiC) is found mostly in meteorites. The company makes gemstones from SiC crystals grown by Cree Research and sells them as loose stones, costing about 5%-10% of the price of natural diamonds. The company also sells an instrument that can distinguish between a fake diamond and the real thing. C3 distributes through more than 70 retailers in the US.

Embrex, Inc.

1035 Swabia Ct., Durham, NC 27703

Telephone: 919-941-5185 **Fax:** 919-941-5186 **Other address:** PO Box 13989, Research Triangle Park, NC 27709 **Metro area:** Raleigh-Durham, NC **Human resources contact:** Pam Rose **Sales:** $28.6 million **Number of employees:** 121 **Number of employees for previous year:** 106 **Industry designation:** Biomedical & genetic products **Company type:** Public

Embrex develops and markets bioscience and bioengineering-based products designed to increase the productivity and profitability of the poultry industry. The company has developed and commercialized the only in ovo (in the egg) automated egg injection system, eliminating the need for manual vaccination of newly hatched broiler chicks. Its patented INOVOJECT system inoculates 100% of chicks three days prior to hatch versus the post-hatch injection method. This sanitized injection system inoculates 20,000-30,000 chicks, and the system is used to inject more than 80% of birds raised in the US. Embrex has entered China via a contract with the Great Wall Food Company, Ltd., a major Chinese poultry producer.

Glaxo Wellcome Inc.

5 Moore Dr., Research Triangle Park, NC 27709

Telephone: 919-483-2100 **Fax:** 919-483-0084 **Other address:** PO Box 133998, Research Triangle Park, NC 27709 **Metro area:** Raleigh-Durham, NC **Web site:** http://www.glaxowellcome.com **Number of employees:** 8,500 **Industry designation:** Drugs **Company type:** Subsidiary **Parent company:** Glaxo Wellcome plc **Top competitors:** Johnson & Johnson; Merck & Co., Inc.; Bristol-Myers Squibb Company

When patients thank their doctors for helping heal them, the response is probably "wellcome" —Glaxo Wellcome. The eponymous US subsidiary of the UK-based pharmaceutical giant, Glaxo Wellcome develops and markets medicines. With research facilities in North Carolina, the company works to find new treatments cancer, diabetes, obesity, osteoporosis, viral diseases, and urological and sexually transmitted diseases. Among the pharmaceuticals manufactured at its North Carolina and Rhode Island plants are allergy treatment Flonase and migraine tablets Imitrex. Glaxo Wellcome also makes HIV therapies Ziagen, Epivir, Retrovir, and Combivir.

Intercardia, Inc.

3200 E. Hwy. 54, Cape Fear Bldg., Ste. 300, Research Triangle Park, NC 27709

Telephone: 919-558-8688 **Fax:** 919-558-8686 **Other address:** PO Box 14287, Research Triangle Park, NC 27709 **Metro area:** Raleigh-Durham, NC **Web site:** http://www.intercardia.com **Human resources contact:** Ann Redick **Sales:** $6.1 million **Number of employees:** 55 **Number of employees for previous year:** 19 **Industry designation:** Drugs **Company type:** Public **Top competitors:** Forest Laboratories, Inc.; SmithKline Beecham plc; Merck & Co., Inc.

Intercardia develops cardiovascular and pulmonary therapeutics. Through 80%-owned subsidiary CPEC, Intercardia is developing beta-blocker BEXTRA (bucindolol), which is in Phase III clinical trials, to treat congestive heart failure. Intercardia's other publicly owned subsidiaries are Aeolus Pharmaceuticals (66%), which develops treatments for respiratory ailments and arthritis, and Renaissance Cell Technologies (80%), which conducts liver-cell research. The Intercardia Research Laboratories division (formerly Transcell Technologies) develops products based on synthetic carbohydrate chemistry. Interneuron Pharmaceuticals owns more than 60% of Intercardia.

Krispy Kreme Doughnut Corporation

370 Knollwood, Ste. 500, Winston-Salem, NC 27103

Telephone: 336-725-2981 **Fax:** 336-733-3794 **Other address:** PO Box 83, Winston-Salem, NC 27102 **Metro area:** Greensboro, NC **Web site:** http://www.krispykreme.com **Human resources contact:** Barbara Thornton **Sales:** $202 million (Est.) **Number of employees:** 2,200 **Industry designation:** Food—confectionery **Company type:** Private **Top competitors:** Allied Domecq PLC; McDonald's Corporation; Winchell's Donut Houses Operating Co. L.L.P.

Sinkers anyone? Krispy Kreme makes a variety of doughnuts (including the original glazed that generates half its sales) at 1950s-styled stores that offer views of the doughnut-making process. About half of its 130-plus stores are franchised. Although increasingly focused on the retail market, Krispy Kreme gets some 65% of its sales from wholesale distribution to grocery and convenience stores. The company, which is capitalizing on its cult status with merchandise tie-ins and a brand of coffee, makes its own machines and still uses Cajun chef Joe LeBeau's original recipe. A Southeastern institution, the company is expanding nationwide. The McAleer family owns 50% of Krispy Kreme, which was founded in 1937.

Laboratory Corporation of America Holdings

358 S. Main St., Burlington, NC 27215

Telephone: 336-229-1127 **Fax:** 336-222-1568 **Metro area:** Greensboro, NC **Web site:** http://www.labcorp.com **Human resources contact:** Robert Elder **Sales:** $1.6 billion **Number of employees:** 18,800 **Number of employees for previous year:** 18,600 **Industry designation:** Medical services **Company type:** Public **Top competitors:** Quest Diagnostics Incorporated; SmithKline Beecham plc; LabOne, Inc.

Following SmithKline Beecham and Quest Diagnostics, Laboratory Corporation of America Holdings (LabCorp) is the #3 clinical lab service in the US. LabCorp was formed by the merger of National Health Laboratories and Roche Biomedical Laboratories. The laboratory performs diagnostic tests for a wide range of health care providers and other institutions in 25 major laboratories and 1,200 service sites nationwide. It performs more than 1,700 different clinical tests (from routine blood analyses to molecular diagnostics) for over 130,000 clients. LabCorp emphasizes its specialty and niche testing business (allergy tests, HIV viral load tests, and others).

MedCath Incorporated

7621 Little Ave., Ste. 106, Charlotte, NC 28226

Telephone: 704-541-3228 **Fax:** 704-541-2615 **Metro area:** Charlotte, NC **Web site:** http://www.medcath.com/ **Sales:** $200 million (Est.) **Number of employees:** 2,000 **Number of employees for previous year:** 1,630 **Industry designation:** Medical services **Company type:** Private **Top competitors:** Columbia/HCA Healthcare Corporation; Tenet Healthcare Corporation; MedPartners, Inc.

MedCath owns and manages medical facilities specializing in cardiology and cardiovascular services. The company operates heart hospitals in Austin and McAllen, Texas; Tucson and Phoenix, Arizona; and Little Rock, Arkansas. Hospitals in California, New Mexico, and Ohio are thumping along, too. MedCath also leases mobile cardiac catheterization labs to 250 hospitals across the US and provides physician practice management services to heart specialists. MedCath enters new markets through acquisitions and by partnering with local heart specialists and offering them a piece of the business. Along with Medcath's management, investment firms Kohlberg Kravis Roberts and Welsh, Carson, Anderson & Stowe own the company.

Medco Research, Inc.

PO Box 13886, Research Triangle Park, NC 27709

Telephone: 919-653-7001 **Fax:** 919-653-7099 **Other address:** PO Box 13886, Research Triangle Park, NC 27709 **Metro area:** Raleigh-Durham, NC **Web site:** http://www.medcores.com **Human resources contact:** Jody Slater **Sales:** $27.5 million **Number of employees:** 27 **Number of employees for previous year:** 23 **Industry designation:** Drugs **Company type:** Public

Medco Research, a drug development company, specializes in treatments for heart disease. Rather than investing in basic research, the company typically buys potential products and sponsors testing needed to bring them to market. Medco then licenses the manufacturing and marketing rights to a corporate partner in exchange for fees and royalties. The company's products include Adenocard, a syringe-administered drug used to treat rapid heartbeats, and Adenoscan, a drug used to diagnose damage from coronary artery disease. Another product in development, Adenosine for Cardioprotection, is designed to reduce damage following a heart attack.

Murphy Family Farms

4134 S. US Hwy. 117, Rose Hill, NC 28458

Telephone: 910-289-2111 **Fax:** 910-289-6400 **Metro area:** Wilmington, NC **Sales:** $650 million (Est.) **Number of employees:** 1,900 **Number of employees for previous year:** 1,000 **Industry designation:** Agricultural operations **Company type:** Private **Top competitors:** Carroll's Foods, Inc.; Smithfield Foods, Inc.; Premium Standard Farms, Inc.

Murphy Family Farms brings home the bacon, pig time. The #1 hog farmer in the US (it will drop to #2 when Smithfield Foods buys Carroll's Foods) is two-thirds owned by pork potentate Wendell Murphy, who founded the operation in 1962 (family members own the rest). Piglets are bred at more than 125 farms in North Carolina and the Midwest, with about 335,000 sows total. (The farms play country music in the nursing rooms to calm piglets.) Piglets are raised by contract farmers paid to keep them until they reach a slaughtering weight of 250 pounds; they are then delivered to packers. Murphy Family Farms owns six million pigs in various growth stages.

Novant Health, Inc.

3333 Silas Creek Pkwy., Winston-Salem, NC 27103

Telephone: 336-718-5000 **Fax:** 336-718-9258 **Metro area:** Greensboro, NC **Web site:** http://www.novanthealth.org **Human resources contact:** Mel Asbury **Sales:** $1.1 billion **Number of employees:** 13,000 **Number of employees for previous year:** 5,109 **Industry designation:** Hospitals **Company type:** Not-for-profit **Top competitors:** Bon Secours Health System, Inc.; Sentara Health System; Mid Atlantic Medical Services, Inc.

A not-for-profit health care system with facilities in North and South Carolina and Virginia, Novant Health was formed in 1997 by the merger of Carolina Medicorp and Presbyterian Health Services. The system includes nine inpatient facilities with about 2,150 beds, three long-term-care facilities, a women's health and wellness center, and more than 60 outpatient offices. Novant Health also includes the for-profit PARTNERS National Health Plans of North Carolina, an HMO covering 275,000 members. Affiliates of the system include Community General Health Partners of Thomasville, North Carolina, and Nash Health Care System of Rocky Mount, North Carolina.

Pharmaceutical Product Development, Inc.

3151 17th St. Ext., Wilmington, NC 28412

Telephone: 910-251-0081 **Fax:** 910-762-5820 **Metro area:** Wilmington, NC **Web site:** http://www.ppdi.com/HOMEPAGE.HTM **Human resources contact:** David Williams **Sales:** $235.6 million **Number of employees:** 3,100 **Number of employees for previous year:** 2,470 **Industry designation:** Medical services **Company type:** Public

Human guinea pigs and newfangled drugs are Pharmaceutical Product Development, Inc.'s focus. As a contract research firm for drug and biotechnology companies around the world, it performs clinical testing, laboratory operations, clinical trial and data management, statistical analysis, and medical writing; it also recruits patients that it pays to be test subjects for new drugs. Contracts last from a few months to several years. One subsidiary offers scientific, technical, and strategic consulting services, including evaluating hazardous-waste contamination and proposing remedies. Clinical trials and some specialized services are routinely outsourced.

Quintiles Transnational Corp.

4709 Creekstone Dr., Ste. 200, Durham, NC 27703

Telephone: 919-941-2000 **Fax:** 919-941-9113 **Other address:** PO Box 13979, Research Triangle Park, NC 27709 **Metro area:** Raleigh-Durham, NC **Web site:** http://www.quintiles.com **Human resources contact:** Phil Newton **Sales:** $1.2 billion **Number of employees:** 10,900 **Number of employees for previous year:** 7,375 **Industry designation:** Medical services **Company type:** Public **Top competitors:** ClinTrials Research Inc.; PAREXEL International Corporation; Covance Inc.

Quintiles Transnational is in the top percentile. In fact, it's the world's largest contract research and marketing organization, providing testing and marketing services that help major pharmaceutical companies bring their drugs to market. Quintiles carries out clinical (testing the efficacy of drugs and devices on human subjects) and preclinical studies (testing product risk) and offers biostatistical analysis, health economics studies, data management, and research. The company, which operates in 30 countries, also markets medical products through late-phase and post-approval trials that compare different drugs of the same type and find new uses for existing drugs. Quintiles has grown through acquisitions.

Royster-Clark, Inc.

409 Main St., Tarboro, NC 27886

Telephone: 252-823-2101 **Fax:** 252-641-9234 **Web site:** http://www.roysterclark.com **Human resources contact:** Thomas A. Ergish **Sales:** $1.1 billion (Est.) **Number of employees:** 2,650 **Industry designation:** Fertilizers **Company type:** Private **Top competitors:** Agrium Inc.; IMC Global Inc.; Terra Industries Inc.

To grow a good crop, many farmers rely on a good rain and a lot of help from Royster-Clark, producer of fertilizer, seed, crop nutrients, pesticides and herbicides. The company also provides crop management, blending, spreading, and delivery services. The crop management services use global positioning satellite systems and software to provide statistics on crop yields, as well as satellite-linked equipment that can apply precise amounts of fertilizer or crop-protection products to a particular site. Royster-Clark's genetically engineered seeds include Roundup Ready soybeans. The company has more than 130 retail supply and service centers in seven states in the southeastern US, and it distributes to 27 states.

Source Technologies, Inc.

628 Griffith Rd., Charlotte, NC 28217

Telephone: 704-522-8500 **Fax:** 704-522-7533 **Metro area:** Charlotte, NC **Web site:** http://www.sourcetech.com **Human resources contact:** Gordon Friedrich **Sales:** $28.5 million (Est.) **Number of employees:** 60 **Number of employees for previous year:** 50 **Industry designation:** Computers—peripheral equipment **Company type:** Private **Top competitors:** Printronix, Inc.; Zebra Technologies Corporation; Troy Group, Inc.

Source Technologies makes printers, retail and financial self-service kiosks, electronic forms generation systems, and software to integrate its products into host networks. The company's products include laser printers that produce electronic forms, Magnetic Ink Character Recognition printers for secure printing of negotiable documents like cashiers checks and money orders, dot and line matrix printers, and specialty bar code printers. Source Technologies' financial kiosk systems handle remote banking transactions such as account inquiries, fund transfers, ATM access, and loan applications, and also distribute products including hotel room keys, stamps, and ATM cards.

Speedway Motorsports, Inc.

US Hwy. 29 North, Concord, NC 28026

Telephone: 704-455-3239 **Fax:** 704-455-2547 **Other address:** PO Box 600, Concord, NC 28026 **Metro area:** Charlotte, NC **Web site:** http://www.speedwaymotorsports.com **Human resources contact:** Cynthia Mankus **Sales:** $229.8 million **Number of employees:** 700 **Number of employees for previous year:** 452 **Industry designation:** Leisure & recreational services **Company type:** Public **Top competitors:** International Speedway Corporation; Dover Downs Entertainment, Inc.; Penske Motorsports, Inc.

Speedway Motorsports promotes, markets, and sponsors motorsports activities in the US. The company owns and operates six racing venues: the Lowe's Motor Speedway in North Carolina, Atlanta Motor Speedway, Bristol Motor Speedway in Tennessee, Las Vegas Motor Speedway, Sears Point Raceway in California, and Texas Motor Speedway in Fort Worth. The company sponsors 15 major racing events annually that are sanctioned by NASCAR. It also owns, operates, and sanctions the Legends Car and Bandolero Racing Circuits, an entry-level stock car racing series. Speedway manufactures and sells 5/8-scale modified cars for use on its circuits. Chairman and CEO Bruton Smith owns about 68% of the company.

Tangram Enterprise Solutions, Inc.

11000 Regency Pkwy. Ste. 401, Cary, NC 27511

Telephone: 919-653-6000 **Fax:** 919-653-6004 **Metro area:** Raleigh-Durham, NC **Web site:** http://www.tesi.com **Human resources contact:** Susan Barbee **Sales:** $20.7 million **Number of employees:** 141 **Number of employees for previous year:** 136 **Industry designation:** Computers—corporate, professional & financial software **Company type:** Public **Top competitors:** Microsoft Corporation; Intel Corporation; International Business Machines Corporation

Tangram Enterprise Solutions develops and sells asset-tracking software. Its Asset Insight software allows companies to automatically track and analyze enterprisewide information technology assets and Year 2000 problems. Its Internet Subsystem add-on allows Internet-usage tracking. Tangram also offers products for managing heterogeneous computer resources throughout entire organizations (AM:PM software) and asset-tracking consulting and implementation services. Tangram markets its products to "FORTUNE" 1000 companies and government agencies through more than 25 value-added resellers, system integrators, and information technology service providers. Safeguard Scientifics owns more than 65% of the company.

Triangle Pharmaceuticals, Inc.

4 University Place, 4611 University Dr., Durham, NC 27707

Telephone: 919-493-5980 **Fax:** 919-493-5925 **Metro area:** Raleigh-Durham, NC **Web site:** http://www.tripharm.com **Human resources contact:** Dan Giannini **Sales:** $100,000 **Number of employees:** 120 **Number of employees for previous year:** 70 **Industry designation:** Drugs **Company type:** Public **Top competitors:** BioQuest, Inc.; Agouron Pharmaceuticals, Inc.; Vertex Pharmaceuticals Incorporated

Triangle Pharmaceuticals develops new drug candidates, primarily antiviral therapies. Triangle's emphasis is on treating HIV, AIDS, and the hepatitis B virus using combinations of drugs, a method that shows promise in treating HIV. The company also develops drugs to treat brain, lung, and other cancers. Triangle Pharmaceuticals focuses on drug development rather than the time-consuming, expensive process of drug discovery. All of its drugs are in the clinical or preclinical trial stages. The company has license agreements with Emory University and the University of Georgia Research Foundation for various drug candidates.

Trimeris, Inc.

4727 University Dr., Ste. 100, Durham, NC 27707

Telephone: 919-419-6050 **Fax:** 919-419-1816 **Metro area:** Raleigh-Durham, NC **Web site:** http://www.trimeris.com **Sales:** $400,000 **Number of employees:** 38 **Number of employees for previous year:** 37 **Industry designation:** Drugs **Company type:** Public **Top competitors:** Merck & Co., Inc.; Abbott Laboratories; Glaxo Wellcome plc

Trimeris is a development-stage company working on drugs that prevent viruses from fusing to a host cell, keeping cells safe. The company's lead product, T-20, is in Phase II clinical trials to test its ability to inhibit fusion of HIV with human cells. Trimeris' product differs from existing offerings in that it seeks to prevent infection as opposed to attacking reproducing viruses. The company has an agreement with MiniMed to utilize their pump that attaches to a patient's belt and continuously delivers T-20 intravenously. Trimeris is also developing orally-administered products to prevent other types of viral infections. Chairman Jesse Treu and director Brian Dovey together own 25% of the company.

Wake Forest University Baptist Medical Center

Medical Center Blvd., Winston-Salem, NC 27157

Telephone: 336-716-2011 **Fax:** 336-716-6841 **Metro area:** Greensboro, NC **Web site:** http://www.wfubmc.edu **Human resources contact:** Ron Hoth **Sales:** $959.7 million **Number of employees:** 9,400 **Number of employees for previous year:** 9,266 **Industry designation:** Hospitals **Company type:** Not-for-profit **Top competitors:** Novant Health, Inc.; UnitedHealth Group; Columbia/HCA Healthcare Corporation

The mind-body connection is clear at Wake Forest University Baptist Medical Center. Formerly known as Bowman Gray/Baptist Hospital Medical Center, the non-profit is comprised of Wake Forest University School of Medicine and The North Carolina Baptist Hospitals, including the Sticht Center on Aging and Rehabilitation, the Comprehensive Cancer Center, the Heart Center, Brenner Children's Hospital, CompRehab, the Nursing Center at Oak Summit, and three home care services. The not-for-profit system has also developed QualChoice, a health maintenance organization (HMO) with over 75,000 members and 1,400 physicians, and a practice management service for more than 1,000 physicians.

NORTH DAKOTA

Great Plains Software, Inc.

1701 SW 38th St., Fargo, ND 58103

Telephone: 701-281-0550 **Fax:** 701-281-3752 **Metro area:** Fargo-Moorhead, ND **Web site:** http://www.greatplains.com **Human resources contact:** Michael A. Slette **Sales:** $85.7 million **Number of employees:** 755 **Number of employees for previous year:** 561 **Industry designation:** Computers—corporate, professional & financial software **Company type:** Public **Top competitors:** Computer Associates International, Inc.; The Sage Group plc; Platinum Software Corporation

Great Plains Software can use its own line of software to account for its success. The company's Dynamics financial software line is designed for small to midsized businesses, with Dynamics C/S+ designed for the more complex needs of larger companies. The software's modules also manage processes such as reporting, manufacturing, payroll, and electronic commerce. About two-thirds of Great Plains' sales come from software licensing, and the balance comes from training and software support services. A network of resellers markets Great Plains' products worldwide. Members of the Burgum family own more than 35% of the company.

OHIO

The Andersons, Inc.

480 W. Dussel Dr., Maumee, OH 43537

Telephone: 419-893-5050 **Fax:** 419-891-6670 **Other address:** PO Box 119, Maumee, OH 43537 **Metro area:** Toledo, OH **Web site:** http://www.andersonsinc.com **Human resources contact:** Joseph C. Christen **Sales:** $1.1 billion **Number of employees:** 3,035 **Number of employees for previous year:** 2,962 **Industry designation:** Agricultural operations **Company type:** Public

The Andersons operates grain elevators and markets grain in the Midwest. The company purchases, processes, stores, and sells yellow corn, yellow soybeans, and soft red-and-white wheat in Ohio, Michigan, Indiana, and Illinois. Domestic processors and feeders buy more than 70% of its grain. The company also makes and sells granular lawn fertilizer, which is sold to professional lawn care companies and retailers, and sells corncob-based products for use in feed, chemicals, and animal litter. The company operates six "The Andersons" home-center stores in Ohio and nine retail farm centers in the Midwest. It also buys, repairs, sells, and leases railcars and provides auto fleet management services.

A. Schulman, Inc.

3550 W. Market St., Akron, OH 44333

Telephone: 330-666-3751 **Fax:** 330-668-7204 **Metro area:** Cleveland, OH **Web site:** http:// www.aschulman.com **Human resources contact:** Toy Friedberg **Sales:** $993.4 million **Number of employees:** 2,250 **Number of employees for previous year:** 2,181 **Industry designation:** Chemicals—plastics **Company type:** Public **Top competitors:** BASF Aktiengesellschaft; GE Plastics; The Dow Chemical Company

A. Schulman puts its plastic resins and compounds in products ranging from toothbrush handles to car bumper guards. Sold under brand names, including Polyman and Polyflam, the firm's products are used in the making of such items as steering wheels, plastic bags, lawn sprinklers, telephone components, and videocassettes. The company sells to manufacturers and suppliers in the agriculture, automotive, consumer products, electronics, packaging, and office equipment markets. A. Schulman also produces specialty color concentrates widely used in products such as plastic packaging films. More than half of its sales are generated in Europe.

Austin Powder Company

25800 Science Park Dr., Cleveland, OH 44122

Telephone: 216-464-2400 **Fax:** 216-464-4418 **Metro area:** Cleveland, OH **Human resources contact:** Linda Manendez **Sales:** $190 million (Est.) **Number of employees:** 1,200 **Industry designation:** Chemicals—diversified **Company type:** Private **Top competitors:** Dyno Industrier A.S.; Mining Services International Corporation; Anglo American Industrial Corporation Limited

Business is a blast at Austin Powder. The firm manufactures commercial explosives such as ammonium nitrate, dynamite, and nitroglycerins, primarily for the construction, mining, and oil and gas industries. It also makes a host of explosive support equipment, including blasthole dewatering pumps, explosive carriers, detonators, fuses, primers, and magazines for storing explosives. Five brothers founded Austin Powder in 1833 to supply explosives for construction of the Ohio and Erie Canal. Contracts to provide explosives to the US military spurred the company's growth in the past century. Despite this high-powered customer, government charges of price fixing have hounded Austin Powder for several years.

Bigmar, Inc.

9711 Sportsman Club Rd., Johnstown, OH 43031

Telephone: 740-966-5800 **Fax:** 614-842-4290 **Metro area:** Columbus, OH **Sales:** $6.5 million **Number of employees:** 80 **Number of employees for previous year:** 66 **Industry designation:** Drugs **Company type:** Public **Top competitors:** Pharmacia & Upjohn, Inc.; Bristol-Myers Squibb Company; Fresenius Medical Care Aktiengesellschaft

Bigmar, through its subsidiaries, makes pharmaceutical products in Switzerland and Germany, including 18 intravenous infusion solutions sold directly to health care providers in Switzerland. Through an agreement with AB Cernelle, Bigmar has exclusive worldwide distribution rights to some 20 generic oral oncological products, including calcium leucovorin. Its alliance with Graminex gives it access to botanical raw materials containing drug substances. Bigmar is awaiting FDA approval for eight new drug applications; once approved, these eight will be distributed by IVAX. The company went public in 1996; John Tramontana (chairman, president, and CEO) controls more than 55% of the company's stock.

Broughton Foods Company

210 N. Seventh St., Marietta, OH 45750

Telephone: 740-373-4121 **Fax:** 614-373-2475 **Metro area:** Parkersburg, WV **Human resources contact:** Brooks Harper **Sales:** $179.4 million **Number of employees:** 883 **Number of employees for previous year:** 719 **Industry designation:** Food—dairy products **Company type:** Public **Top competitors:** Dairy Farmers of America; Land O'Lakes, Inc.; Country Fresh Inc.

Mountain mamas get their milk from Broughton Foods. The dairy company processes raw milk and makes a variety of dairy products (cottage cheese, eggnog, ice cream), beverages (orange juice, iced tea), and extended-life products (half-and-half, whipped toppings) sold under its Broughton, Southern Belle, and Dairylane labels, as well as under private labels. Broughton markets its products to retail and food service customers such as schools and Dairy Queen restaurants, mainly in Kentucky, Michigan, Ohio, Tennessee, and West Virginia. Chairman Marshall Reynolds, who also controls printer Champion Industries, owns 22% of Broughton. Founded in 1910, Broughton is being acquired by Dallas milk processor Suiza Foods.

Cardinal Health, Inc.

5555 Glendon Ct., Dublin, OH 43016

Telephone: 614-717-5000 **Fax:** 614-717-8871 **Metro area:** Columbus, OH **Web site:** http:// www.cardinal-health.com **Human resources contact:** Carole W. Tomko **Sales:** $15.9 billion **Number of employees:** 11,200 **Number of employees for previous year:** 11,000 **Industry designation:** Drugs & sundries—wholesale **Company type:** Public **Top competitors:** AmeriSource Health Corporation; McKesson HBOC, Inc.; Bindley Western Industries, Inc.

Cardinal Health's cardinal number is two—it's the second-largest US wholesaler (behind McKesson HBOC) of pharmaceuticals, surgical and hospital supplies, therapeutic plasma, and other specialty pharmaceutical, health, and beauty products. Its customer-support services include computerized order entry and confirmation systems; customized invoicing; generic sourcing programs; product movement and management reports; and consultation on store operation and merchandising. Its Medicine Shoppe subsidiary is the largest franchisor of independent retail pharmacies; the R.P. Scherer unit is the #1 maker of gelatin capsules for drugs and vitamins; subsidiary Allegiance is the top US medical products distributor.

Cavs/Gund Arena Company

One Center Ct., Cleveland, OH 44115

Telephone: 216-420-2000 **Fax:** 216-420-2101 **Metro area:** Cleveland, OH **Web site:** http:// www.nba.com/cavs **Human resources contact:** Farrell Finnin **Sales:** $61.9 million (Est.) **Number of employees:** 100 **Industry designation:** Leisure & recreational services **Company type:** Private **Top competitors:** Pacers Basketball Corporation; Charlotte Hornets; Chicago Bulls

The Cavs/Gund Arena Company has far from a cavalier attitude toward round-ball; it owns two Cleveland basketball teams and operates the arena in which they play. Its Cleveland Cavaliers joined the NBA in 1970 as part of an expansion that included the Portland Trail Blazers and Buffalo Braves (now the Los Angeles Clippers). Although the team spent much of the 1990s providing highlight footage for Michael Jordan, the Cavaliers remain a competitive unit with a horde of young talent, sending four players to the 1998 All-Star Rookie team. The company, which is owned by chairman Gordon Gund, also brought to town one of the eight original Women's National Basketball Association teams, the Cleveland Rockers.

Cedar Fair, L.P.

One Causeway Dr., Sandusky, OH 44871

Telephone: 419-626-0830 **Fax:** 419-627-2260 **Other address:** PO Box 5006, Sandusky, OH 44871 **Metro area:** Mansfield, OH **Web site:** http://www.cedarfair.com **Human resources contact:** Katja Rall-Koepke **Sales:** $419.5 million **Number of employees:** 1,200 **Number of employees for previous year:** 600 **Industry designation:** Leisure & recreational services **Company type:** Public **Top competitors:** Anheuser-Busch Companies, Inc.; The Walt Disney Company; Premier Parks, Inc.

Cedar Fair is a scream. One of the world's leading amusement park chains, the firm offers thrill and water rides, children's rides, live shows, shops, and other attractions to more than 13 million visitors annually. Its parks include Cedar Point/Soak City (Ohio), Valleyfair (Minnesota), Dorney Park/Wildwater Kingdom (Pennsylvania), Worlds of Fun/Oceans of Fun (Missouri), and Knott's Berry Farm (California). The company bought Knott's Berry Farm in 1997, Cedar Fair's first foray into year-round parks; the other four parks are open daily from about mid-May through Labor Day and then on weekends in September and October. Cedar Fair also owns a handful of hotels and restaurants, a marina, and an RV park.

The Cincinnati Reds

100 Cinergy Field, Cincinnati, OH 45202

Telephone: 513-421-4510 **Fax:** 513-421-7342 **Metro area:** Cincinnati, OH **Web site:** http:// www.cincinnatireds.com **Human resources contact:** Cathy Secor **Sales:** $50.2 million (Est.) **Number of employees:** 290 **Industry designation:** Leisure & recreational services **Company type:** Private **Top competitors:** St. Louis Cardinals, L.P.; Chicago National League Ball Club, Inc.; Houston Astros Baseball Club

America's game got its start in Cincinnati, home of the first professional baseball team, the Red Stockings. Founded in 1869, the team now known as the Cincinnati Reds is a charter member of baseball's National League (NL). The Reds dominated the 1970s with six division titles, four NL pennants, and back-to-back World Series championships in 1975 and 1976. Among that era's standout players was Pete Rose, who became baseball's all-time leading hitter in 1985. The team's controversial owner Marge Schott came under fire from civil rights organizations and received suspensions from baseball in 1993 and 1996 for making racial and ethnic slurs. MLB officials are forcing Schott to sell her interest in the team.

Cincom Systems, Inc.

55 Merchant St., Cincinnati, OH 45246

Telephone: 513-612-2300 **Fax:** 513-612-2000 **Metro area:** Cincinnati, OH **Web site:** http://www.cincom.com **Human resources contact:** Bill Ohr **Sales:** $174 million (Est.) **Number of employees:** 1,180 **Number of employees for previous year:** 1,120 **Industry designation:** Computers—corporate, professional & financial software **Company type:** Private **Top competitors:** Informix Corporation; System Software Associates, Inc.; J.D. Edwards & Company

Cincom Systems has been making business software since the 1960s—before most people knew what software was. Cincom sells tools for manufacturing, financial, and sales automation applications. Its products include software for application development, call center management, customer support management, database management, and product manufacturing management. Customers include Chase Manhattan, Blue Cross and Blue Shield Association, and the US Department of Labor. Cincom has offices in 24 countries and sells worldwide. Thomas Nies has been president, CEO, and owner since he founded the company in 1968; his is the longest tenure in the industry.

The Cleveland Browns

76 Lou Groza Blvd., Berea, OH 44017

Telephone: 440-891-5050 **Fax:** 440-891-5009 **Web site:** http://www.clevelandbrowns.com **Human resources contact:** Jackie Skalba **Number of employees:** 140 **Industry designation:** Leisure & recreational services **Company type:** Private **Top competitors:** Pittsburgh Steelers; Tennessee Titans Inc.; Jacksonville Jaguars

The new Cleveland Browns have yet to lose a game. OK, they have yet to play a game either. In 1995 Cleveland pariah and former Browns owner Art Modell announced plans to move the team to Baltimore, citing financial reasons—despite the fact that Browns home games sold out on a regular basis. However, the NFL let the City of Cleveland keep the team name and colors and awarded the city an NFL franchise scheduled to start play in 1999. Alfred Lerner, CEO of credit card giant MBNA Corporation, and former San Francisco 49ers president Carmen Policy are co-owners of the expansion franchise.

Cleveland Indians Baseball Company, Inc.

2401 Ontario St., Cleveland, OH 44115

Telephone: 216-420-4200 **Fax:** 216-420-4396 **Metro area:** Cleveland, OH **Web site:** http://www.indians.com **Human resources contact:** Sara Lehrke **Sales:** $140 million **Number of employees:** 2,447 **Industry designation:** Leisure & recreational services **Company type:** Public **Top competitors:** Kansas City Royals Baseball Corporation; Minnesota Twins; Chicago White Sox Ltd.

The Cleveland Indians Baseball Company owns the Cleveland Indians baseball team and manages its home ballpark, Jacobs Field. The Indians date to the turn of the century, when the team became a charter member of the American League. After years of poor performance both on the field and off, the Indians were acquired by brothers Richard and David Jacobs in 1986. The Jacobses' turnaround strategy led the team to American League pennants in 1995 and 1997. In 1998 the Indians won the AL Central division but lost their bid for the pennant to the New York Yankees. Chairman, president, and CEO Richard Jacobs, through his ownership of Class B common shares, controls 99.9% of the company's voting power.

Conley, Canitano & Associates, Inc.

5800 Landerbrook Dr., Mayfield Heights, OH 44124

Telephone: 440-684-6600 **Fax:** 440-684-6700 **Metro area:** Cleveland, OH **Web site:** http://www.ccai.net **Human resources contact:** Susan V. Lebas **Sales:** $50.5 million (Est.) **Number of employees:** 339 **Number of employees for previous year:** 289 **Industry designation:** Computers—services **Company type:** Private

Conley, Canitano & Associates, Inc. (CCAi) provides information technology services primarily for midsized organizations or divisions of larger corporations. CCAi customizes, installs, and supports corporate-wide project management software, known as enterprise resource planning. The company serves clients in a variety of industries, including aerospace, automotive, chemical, communications, and financial. The company also provides services for mainframe and legacy applications, year 2000 compliance, and remote support. CCAi sells its services directly in the US and Canada to customers who include Alcoa, Keebler Foods, Oracle, and Procter & Gamble. Venture capital firm TA Associates owns 38% of the company.

Discount Drug Mart Inc.

211 Commerce Dr., Medina, OH 44256

Telephone: 330-725-2340 **Fax:** 330-722-2990 **Metro area:** Cleveland, OH **Human resources contact:** Michael Eby **Sales:** $327 million (Est.) **Number of employees:** 1,250 **Industry designation:** Retail—drugstores **Company type:** Private **Top competitors:** Rite Aid Corporation; CVS Corporation; Walgreen Co.

Drugs are just part of the story at Discount Drug Mart. The largest drugstore chain in northeast Ohio offers pharmacy services, home health care goods, over-the-counter medications and medical goods, food, liquor, home maintenance supplies, and greeting cards. Its approximately 45 stores offer about 22,500 sq. ft. of selling space, and the company sells home health care equipment such as wheelchairs, hospital beds, and walkers from fellow Ohio firm Invacare and Newell Rubbermaid through touch-screen kiosks. It also offers catalogs. Discount Drug Mart runs a pharmacy-by-mail program, IPS Network, in partnership with other local chains. CEO Parviz Boodjeh owns the company, which was founded in 1970.

Duramed Pharmaceuticals, Inc.

7155 E. Kemper Rd., Cincinnati, OH 45249

Telephone: 513-731-9900 **Fax:** 513-731-5270 **Metro area:** Cincinnati, OH **Web site:** http://www.duramed.com **Human resources contact:** Judy Hattendorf **Sales:** $44.3 million **Number of employees:** 327 **Number of employees for previous year:** 303 **Industry designation:** Drugs—generic **Company type:** Public

Duramed Pharmaceuticals makes generic prescription and over-the-counter drugs. Products include the hormone-replacement therapy Estradiol, the diabetes medication Glipizide, and the antiemetic drug Prochlorperazine. It has also received approval to market a hydroxyurea capsule for treating cancer. Duramed hopes to become a global leader in hormone products for women. The company has received FDA approval for an estrogen-replacement drug under the name Cenestin. The FDA had rejected a generic version of the drug, prompting Duramed to consider developing more branded products. The company sells to more than 200 drugstore chains, wholesalers, private-label distributors, and other US outlets.

EPI Technologies, Inc.

810 Chicago St., Toledo, OH 43611

Telephone: 419-727-0495 **Fax:** 419-727-0595 **Metro area:** Toledo, OH **Sales:** $3.4 million **Number of employees:** 34 **Industry designation:** Pollution control equipment & services **Company type:** Subsidiary **Top competitors:** Waste Management, Inc.; Safety-Kleen Corp.; Detrex Corporation

Where some see paint sludge, EPI Technologies sees a recycling opportunity. The company offers car manufacturers and other industrial customers with spray painting operations a more environmentally sound option than shipping paint waste to landfills. EPI Technologies pulverizes paint sludge to produce a coarse powder that can be used in much the same way as sand or calcium carbonate to make bricks, low-strength concrete, and roofing and road-building materials. The company is paid not only for the end product, but also for picking up the waste. EPI is a subsidiary of Meridian National, a maker and distributor of steel products. A planned IPO has been on hold since 1997.

Essef Corporation

220 Park Dr., Chardon, OH 44024

Telephone: 440-286-2200 **Fax:** 440-286-2206 **Metro area:** Cleveland, OH **Web site:** http://www.essef.com **Human resources contact:** David Hillyer **Sales:** $436 million **Number of employees:** 2,700 **Number of employees for previous year:** 2,100 **Industry designation:** Rubber & plastic products **Company type:** Public **Top competitors:** Ionics, Incorporated; Amtrol Inc.; Hayward Industries, Inc.

Taking a dip is all part of a day's work at Essef, a leading manufacturer of filters, pumps, heaters, lights, and other equipment for swimming pools and spas. Essef sells and installs concrete swimming pools through its Anthony & Sylvan Pools subsidiary. The company also produces water treatment and filtration equipment for commercial, municipal, residential, and industrial applications. Essef also makes filters and other equipment for aquariums. It also operates through subsidiaries in Belgium, China, India, Italy, Taiwan, and the US. CEO Thomas Waldin owns more than 17% of the company.

The Geon Company

One Geon Center, Avon Lake, OH 44012

Telephone: 440-930-1000 **Fax:** 440-930-1002 **Metro area:** Cleveland, OH **Web site:** http://www.geon.com **Human resources contact:** Diane Davie **Sales:** $1.3 billion **Number of employees:** 2,000 **Number of employees for previous year:** 1,683 **Industry designation:** Chemicals—plastics **Company type:** Public **Top competitors:** Occidental Petroleum Corporation; Formosa Plastics Corporation; Borden Chemicals and Plastics Limited Partnership

Into vinyl even before Alan Freed, Geon is a leading producer of vinyl compounds. The company makes polyvinyl chloride (PVC) resins for sale to third parties that make the widely used chemical alternative to wood, metal, and other plastics. Because of its high durability and low cost, PVC is used in building products such as piping, siding, and windows, and in components for appliances and automobiles. Geon also produces vinyl chloride monomer (VCM), a raw material used in PVC. It operates plants in Australia, Canada, and the US. Geon is combining its PVC and VCM operations with Occidental Petroleum. Geon also formed a joint venture (Decillion) with Owens Corning to make glass fiber and PVC composites.

Gliatech, Inc.

23420 Commerce Park Rd., Cleveland, OH 44122

Telephone: 216-831-3200 **Fax:** 216-831-4220 **Metro area:** Cleveland, OH **Web site:** http://www.gliatech.com **Sales:** $17.3 million **Number of employees:** 67 **Number of employees for previous year:** 62 **Industry designation:** Medical products **Company type:** Public **Top competitors:** Focal, Inc.; Cohesion Technologies, Inc.; Johnson & Johnson

Think of it as a disappearing Band-Aid for your innards. Using glial cell technology, Gliatech develops and sells absorbable medical devices of carbohydrate polymer designed to inhibit excessive surgical scarring and adhesions after surgery. The company's ADCON products protect a patient's internal tissues from scarring following gynecologic, lumbar, pelvic, peripheral nerve, and tendon surgeries. These products are sold in Africa, the Americas, Asia, Australia, and Europe. The company has also developed its glial cell technology to find possible drugs to treat attention deficit hyperactivity disorder, sleep disorders, and Alzheimer's disease (with partner Janssen Pharmaceutica, a Johnson & Johnson subsidiary).

Great Lakes Cheese Company, Inc.

17825 Great Lakes Pkwy., Hiram, OH 44234

Telephone: 440-834-2500 **Fax:** 440-834-1002 **Metro area:** Cleveland, OH **Web site:** http://www.greatlakescheese.com **Human resources contact:** Beth Wendell **Sales:** $625 million (Est.) **Number of employees:** 950 **Number of employees for previous year:** 900 **Industry designation:** Food—dairy products **Company type:** Private **Top competitors:** Schreiber Foods, Inc.; Land O'Lakes, Inc.; ConAgra, Inc.

Great Lakes Cheese makes, buys, packages, and distributes natural and process cheese, primarily for the the private-label market. However, it also sells a small number of products under its own name, including an award-winning cheddar, which it makes at its plant in New York. The company's Ohio and Wisconsin plants primarily process and package cheese. Great Lakes Cheese also imports cheeses from several countries in Europe. President and CEO Hans Epprecht, a Swedish immigrant, founded the company in 1959 as a small distributor in Cleveland. Epprecht owns the majority of Great Lakes Cheese.

HCR Manor Care, Inc.

One SeaGate, Toledo, OH 43604

Telephone: 419-252-5500 **Fax:** 419-252-5510 **Metro area:** Toledo, OH **Web site:** http://www.hcr-manorcare.com **Human resources contact:** Wade B. O'Brian **Sales:** $2.2 billion **Number of employees:** 55,000 **Number of employees for previous year:** 22,000 **Industry designation:** Hospitals **Company type:** Public **Top competitors:** Beverly Enterprises, Inc.; Vencor, Inc.

Long-term care provider HCR Manor Care, product of a merger of Health Care and Retirement Corporation and Manor Care, operates some 300 nursing homes (some under the Heartland name) and assisted living facilities as well as more than 110 specialty health care units that provide subacute medical care, intensive rehabilitation, and Alzheimer's care. It also operates more than 70 outpatient therapy clinics, offers in-home health care services, and sells program management services to hospitals and nursing homes. Through Manor Care it also owns about two-thirds of In Home Health, which provides home nursing and rehabilitation services. The company operates in some 30 states. Manor Care shareholders own 59% of the company.

Health Power, Inc.

560 E. Town St., Columbus, OH 43215

Telephone: 614-461-9900 **Fax:** 614-461-6683 **Metro area:** Columbus, OH **Human resources contact:** Peggy Wible **Sales:** $75.8 million **Number of employees:** 435 **Number of employees for previous year:** 360 **Industry designation:** Health maintenance organization **Company type:** Public

Health Power is a managed care holding company hoping to keep Ohio's Buckeyes feeling good through its several health care subsidiaries. The company's Health Power HMO serves 19 of Ohio's 88 counties, including the Columbus, Cincinnati, and Cleveland metro areas. Of Health Power HMO's 30,000-plus members, more than 90% are Medicaid recipients, who together account for nearly 60% of total revenues. The company's provider network consists of more than 1,000 primary care physicians, 4,000 specialists, and 61 hospitals. Five other Health Power subsidiaries provide workers' comp, life insurance, and third-party administrative services. Chairman and CEO Dr. Bernard Master owns 33% of the company.

International Total Services, Inc.

5005 Rockside Rd., Crown Centre, Cleveland, OH 44131

Telephone: 216-642-4522 **Fax:** 216-642-4539 **Metro area:** Cleveland, OH **Human resources contact:** Sonja Boardman **Sales:** $173.2 million **Number of employees:** 15,000 **Number of employees for previous year:** 10,690 **Industry designation:** Protection—safety equipment & services **Company type:** Public **Top competitors:** AHL Services, Inc.; Ogden Corporation; Borg-Warner Security Corporation

International Total Services (ITS) provides airport security for more than 60 airlines at about 140 airports. The company's aviation security services include prescreening of baggage (using X-ray and manual searches) and security for parked airplanes, airport entrances, and parking lots. About 80% of its sales come from outsourcing services such as preboard screening and baggage handling. The rest of its business comes from offering staffing services to various industries, including banking and warehousing. Primarily a domestic company (about 94% of sales), ITS continues to grow through acquisitions; its largest airline account, Delta, came with ITS's purchase of aviation services provider Intex.

Invacare Corporation

One Invacare Way, Elyria, OH 44036

Telephone: 440-329-6000 **Fax:** 440-366-9008 **Metro area:** Cleveland, OH **Web site:** http://www.invacare.com **Human resources contact:** Larry Seward **Sales:** $797.5 million **Number of employees:** 4,550 **Number of employees for previous year:** 4,470 **Industry designation:** Medical products **Company type:** Public **Top competitors:** Graham-Field Health Products, Inc.; Sunrise Medical Inc.; Suzuki Motor Corporation

Invacare makes medical equipment for the home health care and extended care markets. The company is the #1 maker of wheelchairs, with about 40% of the market. It also makes motorized scooters, crutches, walkers, home care beds, respiratory equipment, and seating and positioning products. Invacare distributes disposable products made by others, including specialty bedding and incontinence and ostomy products. The company's products are sold to more than 10,000 home health care and medical equipment dealers in Australia, Canada, Europe, New Zealand, and the US, as well as to government agencies and distributors. The company has manufacturing plants in North America, Australia, Europe, and New Zealand.

Karrington Health, Inc.

919 Old Henderson Rd., Columbus, OH 43220

Telephone: 614-451-5151 **Fax:** 614-451-5199 **Metro area:** Columbus, OH **Web site:** http://www.karrington.com **Human resources contact:** Kirk McCoy **Sales:** $19.2 million **Number of employees:** 1,300 **Number of employees for previous year:** 476 **Industry designation:** Nursing homes **Company type:** Public

To help meet the needs of the growing older population, Karrington Health owns and operates more than 45 private-pay, assisted-living residences in 11 states, mostly in the midwestern US. Each property houses 30 to 80 residents and offers care and assistance with housekeeping, grooming, nutrition, and transportation. The focus of each residence can range from simple assisted living to full care for persons with Alzheimer's disease. Karrington Health has joint operating agreements with Catholic Health Initiatives for six facilities. Chairman of the Board John McConnell owns about 33% of the company.

Kendle International Inc.

700 Carew Tower, Cincinnati, OH 45202

Telephone: 513-381-5550 **Fax:** 513-381-5870 **Metro area:** Cincinnati, OH **Web site:** http://www.kendle.com **Human resources contact:** Stephen G. Scheurer **Sales:** $89.5 million **Number of employees:** 1,069 **Number of employees for previous year:** 865 **Industry designation:** Medical services **Company type:** Public **Top competitors:** Quintiles Transnational Corp.; PAREXEL International Corporation; Covance Inc.

When it comes to R&D, Kendle can do. The firm provides contract research and development services for biotechnology and pharmaceutical companies. Kendle International specializes in conducting Phase II to Phase IV clinical trials, but it also provides such services as medical writing, statistical analysis, and regulatory consultation and representation. Kendle's TrialWare software manages research and trial data. The acquisitive company operates in the US and Europe. Its clients include G.D. Searle, which accounts for more than half of Kendle's sales. Founder and CEO Candace Kendle Bryan and her husband, president and COO Christopher Bergen, own approximately 40% of the company.

The Kroll-O'Gara Company

9113 Le Saint Dr., Fairfield, OH 45014

Telephone: 513-874-2112 **Fax:** 513-874-2558 **Metro area:** Cincinnati, OH **Human resources contact:** Carol Pelosi **Sales:** $264.8 million **Number of employees:** 913 **Number of employees for previous year:** 581 **Industry designation:** Protection—safety equipment & services **Company type:** Public **Top competitors:** Pinkerton's, Inc.; Borg-Warner Security Corporation; DaimlerChrysler AG

The Kroll-O'Gara Company makes armored vehicles and provides corporate intelligence services. It also offers advanced driver training, specialized armor for the US Army's "Humvee," and high-end satellite phones. The Kroll Associates subsidiary offers services ranging from the mundane background check to more scintillating intelligence services for crisis management and hostile takeovers. Its Laboratory Specialists of America subsidiary provides employee drug testing services. The O'Gara Hess & Eisenhardt subsidiary makes armored vehicles for private citizens as well as high-ranking diplomats (its armor has protected every US president since Harry Truman).

LanVision Systems, Inc.

One Financial Way, Ste. 400, Cincinnati, OH 45242

Telephone: 513-794-7100 **Fax:** 513-794-7272 **Metro area:** Cincinnati, OH **Web site:** http://www.lanvision.com **Sales:** $8.7 million **Number of employees:** 124 **Number of employees for previous year:** 101 **Industry designation:** Computers—corporate, professional & financial software **Company type:** Public **Top competitors:** MedPlus, Inc.; American Management Systems, Incorporated; McKesson HBOC, Inc.

It's all a matter of record. LanVision Systems makes medical records software that combines patient information into a single, keyword-searchable, indexed online database for the hospital and health care provider. Its ChartVision software stores patients' clinical records, including digitized images; AccountVision handles billing. LanVision's Virtual Healthware Services division offers secure, transaction-based document imaging and management services over the Web. LanVision also provides consulting services such as training, project management, and custom software development. Founders Brian Patsy (chairman, president, and CEO) and Eric Lombardo (EVP) each own about 25% of the company.

LESCO, Inc.

20005 Lake Rd., Rocky River, OH 44116

Telephone: 440-333-9250 **Fax:** 440-356-3909 **Metro area:** Cleveland, OH **Web site:** http://www.lesco.com **Human resources contact:** Rhonda P. Lawson **Sales:** $416.7 million **Number of employees:** 1,244 **Number of employees for previous year:** 1,157 **Industry designation:** Fertilizers **Company type:** Public **Top competitors:** The Scotts Company; Monsanto Company; IMC Global Inc.

LESCO wants you to see green—turf, that is. The firm is a leading producer of turf-care products and equipment for golf courses, lawn-care firms, landscapers, nurseries, and municipalities, among other clients. The firm's fleet of about 70 LESCO Stores-on-Wheels and about 240 LESCO Service Centers offer a range of turf-care products, including the Poly Plus slow-release and Elite fertilizers, turf-protection products (such as herbicides), and turf-grass seed. LESCO also makes rotary mowers, spreaders, sprayers, and other related equipment and replacement parts. It sells a limited assortment of lawn-care products to nonprofessional users through Home Depot stores and worldwide distributors.

LEXIS-NEXIS

9393 Springboro Pike, Miamisburg, OH 45342

Telephone: 937-865-6800 **Fax:** 937-865-7476 **Metro area:** Dayton, OH **Web site:** http://www.lexis-nexis.com **Human resources contact:** Larry Fultz **Sales:** $1.1 billion **Number of employees:** 6,200 **Industry designation:** Computers—online services **Company type:** Subsidiary **Parent company:** Reed Elsevier PLC **Top competitors:** The Dialog Corporation plc; West Group; Dow Jones & Company, Inc.

For info junkies, LEXIS-NEXIS is the ultimate pusher. A subsidiary of publishing giant Reed Elsevier, the company deals the dope via its online, Internet, CD-ROM, and print services. Its three divisions—LEXIS, NEXIS, and Martindale Hubbell—cover the legal, business, government, academic, and general news beats. Selected units include Shepard's (a legal case history reference service), Congressional Information Service (abstracts and indices to hearings and other government documents), and Reed Technology and Information Services (third-party content management). The company serves customers worldwide from 50 US cities and overseas offices that include London, Frankfurt, Toronto, and Hong Kong.

The Lubrizol Corporation

29400 Lakeland Blvd., Wickliffe, OH 44092

Telephone: 440-943-4200 **Fax:** 440-943-5337 **Metro area:** Cleveland, OH **Web site:** http://www.lubrizol.com **Human resources contact:** Mark W. Meister **Sales:** $1.6 billion **Number of employees:** 4,324 **Number of employees for previous year:** 4,291 **Industry designation:** Chemicals—specialty **Company type:** Public **Top competitors:** Shell Oil Company; Ethyl Corporation; Exxon Corporation

Lubrizol is more slippery than an Arkansas politician. The slick company is the world's #1 maker of lubricants and fuel additives, with a market share approaching 40%. Its fuel additives control deposits and improve combustion; its engine oil additives (about 50% of sales) fight sludge buildup, viscosity breakdown, and component wear. Lubrizol markets about 1,100 products—primarily to oil refiners and blenders—in more than 100 countries (some 60% of sales are outside North America). Lubrizol also makes additives for paints, inks, greases, metalworking, and other industrial markets. Lubrizol has research facilities and testing labs in Japan, the UK, and the US.

M. A. Hanna Company

200 Public Sq., Ste. 36-5000, Cleveland, OH 44114

Telephone: 216-589-4000 **Fax:** 216-589-4200 **Metro area:** Cleveland, OH **Web site:** http://www.mahanna.com **Human resources contact:** Lani L. Beach **Sales:** $2.3 billion **Number of employees:** 7,130 **Number of employees for previous year:** 7,016 **Industry designation:** Chemicals—plastics **Company type:** Public

Specialty chemical firm M. A. Hanna is the largest plastics- and rubber-compounding business in North America. The firm and its subsidiaries concentrate on processing (nearly 60% of sales) and distributing compounds, colorants and color additives, resins, and specialty products. In addition to serving the plastics, film and fiber, wire and cable, automotive, and construction markets, the former mining company manages marine terminals; it also has formed an international nylon-compound production and distribution joint venture with Japanese plastics giant Ube. M. A. Hanna serves markets in Asia, Europe, North America, and South America from its facilities worldwide.

Manhattan Life Insurance Co.

1876 Waycross Rd., Cincinnati, OH 45240

Telephone: 513-595-2119 **Fax:** 513-595-2206 **Metro area:** Cincinnati, OH **Human resources contact:** Steve Johnston **Industry designation:** Insurance—life **Company type:** Subsidiary

Manhattan Life Insurance is a guarantee capital life insurance company that concentrates on individual life insurance policies, mostly to high-risk and older (age 50-85) clients. The company writes ordinary, universal, and term life policies. A subsidiary of Union Central Life Insurance Company, Manhattan Life Insurance also provides investment services and pension administration services. The company is licensed to operate in all 50 states; it conducts all sales through about 90 independent agency relationships and about 8,300 contracted brokers.

Marathon Ashland Petroleum LLC

539 S. Main St., Findlay, OH 45840

Telephone: 419-422-2121 **Fax:** 419-421-3837 **Metro area:** Lima, OH **Web site:** http://www.mapllc.com **Human resources contact:** Randy K. Lohoff **Sales:** $19.3 billion **Number of employees:** 30,000 **Industry designation:** Oil refining & marketing **Company type:** Joint venture **Top competitors:** CITGO Petroleum Corporation; Sunoco, Inc.; Tosco Corporation

Marathon Ashland Petroleum (MAP) has found its place on the map as one of US's leading oil refiners. A joint venture between 62%-owner USX-Marathon and 38%-owner Ashland, MAP operates seven refineries in the Midwest and Texas, which handle about 935,000 barrels of oil a day, accounting for 6% of US capacity. MAP sells refined products through its retail subsidiary, Speedway SuperAmerica LLC, which has about 5,400 outlets in 20 states. The company is phasing out the Ashland brand name in favor of Marathon, in part to cash in on Marathon's bigger credit card program. MAP also holds stakes in 10,500 miles of pipeline and operates a terminal network in the Midwest and Southeast.

Meridian Diagnostics, Inc.

3471 River Hills Dr., Cincinnati, OH 45244

Telephone: 513-271-3700 **Fax:** 513-271-3762 **Metro area:** Cincinnati, OH **Human resources contact:** Marlene Cook **Sales:** $33.2 million **Number of employees:** 192 **Number of employees for previous year:** 181 **Industry designation:** Medical products **Company type:** Public **Top competitors:** Abbott Laboratories; Becton, Dickinson and Company; Diagnostic Products Corporation

Meridian Diagnostics' high point is detecting parasitic, gastrointestinal, respiratory, urogenital, and viral diseases. The company's test kits are used to analyze blood, urine, and other bodily fluids and tissues and can detect antibodies produced in response to the presence of bacteria, viruses, and foreign substances. The kits aid in the diagnosis of such maladies as gastrointestinal infections, mononucleosis, and strep throat, as well as in the detection of diseases that affect patients with cancer, AIDS, and other immunosuppressive conditions. All of the firm's products are used in procedures performed in vitro (outside the body). Cofounder and chairman William Motto owns almost one-third of the company.

MPW Industrial Services Group, Inc.

9711 Lancaster Rd., SE, Hebron, OH 43025

Telephone: 740-927-8790 **Fax:** 740-928-8033 **Metro area:** Columbus, OH **Web site:** http://www.mpwgroup.com **Human resources contact:** Vanessa Treadway **Sales:** $93.4 million **Number of employees:** 1,400 **Number of employees for previous year:** 1,300 **Industry designation:** Pollution control equipment & services **Company type:** Public **Top competitors:** Airtech International Group, Inc.; Met-Pro Corporation; C. H. Heist Corp.

MPW Industrial Services Group operates best under pressure. The company's industrial cleaning services include power washing, water-blasting, dry and wet vacuum services, and cryojetic cleaning (which uses dry ice instead of chemicals or abrasives). Applications of MPW's services include scouring off-road heavy equipment, removing water scale and rust from boilers, and water-blasting grooves in cement pipes. The company also offers industrial filtration management and process water purification. Founder, chairman, and CEO Monte Black owns nearly 60% of MPW, which operates from facilities in 19 US states and in Canada and Mexico.

Myers Industries, Inc.

1293 S. Main St., Akron, OH 44301

Telephone: 330-253-5592 **Fax:** 330-253-6568 **Metro area:** Cleveland, OH **Human resources contact:** Thomas A. Bruser **Sales:** $392 million **Number of employees:** 2,503 **Number of employees for previous year:** 2,083 **Industry designation:** Rubber & plastic products **Company type:** Public

Myers Industries makes reusable plastic and metal storage and handling containers. The company also produces molded rubber products used in tire manufacturing and repair. The company's reusable containers (manufactured in US and Europe) are marketed under the names NesTier, Akro-Bins, and Buckhorn and are used to distribute poultry, meat, baked goods, and various nonfood items. Myers also makes Keepbox brand household storage containers and recycling bins that are marketed to residential consumers through stores such as Wal-Mart and Target. Its Myers Tire Supply division distributes air compressors, mechanic's tools, and tire equipment to tire dealers, retreaders, and service centers.

NCS HealthCare, Inc.

3201 Enterprise Pkwy., Cleveland, OH 44122

Telephone: 216-514-3350 **Fax:** 216-464-8376 **Metro area:** Cleveland, OH **Web site:** http://www.ncshealth.com **Human resources contact:** Judy Fimiani **Sales:** $509.1 million **Number of employees:** 3,900 **Number of employees for previous year:** 2,350 **Industry designation:** Medical services **Company type:** Public **Top competitors:** Omnicare, Inc.; Iatros Health Network, Inc.; PharMerica Inc.

NCS HealthCare is building a drug empire across the US—legitimately. The highly acquisitive company provides pharmacy services to nursing homes, assisted-living facilities, and other long-term care facilities in 34 states. NCS HealthCare's pharmacy and pharmacy consultant services (about 75% of company revenues) include prescription and nonprescription drug purchasing and dispensing; automated record keeping; drug therapy evaluation; and regulatory assistance. NCS HealthCare also provides nutrition management and physical, speech, and occupational therapy services. Chairman Jon Outcalt owns more than 55% of NCS, which included in its 1998 acquisitions the long-term care pharmacy units of Eckerd and Walgreen.

North Coast Energy, Inc.

1993 Case Pkwy., Twinsburg, OH 44087

Telephone: 330-425-2330 **Fax:** 330-405-3298 **Metro area:** Cleveland, OH **Web site:** http://www.northcoastenergy.com **Human resources contact:** Michelle Harris **Sales:** $8.6 million **Number of employees:** 40 **Number of employees for previous year:** 38 **Industry designation:** Oil & gas—exploration & production **Company type:** Public **Top competitors:** Energy Search, Incorporated; Petroleum Development Corporation; Cabot Oil & Gas Corporation

Independent oil and gas exploration and production company North Coast Energy sees beaches only on vacations. The company operates in the Appalachian Basin (principally in eastern Ohio and western Pennsylvania), where it acquires undeveloped properties with proved reserves and manages drilling and production programs. North Coast manages more than 1,600 wells, including about 370 for partnerships in which the company acts as managing general partner. The company also operates 200 miles of pipeline for gathering natural gas from more than 600 wells. Dutch utility Nuon owns 51% of North Coast Energy.

OhioHealth

3555 Olentangy River Rd., Columbus, OH 43214

Telephone: 614-566-5424 **Fax:** 614-447-8244 **Metro area:** Columbus, OH **Web site:** http://www.ohiohealth.com **Human resources contact:** John Boswell **Sales:** $828 million **Number of employees:** 13,400 **Number of employees for previous year:** 10,000 **Industry designation:** Hospitals **Company type:** Not-for-profit **Top competitors:** Catholic Healthcare Partners; Catholic Health Initiatives; Holy Cross Health System Corporation

With some 2,500 affiliated physicians in more than half of the state's 88 counties, OhioHealth aims to keep Buckeyes healthy. The system's member hospitals include Grant Medical Center and Riverside Methodist Hospital in Columbus, Southern Ohio Medical Center in Portsmouth, and Hardin Memorial in Kenton. A network including imagery, surgery, and physical therapy and neurological rehabilitation centers supports OhioHealth. The system also manages three community hospitals in Morrow County, Bucyrus, and Galion, and it operates the OhioHealth Group managed care plan, a 50-50 joint venture with an independent physicians' association. OhioHealth is buying Doctors Hospital, which will add three new facilities.

OM Group, Inc.

50 Public Sq., 3800 Terminal Tower, Cleveland, OH 44113

Telephone: 216-781-0083 **Fax:** 216-781-1502 **Metro area:** Cleveland, OH **Web site:** http://www.omgi.com **Human resources contact:** Michael J. Scott **Sales:** $521.2 million **Number of employees:** 988 **Number of employees for previous year:** 758 **Industry designation:** Chemicals—specialty **Company type:** Public

OM Group is an international producer of value-added metal-based specialty chemicals, including metal carboxylates, metal salts, and metal powders. The company's products are used for custom catalysts, liquid detergents, lubricants, specialty additives to accelerate the drying of inks, and bonding agents for rubber tires. It also makes coloring agents used in pigments, ceramics, and glass and specialty powders used to make machine, mining, and drilling tools. OM Group operates manufacturing facilities in North America, Europe, and Asia. The company has acquired Dussek Campbell, a Canadian metal carboxylates manufacturer.

Owens-Illinois, Inc.

One SeaGate, Toledo, OH 43666

Telephone: 419-247-5000 **Fax:** 419-247-1132 **Metro area:** Toledo, OH **Web site:** http://www.o-i.com **Human resources contact:** Gary Benjamin **Sales:** $5.3 billion **Number of employees:** 32,400 **Number of employees for previous year:** 30,800 **Industry designation:** Glass products **Company type:** Public **Top competitors:** Compagnie de Saint-Gobain; Alcoa Inc.; Continental Can Company, Inc.

If it holds liquid, chances are Owens-Illinois makes it. Owens-Illinois manufactures about one of every two glass containers worldwide and is a US market leader in plastic containers and closures, labels, trigger sprayers, prescription containers, multipack beverage carriers, and packaging material. The company's plastic containers are used for household, personal care, health care, chemical, automotive, and food products. Owens-Illinois' plastics and international operations are contributing an increasingly larger portion of the company's sales. Kohlberg Kravis Roberts owns about 26% of the company.

The Procter & Gamble Company

One Procter & Gamble Plaza, Cincinnati, OH 45202

Telephone: 513-983-1100 **Fax:** 513-983-9369 **Other address:** PO Box 599, Cincinnati, OH 45201 **Metro area:** Cincinnati, OH **Web site:** http://www.pg.com **Human resources contact:** Richard Antoine **Sales:** $37.2 billion **Number of employees:** 110,000 **Number of employees for previous year:** 106,000 **Industry designation:** Soap & cleaning preparations **Company type:** Public **Top competitors:** Unilever; Kimberly-Clark Corporation; Johnson & Johnson

The Tide is in at Procter & Gamble (P&G), as are Folgers, Pampers, Cover Girl, and fake fat. P&G is the #1 US manufacturer of household products, with five main categories: laundry and cleaning (detergents, bleaches), paper goods (toilet paper, feminine protection products), beauty care (lotions, shampoos), food and beverage (coffee, snacks), and health care (toothpaste, medicine). The company developed olestra, a fat substitute used in snacks and crackers. It also produces soap operas "As the World Turns," "Another World," and "Guiding Light." P&G has shifted its strategy, reorganizing around global business units instead of by geographic regions. About half of its sales come from outside the US.

RPM, Inc.

2628 Pearl Rd., Medina, OH 44258

Telephone: 330-273-5090 **Fax:** 330-225-8743 **Other address:** PO Box 777, Medina, OH 44258 **Metro area:** Cleveland, OH **Web site:** http://www.rpminc.com **Human resources contact:** Ronald A. Rice **Sales:** $1.6 billion **Number of employees:** 6,926 **Number of employees for previous year:** 6,651 **Industry designation:** Paints & related products **Company type:** Public **Top competitors:** The Sherwin-Williams Company; E. I. du Pont de Nemours and Company; PPG Industries, Inc.

RPM knows the ABCs of sealants. It makes more than 100 brand-name coatings and specialty chemicals, including Rust-Oleum rust preventative and Day-Glo fluorescent paint. Industrial products make up about 60% of sales and include coatings for waterproofing, floor maintenance, and wall finishing. RPM also makes do-it-yourself auto and home decoration and protection products, marine coatings, and hobby paints. The family-run business (CEO Thomas Sullivan is the founder's son, and has sons of his own at RPM) has enjoyed 51 profitable years of growth, thanks to a strategy of buying successful companies and allowing them to retain their autonomy. Retail investors own 58% of RPM.

Safelite AutoGlass Corp.

1105 Schrock Rd., Columbus, OH 43229

Telephone: 614-842-3000 **Fax:** 614-842-3180 **Other address:** PO Box 2000, Columbus, OH 43216 **Metro area:** Columbus, OH **Web site:** http://www.safelite.com **Human resources contact:** Jack Warren **Sales:** $213.8 million (Est.) **Number of employees:** 6,800 **Number of employees for previous year:** 6,500 **Industry designation:** Glass products **Company type:** Private **Top competitors:** Apogee Enterprises, Inc.; Guardian Industries Corp.; PPG Industries, Inc.

Safelite AutoGlass repairs shattered dreams—or at least shattered windshields. The #1 US auto-glass repair and replacement company has some 75 warehouses that supply a nationwide network of company-owned service centers and independent contractors. Safelite makes windshields at its Kansas and North Carolina facilities. Its aftermarket services include window tinting and sales and installation of sunroofs, windshield wipers, and truck backslider windows. It serves auto dealers, car-rental agencies, and body shops, as well as insurance and fleet companies. Private equity firm Thomas H. Lee Company controls the company, which changed its name from Safelite Glass Corp. following its merger with rival Vistar.

SARCOM, Inc.

8405 Pulsar Place, Columbus, OH 43240

Telephone: 614-854-1000 **Fax:** 614-854-1074 **Metro area:** Columbus, OH **Web site:** http://www.sarcom.com **Human resources contact:** Sharon Dunn **Sales:** $400 million (Est.) **Number of employees:** 1,400 **Number of employees for previous year:** 800 **Industry designation:** Computers—services **Company type:** Private **Top competitors:** InaCom Corp.; Hartford Computer Group, Inc.; En Pointe Technologies, Inc.

The acronym SITCOM stands for Single Income, Two Children, Oppressive Mortgage. SARCOM stands for information technology services, hoping to satisfy your computer needs. The company offers consulting and engineering services, procures hardware and software, and designs and implements networks. It also supports company Internet/intranet applications, manages projects, provides technology staffing, training and education, licenses software, and rents and leases systems. SARCOM has helped Cincinnati schools switch from a paper-based spreadsheet inventory of textbooks to a computerized system. The company is expanding its technological capabilities through acquisitions in the mid-Atlantic and West Coast regions.

Seiler Pollution Control Systems, Inc.

211 Blue Jay Dr., Columbus, OH 43235

Telephone: 614-846-9966 **Metro area:** Columbus, OH **Number of employees:** 29 **Number of employees for previous year:** 22 **Industry designation:** Pollution control equipment & services **Company type:** Public **Top competitors:** GTS Duratek, Inc.

Seiler Pollution Control Systems has a burning desire that is hazardous. The company uses High Temperature Vitrification (HTV), a high heat conversion process, to recycle hazardous waste materials into inert nonhazardous materials, mainly glass ceramic. The glass ceramic produced is then sold as building materials, blast abrasives, and insulating glass. To reduce transportation cost and liability associated with offsite management, the company prefers to install HTV systems at or near the site where the waste is generated. Seiler also owns 60% of Seiler Nuclear Control Systems (formerly N.W. Technology), which plans to develop a similar system for treating low-level nuclear waste.

Specialty Chemical Resources, Inc.

9055 S. Freeway Dr., Macedonia, OH 44056

Telephone: 330-468-1380 **Fax:** 330-468-0287 **Metro area:** Cleveland, OH **Human resources contact:** Dorne J. Chadsey **Sales:** $40.3 million **Number of employees:** 219 **Number of employees for previous year:** 187 **Industry designation:** Chemicals—specialty **Company type:** Public **Top competitors:** Airgas, Inc.; Arrow-Magnolia International, Inc.; Evans Systems, Inc.

Janitors and mechanics rely on Specialty Chemical Resources, a manufacturer of specialty chemical products for the automotive service, janitorial, and industrial maintenance markets. The company's products, sold almost exclusively in aerosol containers, include cleaners, sealants, lubricants, waxes, adhesives, paints, degreasers, polishes, and a nonflammable tire inflator. Specialty Chemical develops proprietary chemical formulations that are sold primarily under its customers' brand names, but also under the company's own brands, including Taylor Made Products and Aerosol Maintenance Products. The company also offers its customers design, marketing, filling and packaging, and management services, among others.

STERIS Corporation

5960 Heisley Rd., Mentor, OH 44060

Telephone: 440-354-2600 **Fax:** 440-354-7043 **Metro area:** Cleveland, OH **Human resources contact:** Sid Booker **Sales:** $719.7 million **Number of employees:** 4,500 **Number of employees for previous year:** 4,000 **Industry designation:** Medical instruments **Company type:** Public **Top competitors:** Maxxim Medical, Inc.; Johnson & Johnson; Aesculap AG

STERIS is the world's largest provider of infection-prevention systems for the health care, research, food, and industrial markets. Using the company's main product, STERIS SYSTEM 1, health care professionals can sterilize immersible surgical and diagnostic devices. STERIS also makes high- and low-temperature gaseous sterilizers and decontamination systems. The firm makes surgical support products such as exam lights, warming cabinets, and scrub sinks. Subsidiary Isomedix focuses on gamma irradiation processes to eliminate possible contaminants (such as "E. coli") in red meat. Isomedix already uses STERIS gamma irradiation devices to sterilize medical products.

Sterling Commerce, Inc.

4600 Lakehurst Ct., Dublin, OH 43016

Telephone: 614-793-7000 **Fax:** 614-793-4040 **Other address:** P.O. Box 8000, Dublin, OH 43016 **Metro area:** Columbus, OH **Web site:** http://www.sterlingcommerce.com **Human resources contact:** Richard Needles **Sales:** $490.3 million **Number of employees:** 2,300 **Number of employees for previous year:** 1,700 **Industry designation:** Computers—corporate, professional & financial software **Company type:** Public **Top competitors:** Elcom International, Inc.; Harbinger Corporation; CheckFree Holdings Corporation

Sterling is a Web alloy (and ally). Sterling Commerce offers e-commerce software and networking support (including e-mail, electronic business transactions, and electronic libraries) to over 42,000 business customers worldwide in such industries as banking, transportation, retail, and telecommunications. The company's electronic payment software (VECTOR) is used by most of the largest banks in the US. Sterling Commerce's other products include software for automated file transfer (CONNECT) and messaging management and electronic data interchange translation software (GENTRAN). The company was spun off from parent Sterling Software in 1996.

Structural Dynamics Research Corporation

2000 Eastman Dr., Milford, OH 45150

Telephone: 513-576-2400 **Fax:** 513-576-2922 **Metro area:** Cincinnati, OH **Web site:** http://www.sdrc.com **Human resources contact:** Bryan M. Valentine **Sales:** $403 million **Number of employees:** 2,366 **Number of employees for previous year:** 2,067 **Industry designation:** Computers—engineering, scientific & CAD-CAM software **Company type:** Public **Top competitors:** Parametric Technology Corporation; International Business Machines Corporation; Dassault Systemes S.A.

Structural Dynamics Research develops software for mechanical design automation and product data management for computer-aided design, manufacturing, and engineering. The company's I-DEAS Master and Artisan Series software allows development teams to work simultaneously on a project while sharing a common master model. The company's Metaphase Enterprise software enables companywide management and control of product information, configuration, and work flow throughout the product's life cycle. The software runs on Unix or Microsoft NT operating systems and is sold directly and through distributors and value-added resellers worldwide. Customers include Ford and Information Services International-Dentsu Ltd.

Symix Systems, Inc.

2800 Corporate Exchange Dr., Columbus, OH 43231

Telephone: 614-523-7000 **Fax:** 614-895-2504 **Metro area:** Columbus, OH **Web site:** http://www.symix.com **Human resources contact:** Robert D. Williams **Sales:** $97.6 million **Number of employees:** 623 **Number of employees for previous year:** 488 **Industry designation:** Computers—corporate, professional & financial software **Company type:** Public **Top competitors:** DataWorks Corporation; System Software Associates, Inc.; MAPICS, Inc.

Symix Systems mixes it up and sorts it out. The company makes enterprise resource planning software that integrates a company's management, manufacturing, and financial operations. Its products, designed for midsize companies, include core software SyteLine, plus SyteEDI (e-commerce), SytePower (data analysis), and SyteService (customer service). Symix products are geared primarily to users of Windows NT operating systems (70% of sales). About 20% of its sales come from outside North America. The bulk of Symix customers are in the industrial equipment, furniture, electronics, fabricated metals, and packaging markets. Founder and chairman Larry Fox owns 33% of the company, which is growing through acquisitions.

The Union Central Life Insurance Company

1876 Waycross Rd., Cincinnati, OH 45240

Telephone: 513-595-2200 **Fax:** 513-595-5418 **Other address:** PO Box 40888, Cincinnati, OH 45240 **Metro area:** Cincinnati, OH **Web site:** http://www.unioncentral.com **Human resources contact:** Stephen K. Johnston **Sales:** $1.2 billion **Number of employees:** 755 **Number of employees for previous year:** 743 **Industry designation:** Insurance—life **Company type:** Mutual company **Top competitors:** New York Life Insurance Company; Metropolitan Life Insurance Company; The Prudential Insurance Company of America

Union Central Life Insurance Company is a mutual life insurance company that operates in all 50 states and the District of Columbia. The company offers a range of individual life and disability insurance, investment products, annuities, group retirement plans, and group insurance. Union Central also offers employee and executive benefit planning, estate planning, and retirement planning. One-third of Union Central's investments are in collateralized mortgage obligations, of which mortgage investments accounted for about 18%. Union Central was founded in 1867 in Cincinnati, Ohio, and is owned by its policyholders.

United Air Specialists, Inc.

4440 Creek Rd., Cincinnati, OH 45242

Telephone: 513-891-0400 **Fax:** 513-891-4882 **Metro area:** Cincinnati, OH **Web site:** http://www.uasinc.com **Human resources contact:** Rich Spence **Sales:** $40.8 million **Industry designation:** Pollution control equipment & services **Company type:** Subsidiary **Top competitors:** Met-Pro Corporation; Crown Andersen Inc.; Environmental Elements Corporation

United Air Specialists (UAS) has ESP and causes static almost everywhere it goes. The company makes electrostatic precipitators (ESP) that electrify airborne particles and remove them from the air. It also makes industrial air cleaning systems, electrostatic fluid contamination control equipment, and high-precision spraying equipment. The company's products are used in offices, hospitals, bars, schools, and industrial settings. Trade names include SMOKEETER, SMOG-HOG, DUST-HOG, DUST-CAT, CRYSTAL-AIRE, FRESH-X-CHANGER, TOTALSTAT, and KLEENTEK. A subsidiary of CLARCOR, UAS sells its products in Australia, Canada, China, Germany, Japan, the UK, and the US.

Wastequip, Inc.

25800 Science Park Dr., Ste. 140, Beachwood, OH 44122

Telephone: 216-292-2554 **Fax:** 216-292-0625 **Metro area:** Cleveland, OH **Web site:** http://www.wastequip.com **Human resources contact:** Page Farinatca **Sales:** $94.9 million (Est.) **Number of employees:** 798 **Industry designation:** Pollution control equipment & services **Company type:** Private

You can't call Wastequip wasteful—it's mopping up all the small waste-equipment makers it can get. Wastequip is a consolidator; since its founding in 1989, it has acquired eight waste-handling equipment manufacturers in the southern, midwestern, northeastern, and Rocky Mountain regions of the US. The company provides a range of metal containers for on-site waste collection; balers and compactors for waste processing; and containers, trailers, hoists, and other mechanical equipment used for transporting solid, liquid, semiliquid, and hazardous waste. Its customers include solid-waste disposal firms, commercial businesses, and government agencies; Waste Management accounts for about 14% of sales.

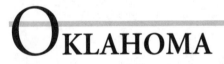

Oklahoma

Advantage Marketing Systems, Inc.

2601 Northwest Expwy., Ste. 1210W, Oklahoma City, OK 73112

Telephone: 405-842-0131 **Fax:** 405-843-4935 **Metro area:** Oklahoma City, OK **Web site:** http://www.amsonline.com **Human resources contact:** Marcy Bickers **Sales:** $13.3 million **Number of employees:** 46 **Number of employees for previous year:** 43 **Industry designation:** Cosmetics & toiletries **Company type:** Public **Top competitors:** Herbalife International, Inc.; Nu Skin USA, Inc.; Sunrider International

If it weren't for multilevel marketing, how would anyone ever buy vitamins? Advantage Marketing Systems follows that sales model—in which its more than 23,000 independent distributors both sell products and recruit other distributors—to market more than 100 dietary supplements, weight-management products, and personal-care items. Advantage Marketing Systems' product line (which includes appetite suppressant Choc-Quilizer; cosmetics; and dietary supplements Shark Cartilage Complex and Chlorella) has been expanded through acquisitions. Advantage Marketing Systems also offers a consumer-benefits program that gives customers discounts on groceries, merchandise, travel, and legal services.

Avalon Correctional Services, Inc.

13401 Railway Dr., Oklahoma City, OK 73114

Telephone: 405-752-8802 **Fax:** 405-752-8852 **Other address:** PO Box 57012, Oklahoma City, OK 73157 **Metro area:** Oklahoma City, OK **Web site:** http://www.avaloncomsvs.com **Human resources contact:** Gayle Smith **Sales:** $5.8 million **Number of employees:** 261 **Number of employees for previous year:** 158 **Industry designation:** Protection—safety equipment & services **Company type:** Public **Top competitors:** Cornell Corrections, Inc.; Prison Realty Corporation; Wackenhut Corrections Corporation

Avalon is the mythical isle of dead heroes, but the tenants of Avalon Correctional Services are alive and kickin'—although not exactly heroes. The company owns and operates four private prisons and provides therapy and rehabilitation for inmates in minimum- and medium-security prisons. The company runs one medium-security facility in El Paso, Texas, and three minimum-security prisons in Oklahoma (more than half of its revenue comes from its prisons). It also offers substance abuse programs in six prisons in Nebraska and one prison in Missouri. Other services include educational programs, reintegration services, and vocational training. CEO Donald Smith owns about 36% of Avalon.

Chesapeake Energy Corporation

6100 N. Western Ave., Oklahoma City, OK 73118

Telephone: 405-848-8000 **Fax:** 405-879-9570 **Metro area:** Oklahoma City, OK **Web site:** http://www.chesapeake-energy.com **Human resources contact:** Martha A. Burger **Sales:** $381.9 million **Number of employees:** 362 **Number of employees for previous year:** 344 **Industry designation:** Oil & gas—exploration & production **Company type:** Public **Top competitors:** Adams Resources & Energy, Inc.; Helmerich & Payne, Inc.; Nuevo Energy Company

Just a peek at its annual report will reveal that Chesapeake Energy Corporation is an independent oil and natural gas exploration company that drills primarily in Louisiana, Oklahoma, and Texas. Chesapeake expands its holdings by drilling new wells and is among the five most active drillers of new wells in the US. It has drilled about 750 wells since it was formed in 1989. Aquila Southwest Pipeline, GPM Gas, and Koch Oil account for 57% of its oil and gas sales. Subsidiary Hugoton Energy explores for and produces gas and oil in the central US. Co-founders and top executives Tom Ward and Aubrey McClendon each own 16% of the company.

Devon Energy Corporation

20 N. Broadway, Ste. 1500, Oklahoma City, OK 73102

Telephone: 405-235-3611 **Fax:** 405-552-4667 **Metro area:** Oklahoma City, OK **Web site:** http://www.devonenergy.com **Human resources contact:** Merla Wells **Sales:** $387.5 million **Number of employees:** 383 **Number of employees for previous year:** 231 **Industry designation:** Oil & gas—exploration & production **Company type:** Public **Top competitors:** Vastar Resources, Inc.; Chesapeake Energy Corporation; Apache Corporation

Devon Energy is engaged in oil and gas acquisition, exploration, and production, with stakes in oil and gas properties in New Mexico, Texas, Oklahoma, Wyoming, and Alberta, Canada. It has proved reserves of more than 616 billion cu. ft. of natural gas and about 70 million barrels of oil. The company sells its natural gas to pipelines, utilities, gas marketing firms, industrial users, and local distribution companies such as Aquila Energy Marketing. Devon has holdings split almost evenly between oil and natural gas and between the US and Canada since its purchase of Alberta-based Northstar Energy. Oklahoma-based energy firm Kerr-McGee owns 31% of Devon.

Foodbrands America, Inc.

1601 Northwest Expwy., Ste. 1700, Oklahoma City, OK 73118

Telephone: 405-879-4100 **Fax:** 405-879-4173 **Other address:** PO Box 26724, Oklahoma City, OK 73126 **Metro area:** Oklahoma City, OK **Web site:** http://www.foodbrands.com **Human resources contact:** Robert E. Hedrick **Sales:** $835.2 million **Number of employees:** 3,400 **Number of employees for previous year:** 3,193 **Industry designation:** Food—meat products **Company type:** Subsidiary **Parent company:** IBP, inc.

Foodbrands America makes and sells branded and processed perishable foods for food service, delicatessen, and retail clients. The firm's Doskocil Food Service segment is a leading US supplier of branded and private-label pepperoni and pizza toppings for the food service industry. The Specialty Brands division produces more than 720 frozen prepared foods, including ethnic foods and appetizers. Custom soups, sauces, and side dishes as well as pizza toppings are made and packaged by the firm's KPR Foods segment. The Continental Deli Foods division offers more than 150 products to the deli market under several brand names. Foodbrands America is a subsidiary of IBP, a leading producer of beef and pork.

Gothic Energy Corporation

5727 S. Lewis Ave., Ste. 700, Tulsa, OK 74105

Telephone: 918-749-5666 **Fax:** 918-749-5882 **Metro area:** Tulsa, OK **Web site:** http://www.gothicenergy.com **Human resources contact:** Linda Esley **Sales:** $53 million **Number of employees:** 25 **Number of employees for previous year:** 18 **Industry designation:** Oil & gas—exploration & production **Company type:** Public **Top competitors:** Belco Oil & Gas Corporation; The Wiser Oil Company; Santa Fe Energy Resources, Inc.

Gothic Energy could probably tell some horror stories about the ups and downs of the cyclical oil and gas market. The exploration and production company operates primarily in Oklahoma, New Mexico, and Texas, in the Anadarko, Arkoma and Delaware/Permian basins. Gothic Energy has pursued a strategy of acquiring older, producing properties with significant potential for development and exploitation. The company has proved reserves of more than 300 billion cu. ft. of natural gas and 3.5 million barrels of oil. It has interests in about 1,200 wells and operates more than 600 properties.

The Home-Stake Oil & Gas Company

15 E. Fifth St., Ste. 2800, Tulsa, OK 74103

Telephone: 918-583-0178 **Fax:** 918-583-0237 **Metro area:** Tulsa, OK **Web site:** http://www.home-stake.com **Sales:** $10 million **Number of employees:** 17 **Industry designation:** Oil & gas—exploration & production **Company type:** Public

There was gold in them thar plains in 1905. That's when O. D. Strother bought the mineral rights to land in Oklahoma that formed the basis for the Home-Stake Oil & Gas Company. Today the company, which is still managed by a Strother descendant, owns and develops oil, gas, and mineral properties and has interests in 50 producing wells and seven service wells in 10 fields in Oklahoma, Texas, Montana, and Pennsylvania. In addition, Home-Stake owns more than 1,500 active properties and nearly 3,300 nonproducing properties, some of which are licensed for a royalty interest. The Home-Stake Oil & Gas Company is a product of a merger between Home-Stake and the related Home-Stake Royalty Corporation.

Kinark Corporation

2250 E. 73rd. St., Tulsa, OK 74136

Telephone: 918-494-0964 **Fax:** 918-494-3999 **Metro area:** Tulsa, OK **Sales:** $48 million **Number of employees:** 493 **Number of employees for previous year:** 453 **Industry designation:** Chemicals—specialty **Company type:** Public **Top competitors:** Aztec Manufacturing Co.; Evans Systems, Inc.; Dofasco Inc.

Kinark knows that rust never sleeps. The company's North American Galvanizing subsidiary provides corrosion protection for fabricated structural steel components by hot-dip galvanizing. Its galvanizing products are used in the petrochemical, highway and transportation, and energy and utilities industries, among others. Kinark also has a chemical storage and distribution subsidiary, Lake River, that provides liquid bulk storage via more than 200 tanks with 44 million gallons of on-site storage capacity. Kinark's North American Warehousing subsidiary operates 410,000 sq. ft. of warehouse storage space for petrochemicals and construction wares. Director Joseph Morrow and his wife own more than 25% of Kinark.

Laboratory Specialists of America, Inc.

101 Park Ave., Ste. 810, Oklahoma City, OK 73102

Telephone: 405-232-9800 **Fax:** 405-232-9801 **Metro area:** Oklahoma City, OK **Human resources contact:** Sheri Harrison **Sales:** $12.8 million **Number of employees:** 111 **Number of employees for previous year:** 98 **Industry designation:** Medical services **Company type:** Subsidiary **Top competitors:** SmithKline Beecham plc; LabOne, Inc.; Laboratory Corporation of America Holdings

Laboratory Specialists of America, through its Laboratory Specialists subsidiary, owns and operates an independent laboratory that provides employee drug testing services to institutional and corporate clients. The company aids customers in designing and implementing drug testing programs; trains client personnel; collects and tests samples; analyzes test results; and provides expert testimony when test results are challenged. All of Laboratory Specialists of America's services are customized to meet individual clients' needs and are aimed at detecting and deterring the use of illegal drugs in the workplace. The company is a subsidiary of The Kroll-O'Gara Company, a maker of safety equipment.

Lopez Foods Inc.

9500 NW Fourth St., Oklahoma City, OK 73127

Telephone: 405-789-7500 **Fax:** 405-499-0114 **Metro area:** Oklahoma City, OK **Human resources contact:** Dee Bithell **Sales:** $161.3 million (Est.) **Number of employees:** 297 **Number of employees for previous year:** 266 **Industry designation:** Food—meat products **Company type:** Private

Lopez Foods (formally Normac) could be the Hamburglar's Fort Knox. The company's plant grinds, blends, molds, and quick-freezes more than 650,000 pounds of Big Mac hamburger patties and breakfast sausage patties a day. The company has been a major supplier for McDonald's since 1968. Lopez Foods is scrupulous about safety. Technicians at the company's on-site lab test meat for "E. coli" and other dangerous bacteria before and after processing. Lopez Foods has also developed a Hazard Analysis Critical Control Points program to train employees and suppliers in safe food handling. The company generates more than $150 million in revenues annually for its owners, the Lopez family.

National Environmental Service Co.

12331 E. 60th St., Tulsa, OK 74146

Telephone: 918-250-2227 **Fax:** 918-250-1418 **Metro area:** Tulsa, OK **Web site:** http://Nesco-USA.com **Human resources contact:** Judy Learie **Sales:** $18.3 million **Number of employees:** 131 **Number of employees for previous year:** 97 **Industry designation:** Pollution control equipment & services **Company type:** Public **Top competitors:** Southern Cathodic Protection Company; Tanknology-NDE International, Inc.; USTMAN Technologies, Inc.

Legislation to prevent underground fuel leaks has helped fuel the business of the National Environmental Service Co. (NESCO), which installs and maintains underground storage tanks and fueling systems. The company's services include site assessment, testing, cathodic protection (corrosion prevention), spill protection, soil and water remediation, and tank removal. NESCO also distributes cathodic protection systems. Customers include service stations and convenience stores, trucking firms, railroads, airports, oil producers and refiners, pipeline operators, and government entities. The company maintains regional offices in Dallas and San Antonio.

Noble Affiliates, Inc.

110 W. Broadway, Ardmore, OK 73401

Telephone: 580-223-4110 **Fax:** 580-221-1386 **Other address:** PO Box 1967, Ardmore, OK 73401 **Human resources contact:** Calvin Burton **Sales:** $893.6 million **Number of employees:** 630 **Number of employees for previous year:** 614 **Industry designation:** Oil & gas—exploration & production **Company type:** Public

Noble Affiliates explores for and produces oil and natural gas onshore across the US and offshore in the Gulf of Mexico. Its exploration areas include the Gulf Coast, California, Colorado, Kansas, Louisiana, Montana, North Dakota, Oklahoma, Texas, and Wyoming. Noble also has wells in Argentina, China, Ecuador, Equatorial Guinea, and the North Sea. Much of the company's exploration and production is conducted by its Samedan subsidiary. Noble markets its own natural gas and oil and third-party gas and oil through its Noble Gas Marketing and Noble Trading subsidiaries.

Premier Parks, Inc.

11501 Northeast Expwy., Oklahoma City, OK 73131

Telephone: 405-475-2500 **Fax:** 405-475-2555 **Metro area:** Oklahoma City, OK **Web site:** http://www.sixflags.com **Sales:** $813.6 million **Number of employees:** 40,300 **Number of employees for previous year:** 11,142 **Industry designation:** Leisure & recreational services **Company type:** Public **Top competitors:** Anheuser-Busch Companies, Inc.; Cedar Fair, L.P.; The Walt Disney Company

Premier Parks owns and operates 31 family-oriented theme parks and water parks throughout the US and Europe. Its parks include Frontier City, White Water Bay, Geauga Lake, Wyandot Lake, Adventure World, Paradise Island, and Elitch Gardens and feature thrill rides, water slides, animal attractions, shows, food, games, and merchandise outlets. The company's 1998 purchase of Six Flags Theme Parks made it the nation's #2 amusement park operator (behind Walt Disney). Premier Parks owns 94% of Walibi, which operates six amusement parks in Belgium, France, and the Netherlands. The company plans to incorporate the Six Flags brand name at most of its parks.

ViaGrafix Corporation

One American Way, Pryor, OK 74361

Telephone: 918-825-6700 **Fax:** 918-825-6744 **Web site:** http://www.viagrafix.com **Human resources contact:** Rick Ogg **Sales:** $18.8 million **Number of employees:** 216 **Number of employees for previous year:** 145 **Industry designation:** Computers—services **Company type:** Public **Top competitors:** CBT Group PLC; Autodesk, Inc.; Gartner Group, Inc.

ViaGrafix produces information technology training courses for popular software packages and makes computer-aided design graphics software. The company has more than 650 training courses available on video and CD-ROM, as well as through local-area networks, intranets, and the Internet. Its principal graphics software product is DesignCAD. The company's software is designed for Microsoft platforms such as Windows NT and Windows 3.1. ViaGrafix sells its products through distributors and resellers and directly to end users through its 800 number, Web site, and catalog. Michael Webster, CEO, owns 33% of the company; his brother, Robert (an EVP), owns about 21%.

ZymeTx, Inc.

800 Research Pkwy., Ste. 100, Oklahoma City, OK 73104

Telephone: 405-271-1314 **Fax:** 405-271-1944 **Metro area:** Oklahoma City, OK **Web site:** http://www.zymetx.com **Human resources contact:** G. Carl Gibson **Sales:** $100,000 **Number of employees:** 32 **Number of employees for previous year:** 22 **Industry designation:** Biomedical & genetic products **Company type:** Public **Top competitors:** Roche Holding Ltd; Quidel Corporation; Glaxo Wellcome plc

ZymeTx is a development-stage biotechnology company that specializes in the diagnosis and treatment of viruses, particularly influenza, HIV, and herpes simplex. The company has received FDA approval for several diagnostic products and is awaiting approval for several others. These products provide quick diagnosis for patients most at risk of contracting the flu, including babies, the elderly, and those with immune-system impairments. ZymeTx is affiliated with the Oklahoma Medical Research Foundation and maintains licensing agreements for the use of the foundation's research results. The company also intends to develop enzyme-blocking treatments for viral diseases.

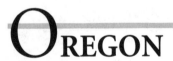

OREGON

Agritope, Inc.

16160 SW Upper Boones Ferry Rd., Portland, OR 97224

Telephone: 503-670-7702 **Fax:** 503-670-7703 **Metro area:** Portland, OR **Web site:** http://www.agritope.com **Human resources contact:** Paige Khan **Sales:** $2.8 million **Number of employees:** 56 **Number of employees for previous year:** 46 **Industry designation:** Agricultural operations **Company type:** Public **Top competitors:** Calgene, Inc.; The Dow Chemical Company; DNAP Holding Corporation

Agritope's ideas don't wither on the vine. The company, a spinoff of medical diagnostics developer Epitope, has developed a gene that slows produce spoilage by inhibiting the production of ethylene. Agritope is focusing this technology on highly perishable crops such as melons, tomatoes, and raspberries. It has conducted successful field tests with modified cantaloupe and is requesting commercial distribution clearance from the FDA and USDA. Under an agreement with the Salk Institute for Biological Studies, Agritope has received rights to five proprietary genes with potential to boost such traits as disease resistance and yield. Subsidiary Vinifera grows grapevines and markets them to the wine grape industry.

Analogy, Inc.

9205 SW Gemini Dr., Beaverton, OR 97008

Telephone: 503-626-9700 **Fax:** 503-643-3361 **Metro area:** Portland, OR **Web site:** http://www.analogy.com **Human resources contact:** Nancy Martell **Sales:** $25.8 million **Number of employees:** 218 **Number of employees for previous year:** 181 **Industry designation:** Computers—engineering, scientific & CAD-CAM software **Company type:** Public **Top competitors:** IKOS Systems, Inc.; Summit Design, Inc.; Avant! Corporation

You don't need a card to check out the simulation software and component model libraries made by Analogy. Analogy simulation products are used by designers and engineers to predict the behavior of specific devices (diodes, transistors, fuses, and fiber-optic devices) under a variety of conditions, such as variations in voltage, current, and temperature. Customers include aircraft and automotive makers; government entities account for 11% of sales. Analogy develops its Express packages a la carte, customized for power supply engineers (PowerExpress), telecom designers, and consumer electronics makers. The company continues to focus efforts on its international business, which accounts for more than 40% of sales.

Assisted Living Concepts Inc.

9955 SE Washington, Ste. 300, Portland, OR 97216

Telephone: 503-252-6233 **Fax:** 503-252-6597 **Metro area:** Portland, OR **Human resources contact:** Diane Schander **Sales:** $48.7 million **Number of employees:** 2,100 **Number of employees for previous year:** 1,395 **Industry designation:** Nursing homes **Company type:** Public **Top competitors:** Beverly Enterprises, Inc.; Marriott International, Inc.; Life Care Centers of America

Assisted Living Concepts runs residences for elderly people who do not need full-time nursing care. The residences, which include apartment units with kitchen facilities, allow seniors to maintain a fairly independent lifestyle while having access to staff help, as required, for such activities as bathing, dressing, and laundry. Each residence also has a common lounge, dining hall, and laundry facility. Assisted Living is targeting Medicaid and private-pay clients in communities with populations of 10,000 to 40,000. It runs about 140 assisted living centers in 12 states.

AVI BioPharma Inc.

One SW Columbia, Ste. 1105, Portland, OR 97201

Telephone: 503-227-0554 **Fax:** 503-227-0751 **Metro area:** Portland, OR **Web site:** http://www.antivirals.com **Human resources contact:** Connie Hensley-Jones **Sales:** $100,000 **Number of employees:** 54 **Number of employees for previous year:** 48 **Industry designation:** Drugs **Company type:** Public

AVI BioPharma (formerly Antivirals Inc.) develops gene-inactivating compounds for treatment of cancer and cardiovascular diseases. The company's NEUGENE compound is in preclinical development and is intended to treat cellular proliferative disorders, such as cancer, and restenosis, a cardiovascular disease. Its lead cancer vaccine candidate Avicine is in clinical trials. AVI BioPharma is also developing CYTOPORTER, a drug delivery engine intended to improve delivery of two approved drugs with delivery problems, paclitaxel (Taxol) and cyclosporin. CYTOPORTER is also in the preclinical test stage. The company enlarged its business by buying ImmunoTherapy Corporation.

CFI ProServices, Inc.

400 SW Sixth Ave., Portland, OR 97204

Telephone: 503-274-7280 **Fax:** 503-274-7284 **Metro area:** Portland, OR **Web site:** http://www.cfipro.com **Human resources contact:** Shannon Lynch **Sales:** $85.6 million **Number of employees:** 613 **Number of employees for previous year:** 530 **Industry designation:** Computers—corporate, professional & financial software **Company type:** Public **Top competitors:** Pegasystems Inc.; Phoenix International Ltd., Inc.; Jack Henry & Associates, Inc.

CFI ProServices makes software that automates customer transactions for financial institutions. The company's systems, including its Laser Pro and Encore! product lines, simplify transactions such as lending, opening new accounts, account inquiries, and product cross-selling by making information accessible across platforms. The systems also allow financial institutions and their customers to conduct transactions through a choice of contact methods, whether in person, over the telephone, or through electronic banking. The company provides its products to more than 5,000 banks and financial institutions in the US through a direct sales force.

International Yogurt Company

5858 NE 87th Ave., Portland, OR 97220

Telephone: 503-256-3754 **Fax:** 503-256-3976 **Metro area:** Portland, OR **Web site:** http://www.yocream.com **Human resources contact:** Ken McClain **Sales:** $10.2 million **Number of employees:** 50 **Number of employees for previous year:** 42 **Industry designation:** Food—dairy products **Company type:** Public **Top competitors:** Yogen Fruz World-Wide Inc.; Groupe Danone; General Mills, Inc.

When action on the basketball court heats up for the Portland Trail Blazers, fans can cool off with a Blazers Swirl, one of many frozen treats made by hometown firm International Yogurt. Sold under the YOCREAM name, the company's products include premium, low-fat, nonfat, and sugar-free frozen yogurt; smoothies; nondairy sorbet; and organic yogurt and ice cream. Its products are distributed to retailers, restaurants, and institutions such as hospitals, schools, and military bases in 35 states, Australia, Canada, Italy, Mexico, and the Pacific Rim. Brothers and executives John, David, and James Hanna together own 36% of the company, which they founded in 1977 and plan to rename YOCREAM INTERNATIONAL.

Legacy Health System

1919 NW Lovejoy St., Portland, OR 97209

Telephone: 503-415-5600 **Fax:** 503-415-5777 **Metro area:** Portland, OR **Web site:** http://www.legacyhealth.org **Human resources contact:** Barbara A. Zappas **Sales:** $486.6 million **Number of employees:** 6,731 **Number of employees for previous year:** 5,055 **Industry designation:** Hospitals **Company type:** Not-for-profit

Legacy Health System is a not-for-profit group of hospitals and home health agencies. Its hospitals include Emanuel Children's Hospital, Emanuel Hospital & Health Center (established in 1912 by the Lutheran church), Good Samaritan Hospital & Medical Center (founded in 1875 by the Episcopal Diocese), Meridian Park Hospital, and Mount Hood Medical Center. Legacy Visiting Nurse Association, which dates back to 1902, is one of Oregon's oldest home care providers. Other services include forensic and substance-abuse testing, postgraduate physician training and continuing education programs, minimally invasive surgery, and cancer support.

Mentor Graphics Corporation

8005 SW Boeckman Rd., Wilsonville, OR 97070

Telephone: 503-685-7000 **Fax:** 503-685-1202 **Metro area:** Portland, OR **Web site:** http://www.mentorg.com **Human resources contact:** Gary Rebello **Sales:** $490.4 million **Number of employees:** 2,570 **Number of employees for previous year:** 2,500 **Industry designation:** Computers—engineering, scientific & CAD-CAM software **Company type:** Public **Top competitors:** Cadence Design Systems, Inc.; Parametric Technology Corporation; Intergraph Corporation

Mentor Graphics software helps computers design computers. One of the world's leading suppliers of electronic design software, Mentor makes products that model electronic components such as integrated circuits and the systems that encompass them. Primarily for engineering- and science-geared UNIX computers, Mentor software is increasingly available for Windows NT-based systems. Mentor's customers include aerospace, computer, consumer electronics, telecommunications, and semiconductor companies. Mentor has manufacturing and distribution operations in Asia, Europe, and North America. About 45% of its sales come from outside the US.

Portland Trail Blazers

One Center Ct., Ste. 200, Portland, OR 97227

Telephone: 503-234-9291 **Fax:** 503-736-2187 **Metro area:** Portland, OR **Web site:** http://www.nba.com/blazers **Human resources contact:** Traci Reandeau **Sales:** $94.1 million (Est.) **Number of employees:** 1,425 **Number of employees for previous year:** 1,420 **Industry designation:** Leisure & recreational services **Company type:** Private **Top competitors:** California Sports, Inc.; Seattle SuperSonics; Phoenix Suns

After entering the NBA as an expansion team in 1970, the Portland Trail Blazers blazed a trail to the championship title in just seven years. The 1976-77 team was coached by Jack Ramsay and led by center Bill Walton. The Trail Blazers have had only three losing seasons since then and have made the playoffs 16 consecutive times, but without another championship. With Clyde Drexler, Terry Porter, Jerome Kersey, and Buck Williams, the team made the NBA Finals twice between 1989 and 1992. The team continues to blaze new trails in its 20,000 seat Rose Garden arena under coach Mike Dunleavy. Microsoft co-founder Paul Allen owns the Trail Blazers.

Protocol Systems, Inc.

8500 SW Creekside Place, Beaverton, OR 97008

Telephone: 503-526-8500 **Fax:** 503-526-4200 **Metro area:** Portland, OR **Web site:** http://www.protocol.com **Human resources contact:** Allen L. Oyler **Sales:** $67.3 million **Number of employees:** 409 **Number of employees for previous year:** 401 **Industry designation:** Medical instruments **Company type:** Public **Top competitors:** Datascope Corp.; Siemens AG; Novametrix Medical Systems Inc.

Protocol Systems keeps an eye on you. The company makes patient monitoring systems that allow hospitals and clinics to track their patients' vital signs. Protocol's products include its Propaq, Modem Propaq, and Propaq Encore mobile patient monitoring systems that can measure heartbeat, blood pressure, blood oxygen and carbon dioxide levels, and body temperature. Protocol's cordless telemetry products let doctors monitor ambulatory heart patients via radio waves. The company's networked Acuity System combines Propaq monitors, Sun Microsystems workstations, and Protocol's cordless telemetry devices to allow hospitals to monitor the vital signs of up to 60 patients simultaneously.

R-B Rubber Products, Inc.

904 E. 10th Ave., McMinnville, OR 97128

Telephone: 503-472-4691 **Fax:** 503-434-4455 **Metro area:** Portland, OR **Sales:** $8.6 million **Number of employees:** 72 **Number of employees for previous year:** 62 **Industry designation:** Rubber & plastic products **Company type:** Public **Top competitors:** Vulcan International Corporation; North West Rubber Mats Ltd.; Double D Family Mat Shop

Old tires don't die—R-B Rubber Products recycles them into rubber matting and other protective surfaces. The company produces rubber matting primarily as flooring for horse and livestock trailers and for weight-room floors in gyms. Secondary product lines include truck bed liners, rubber edging, and drain tiles. It added rubber paving tiles and molded rubber barbell plates to its product line with the 1998 acquisition of Iowa Mat Co. The company sells more than 85% of its products to distributors and retailers, with OEMs of horse trailers and farm implements buying the rest. Chairman and president Ronald Bogh owns 25% of R-B Rubber Products.

Regent Assisted Living, Inc.

121 SW Morrison St., Ste 1000, Portland, OR 97204

Telephone: 503-227-4000 **Fax:** 503-274-4685 **Metro area:** Portland, OR **Web site:** http://www.rgnt.com **Human resources contact:** Janette Angus **Sales:** $30.4 million **Number of employees:** 1,400 **Number of employees for previous year:** 542 **Industry designation:** Nursing homes **Company type:** Public

Regent Assisted Living owns, operates, and develops private-pay assisted-living communities that offer housing and support services for senior citizens who are not fully independent but don't require 24-hour skilled medical care. The firm has two types of facilities: housing devoted to assisting residents at their independence levels (Regent) and housing specifically for special-needs clients such as Alzheimer's patients (Regent Court). Services include housekeeping, laundry, medication management, personal care (bathing, feeding, grooming), transportation, and pet care. Chairman and CEO Walter Bowen owns nearly 70% of the firm, which has more than 2,000 beds in about 20 facilities in eight states.

Sonus Corp.

111 SW Fifth Ave., Ste. 2390, Portland, OR 97204

Telephone: 503-225-9152 **Fax:** 503-225-9309 **Metro area:** Portland, OR **Web site:** http://www.sonus.com **Human resources contact:** Nancy Sayles **Sales:** $22.4 million **Number of employees:** 353 **Number of employees for previous year:** 210 **Industry designation:** Medical services **Company type:** Public **Top competitors:** Sight Resource Corporation; Bausch & Lomb Incorporated; HEARx Ltd.

Sonus is making itself heard in the hearing care industry. An acquisitive provider of audiological products and services, the company operates about 90 clinics in the US and western Canada through its Sonus-USA and Sonus-Canada subsidiaries. About 10% of the clinics are franchises licensed via The Sonus Network. Sonus' clinics offer such diagnostic services as testing, evaluation, and rehabilitation, and the company also services and sells hearing aids, batteries, ear plugs, and other types of hearing assistance devices, some under its own private-label Sonus Digital Hearing System brand. The company provides group and managed care benefit contracts through subsidiary Hear PO Corp.

StanCorp Financial Group, Inc.

1100 SW Sixth Ave., Portland, OR 97204

Telephone: 503-321-7000 **Fax:** 503-321-6776 **Other address:** PO Box 711, Portland, OR 97207 **Metro area:** Portland, OR **Web site:** http://www.standard.com **Human resources contact:** Gayle M. Evans **Sales:** $1.2 billion **Number of employees:** 1,849 **Number of employees for previous year:** 1,725 **Industry designation:** Insurance—accident & health **Company type:** Mutual company **Top competitors:** Provident Companies, Inc.; Golden Rule Insurance Company; Aon Corporation

In a move it hopes will be mutually beneficial to all concerned, Standard Insurance Company is demutualizing and making StanCorp Financial Group the holding company for its operations. Standard Insurance offers a wide range of insurance products, including both individual and group life, disability, and retirement plans, as well as group dental insurance and life reinsurance. The company provides coverage for more than four million employees in the US through about 65 sales offices and also has mortgage lending and real estate management subsidiaries. StanCorp's demutualization plan, which has been approved by Oregon insurance regulators, must be approved by policyholders before a public offering can proceed.

Synthetech, Inc.

1290 Industrial Way, Albany, OR 97321

Telephone: 541-967-6575 **Fax:** 541-967-9424 **Metro area:** Salem, OR **Web site:** http://www.synthetech.com **Human resources contact:** Charles B. Williams **Sales:** $8.3 million **Number of employees:** 43 **Number of employees for previous year:** 34 **Industry designation:** Chemicals—specialty **Company type:** Public

Synthetech makes chemically modified amino acids called peptide building blocks (PBBs) for the pharmaceutical industry. PBBs are used as raw material in peptide-based drugs developed by other companies to treat AIDS, cardiovascular diseases, and disorders related to immunology and endocrinology. The company sells PBBs to more than 250 firms in the US, Japan, and Europe. Synthetech buys amino acids from outside vendors and also produces its own synthetic amino acids for modification at its two Oregon production facilities. The company has produced more than 400 PBB products, with almost half of its sales related to drugs already on the market.

ThrustMaster, Inc.

7175 NW Evergreen Pkwy., Ste. 400, Hillsboro, OR 97124

Telephone: 503-615-3200 **Fax:** 503-615-3300 **Metro area:** Portland, OR **Web site:** http://www.thrustmaster.com **Human resources contact:** Allen Robison **Sales:** $25.9 million **Number of employees:** 117 **Number of employees for previous year:** 99 **Industry designation:** Computers—peripheral equipment **Company type:** Public **Top competitors:** Labtec Inc.; Logitech International SA; Microsoft Corporation

ThrustMaster is saving the world from evil sorcerers and aliens bent on world domination. The company makes high-end PC game controllers, such as joysticks and steering wheels for driving games, including its NASCAR Pro Digital model that comes with a separate gas and brake pedal unit. Flight control devices range from simple flight sticks to units which replicate controls on military aircraft featuring rudder pedals and throttle controls. ThrustMaster makes first person shooter controls for games designed from the player's point of view. A new line of less expensive controls targets the much larger video game market.

Timberline Software Corporation

15195 NW Greenbrier Pkwy., Beaverton, OR 97006

Telephone: 503-690-6775 **Fax:** 503-439-5700 **Metro area:** Portland, OR **Web site:** http://www.timberline.com **Human resources contact:** Judith Ratnieks **Sales:** $44.3 million **Number of employees:** 367 **Number of employees for previous year:** 312 **Industry designation:** Computers—corporate, professional & financial software **Company type:** Public **Top competitors:** Timeline, Inc.; SVI Holdings, Inc.; Lawson Software

No trees were destroyed to make Timberline Software's products. Construction companies, contractors, residential builders/remodelers, and property managers use Timberline's Gold Collection accounting software to manage financial information. Timberline designs products for companies of all sizes to include accounts payable, estimates, general ledger, and payroll applications. Its property management software generates reports containing tenant and lease information. Timberline also provides customer service (which accounts for more than 40% of sales), including maintenance and support, classroom training, and on-site training and consulting.

WebTrends Corporation

621 SW Morrison, Ste. 1300, Portland, OR 97205

Telephone: 503-294-7025 **Fax:** 503-294-7130 **Metro area:** Portland, OR **Web site:** http://www.webtrends.com **Sales:** $8 million **Number of employees:** 78 **Number of employees for previous year:** 76 **Industry designation:** Computers—corporate, professional & financial software **Company type:** Public **Top competitors:** net.Genesis; Network Associates, Inc.; AXENT Technologies, Inc.

WebTrends Corporation (formerly e.g. Software) answers the who, what, when, where, and how of corporate Web sites. Its flagship WebTrends Professional Suite enables businesses to profile and fine-tune their sites by determining who is accessing a site, what pages visitors view most, and when a problem is about to occur. It can also track where employees go on the Internet and how users access a company's site. WebTrends Enterprise analyzes e-commerce functions and allows users to combine site analysis data with existing company databases. Customers include AT&T, Boeing, IBM, Playboy Enterprises, and NASA. Co-founders Elijahu Shapira and Glen Boyd each own about 33% of WebTrends.

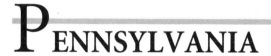

PENNSYLVANIA

Air Products and Chemicals, Inc.

7201 Hamilton Blvd., Allentown, PA 18195

Telephone: 610-481-4911 **Fax:** 610-481-5900 **Metro area:** Allentown, PA **Web site:** http://www.airproducts.com **Human resources contact:** Joseph P. McAndrew **Sales:** $4.9 billion **Number of employees:** 16,700 **Number of employees for previous year:** 16,400 **Industry designation:** Chemicals—specialty **Company type:** Public **Top competitors:** Praxair, Inc.; The BOC Group plc; L'Air Liquide SA

Passing gas is not a faux pas at Air Products and Chemicals. The company produces industrial gases and chemicals. Air Products provides argon, helium, hydrogen, nitrogen, and oxygen for industrial applications (gases account for nearly 60% of sales). Its chemicals unit produces a range of industrial and specialty chemicals, including polyurethane, amines, emulsions, and surfactants. Air Products supplies industrial gases in two ways: for large-volume customers it builds plants adjacent to customer facilities, and for smaller customers Air Products delivers gas by truck. The company has operations in 30 countries and exports to more than 100.

Allin Corporation

400 Greentree Commons, 381 Mansfield Ave., Pittsburgh, PA 15220

Telephone: 412-928-8800 **Fax:** 412-928-0887 **Metro area:** Pittsburgh, PA **Web site:** http://www.allin.com **Human resources contact:** Frank DiVito **Sales:** $15.3 million **Number of employees:** 170 **Number of employees for previous year:** 85 **Industry designation:** Leisure & recreational services **Company type:** Public **Top competitors:** NTN Communications, Inc.; LodgeNet Entertainment Corporation; On Command Corporation

Allin (formerly Allin Communications) provides interactive television (ITV), digital imaging, and consulting services through its operating units. Its Allin Systems business unit offers ITV services such as pay-per-view movies and video games to cruise lines, as well as digital imaging integration and support to the professional photography industry. It also offers its integrated ITV services to hospitals and educational institutions. Allin Consulting provides Windows NT software design, integration, and support to worldwide clients.

Aloette Cosmetics, Inc.

1301 Wright's Ln. East, West Chester, PA 19380

Telephone: 678-444-2563 **Fax:** 678-444-2564 **Metro area:** Philadelphia, PA **Web site:** http://www.aloettecosmetics.com **Human resources contact:** Janet Bical **Sales:** $10 million (Est.) **Number of employees:** 31 **Number of employees for previous year:** 25 **Industry designation:** Cosmetics & toiletries **Company type:** Private **Top competitors:** Mary Kay Inc.; Avon Products, Inc.; ThermoLase Corporation

Aloette Cosmetics sells skin care products, cosmetics, and other personal care items through a network of about 85 franchises in the US and Canada. The company offers more than 100 aloe vera-based products that are not sold in stores. Skin care accounts for more than half of sales; makeup and accessories account for about 25%. The rest is generated by fragrances and the sale of promotional items to the franchises. Aloette also sells its products through distributors in Australia, Taiwan, and Europe. The company was taken private in 1998 by an investor group led by franchisee Robert Cohen.

Analytical Graphics, Inc.

325 Technology Dr., Malvern, PA 19355

Telephone: 610-578-1000 **Fax:** 610-578-1001 **Metro area:** Philadelphia, PA **Web site:** http://www.analyticalgraphics.com **Human resources contact:** Lisa Velte **Sales:** $12.9 million (Est.) **Number of employees:** 130 **Industry designation:** Computers—engineering, scientific & CAD-CAM software **Company type:** Private **Top competitors:** L-3 Communications Holdings, Inc.

Analytical Graphics' Satellite Tool Kit (STK) helps government contractors, commercial firms, and government agencies design and monitor satellite systems. The software has been used in such high-profile projects as the Iridium network and the tracking and rescue of the space station "Mir." Analytical Graphics gives away STK, but it charges for its more than 20 add-on application tools, which expand STK's abilities in areas such as 3-D visualization and orbit simulation. The base software, which runs on Windows, Windows NT, and UNIX systems, evaluates relationships between satellites and ground stations. Add-ons can figure the effects of gravity, predict fuel needs, and help select ground station sites.

Ansoft Corporation

4 Station Sq., Ste. 660, Pittsburgh, PA 15219

Telephone: 412-261-3200 **Fax:** 412-471-9427 **Metro area:** Pittsburgh, PA **Web site:** http://www.ansoft.com **Human resources contact:** Ellen Allston **Sales:** $26.3 million **Number of employees:** 198 **Number of employees for previous year:** 154 **Industry designation:** Computers—engineering, scientific & CAD-CAM software **Company type:** Public **Top competitors:** Synopsys, Inc.; Cadence Design Systems, Inc.; Parametric Technology Corporation

Engineers use Ansoft's software to design hardware, including high-performance electrical devices and systems like cellular phones, satellite communications, computer circuit boards, and motors. The company's products, most of which are marketed under the Maxwell name (after James Clerk Maxwell, whose equations describe electric and magnetic fields over time and space), analyze electromagnetic interaction, determine signal degradation, and help design high-performance electrical devices such as antenna, radar, and microwave systems. Ansoft's tools support UNIX and Windows platforms. They are sold worldwide to such customers as Boeing, Ford, and Intel. Founder and director Thomas Miller owns about 20% of Ansoft.

ANSYS, Inc.

275 Technology Dr., Canonsburg, PA 15317

Telephone: 724-746-3304 **Fax:** 724-746-9494 **Metro area:** Pittsburgh, PA **Web site:** http://www.ansys.com **Human resources contact:** Karen Harker **Sales:** $56.6 million **Number of employees:** 260 **Number of employees for previous year:** 243 **Industry designation:** Computers—engineering, scientific & CAD-CAM software **Company type:** Public **Top competitors:** Structural Dynamics Research Corporation; Parametric Technology Corporation; The MacNeal-Schwendler Corporation

ANSYS has the "an-sas" when it comes to design. The company makes CAD and CAE software that helps engineers and designers test their computer-made designs. The ANSYS/Multiphysics programs (about 69% of sales), available in modular components or suites, have database and modeling capabilities that enable users to test a design's performance and response to such variables as stress, pressure, temperature, and velocity. More than 20% of revenues go to research and development. Investment group TA Associates owns about 40% of the firm, which sells its products through independent distributors in more than 30 countries.

Arrow International, Inc.

2400 Bernville Rd., Reading, PA 19605

Telephone: 610-378-0131 **Fax:** 610-374-5360 **Metro area:** Reading, PA **Web site:** http://www.arrowintl.com **Human resources contact:** Philip Jacobelli **Sales:** $260.9 million **Number of employees:** 2,551 **Number of employees for previous year:** 2,264 **Industry designation:** Medical & dental supplies **Company type:** Public **Top competitors:** Becton, Dickinson and Company; C. R. Bard, Inc.; Medtronic, Inc.

Arrow International makes cardiac and critical care products to diagnose and treat critically ill patients. The company's critical care products (about 85% of sales) consist mostly of disposable catheters used to access the central vascular system to diagnose and monitor patients and administer fluids, pain-relieving drugs, and blood products. Arrow's cardiac care products are mostly intra-aortic balloon pumps and catheters used to temporarily aid the heart's pumping ability following heart surgery, heart attacks, or balloon angioplasty. The company's products are marketed to doctors and hospitals through direct sales and independent distributors.

Balanced Care Corporation

5021 Louise Dr., Ste. 200, Mechanicsburg, PA 17055

Telephone: 717-796-6100 **Fax:** 717-796-6150 **Metro area:** Harrisburg, PA **Web site:** http://www.balancedcare.com **Human resources contact:** Brad Witmer **Sales:** $90.7 million **Number of employees:** 2,400 **Number of employees for previous year:** 2,000 **Industry designation:** Nursing homes **Company type:** Public **Top competitors:** Beverly Enterprises, Inc.; Alternative Living Services, Inc.; Sentara Health System

Balanced Care wants to meet the needs of the aged with its assisted-living, skilled nursing, and independent-living facilities in nonurban areas. The acquisitive company operates more than 60 facilities in Arkansas, Missouri, North Carolina, Ohio, Pennsylvania, Virginia, and Wisconsin. The company's Outlook Pointe facilities provide community-like living for more affluent residents. Its assisted-living facilities offer 24-hour personal support services to residents, including help with bathing, eating, and dressing. Balanced Care also operates a home health care agency in Missouri that provides nursing, therapy, and personal care services to patients in assisted- and independent-living centers.

Bentley Systems, Incorporated

690 Pennsylvania Dr., Exton, PA 19341

Telephone: 610-458-5000 **Fax:** 610-458-1060 **Metro area:** Philadelphia, PA **Web site:** http://www.bentley.com **Sales:** $155 million (Est.) **Number of employees:** 950 **Number of employees for previous year:** 604 **Industry designation:** Computers—engineering, scientific & CAD-CAM software **Company type:** Private **Top competitors:** Eagle Point Software Corporation; Parametric Technology Corporation; Dassault Systemes S.A.

If it's a big building, it probably began with Bentley Systems. The company and its affiliates, which make computer-aided design software for large-scale engineering projects, have a customer list that includes AT&T, Exxon, Ford, and the US Air Force. Bentley products such as MicroStation and ModelServer have helped kick off the designs of roadways, machines, and well-known buildings for the geoengineering, construction, and mechanical engineering industries worldwide. In addition, Bentley SELECT is the engineering software industry's first technology and service subscription program. Founded by brothers Keith and Barry Bentley in 1984, Bentley Systems has offices in Australia, the Netherlands, and the US.

Bionx Implants, Inc.

1777 Sentry Pkwy. West, Gwynedd Hall, Ste. 400, Blue Bell, PA 19422

Telephone: 215-643-5000 **Fax:** 610-296-2249 **Metro area:** Philadelphia, PA **Sales:** $16 million **Number of employees:** 154 **Number of employees for previous year:** 70 **Industry designation:** Medical products **Company type:** Public

Bionx Implants develops and manufactures variable-strength polymer implants, including screws, pins, arrows, and stents, for use in orthopedic surgery, urology, dentistry, and maxillofacial surgery. The company's self-reinforced, resorbable polymer implants improve bone and soft tissue healing, lower implant failure rate, and reduce the need for repeat surgery. The company's pins and screws are used for repairing fractures, while the resorbable stents are used in urological procedures. Its Meniscus Arrow is used to repair tears of the medial and lateral meniscus of the knee, and its Bankart Tack helps surgeons repair shoulder injuries.

Catholic Health East

14 Campus Blvd., Ste. 300, Newtown Square, PA 19073

Telephone: 610-355-2000 **Fax:** 610-355-2050 **Metro area:** Philadelphia, PA **Web site:** http://www.chenet.org **Human resources contact:** Maria Butz **Sales:** $3 billion **Number of employees:** 31,838 **Industry designation:** Hospitals **Company type:** Not-for-profit **Top competitors:** Columbia/HCA Healthcare Corporation; Foundation Health Systems, Inc.; Daughters of Charity National Health System

Catholic Health East is the #3 religious health system in the US (behind #1 Daughters of Charity National Health System and #2 Catholic Health Initiatives). The network is a product of the consolidation of Eastern Mercy Health System of Pennsylvania, Franciscan Sisters of Allegheny Health System of Florida, and Sisters of Providence Health System of Massachusetts. These nuns are on the run to merge, in part because fewer women are wearing the habit these days, creating concern about the future of Catholic health care systems. The system offers health care through more than 30 hospitals, 30 nursing homes, and 20 independent- and assisted-living facilities.

Cell Pathways, Inc.

702 Electronic Dr., Horsham, PA 19044

Telephone: 215-706-3800 **Fax:** 215-706-3801 **Metro area:** Philadelphia, PA **Web site:** http://www.cellpathways.com **Human resources contact:** Susan Little **Number of employees:** 27 **Industry designation:** Drugs **Company type:** Public **Top competitors:** OSI Pharmaceuticals, Inc.; Vertex Pharmaceuticals Incorporated; Repligen Corporation

Cell Pathways (CPI) develops drugs to prevent and treat cancer. Lead drug candidates CP 461 and Prevatac are in the clinical trials (the latter suffered some disappointing late-stage trial results). The drugs were developed to treat such conditions as precancerous polyps of the colon, prostate cancer, and breast cancer. CPI plans to develop more drugs based on a mechanism that may induce selective cell death in precancerous and cancerous cells without affecting normal cells. The firm has collaborative agreements with the National Cancer Institute and the University of Arizona. On its path to going public, CPI bought semiconductor maker Tseng Labs in 1998.

Centeon L.L.C.

1020 First Ave., King of Prussia, PA 19406

Telephone: 610-878-4000 **Fax:** 610-878-4009 **Metro area:** Philadelphia, PA **Web site:** http://www.centeon.com/na/index.htm **Human resources contact:** Ray Reagan **Sales:** $1 billion **Number of employees:** 4,700 **Number of employees for previous year:** 4,500 **Industry designation:** Biomedical & genetic products **Company type:** Joint venture **Parent company:** Hoechst Group; Rhone-Poulenc Rorer Inc. **Top competitors:** Baxter International Inc.; Serologicals Corporation; NABI

Take away the red and white blood cells from blood and you get plasma, a protein-rich fluid. Centeon, through its Centeon Bio-Services unit, is among the world's largest fully integrated plasma collection companies. Centeon's plasma protein products are used routinely during surgery, in dialysis, and in the treatment of a range of other disorders, including immune deficiencies, trauma, and burns. As a US-based joint venture between Franco-American company Rhone-Poulenc Rorer and German chemical giant Hoechst AG, Centeon has the critical mass to keep rolling while increasing its research.

Centocor Diagnostics, Inc.

244 Great Valley Pkwy., Malvern, PA 19355

Telephone: 610-651-6000 **Fax:** 610-651-6100 **Metro area:** Philadelphia, PA **Human resources contact:** Mike Melore **Sales:** $40.1 million **Number of employees:** 130 **Industry designation:** Medical products **Company type:** Subsidiary **Top competitors:** Abbott Laboratories

Centocor Diagnostics is serious as a heart attack about the rapid diagnoses of chest pains. Heart attack symptoms are often difficult to differentiate from those of unstable angina or from less serious ailments. The company's test, still in the trial stage, detects the presence of P-selectin, an indicator of platelet activity related to heart attacks. This point-of-care test is intended to diagnose heart attacks quickly, when early treatment can prevent some heart damage from becoming irreversible. The company also makes a test that measures cancer-related antigens in blood cells, which may help determine the efficacy of therapies. Centocor Diagnostics is a subsidiary of Centocor.

Centocor, Inc.

200 Great Valley Pkwy., Malvern, PA 19355

Telephone: 610-651-6000 **Fax:** 610-651-6100 **Metro area:** Philadelphia, PA **Web site:** http://www.centocor.com **Human resources contact:** Mike Melore **Sales:** $338.1 million **Number of employees:** 640 **Number of employees for previous year:** 545 **Industry designation:** Biomedical & genetic products **Company type:** Public **Top competitors:** Rhone-Poulenc S.A.; Zeneca Group PLC; Genentech, Inc.

Centocor makes therapeutic and diagnostic drugs for cancer, cardiovascular problems, and other diseases. Three of the company's products are approved for sale in the US: ReoPro prevents blood clots during angioplasty, Remicade treats the bowel disorder Crohn's disease (and is being tested for efficacy against rheumatoid arthritis), and Panorex treats cancer. ReoPro is sold in the US and Europe by Eli Lilly. Centocor's drug Avakine is in the final US testing stages for treatment of Crohn's disease. The company owns the US and Canadian marketing rights for Retavase, a cardiovascular drug developed by Roche Holding. Centocor is selling its oncology diagnostics business to focus on therapeutics.

Cephalon, Inc.

145 Brandywine Pkwy., West Chester, PA 19380

Telephone: 610-344-0200 **Fax:** 610-344-0065 **Metro area:** Philadelphia, PA **Web site:** http://www.cephalon.com **Human resources contact:** Carl A. Savini **Sales:** $15.7 million **Number of employees:** 295 **Number of employees for previous year:** 282 **Industry designation:** Drugs **Company type:** Public **Top competitors:** Synthelabo; Amgen Inc.; Rhone-Poulenc S.A.

"Cephalon" means head of the extinct trilobite, but the biotechnology company is alive and well. Cephalon discovers and develops drugs for treating neurological disorders, such as Alzheimer's and multiple sclerosis, as well as prostate cancer. The company has several product candidates in the pipeline in various phases of research, development, and clinical trials. Its Myotrophin compound was jointly developed with Chiron to treat amyotrophic lateral sclerosis (ALS, or Lou Gehrig's disease). Rejected by the FDA's advisory panel in 1997, Myotrophin is still under review, pending more data. Cephalon's Provigil, a nonamphetamine treatment for narcolepsy, is marketed in the US and abroad.

CollaGenex Pharmaceuticals, Inc.

301 S. State St., Newtown, PA 18940

Telephone: 215-579-7388 **Fax:** 215-579-8577 **Metro area:** Philadelphia, PA **Web site:** http://www.collagenex.com **Sales:** $3.5 million **Number of employees:** 134 **Number of employees for previous year:** 14 **Industry designation:** Drugs **Company type:** Public **Top competitors:** Creative BioMolecules, Inc.; Atrix Laboratories, Inc.; Biora AB

CollaGenex develops drugs for dental diseases. The company's first product is Periostat, which is based on doxycycline, a form of tetracycline whose antibiotic properties have been eliminated but which inhibits the tissue damage that results from periodontal infections. Other applications of the drug technology include cancer, wounds, and arthritis. CollaGenex also markets SmithKline Beecham's cold sore treatment Denavir to dentists. The firm has no research personnel or facilities and contracts out all such activities. It licensed the doxycycline technology from the State University of New York. The company has licensed Periostat to Boehringer Mannheim Italia to produce the drug for sale in Italy.

Covalent Group, Inc.

One Glenhardie Corporate Center, 1275 Drummers Ln., Ste. 100, Wayne, PA 19087

Telephone: 610-975-9533 **Fax:** 610-975-9556 **Metro area:** Philadelphia, PA **Web site:** http://www.taraonline.com/cracorp **Human resources contact:** Diane Paretchan **Sales:** $9.4 million **Number of employees:** 30 **Number of employees for previous year:** 20 **Industry designation:** Medical services **Company type:** Public

Covalent Group has some strong bonds with its clients. The company, through its Covalent Research Alliance (CRA) subsidiary, manages drug and medical device clinical trials for pharmaceutical, managed care, and insurance firms. CRA uses both full-time and contract personnel to provide clinical trial and data management, biostatistical analysis, medical and regulatory services, and health economics and outcomes research. CRA also has developed Virtual HouseCall, an interactive voice recognition system for collecting and reporting patient information, and for use in disease management. President and CEO Bruce LaMont owns more than half the company.

DENTSPLY International Inc.

570 W. College Ave., York, PA 17405

Telephone: 717-845-7511 **Fax:** 717-854-2343 **Other address:** PO Box 872, York, PA 17405 **Metro area:** York, PA **Web site:** http://www.dentsply.com **Human resources contact:** Glenn K. Weingarth **Sales:** $795.1 million **Number of employees:** 5,300 **Number of employees for previous year:** 5,100 **Industry designation:** Medical products **Company type:** Public **Top competitors:** Henry Schein, Inc.; Sybron International Corporation; Patterson Dental Company

DENTSPLY International makes dental consumable and laboratory products and dental equipment. Products include artificial teeth, crown and bridge materials, dental sealants, and dental implants. DENTSPLY makes dental equipment, such as dental X-ray systems, handpieces, cutting instruments, and ultrasonic scalers and polishers. The company manufactures approximately 1,200 different consumable and laboratory products marketed under more than 70 brand names, including TRUBYTE (artificial teeth), JELTRATE (impression material), and CERAMCO (castable ceramic material). DENTSPLY markets its goods to dentists, dental labs, and dental schools in more than 100 countries.

Dialysis Corporation of America

27 Miller Ave., Lemoyne, PA 17043

Telephone: 717-730-7399 **Metro area:** Harrisburg, PA **Sales:** $4.4 million **Number of employees:** 42 **Number of employees for previous year:** 31 **Industry designation:** Medical services **Company type:** Public **Top competitors:** Fresenius Medical Care Aktiengesellschaft; Gambro AB; Total Renal Care Holdings, Inc.

This company's officers pledge allegiance to the Dialysis Corporation of America (and to the three kidney dialysis centers for which it stands), a 66%-owned subsidiary of Medicore offering outpatient dialysis and related services to all with end-stage renal failure. Related services include bone-density testing; electrocardiogram administration; nerve-conduction study; and administration of erythropoietin, which stimulates red blood cell growth for those with anemia. The company also provides inpatient dialysis to three Pennsylvania hospitals. Dialysis Corporation of America's centers are located in the Pennsylvania communities of Carlisle, Lemoyne, and Wellsboro.

Foamex International Inc.

1000 Columbia Ave., Linwood, PA 19061

Telephone: 610-859-3000 **Fax:** 800-356-0740 **Metro area:** Philadelphia, PA **Web site:** http://www.foamex.com **Human resources contact:** Donald Mallo **Sales:** $1.3 billion **Number of employees:** 6,414 **Number of employees for previous year:** 4,453 **Industry designation:** Rubber & plastic products **Company type:** Public

Foamex International produces and distributes flexible polyurethane foam and polymer foam products for bedding and furniture, automotive uses, and filtration. Foamex sells its products through a network of independent fabrication and distribution companies in North America, the UK, and South Korea. The company's products also include Plushlife carpet cushioning, Latex Plus bedding, and Reflex cushion wraps and cores. Its automotive foam products are used in auto door panels and headliners and for acoustical purposes. Chairman Marshall Cogan's Trace International Holdings owns about 46% of the company. Cogan has abandoned plans to buy the remainder of Foamex and is seeking a buyer for his stake.

Genesis Health Ventures, Inc.

148 W. State St., Kennett Square, PA 19348

Telephone: 610-444-6350 **Fax:** 610-444-3365 **Metro area:** Philadelphia, PA **Web site:** http://www.ghv.com **Human resources contact:** James W. Tabak **Sales:** $1.4 billion **Number of employees:** 45,000 **Number of employees for previous year:** 43,400 **Industry designation:** Nursing homes **Company type:** Public **Top competitors:** Integrated Health Services, Inc.; Beverly Enterprises, Inc.; Mariner Post-Acute Network, Inc.

Genesis Health Ventures provides basic and specialty health care for the elderly. The aggressively acquisitive company, which offers services under the Genesis ElderCare brand name, owns or manages about 325 geriatric care facilities. Its network includes primary care physician clinics, institutional and community-based pharmacies, medical supply distribution centers, certified rehabilitation clinics, and infusion therapy services. Its facilities are located in 16 eastern and midwestern states. Genesis also provides such specialty care as skilled, intermediate, and personal nursing; rehabilitation; respiratory therapy; and wound management.

Gen Trak, Inc.

5100 Campus Dr., Plymouth Meeting, PA 19462

Telephone: 610-825-5115 **Fax:** 610-941-9498 **Metro area:** Philadelphia, PA **Human resources contact:** Donald O. Nichols **Sales:** $2.7 million (Est.) **Number of employees:** 15 **Industry designation:** Medical products **Company type:** Private **Top competitors:** Hyseq, Inc.; Sangstat Medical Corporation; Abbott Laboratories

Gen Trak is the bloodhound of gene marking. The company's cellular diagnostic, paternity, and genetic testing kits create genetic maps using human leukocyte antigens. Hospitals, laboratories, and research facilities use these tests to determine a donor's organ or bone marrow compatibility, diagnose infectious diseases, or conduct other research. In addition to its genetic testing kits, Gen Trak is also developing a test doctors can use in their offices to diagnose infectious diseases; the test uses a technology that amplifies the presence of infection-fighting antibodies produced by the patient's immune system. Gen Trak markets its testing kits around the world, with 80% of its sales in the US.

Great Expectations International, Inc.

PO Box 918, Spring House, PA 19477

Telephone: 215-444-7700 **Fax:** 215-444-5650 **Metro area:** Philadelphia, PA **Human resources contact:** Candy Krier **Sales:** $5 million (Est.) **Industry designation:** Leisure & recreational services **Company type:** Private **Top competitors:** It's Just Lunch!, Inc.; MatchMaker International Development Corp.

Dating service Great Expectations International helps single people avoid the Ms. Havishams of the world. After going through an initial interview and paying a fee, the company's more than 165,000 members are asked to fill out a profile describing themselves and what they are looking for in a potential mate. The members are then photographed and videotaped so that other members can take a look. The company has about 50 offices in 25 states and the District of Columbia. Great Expectations International is owned by Advanta Partners LP, a venture capital subsidiary of Advanta Corp.

Hemispherx BioPharma, Inc.

1617 JFK Blvd., Philadelphia, PA 19103

Telephone: 215-988-0080 **Fax:** 215-988-1739 **Metro area:** Philadelphia, PA **Web site:** http://www.hemispherx.com **Human resources contact:** Josephine M. Dolhancryk **Sales:** $400,000 **Number of employees:** 45 **Number of employees for previous year:** 17 **Industry designation:** Drugs **Company type:** Public **Top competitors:** Gilead Sciences, Inc.; Isis Pharmaceuticals, Inc.; Genentech, Inc.

Hemispherx Biopharma is doing a world of good with its RNA drugs. The development-stage company is working with Bioclones (a subsidiary of South African Breweries) to develop Ampligen, an intravenously administered RNA drug, to treat hepatitis B, HIV, chronic fatigue syndrome, and such cancers as kidney and skin cancer. Hemispherx is also working on Oragen, a group of orally administered RNA drugs, to treat HIV, hepatitis B, and other infections. In addition to its RNA drugs, the company is developing laboratory tests using RNA to detect viral infections. Subsidiary BioPro is working to use RNA technology in tobacco filters to create cleaner cigarettes and other products. Officers own nearly 25% of the company.

Henkel of America, Inc.

2200 Renaissance Blvd., Ste. 200, Gulph Mills, PA 19406

Telephone: 610-270-8100 **Fax:** 610-270-8165 **Metro area:** Philadelphia, PA **Web site:** http://www.henkelcorp.com **Human resources contact:** Martin Brown **Industry designation:** Chemicals—diversified **Company type:** Subsidiary **Parent company:** Henkel KGaA **Top competitors:** The Dow Chemical Company; E. I. du Pont de Nemours and Company; Hoechst AG

It's a dirty world, and chemical manufacturer Henkel of America, subsidiary of German chemical giant Henkel, wants to clean as much of it as it can. While the company makes both household and institutional cleaners, it also produces oleochemicals used in soap production. The company also manufactures pesticides; health products such as vitamin E; adhesives (sold under the Macromelt, Purmelt, and Sicomet brands); chemicals used to recover precious and base metals; high-quality fatty alcohols used in cosmetics and lubricants; synthetic ester lubricants for automotive, aviation, and industrial use; coatings and inks; and chemicals for the textile industry. The company operates facilities in the US and Canada.

Highmark Inc.

120 Fifth Ave., Pittsburgh, PA 15222

Telephone: 412-544-7000 **Fax:** 412-544-8368 **Metro area:** Pittsburgh, PA **Web site:** http://www.highmark.com **Human resources contact:** Thomas C. Sommers **Sales:** $7.4 billion **Number of employees:** 12,000 **Number of employees for previous year:** 10,500 **Industry designation:** Health maintenance organization **Company type:** Not-for-profit **Top competitors:** The Guardian Life Insurance Company of America; Humana Inc.; Aetna Inc.

Highmark aims to be at the acme of HMOs. Formed by the merger of Pennsylvania Blue Shield with Veritus (formerly Blue Cross of Western Pennsylvania), Highmark provides health-related coverage (such as Keystone Health Plan West and HealthGuard), Medicare claims processing (Veritus Medicare and Xact Medicare), and administrative and information services (Synertech and Alliance Ventures). Its Trans-General Group offers group life, disability, and employer stop loss insurance. The company also provides community service programs such as the Western Pennsylvania Caring Foundation. Highmark serves some 18 million Americans throughout the US.

Home Health Corporation of America, Inc.

2200 Renaissance Blvd., Ste. 300, King of Prussia, PA 19406

Telephone: 610-272-1717 **Fax:** 610-272-6809 **Metro area:** Philadelphia, PA **Web site:** http://www.hhcainc.com **Human resources contact:** Bob Simon **Sales:** $174.3 million **Number of employees:** 3,069 **Number of employees for previous year:** 3,068 **Industry designation:** Health care—outpatient & home **Company type:** Public **Top competitors:** Coram Healthcare Corporation; Apria Healthcare Group Inc.; National HealthCare Corp.

Home Health Corporation of America provides home health care services and products. Among its offerings are nursing and related services (registered nurses, personal and homemaking assistants, and speech, occupational, and physical therapists), infusion and respiratory therapy and supplies, and medical equipment rentals (beds, wheelchairs, and lifts). The company provides its roster of services to managed care companies on a contract basis. Medicare and Medicaid reimbursements have forced Home Health Corporation of America to cut costs and restructure its operations. The company has more than 40 branches in Delaware, Florida, Illinois, Maryland, Massachusetts, New Hampshire, New Jersey, Pennsylvania, and Texas.

IBAH, Inc.

4 Valley Sq., 512 Township Line Rd., Blue Bell, PA 19422

Telephone: 215-283-0770 **Fax:** 215-283-0733 **Metro area:** Philadelphia, PA **Web site:** http://www.ibah.com **Human resources contact:** Mari-Lou Biancarelli **Sales:** $88.1 million **Number of employees:** 908 **Number of employees for previous year:** 755 **Industry designation:** Biomedical & genetic products **Company type:** Subsidiary **Top competitors:** Pharmaceutical Product Development, Inc.; Covance Inc.; Quintiles Transnational Corp.

IBAH provides product development services to pharmaceutical, biotechnology, medical-device, and diagnostics companies. It is a subsidiary of Omnicare, which provides pharmaceutical services to long-term care facilities. The core of IBAH is the Bio-Pharm Clinical Service Division, which designs product development programs, manages preclinical studies, designs and conducts clinical trials, and prepares filings for regulatory approval. The company's other operating unit, the Bio-Pharm Pharmaceuticals Division, provides traditional product formulation services, process development, pilot plant manufacturing, and packaging of supplies for clinical trials.

Kensey Nash Corporation

Marsh Creek Corporate Center, 55 E. Uwchlan Ave., Ste. 204, Exton, PA 19341

Telephone: 610-524-0188 **Fax:** 610-524-0265 **Metro area:** Philadelphia, PA **Web site:** http://www.kenseynash.com **Human resources contact:** June E. Sheets **Sales:** $8.3 million **Number of employees:** 100 **Number of employees for previous year:** 90 **Industry designation:** Medical products **Company type:** Public **Top competitors:** Perclose, Inc.; Datascope Corp.; Guidant Corporation

Kensey Nash works not in vain—rather, in arteries. The firm's Angio-Seal is made of absorbable material and is designed to seal arterial punctures (that can occur during cardiovascular procedures) faster and more effectively than conventional methods. Kensey Nash, which makes collagen products for other manufacturers, is also developing the Aegis Vortex system, which clears blocked veins without causing embolisms. A Tyco International subsidiary (which accounts for nearly 90% of Kensey Nash's sales) is selling to St. Jude Medical's Daig division its worldwide rights to make and market Angio-Seal. Co-founders Kenneth Kensey (chairman) and John Nash (vice chairman) own 30% and 13% of the company, respectively.

Keystone Foods Corp.

401 City Ave., Ste. 800, Bala Cynwyd, PA 19004

Telephone: 610-667-6700 **Fax:** 610-667-1460 **Metro area:** Philadelphia, PA **Web site:** http://www.keystonefoods.com **Human resources contact:** Robert S. Weinberg **Sales:** $2.2 billion (Est.) **Number of employees:** 4,300 **Number of employees for previous year:** 4,000 **Industry designation:** Food—meat products **Company type:** Private **Top competitors:** IBP, inc.; ConAgra, Inc.; The Martin-Brower Company

Keystone Foods is one of the nation's largest makers of hamburger, sausage, and processed poultry. A major supplier to McDonald's restaurants, Keystone developed a new method of freezing meat patties in the 1970s and persuaded the fast-food giant to switch to frozen beef, greatly reducing the health risks associated with fresh beef. The company was also instrumental in developing Chicken McNuggets for McDonald's. Keystone's other operations include selling restaurant supplies through M&M Restaurant Supply. Chairman, CEO, and president Herbert Lotman is the sole owner of the company.

Leak-X Environmental Corporation

790 E. Market St., Ste. 270, West Chester, PA 19382

Telephone: 610-344-3380 **Fax:** 610-344-3388 **Metro area:** Philadelphia, PA **Human resources contact:** Eileen E. Bartoli **Sales:** $10.1 million **Number of employees:** 45 **Number of employees for previous year:** 41 **Industry designation:** Pollution control equipment & services **Company type:** Public **Top competitors:** Omega Environmental, Inc.; Thermo TerraTech Inc.; CET Environmental Services, Inc.

Leak-X Environmental wants to keep groundwater clean and underground storage tanks sealed tight. The company operates two businesses: environmental consulting, through Lexicon Environmental Associates, and groundwater remediation, through Groundwater Recovery Systems (GRS). Lexicon's services include environmental engineering, hydrogeological and remedial consulting services, and storage tank-related construction management services. GRS's groundwater pollution control services include the design and manufacture of site-specific remediation systems, which it installs and maintains worldwide.

Mastech Corporation

1004 McKee Rd., Oakdale, PA 15071

Telephone: 412-787-2100 **Fax:** 412-787-7451 **Metro area:** Pittsburgh, PA **Web site:** http://www.mastech.com **Human resources contact:** Murali Balasubamanyam **Sales:** $390.9 million **Number of employees:** 4,700 **Number of employees for previous year:** 3,125 **Industry designation:** Computers—services **Company type:** Public **Top competitors:** Control Data Systems, Inc.; Computer Sciences Corporation; Computer Horizons Corp.

Mastech provides large organizations with a wide selection of information technology consultants offering services including computer network design and development, system conversion, year 2000 date conversion, and maintenance outsourcing. It stays on top of industry changes through business alliances with software makers like Baan, Oracle, and PeopleSoft. Mastech sells direct to customers both in the US and overseas, including AT&T, Citibank, Intel, NIKE, Wal-Mart, and EDS (which accounts for 13% of sales). The company continues to expand internationally through acquisitions. Co-founders Sunil Wadhwani (CEO) and Ashok Trivedi (president) each own about 37% of the company.

Molecular Circuitry, Inc.

321 Spruce St., Ste. 525, Scranton, PA 18503

Telephone: 717-207-7200 **Fax:** 717-347-1734 **Metro area:** Scranton, PA **Human resources contact:** George W. Ginader **Number of employees:** 6 **Industry designation:** Medical products **Company type:** Private **Top competitors:** The Perkin-Elmer Corporation; Neogen Corporation; Meridian Diagnostics, Inc.

Vile microbes beware—Molecular Circuitry "will" find you. The company was founded in 1994 to develop an immunoassay system that detects pathogens in food. The system, MC-18, detects the "Gang of Four" pathogens most feared by US food producers: salmonella, "E. coli," listeria, and campylobacter. The company intends to market the MC-18 to food producers and distributors worldwide through VWR Scientific Products. Upon completion of the IPO (and a concurrent reorganization of debt), chairman and CEO Herbert Lotman's interest in the company will rise from 15% to about half. Lotman founded Keystone Foods, a major supplier for McDonald's, and gained an interest in the company following its 1996 bankruptcy.

Moyco Technologies, Inc.

200 Commerce Dr., Montgomeryville, PA 18936

Telephone: 215-855-4300 **Fax:** 215-362-3809 **Other address:** PO Box 505, Montgomeryville, PA 18936 **Metro area:** Philadelphia, PA **Web site:** http://www.moycotech.com/moyco **Human resources contact:** Drew Lipkin **Sales:** $15.3 million **Number of employees:** 161 **Number of employees for previous year:** 145 **Industry designation:** Medical & dental supplies **Company type:** Public **Top competitors:** DENTSPLY International Inc.; Sybron International Corporation; Minnesota Mining and Manufacturing Company

Moyco Technologies gets to the root of the problem and makes it shine with its dental instruments and precision abrasives. The dental side of the business makes instruments, mirrors, waxes, and other items, in addition to repackaging and distributing dental products from other makers. Root-canal instruments account for about 25% of total sales. The precision abrasives segment makes abrasives (Flex-I-Grit) and slurries (Ultralap) used not only in the dental industry but also in the making of such products as fiber optics, semiconductors, and fingernail files. Moyco Technologies' products are sold internationally to distributors and end users. Chairman and president Marvin Sternberg owns some 58% of the company.

Moyer Packing Co.

249 Allentown Rd., Souderton, PA 18964

Telephone: 215-723-5555 **Fax:** 215-723-1018 **Other address:** PO Box 395, Souderton, PA 18964 **Metro area:** Philadelphia, PA **Web site:** http://www.mopac.com **Human resources contact:** Robert Daubenspeck **Sales:** $553 million (Est.) **Number of employees:** 1,600 **Number of employees for previous year:** 1,550 **Industry designation:** Food—meat products **Company type:** Private **Top competitors:** Packerland Packing Company; Rosen's Diversified, Inc.; IBP, inc.

Cattle meet their maker through Moyer Packing (MOPAC). Every week MOPAC processes more than 10,000 of the hapless (if tasty) animals; its yearly output is 330 million pounds of beef products. The company markets fresh, frozen, or vacuum-packed boxed beef, ground beef, and "variety meats" to chain stores, processors, wholesalers, and distributors to hotels and restaurants. It also sells otherwise-inedible by-products for use in the production of such items as animal feed, chemicals, and soap. The company has three plants in Pennsylvania and one each in Delaware and Virginia. About half of MOPAC's sales are exports. The Moyer family owns the company, which was started as a one-person meat business in 1877.

Mylan Laboratories Inc.

1030 Century Bldg., 130 Seventh St., Pittsburgh, PA 15222

Telephone: 412-232-0100 **Fax:** 412-232-0123 **Metro area:** Pittsburgh, PA **Web site:** http://www.mylan.com **Human resources contact:** Robert Myers **Sales:** $528.6 million **Number of employees:** 1,946 **Number of employees for previous year:** 1,750 **Industry designation:** Drugs—generic **Company type:** Public **Top competitors:** Merck & Co., Inc.; Novartis AG; American Home Products Corporation

Mylan Laboratories knows you may not recognize the names of its drugs, but it hopes you'll appreciate their prices. Mylan is one of the largest manufacturers and marketers of prescription generic drugs in the US. The company's pharmaceuticals include antibiotics, anti-inflammatories, cardiovascular drugs, and central nervous system agents as well as antipsychotics, diuretics, antianxiety drugs, antidepressants, beta-blockers, and antihypertensive agents. The company also owns 50% of research joint venture Somerset Pharmaceuticals (with Watson Pharmaceuticals). The Federal Trade Commission has accused Mylan of illegally raising prices on lorazepam (generic Ativan).

NovaCare, Inc.

1016 W. Ninth Ave., King of Prussia, PA 19406

Telephone: 610-992-7200 **Fax:** 610-992-3328 **Metro area:** Philadelphia, PA **Web site:** http://www.novacare.com **Human resources contact:** Kathryn P. Kehoe **Sales:** $1.7 billion **Number of employees:** 53,000 **Number of employees for previous year:** 39,800 **Industry designation:** Medical services **Company type:** Public **Top competitors:** Columbia/HCA Healthcare Corporation; HEALTHSOUTH Corporation; Staff Leasing, Inc.

A stellar performer, NovaCare is the #2 provider of rehabilitation services in the US (behind HEALTHSOUTH) and the top provider of orthotic and prosthetic (O&P) products and services. The company provides contract rehabilitation (physical, occupational, and speech therapy) to 2,700 nursing homes and hospitals in 44 states. It also fixes the aches and sprains of athletes on some 20 pro sports teams. NovaCare Employee Services, in which it holds a 71% stake, is one of the largest professional employer organizations in the US, providing a full range of employee services such as benefits administration, risk management, and workers' compensation.

Orthovita, Inc.

45 Great Valley Pkwy., Malvern, PA 19355

Telephone: 610-640-1775 **Fax:** 610-640-1714 **Metro area:** Philadelphia, PA **Web site:** http://www.orthovita.com **Human resources contact:** Colleen Hamilton **Sales:** $3.3 million (Est.) **Number of employees:** 39 **Industry designation:** Medical products **Company type:** Private

Orthovita is developing new materials for physicians and dentists to use as bone substitutes and bone cements. The company is focusing on developing products that interface with tissue on a biological level, mimic natural bone characteristics, are easier to use, and harden more quickly than products currently in use. BioGran, which is used in oral surgery, is on the market in the US and in Europe. Two other products—OrthoComp and VitaGraft—are in testing for use in bone and vertebrae repair and in facial reconstruction. Orthovita has filed an IPO in Belgium on Europe's EASDAQ exchange. Chairman Paul Ducheyne, a scientist on the University of Pennsylvania faculty, founded the company in 1993.

PDG Environmental, Inc.

300 Oxford Dr., Monroeville, PA 15146

Telephone: 412-856-2200 **Fax:** 412-856-6914 **Metro area:** Pittsburgh, PA **Web site:** http://www.pdge.com **Human resources contact:** Dulcia Maire **Sales:** $24.6 million **Number of employees:** 235 **Number of employees for previous year:** 216 **Industry designation:** Pollution control equipment & services **Company type:** Public

PDG Environmental, through its subsidiaries, provides asbestos abatement services to private and public customers. Asbestos, once widely used as insulation and as a fire-retardant material, was banned by the Environmental Protection Agency in 1973 after it was found to cause lung cancer and related disorders. PDG's services include removing and disposing of asbestos, constructing enclosures around asbestos-filled areas, and spraying sealants on materials that contain asbestos. The company offers its services primarily for commercial and government buildings, schools, and industrial facilities in the eastern and southwestern US. Chairman John Regan owns approximately 30% of the company.

Penn Mutual Life Insurance Co.

600 Dresher Rd., Horsham, PA 19044

Telephone: 215-956-8000 **Fax:** 215-956-8347 **Metro area:** Philadelphia, PA **Web site:** http://www.pennmutual.com **Human resources contact:** Michael Biondolillo **Sales:** $1.1 billion **Number of employees:** 848 **Industry designation:** Insurance—life **Company type:** Mutual company **Top competitors:** New York Life Insurance Company; The Prudential Insurance Company of America; Metropolitan Life Insurance Company

Founded in 1847, Penn Mutual Life Insurance is the fourth-oldest US life insurer. The company has five main subsidiaries, including Penn Insurance and Annuity and brokerages Janney Montgomery Scott and Hornor, Townsend & Kent. Penn tailors its selling to the affluent: business owners, entrepreneurs, executives, and professionals. Products include term, whole life, universal life, variable universal life, and disability income insurance policies, as well as a full range of deferred and immediate annuity products. The company has prospered by focusing on the individual life and individual and group pension markets.

Penn National Gaming, Inc.

Wyomissing Professional Center, 825 Berkshire Blvd., Ste. 200, Wyomissing, PA 19610

Telephone: 610-373-2400 **Fax:** 610-376-2842 **Metro area:** Reading, PA **Web site:** http://www.pennnational.com **Human resources contact:** George Connolly **Sales:** $154.1 million **Number of employees:** 1,654 **Number of employees for previous year:** 1,629 **Industry designation:** Leisure & recreational services **Company type:** Public **Top competitors:** Penske Motorsports, Inc.; Greenwood Racing, Inc.; The Pennsylvania Lottery

Every day is a day at the races for Penn National Gaming. The company's Penn National Race Course features live horse racing, and its Pocono Downs Racetrack offers live harness racing. Both facilities are located in Pennsylvania and offer simulcast races and phone betting. Gamblers not at the track can place bets at one of Penn's 10 Pennsylvania off-track facilities. Penn owns 89% of Charles Town Entertainment Complex, a West Virginia facility featuring live and simulcast horse racing and more than 740 video gaming machines. Through a joint venture with Greenwood Racing, Penn also owns interests in Freehold Raceway and the lease on Garden State Park, both of New Jersey. CEO Peter Carlino owns 42% of Penn.

Penn Treaty American Corporation

3440 Lehigh St., Allentown, PA 18103

Telephone: 610-965-2222 **Fax:** 610-967-4616 **Metro area:** Allentown, PA **Web site:** http://www.penntreaty.com **Human resources contact:** Gary Koontz **Sales:** $254.2 million **Number of employees:** 322 **Number of employees for previous year:** 253 **Industry designation:** Insurance—accident & health **Company type:** Public **Top competitors:** AFLAC Incorporated; Washington National Corporation; New York Life Insurance Company

Penn Treaty American provides long-term nursing home and health care insurance to people age 65 and over. Long-term-care policies account for nearly 92% of its business. The firm's products include accident and health insurance policies covering nursing home care, home health care, hospital care, and policies that supplement Medicare benefits. The company also offers disability and life insurance policies. Its policies are marketed nationwide via a network of 25,000 independent agents. Penn Treaty American's three subsidiaries—Penn Treaty Life Insurance, Network America Life Insurance, and American Network—underwrite its insurance products.

Philadelphia Eagles

3501 S. Broad St., Veterans Stadium, Philadelphia, PA 19148

Telephone: 215-463-2500 **Fax:** 215-339-5464 **Metro area:** Philadelphia, PA **Web site:** http://www.eaglesnet.com **Human resources contact:** Vicki Chatley **Sales:** $83 million (Est.) **Number of employees:** 500 **Industry designation:** Leisure & recreational services **Company type:** Private **Top competitors:** Dallas Cowboys Football Club, Ltd.; New York Giants; Arizona Cardinals

The Philadelphia Eagles have been battling in the National Football League since 1933, but without a lot of success. The team has an overall losing record over that time span, although it did make it to the Super Bowl during the 1979-80 season (losing to the Oakland Raiders). Still, the team has an estimated value of about $209 million, putting it ahead of most other NFL teams. Eagles owner Jeff Lurie has made it clear that he wants a new stadium to replace Veterans Stadium, which first opened in 1971. Lurie has called the stadium one of the worst facilities in all of sports.

Philadelphia Flyers

First Union Center, 3601 S. Broad St., Philadelphia, PA 19148

Telephone: 215-465-4500 **Fax:** 215-389-9403 **Metro area:** Philadelphia, PA **Web site:** http://www.philadelphiaflyers.com **Human resources contact:** Alice Marini **Sales:** $74.6 million (Est.) **Number of employees:** 100 **Industry designation:** Leisure & recreational services **Company type:** Private **Top competitors:** New York Rangers; New Jersey Devils; Pittsburgh Penguins

The Philadelphia Flyers, once nicknamed the Broad Street Bullies for the high number of "enforcers" on their roster, joined the National Hockey League in 1967. This back-to-back winner of the Stanley Cup (1974 and 1975 seasons) also came out on the losing end of the Stanley Cup finals in 1976, 1980, 1985, and 1987. The team boasts high-dollar, high-scoring center Eric Lindros and has the First Union Center as its new home. Flyers ex-center Bobby Clarke is president and general manager of the team. Chairman Ed Snider and Comcast are majority owners of the team.

The Philadelphia Phillies

3501 S. Broad St., Philadelphia, PA 19148

Telephone: 215-463-6000 **Fax:** 215-389-3050 **Metro area:** Philadelphia, PA **Web site:** http://www.phillies.com **Sales:** $57.1 million (Est.) **Number of employees:** 208 **Number of employees for previous year:** 195 **Industry designation:** Leisure & recreational services **Company type:** Private **Top competitors:** The Atlanta Braves; Montreal Baseball Club Inc.; Metropolitan Baseball Club Inc.

Many fans of the Philadelphia Phillies wish for two things: a new stadium and the return of Mike Schmidt. One wish was granted in 1999, when the Pennsylvania legislature approved plans to replace aging Veterans Stadium with a new baseball-only park in 2002. As for the other wish, today the club is far removed from its glory days of the late 1970s, when Hall of Famer Schmidt led the Phillies to three consecutive division titles, a feat soon followed by a 1980 World Series championship. Bill Giles, one of four owners, has a controlling interest in the Phillies. One of baseball's older teams, the Phillies began play in 1883 as the Brown Stockings of Worcester, Massachusetts.

Philadelphia 76ers

First Union Center, 3601 S. Broad St., Philadelphia, PA 19148

Telephone: 215-339-7600 **Fax:** 215-339-7632 **Metro area:** Philadelphia, PA **Web site:** http://www.nba.com/sixers **Human resources contact:** Curt Wilson **Sales:** $69.9 million (Est.) **Number of employees:** 100 **Industry designation:** Leisure & recreational services **Company type:** Private **Top competitors:** New York Knickerbockers; Miami Heat; New Jersey Nets

It's a good thing the NBA's Philadelphia 76ers play in the City of Brotherly Love. Despite a notable lack of success, the 76ers set an all-time attendance record in the 1997-98 season. Originally the Syracuse Nationals, the team moved to Philadelphia in 1963 and signed hometown legend Wilt Chamberlain the next year. The 76ers became NBA champs in 1967 with Chamberlain leading the way, and again in 1983, paced by Julius "Dr. J" Erving. Former strength and conditioning coach Pat Croce bought the team in 1996 and established the new First Union Center as home court. Future Philly fortunes rest in the hands of veteran coach Larry Brown and explosive point guard Allen Iverson.

Pittsburgh Penguins

One Chatham Center, Ste. 400, Pittsburgh, PA 15219

Telephone: 412-642-1800 **Fax:** 412-642-1859 **Metro area:** Pittsburgh, PA **Web site:** http://www.pittsburghpenguins.com **Human resources contact:** Elaine Heufelder **Sales:** $52.6 million (Est.) **Number of employees:** 196 **Industry designation:** Leisure & recreational services **Company type:** Private **Top competitors:** New Jersey Devils; Philadelphia Flyers; New York Rangers

The Pittsburgh Penguins professional hockey team is skating on thin ice. It is operating under Chapter 11 bankruptcy protection for the second time (the first was in 1975), having lost about $40 million since 1996. The team owes legendary player Mario Lemieux (who unofficially retired in 1997) nearly $30 million. However, the Penguins' co-owners, Roger Marino and Howard Baldwin, have decided to sell the team with Lemieux a possible buyer. Founded in 1967, the Pittsburgh Penguins went through a string of owners, coaches, and bad luck (including the deaths of center Michel Briere and general manager Baz Bastien) before winning back-to-back Stanley Cup championships in 1991 and 1992.

Pittsburgh Pirates

Three Rivers Stadium, 600 Stadium Circle, Pittsburgh, PA 15212

Telephone: 412-323-5000 **Fax:** 412-323-9133 **Other address:** PO Box 7000, Pittsburgh, PA 15212 **Metro area:** Pittsburgh, PA **Web site:** http://www.pirateball.com **Human resources contact:** Linda Yenerall **Sales:** $49.3 million (Est.) **Industry designation:** Leisure & recreational services **Company type:** Private **Top competitors:** Chicago National League Ball Club, Inc.; Houston Astros Baseball Club; St. Louis Cardinals, L.P.

By building a new ballpark, the Pirates are hoping to steal a page on how to remain competitive against the big boys and their larger galleons of gold. The Pittsburgh Pirates, dating back to 1891, have given the city several World Series Championships (1909, 1925, 1960, 1971, and 1979) as well as such great players as Honus Wagner, Bill Mazeroski, Willie Stargell, and Roberto Clemente. In the 1990s, however, a tight team budget has hurt the Pirates' ability to attract and retain high-dollar players. In 1999 the Pennsylvania state legislature agreed to fund about a third of the Pirates' 38,000-seat baseball-only stadium, scheduled to open in 2001. CEO Kevin McClatchy is the controlling owner of the team.

Pittsburgh Steelers

300 Stadium Circle, Three Rivers Stadium, Pittsburgh, PA 15212

Telephone: 412-323-0300 **Fax:** 412-323-1393 **Metro area:** Pittsburgh, PA **Web site:** http://steelerslive.com **Sales:** $75.1 million (Est.) **Number of employees:** 125 **Industry designation:** Leisure & recreational services **Company type:** Private **Top competitors:** Jacksonville Jaguars; Cincinnati Bengals; Baltimore Ravens

Founded in 1933 as the Pirates, the Pittsburgh Steelers (renamed in 1940) embarked on a 40-year stretch of losing seasons. In the 1970s, with such greats as Terry Bradshaw, Lynn Swan, and a defense known as the "Steel Curtain," the team got its first taste of victory; it won its first of four Super Bowl titles (over a six-year period) in 1974. In the 1990s the Steelers, with the third-lowest franchise value in the NFL, continue to play fiercely, often ranking as AFC contenders. In 1999 the Pennsylvania state legislature agreed to fund one-third of a new $230 million stadium for the team. Three Rivers Stadium, the Steelers' current home, will be demolished. Dan Rooney (son of the late Art Rooney) owns the team.

PPG Industries, Inc.

One PPG Place, Pittsburgh, PA 15272

Telephone: 412-434-3131 **Fax:** 412-434-2448 **Metro area:** Pittsburgh, PA **Web site:** http://www.ppg.com **Human resources contact:** Russell L. Crane **Sales:** $7.5 billion **Number of employees:** 32,500 **Number of employees for previous year:** 31,900 **Industry designation:** Chemicals—diversified **Company type:** Public **Top competitors:** E. I. du Pont de Nemours and Company; Akzo Nobel N.V.; Corning Incorporated

PPG Industries helps do-it-yourself homeowners brighten up dingy rooms with its Lucite brand of house paints. PPG also makes the Olympic line of stains and other protective and decorative coatings for architectural, automotive, industrial, and other uses. Coatings account for almost half of sales. PPG also produces glass products such as car windshields, flat glass for buildings, and continuous-strand fiberglass. PPG's chemicals segment makes optical lenses that change tint, chlorine and chlorine derivatives, silica products, and fine chemicals. PPG operates more than 75 manufacturing facilities in 16 countries, but North America accounts for some 70% of sales.

Premier Research Worldwide, Ltd.

124 S. 15th St., Philadelphia, PA 19102

Telephone: 215-972-0420 **Fax:** 215-972-0352 **Metro area:** Philadelphia, PA **Web site:** http://www.premier-research.com **Human resources contact:** Marian Wissman **Sales:** $31.8 million **Number of employees:** 201 **Number of employees for previous year:** 130 **Industry designation:** Medical services **Company type:** Public **Top competitors:** Covance Inc.; PAREXEL International Corporation; Quintiles Transnational Corp.

Premier Research Worldwide gives drugs their debut. The company is a clinical research organization (CRO) that provides product development services to customers in the pharmaceutical, biotechnology, and medical device industries. Premier services include centralized diagnostic testing, clinical trial management, clinical data management, biostatistical analysis, Phase I clinical research, and health care economics. The company's computer-assisted new drug application system simplifies the collection, transfer, analysis, and preparation of clinical trial data. The company is affiliated with PREMIER, a health care alliance and trial management organization.

Prophet 21, Inc.

19 W. College Ave., Yardley, PA 19067

Telephone: 215-493-8900 **Fax:** 215-321-8001 **Metro area:** Philadelphia, PA **Web site:** http://www.p21.com **Human resources contact:** Carol Frymire **Sales:** $46.6 million **Number of employees:** 305 **Number of employees for previous year:** 278 **Industry designation:** Computers—corporate, professional & financial software **Company type:** Public **Top competitors:** System Software Associates, Inc.; J.D. Edwards & Company; PeopleSoft, Inc.

Prophet 21 knows the busy distributor can't rely on clairvoyance or luck. The company provides business application software and support services to distributors and wholesalers. Its primary products, Prophet 21 System, Prophet 21 Acclaim (for use with UNIX), and Prophet 21 Servant (for use with Windows/NT), provide functions such as purchasing, order and inventory management, and e-commerce. The company also offers services such as system design, training, installation, support, and maintenance. Prophet 21 markets to about 45,000 distributors, wholesalers, and dealers in the automotive, electronics, defense, and medical industries, among others. The company has sold nearly 2,000 systems in the US and Canada.

Quaker Chemical Corporation

Elm and Lee Sts., Conshohocken, PA 19428

Telephone: 610-832-4000 **Fax:** 610-832-8682 **Metro area:** Philadelphia, PA **Web site:** http://www.quakerchem.com **Human resources contact:** James A. Geier **Sales:** $257.1 million **Number of employees:** 923 **Number of employees for previous year:** 871 **Industry designation:** Chemicals—specialty **Company type:** Public

Quaker Chemical Corporation makes industrial specialty chemicals and is the global market leader in the production of lubricants used in the hot and cold rolling of steel. The company's other products for the metals industry include corrosion inhibitors, finishing compounds, sealants, coatings, and hydraulic fluids. The firm also makes chemicals for the paper industry and milling compounds for the aerospace sector. In addition, Quaker Chemical provides recycling and chemical management services. The company serves the steel, packaging, automotive, aerospace, pulp and paper, and appliance industries with manufacturing facilities in Europe and North America and a joint venture in Brazil.

The Quigley Corporation

10 S. Clinton St., Doylestown, PA 18901

Telephone: 215-345-0919 **Fax:** 215-345-5920 **Other address:** PO Box 1349, Doylestown, PA 18901 **Metro area:** Philadelphia, PA **Web site:** http://www.quigleyco.com **Human resources contact:** Guy J. Quigley **Sales:** $36.4 million **Number of employees:** 16 **Number of employees for previous year:** 10 **Industry designation:** Drugs **Company type:** Public

Quigley wants cold sufferers to put away their tissues and tonics and pop in a Cold-Eeze lozenge. The company contends its zinc gluconate lozenges lessen the length and severity of the common cold. Cold-Eeze and Cold-Eezer Plus (a higher-dosage zinc lozenge), and Kids-Eeze (bubblegum with zinc) aren't sold at independent and chain drug and discount stores such as Walgreen and Wal-Mart, as well as through the QVC cable shopping network and several Internet venues. Next on the agenda is Bodymate, a lozenge designed to suppress appetites and burn body fat. Founder and CEO Guy Quigley, who acquired manufacturing and distribution rights to Cold-Eeze in 1992, owns 26% of the company.

Respironics, Inc.

1501 Ardmore Blvd., Pittsburgh, PA 15221

Telephone: 412-731-2100 **Fax:** 412-473-5010 **Metro area:** Pittsburgh, PA **Web site:** http://www.respironics.com **Human resources contact:** Steven P. Fulton **Sales:** $351.6 million **Number of employees:** 2,045 **Number of employees for previous year:** 1,565 **Industry designation:** Medical instruments **Company type:** Public **Top competitors:** Mallinckrodt Inc.; ResMed Inc.; Sunrise Medical Inc.

Products from Respironics make respites more restful. The company makes respiratory products for use at home, in hospitals, and in emergency situations. About half the company's sales come from devices that treat obstructive sleep apnea, including its REMstar CPAP system, which treats irregular snoring and sleep apnea (disrupted sleep caused by blocked breathing passages). It also makes ventilation products for individuals who have trouble breathing but are not dependent on a ventilator for life support. Respironics also makes face masks for administering anesthesia and for use during surgery. The company is branching into infant and fetal care with its monitors for SIDS, bilirubin, and fetal oxygen levels.

Rite Aid Corporation

30 Hunter Ln., Camp Hill, PA 17011

Telephone: 717-761-2633 **Fax:** 717-975-5871 **Metro area:** Harrisburg, PA **Web site:** http://www.riteaid.com **Human resources contact:** Robert R. Sounder **Sales:** $12.7 billion **Number of employees:** 83,000 **Number of employees for previous year:** 73,000 **Industry designation:** Retail—drugstores **Company type:** Public **Top competitors:** J. C. Penney Company, Inc.; CVS Corporation; Walgreen Co.

Rite Aid is bulking up, and drugs are partly to blame. The company is the nation's third-largest drugstore chain (behind #1 Walgreen and #2 CVS, based on sales), with about 3,900 drugstores in 32 states. In addition to filling prescriptions, its stores sell cards, film, vitamins, and other general merchandise. Rite Aid is remodeling many of the stores it has recently acquired (including Thrifty PayLess and New Orleans' favorite K&B) and will open General Nutrition Companies (GNC) stores within 1,500 Rite Aid locations. It is also expanding the size of its older stores in the East and adding new stores. Rite Aid's wholly owned Eagle Managed Care sells prescription benefit programs.

Sanchez Computer Associates, Inc.

40 Valley Stream Pkwy., Malvern, PA 19355

Telephone: 610-296-8877 **Fax:** 610-296-7371 **Metro area:** Philadelphia, PA **Web site:** http://www.sanchez.com **Human resources contact:** Anne Novak **Sales:** $44.1 million **Number of employees:** 307 **Number of employees for previous year:** 241 **Industry designation:** Computers—corporate, professional & financial software **Company type:** Public **Top competitors:** Andersen Consulting; Fiserv, Inc.

Sanchez Computer Associates' PROFILE banking software is a multicurrency bank production system that supports bank and customer transactions through a variety of distribution channels, including the Internet. Sanchez targets three market segments: emerging banking markets in developing and emerging economies (as in Central Europe, Asia/Pacific, and Russia), direct-banking markets that offer services over the Internet and other electronic commerce, and top-tier banking markets, or the top 1,000 worldwide banks. Sanchez has strategic alliances to market its software with Digital Equipment, Hewlett Packard, Oracle, IBM, and Price Waterhouse. Safeguard Scientifics owns more than 25% of the company.

Scan-Graphics, Inc.

649 N. Lewis Rd., Ste. 220, Limerick, PA 19468

Telephone: 610-495-3003 **Fax:** 732-528-9065 **Metro area:** Philadelphia, PA **Web site:** http://www.scangraphics.com **Human resources contact:** Victoria Franchetti **Sales:** $4.8 million **Number of employees:** 79 **Number of employees for previous year:** 68 **Industry designation:** Computers—peripheral equipment **Company type:** Public **Top competitors:** Scitex Corporation Ltd.; BARCO N.V.; Isomet Corporation

Scan-Graphics is expanding its field of vision. The company, originally a maker of military- and government-marketed scanners for digitizing illustrations, encompasses three imaging-centric divisions. Sedona GeoServices develops software that visually organizes and displays database information, Tangent Imaging Systems makes large-format color scanners, and Technology Resource Centers offers document conversion and management services. Scan-Graphics' products are marketed internationally by integrators and distributors. The company has strategic alliances with Oracle, Sun Microsystems, and other firms. Founder and former chairman Andrew Trolio owns 13% of the company.

Shared Medical Systems Corporation

51 Valley Stream Pkwy., Malvern, PA 19355

Telephone: 610-219-6300 **Fax:** 610-219-3124 **Metro area:** Philadelphia, PA **Web site:** http://www.smed.com **Human resources contact:** Paul Yakulis **Sales:** $1.1 billion **Number of employees:** 5,984 **Number of employees for previous year:** 5,420 **Industry designation:** Computers—corporate, professional & financial software **Company type:** Public **Top competitors:** IDX Systems Corporation; National Data Corporation; McKesson HBOC, Inc.

Shared Medical Systems (SMS), the nation's #2 health care information systems and services provider (after McKesson HBOC), offers outsourced computer services, allowing clients to share its powerful mainframe computers and extensive databases. SMS also sets up distributed processing systems and on-site systems. Customers include hospitals, physician groups, and managed services organizations. SMS has online connections to more than 900 customers. The company has formed alliances with other technology companies, including Microsoft and Cisco Systems, to help it stay ahead of the competition. SMS has operations throughout the US and in Europe. Customers in North America account for about 90% of sales.

Sklar Instruments

889 S. Matlack St., West Chester, PA 19382

Telephone: 610-430-3200 **Fax:** 610-696-9007 **Metro area:** Philadelphia, PA **Web site:** http://www.sklarcorp.com **Human resources contact:** Janice Terry Russell **Sales:** $13.8 million (Est.) **Number of employees:** 63 **Number of employees for previous year:** 60 **Industry designation:** Instruments—scientific **Company type:** Private **Top competitors:** BEI Medical Systems Company, Inc.

Sklar Instruments sells and distributes more than 15,000 different handheld surgical and medical instruments, made primarily by German and Pakistani manufacturers. The company also provides instrument care and cleaning products, sterilizing kits, scalpels, and disposable blades to hospitals, clinics, and physicians. Other clients include dentists and veterinarians. It sells specialty instruments and equipment for use in endoscopy, arthroscopy, dermatology, obstetrics/gynecology, podiatry, and orthodontics. The company traces its roots back to 1892. President Don Taylor holds more than 30% of Sklar Instruments' common stock; CFO Michael Malinowski holds more than 15%.

SmithKline Beecham Corporation

One Franklin Plaza, Philadelphia, PA 19101

Telephone: 215-751-4000 **Fax:** 215-751-7655 **Other address:** PO Box 7929, Philadelphia, PA 19101 **Metro area:** Philadelphia, PA **Human resources contact:** Daniel Phelan **Industry designation:** Drugs **Company type:** Subsidiary **Parent company:** SmithKline Beecham PLC **Top competitors:** Merck & Co., Inc.; Glaxo Wellcome plc; Amgen Inc.

SmithKline Beecham Corporation, the US-based subsidiary of SmithKline Beecham plc, manufactures pharmaceuticals and consumer health products. The company makes Denavir, a treatment for the herpes virus that causes cold sores; Famvir, a genital herpes drug; Relafen, an anti-inflammatory drug for the treatment of osteoarthritis and rheumatoid arthritis; and other drugs. SmithKline Beecham Corporation also has alliances with other companies, including a research collaboration with Cadus Pharmaceutical to develop small-molecule drugs and a joint venture with a subsidiary of Q-Med that is developing a medical system to help identify heart attack risks.

Stadtlanders Drug Distribution Co., Inc.

600 Penn Center Blvd., Ste. 300, Pittsburgh, PA 15235

Telephone: 412-824-2487 **Fax:** 412-824-1419 **Metro area:** Pittsburgh, PA **Web site:** http://www.stadtlander.com **Human resources contact:** Diana Long **Sales:** $400 million **Number of employees:** 750 **Number of employees for previous year:** 700 **Industry designation:** Medical services **Company type:** Subsidiary **Top competitors:** Express Scripts, Inc.; Walgreen Co.

Sometimes the corner drugstore is a mailbox. Stadtlanders Drug Distribution provides mail-order pharmaceuticals for special needs customers, including those with HIV and AIDS or cancer, or those undergoing infertility treatment. The company provides customer monitoring and counseling, as well as outcome data. The company was founded in the 1950s as a neighborhood drugstore and has returned to its retail roots by opening stores in areas where potential customers are concentrated, including one in San Francisco's Castro district. Counsel Corporation, Stadtlanders' former owner, sold the company to drug supply giant Bergen Brunswig in 1999. The company also has a relationship with drugmaker Novartis.

SunGard Data Systems Inc.

1285 Drummers Ln., Wayne, PA 19087

Telephone: 610-341-8700 **Fax:** 610-341-8739 **Metro area:** Philadelphia, PA **Web site:** http://www.sungard.com **Human resources contact:** Donna J. Pedrick **Sales:** $1.2 billion **Number of employees:** 4,500 **Number of employees for previous year:** 3,700 **Industry designation:** Computers—services **Company type:** Public **Top competitors:** General Automation, Inc.; Applix, Inc.; Strategia Corporation

SunGard Data Systems is a computer services and software company specializing in investment support systems, computer disaster-recovery services, and health care information systems. Its investment support systems for the financial services industry supply calculations, record keeping, and reporting for investment operations. SunGard Data Systems' disaster-recovery services help businesses function when their own systems are down. Health care information systems provide workflow management and document imaging for health care and financial institutions. The company has more than 30 subsidiaries located throughout Australia, Europe, Japan, and the US; about 80% of its sales are in the US.

Sunoco, Inc.

10 Penn Center, 1801 Market St., Philadelphia, PA 19103

Telephone: 215-977-3000 **Fax:** 215-977-3409 **Metro area:** Philadelphia, PA **Web site:** http://www.sunocoinc.com **Human resources contact:** David C. Shanks **Sales:** $6.9 billion **Number of employees:** 11,100 **Number of employees for previous year:** 10,900 **Industry designation:** Oil refining & marketing **Company type:** Public **Top competitors:** Clark USA, Inc.; Ultramar Diamond Shamrock Corporation; Tosco Corporation

The #3 independent oil refiner and marketer in the US (after Tosco and Ultramar Diamond Shamrock), Sunoco operates five refineries. It markets gasoline through about 3,800 service stations in 17 states, primarily in the Northeast, through its Sunoco and Ultra Service Center gas stations and its APlus convenience stores. Sunoco has no exploration and production activities. Its core refining and marketing operations produce lubricants and other petrochemicals (including aromatics and olefins for use in plastics and other industries). Sunoco also has coal and coke businesses located in Indiana, Kentucky, and Virginia.

Sylvan Inc.

333 Main St., Saxonburg, PA 16056

Telephone: 724-352-7520 **Fax:** 724-352-7550 **Other address:** PO Box 249, Saxonburg, PA 16056 **Web site:** http://www.sylvaninc.com **Human resources contact:** Louise Allen **Sales:** $89.6 million **Number of employees:** 925 **Number of employees for previous year:** 910 **Industry designation:** Agricultural operations **Company type:** Public **Top competitors:** Campbell Soup Company; Seneca Foods Corporation; Monterey Mushrooms, Inc.

When Sylvan says it has an idea that's mushrooming, you can interpret it literally. The firm is a leading global supplier of mushroom spawn (or mushroom "seed") and related products to growers. Besides producing and distributing spawn, the company sells Sylvan Casing Inoculum, a production additive that accelerates mushroom growth. Sylvan also produces fresh mushrooms under the Prime brand, which it sells to supermarkets, food processors, and distributors in the US. The company distributes its mushroom spawn primarily in North America, Europe, and Australia.

Systems & Computer Technology Corporation

4 Country View Rd., Malvern, PA 19355

Telephone: 610-647-5930 **Fax:** 610-578-5102 **Metro area:** Philadelphia, PA **Web site:** http://www.sctcorp.com **Human resources contact:** Mark A. Cochran **Sales:** $398.3 million **Number of employees:** 3,400 **Number of employees for previous year:** 2,700 **Industry designation:** Computers—corporate, professional & financial software **Company type:** Public **Top competitors:** PeopleSoft, Inc.; Oracle Corporation; Electronic Data Systems Corporation

Systems & Computer Technology (SCT) helps its customers keep track of those pesky details. The company offers information technology services and administrative software to universities (40% of sales), local governments, utilities, and manufacturers. SCT generates about a third of its revenue through its outsourcing services. It also offers other services that include system support, implementation, and training. SCT's product line includes BANNER software (an administrative package available in versions tailored to higher-education, utility, and government customers) and ADAGE supply chain management software. SCT's 2,500 clients include Villanova University and SmithKline Beecham.

Teleflex Incorporated

630 W. Germantown Pike, Ste. 450, Plymouth Meeting, PA 19462

Telephone: 610-834-6301 **Fax:** 610-834-8307 **Metro area:** Philadelphia, PA **Web site:** http://www.teleflex.com **Human resources contact:** Ronald D. Boldt **Sales:** $1.4 billion **Number of employees:** 13,500 **Number of employees for previous year:** 11,700 **Industry designation:** Medical products **Company type:** Public

With goods from steering systems to skin staples, Teleflex is a diversified provider of products and services in three segments: aerospace, commercial, and medical. Its aerospace segment manufactures equipment such as controls and components for flight cargo systems and turbine engines. The commercial segment makes products for the automotive industry, including accelerators and fuel lines, and hydraulic control products and Humminbird fish locators for the marine industry. Medical products include devices such as catheters and face masks for urology, gastroenterology, anesthesiology, and respiratory care. Teleflex primarily sells to original equipment manufacturers, both directly and through distributors.

UBICS, Inc.

333 Technology Dr., Ste. 210, Southpointe, Canonsburg, PA 15317

Telephone: 724-746-6001 **Fax:** 724-746-9597 **Metro area:** Pittsburgh, PA **Web site:** http://www.ubics.com **Human resources contact:** Vijay P. Reddy **Sales:** $30.2 million **Number of employees:** 154 **Industry designation:** Computers—services **Company type:** Public

UBICS provides information technology (IT) professional services to large and medium-sized companies, primarily in the US. Its services include client/server design and development, enterprise resource planning, and database administration. The company, which recruits IT professionals worldwide (primarily from India), provides its services on a time-and-materials basis. Its customers include El Paso Energy, The Hartford, Access Graphics, Advance Auto Parts, and CompUSA, which combined account for 31% of total sales. UBICS is affiliated with the UB International Group, an India-based industrial group of companies under the control of chairman Vijay Mallya. Mallya owns approximately 67% of UBICS.

Unisys Corporation

Unisys Way, Blue Bell, PA 19424

Telephone: 215-986-4011 **Fax:** 215-986-2312 **Metro area:** Philadelphia, PA **Web site:** http://www.unisys.com **Human resources contact:** David O. Aker **Sales:** $7.2 billion **Number of employees:** 33,200 **Number of employees for previous year:** 32,600 **Industry designation:** Computers—services **Company type:** Public **Top competitors:** Hewlett-Packard Company; International Business Machines Corporation; Compaq Computer Corporation

Computer server and services firm Unisys provides hardware and software, and systems integration other services to clients such as Lufthansa Airlines, Pacific Bell, and the US Department of Justice. Federal entities account for 12% of sales. As the market has moved to network computing, Unisys (formerly a mainframe and defense electronics manufacturer) has scrambled to reinvent itself with new products, including its ClearPath servers (which combine mainframe, Microsoft Windows NT, and UNIX systems on a single platform). The company is also repositioning itself as a major provider of systems integration and support services (now nearly two-thirds of sales).

Universal Health Services, Inc.

367 S. Gulph Rd., King of Prussia, PA 19406

Telephone: 610-768-3300 **Fax:** 610-768-3336 **Other address:** P.O. Box 61558, King of Prussia, PA 19406 **Metro area:** Philadelphia, PA **Web site:** http://www.uhsinc.com **Human resources contact:** Eileen Bove **Sales:** $1.9 billion **Number of employees:** 19,200 **Number of employees for previous year:** 17,800 **Industry designation:** Hospitals **Company type:** Public **Top competitors:** Tenet Healthcare Corporation; Gambro AB; Columbia/HCA Healthcare Corporation

Universal but not ubiquitous, Universal Health Services (UHS) is the #3 for-profit hospital operator in the US, behind Columbia/HCA Healthcare and Tenet Healthcare. UHS owns and operates more than 40 acute care hospitals and behavioral health centers and more than 25 ambulatory surgical and radiation therapy centers in the US and Puerto Rico. It also operates three women's specialty health centers. UHS provides laboratory services, mobile computerized tomography (CT) and magnetic resonance imaging (MRI) services, and administrative services such as finance, facilities planning, personnel management, physician recruitment, and public relations. Chairman and CEO Alan Miller owns more than 70% of the company.

U.S. Bioscience, Inc.

One Tower Bridge, 100 Front St., West Conshohocken, PA 19428

Telephone: 610-832-0570 **Fax:** 610-832-4500 **Metro area:** Philadelphia, PA **Web site:** http://www.usbio.com **Human resources contact:** Chuck Ford **Sales:** $20.7 million **Number of employees:** 158 **Number of employees for previous year:** 150 **Industry designation:** Drugs **Company type:** Public **Top competitors:** Schering-Plough Corporation; Pharmacia & Upjohn, Inc.; Bristol-Myers Squibb Company

Pharmaceutical firm U.S. Bioscience develops and markets drugs that treat cancer, AIDS, and other conditions. Its three marketed drugs, which account for nearly half of revenues, are Hexalen, a treatment for advanced ovarian cancer; NeuTrexin, a drug to treat a form of pneumonia infection associated with AIDS; and Ethyol, which reduces kidney toxicity in patients being treated for advanced ovarian cancer. U.S. Bioscience's products are co-promoted in the US with drug-delivery firm ALZA. The company has three drugs in various stages of clinical trials: AZQ is an anticancer agent, lodenosine is an anti-HIV agent, and PALA enhances some cancer treatments. It also has three drugs in preclinical testing.

VerticalNet, Inc.

2 Walnut Grove Dr., Ste. 150, Horsham, PA 19044

Telephone: 215-328-6100 **Fax:** 215-443-3336 **Metro area:** Philadelphia, PA **Web site:** http://www.verticalnet.com **Human resources contact:** Melissa Fullerton **Sales:** $792,000 **Number of employees:** 80 **Industry designation:** Computers—online services **Company type:** Public **Top competitors:** Perot Systems Corporation; Penton Media, Inc.; MiningCo.com, Inc.

VerticalNet is one of the largest operators of online vertical trade communities. Its string of about 30 Web sites focuses on a variety of industries (including electronics and utilities) and features buyer's guides, news, discussion forums, career centers, and auctions. Among its fastest-growing Web sites are Water Online, which focuses on the water and wastewater industry and boasts more than 80,000 visits each month; and Chemical Online, a Web site dedicated to the chemical processing industry. VerticalNet generates most of its revenue from "storefronts" featuring detailed information about advertisers. Internet Capital Group owns 38% of the company.

ViroPharma Incorporated

405 Eagleview Blvd., Exton, PA 19341

Telephone: 610-458-7300 **Fax:** 610-458-7380 **Metro area:** Philadelphia, PA **Web site:** http://www.viropharma.com **Human resources contact:** Michael Kelly **Sales:** $1.5 million **Number of employees:** 84 **Number of employees for previous year:** 59 **Industry designation:** Drugs **Company type:** Public

Pharmaceutical company ViroPharma is focusing its drug discovery efforts on fighting diseases caused by RNA viruses. (Rabies, Ebola, and measles all are caused by RNA viruses.) ViroPharma's oral compound pleconaril is in clinical trials for treating viral meningitis, hand-foot-mouth disease, and the common cold. The company also is researching compounds to fight other viruses. ViroPharma licensed the exclusive rights to develop and market pleconaril and related compounds in the US and Canada from Sanofi. Boehringer Ingelheim has exclusive worldwide rights to develop and market ViroPharma's compounds targeting hepatitis C.

Worldgate Communications, Inc.

3220 Tillman Dr., Ste. 300, Bensalem, PA 19020

Telephone: 215-633-5100 **Fax:** 215-633-9590 **Metro area:** Philadelphia, PA **Web site:** http://www.wgate.com **Human resources contact:** Ed Bamford **Sales:** $1 million (Est.) **Number of employees:** 131 **Number of employees for previous year:** 100 **Industry designation:** Computers—online services **Company type:** Private **Top competitors:** NetChannel Inc.; America Online, Inc.; WebTV Networks, Inc.

The race to send the Internet through the TV is on, and WorldGate Communications is running hard; it has signed on Charter Communications and four other cable companies to launch services. WorldGate delivers full Internet access over cable lines through a set-top box hooked to the TV, delivering data at 128,000 bps (faster than conventional phone modems). Its Channel HyperLinking allows TV viewers to go directly to Web sites associated with TV programs; about 70 TV programmers are HyperLinking partners. WorldGate has received equity investments from its set-top providers, General Instrument and Scientific-Atlanta, as well as from other large and influential investors. CEO Hal Krisbergh owns about 42% of the firm.

Puerto Rico

Margo Caribe Inc.

Rd. 690, Kilometer 5.8, Vega Alta, PR 00692

Telephone: 787-883-2570 **Fax:** 787-883-3244 **Human resources contact:** Lillian Fuentes **Sales:** $5.3 million **Number of employees:** 138 **Number of employees for previous year:** 122 **Industry designation:** Agricultural operations **Company type:** Public

Margo Caribe, formerly Margo Nursery Farms, operates two nurseries in Puerto Rico. Its nurseries specialize in the production and distribution of tropical and flowering plants for the commercial interior and exterior landscape market in Puerto Rico and the Caribbean. In addition to its nursery business, the company provides commercial and residential landscaping; sells lawn and garden products (pottery, mulch); and produces soil, mulch, growing mixes, river rock, and gravel. Margo Caribe sold its Florida-based nurseries and operations. CEO Michael Spector and secretary Margaret Spector together own almost 67% of the company.

Rhode Island

Astro-Med, Inc.

600 E. Greenwich Ave., West Warwick, RI 02893

Telephone: 401-828-4000 **Fax:** 401-822-2430 **Metro area:** Providence, RI **Web site:** http://www.astro-med.com/index.html **Human resources contact:** Cathy Barlow **Sales:** $41.6 million **Number of employees:** 365 **Number of employees for previous year:** 356 **Industry designation:** Computers—peripheral equipment **Company type:** Public **Top competitors:** Axiohm Transaction Solutions, Inc.; Eltron International, Inc.; Source Technologies, Inc.

Astro-Med makes specialty printing systems and data recording devices used for industrial, medical, and scientific applications. The company's test and measurement product line prints scientific signals on charts or electronic media products that record scientific data. Astro-Med's QuickLabel Systems division makes bar code printer products including color and monochrome printers for packaging labels and tags made of nylon, paper, polyester, and PVC. Its Grass Instruments division makes devices, such as EEG equipment and polysomnographs, used to record the physiological signals of living organisms. Customers include AT&T, Boeing, and General Motors. Chairman and CEO Albert Ondis owns 25% of the company.

Bacou USA, Inc.

10 Thurber Blvd., Smithfield, RI 02917

Telephone: 401-233-0333 **Fax:** 401-232-0547 **Metro area:** Providence, RI **Web site:** http://www.bacouusa.com **Human resources contact:** J. Michael Vittoria **Sales:** $219.6 million **Number of employees:** 1,942 **Number of employees for previous year:** 940 **Industry designation:** Protection—safety equipment & services **Company type:** Public **Top competitors:** Aearo Corporation; Norcross Safety Products LLC; Minnesota Mining and Manufacturing Company

Safeguarding every kid who owns a junior chemistry set, Bacou USA manufactures equipment for protecting vision, hearing, and respiratory systems. The company's products are sold under six brand names: Uvex (nonprescription and laser protective eyewear), Titmus (safety frames for protective prescription eyewear), Survivair and Pro-Tech (air-purifying respirators), Biosystems (gas-detection systems), and Howard Light (earplugs and earmuffs). The company's products are sold internationally, primarily through industrial-safety distributors and optical retailers.

CVS Corporation

One CVS Dr., Woonsocket, RI 02895

Telephone: 401-765-1500 **Fax:** 401-766-2917 **Metro area:** Providence, RI **Web site:** http://www.cvs.com **Human resources contact:** Rosemary Mede **Sales:** $15.3 billion **Number of employees:** 90,000 **Number of employees for previous year:** 44,000 **Industry designation:** Retail—drugstores **Company type:** Public **Top competitors:** Walgreen Co.; Rite Aid Corporation; Wal-Mart Stores, Inc.

CVS Corporation interprets the bad handwriting of more doctors than almost anybody. The company operates about 4,000 Arbor and CVS drugstores in 24 states and the District of Columbia. Thanks to its acquisitions of Revco and Arbor Drugs, CVS is the #2 drugstore chain in the US (trailing only Walgreen). More than 50% of sales come from pharmacies; general merchandise, including cards and cosmetics, accounts for the rest. The company also provides managed-care drug programs through PharmaCare Management Services. CVS is remodeling the former Revco stores, a conversion that includes stocking the stores with hundreds of CVS' private-label products.

Log On America, Inc.

3 Regency Plaza, Providence, RI 02903

Telephone: 401-459-6298 **Fax:** 401-459-6222 **Metro area:** Providence, RI **Web site:** http://www.loa.com **Human resources contact:** Raymond Paolo **Sales:** $760,000 (Est.) **Number of employees:** 13 **Number of employees for previous year:** 12 **Industry designation:** Computers—online services **Company type:** Private **Top competitors:** NETCOM On-Line Communication Services, Inc.; UUNET WorldCom; America Online, Inc.

Log On America (LOA) wants to sign on America—or at least the Northeast. The company provides Internet access in about 230 cities nationwide; most of its business is with businesses (dedicated access lines for commercial accounts). It plans to become a communications convenience store for consumers by adding telephone, cable TV, and data services to its product line, through company acquisitions. The company also provides Web hosting, network consulting, and other services. A competitive local-exchange carrier in Rhode Island, LOA focuses on cities in the northeastern US with populations of 200,000 to one million. Founder and CEO David Paolo owns 53% of the company (falling to 35% after LOA's planned IPO).

Network Six, Inc.

475 Kilvert St., Warwick, RI 02886

Telephone: 401-732-9000 **Fax:** 401-732-9009 **Metro area:** Providence, RI **Web site:** http://www.networksix.com **Human resources contact:** Gail Stahr **Sales:** $10.4 million **Number of employees:** 100 **Number of employees for previous year:** 74 **Industry designation:** Computers—services **Company type:** Public **Top competitors:** Andersen Worldwide; Electronic Data Systems Corporation; TRW Inc.

State human services agencies from Arizona to Maine are tuning in to Network Six. The company provides information technology consulting services to data-heavy agencies overseeing such services as child support, food stamps, Medicaid, and welfare. Network Six provides hardware and software procurement; system design, installation, customization, testing, and management; programming; and strategic planning and training services. The company's Network Services Division offers LAN, WAN, Internet/intranet, and remote communications technology services. Rhode Island is one of Network Six's biggest customers. Other customers include health care providers, pharmacy benefit managers, and higher education institutions.

SOUTH CAROLINA

Glassmaster Company

126 Glassmaster Rd., Lexington, SC 29072

Telephone: 803-359-2594 **Fax:** 803-359-0897 **Other address:** PO Box 788, Lexington, SC 29071 **Metro area:** Columbia, SC **Web site:** http://www.glassmasterco.com **Human resources contact:** Neil A. McLeod Jr. **Sales:** $24.5 million **Number of employees:** 218 **Number of employees for previous year:** 192 **Industry designation:** Chemicals—plastics **Company type:** Public **Top competitors:** Cambridge Industries, Inc.; Hoffer Plastics Corporation; Scapa Group PLC

Glassmaster helps take care of life's necessities: fishing and yard work. Glassmaster makes monofilaments, wires, and plastic control panels. Its monofilaments are made from nylon, polyester, and other engineering resins, account for nearly 70% of sales, and have such varied uses as sewing thread, lawn-trimmer and fishing line, and industrial weaving. Glassmaster also makes modular building systems and fiberglass marine and CB antennas for commercial and recreational boats. Its wire controls and molded plastic control panels are used in trucks, cars, farm equipment, and boats. The company sells its products in North and South America, Europe, and the Pacific Rim. The Trewhella family owns 36% of Glassmaster.

Greenville Hospital System

701 Grove Rd., Greenville, SC 29605

Telephone: 864-455-7000 **Fax:** 864-455-6218 **Metro area:** Greenville, SC **Web site:** http://www.ghs.org **Human resources contact:** Douglas Dorman **Sales:** $494.3 million **Number of employees:** 5,700 **Industry designation:** Hospitals **Company type:** Not-for-profit **Top competitors:** Novant Health, Inc.; Health Management Associates, Inc.; Bon Secours Health System, Inc.

Greenville Hospital System is a not-for-profit community hospital system serving South Carolina's "Golden Strip" —the area between Charlotte, North Carolina, and Atlanta. The system consists of a regional medical, teaching, and research hospital; three community hospitals; a rehabilitation hospital; a children's hospital; a cancer center; and a mental health hospital. Directed by a board of appointed volunteer representatives, the health provider offers a full range of services including a primary-care physician network; health and behavioral health services; prevention and wellness programs; and health education and training.

The Liberty Corporation

2000 Wade Hampton Blvd., Greenville, SC 29615

Telephone: 864-609-8111 **Fax:** 864-609-3120 **Other address:** POBox 789, Greenville, SC **Metro area:** Greenville, SC **Web site:** http://www.libertycorp.com **Human resources contact:** Jan Haubenreich **Sales:** $584.3 million **Number of employees:** 2,930 **Number of employees for previous year:** 2,754 **Industry designation:** Insurance—life **Company type:** Public

The Liberty Corporation is the holding company for Liberty Life Insurance and Cosmos Broadcasting, which owns 11 television stations. Liberty Life's agency division generates more than half of the company's premiums; agents sell individual life and health insurance, primarily in the Southeast. The insurer writes mortgage-protection policies as well; these pay mortgages in the case of a policyholder's death or disability. Subsidiary Cosmos Broadcasting has TV stations in Alabama, Arkansas, Georgia, Indiana, Kentucky, Louisiana, Mississippi, Ohio, North and South Carolina, and Texas. All of the stations are affiliated with a major broadcasting network. The company is eyeing a spin-off of its media business.

Martin Color-Fi, Inc.

306 Main St., Edgefield, SC 29824

Telephone: 803-637-7000 **Fax:** 803-637-7117 **Metro area:** Augusta, GA **Human resources contact:** Kim Saxton **Sales:** $120.5 million **Number of employees:** 1,012 **Number of employees for previous year:** 991 **Industry designation:** Chemicals—fibers **Company type:** Public **Top competitors:** Wellman, Inc.; Carpenter Co.; Reliance Industries Limited

Martin Color-Fi makes polyester fiber and pellets from recycled plastic such as soft-drink bottles, film waste, and packaging resin. The company uses the fiber to make a variety of products, including retail and commercial carpet (Forum Contract Carpet), manufactured housing and vehicle carpet (Condor), and yarns. Martin's plastic pellets are consumed internally and sold to manufacturers of nonfood containers, plastic trays, and paint roller trays. The company also makes pigments and additives used to manufacture fiber and pellets. Its direct sales force markets its products in the US; sales agents represent Martin in international markets. James Martin, chairman and CEO, owns about 40% of the company.

Polymer Group, Inc.

4838 Jenkins Ave., North Charleston, SC 29405

Telephone: 843-566-7293 **Fax:** 843-747-4092 **Metro area:** Charleston, SC **Human resources contact:** Jay Tiedemann **Sales:** $802.9 million **Number of employees:** 3,600 **Number of employees for previous year:** 2,300 **Industry designation:** Medical & dental supplies **Company type:** Public **Parent company:** InterTech Group **Top competitors:** Kimberly-Clark Corporation; Unternehmensgruppe Freudenberg; E. I. du Pont de Nemours and Company

Polymer Group is the world's #3 producer of nonwoven polyolefin materials (flat porous sheets made of interlocking fibers, filaments, or perforating films). The company supplies customers who make disposable wiping, medical, and hygiene products. These include hospital surgical gowns and drapes, cloths and towels, filters, flexible industrial packaging, diapers, tampons, and automotive insulation products. Polymer Group's major customers include Johnson & Johnson and Procter & Gamble. The company has developed a more durable nonwoven fabric, Miratec, which WestPoint Stevens will use to make sheets and towels. Polymer Group has 22 plants in eight countries in North America, South America, and Europe.

UCI Medical Affiliates, Inc.

1901 Main St., Ste. 1200, Mail Code 1105, Columbia, SC 29201

Telephone: 803-252-3661 **Fax:** 803-252-8077 **Metro area:** Columbia, SC **Human resources contact:** Susan Scaffe **Sales:** $37.6 million **Number of employees:** 612 **Number of employees for previous year:** 384 **Industry designation:** Medical practice management **Company type:** Public **Top competitors:** MedPartners, Inc.; Complete Management, Inc.; PhyCor, Inc.

UCI Medical Affiliates (UCI), through subsidiaries UCI Medical Affiliates of South Carolina and UCI Medical Affiliates of Georgia, provides practice management services to about 40 medical centers in Georgia, South Carolina, and Tennessee. The centers operate primarily under the Doctor's Care name. UCI provides such services as contracting with and the billing of third-party payors, collecting and managing accounts receivable, non-medical staffing, and administrative services. Since UCI is legally prevented from providing actual medical services, its Doctor's Care centers provide care through companies wholly owned by UCI officers. Blue Cross and Blue Shield of South Carolina owns about 40% of the company.

SOUTH DAKOTA

Daktronics, Inc.

331 32nd Ave., Brookings, SD 57006

Telephone: 605-697-4000 **Fax:** 605-697-4700 **Other address:** PO Box 5128, Brookings, SD 57006 **Metro area:** Sioux Falls, SD **Web site:** http://www.daktronics.com **Human resources contact:** Nancy Bohlen **Sales:** $69.9 million **Number of employees:** 878 **Number of employees for previous year:** 816 **Industry designation:** Computers—peripheral equipment **Company type:** Public **Top competitors:** Display Technologies, Inc.; Trans-Industries, Inc.; Trans-Lux Corporation

Keep track of the score with Daktronics, a company that designs and manufactures computer-programmable information display systems. Its products include scoreboards, game timers, shot clocks, and animation displays for sports facilities; advertising and information displays for businesses; and data display systems used by the government for road condition alerts and legislative votes. Other applications include airport information and time and temperature signs. Daktronics system installations include Times Square, Olympics venues, and professional sports facilities.

TENNESSEE

American Healthcorp, Inc.

One Burton Hills Blvd., Nashville, TN 37215

Telephone: 615-665-1122 **Fax:** 615-665-7697 **Metro area:** Nashville, TN **Human resources contact:** Rita R. Sailer **Sales:** $41.2 million **Number of employees:** 527 **Number of employees for previous year:** 452 **Industry designation:** Health care—outpatient & home **Company type:** Public **Top competitors:** Gambro AB; Total Renal Care Holdings, Inc.; Fresenius Medical Care Aktiengesellschaft

When managed care needs diabetes care, they call in the corps—American Healthcorp. The company provides outsourced diabetes treatment programs to hospitals and health maintenance organizations (HMOs) through its subsidiary Diabetes Treatment Centers of America. The company contracts with 17 HMOs, operating on-site diabetes care programs using a combination of hospital and company staffs in more than 70 hospitals in 24 states. The program features aggressive preventive treatment to minimize expensive hospitalization. Contracts with Columbia/HCA account for more than 10% of sales, but the company is increasingly targeting HMOs as clients. It also runs two arthritis and osteoporosis care centers.

American HomePatient, Inc.

5200 Maryland Way, Ste. 400, Brentwood, TN 37027

Telephone: 615-221-8884 **Fax:** 615-373-9932 **Metro area:** Nashville, TN **Human resources contact:** Sandy Irvin **Sales:** $387.3 million **Number of employees:** 4,800 **Number of employees for previous year:** 4,150 **Industry designation:** Medical services **Company type:** Public **Top competitors:** Apria Healthcare Group Inc.; Coram Healthcare Corporation; National HealthCare Corp.

There are more American home patients than ever before, and American HomePatient provides them with health care services and medical equipment. The company, whose main services include respiratory and infusion therapies and enteral and parenteral feeding, operates about 300 branches in 35 states, and it has gained a foothold in many midsized and small communities, with the bulk of its home centers located in towns of fewer than 100,000 residents. The company, which is heavily dependent on the whims of Medicare, also provides home care through joint ventures with particular hospitals.

American Retirement Corporation

111 Westwood Place, Ste. 402, Brentwood, TN 37027

Telephone: 615-221-2250 **Fax:** 615-221-2269 **Metro area:** Nashville, TN **Web site:** http://www.arclp.com **Human resources contact:** Joseph H. Baron **Sales:** $142.4 million **Number of employees:** 5,175 **Number of employees for previous year:** 2,620 **Industry designation:** Health care—outpatient & home **Company type:** Public

American Retirement provides the elderly with health care and senior-living services, including independent and assisted living, skilled nursing, and home health care services. The company operates more than 20 senior-living communities in 12 states, including Florida, Texas, and Virginia; 10 of these communities are traditional nursing homes. American Retirement also owns 11 home health care agencies and manages four more. The company targets its services at seniors age 75 and older. American Retirement plans to expand by developing freestanding assisted-living residences and by acquiring other senior-living communities and home health care agencies.

America Service Group Inc.

105 Westpark Dr., Ste. 300, Brentwood, TN 37027

Telephone: 615-373-3100 **Fax:** 931-376-9862 **Metro area:** Nashville, TN **Web site:** http://www.asgr.com **Human resources contact:** Mike Cassity **Sales:** $113.9 million **Number of employees:** 2,950 **Number of employees for previous year:** 1,645 **Industry designation:** Health care—outpatient & home **Company type:** Public

America Service Group (ASG) is a holding company for subsidiaries that provide health care to inmates in state prisons and county and local jails. Through Prison Health Services (PHS), the company contracts with government agencies to provide physical and mental health screenings and treatment, dental care, and OB/GYN testing and care. PHS also provides off-site testing, surgery, and emergency room services. ASG, which focuses on facilities that maintain an average population of over 300 inmates per day, serves customers in more than a dozen states. Subsidiaries Harbor Insurance, Inc., and UniSource, Inc., sell insurance and pharmaceuticals to PHS.

AmSurg Corp.

One Burton Hills Blvd., Ste. 350, Nashville, TN 37215

Telephone: 615-665-1283 **Fax:** 615-665-0755 **Metro area:** Nashville, TN **Web site:** http://www.amsurg.com **Human resources contact:** Carolyn Heaton **Sales:** $80.3 million **Number of employees:** 300 **Number of employees for previous year:** 250 **Industry designation:** Medical services **Company type:** Public **Top competitors:** Physicians Resource Group, Inc.; HEALTHSOUTH Corporation; Laser Vision Centers, Inc.

Focusing on a narrow range of high volume, lower-risk surgical procedures, AmSurg operates practice-based ambulatory surgery centers, typically near the specialty medical practice of a physician group office (centers are partnerships between majority-owner AmSurg and the doctors' practice). There are about 35 such AmSurg facilities in 15 states and Washington, DC, and about a dozen more in development. It is using the centers as a base to develop specialty physician networks, adding to three it operates in the Southeast. AmSurg focuses on such specialties as gastroenterology and ophthalmology, marketing to third-party payors, employers, and patients. The company was spun off from American Healthcorp in 1997.

Chattem, Inc.

1715 W. 38th St., Chattanooga, TN 37409

Telephone: 423-821-4571 **Fax:** 423-821-0395 **Metro area:** Chattanooga, TN **Web site:** http://www.chattem.com **Human resources contact:** Bruce Long **Sales:** $220.1 million **Number of employees:** 364 **Number of employees for previous year:** 340 **Industry designation:** Drugs **Company type:** Public **Top competitors:** The Procter & Gamble Company; Unilever; Johnson & Johnson

Chattem makes over-the-counter (OTC) pharmaceuticals, personal care products, and dietary supplements. The company is an international seller of leading niche market OTC drugs (more than half of all sales), toiletries, cosmetics, and supplements; products include Flexall joint and muscle pain reliever, Pamprin menstrual symptom reliever, Melatonex sleep aid, and Mudd clay-based facial mask. Chattem continues to bolster its leading market positions through acquisitions, such as those of skin cleanser pHisoderm, dental analgesic Benzodent, medicated powder Gold Bond, and antiperspirant Ban. Appetite suppressant Dexatrim and Aspercreme have also been added to Chattem's product line.

Columbia/HCA Healthcare Corporation

One Park Plaza, Nashville, TN 37203

Telephone: 615-344-9551 **Fax:** 615-344-2266 **Metro area:** Nashville, TN **Web site:** http://www.columbia.net **Human resources contact:** Philip Patton **Sales:** $18.7 billion **Number of employees:** 295,000 **Number of employees for previous year:** 285,000 **Industry designation:** Hospitals **Company type:** Public **Top competitors:** Tenet Healthcare Corporation; Daughters of Charity National Health System; Kaiser Foundation Health Plan, Inc.

The largest hospital company in the US (ahead of Tenet Healthcare by a wide margin), Columbia/HCA Healthcare operates some 345 hospitals and surgery centers nationwide. It also has operations in Spain, Switzerland, and the UK. Columbia/HCA, which also offers rehabilitation and home health care, is in turmoil: There is a wide-ranging federal investigation into its Medicare and patient-referral procedures, causing several top executives to leave the company. In addition, Columbia/HCA has halted the aggressive expansion responsible for its growth. It has sold its prescription benefit management unit and plans to sell its home care operations, about one-third of its hospitals, and some of its surgery centers.

Community Health Systems, Inc.

155 Franklin Rd., Ste. 400, Brentwood, TN 37027

Telephone: 615-373-9600 **Fax:** 615-371-1068 **Other address:** PO Box 217, Brentwood, TN 37024
Metro area: Nashville, TN **Human resources contact:** Linda K. Parsons **Sales:** $745.9 million (Est.)
Number of employees: 10,929 **Number of employees for previous year:** 10,575 **Industry
designation:** Hospitals **Company type:** Private **Top competitors:** Health Management Associates, Inc.;
Quorum Health Group, Inc.; Columbia/HCA Healthcare Corporation

Community Health Systems (CHS) owns and operates full-service, acute-care hospitals in nonurban communities
where the CHS hospitals typically are the prominent providers of primary health care services. CHS operates about
40 acute-care hospitals in 15 states, primarily in the southeastern and southwestern US, and offers a variety of
inpatient and outpatient medical, surgical, and emergency services. Some offer other services, including obstetrics,
psychiatric care, and chemical-dependency treatment. CHS's multi-hospital structure provides greater leverage in
negotiating purchasing agreements (including one with Tenet Healthcare's BuyPower) and HMO contracts.
Investment firm Forstmann Little & Co. owns CHS.

King Pharmaceuticals, Inc.

501 Fifth St., Bristol, TN 37620

Telephone: 423-989-8000 **Fax:** 423-274-8677 **Metro area:** Johnson City, TN **Web site:** http://
www.kingpharm.com **Human resources contact:** Diane Holbrook **Sales:** $163.5 million **Number of
employees:** 918 **Number of employees for previous year:** 320 **Industry designation:** Drugs
Company type: Public

King Pharmaceuticals makes and markets generic and brand name drugs. The company sells its branded products
through subsidiary Monarch Pharmaceuticals. King Pharmaceuticals' branded products, which account for almost
80% of its sales, include Anusol, Cortisporin, Thalitone, and Viroptic. King Pharmaceuticals also makes health care
products for animals under the Royal Vet and Show Winner trade names. The company contracts its excess
manufacturing capabilities to outside pharmaceutical companies. Run by the Gregory brothers, the company more
than doubled its sales with its 1998 purchase of several product lines from Warner-Lambert; it also acquired
additional products from Hoechst Marion Roussel.

Miller Petroleum, Inc.

3651 Baker Hwy., Huntsville, TN 37756

Telephone: 423-663-9457 **Fax:** 423-663-9461 **Other address:** PO Box 130, Huntsville, TN 37756
Metro area: Knoxville, TN **Web site:** http://www.millerpetroleum.com **Human resources contact:**
Theresa Cotton **Sales:** $1.7 million **Number of employees:** 21 **Number of employees for
previous year:** 14 **Industry designation:** Oil & gas—exploration & production **Company type:**
Public **Top competitors:** The Wiser Oil Company; American Rivers Oil Company; Columbia Energy Group

"Gas Man's Daughter" doesn't have the same ring to it, but Miller Petroleum digs for oil and gas in the
Appalachian region that brought forth Loretta Lynn. In addition to operating wells, the firm organizes joint drilling
ventures with partners and rebuilds and sells oil field equipment. Miller Petroleum owns active wells in five
Tennessee counties and some 80,000 acres of promising land in Tennessee and Kentucky (192,000 barrels of oil and
7.3 million cu. ft. of natural gas). Few pipelines serve its drilling area, so it relies on Delta Natural Gas to purchase
its products for distribution. President and founder Deloy Miller owns 72% of its stock.

Nashville Predators

501 Broadway, Nashville, TN 37203

Telephone: 615-770-2300 **Fax:** 615-770-2309 **Metro area:** Nashville, TN **Web site:** http://
www.nashvillepredators.com **Human resources contact:** Kim Marrone **Number of employees:** 75
Industry designation: Leisure & recreational services **Company type:** Private **Top competitors:**
Chicago Blackhawk Hockey Team, Inc.; St. Louis Blues Hockey Club L.L.C.; Detroit Red Wings

Forget broken hearts, this year's honky-tonk hits could be about broken bones. Bringing hockey to the country
music capital of the world, the Nashville Predators joined the NHL as an expansion team in 1997. It is part of the
city's sports franchise boom, which includes the Tennessee Titans (formerly the Oilers) professional football team,
as well as arena football and women's basketball teams. Fighting for the sports dollar in a nontraditional hockey
market, the Predators are pinning their hopes on country music's elite; Garth Brooks, Barbara Mandrell, and Trisha
Yearwood are just a few of the artists who have lent their support to the team. The Predators are owned by
Wisconsin businessman Craig Leipold.

National HealthCare Corp.

100 Vine St., Murfreesboro, TN 37130

Telephone: 615-890-2020 **Fax:** 615-890-0123 **Metro area:** Nashville, TN **Human resources contact:** Dave Luster **Sales:** $441.2 million **Number of employees:** 16,017 **Number of employees for previous year:** 16,000 **Industry designation:** Health care—outpatient & home **Company type:** Public **Top competitors:** Home Health Corporation of America, Inc.; RoTech Medical Corporation; Continucare Corporation

National HealthCare Corporation, formerly National Healthcare L.P., operates more than 110 long-term health care centers and 36 home health care programs in the southeastern US. The company's centers provide skilled and intermediate nursing; rehabilitative care such as speech, physical, and occupational therapy; and specialized services such as care programs for Alzheimer's patients. Its home health care programs provide rehabilitative care in patients' homes. National Healthcare also manages assisted living units and retirement centers. The company has spun off its property interests, which are now owned by National Health Realty, a real estate investment trust (REIT).

NetCare Health Systems, Inc.

424 Church St., Ste. 2100, Nashville, TN 37219

Telephone: 615-742-8500 **Fax:** 615-742-8505 **Metro area:** Nashville, TN **Web site:** http://www.netcarehealthsystems.com **Sales:** $130.3 million (Est.) **Number of employees:** 1,210 **Industry designation:** Hospitals **Company type:** Private

NetCare Health Systems operates 10 community hospitals in rural California, Georgia, Mississippi, and Texas, offering acute care, skilled nursing, rehabilitation, and psychiatric care. It also operates four nursing homes and plans to buy three hospitals from a slimming Columbia/HCA. The company was founded by Charterhouse Equity Partners and executives from Healthtrust in 1996 to buy hospitals in rural areas, where there is greater customer loyalty and less competition from national hospital giants. Its initial purchase was Southern Health Corporation, operator of four hospitals and three nursing homes in Georgia. The company intends to use the proceeds from its IPO to become a consolidator in its field.

New American Healthcare Corporation

109 Westpark Dr., Ste. 440, Brentwood, TN 37027

Telephone: 615-221-5070 **Fax:** 615-221-5009 **Metro area:** Nashville, TN **Web site:** http://www.nahcorp.com **Sales:** $75.6 million **Number of employees:** 1,723 **Industry designation:** Hospitals **Company type:** Public

New American Healthcare operates eight acute care hospitals in nonurban markets in Iowa, Missouri, Oregon, Tennessee, Texas, and Wyoming. The company was formed by hospital industry veterans to acquire nonurban hospitals, which the company sees as less subject to competition from national consolidators or to penetration by national managed care companies. New American Healthcare seeks to make its hospitals the focus of community health care by adding inpatient and outpatient services tailored to the needs of each community, seeking alliances with other area caregivers, and building physician networks, with an emphasis on primary care providers. The company reduces costs by standardizing management systems.

Omega Health Systems, Inc.

5100 Poplar Ave., Ste. 2100, Memphis, TN 38137

Telephone: 901-683-7868 **Fax:** 901-683-5343 **Metro area:** Memphis, TN **Web site:** http://www.omegahealth.com **Human resources contact:** Lori Jennings **Sales:** $97.8 million **Number of employees:** 576 **Number of employees for previous year:** 329 **Industry designation:** Medical practice management **Company type:** Public **Top competitors:** Vision Twenty-One, Inc.; Omega Health Systems, Inc.; Physicians Resource Group, Inc.

Omega Health Systems manages eye care offices so optometrists and ophthalmologists can optimize their time in patient care. Omega supplies facilities, support staff, and financial and purchasing services to the network's 700 optometrists and about 50 ophthalmologists in 100 service locations and seven surgical centers. Network primary-care optometrists refer patients to affiliated ophthalmologists for surgical procedures for such problems as cataracts, glaucoma, and retinal conditions. Omega operates in cities; it has satellite offices and offers use of mobile surgical equipment in rural areas. The company contracts with managed care and insurance companies and receives 40% to 70% of affiliates' earnings.

Phycor, Inc.

30 Burton Hills Blvd., Ste. 400, Nashville, TN 37215

Telephone: 615-665-9066 **Fax:** 615-665-9088 **Metro area:** Nashville, TN **Web site:** http://www.phycor.com **Human resources contact:** Brandon Dyson **Sales:** $1.5 billion **Number of employees:** 19,000 **Number of employees for previous year:** 15,000 **Industry designation:** Medical practice management **Company type:** Public **Top competitors:** Coastal Physician Group, Inc.; MedPartners, Inc.; FPA Medical Management, Inc.

PhyCor is tied with FPA Medical Management for the #2 spot among physician practice management companies, after #1 MedPartners. The company runs the business end of multi-specialty medical clinics, provides practices with expansion capital, and uses its bargaining power to negotiate contracts with managed care providers. PhyCor acquires and manages a clinic's operating assets under long-term service agreements. The company also develops and manages independent practice associations (IPAs) of physicians who contract with health care entities for their services. PhyCor operates nearly 60 clinics with about 4,000 physicians in 29 states and manages IPAs with more than 20,000 physicians.

Provident Companies, Inc.

One Fountain Sq., Chattanooga, TN 37402

Telephone: 423-755-1011 **Fax:** 423-755-7013 **Metro area:** Chattanooga, TN **Web site:** http://www.providentcompanies.com **Human resources contact:** Kathy Schoeffler **Sales:** $3.9 billion **Number of employees:** 4,039 **Number of employees for previous year:** 1,964 **Industry designation:** Insurance—accident & health **Company type:** Public **Top competitors:** The Prudential Insurance Company of America; Metropolitan Life Insurance Company; CIGNA Corporation

Is it fate or Provident? An insurance holding company, Provident Companies sells life and disability insurance in the US, Puerto Rico, and Canada. Through its seven subsidiaries, some of which it acquired when it bought The Paul Revere Corporation in 1997, Provident offers insurance such as accident, accidental death and dismemberment, cancer, disability, and life to individuals or groups. The company's GENEX Services provides case management and vocational rehabilitation to corporations, third-party administrators, and insurance companies. Members of the Mclellan family own about half of the company. Provident is merging with Unum Corporation to become the largest worker-disability insurer in the US.

Quorum Health Group, Inc.

103 Continental Place, Brentwood, TN 37027

Telephone: 615-371-7979 **Fax:** 615-371-4853 **Metro area:** Nashville, TN **Web site:** http://www.quorumhealth.com **Human resources contact:** Ray Langham **Sales:** $1.6 billion **Number of employees:** 18,000 **Number of employees for previous year:** 17,935 **Industry designation:** Hospitals **Company type:** Public **Top competitors:** Columbia/HCA Healthcare Corporation; Daughters of Charity National Health System; Tenet Healthcare Corporation

Quorum Health Group knows that even hicks in the sticks need health care. The group owns and runs 18 hospitals in rural and midsized communities. Subsidiary Quorum Health Resources, the largest contract manager of not-for-profit hospitals in the US, manages about 240 hospitals and provides consulting services to more than 180 hospitals. In addition to its own hospitals, Quorum has joint ventures with Universal Health Systems and Columbia/HCA to operate hospital systems in Las Vegas and Macon, Georgia, respectively. The company has operations in 44 states and the District of Columbia.

Renal Care Group, Inc.

2100 W. End Ave., Ste. 800, Nashville, TN 37203

Telephone: 615-345-5500 **Fax:** 931-320-3644 **Metro area:** Nashville, TN **Human resources contact:** John Anderson **Sales:** $369.4 million **Number of employees:** 3,454 **Number of employees for previous year:** 2,904 **Industry designation:** Medical services **Company type:** Public **Top competitors:** Fresenius Medical Care Aktiengesellschaft; Total Renal Care Holdings, Inc.; Gambro AB

Renal Care Group keeps kidneys clean by providing dialysis and related nephrology services to patients suffering from kidney disease, including chronic kidney failure. The company offers such ancillary services as electrocardiograms, Doppler flow tests, blood transfusions, and erythropoietin anti-anemia injections. Created by the merger of a number of smaller dialysis companies, the acquisitive Renal Care Group owns and operates more than 170 kidney dialysis outpatient centers in 21 states. It also provides acute dialysis services to more than 100 hospitals. In addition to dialysis services, the company provides physician practice management services.

ResortQuest International, Inc.

530 Oak Ct. Dr., #360, Memphis, TN 38117

Telephone: 901-762-0600 **Fax:** 901-762-0678 **Metro area:** Memphis, TN **Sales:** $69.4 million **Number of employees:** 2,800 **Number of employees for previous year:** 1,300 **Industry designation:** Leisure & recreational services **Company type:** Public

ResortQuest International owns vacation rental and property management companies that operate about 14,400 condos and homes in 14 states and in Canada. The company's properties are located in beach and island resort locations such as Hawaii and Nantucket, Massachusetts, and mountain resorts such as Aspen, Colorado. ResortQuest provides its customers with furnished, privately owned condos and houses. Other services include housekeeping, maintenance, restaurant reservations, ski lift tickets, and golf tee times. Through its First Resort Software subsidiary, the company provides property management software and services to about 650 resort management companies worldwide.

Response Oncology, Inc.

1775 Moriah Woods Blvd., Memphis, TN 38117

Telephone: 901-761-7000 **Fax:** 901-763-7045 **Metro area:** Memphis, TN **Web site:** http:// www.responseoncology.com **Human resources contact:** Cindy Dill **Sales:** $128.2 million **Number of employees:** 700 **Number of employees for previous year:** 550 **Industry designation:** Medical services **Company type:** Public **Top competitors:** Cancer Treatment Holdings, Inc.; Physician Reliance Network, Inc.; American Oncology Resources, Inc.

You've been diagnosed with cancer: Response Oncology hopes that after the initial panic, you'll call one of the 11 oncology practices it manages in Florida and Tennessee. They may refer you to one of the 53 IMPACT (short for implementing advanced cancer treatments) Centers that the company owns or manages. Practice management accounts for about half of the company's sales. The company also sells cancer treatment drugs to its member practices and conducts treatment outcomes research for major pharmaceutical companies. Seafield Capital Corporation, now known as Lab One (a provider of clinical tests for the life and health insurance industry), spun the company off to shareholders in 1998.

Sofamor Danek Group, Inc.

1800 Pyramid Place, Memphis, TN 38132

Telephone: 901-396-2695 **Fax:** 901-396-2699 **Metro area:** Memphis, TN **Web site:** http:// www.sofamordanek.com **Human resources contact:** Arnold Malone **Sales:** $312.9 million **Number of employees:** 1,000 **Number of employees for previous year:** 810 **Industry designation:** Medical products **Company type:** Subsidiary **Top competitors:** Sulzer Medica Ltd.; DePuy, Inc.; Biomet, Inc.

It takes backbone to be the world's #1 maker of spinal implants. Now a Medtronic subsidiary, Sofamor Danek Group's products treat degenerative diseases, deformities, and spine trauma, as well as stabilize and promote vertebrae fusion. Products include the TSRH Spinal System (support rods and locking bolts), the Cotrel-Dubousset system (spinal rods, hooks, and traction devices), and the ORION Anterior Cervical Plate System (spinal plate and screws for the neck). It also makes a computer-assisted surgical guidance system and surgical instruments. Sofamor Danek is developing regenerative replacement bone tissue. The firm's products are sold by 200 agents in more than 70 countries.

Tennessee Farmers Cooperative

200 Waldron Rd., La Vergne, TN 37086

Telephone: 615-793-8011 **Fax:** 615-793-8343 **Other address:** PO Box 3003, La Vergne, TN 37086 **Metro area:** Nashville, TN **Web site:** http://www.tncoop.com **Human resources contact:** Carole Hopkins **Sales:** $450 million **Number of employees:** 650 **Number of employees for previous year:** 600 **Industry designation:** Agricultural operations **Company type:** Cooperative **Top competitors:** Cenex Harvest States Cooperatives; Ag Processing Inc; Farmland Industries, Inc.

Tennessee Farmers Cooperative (TFC) keeps the cows fat, the bugs away, and the tractors running. Serving more than 70 member co-ops, TFC supplies about 40,000 products, including chemicals, animal health products, feed, fertilizer, home and lawn care products, seeds, fuel, and machine accessories to some 70,000 Tennessee farmers. It also has research and supply joint ventures with other co-ops, including CF Industries, Universal Cooperatives, and CoBank. Founded in 1945, TFC operates in a pyramid structure in which farmers own local co-ops that, in turn, own TFC. It also operates about 150 retail outlets serving the public as well as co-op members.

Tennessee Titans Inc.

115 S. First St., Nashville, TN 37213

Telephone: 615-733-3000 **Fax:** 615-251-0181 **Other address:** PO Box 198497, Nashville, TN 37219 **Metro area:** Nashville, TN **Web site:** http://www.titansonline.com **Human resources contact:** Jeanene Dainwood **Sales:** $71.5 million (Est.) **Number of employees:** 75 **Industry designation:** Leisure & recreational services **Company type:** Private **Top competitors:** Baltimore Ravens; Pittsburgh Steelers; Jacksonville Jaguars

Relocating his business, the NFL's Tennessee Titans, has not been easy for owner Bud Adams. The Titans, which was known as the Houston Oilers since its 1959 founding, moved to Nashville in 1997. Playing in Memphis (its Nashville stadium is scheduled for completion in 1999), the team attracted an average of merely 28,000 fans, an NFL low. Fan apathy and downright anger led Adams to hire a public relations firm to boost support and reshape the old Oilers' image. Things are not all bad, however, as the team will share in the NFL's new $2.2 billion-a-year TV contract.

TEXAS

Abatix Environmental Corp.

8311 Eastpoint Dr., Ste. 400, Dallas, TX 75227

Telephone: 214-381-1146 **Fax:** 214-381-9513 **Metro area:** Dallas-Fort Worth, TX **Web site:** http://www.Abatix.com **Human resources contact:** Frank J. Cinatl **Sales:** $37.3 million **Number of employees:** 103 **Number of employees for previous year:** 78 **Industry designation:** Pollution control equipment & services **Company type:** Public **Top competitors:** Vallen Corporation; Lakeland Industries, Inc.

Abatix Environmental markets and distributes personal protection gear, safety equipment, and supplies to clients who deal in hazardous materials, industrial safety, and asbestos and lead abatement. The company also sells tools to customers in the construction industry. Abatix Environmental's eight distribution centers (in Arizona, California, Colorado, Nevada, Texas, and Washington) handle more than 9,000 products and serve some 4,000 customers, primarily in the Southwest, Midwest, and Pacific Coast. More than half of the company's sales are related to asbestos and lead abatement; the industrial safety market accounts for another 25%. President and CEO Terry Shaver owns nearly a third of the company.

Abraxas Petroleum Corporation

500 N. Loop 1604 East, Ste. 100, San Antonio, TX 78232

Telephone: 210-490-4788 **Fax:** 210-490-8816 **Other address:** P.O. Box 701007, San Antonio, TX 78270 **Metro area:** San Antonio, TX **Web site:** http://www.abraxaspetroleum.com **Human resources contact:** Dixie Bane **Sales:** $60.1 million **Number of employees:** 74 **Number of employees for previous year:** 64 **Industry designation:** Oil & gas—exploration & production **Company type:** Public **Top competitors:** Royal Dutch/Shell Group; Mobil Corporation; Exxon Corporation

Abraxas is an independent energy company engaged mainly in crude oil and natural gas exploration, development, and production in Texas (along the Gulf Coast and in the Permian Basin of West Texas), Wyoming, and western Canada. The company's strategy is based on buying the underexploited properties of other oil companies. Abraxas' holdings include about 350 operating wells, more than 200 miles of gas gathering lines in Canada and Texas, and proved reserves of more than 55 million barrels of oil equivalent. Following a plan to increase production while cutting operating costs, CEO Robert Watson is focusing on exploiting the company's recent acquisitions, which have tripled the size of his firm.

Access Pharmaceuticals, Inc.

2600 Stemmons Frwy., Ste. 176, Dallas, TX 75207

Telephone: 214-905-5100 **Fax:** 214-905-5101 **Metro area:** Dallas-Fort Worth, TX **Human resources contact:** Stephen B. Thompson **Sales:** $435,000 **Number of employees:** 18 **Number of employees for previous year:** 15 **Industry designation:** Drugs **Company type:** Public **Top competitors:** NeXstar Pharmaceuticals, Inc.; ALZA Corporation; The Liposome Company, Inc.

Access Pharmaceuticals looks for ways to send drugs directly and effectively to the parts of the body that need treatment. The company develops drug-delivery systems for application in cancer treatment, dermatology, and MRI imaging diagnosis. Access Pharmaceuticals developed a canker sore treatment sold in the US under a royalty agreement with Block Drug. Products in development include a chemotherapy drug designed to more effectively target tumors, a dermatological drug, and an MRI imaging agent designed to better detect small tumors. The company has licensed its dermatological and imaging products to Strakan Limited and Dow Chemical, respectively. It is buying biopharmaceutical company Virologix.

Acuity Corporation

11100 Metric Blvd., Bldg. 7, Austin, TX 78758

Telephone: 512-425-2200 **Fax:** 512-719-8225 **Metro area:** Austin, TX **Web site:** http://www.acuity.com **Human resources contact:** Neal Fuller **Sales:** $5 million (Est.) **Number of employees:** 100 **Number of employees for previous year:** 72 **Industry designation:** Computers—online services **Company type:** Private **Top competitors:** International Business Machines Corporation; NetObjects, Inc.; Lucent Technologies Inc.

Looking for instant answers? Acuity (formerly iChat) makes software that lets call center representatives chat with customers over the Internet and respond instantaneously to questions via the same technology used to facilitate chat rooms. Its WebCenter Enterprise manages Internet-based customer service sessions by offering self-help, queuing calls to be handled by representatives, and responding to routine questions by e-mail. Founded in 1995, the company initially focused on consumer chat programs, but redesigned its technology for corporate customer service use. Customers include Ascend Communications, Lucent, and Amazon.com spinoff drugstore.com.

Advanced Neuromodulation Systems, Inc.

201 Allentown Pkwy., Allen, TX 75002

Telephone: 972-390-9800 **Fax:** 972-390-2881 **Metro area:** Dallas-Fort Worth, TX **Web site:** http://www.ans-medical.com **Human resources contact:** James P. Calhoun **Sales:** $14.7 million **Number of employees:** 103 **Number of employees for previous year:** 100 **Industry designation:** Medical products **Company type:** Public **Top competitors:** CytoTherapeutics, Inc.; Cardiac Control Systems, Inc.; Medtronic, Inc.

Of all the nerve. Advanced Neuromodulation Systems (formerly Quest Medical) makes products for treatment of neurology-related health problems and chronic pain. Its Advanced Neuromodulation System uses probes to disrupt pain signals in the nervous system. The company also makes drug pumps that deliver medication directly to the spinal cord. The firm markets its products to hospitals and other end users. It has a distribution and development alliance with Tricumed Medizointechnik GmbH. Advanced Neuromodulation Systems has sold its cardiovascular products and intravenous fluid-delivery products operations to medical product maker Atrion.

Advance Paradigm, Inc.

545 E. John Carpenter Fwy., Ste. 1570, Irving, TX 75062

Telephone: 972-830-6199 **Fax:** 972-830-6196 **Metro area:** Dallas-Fort Worth, TX **Web site:** http://www.advparadigm.com **Human resources contact:** Toni Sircely **Sales:** $476.7 million **Number of employees:** 697 **Number of employees for previous year:** 336 **Industry designation:** Medical practice management **Company type:** Public **Top competitors:** Express Scripts, Inc.; MedPartners, Inc.; Walgreen Co.

Advance Paradigm may have an '80s name, but it fills a '90s need, providing pharmacy benefit management services to health plans covering 12 million members. It works with providers on program design and formularies of the most appropriate and cost-effective drugs and processes claims for more than 50,000 pharmacies. Advance Paradigm also offers mail-order pharmacy programs. Its health benefit management services include disease-specific care management programs. Subsidiary Innovative Medical Research provides clinical trials and survey research. Blue Cross and Blue Shield of Texas owns 11% of the company, investment firm J.H. Whitney owns 5%, and founder David Halbert and his brother Jon own another 10%.

Affiliated Computer Services, Inc.

2828 N. Haskell Ave., Dallas, TX 75204

Telephone: 214-841-6111 **Fax:** 214-821-8315 **Metro area:** Dallas-Fort Worth, TX **Web site:** http://www.acs-inc.com **Human resources contact:** Lora Villarreal **Sales:** $1.2 billion **Number of employees:** 12,300 **Number of employees for previous year:** 7,030 **Industry designation:** Computers—services **Company type:** Public **Top competitors:** International Business Machines Corporation; Electronic Data Systems Corporation; Computer Sciences Corporation

The "C" in ACS should stand for "cash." Affiliated Computer Services is the second-largest nonbank operator of ATMs in the US (behind Electronic Data Systems), boasting more than 13,200 MoneyMaker machines in its ATM network. In addition to its electronic commerce services, ACS also provides professional services and business process and technology outsourcing. About one-third of its sales come from contracts with the US government. The company's aggressive growth strategy has resulted in its acquisition of more than 40 companies since its 1988 inception, which combined make it the one of the largest information technology services companies in the US.

Airtech International Group, Inc.

15400 Knoll Trail, Ste. 106, Dallas, TX 75248

Telephone: 972-960-9400 **Fax:** 972-960-9395 **Metro area:** Dallas-Fort Worth, TX **Web site:** http://www.airtechgroup.com **Sales:** $1.1 million **Number of employees:** 32 **Number of employees for previous year:** 30 **Industry designation:** Pollution control equipment & services **Company type:** Public **Top competitors:** MPW Industrial Services Group, Inc.; Thermatrix Inc.; Met-Pro Corporation

Airtech International Group, formerly Interactive Technologies Corporation (ITC), makes air purification products for commercial and residential use. The company's Airsopure product line removes up to 99% of hazardous gases and airborne particles, such as smoke, dust, fungi, and animal dander. Its products are sold across the US through franchises, auto dealers, and medical equipment suppliers for use in restaurants, hospitals, homes, and cars. Airtech also offers heating, ventilation, and air conditioning (HVAC) services in the Dallas area through subsidiary MSS. Before purchasing Airtech International Corporation, ITC operated in the interactive programming industry. Its remnant product, Rebate TV, is up for sale.

Amarillo Biosciences, Inc.

800 W. Ninth Ave., Amarillo, TX 79101

Telephone: 806-376-1741 **Fax:** 806-376-9301 **Metro area:** Amarillo, TX **Web site:** http://www.amacell.com **Sales:** $600,000 **Number of employees:** 13 **Number of employees for previous year:** 8 **Industry designation:** Biomedical & genetic products **Company type:** Public **Top competitors:** Interferon Sciences, Inc.; Biogen, Inc.; Genentech, Inc.

Little. Yellow. Different. Better? Amarillo Biosciences hopes its low-dose oral interferon alpha (IFNa) will make a difference for people suffering from hepatitis B and C and Sjogren's syndrome, a chronic autoimmune disease that leaves tissues painfully dry. The development-stage company believes that patients taking its IFNa lozenges (which help modulate the immune system) will not suffer the side effects that higher doses of IFNa can induce. While its drugs are in various stages of development in the US, Amarillo Biosciences has received clearance to sell its Veldona lozenges in Ghana to treat hepatitis B.

American Oncology Resources, Inc.

16825 Northchase Dr., Ste. 1300, Houston, TX 77060

Telephone: 281-873-2674 **Fax:** 281-775-0333 **Metro area:** Houston, TX **Web site:** http://www.aori.com **Human resources contact:** Paul Howell **Sales:** $456 million **Number of employees:** 1,293 **Number of employees for previous year:** 1,162 **Industry designation:** Medical practice management **Company type:** Public

American Oncology Resources manages more than 300 physicians' cancer-treatment practices in 16 states. Specialties include gynecological oncology, hematology, radiation oncology, diagnostic radiology, and stem cell transplantation. Under its management agreements with affiliated practices, American Oncology develops strategic plans for the practices, conducts financial analyses, implements management information systems, and manages facilities. The firm purchases supplies, manages nonmedical personnel, and markets its physicians' services for clinical trials. American Oncology Resources and former competitor Physician Reliance Network are merging to form a firm that will manage about 13% of new US cancer cases.

American Physician Partners, Inc.

2301 Nationsbank Plaza, 901 Main St., Dallas, TX 75202

Telephone: 214-761-3100 **Fax:** 214-761-3175 **Metro area:** Dallas-Fort Worth, TX **Human resources contact:** Karen Walker **Sales:** $135.6 million **Number of employees:** 1,600 **Number of employees for previous year:** 1,230 **Industry designation:** Medical practice management **Company type:** Public

American Physician Partners (APP) is a practice management company for doctors with X-ray vision. The company operates and manages ten practices that employ more than 250 radiologists in California, Florida, Kansas, Maryland, New York, Texas, Virginia, and Washington, DC. The company purchases the nonmedical assets of each practice and in return provides administrative services, including billing, insurance claims filing, accounting, and marketing. Participating practices sign service agreements that involve paying APP either a flat fee or a percentage of sales (usually 20% to 30%) or both. The company also owns and operates more than 70 imaging centers used by its practices.

American Rice, Inc.

411 N. Sam Houston Pkwy. East, Ste. 600, Houston, TX 77060

Telephone: 281-272-8800 **Fax:** 281-272-9707 **Metro area:** Houston, TX **Web site:** http://www.amrice.com **Human resources contact:** Marsha Donaghe **Sales:** $515.5 million **Number of employees:** 1,500 **Industry designation:** Food—flour & grain **Company type:** Public **Top competitors:** Riceland Foods, Inc.; Riviana Foods Inc.; Producers Rice Mills

Pitting olives against rice, American Rice goes with the grain. The company, 81%-owned by ERLY Industries, is one of the US's largest rice millers. It sold its olive producing operations (it was the second-largest producer in the US) to industry leader Musco Olive Products in late 1998. Formed in 1969 as a marketing cooperative, American Rice produces and markets white, brown, and instant rices under the US brands Comet, Adolphus, Blue Ribbon, and AA. The company also has international brands and exports to Africa, Asia, Europe, and the Middle East. American Rice is operating under Chapter 11 bankruptcy.

AMX Corporation

11995 Forestgate Dr., Dallas, TX 75243

Telephone: 972-644-3048 **Fax:** 972-907-2053 **Metro area:** Dallas-Fort Worth, TX **Web site:** http://www.amx.com **Human resources contact:** Holly Hawk **Sales:** $58.8 million **Number of employees:** 317 **Number of employees for previous year:** 266 **Industry designation:** Computers—peripheral equipment **Company type:** Public **Top competitors:** Dukane Corporation; Universal Electronics Inc.; Rauland-Borg Corporation

AMX Corporation can make things happen at the push of a button. The company makes remote-control systems that help corporations open drapes, switch off lights, start the air conditioner, and run closed-circuit cameras, among other functions. Its systems are used in corporate, educational, entertainment, government, and residential settings, including Epcot Center, the Library of Congress, and The Ballpark in Arlington, Texas. The company distributes its products through more than 1,600 electronics dealers in the US and to about 45 other countries. AMX continues to make inroads into the residential market.

Anadarko Petroleum Corporation

17001 Northchase Dr., Houston, TX 77060

Telephone: 281-875-1101 **Fax:** 281-874-3316 **Other address:** PO Box 1330, Houston, TX 77251 **Metro area:** Houston, TX **Web site:** http://www.anadarko.com **Human resources contact:** Richard A. Lewis **Sales:** $560.2 million **Number of employees:** 1,476 **Number of employees for previous year:** 1,386 **Industry designation:** Oil & gas—exploration & production **Company type:** Public **Top competitors:** Exxon Corporation; Apache Corporation; Pioneer Natural Resources Company

Anadarko Petroleum is one of the world's largest independent oil and gas companies. It is engaged in exploring for, developing, producing, and marketing natural gas, crude oil, condensate, and natural gas liquids. Anadarko conducts its explorations in the central US, the Gulf of Mexico, Alaska, Algeria's Sahara Desert, Eritrea, Jordan, and Peru. The company has proved reserves of more than 700 million barrels of crude oil, condensate, natural gas liquids (about 60% of total), and natural gas (about 40%), most of which is in the US. All of the company's production is in the US, where it owns interests in 13 gas-gathering systems and four gas-processing plants.

Apache Corporation

2000 Post Oak Blvd., Ste. 100, Houston, TX 77056

Telephone: 713-296-6000 **Fax:** 713-296-6496 **Metro area:** Houston, TX **Web site:** http://www.apachecorp.com **Human resources contact:** Dan Schaeffer **Sales:** $876.4 million **Number of employees:** 1,287 **Number of employees for previous year:** 1,256 **Industry designation:** Oil & gas—exploration & production **Company type:** Public **Top competitors:** Sonat Inc.; Burlington Resources Inc.; Unocal Corporation

Neither rain, sleet, nor nations' boundaries can keep Apache from an oil well. Apache is an oil and gas exploration and production company with onshore and offshore operations in Australia, China, Egypt, Indonesia, the Ivory Coast, Poland, and North America. The company has proved reserves of 586 million barrels of oil equivalent, mostly from its five North American regions: the midcontinent, the Gulf of Mexico, the Gulf Coast of Texas and Louisiana, the western US, and Canada. More than 50% of these reserves are natural gas. The company has been aggressively targeting overseas drilling opportunities, especially in Australia and Egypt.

Apple Orthodontix, Inc.

2777 Allen Pkwy., Ste. 700, Houston, TX 77019

Telephone: 713-852-2500 **Fax:** 713-852-2550 **Metro area:** Houston, TX **Web site:** http://www.appleorthodontix.com **Human resources contact:** Becky Curtis **Sales:** $19.2 million **Number of employees:** 481 **Number of employees for previous year:** 10 **Industry designation:** Medical practice management **Company type:** Public **Top competitors:** Orthodontic Centers of America, Inc.; Omega Orthodontics, Inc.; Castle Dental Centers, Inc.

Apple Orthodontix manages orthodontic practices. The company provides services such as staffing, education and training, billing and collections, payroll processing, patient scheduling, purchasing, inventory management, advertising production, and new-site development. The company offers service contracts to its practices for periods of 20-40 years with a variety of options related to service-fee payment. In addition, Apple Orthodontix requires its practices to provide affordable payment plans featuring small downpayments with monthly installments spread over periods of 26-34 months. The firm provides dental management services to about 70 orthodontists in 15 states and three Canadian provinces.

Aronex Pharmaceuticals, Inc.

8707 Technology Forest Place, The Woodlands, TX 77381

Telephone: 281-367-1666 **Fax:** 281-367-1676 **Metro area:** Houston, TX **Web site:** http://www.aronex.com **Human resources contact:** Marsha Kane **Sales:** $8 million **Number of employees:** 93 **Number of employees for previous year:** 72 **Industry designation:** Drugs **Company type:** Public

Aronex Pharmaceuticals is a development-stage biopharmaceutical company targeting cancer and infectious diseases. Through collaborations and strategic alliances with Boehringer Hannheim, Genzyme, Grupo Ferrer Internacional, and the University of Texas MD Anderson Cancer Center, Aronex is developing four products. NYOTRAN, which treats systemic fungal infections (including those related to AIDs), is in Phase II and Phase III clinical trials. Its HIV infection drug, Zintevir, is in Phase I and II clinical trials. ATRAGEN, which treats acute promyelocytic leukemia, is in Phase II clinical trials, and the breast-cancer drug Annamycin is in Phase II clinical trials.

Atrion Corporation

One Allentown Pkwy., Allen, TX 75002

Telephone: 972-390-9800 **Fax:** 205-381-2858 **Metro area:** Dallas-Fort Worth, TX **Web site:** http://www.atrioncorp.com **Sales:** $43.4 million **Number of employees:** 461 **Number of employees for previous year:** 386 **Industry designation:** Medical instruments **Company type:** Public **Top competitors:** Baxter International Inc.; Coherent, Inc.; Alcon Laboratories, Inc.

The metamorphosis is nearly complete: Atrion is almost out of the energy business. The company now makes such medical products as ophthalmic, diagnostic, and cardiovascular equipment; its Myocardal Protection System (which manages fluid delivery to the heart) has been used in more than 13,000 open-heart surgeries. Subsidiary Halkey-Roberts makes valves and clamps that regulate fluids and gases used in both hospital and outpatient care; its fluid control technology also has marine and aviation safety equipment applications. Another subsidiary, QMI, makes cardiovascular and intravenous fluid delivery products. Atrion's lone link to its past is a 22-mile pipeline that transports gaseous oxygen in Alabama.

Aviva Petroleum Inc.

8235 Douglas Ave., Ste. 400, Dallas, TX 75225

Telephone: 214-691-3464 **Fax:** 214-361-0010 **Metro area:** Dallas-Fort Worth, TX **Human resources contact:** Deena Pluto **Sales:** $3.3 million **Number of employees:** 65 **Number of employees for previous year:** 10 **Industry designation:** Oil & gas—exploration & production **Company type:** Public **Top competitors:** Triton Energy Limited; Atlantic Richfield Company; Abraxas Petroleum Corporation

Aviva Petroleum may explore for oil and gas, but it has found a jewel. The small independent has merged with Garnet Resources, doubling its proved reserves to more than three million barrels of oil. It has operations in Colombia, Papua New Guinea, and the US. In Colombia, through a long-term contract granted by national oil company Empresa Colombiana de Petroleos, it operates mainly in the southwestern part of the country. However, falling oil prices and guerrilla attacks on its facilities there have hurt the firm. Subsidiary Aviva America conducts its US operations, which include interests in 17 wells in the Gulf of Mexico offshore Louisiana. Aviva Petroleum also has 1.1 billion cu. ft. of natural gas reserves.

BancTec, Inc.

4851 LBJ Fwy., Dallas, TX 75244

Telephone: 972-341-4000 **Fax:** 972-341-4867 **Metro area:** Dallas-Fort Worth, TX **Web site:** http://www.banctec.com **Human resources contact:** James R. Wimberley **Sales:** $597.9 million **Number of employees:** 4,000 **Number of employees for previous year:** 3,650 **Industry designation:** Optical character recognition **Company type:** Public

BancTec markets electronic processing systems, software, and services for financial-transaction documentation. Products include ImageFIRST systems, which are used to capture, digitize, and process checks, utility bills, mortgage coupons, and other documents. BancTec's OpenARCHIVE is designed for high-speed archiving of financial document images and related transaction data. BancTec also makes software for electronically processing credit, debit, and courtesy cards and for electronic check authorization. Support services account for about 45% of sales. The firm, which an affiliate of investment firm Welsh Carson Anderson & Stowe is buying, also does warranty repairs for Dell, Compaq, and Toshiba.

Baylor Health Care System

3500 Gaston Ave., Dallas, TX 75246

Telephone: 214-820-0111 **Fax:** 214-820-7499 **Metro area:** Dallas-Fort Worth, TX **Web site:** http://www.baylordallas.edu **Human resources contact:** Beverly Bradshaw **Sales:** $993.2 million **Number of employees:** 12,900 **Number of employees for previous year:** 12,736 **Industry designation:** Hospitals **Company type:** Not-for-profit **Top competitors:** Parkland Health & Hospital System; Columbia/HCA Healthcare Corporation; Texas Health Resources

The Baylor Health Care System (BHCS) offers a bundle of services. Founded in 1981, it is governed by Baylor University and supported by the Baptist General Convention of Texas. The not-for-profit regional medical network includes the five-hospital Baylor University Medical Center complex, one of the state's major teaching and referral facilities. Other system members include an acute care rehabilitation facility, a restorative care facility, thirteen senior health centers, five family health centers, community hospitals, medical centers, and a cancer center. The system also provides home health care and specialty pediatric services. BHCS is working out a possible merger with Texas Health Resources.

Bellwether Exploration Company

1331 Lamar, Ste. 1455, Houston, TX 77010

Telephone: 713-650-1025 **Fax:** 713-652-2916 **Metro area:** Houston, TX **Web site:** http://www.bellwetherexp.com **Sales:** $75.8 million **Number of employees:** 17 **Number of employees for previous year:** 8 **Industry designation:** Oil & gas—exploration & production **Company type:** Public **Top competitors:** Maynard Oil Company; Abraxas Petroleum Corporation; Remington Oil & Gas Corporation

Bellwether Exploration likes to be in on a trend (especially if there's oil in it). The company explores for oil and gas, develops oil and gas properties, and gathers and processes natural gas. It has interests in producing properties in Texas, Louisiana, Alabama, off the coast of California, and in the Gulf of Mexico. In addition, the company holds interests in gas processing plants in California and West Texas and wholly owns a gas gathering system in northern Louisiana. Bellwether uses 3-D seismic and computer-aided exploration technology. It seeks to acquire producing properties that can be exploited using advanced recovery techniques including seismic modeling, well workovers, and horizontal drilling.

Blue Bell Creameries L.P.

1101 S. Horton, Brenham, TX 77833

Telephone: 409-836-7977 **Fax:** 409-830-2198 **Metro area:** College Station, TX **Web site:** http://www.bluebell.com **Human resources contact:** Darrell Winkelmann **Sales:** $225 million (Est.) **Number of employees:** 2,300 **Number of employees for previous year:** 2,000 **Industry designation:** Food—dairy products **Company type:** Private **Top competitors:** Dreyer's Grand Ice Cream, Inc.; Ben & Jerry's Homemade, Inc.; Unilever

Texas ice-cream maker Blue Bell Creameries says it all started with a "little creamery in Brenham." Despite its bucolic trademark of a barefoot country girl leading a milk cow, Blue Bell means big business. With plants in three states, it cranks out about 100,000 gallons of ice cream per day, making Blue Bell the #3 ice-cream maker in the country. Although the company is slowly expanding from its strong regional base surrounding Texas, it is trying to maintain strict control over the production process. CEO Howard Kruse and his family maintain control of the creamery, which was started in an abandoned cotton gin in 1907.

Blue Cross and Blue Shield of Texas Inc.

901 S. Central Expwy., Richardson, TX 75080

Telephone: 972-766-6900 **Fax:** 972-766-6234 **Metro area:** Dallas-Fort Worth, TX **Web site:** http://www.bcbstx.com **Human resources contact:** Paulette Smith **Sales:** $2.6 billion **Number of employees:** 5,039 **Number of employees for previous year:** 4,595 **Industry designation:** Insurance—accident & health **Company type:** Not-for-profit **Top competitors:** UnitedHealth Group; The Prudential Insurance Company of America; Aetna Inc.

If an apple a day kept the doctor away, Blue Cross and Blue Shield of Texas would supply a daily Red Delicious one to its 1.7 million health plan customers. The not-for-profit association emphasizes the use of preventive medicine to hold down the costs of operating its HMO, PPO, point-of-service, and indemnity insurance health care plans in Texas. The company also operates in Colorado, Maryland, and New Mexico through Medicare claims administration contracts. The company is attempting to merge with Health Care Service Corporation (Blue Cross' Illinois licensee), but despite court approval, Texas regulators oppose the deal because the Texas company has received tax breaks as a quasi-charitable organization.

Blue Dolphin Energy Company

11 Greenway Plaza, Ste. 1606, Houston, TX 77046

Telephone: 713-621-3993 **Fax:** 713-621-4687 **Metro area:** Houston, TX **Web site:** http://www.blue-dolphin.com **Sales:** $5 million **Number of employees:** 20 **Number of employees for previous year:** 14 **Industry designation:** Oil & gas—exploration & production **Company type:** Public **Top competitors:** Leviathan Gas Pipeline Partners, L.P.; Tejas Energy, LLC; El Paso Energy Corporation

Blue Dolphin is fishing out oil prospects in the deep blue Gulf waters. Blue Dolphin Energy explores for and acquires, develops, and operates oil and gas properties in the Gulf of Mexico and along the Texas Gulf Coast. The firm has proved reserves of 184 thousand barrels of oil and 31.4 million cu. ft. of natural gas. The firm also owns offshore pipeline operations and, through subsidiary Petroport, develops deep-water terminals and storage facilities (16 million barrels of capacity) for both crude oil and refined products in natural salt dome caverns. Supertankers can dock and discharge oil to avoid unloading, called lightering, into smaller vessels close to environmentally sensitive shorelines.

Brigham Exploration Company

6300 Bridge Point Pwky., Bldg. 2, Ste. 500, Austin, TX 78730

Telephone: 512-427-3300 **Fax:** 512-427-3400 **Metro area:** Austin, TX **Web site:** http://www.bog3d.com **Human resources contact:** Anne L. Brigham **Sales:** $9.8 million **Number of employees:** 66 **Number of employees for previous year:** 57 **Industry designation:** Oil & gas—exploration & production **Company type:** Public **Top competitors:** Chesapeake Energy Corporation; Apache Corporation; KCS Energy, Inc.

Brigham Exploration is riding the waves—sound waves, that is. The independent oil and gas firm relies on 3-D seismic imaging (using sound waves to record geologic formations) for onshore exploration. It explores mainly in Oklahoma-Texas' Anadarko Basin, the Gulf Coast, and West Texas, but also in Colorado, Kansas, Louisiana, and Montana. Since 1990 the company has drilled some 370 wells (with a 63% success rate), acquired more than 4,000 sq. mi. of 3-D seismic data, and identified about 1,200 potential drilling locations; it has estimated proved reserves of 72 billion cu. ft. of natural gas equivalent. Brigham Exploration has agreed to give Enron about a 14% stake in exchange for drilling financing.

BrightStar Information Technology Group, Inc.

10375 Richmond Ave., Ste. 1620, Houston, TX 77042

Telephone: 713-361-2500 **Fax:** 713-361-2501 **Metro area:** Houston, TX **Web site:** http://www.brightstar-it.com **Sales:** $59.5 million **Number of employees:** 840 **Number of employees for previous year:** 690 **Industry designation:** Computers—services **Company type:** Public **Top competitors:** Computer Management Sciences, Inc.; Cambridge Technology Partners (Massachusetts), Inc.; PRT Group Inc.

BrightStar Information Technology provides large corporations with information technology (IT) services ranging from consulting and software implementation to Web site design. Its more than 800 IT professionals in 16 US cities and seven more abroad provide such services as database design and development, IT outsourcing and training, systems integration, project management, year 2000 compliance, and enterprise resource planning software implementation. BrightStar's software tools are geared for SAP and PeopleSoft products, Web-enabled ERP applications, and custom software development. About 28% of sales originate overseas, and clients include ALLTEL, General Electric, SAP, Ernst & Young, and PepsiCo.

broadcast.com inc.

2914 Taylor St., Dallas, TX 75226

Telephone: 214-748-6660 **Fax:** 214-748-6657 **Metro area:** Dallas-Fort Worth, TX **Web site:** http://www.broadcast.com **Human resources contact:** Kathy Shunatona **Sales:** $22.4 million **Number of employees:** 170 **Industry designation:** Computers—online services **Company type:** Public **Top competitors:** RealNetworks, Inc.; SportsLine USA, Inc.; audiohighway.com

Media company broadcast.com (formerly AudioNet) provides Internet users access to a variety of programming, including live music and sports broadcasts. broadcast.com offers access to more than 425 radio and television stations, and cable networks through its Web site. Customers may follow the play-by-play of college and professional sporting events, indulge in police scanner eavesdropping, catch the BBC News, or enjoy a live concert. The company also provides on-demand access to music CDs and transmission services for company meetings and promotions. Co-founder and chairman Mark Cuban owns about 28% of the company. Internet search giant Yahoo! has agreed to buy broadcast.com.

Cabot Oil & Gas Corporation

15375 Memorial Dr., Houston, TX 77079

Telephone: 281-589-4600 **Fax:** 281-589-4828 **Metro area:** Houston, TX **Web site:** http://www.cabotog.com **Human resources contact:** Abraham Garza **Sales:** $159.6 million **Number of employees:** 365 **Number of employees for previous year:** 342 **Industry designation:** Oil & gas—exploration & production **Company type:** Public **Top competitors:** Belden & Blake Corporation; Equitable Resources, Inc.; Columbia Energy Group

Cabot Oil & Gas produces and sells natural gas and oil. It operates more than 4,000 wells and has more than 935 billion cu. ft. of total proved reserves, 96% of which are natural gas. Cabot's Appalachian operations are concentrated in Ohio, Pennsylvania, Virginia, and West Virginia and make up 45% of the company's proved reserves. Operations in Kansas, Oklahoma, Texas, and Wyoming make up 55% of its proved reserves. The company also has wells in the Rocky Mountain and Gulf Coast regions and operates about 2,800 miles of pipeline systems. Cabot's products are sold in the North, South, and Midwest, primarily to industry, local distribution companies, and gas marketers.

Caltex Petroleum Corporation

125 E. John Carpenter Fwy., Irving, TX 75062

Telephone: 972-830-1000 **Fax:** 972-830-1081 **Other address:** PO Box 619500, Dallas, TX 75261 **Metro area:** Dallas-Fort Worth, TX **Web site:** http://www.caltex.com **Human resources contact:** Stephen H. Nichols **Sales:** $18.4 billion **Number of employees:** 7,600 **Number of employees for previous year:** 7,300 **Industry designation:** Oil refining & marketing **Company type:** Joint venture **Parent company:** Chevron Corporation; Texaco Inc. **Top competitors:** BP Amoco p.l.c.; Royal Dutch/Shell Group; Exxon Corporation

For more than six decades California and Texas have paired two of their top oil businesses to sell refined petroleum products worldwide. Caltex Petroleum is a 50-50 joint venture between Texaco and Chevron, with operations primarily in Africa, Asia, Australasia, and the Middle East. The company, which will move its headquarters to Singapore in 1999, markets products through more than 7,900 retail outlets, fuels aircraft at 38 airports, and provides marine fuels and lubricants to more than 100 ports in 22 countries. The company has stakes in 13 fuel refineries, two lubricant refineries, 17 lubricant-blending plants, six asphalt plants, six grease plants, and more than 500 ocean terminals and depots.

CanArgo Energy Corporation

1400 Broadfield, Ste. 100, Houston, TX 77084

Telephone: 281-492-6992 **Fax:** 281-492-6673 **Metro area:** Houston, TX **Human resources contact:** Darrell Keller **Sales:** $300,000 **Number of employees:** 34 **Number of employees for previous year:** 31 **Industry designation:** Oil & gas—exploration & production **Company type:** Public

CanArgo Energy Corporation, formerly Fountain Oil, is an independent oil and gas company that primarily acquires, develops, and exploits oil properties with proved reserves in Canada, Eastern Europe, and the US; the firm generally pursues joint-venture agreements. CanArgo Energy has estimated proved reserves of 11 million barrels of oil. The former Fountain Oil was acquired by CanArgo Energy Inc. in a reverse acquisition that gave the acquiring firm about 47% of the company's stock and made CanArgo Energy Inc. a subsidiary of the company.

Capital Senior Living Corporation

14160 Dallas Pkwy., Ste. 300, Dallas, TX 75240

Telephone: 972-770-5600 **Fax:** 972-770-5666 **Metro area:** Dallas-Fort Worth, TX **Human resources contact:** Colleen Landino **Sales:** $42.8 million **Number of employees:** 1,600 **Number of employees for previous year:** 1,558 **Industry designation:** Nursing homes **Company type:** Public **Top competitors:** Regent Assisted Living, Inc.; ARV Assisted Living, Inc.; Greenbriar Corporation

Capital Senior Living owns or manages 33 senior residential properties in 17 states. Formed to consolidate the operations of several partnerships that previously owned its facilities, the company provides independent-living, assisted-living, and nursing services. Capital also operates a home health care agency that manages the health care needs of residents in certain communities. Specialized care units for treatment of Alzheimer's patients are also available. Capital has a joint venture agreement with New World Development Company to develop and manage senior living communities in China. To accommodate more new residents, Capital is developing 20 new communities and expanding 11 existing ones.

Carrington Laboratories, Inc.

2001 Walnut Hill Ln., Irving, TX 75038

Telephone: 972-518-1300 **Fax:** 972-518-1020 **Metro area:** Dallas-Fort Worth, TX **Web site:** http://www.carringtonlabs.com **Human resources contact:** Carol Kitchell **Sales:** $23.6 million **Number of employees:** 278 **Number of employees for previous year:** 252 **Industry designation:** Drugs **Company type:** Public **Top competitors:** Alpha-Beta Technology, Inc.; Lifecore Biomedical, Inc.; Cytel Corporation

Carrington Laboratories promotes a high-carbo lifestyle, with its carbohydrate-based therapeutics for major illnesses and wounds (the firm's products keep wounds moist to promote healing). It is also working on a tumor treatment. In addition to professional-use products, Carrington Laboratories sells consumer and veterinary products through a worldwide distributor network. Subsidiary Caraloe sells aloe-based nutrition and skin-care consumer products under the Aloe Nutritional name; it also sells bulk aloe extracts to manufacturers. The Carrington Veterinary Medical Division sells wound and skin-care products and Acemannan Immunostimulant, a substance used in anticancer vaccines for cats and dogs.

Carrizo Oil & Gas, Inc.

14811 St. Mary's Ln., Ste. 148, Houston, TX 77079

Telephone: 281-496-1352 **Metro area:** Houston, TX **Sales:** $7.9 million **Number of employees:** 22 **Number of employees for previous year:** 15 **Industry designation:** Oil & gas—exploration & production **Company type:** Public **Top competitors:** Coho Energy, Inc.; Columbus Energy Corp.; Chesapeake Energy Corporation

Carrizo Oil & Gas sees its future in 3-D. An independent exploration and production company that drills in proven onshore fields along the Gulf Coast of Texas and Louisiana, Carrizo aggressively acquires 3-D seismic data and arranges land lease options in conjunction with conducting seismic surveys. The company typically exploits the shallow reservoirs in its fields and sells the deeper prospects. Carrizo operates about 55 producing oil wells and more than 10 natural gas wells, and has interests in two dozen others. The company's total proved reserves stand at 43 billion cu. ft. of natural gas equivalent.

Castle Dental Centers, Inc.

1360 Post Oak Blvd., Ste. 1300, Houston, TX 77056

Telephone: 713-479-8000 **Fax:** 713-513-1401 **Metro area:** Houston, TX **Human resources contact:** Richard O'Connor **Sales:** $74.8 million **Number of employees:** 1,220 **Number of employees for previous year:** 750 **Industry designation:** Medical practice management **Company type:** Public **Top competitors:** Coast Dental Services, Inc.; Monarch Dental Corporation; Orthodontic Centers of America, Inc.

Castle Dental Centers manages and operates dental practice networks in Florida, Tennessee, and Texas. The company provides nondental management services to 55 dental centers, including general, orthodontic, and multispecialty dental practices. Its administrative management services include human resources services, equipment supply, insurance services, and financial and accounting reporting and administration. Castle Dental intends to continue to add dental practices to its networks, and thereby enhance its position as a contractor for health care management companies. Cofounder and CEO Jack H. Castle, Jr. owns about 22% of the company.

Chaparral Resources, Inc.

2211 Norfolk, Ste. 1150, Houston, TX 77098

Telephone: 713-807-7100 **Fax:** 713-807-7561 **Metro area:** Houston, TX **Sales:** $200,000 **Number of employees:** 8 **Number of employees for previous year:** 5 **Industry designation:** Oil & gas—exploration & production **Company type:** Public

Chaparral Resources, an independent oil and gas exploration and production company, pursues international oil and gas projects, primarily in the former Soviet Union state of Kazakhstan. The company sold its US exploration and production interests to purchase a half-interest in Karakuduk-Munay, which has the rights to develop the Karakuduk Field oil property in Kazakhstan. Exploratory wells built to delineate Karakuduk have produced oil, but future production value remains uncertain for the 17,000-acre field, which has not been commercially drilled.

Cheniere Energy, Inc.

1200 Smith St., Ste. 1740, Houston, TX 77002

Telephone: 713-659-1361 **Fax:** 713-659-5459 **Metro area:** Houston, TX **Human resources contact:** Don A. Tukleson **Sales:** $100,000 **Number of employees:** 9 **Number of employees for previous year:** 2 **Industry designation:** Oil & gas—exploration & production **Company type:** Public **Top competitors:** Vastar Resources, Inc.; Apache Corporation; Union Pacific Resources Group Inc.

Shhhh. Cheniere Energy is tiptoeing its way into the oil business. A development-stage company, Cheniere Energy is the holding company for Cheniere Energy Operating Company, engaged in exploration for oil and gas. The operating company has a 50% participation right in a joint exploration project with sometimes contentious partner Zydeco Energy, along the coast of Louisiana, both onshore and in the shallow waters of the Gulf of Mexico. Data collection and processing from the 3-D seismic survey covering most of the 310-sq.-mi. project is complete. The company plans to keep a significant working interest in the project, though not to become an operator in the venture.

ClubCorp International, Inc.

3030 LBJ Fwy., Ste. 700, Dallas, TX 75234

Telephone: 972-243-6191 **Fax:** 972-888-7700 **Metro area:** Dallas-Fort Worth, TX **Web site:** http://www.clubcorp.com **Human resources contact:** Albert Chew **Sales:** $840.3 million (Est.) **Number of employees:** 21,000 **Number of employees for previous year:** 20,000 **Industry designation:** Leisure & recreational services **Company type:** Private **Top competitors:** Club Mediterranee S.A.; Hyatt Corporation; American Golf Corporation

Through its subsidiaries, holding company ClubCorp International is the world's largest operator of private clubs and resorts. Operating 220 private clubs, resorts, and public and private golf courses worldwide, the company's properties include Mission Hills Country Club and Pinehurst Resort and Country Club (the world's largest golf resort and site of the 1999 US Open). Founded by chairman Robert Dedman in 1957, ClubCorp has a 30% stake in PGA European Tour Courses. The company also offers an Associate Clubs program (allowing club members to use the facilities of other clubs operated by the company), ClubHaven.com (a virtual private club on the Internet), and club member magazine "Private Clubs."

Coho Energy, Inc.

14785 Preston Rd., Ste. 860, Dallas, TX 75240

Telephone: 972-774-8300 **Fax:** 972-991-8514 **Metro area:** Dallas-Fort Worth, TX **Human resources contact:** R. Lynn Guillory **Sales:** $68.8 million **Number of employees:** 166 **Number of employees for previous year:** 134 **Industry designation:** Oil & gas—exploration & production **Company type:** Public

Just like the salmon its named after, Coho Energy swims upstream but in oil. The independent oil and gas company develops, produces, and explores for crude oil and natural gas in low-risk activities such as development drilling, multi-zone completions, recompletions, enhancement of production facilities, and secondary recovery projects. Mississippi, Oklahoma, and Louisiana make up its principal interests. It also owns and operates more than 1,000 miles of gas-gathering systems and pipeline in Louisiana. The company more than doubled its proved reserves through its 1997 purchase from Amoco (now BP Amoco) of oil and gas properties in southern Oklahoma.

CompuTrac, Inc.

222 Municipal Dr., Richardson, TX 75080

Telephone: 972-234-4241 **Fax:** 972-234-6280 **Metro area:** Dallas-Fort Worth, TX **Web site:** http://www.computrac.com **Human resources contact:** Lynda K. Thomas **Sales:** $4.8 million **Number of employees:** 62 **Number of employees for previous year:** 61 **Industry designation:** Computers—corporate, professional & financial software **Company type:** Public **Top competitors:** Eltrax Systems, Inc.; Broadway & Seymour, Inc.; PC DOCS Group International Inc.

Not every Perry Mason has a Della Street, but many an attorney has a CompuTrac computer system. The company's systems include hardware and software that help law firms handle such tasks as timekeeping, disbursement tracking, billing, accounting, management, and financial reporting. Traditionally, CompuTrac systems used the company's flagship CompuTrac Law Firm Management System (LFMS) software and Hewlett-Packard hardware (the company is an authorized HP reseller). However, CompuTrac's newest version of LFMS is Windows-compatible. CompuTrac offers such services as maintenance, conversions, training, support, and software upgrades. Chairman and CEO Harry Margolis, a company founder, owns 31% of CompuTrac.

CONDEA Vista Company

900 Threadneedle, Houston, TX 77079

Telephone: 281-588-3000 **Fax:** 281-588-3236 **Metro area:** Houston, TX **Web site:** http://www.condea.com/vista/index.html **Human resources contact:** Crystal Wright **Number of employees:** 1,450 **Number of employees for previous year:** 1,440 **Industry designation:** Chemicals—diversified **Company type:** Subsidiary **Parent company:** RWE-DEA **Top competitors:** Great Lakes Chemical Corporation; Velsicol Chemical Corporation; Albemarle Corporation

CONDEA Vista is the US affiliate of CONDEA, the global chemical arm of RWE-AG, a 100-year-old German holding company. Among the chemicals produced are aluminas and aluminum oxides used in polishes and synthetic gemstone production; alcohols, used to make household cleaners, lubes, and greases; and paraffins for printing inks and insecticides. CONDEA's chemicals are also included in the manufacture of everyday products such as shampoos, cosmetics, handcreams, and automobile interior trim. CONDEA Vista operates six manufacturing plants and one research and development facility in the US.

Cornell Corrections, Inc.

1700 W. Loop South, Ste. 1500, Houston, TX 77027

Telephone: 713-623-0790 **Fax:** 713-623-2853 **Metro area:** Houston, TX **Web site:** http://cornellcorrections.com **Human resources contact:** Patrick Perrin **Sales:** $123.1 million **Number of employees:** 2,954 **Number of employees for previous year:** 1,965 **Industry designation:** Protection—safety equipment & services **Company type:** Public **Top competitors:** Wackenhut Corrections Corporation; Youth Services International, Inc.; Prison Realty Corporation

As an operator of detention and correction centers for state and federal agencies, Cornell Corrections has contracts to operate more than 40 programs in 11 states. The adult and juvenile correction and detention centers it runs contain nearly 8,000 beds. The company's prerelease facilities (including halfway houses) provide such services as job training and transition planning for inmates serving the last three months of their sentences. The company's facilities generally offer food services, education programs, health care, work and recreational programs, and chemical-dependency and substance-abuse programs. Cornell Corrections also provides consultation services for facility design and construction.

Costilla Energy, Inc.

400 W. Illinois, Ste. 1000, Midland, TX 79701

Telephone: 915-683-3092 **Fax:** 915-686-6080 **Metro area:** Odessa, TX **Human resources contact:** Nancy Christmas **Sales:** $72.3 million **Number of employees:** 139 **Number of employees for previous year:** 114 **Industry designation:** Oil & gas—exploration & production **Company type:** Public

Costilla Energy explores for, develops, and acquires oil and gas properties in South and East Texas, the Rocky Mountain region, and the Permian Basin of Texas and New Mexico. The company has estimated proved reserves of about 15 million barrels of oil, 148.6 million cu. ft. of gas, and 39.7 million barrels of oil equivalent. Its in-house exploration efforts primarily use 3-D seismic technology to identify drilling opportunities. Costilla Energy has interests in almost 2,000 productive oil and gas wells and sells its production at the well site. In a $410 million deal, Costilla Energy agreed to buy 425 oil and gas fields in Texas and Oklahoma from Pioneer Natural Resources.

Cotton Valley Resources Corporation

6510 Abrams, Ste. 300, Dallas, TX 75231

Telephone: 214-221-6500 **Fax:** 214-221-6510 **Metro area:** Dallas-Fort Worth, TX **Web site:** http://www.cottonvalley.com **Human resources contact:** Diana Campbell **Sales:** $1.8 million **Number of employees:** 20 **Number of employees for previous year:** 9 **Industry designation:** Oil & gas—exploration & production **Company type:** Public **Top competitors:** Maynard Oil Company; Magnum Hunter Resources, Inc.; Sonat Inc.

Cotton Valley Resources is looking for oil and gas pickings in its own backyard. The exploration and production company and its subsidiaries operate in Texas and Oklahoma. Holdings include the Cheneyboro Field, the Means (Queen Sand) Unit, and the Sears Ranch Prospect in Texas and the N.E. Alden Field in Oklahoma. The company's proved reserves include 5.7 million barrels of oil and 12.7 billion cu. ft. of gas. Through its Mustang subsidiaries, the company also provides horizontal drilling services and purchases used oilfield equipment for resale. CEO Eugene Soltero owns 25% of Cotton Valley Resources, and COO James Hogue owns 26%.

Cross Timbers Oil Company

810 Houston St., Ste. 2000, Fort Worth, TX 76102

Telephone: 817-870-2800 **Fax:** 817-870-1671 **Metro area:** Dallas-Fort Worth, TX **Web site:** http://www.crosstimbers.com **Sales:** $249.5 million **Number of employees:** 521 **Number of employees for previous year:** 349 **Industry designation:** Oil & gas—exploration & production **Company type:** Public

Cross Timbers Oil Company acquires, exploits, and develops quality, long-lived producing oil and gas properties. The company's properties are located in Alaska, East and West Texas, Kansas, Louisiana, New Mexico, Oklahoma, and Wyoming. The company also owns and operates a 295-mile gas gathering system in Oklahoma, markets natural gas, and trades crude oil. Most of the company's gas is sold to purchasers at the wellhead at market prices. Cross Timbers has proved reserves of about 50 million barrels of oil and about 1.05 trillion cu. ft. of natural gas. The company also owns about 13,000 acres of undeveloped land in Texas.

Cyberonics, Inc.

16511 Space Center Blvd., #600, Houston, TX 77058

Telephone: 281-228-7200 **Fax:** 281-218-9332 **Metro area:** Houston, TX **Web site:** http://www.cyberonics.com **Human resources contact:** Freddie Marcussen **Sales:** $14.9 million **Number of employees:** 185 **Number of employees for previous year:** 69 **Industry designation:** Medical instruments **Company type:** Public **Top competitors:** Novo Nordisk A/S; Medtronic, Inc.; Pace Medical, Inc.

Cyberonics makes the first medical device to be cleared by the FDA for treating epilepsy. The NeuroCybernetic Prosthesis (NCP) is a pacemaker-like device implanted under the collarbone, with a lead attached to the vagus nerve in the neck; the device delivers intermittent signals to the brain to control epileptic seizures. Patients can activate additional signals with a magnet if they feel a seizure coming on; the NCP's generator can be programmed by a wand connected to a personal computer. The NCP System is also approved for use in Canada, the European Union, and other countries. The company has received FDA approval to build a manufacturing facility with laser capabilities.

Cytoclonal Pharmaceutics, Inc.

9000 Harry Hines Blvd., Ste. 330, Dallas, TX 75235

Telephone: 214-353-2922 **Fax:** 214-350-9514 **Metro area:** Dallas-Fort Worth, TX **Human resources contact:** Daniel Shusterman **Sales:** $100,000 **Number of employees:** 19 **Number of employees for previous year:** 13 **Industry designation:** Drugs **Company type:** Public **Top competitors:** Hauser, Inc.; ImClone Systems Incorporated; Vion Pharmaceuticals, Inc.

Yew'd better believe Cytoclonal Pharmaceutics wants to make cheaper paclitaxel. The development-stage company owns rights to a technology to produce the breast cancer drug from a fungus derived from Pacific yew trees (instead of the bark and needles). It has licensed the technology to Bristol-Myers Squibb, the exclusive US distributor of TAXOL (paclitaxel). Cytoclonal also owns the rights to a gene isolated from the yew that is critical in paclitaxel production. In addition to its fungal work, Cytoclonal has developed a kidney disease treatment using paclitaxel and is researching a specific gene that can be used to diagnose lung cancer. Its partners include a number of academic research centers, Enzon, and Helm.

DA Consulting Group, Inc.

5847 San Felipe Rd., Ste. 3700, Houston, TX 77057

Telephone: 713-361-3000 **Fax:** 713-361-3001 **Metro area:** Houston, TX **Web site:** http://www.dacg.com **Human resources contact:** Eric J. Fernette **Sales:** $80.1 million **Number of employees:** 863 **Number of employees for previous year:** 568 **Industry designation:** Computers—services **Company type:** Public **Top competitors:** Intelligroup, Inc.; Andersen Consulting

Give employees a new software program and they're likely to ask, "What do I do with it?" DA Consulting helps answer that question for companies that are installing enterprise resource planning (ERP) software—complex systems that enable companies to manage their operations more easily. DA Consulting smooths the transition by developing customized implementation programs that include employee focus groups, presentations, newsletters, computer-based or instructor-led training, and reference guides. The company, which operates about 15 offices around the globe, supports ERP software applications from companies such as SAP, J.D. Edwards, Baan, and Oracle.

Denali Incorporated

1360 Post Oak Blvd., Ste. 2250, Houston, TX 77056

Telephone: 713-627-0933 **Fax:** 713-627-0937 **Metro area:** Houston, TX **Web site:** http://www.denaliincorporated.com **Human resources contact:** Janice McCormick **Sales:** $99.9 million **Number of employees:** 930 **Number of employees for previous year:** 612 **Industry designation:** Pollution control equipment & services **Company type:** Public **Top competitors:** ITEQ, Inc.; Matrix Service Company

Denali tanks its job seriously, making underground and aboveground storage tanks and fiberglass-reinforced composites used to handle hazardous fluids. Formed to acquire Owens Corning's fiberglass composite underground storage tank operations, Denali makes products for petroleum, chemical, pulp and paper, electric power, and other industrial process plants. Its products include underground storage tanks, manhole products, oil and water separators, steel rectangular aboveground storage tanks, and fiberglass-reinforced plastic products for handling corrosive fluids. Denali operates manufacturing plants in eight states. Denali is buying Welna (The Netherlands) to expand into Europe, South America, and Asia.

Denbury Resources Inc.

17304 Preston Rd., Ste. 200, Dallas, TX 75252

Telephone: 972-673-2000 **Fax:** 972-673-2150 **Metro area:** Dallas-Fort Worth, TX **Web site:** http://www.denbury.com **Human resources contact:** Kandy Griffin **Sales:** $81.9 million **Number of employees:** 205 **Number of employees for previous year:** 157 **Industry designation:** Oil & gas—exploration & production **Company type:** Public **Top competitors:** FINA, Inc.; Burlington Resources Inc.; The Meridian Resource Corporation

Denbury Resources, which buried its hopes of striking it rich in its native Canadian soil, is searching for a warmer economic climate in the US Gulf Coast states of Louisiana and Mississippi. The small independent exploration and production company has onshore interests in more than 40 fields in Louisiana and nearly 40 in Mississippi. It has proved reserves of nearly 65 million barrels of oil equivalent. Customers include Hunt Refining (42% of sales), Dynegy (22%), and Columbia Energy Services (10%). Led by David Bonderman, buyout firm Texas Pacific Group owns a 60% stake in the company.

DocuCorp International, Inc.

5910 N. Central Expwy., Ste. 800, Dallas, TX 75206

Telephone: 214-891-6500 **Fax:** 214-987-8187 **Metro area:** Dallas-Fort Worth, TX **Web site:** http://www.docucorp.com **Human resources contact:** Pat Jones **Sales:** $45.2 million **Number of employees:** 315 **Number of employees for previous year:** 285 **Industry designation:** Computers—corporate, professional & financial software **Company type:** Public **Top competitors:** Cincom Systems, Inc.; Document Sciences Corporation; Mobius Management Systems, Inc.

DocuCorp International has thousands of work policies. More than half of the 200 largest North American insurance companies (three-fourths of sales), including Prudential (13% of sales) and American International Group, use DocuCorp's document automation software and printing services for high-volume processing of documents such as insurance policies. DocuCorp also helps about 700 other clients, including Consolidated Edison of New York and the University of Texas, process telephone bills; direct-mail correspondence; and bank, mutual fund, and utility statements. Safeguard Scientifics and Xerox each own about 11% of the company.

drkoop.com, Inc.

8920 Business Park Dr., Ste. 200, Austin, TX 78759

Telephone: 512-726-5110 **Fax:** 512-726-5130 **Metro area:** Austin, TX **Web site:** http://www.drkoop.com **Sales:** $43,000 (Est.) **Number of employees:** 63 **Industry designation:** Computers—online services **Company type:** Private **Top competitors:** iVillage Inc.; OnHealth Network Company; WebMD, Inc.

Former US Surgeon General C. Everett Koop has written a prescription for good health in the new millennium: Surf the Net. Boasting more than 2.6 million visitors, the drkoop.com Web site offers eight interactive communities dispensing information on topics ranging from addiction to children's health. The Web site also features interactive health tools (polls, questionnaires, information searches) and more than 100 health-related chat support groups. drkoop.com generates revenue through advertising, content syndication, and e-commerce. Chairman Koop, VC John Zaccaro, and president and CEO Donald Hackett founded drkoop.com in 1997. Hackett owns 30% of the company.

Edge Petroleum Corporation

Texaco Heritage Plaza, 1111 Bagby, Ste. 2100, Houston, TX 77002

Telephone: 713-654-8960 **Fax:** 713-654-7722 **Metro area:** Houston, TX **Human resources contact:** Diane Sheppard **Sales:** $15.5 million **Number of employees:** 48 **Number of employees for previous year:** 43 **Industry designation:** Oil & gas—exploration & production **Company type:** Public **Top competitors:** Enron Corp.; Conoco Inc.; Texaco Inc.

Edge Petroleum hopes to gain an edge on its rivals in the oil and gas exploration, development, and production business by pairing sophisticated visualization software with computerized 3-D seismic data analysis to find petroleum prospects. The firm maintains a large database of 3-D seismic data for onshore coastal South Texas and has interests in more than 150 productive wells. It is active mainly in Texas, as well as in Louisiana and Mississippi. It has proved reserves of 29 billion cu. ft. of gas and almost a million barrels of oil. The company has also teamed with larger firms such as Texaco and Carrizo in onshore Gulf Coast exploration activities.

Electronic Transmission Corporation

5025 Arapahoe Rd., Ste. 501, Dallas, TX 75248

Telephone: 972-980-0900 **Fax:** 972-980-0929 **Metro area:** Dallas-Fort Worth, TX **Sales:** $3.2 million **Number of employees:** 66 **Industry designation:** Computers—corporate, professional & financial software **Company type:** Public **Top competitors:** Careflow Net, Inc.; Medical Manager Corporation; CITATION Computer Systems, Inc.

Electronic Transmission provides automated processes and systems, including electronic data interchange (EDI) services for non-providers in the health care industry. The company handles claims automation for managed care organizations and third-party administrators (TPAs), but most of its clients are self-insured businesses. It provides EDI to physician provider and physician hospital organizations, as well as independent physician associations. It also offers TPA services to self-insuring companies, handling everything from medical-claims scanning to provider payment. Wal-Mart is the company's largest client, generating more than half of its revenues. President and CEO Robert Fortier owns 42% of the company.

EmCare Holdings Inc.

1717 Main St., Ste. 5200, Dallas, TX 75201

Telephone: 214-712-2000 **Fax:** 214-712-2444 **Metro area:** Dallas-Fort Worth, TX **Web site:** http://www.emcare.com **Human resources contact:** Michael Lane **Sales:** $196.3 million **Number of employees:** 583 **Number of employees for previous year:** 380 **Industry designation:** Medical practice management **Company type:** Subsidiary **Top competitors:** Med-Emerg International Inc.; Coastal Physician Group, Inc.; FPA Medical Management, Inc.

EmCare provides emergency department management in some 400 hospitals and related urgent-care centers in 42 states. The subsidiary of Laidlaw (North America's top ambulance company) has nearly 5,000 physicians on its employee rolls. EmCare manages emergency services for hospitals—scheduling physicians and other staff members, monitoring performance, handling clinical and administrative tasks. The firm, which has become a major consolidator in its industry, has expanded the marketing of its services to include suburban and small-town hospitals, as well as the urban facilities it initially targeted.

Encore Medical Corporation

9800 Metric Blvd., Austin, TX 78758

Telephone: 512-832-9500 **Fax:** 512-834-6300 **Metro area:** Austin, TX **Web site:** http://www.encoremed.com **Human resources contact:** Kathy Wiederkehr **Sales:** $29 million **Number of employees:** 95 **Number of employees for previous year:** 82 **Industry designation:** Medical products **Company type:** Public

Encore Medical, through its subsidiary Encore Orthopedics, designs and sells more than 5,700 products used to treat and reconstruct joints and bones damaged by degenerative diseases, deformities, traumatic events, and sports injuries. The company's top-selling product, the Foundation Knee System, closely duplicates the function of the human knee and accounts for about 70% of total sales. Other products include reconstructive hip and shoulder implants and trauma devices used to repair bone fractures. Through internal development and acquisitions, the company plans to expand its trauma line and enter the spinal implant market. Encore Medical's products are sold in Canada, Japan, the US, and Europe.

Enron Oil & Gas Company

1400 Smith St., Houston, TX 77002

Telephone: 713-853-6161 **Fax:** 713-853-3129 **Other address:** PO Box 4362, Houston, TX 77210 **Metro area:** Houston, TX **Web site:** http://www.eog.enron.com **Human resources contact:** Patricia L. Edwards **Sales:** $769.2 million **Number of employees:** 1,190 **Number of employees for previous year:** 825 **Industry designation:** Oil & gas—exploration & production **Company type:** Public **Top competitors:** Union Texas Petroleum Holdings, Inc.; Apache Corporation; Shell Oil Company

Enron Oil & Gas is an independent oil and gas company engaged in exploring for, developing, producing, and marketing natural gas and crude oil. The company operates in major production basins in Canada, India, Trinidad, and the US. Subsidiary Enron Oil & Gas Marketing negotiates short- and long-term sales contracts with third-party producers, pipelines, and other marketing companies. Enron has net proved natural gas reserves of four trillion cu. ft. and net proved crude oil, condensate, and natural gas liquids reserves of 78 million barrels. Energy company Enron Corporation owns 55% of the company's outstanding common stock.

Environmental Safeguards, Inc.

2600 South Loop West, Ste. 645, Houston, TX 77054

Telephone: 713-641-3838 **Fax:** 713-641-0756 **Metro area:** Houston, TX **Human resources contact:** Dolores Casas **Sales:** $10.7 million **Number of employees:** 20 **Number of employees for previous year:** 18 **Industry designation:** Pollution control equipment & services **Company type:** Public

Environmental Safeguards, Inc. (ESI), provides remediation services for the removal of contaminants left in the soil at oil and gas drilling sites. The company, which conducts business through its National Fuel & Energy and OnSite Technologies subsidiaries, vaporizes hydrocarbon contaminants by passing the soil through a rotating drum in which temperatures range from 300 to 1200 degrees Fahrenheit. The company then condenses the hydrocarbon to a liquid state for reuse or disposal. The company-developed remediation systems are transported from site to site. ESI's primary customers are energy companies in the western US, but the company is expanding its customer base internationally, including in South America.

Equistar Chemicals, LP

One Houston Center, 1221 McKinney St., Ste. 1600, Houston, TX 77010

Telephone: 713-652-7300 **Fax:** 713-652-4151 **Other address:** PO Box 2583, Houston, TX 77252 **Metro area:** Houston, TX **Web site:** http://www.equistarchem.com **Human resources contact:** Myra Perkinson **Sales:** $365 million **Number of employees:** 4,000 **Industry designation:** Chemicals— plastics **Company type:** Partnership **Top competitors:** Formosa Plastics Corp., U.S.A.; The Geon Company; M. A. Hanna Company

Credit good chemistry, but Equistar Chemical—a partnership of Lyondell (41%), Millennium, and Occidental (29.5% each)—is one of the world's largest producers of olefins, polymers, ethylene and its derivatives. Equistar's olefin products are used to make food packaging, adhesives, anti-freeze, nylon clothing, and paint. The company also makes oxygenated products such as automobile starting fluid, gunpowder, hair spray, cosmetics, and polishes. Its polymer products include trash bags, grocery bags, milk crates, and disposable cups. Equistar's plants are mostly in the Gulf Coast area, and the company has a technology center in Cincinnati.

EXCO Resources, Inc.

5735 Pineland Dr., Ste. 235, Dallas, TX 75231

Telephone: 214-368-2084 **Fax:** 214-368-2087 **Metro area:** Dallas-Fort Worth, TX **Web site:** http://www.excoresources.com **Human resources contact:** J. Douglas Ramsey **Sales:** $1.4 million **Number of employees:** 19 **Number of employees for previous year:** 7 **Industry designation:** Oil & gas—exploration & production **Company type:** Public **Top competitors:** Pease Oil and Gas Company; Texoil, Inc.; Alliance Resources PLC

EXCO Resources has high expectations for Texas and Louisiana, where the onshore oil and gas exploration and production company has its primary operations. The company's proved reserves consist of nearly 60,000 barrels of oil and more than four million cu. ft. of natural gas. EXCO Resources oversees production from most of its properties, but its wells are drilled by independent contractors. Scurlock Permian, Delhi Gas Pipeline, and Aurora Natural Gas together account for more than half of the company's sales. Chairman and CEO Doug Miller owns a 41% stake in EXCO Resources.

EXE Technologies, Inc.

12740 Hillcrest Rd., Dallas, TX 75230

Telephone: 972-233-3761 **Fax:** 972-788-4208 **Metro area:** Dallas-Fort Worth, TX **Web site:** http://www.exe.com **Human resources contact:** Pat Pyle **Sales:** $26.8 million (Est.) **Number of employees:** 750 **Number of employees for previous year:** 615 **Industry designation:** Computers—corporate, professional & financial software **Company type:** Private **Top competitors:** SAP AG; Manhattan Associates, Inc.; Catalyst International, Inc.

EXE Technologies's inventory software tracks what, where, and how much. The company makes supply chain execution software primarily for retail and wholesale companies, manufacturing and consumer packaged goods firms, and third-party logistics providers. The company's EXceed software package, which is designed for use on mainframe, UNIX, and Windows NT platforms, includes a core warehouse management system and optional extensions such as labor and transportation management and performance monitoring. EXE markets its products through direct sales in Asia, Europe and North America. Customers include BAX Global CompUSA, Ford, and Logistics. Venture capital firm General Atlantic Partners owns about 32% of EXE.

The Exploration Company

500 N. Loop 1604 East, Ste. 250, San Antonio, TX 78232

Telephone: 210-496-5300 **Fax:** 210-496-3232 **Metro area:** San Antonio, TX **Human resources contact:** Mary Black **Sales:** $3 million **Number of employees:** 12 **Number of employees for previous year:** 11 **Industry designation:** Oil & gas—exploration & production **Company type:** Public **Top competitors:** Conoco Inc.; Texaco Inc.; Mobil Corporation

The Exploration Company isn't looking to go where no man has gone before—only where no other oil and gas drillers have gone. Through its direct efforts and joint ventures with Continental Resources, Union Pacific Resources, and Eagle Oil & Gas, the company explores for oil and natural gas and drills wells in the Dakotas, Montana, and South Texas. It has estimated proved reserves of more than 100,000 barrels of oil and 6 billion cu. ft. of natural gas. The Exploration Company, whose use of 3-D seismic surveys have helped increase its drilling success rate, sells its oil and gas under short-term contracts to the highest bidders.

FlashNet Communications, Inc.

1812 N. Forest Park Blvd., Fort Worth, TX 76102

Telephone: 817-332-8883 **Fax:** 817-332-3934 **Metro area:** Dallas-Fort Worth, TX **Web site:** http://www.flash.net **Sales:** $26.9 million **Number of employees:** 248 **Number of employees for previous year:** 225 **Industry designation:** Computers—online services **Company type:** Public **Top competitors:** America Online, Inc.; Internet America, Inc.; EarthLink Network, Inc.

FlashNet Communications exploded from being a small operation in Texas to providing Internet access to about 170,000 customers in more than 450 cities across the US. FlashNet's services include Web access, e-mail, newsgroup access, and Web pages. FlashNet offers its 2,900 small and medium-sized business clients high-speed dedicated and broadband access, Web hosting, and e-commerce opportunities. It plans to add long-distance access and advanced data services. The company uses radio, television, and direct advertising to promote its products and sells several service packages through a direct sales force and independent representatives.

Friona Industries, L.P.

900 Amarillo National Bank Bldg., Amarillo, TX 79105

Telephone: 806-374-1811 **Fax:** 806-374-1324 **Metro area:** Amarillo, TX **Web site:** http://www.frionaind.com **Sales:** $240 million (Est.) **Number of employees:** 400 **Industry designation:** Agricultural operations **Company type:** Private **Top competitors:** Cactus Feeders, Inc.; AZTX Cattle Co.

Friona Industries' business isn't chicken feed—it's cattle feed. Founded in 1962, Friona Industries owns five feedyards for about 189,000 head of cattle in the Texas Panhandle. The firm also owns a feed plant and distribution center that serves Texas, Oklahoma, Colorado, New Mexico, and Arizona, and its Hi-Pro Animal Health division distributes pharmaceuticals through 12 retail outlets and about 50 sales representatives. Friona Agricultural Credit helps ranchers finance and market feeding programs, and the company is partners with two other cattle firms and burger-maker McDonald's in BAP Management, which focuses on beef quality control. Private investment firm Edwin L. Cox Co. controls Friona Industries.

Gamma Biologicals, Inc.

3700 Mangum Rd., Houston, TX 77092

Telephone: 713-681-8481 **Fax:** 713-956-3333 **Other address:** PO Box 41027, Houston, TX 77240 **Metro area:** Houston, TX **Web site:** http://www.gammabio.com **Human resources contact:** Tina Sullivan **Sales:** $18.3 million **Number of employees:** 134 **Number of employees for previous year:** 126 **Industry designation:** Medical products **Company type:** Subsidiary **Top competitors:** TECHNE Corporation; Abaxis, Inc.; Hemagen Diagnostics, Inc.

Gamma Biologicals, a subsidiary of blood test kit maker Immucor, manufactures and sells reagents and systems for testing human blood. The company's reagents are sold to hospitals, blood banks, and medical laboratories for use in testing blood compatibility before transfusions, identifying antibodies and blood group antigens, and detecting hemolytic disease in newborns. The firm markets its products to more than 3,500 customers in the US and Canada and to dealers in about 50 other countries. Gamma sells its products directly in North America; independent distributors and a Dutch subsidiary market its wares internationally.

Genesis Energy, L.P.

500 Dallas, Ste. 2500, Houston, TX 77002

Telephone: 713-860-2500 **Fax:** 713-860-2640 **Metro area:** Houston, TX **Human resources contact:** Joe Mueller **Sales:** $2.2 billion **Number of employees:** 290 **Number of employees for previous year:** 240 **Industry designation:** Oil refining & marketing **Company type:** Public **Top competitors:** EOTT Energy Partners, L.P.; Koch Industries, Inc.

In the beginning, there was Basis and Howell ... and then there was Genesis. Genesis Energy is an independent crude-oil gatherer and marketer formed from the oil gathering and marketing operations of Basis Petroleum and the marketing and pipeline operations of Howell Corporation. Genesis Energy purchases and aggregates crude oil at the wellhead and makes bulk buys at pipeline and terminal facilities for resale. It transports crude oil via its tanker trucks and through its five pipeline systems: a 553-mi. system in Texas, and another 200-mi. one in the same state; 117-mi. system between Florida and Alabama; a 281-mi. system between Mississippi and Louisiana; and an offshore pipeline in the Gulf of Mexico.

Grand Adventures Tour & Travel Publishing Corporation

211 E. Seventh St., 11th Fl., Austin, TX 78701

Telephone: 512-391-2000 **Fax:** 512-391-2092 **Metro area:** Austin, TX **Web site:** http://perx.com **Sales:** $12.8 million **Number of employees:** 51 **Industry designation:** Leisure & recreational services **Company type:** Public

Grand Adventures Tour & Travel Publishing publishes "Interline Adventures," a color magazine that offers cruise and tour opportunities for interliners. Interliners are active employees or retirees of the airline industry who can fly for free or at a reduced rate. The company sells some subscriptions, but distributes the bulk of its magazines for free to airline representatives and past customers. It earns revenues by selling advertising space in the magazine to cruise and tour operators. In addition, its marketing division books hotel and resort accommodations and cruise tours in the US and abroad. The company operates in Austin, Texas, and Boca Raton, Florida.

Greenbriar Corporation

4265 Kellway Circle, Dallas, TX 75244

Telephone: 972-407-8400 **Fax:** 972-407-8420 **Metro area:** Dallas-Fort Worth, TX **Web site:** http://www.greenbriar.com **Human resources contact:** Jerry Ransdale **Sales:** $39 million **Number of employees:** 1,834 **Number of employees for previous year:** 1,384 **Industry designation:** Nursing homes **Company type:** Public

Greenbriar provides residential retirement and personal assistance services to the growing senior-citizen market. The company operates more than 50 assisted-living communities in 12 states. Its communities have a capacity of about 4,300 residents and provide basic, personal, and supplemental care, with services including dining, laundry, housekeeping, bathing, ambulation, and shopping. Greenbriar also offers special care services for Alzheimer's patients and those needing 24-hour assistance. The Gilley family owns 43% of Greenbriar. Floyd Rhoades received a 13% stake and Victor Lund received a 19% stake with the purchase of the American Care and Wedgwood subsidiaries, respectively.

H & H Meat Products Co., Inc.

Mile One E. Expwy. 83, Mercedes, TX 78570

Telephone: 956-565-6363 **Fax:** 956-565-0227 **Other address:** PO Box 358, Mercedes, TX 78570 **Metro area:** McAllen, TX **Web site:** http://www.rgv.net/hhfoods **Human resources contact:** Fred Gonzalez **Sales:** $39.7 million (Est.) **Number of employees:** 375 **Number of employees for previous year:** 350 **Industry designation:** Food—meat products **Company type:** Private **Top competitors:** Hormel Foods Corporation; Delimex; Authentic Specialty Foods, Inc.

H & H Meat Products, operating under the H & H Foods name, puts meat and potatoes on the table in the form of breakfast tacos. Formed in 1947, the company produces processed meats, specialty foods, and the La Rancherita brand of prepared Mexican foods. Products from the company's meat-processing plant include burgers, pork patties, and chorizo sausage. The La Rancherita line includes breakfast tacos, tamales, fajita strips, and entrees such as arroz con pollo. H&H also makes soups, side dishes, and condiments. It sells its products by the trailerload to retail stores, food-service distribution centers, and school districts throughout the US. The Hinojosa family owns the company.

Harken Energy Corporation

5605 N. MacArthur Blvd., Ste. 400, Irving, TX 75038

Telephone: 972-753-6900 **Fax:** 972-753-6944 **Metro area:** Dallas-Fort Worth, TX **Web site:** http://www.harkenenergy.com **Human resources contact:** Roger Ehrlish **Sales:** $19.8 million **Number of employees:** 132 **Number of employees for previous year:** 106 **Industry designation:** Oil & gas—exploration & production **Company type:** Public

Harken Energy explores for, develops, and produces natural gas and oil in the US and Colombia. The company's domestic operations consist of about 425 wells located on more than 60,000 developed and undeveloped acres in Arizona, Arkansas, New Mexico, Texas, and Utah. Harken's international operations consist of exploratory operations in Colombia. The company has six contracts with Colombia's state-owned oil company, Empresa Colombiana de Petroleos (Ecopetrol). Harken annually produces about 416,000 barrels of oil and 1.9 million cu. ft. of natural gas.

Helen of Troy Limited

6827 Market Ave., El Paso, TX 79915

Telephone: 915-779-6363 **Fax:** 915-774-4793 **Metro area:** El Paso, TX **Web site:** http://www.hotus.com **Human resources contact:** Monica Draper **Sales:** $248.1 million **Number of employees:** 318 **Number of employees for previous year:** 260 **Industry designation:** Cosmetics & toiletries **Company type:** Public **Top competitors:** Conair Corporation; Windmere-Durable Holdings, Inc.; Remington Products Company, L.L.C.

Need help battling your hair? You might call on the warrior Helen of Troy. The firm sells personal care products and accessories under the Vidal Sassoon and Revlon brand names (licensed from Procter & Gamble and Revlon, respectively) and under other brands, including WIGO, Karina, and its own Helen of Troy. Hair care items include hair dryers, curling irons, brushes, and mirrors; other products include women's shavers, artificial nails, and foot massagers (the latter under Dr. Scholl's). Helen of Troy products are made under contract by manufacturers in Asia and are marketed primarily to retailers—such as warehouse clubs and grocery stores—and salons in the US (its main market) and abroad.

Henley Healthcare, Inc.

120 Industrial Blvd., Sugar Land, TX 77478

Telephone: 281-276-7000 **Fax:** 281-276-7176 **Metro area:** Houston, TX **Web site:** http://www.henleyhealth.com **Human resources contact:** Angela Murphy **Sales:** $24.3 million **Number of employees:** 381 **Number of employees for previous year:** 173 **Industry designation:** Medical products **Company type:** Public **Top competitors:** Dynatronics Corporation; Empi, Inc.; Rehabilicare Inc.

Henley Healthcare produces noninvasive physical medicine and rehabilitation products used to control acute or chronic pain. Its Microlight division develops handheld, low-energy laser devices to treat repetitive stress injuries. Henley provides training, safety products, and technical support designed to meet federal Occupational Safety and Health Act (OSHA) compliance through its Health Career Learning Systems division. Maxxim Medical controls about 45% of the company's stock. The company has sold its Homecare division, which makes physical therapy and rehabilitation products, to home healthcare products maker Rehabilicare.

Holly Corporation

100 Crescent Ct., Ste. 1600, Dallas, TX 75201

Telephone: 214-871-3555 **Fax:** 214-871-3560 **Metro area:** Dallas-Fort Worth, TX **Web site:** http://www.hollycorp.com **Human resources contact:** Pam Reese **Sales:** $589.6 million **Number of employees:** 588 **Number of employees for previous year:** 572 **Industry designation:** Oil refining & marketing **Company type:** Public **Top competitors:** Exxon Corporation; Ultramar Diamond Shamrock Corporation; Texaco Inc.

Don't strike a match after decking the halls with boughs of this Holly. Holly is an independent refiner of petroleum, producing gasoline, diesel fuel, and jet fuel that is sold primarily in the southwestern US, northern Mexico, and Montana. Principal gasoline customers include other refiners, convenience store chains, independent marketers, an affiliate of Mexican energy company PEMEX, and other retailers. Its diesel fuel is sold to other refiners, wholesalers, independent dealers, and railroads. Jet fuel is sold primarily to the military. The company also conducts small-scale oil and gas exploration. Subsidiaries Navajo Refining and Montana Refining operate refineries in New Mexico and Montana, respectively.

Horizon Health Corporation

1500 Waters Ridge Dr., Lewisville, TX 75057

Telephone: 972-420-8200 **Fax:** 972-420-8252 **Metro area:** Dallas-Fort Worth, TX **Human resources contact:** Dan Perkins **Sales:** $123.8 million **Number of employees:** 1,485 **Number of employees for previous year:** 1,208 **Industry designation:** Medical practice management **Company type:** Public **Top competitors:** Integra, Inc.; Magellan Health Services, Inc.; Ramsay Youth Services, Inc.

Horizon Health (formerly Horizon Mental Health Management) manages about 150 mental health and physical rehabilitation programs offered by general hospitals in 37 states; Horizon Health handles licensing, accreditation, certificates of need approval, and Medicare certification. Its programs provide inpatient hospitalization, day treatment, outpatient treatment, and home health services (70% of its managed programs are in psychiatric care for the elderly). Horizon Health also has about 200 contracts to provide employee assistance programs and mental health services to businesses and managed-care organizations. The acquisitive company has offices in Boston, Chicago, Dallas, Los Angeles, and Tampa.

HORIZON Pharmacies, Inc.

531 W. Main St., Denison, TX 75020

Telephone: 903-465-2397 **Fax:** 903-465-8922 **Metro area:** Dallas-Fort Worth, TX **Web site:** http://www.horizonrx.com **Human resources contact:** Fae Landrum **Sales:** $28.4 million **Number of employees:** 394 **Number of employees for previous year:** 180 **Industry designation:** Retail—drugstores **Company type:** Public **Top competitors:** Walgreen Co.; Eckerd Corporation; Wal-Mart Stores, Inc.

HORIZON Pharmacies has acquisitions on its horizon. It owns and operates about 50 pharmacies in small communities in the Midwest, West, and Southwest. The stores' offerings include prescription and over-the-counter drugs, health supplies and equipment, beauty aids, greeting cards, snack foods, and film and photo-finishing services. Sales of prescription drugs account for about 75% of the company's sales. HORIZON also has 12 home medical equipment (HME) locations, five institutional pharmacies, five intravenous infusion operations, two home health care operations, and a wholesale operation. HORIZON plans to add 20 or so pharmacies and HME locations per year by acquiring independent stores and small chains.

Houston Astros Baseball Club

8400 Kirby Dr., Houston, TX 77054

Telephone: 713-799-9500 **Fax:** 713-799-9562 **Other address:** PO Box 288, Houston, TX 77001 **Metro area:** Houston, TX **Web site:** http://www.astros.com **Human resources contact:** Kevin Ward **Sales:** $68 million (Est.) **Number of employees:** 67 **Number of employees for previous year:** 65 **Industry designation:** Leisure & recreational services **Company type:** Private **Top competitors:** Chicago National League Ball Club, Inc.; St. Louis Cardinals, L.P.; The Cincinnati Reds

Originally known as the Colt .45s, the Houston Astros joined the National League (with the New York Mets) in the expansion of 1962. The team became the Astros when it moved into the Astrodome—billed as the Eighth Wonder of the World—in 1965. Despite having such baseball luminaries as pitcher Nolan Ryan, attendance has declined in recent decades. Owner Drayton McLane, whose family made its fortune in grocery distribution, is hoping that consecutive division titles (1997 and 1998) as well as hot-shot players (such as third baseman Ken Caminiti) will revitalize the franchise. The team lost their 1998 division series to the San Diego Padres. The Astros plan to move into a new downtown stadium in 2000.

The Houston Exploration Company

1100 Louisiana, Ste. 2000, Houston, TX 77002

Telephone: 713-830-6800 **Fax:** 713-652-4017 **Metro area:** Houston, TX **Web site:** http://www.houstonexploration.com **Human resources contact:** Christine Teichelman **Sales:** $128.2 million **Number of employees:** 111 **Number of employees for previous year:** 104 **Industry designation:** Oil & gas—exploration & production **Company type:** Public **Top competitors:** British-Borneo Oil & Gas PLC; Shell Oil Company; Texaco Inc.

Houston is a long way from Brooklyn, but it's the place to be if you're looking for oil. Houston Exploration, 64%-owned by Brooklyn Union Gas through subsidiary THEC Holdings, explores for, buys, and develops US natural gas and oil properties. It focuses on offshore properties in the shallow waters of the Gulf of Mexico, but it seeks to mitigate the risk of the high-potential Gulf operations through holdings in lower-risk, more stable onshore properties in Arkansas, East Texas, Oklahoma, southern Louisiana, and West Virginia. Houston Exploration's proved reserves total one billion barrels of oil and about 400 billion cu. ft. of natural gas. Brooklyn Union Gas is a subsidiary of KeySpan Energy.

Houston Rockets

Two Greenway Plaza, Ste. 400, Houston, TX 77046

Telephone: 713-627-3865 **Fax:** 713-963-7315 **Metro area:** Houston, TX **Web site:** http://www.nba.com/rockets **Human resources contact:** Emily Guitierrez **Sales:** $72.1 million (Est.) **Number of employees:** 90 **Industry designation:** Leisure & recreational services **Company type:** Private **Top competitors:** San Antonio Spurs, Ltd.; Minnesota Timberwolves; Utah Jazz

An NBA team, the Houston Rockets took to the court for the first time in 1967 as the San Diego Rockets and fizzled. Despite the playing ability of Elvin Hayes, the Rockets couldn't get it going on the West Coast and moved to Houston after only four years. It wasn't until 1976, when the Rockets picked up center Moses Malone (who bypassed college to play pro ball), that the team became a force in the NBA. Under the leadership of head coach and former Rocket Rudy Tomjanovich, the team won repeat championships in 1994 and 1995. Houston boasts such NBA greats as center Hakeem "The Dream" Olajuwon and fowards Charles Barkley and Scottie Pippen. Former Wall Street securities trader Leslie Alexander owns the team.

Howell Corporation

1111 Fannin St., Ste. 1500, Houston, TX 77002

Telephone: 713-658-4000 **Fax:** 713-658-4007 **Metro area:** Houston, TX **Web site:** http://www.howellcorp.com **Sales:** $51.4 million **Number of employees:** 126 **Number of employees for previous year:** 60 **Industry designation:** Oil & gas—exploration & production **Company type:** Public **Top competitors:** Chesapeake Energy Corporation; Frontier Oil Corporation

Howell looks high (in Wyoming) and low (along the Gulf Coast, both onshore and offshore) for oil and gas. The company has proved reserves of 42 million barrels of oil and 84 billion cu. ft. of natural gas. It conducts its exploration and production operations through subsidiary Howell Petroleum. The company sells its production on the spot market. Howell owns minority interests in the Genesis companies, which purchased Howell's gathering, marketing, and pipeline operations. Howell has completed its exit from the technical fuels and chemical processing business and has sold mineral properties in Alabama, Louisiana, and Mississippi to pay down debt.

Iatros Health Network, Inc.

11910 Greenville Ave., Ste. 300, Dallas, TX 75243

Telephone: 972-889-0843 **Fax:** 972-889-0853 **Metro area:** Dallas-Fort Worth, TX **Sales:** $25.5 million **Number of employees:** 659 **Number of employees for previous year:** 155 **Industry designation:** Medical practice management **Company type:** Public **Top competitors:** MHM Services, Inc.; Lexington Healthcare Group, Inc.; Nyer Medical Group, Inc.

Iatros Health Network provides management and ancillary care programs to long-term health care facilities it owns or operates, primarily in New England and Pennsylvania. The company provides financial and administrative management directly to its own operations; Ancillary services, including pharmacy services, medical equipment supply, infusion and respiratory therapy, and consultation, are provided by Iatros subsidiaries to other long-term-care facilities in its market areas. NewCare Health, which owns and operates nursing homes in the southern US, owns a fifth of Iatros. Plagued by numerous lawsuits, Iatros is seeking ways to maximize profitability to offset legal costs and potential liabilities.

ILEX Oncology, Inc.

11550 IH 10 West, Ste. 300, San Antonio, TX 78230

Telephone: 210-949-8200 **Fax:** 210-949-8210 **Metro area:** San Antonio, TX **Web site:** http://www.ilexoncology.com/index1.html **Human resources contact:** John Barnes **Sales:** $14.3 million **Number of employees:** 185 **Number of employees for previous year:** 130 **Industry designation:** Drugs **Company type:** Public

ILEX Oncology develops pharmaceuticals for the treatment and prevention of cancer. It also provides contract research services to the pharmaceutical and biotechnology industries. Cancer drugs developed by ILEX include Campath-1H for the treatment of chronic lymphocytic leukemia. Campath-1H is in clinical trials, but the company hopes it might be available to the public by 2000. The company also is working on an enzyme inhibitor, DFMO, to treat brain tumors and breast cancer. The company has development and marketing collaborations with LeukoSite for Campath-1H-related products and with Pharma Forschung Kaugbeuen. It also has an alliance with Symphar to develop the latter's cancer-killing compound.

Imperial Sugar Company

One Imperial Sq., Sugar Land, TX 77487

Telephone: 281-491-9181 **Fax:** 281-491-9895 **Other address:** PO Box 9, Sugar Land, TX 77478 **Metro area:** Houston, TX **Web site:** http://www.imperialholly.com **Human resources contact:** R. Martin Thompson **Sales:** $1.8 billion **Number of employees:** 3,800 **Number of employees for previous year:** 1,700 **Industry designation:** Food—sugar & refining **Company type:** Public **Top competitors:** SYSCO Corporation; American Crystal Sugar Company; Tate & Lyle PLC

Imperial Sugar (formerly Imperial Holly Corp.) occupies the sweetest spot in its field—its Imperial, Holly, Spreckels, Pioneer, Wholesome, and Dixie Crystals brands make the firm the largest refined sugar supplier in the US. Imperial makes sugar in 15 refineries in eight states and sells to grocery, food service, and industrial customers. Through subsidiaries Savannah Foods and Diamond Crystal Specialty Foods, Imperial's non-sugar business (about 25% of sales) supplies restaurants and schools with drink mixes, desserts, plastic forks, and related items. It bought Wholesome Foods (organic sweeteners) in 1998. The Kempner family owns about 38% of Imperial and Irish sugar maker Greencore owns 16%.

Incarnate Word Health System

9311 San Pedro Ave., Ste. 1250, San Antonio, TX 78216

Telephone: 210-524-4100 **Fax:** 210-525-8443 **Metro area:** San Antonio, TX **Web site:** http://www.incarnatewordhealth.org **Sales:** $663.6 million **Number of employees:** 7,500 **Number of employees for previous year:** 5,800 **Industry designation:** Hospitals **Company type:** Not-for-profit

Incarnate Word Health System operates primarily in South Texas and includes nine acute-care hospitals, a children's hospital, a rehabilitation hospital, and a psychiatric hospital. The organization also owns 50% of Baptist St. Anthony's Health System in Amarillo, Texas, and has a hospital in St. Louis. Incarnate Word Health System is planning to merge with Sisters of Charity Health Care System, based in Houston, to form Christus Health. In addition to its hospitals, the organization operates a network of clinics, educational centers, hospice services, and physician partnerships.

Integrated Orthopaedics, Inc.

5858 Westheimer, Ste. 500, Houston, TX 77057

Telephone: 713-225-5464 **Fax:** 713-361-2000 **Metro area:** Houston, TX **Web site:** http://www.ioinet.com **Human resources contact:** Jeffrey Stevens **Sales:** $12.2 million **Number of employees:** 129 **Number of employees for previous year:** 119 **Industry designation:** Medical practice management **Company type:** Public

Integrated Orthopaedics (formerly DRCA Medical) manages outpatient medical, diagnostic and rehabilitation centers in four states. The company-run centers provide occupational health care services to prevent and treat on-the-job injuries and illnesses using case management to provide lower-cost treatment than traditional health care providers do. Integrated Orthopaedics operates physical/occupational therapy centers, occupational and urgent care medicine clinics, mobile testing units, work-hardening clinics, and MRI centers. The company is pursuing more business relationships with physician practices to stabilize profits. An investment group led by Texas billionaire Robert Bass owns a 35% stake.

International Isotopes Inc.

3100 Jim Christal Rd., Denton, TX 76207

Telephone: 940-484-9492 **Fax:** 940-484-0877 **Metro area:** Dallas-Fort Worth, TX **Web site:** http://www.intiso.com **Human resources contact:** Lori Faries **Sales:** $2 million **Number of employees:** 100 **Number of employees for previous year:** 41 **Industry designation:** Drugs **Company type:** Public **Top competitors:** Mallinckrodt Inc.; Elscint Limited; ADAC Laboratories

International Isotopes intends to be the first domestic producer of radioactive isotopes for sale to the nuclear medicine industry. To make these isotopes, the company bought the remains of the US Superconducting Super Collider project (terminated 1994), including the proton linear accelerator (LINAC), which will produce radioisotopes that can be used alone or in combinations to diagnose a variety of diseases, including cancer. The company also is developing a nuclear medical imaging camera (based on research by company founder Ira Lon Morgan) with capabilities greater than the industry standard. The company's only revenues to date have been generated from the resale of nonessential Super Collider components.

Interphase Corporation

13800 Senlac, Dallas, TX 75234

Telephone: 214-654-5000 **Fax:** 214-654-5500 **Metro area:** Dallas-Fort Worth, TX **Web site:** http://www.iphase.com **Human resources contact:** Deborah Shute **Sales:** $68.8 million **Number of employees:** 229 **Number of employees for previous year:** 222 **Industry designation:** Computers—peripheral equipment **Company type:** Public

Interphase makes high-performance network (more than 75% of sales) and mass-storage products—network adapters, concentrators, operating system software drivers. Interphase's network adapters consist of printed circuit boards that accept fiber-optic and copper wire network cabling, as well as software that works with various client/server systems. The company's mass-storage devices give stand-alone desktop and notebook computers high-speed access to peripheral devices (disk drives, printers). Products are used in graphic workstations, medical imaging, financial services networks, and online transaction processing. Interphase sells to end users, computer system makers, distributors, and systems integrators.

Introgen Therapeutics, Inc.

301 Congress Ave., Ste. 1850, Austin, TX 78701

Telephone: 512-708-9310 **Fax:** 512-708-9311 **Metro area:** Austin, TX **Web site:** http://www.introgen.com **Human resources contact:** Tia Stovall-Artisst **Sales:** $8.6 million (Est.) **Number of employees:** 62 **Number of employees for previous year:** 57 **Industry designation:** Biomedical & genetic products **Company type:** Private **Top competitors:** Targeted Genetics Corporation; Vical Incorporated; Megabios Corp.

Introgen Therapeutics develops gene-therapy products that treat cancer by introducing therapeutic gene products directly into the body. These gene-therapy products in clinical testing treat cancer by attempting to restore or correct missing or aberrant gene functions. Subsidiary Gendux operates in the UK. Introgen develops both gene replacement products and gene blocking products, which are designed to neutralize the activity of mutant genes. Introgen funds research at the University of Texas M.D. Anderson Cancer Center in Houston and holds a license to commercialize its technologies. It has collaboration agreements with Rhone-Poulenc Rorer to help develop and market gene-therapy products for cancer treatment.

i2 Technologies, Inc.

909 E. Las Colinas Blvd., 16th Fl., Irving, TX 75039

Telephone: 214-860-6000 **Fax:** 214-860-6060 **Metro area:** Dallas-Fort Worth, TX **Web site:** http://www.i2.com **Human resources contact:** Jeanne Durbin **Sales:** $361.9 million **Number of employees:** 2,244 **Number of employees for previous year:** 1,006 **Industry designation:** Computers—corporate, professional & financial software **Company type:** Public **Top competitors:** Manugistics Group, Inc.; Oracle Corporation; SAP AG

i2 Technologies' RHYTHM supply chain management software helps manufacturers plan and schedule production and related operations such as raw materials procurement and product delivery. Companies that use RHYTHM include 3M, Dell, Ford, Johnson & Johnson, Motorola, and USX-U.S. Steel. i2 supports RHYTHM with maintenance, training, and other services. RHYTHM products are available in English, French, German, Japanese, and Spanish, and the company has offices in Asia, Australia, Europe, and the Americas. A third of i2's sales are outside the US. Chairman and CEO Sanjiv Sidhu, who founded the company, owns about 51% of i2.

Kinetic Concepts, Inc.

8023 Vantage Dr., San Antonio, TX 78230

Telephone: 210-524-9000 **Fax:** 210-255-6998 **Metro area:** San Antonio, TX **Web site:** http://www.KCI1.com **Human resources contact:** Larry P. Baker **Sales:** $306.9 million (Est.) **Number of employees:** 2,100 **Number of employees for previous year:** 2,066 **Industry designation:** Medical products **Company type:** Private **Top competitors:** Invacare Corporation; Hillenbrand Industries, Inc.; Sunrise Medical Inc.

Kinetic Concepts makes specialized therapeutic surfaces and provides rental medical equipment for the worldwide health care community. The company's products treat and prevent complications associated with patient immobility, such as pressure sores and the harmful buildup of fluid in the lungs. Kinetic Concepts' overseas market (which includes Australia and Europe) accounts for a quarter of all sales. Equity fund Fremont Partners owns about 37% of the company; founder and former CEO James Leininger, about 31%; and investment concern Richard C. Blum & Associates, roughly 24%.

KMG Chemicals, Inc.

10611 Harwin Dr., Ste. 402, Houston, TX 77036

Telephone: 713-988-9252 **Fax:** 713-988-9298 **Metro area:** Houston, TX **Web site:** http://www.kmgb.com **Sales:** $22.7 million **Number of employees:** 76 **Number of employees for previous year:** 74 **Industry designation:** Chemicals—specialty **Company type:** Public **Top competitors:** Koppers Industries, Inc.; Grupo Mexico S.A.

KMG Chemicals (formerly KMG-B) makes and distributes wood preservatives used to treat railroad ties, utility and telephone poles, and fresh-cut lumber. Its main products include penta, sodium penta, and creosote. Penta is sold in the US, while sodium penta, which is not registered for domestic sale, is sold in Europe, Latin America, and Malaysia. Creosote is supplied by AlliedSignal and German manufacturer VfT. KMG's Alabama plant blends and distributes penta. Hydrochloric acid, a by-product of penta manufacturing, is sold to the oil and steel industries. Texas Electric Cooperatives and Cahaba Wood Preserving each account for about 10% of KMG's sales. Chairman and president David Hatcher owns more than 70% of KMG.

LifeCell Corporation

3606 Research Forest Dr., The Woodlands, TX 77381

Telephone: 281-367-5368 **Fax:** 281-363-3360 **Metro area:** Houston, TX **Web site:** http://www.lifecell.com **Human resources contact:** Judy Colyn **Sales:** $8 million **Number of employees:** 111 **Number of employees for previous year:** 101 **Industry designation:** Biomedical & genetic products **Company type:** Public **Top competitors:** Advanced Tissue Sciences, Inc.; Genzyme Corporation; Organogenesis Inc.

LifeCell Corporation puts new life into the tissue-graft market: The company's sole commercial product is AlloDerm, a skin-graft material processed from cadaver skin. The substance is marketed in the US and abroad for reconstructive plastic, dental, and burn surgery. The company is developing other biomedical products, including an injectable form of AlloDerm, vascular grafts, heart replacement valves, and conduits for bypass surgeries. Its ThromboSol is a storage solution designed to extend the shelf life of blood used in transfusions. LifeCell conducts research under government contract and in collaboration with Medtronic, the leading maker of implantable medical devices.

Lincoln Heritage Corporation

1250 Capital of Texas Hwy., Bldg. 3, Ste. 100, Austin, TX 78746

Telephone: 512-328-0075 **Fax:** 512-328-9290 **Metro area:** Austin, TX **Human resources contact:** Jolene Marsh **Sales:** $46.9 million **Number of employees:** 69 **Industry designation:** Insurance—life **Company type:** Public

Holding company Lincoln Heritage buys, issues, and manages life insurance and annuities through its two subsidiaries, Memorial Service Life Insurance and Lincoln Memorial Life Insurance. Most of the company's premiums are derived from the issuance of insurance policies to fund prearranged funeral contracts sold primarily in Texas and Missouri by National Prearranged Services. Acquisitions are a key component of Lincoln Heritage's growth strategy, and the company is buying Harbourton Reassurance and World Service. The acquisition of World Service will expand the number of states in which Lincoln Heritage is licensed to operate from 29 to 43, plus Washington, DC.

Lucky Lady Oil Company

107 NW 28th St., Fort Worth, TX 76106

Telephone: 817-740-7400 **Fax:** 817-740-0245 **Metro area:** Dallas-Fort Worth, TX **Human resources contact:** Leann Davenport **Sales:** $110 million (Est.) **Number of employees:** 138 **Number of employees for previous year:** 135 **Industry designation:** Oil refining & marketing **Company type:** Private **Top competitors:** Ultramar Diamond Shamrock Corporation; Caltex Petroleum Corporation; CITGO Petroleum Corporation

In Las Vegas or the oil business, luck be a lady, and Lucky Lady Oil is a jobber, reselling name-brand gasoline and lubricants in volume to large businesses. The company buys and stores petroleum products and transports them to its customers. It is among the largest Fina distributors in the US. Lucky Lady Oil also owns 19 gas station-convenience store properties in the Dallas-Fort Worth area, operating four and leasing 15. The company was founded in 1976 by Sue Palmer, then a single mother. CEO Palmer, who is now married, owns the company. She was elected to her second term in the Texas House of Representatives in 1998.

Magnum Hunter Resources, Inc.

600 E. Las Colinas Blvd., Ste. 1200, Irving, TX 75039

Telephone: 972-401-0752 **Fax:** 972-443-6487 **Metro area:** Dallas-Fort Worth, TX **Web site:** http://www.magnumhunter.com **Human resources contact:** Frances Evans **Sales:** $49.9 million **Number of employees:** 67 **Number of employees for previous year:** 37 **Industry designation:** Oil & gas—exploration & production **Company type:** Public **Top competitors:** Devon Energy Corporation; Sonat Inc.; Chesapeake Energy Corporation

For Magnum Hunter Resources, it's always open season on oil and gas. The exploration and production company, which operates primarily in Texas, Oklahoma, and New Mexico, has estimated proved reserves of 208 billion cu. ft. of gas and 21 million barrels of oil. In addition, Magnum Hunter owns more than 500 miles of gas gathering systems in Oklahoma, Texas, and Louisiana and a 50% interest in the McLean Gas Plant, a gas processing facility in the Texas Panhandle. Natural gas distribution giant ONEOK acquired a 31% stake in Magnum Hunter for $50 million in 1999.

Malibu Entertainment Worldwide, Inc.

717 N. Harwood Ave., Ste. 1650, Dallas, TX 75201

Telephone: 214-210-8701 **Fax:** 214-210-8702 **Metro area:** Dallas-Fort Worth, TX **Human resources contact:** Linda Gould **Sales:** $44.6 million **Number of employees:** 1,800 **Number of employees for previous year:** 1,400 **Industry designation:** Leisure & recreational services **Company type:** Public **Top competitors:** AMF Bowling, Inc.; CEC Entertainment, Inc.; Regal Cinemas, Inc.

Malibu Entertainment Worldwide, formerly Mountasia Entertainment, develops, owns, and operates 29 family-oriented entertainment centers under the names Malibu Grand Prix, Mountasia Family Fun Centers, and SpeedZone. Each center offers a combination of attractions, which includes miniature golf, go-cart racing, video arcades, bumper boats, batting cages, and concession stands. The company is focusing on expanding its teen-oriented SpeedZone centers, which offer scaled Grand Prix-style racetracks. The company operates in 10 states, primarily California, Florida, Georgia, and Texas. In 1998 Malibu agreed to merge with Houlihan's Restaurant Group.

Mannatech, Incorporated

600 S. Royal Ln., Ste. 200, Coppell, TX 75019

Telephone: 972-471-7400 **Fax:** 972-471-8135 **Metro area:** Dallas-Fort Worth, TX **Human resources contact:** Gwen Pennington **Sales:** $150.9 million **Number of employees:** 300 **Industry designation:** Vitamins & nutritional products **Company type:** Public **Top competitors:** General Nutrition Companies, Inc.; Weider Nutrition International, Inc.; Twinlab Corporation

Mannatech develops and sells nutritional supplements and topical products in the US and Canada through its network of more than 200,000 salespeople. The company's products are designed for dermal care, sports performance, and the support of the immune, endocrine, and intestinal systems. The products, which are made by third-party manufacturers, include Ambrotose, Em-Pact, Emprizone, Man-Aloe, MannaCleanse, Phyt-Aloe, and Phyto-Bears. Mannatech also sells MannaBAR, a nutritional supplement bar. President Samuel Caster, chairman and CEO Charles Fioretti, and William Fioretti each own nearly 25% of Mannatech.

Massimo Enterprises, Inc.

8643 Grenadier Dr., Dallas, TX 75238

Telephone: 214-340-3506 **Fax:** 214-340-1134 **Metro area:** Dallas-Fort Worth, TX **Number of employees:** 3 **Industry designation:** Cosmetics & toiletries **Company type:** Private **Top competitors:** Carson, Inc.; Revlon, Inc.; Soft Sheen Products Inc.

In today's bustling world, it's difficult to find time to relax. Massimo Enterprises wants to help (with hair, that is). The company has developed and produced, but not yet sold, an applicator for hair relaxer (also known as hair straightener) designed to shorten the time needed for the process from more than 30 minutes to as little as five. Massimo also will offer hair relaxer, hair spray, conditioner, and shampoo, all to be marketed mainly to African-Americans under the Smooth & Easy brand. The company plans to sell its products directly to consumers through TV and print ads. After Massimo's planned IPO, chairman and CEO Jason Romano and VP Joseph Romano will each own about 13% of the company.

Memorial Hermann Healthcare System

7737 Southwest Fwy., Ste. 200, Houston, TX 77074

Telephone: 713-776-5484 **Fax:** 713-776-5665 **Metro area:** Houston, TX **Web site:** http://www.mhcs.org **Human resources contact:** R. Eugene Ross **Sales:** $1.2 billion **Number of employees:** 12,000 **Number of employees for previous year:** 7,500 **Industry designation:** Hospitals **Company type:** Not-for-profit **Top competitors:** Methodist Health Care System; Columbia/HCA Healthcare Corporation; Tenet Healthcare Corporation

Memorial Hermann Healthcare System is a "munster" of an organization. The largest not-for-profit health care system in the Houston area, it consists of 12 hospitals, including a children's hospital, two long-term nursing facilities, and a retirement community. Its subsidiaries include a home health care company, a managed-care company, and a physician practice company. The company's Hermann Hospital is the teaching hospital for The University of Texas-Houston Medical School. Memorial Regional Healthcare Services provides support for health care needs at 16 affiliated hospitals. Memorial Hermann Healthcare was formed in 1997 from the $1 billion merger of Hermann Hospital and Memorial Healthcare System.

The Meridian Resource Corporation

15995 N. Barkers Landing, Ste. 300, Houston, TX 77079

Telephone: 281-558-8080 **Fax:** 281-558-5595 **Metro area:** Houston, TX **Web site:** http://www.tmrc.com **Sales:** $73.3 million **Number of employees:** 98 **Number of employees for previous year:** 68 **Industry designation:** Oil & gas—exploration & production **Company type:** Public **Top competitors:** Forest Oil Corporation; Remington Oil & Gas Corporation; Louis Dreyfus Natural Gas Corp.

The Meridian Resource Corporation (TMRC) finds and develops oil and natural gas properties using 3-D seismic and computer-aided exploration technologies. TMRC concentrates its exploration efforts in the Texas and Louisiana Gulf Coast region in areas known to have potential natural gas reserves of at least 50 billion cu. ft. and in multiple productive zones that can provide 10 million cu. ft. or more of natural gas daily. TMRC acquired Cairn Energy USA and expanded its search area to the offshore waters in the Gulf of Mexico, and it will acquire all of Shell Oil's southern Louisiana exploration properties in exchange for a 40% stake in TMRC.

Methodist Health Care System

6565 Fannin St., Houston, TX 77030

Telephone: 713-790-3311 **Fax:** 713-790-4885 **Metro area:** Houston, TX **Web site:** http://www.methodisthealth.com **Human resources contact:** Donald Benson **Sales:** $721.9 million **Number of employees:** 8,779 **Number of employees for previous year:** 4,991 **Industry designation:** Hospitals **Company type:** Not-for-profit **Top competitors:** The Johns Hopkins Health System Corporation; Mayo Foundation; Daughters of Charity National Health System

Founded in 1919, the Methodist Health Care System owns and operates Methodist Hospital, San Jacinto Methodist Hospital, Diagnostic Center Hospital, and Methodist Health Center-Sugar Land. The not-for-profit flagship Methodist Hospital is known for innovations in cardiology and neurosurgery, among other specialties, as well as for being Baylor College of Medicine's teaching facility. The system's four hospitals have a total of almost 1,900 beds and 1,600 physicians on staff and serve more than 300,000 patients each year. The firm owns and operates MethodistCare, a managed care organization; Visiting Nurse Association of Houston, a home health and hospice services agency; and two physician organizations.

Microelectronics and Computer Technology Corporation

3500 W. Balcones Center Dr., Austin, TX 78759

Telephone: 512-343-0978 **Fax:** 512-338-3898 **Metro area:** Austin, TX **Web site:** http://www.mcc.com **Human resources contact:** Alicia Bogart **Number of employees:** 120 **Number of employees for previous year:** 110 **Industry designation:** Computers—services **Company type:** Consortium **Top competitors:** SEMATECH, Inc.; Science Applications International Corporation; Battelle Memorial Institute

Microelectronics and Computer Technology Corporation (MCC) is a research consortium that focuses on specific technology-related projects as well as speculative R&D. Its areas of expertise include advanced electronics, software and information technology, and the environmental impact of computer and electronics manufacturing. The consortium consists of more than 30 corporations and government agencies (shareholders, associate members, and project participants). In addition to US organizations, MCC members include shareholder Northern Telecom (Canada), associate Nokia (Finland), and project participants Rafael (Israel) and Telefonica (Spain).

Middle Bay Oil Company, Inc.

1221 Lamar St., Ste. 1020, Houston, TX 77010

Telephone: 713-759-6808 **Fax:** 713-650-0352 **Metro area:** Houston, TX **Human resources contact:** Kelly Green **Sales:** $11.2 million **Number of employees:** 17 **Number of employees for previous year:** 8 **Industry designation:** Oil & gas—exploration & production **Company type:** Public **Top competitors:** Chesapeake Energy Corporation; Abraxas Petroleum Corporation; KCS Energy, Inc.

Middle Bay Oil Company has chosen the middle way of expansion through acquisition. The independent oil and gas exploration and production company has operations in the US Gulf Coast and midcontinent regions, primarily in Alabama, Kansas, New Mexico, Oklahoma and Texas. Middle Bay made six purchases in 1997 and 1998—most notably, Enex Resources—that increased its proved reserves by 10.8 million barrels of oil equivalent to 12.3 million barrels of oil equivalent. The company's proved reserves consist of more than four million barrels of oil and 49.2 billion cu. ft. of natural gas. Independent producer Kaiser-Francis Oil owns 38% of Middle Bay.

Monarch Dental Corporation

4201 Spring Valley Rd., Ste. 320, Dallas, TX 75244

Telephone: 972-702-7446 **Fax:** 972-702-0824 **Metro area:** Dallas-Fort Worth, TX **Human resources contact:** Tony Meadows **Sales:** $129.6 million **Number of employees:** 1,157 **Number of employees for previous year:** 641 **Industry designation:** Medical practice management **Company type:** Public **Top competitors:** Castle Dental Centers, Inc.; Orthodontic Centers of America, Inc.

Open wide and say, "Monarch." Monarch Dental manages almost 200 dental practice offices in 21 markets. The practices offer general dentistry and such specialty services as orthodontics, oral surgery, endodontics, periodontics, and pediatric dentistry. Monarch has regional call centers in each of its markets to schedule patient visits, answer patient questions, and remind patients of appointments. The company also maintains patient information, practitioner schedules, insurance information, clinical records, and billing information at the individual offices. Venture capital firm TA Associates Group owns 26% of the company; Chairman Warren Melamed, a dentist who founded Monarch, owns another 20%

MultiMedia Access Corporation

2665 Villa Creek Dr., Ste. 200, Dallas, TX 75234

Telephone: 972-488-7200 **Fax:** 972-488-7299 **Metro area:** Dallas-Fort Worth, TX **Web site:** http://www.mmac.com **Sales:** $8 million **Number of employees:** 65 **Number of employees for previous year:** 55 **Industry designation:** Computers—peripheral equipment **Company type:** Public **Top competitors:** Datapoint Corporation; Intel Corporation; Corel Corporation

The multimedia is the message at MultiMedia Access. The firm develops PC-based desktop video teleconferencing products. Its VBX video distribution and switching system, Osprey video and peripherals line (video peripheral products account for 66% of sales), and ViewCast servers for Web video broadcasting let businesses videoconference from remote locations, do video-based training and distance learning, set up surveillance, perform telemedicine, and offer Internet/intranet video services, among other functions. MultiMedia Access sells its products through resellers, system integrators, manufacturers, and customized application developers.

National Energy Group, Inc.

4925 Greenville Ave., Dallas, TX 75206

Telephone: 214-692-9211 **Fax:** 214-692-9310 **Metro area:** Dallas-Fort Worth, TX **Human resources contact:** Gary Knee **Sales:** $54.6 million **Number of employees:** 74 **Number of employees for previous year:** 58 **Industry designation:** Oil & gas—exploration & production **Company type:** Public

National Energy Group explores for, develops, and produces oil and natural gas. The company, which has grown through more than $170 million worth of acquisitions since 1991, is now focusing its development operations on properties in Texas, Louisiana, Mississippi, and the Gulf of Mexico. It also has extensive properties in Oklahoma and lesser holdings in Arkansas. National Energy has proved reserves of about 169 billion cu. ft. of natural gas equivalent—nearly 25 times the total it had at the end of 1991. Investor Carl Icahn owns about 19% of National Energy.

National Western Life Insurance Company

850 E. Anderson Ln., Austin, TX 78752

Telephone: 512-836-1010 **Fax:** 512-835-2729 **Metro area:** Austin, TX **Web site:** http://www.nwlic.com **Human resources contact:** Carol Jackson **Sales:** $312.3 million **Number of employees:** 237 **Number of employees for previous year:** 230 **Industry designation:** Insurance—life **Company type:** Public

National Western Life Insurance sells individual whole, universal, and term life insurance; endowments; and flexible-premium and single-premium annuities. The company also holds health and accident insurance policies, but it no longer writes new ones. It markets to customers in 43 states and the District of Columbia, as well as in Central and South America, the Caribbean, and the Pacific Rim, mostly through more than 7,900 independent broker/agents. Subsidiary Westcap, a Houston brokerage firm, filed for bankruptcy and has discontinued operations in the wake of numerous lawsuits holding Westcap and parent National Western Life responsible for misrepresentation and other violations in securities sales.

NEON Systems, Inc.

14100 Southwest Fwy., Ste. 500, Sugar Land, TX 77478

Telephone: 281-491-4200 **Fax:** 281-242-3880 **Metro area:** Houston, TX **Web site:** http://www.neonsys.com **Human resources contact:** Cathy Zapalac **Sales:** $12 million **Number of employees:** 71 **Industry designation:** Computers—corporate, professional & financial software **Company type:** Public **Top competitors:** BEA Systems, Inc.; Information Builders Inc.; IONA Technologies PLC

NEON Systems is lighting up the middleware market. The company develops software that lets outdated computer applications connect and communicate with new systems. Its Shadow Web Server offers Web access directly to established mainframe computers without additional programming. Other products let networked computer users access mainframes. Customers include American Express, Exxon, and the U.S. Postal Service. NEON sells its products directly and through independent distributors. The UK accounts for a quarter of the company's sales. JMI Equity Fund and Peter Schaeffer (founder and chief technology officer) own 38% and 24% of the company, respectively.

NetSolve, Incorporated

12331 Riata Trace Pkwy., Austin, TX 78727

Telephone: 512-340-3000 **Fax:** 512-340-3008 **Metro area:** Austin, TX **Web site:** http://www.netsolve.net **Human resources contact:** Michelle Friesenhahn **Sales:** $14.5 million (Est.) **Number of employees:** 116 **Number of employees for previous year:** 110 **Industry designation:** Computers—services **Company type:** Private **Top competitors:** LanOptics Ltd.; Secure Computing Corporation; CyberGuard Corporation

Network bloodhound NetSolve sniffs out intruders. The company provides midsized businesses with a variety of remote network and security management services, including LAN and WAN design and implementation, upgrades, troubleshooting, configuration, and firewall management. NetSolve also sells third-party connectivity hardware and its own software tools for accessing network status reports through standard Web browsers. The company sells its services and products both directly and through telecommunications carriers (including AT&T, which accounts for about 50% of sales), Internet service providers, and other resellers. Venture capitalist and NetSolve director Richard Kramlich owns 33% of the company.

Newfield Exploration Company

363 N. Sam Houston Pkwy. East, Ste. 2020, Houston, TX 77060

Telephone: 281-847-6000 **Fax:** 281-847-6006 **Metro area:** Houston, TX **Web site:** http://www.newfld.com **Human resources contact:** Ronald P. Lege **Sales:** $195.7 million **Number of employees:** 96 **Number of employees for previous year:** 86 **Industry designation:** Oil & gas—exploration & production **Company type:** Public

Independent oil and gas company Newfield Exploration concentrates its activities in the Gulf of Mexico, including the shallow waters off the Louisiana coast. The company owns interests in more than 120 leases and 430 wells and operates about 90 platforms; it added nine natural gas fields to its Gulf Coast operations. Newfield Exploration uses 3-D seismic and other advanced technologies to conduct geophysical and geological analysis for finding new reserves. The company operates most of its properties. It owns a 35% stake in a property off the coast of China and is considering investments in West Africa and Latin America.

Nuevo Energy Company

1331 Lamar, Ste. 1650, Houston, TX 77010

Telephone: 713-652-0706 **Fax:** 713-756-1744 **Metro area:** Houston, TX **Web site:** http://www.nuevoenergy.com **Human resources contact:** Joan Gallagher **Sales:** $252.7 million **Number of employees:** 919 **Number of employees for previous year:** 780 **Industry designation:** Oil & gas—exploration & production **Company type:** Public **Top competitors:** Benton Oil and Gas Company; Chesapeake Energy Corporation; Texaco Inc.

Nuevo Energy engages in oil and natural gas exploration and production. The company accumulates oil and gas assets through the drilling of exploration and developmental wells on acreage it owns. Nuevo Energy has gas pipeline and storage assets, but it plans to sell these in order to focus on exploration and production. The company's drilling and exploration activities take place primarily in Alabama, California, Louisiana, Texas, and the Gulf of Mexico, but it also conducts exploration activities in West Africa. The company has net proved reserves of 292 billion barrels of oil equivalent.

Nutrition For Life International, Inc.

9101 Jameel, Houston, TX 77040

Telephone: 713-460-1976 **Fax:** 713-460-4084 **Metro area:** Houston, TX **Web site:** http://nutritionforlife.com **Human resources contact:** Tammy Mitcham **Sales:** $69.7 million **Number of employees:** 269 **Number of employees for previous year:** 210 **Industry designation:** Vitamins & nutritional products **Company type:** Public **Top competitors:** Nature's Sunshine Products, Inc.; Herbalife International, Inc.; Amway Corporation

Nutrition For Life International sells more than 350 products, including nutritional supplements, weight management foods, cleaning concentrates, and motivational tapes (including Mega Memory), through a multilevel system of more than 75,000 distributors in Canada, Guam, Ireland, The Netherlands, the Philippines, Puerto Rico, the UK, and the US. The company markets its custom-made products under private labels such as Grand Master, Lean Life, and Nutri-Mac. Nutrition For Life has terminated distributor and top recruiter Kevin Trudeau, who had been previously convicted of larceny and fraud, after several years of lawsuits involving Trudeau's recruitment tactics.

O.I. Corporation

151 Graham Rd., College Station, TX 77842

Telephone: 409-690-1711 **Fax:** 409-690-0440 **Other address:** PO Box 9010, College Station, TX 77842 **Metro area:** College Station, TX **Human resources contact:** Sharon Cheatham **Sales:** $23.7 million **Number of employees:** 165 **Number of employees for previous year:** 158 **Industry designation:** Instruments—scientific **Company type:** Public **Top competitors:** The Perkin-Elmer Corporation; Dionex Corporation; Thermo Instrument Systems Inc.

Like a band of faithful awaiting the apocalypse, O.I. Corporation is hunkered down in the compound. The firm makes instruments used to prepare, detect, measure, analyze, and monitor chemical compounds. Products include instruments that separate organic compounds based on their physical and chemical properties, analyzers for measuring carbon and pH levels in water, emissions equipment for testing air quality, and sample preparation equipment. The firm is a value-added reseller of Hewlett-Packard analysis equipment. Federal, state, and municipal governments account for 35% of sales. O.I. continues to expand through acquisitions that complement its product lines.

Owen Healthcare, Inc.

9800 Centre Pkwy., Ste. 1100, Houston, TX 77036

Telephone: 713-777-8173 **Fax:** 713-777-5417 **Metro area:** Houston, TX **Web site:** http://www.owenhealth.com **Human resources contact:** Cathy Cooney **Sales:** $449.3 million **Number of employees:** 4,000 **Number of employees for previous year:** 3,500 **Industry designation:** Medical practice management **Company type:** Subsidiary **Parent company:** Cardinal Health, Inc. **Top competitors:** Omnicare, Inc.; McKesson HBOC, Inc.; Syncor International Corporation

Owen Healthcare, a subsidiary of drug distributor Cardinal Health, is the US's top provider of fully integrated pharmacy management and information services for hospitals, with more than 600 hospital pharmacies under management or otherwise using its services. Owen typically manages all aspects of its clients' pharmacy operations, including staffing, purchasing, inventory control, billing, administration, and information technology. After buying Owen in 1997, Cardinal Health combined its operations with those of its Allied Health hospital pharmacy management subsidiary, adding its 60 contracts to Owen's portfolio.

Paracelsus Healthcare Corporation

515 W. Greens Rd., Ste. 800, Houston, TX 77067

Telephone: 281-774-5100 **Fax:** 281-774-5200 **Metro area:** Houston, TX **Human resources contact:** Randy Stone **Sales:** $659.2 million **Number of employees:** 10,400 **Number of employees for previous year:** 10,100 **Industry designation:** Hospitals **Company type:** Public **Top competitors:** HEALTHSOUTH Corporation

Learned physician Philippus Aureolus Paracelsus would be amazed at today's health care industry. His namesake company, Paracelsus Healthcare, and its subsidiaries own and operate 26 acute-care hospitals in nine states that provide a full range of inpatient services, as well as rehabilitation and home health care. The company also operates four nursing homes in California and provides physician practice management services. Paracelsus generally operates in small to midsized markets with limited competition from major hospital consolidators. As part of this strategy, the company is in the process of selling its operations in the Los Angeles area, as well as its noncore psychiatric care operations.

Parallel Petroleum Corporation

One Marienfeld Place, 110 N. Marienfeld St., Ste. 465, Midland, TX 79701

Telephone: 915-684-3727 **Fax:** 915-684-3905 **Metro area:** Odessa, TX **Human resources contact:** Becky Burrell **Sales:** $12.6 million **Number of employees:** 7 **Number of employees for previous year:** 6 **Industry designation:** Oil & gas—exploration & production **Company type:** Public

Parallel Petroleum explores for, develops, and produces natural gas and oil, primarily on the Gulf Coast of South Texas, including Dewitt, Jackson, Lavaca, Victoria, and Wharton counties. The company also has operations in the Permian Basin of West Texas. Parallel Petroleum owns or has interests in about 70 oil and 110 natural gas wells, with nearly three-quarters of proved reserves being natural gas. As opposed to selling its products on the spot market, Parallel Petroleum sells directly to companies with which it has term contracts, including Cox & Perkins Exploration (over 50% of sales) and Enron (12%).

Pennzoil-Quaker State Company

Pennzoil Place, 700 Milam, Houston, TX 77002

Telephone: 713-546-4000 **Fax:** 713-546-6589 **Metro area:** Houston, TX **Web site:** http://www.pennzoil.com **Sales:** $1.8 billion **Number of employees:** 13,200 **Number of employees for previous year:** 8,970 **Industry designation:** Oil refining & marketing **Company type:** Public **Top competitors:** Burmah Castrol plc; Ashland Inc.; Texaco Inc.

Every three months or 3,000 miles, Pennzoil-Quaker State wants to land your business. Formed by the 1998 merger of Pennzoil and Quaker State, the company makes the US's #1 brand of motor oil (Pennzoil) and venerable brand Quaker State; it controls about 35% of the US motor oil market. It owns the US's largest chain of oil-change centers—Jiffy Lube, which has about 1,500 outlets (more than half are franchised), as well as almost 600 Q Lube centers. It also owns an arsenal of brand-name auto products, including Gumout, Snap, Outlaw fuel additives; Fix-A-Flat tire inflator; and Slick 50 engine and fuel treatments. The new company is 61.5%-owned by Pennzoil shareholders and 38.5%-owned by Quaker State shareholders.

Perot Systems Corporation

12377 Merit Dr., Ste. 1100, Dallas, TX 75251

Telephone: 972-383-5600 **Fax:** 972-455-4100 **Metro area:** Dallas-Fort Worth, TX **Web site:** http://www.perotsystems.com **Human resources contact:** Paul Turevon **Sales:** $781.6 million **Number of employees:** 6,000 **Number of employees for previous year:** 5,500 **Industry designation:** Computers—services **Company type:** Public **Top competitors:** International Business Machines Corporation; Andersen Consulting; Electronic Data Systems Corporation

He didn't win public office, but former presidential candidate Ross Perot runs a public company after years of campaigning. His namesake company, Perot Systems, provides technology consulting and services, including systems management and systems integration. Its customers include Swiss bank UBS (27% of sales), UK utility East Midlands Electricity (10%), Tenet Healthcare, and National Car Rental. Leaving its private status behind (more than 90% of the company's employees are shareholders) has been the biggest in a number of changes for Perot Systems, including the return of Ross as boss. Perot owns about 32% of the firm.

Pervasive Software Inc.

12365 Riata Trace Pkwy., Bldg. II, Austin, TX 78727

Telephone: 512-231-6000 **Fax:** 512-231-6010 **Metro area:** Austin, TX **Web site:** http://www.pervasive.com **Human resources contact:** Yolanda Owens **Sales:** $36.7 million **Number of employees:** 220 **Number of employees for previous year:** 168 **Industry designation:** Computers—corporate, professional & financial software **Company type:** Public **Top competitors:** Sybase, Inc.; Oracle Corporation; Informix Corporation

When Pervasive Software talks about embedded programs, they don't mean that picture-in-a-picture feature you have on your television. The firm makes small databases that software developers embed into more complex software. The products, designed to require little maintenance (the company calls it "zero administration"), are especially tailored for midsized companies that have minimal technical support. About 70% of Pervasive's sales come from licensing fees. Its customers include McKesson HBOC, Great Plains Software, MGM Grand, Dillard's, and Time Warner. Founders Nancy (chairman) and Douglas Woodward own 32% of the company; Austin Ventures, 17%, and CEO Ron Harris, 10%.

PetroCorp Incorporated

16800 Greenspoint Dr., Ste. 300, North Atrium, Houston, TX 77060

Telephone: 281-875-2500 **Fax:** 281-875-5080 **Metro area:** Houston, TX **Web site:** http://www.petrocorp.com **Sales:** $25.2 million **Number of employees:** 57 **Number of employees for previous year:** 55 **Industry designation:** Oil & gas—exploration & production **Company type:** Public **Top competitors:** Pioneer Natural Resources Company; Barnwell Industries, Inc.; Abraxas Petroleum Corporation

Plummeting petroleum prices are prodding PetroCorp to ponder its prospects. The oil and gas exploration and production company, which operates primarily in Kansas, Louisiana, Mississippi, Oklahoma, Texas, and Alberta, Canada, has hired bankers to evaluate its options, including sale or reorganization of the company. PetroCorp concentrates on acquiring and developing proven, long-lived North American onshore gas reserves with a potential for further development. The company operates 40 wells in a dozen fields. PetroCorp's proved reserves consist of five million barrels of oil and 87 million cu. ft. of natural gas. Kaiser-Francis Oil owns 50% of PetroCorp.

Physician Reliance Network, Inc.

2 Lincoln Center, 5420 LBJ Fwy., Ste. 900, Dallas, TX 75240

Telephone: 972-392-8700 **Fax:** 972-387-0128 **Metro area:** Dallas-Fort Worth, TX **Web site:** http://www.prninc.com **Human resources contact:** Jerry McMorrough **Sales:** $398 million **Number of employees:** 2,700 **Number of employees for previous year:** 1,192 **Industry designation:** Medical practice management **Company type:** Public **Top competitors:** EquiMed, Inc.; Response Oncology, Inc.

Physician Reliance Network, which is merging with American Oncology Resources, is an oncology practice management firm that provides financial, clinical, and management services to outpatient cancer centers and physicians. It offers facilities, management, administration, and technical support to 27 outpatient cancer centers and more than 340 physicians in about 125 practices in 13 states. Physician Reliance provides financing to develop and equip cancer centers and doctors' offices; offers billing and accounts-receivable services; buys medical supplies, equipment, and pharmaceuticals; helps administer health care sites; and runs some 20 pharmacies in physicians' offices and cancer centers.

Physicians Resource Group, Inc.

3 Lincoln Centre, 5430 LBJ Fwy., Ste. 1540, Dallas, TX 75240

Telephone: 972-982-8200 **Fax:** 972-982-8296 **Metro area:** Dallas-Fort Worth, TX **Web site:** http://www.physiciansresource.com **Human resources contact:** Lisa Goodoien **Sales:** $403.5 million **Number of employees:** 4,900 **Number of employees for previous year:** 4,200 **Industry designation:** Medical practice management **Company type:** Public **Top competitors:** Vision Twenty-One, Inc.; Sight Resource Corporation; Omega Health Systems, Inc.

With about 600 ophthalmologists and optometrists on staff, troubled Physicians Resource Group (PRG) should have been able to keep an eye on the bottom line. Founded in 1995, it was the largest management company of eye-care practices by 1997. It was also in debt and mired in litigation with many of its 140 practices. In response, PRG is terminating some of its contracts, reselling assets, returning daily operations to its remaining practices, and limiting its services to negotiations with suppliers and care providers, lease and contract administration, and assembling outcomes data. In addition to practice management, the company owns or operates 48 surgery centers and about 170 optical dispensaries.

Physicians Trust, Inc.

1300 Post Oak Blvd., Ste. 1800, Houston, TX 77056

Telephone: 713-622-1818 **Fax:** 713-622-2227 **Metro area:** Houston, TX **Human resources contact:** Suzanne E. Speak **Number of employees:** 125 **Industry designation:** Medical practice management **Company type:** Private

Physicians Trust is a physician practice management company formed to consolidate the business operations of 14 neuromusculoskeletal physician practices in Arizona, California, the District of Columbia, Georgia, Louisiana, Pennsylvania, and Texas. Concurrent with its planned IPO, the company will acquire a sleep disorder treatment operation and a 70% stake in an outpatient surgery center. As a practice management organization, Physicians Trust acquires the nonmedical assets of medical practices and receives a management fee. The company's administrative and management support services include billing, payroll, personnel, and inventory supply services.

Plains Cotton Cooperative Association

3301 E. 50th St., Lubbock, TX 79404

Telephone: 806-763-8011 **Fax:** 806-762-7333 **Metro area:** Lubbock, TX **Web site:** http://www.pcca.com **Human resources contact:** Lee Phenix **Sales:** $1 billion **Number of employees:** 1,350 **Number of employees for previous year:** 800 **Industry designation:** Agricultural operations **Company type:** Cooperative **Top competitors:** Cargill, Incorporated; Dunavant Enterprises Inc.; Calcot, Ltd.

Plainly speaking, the Plains Cotton Cooperative Association (PCCA) is one of the nation's largest cotton handlers. The farmer-owned marketing cooperative has more than 25,000 members in Oklahoma and Texas. PCCA markets about three million bales of cotton each year through TELCOT, its computerized trading system, which continually updates cotton prices, buyer data, and other information. The co-op has cotton warehouses in Texas and Oklahoma and a denim mill in Texas whose primary customer is Levi Strauss. Through its Mission Valley Textiles unit, PCCA makes yarn-dyed woven fabric. The co-op was formed in 1953 to enable cotton farmers to obtain the most competitive price for their cotton.

Plains Resources Inc.

500 Dallas St., Ste. 700, Houston, TX 77002

Telephone: 713-654-1414 **Fax:** 713-654-1523 **Metro area:** Houston, TX **Web site:** http://internet.plainsresources.com **Human resources contact:** Mary O. Peters **Sales:** $1.3 billion **Number of employees:** 230 **Number of employees for previous year:** 201 **Industry designation:** Oil & gas—exploration & production **Company type:** Public **Top competitors:** Bellwether Exploration Company; Chesapeake Energy Corporation; Helmerich & Payne, Inc.

Plainly resourceful, Plains Resources is an independent energy company that acquires, develops, and produces crude oil and natural gas, mainly from underdeveloped, mature fields. The company is also engaged in the downstream activities of marketing, transporting, and storage of crude oil. Plains Resources' oil- and gas-producing activities are concentrated in California, Florida, and Illinois. Subsidiary Plains All American Pipeline owns a 1,233-mile-long crude oil pipeline that runs between California and Texas. Plains Resources has proved oil and natural gas reserves of 162 million barrels of oil equivalent (BOE).

Pogo Producing Company

5 Greenway Plaza, Ste. 2700, Houston, TX 77252

Telephone: 713-297-5000 **Fax:** 713-297-5100 **Other address:** PO Box 2504, Houston, TX 77252 **Metro area:** Houston, TX **Human resources contact:** Kenneth R. Good **Sales:** $202.8 million **Number of employees:** 185 **Number of employees for previous year:** 160 **Industry designation:** Oil & gas—exploration & production **Company type:** Public

It's not what you think. Pogo Producing develops, produces, and explores for crude oil and natural gas in Louisiana, New Mexico, Texas, Thailand, and the Gulf of Mexico. It has more than 460 oil wells and 230 natural gas wells as well as interests in more than 100 federal and state lease blocks in the Gulf of Mexico. Diamond Shamrock accounts for about 60% of the company's sales. Pogo Producing also has interests in eight hydrocarbon production pipelines. The company's purchase of Arch Petroleum expanded its holdings with properties in West Texas, the Permian Basin, and Canada and gave the company total proved reserves of 860.7 billion cu. ft. of natural gas equivalent.

Prime Medical Services, Inc.

1301 Capital of Texas Hwy. South, Ste. C300, Austin, TX 78746

Telephone: 512-328-2892 **Fax:** 512-328-8510 **Metro area:** Austin, TX **Web site:** http://www.primemedical.com **Human resources contact:** Cindy Green **Sales:** $104.6 million **Number of employees:** 350 **Number of employees for previous year:** 270 **Industry designation:** Medical services **Company type:** Public **Top competitors:** Integrated Health Services, Inc.; Mission Pharmacal; Medstone International, Inc.

Kidney stones rock for Prime Medical Services, the top US provider of lithotripsy services. Lithotripsy is an outpatient procedure that uses shock waves to fragment kidney stones, which are then passed from the body. Prime Medical owns and operates more than 60 lithotripters (most are installed in mobile facilities that travel from hospital to hospital), which serve some 450 hospitals and surgery centers in more than 30 states. Prime Medical also operates Prostatron machines (which use heat to shrink enlarged prostate glands) and makes mobile lithotripsy and MRI equipment trailers.

ProMedCo Management Company

801 Cherry St., Ste. 1450, Fort Worth, TX 76102

Telephone: 817-335-5035 **Fax:** 817-335-8321 **Metro area:** Dallas-Fort Worth, TX **Web site:** http://www.promedco.com **Human resources contact:** Charles W. McQueary **Sales:** $222.5 million **Number of employees:** 3,400 **Number of employees for previous year:** 2,000 **Industry designation:** Medical practice management **Company type:** Public

A medical practice management company, ProMedCo Management buys and consolidates physician groups. With about 1,000 providers in 10 states, ProMedCo concentrates on buying practices in areas that have populations between 30,000 and 500,000. The company usually buys the physician groups' non-real-estate assets with cash, common stock, and other securities. About 60% of ProMedCo's doctors are primary care physicians. ProMedCo focuses on primary care physicians because the company believes this group will have increasing control over health care expenditures.

PSW Technologies, Inc.

6300 Bridgepoint Pkwy., Bldg. 3, Ste. 200, Austin, TX 78730

Telephone: 512-343-6666 **Fax:** 512-343-9650 **Metro area:** Austin, TX **Web site:** http://www.psw.com **Human resources contact:** Julie M. Kirk **Sales:** $39.1 million **Number of employees:** 461 **Number of employees for previous year:** 375 **Industry designation:** Computers—services **Company type:** Public **Top competitors:** Unisys Corporation; Electronic Data Systems Corporation; American Management Systems, Incorporated

PSW Technologies has no problem serving two masters. For software developers, PSW provides software research and development services such as development, porting (adapting software to run on a new operating system), testing, and certification. For end users, primarily "FORTUNE" 1000 companies, PSW develops enterprisewide software systems. It also offers system integration services such as custom application development, system management, and technology migration (for example, migrating Unix-based systems to Windows NT-based systems). IBM accounts for nearly 40% of the company's sales. Other clients include AT&T, Compaq, and US Bank. PSW provides its services throughout the US.

Queen Sand Resources, Inc.

3500 Oak Lawn, Ste. 380, Dallas, TX 75219

Telephone: 214-521-9959 **Fax:** 214-521-9960 **Metro area:** Dallas-Fort Worth, TX **Web site:** http://www.qsri.com **Human resources contact:** Robert P. Lindsay **Sales:** $11 million **Number of employees:** 22 **Number of employees for previous year:** 21 **Industry designation:** Oil & gas—exploration & production **Company type:** Public **Top competitors:** Mitchell Energy & Development Corp.; Apache Corporation; Burlington Resources Inc.

Exploration and production company Queen Sand Resources has extended its domain to include more than 1,000 oil and gas wells. It has proved reserves of 224 billion cu. ft. of natural gas equivalent. Queen Sand Resources operates in 114 producing fields, predominantly in Kentucky, Louisiana, Mississippi, New Mexico, Oklahoma, and Texas, and it sells its products on the spot market and under short-term contracts. Subsidiaries include Queen Sand Resources, Northland Operating, and Corrida Resources. An affiliate of petroleum giant Enron owns 33% of Queen Sand Resources.

Range Resources Corp.

500 Throckmorton St., Fort Worth, TX 76102

Telephone: 817-870-2601 **Fax:** 817-870-2316 **Metro area:** Dallas-Fort Worth, TX **Human resources contact:** Sally Hayes **Sales:** $146.6 million **Number of employees:** 390 **Number of employees for previous year:** 367 **Industry designation:** Oil & gas—exploration & production **Company type:** Public **Top competitors:** Vintage Petroleum, Inc.; Burlington Resources Inc.; Apache Corporation

Range Resources, formerly Lomak Petroleum, is an independent oil and gas company that explores for oil and gas and acquires and develops oil and gas properties in the US. The company concentrates on long-life established properties and has major development areas in the Appalachian (40% of reserves), Permian (West Texas), midcontinent (western Oklahoma, Texas Panhandle), and Gulf Coast regions. Natural gas accounts for about 76% of Range Resources proved reserves: 960 billion cu. ft. of natural gas and 30 million barrels of oil. The company operates 98% of its own wells and has grown rapidly through acquisitions, which almost doubled its reserves in 1997.

Remington Oil & Gas Corporation

8201 Preston Rd., Ste. 600, Dallas, TX 75225

Telephone: 214-890-8000 **Fax:** 214-890-8025 **Metro area:** Dallas-Fort Worth, TX **Human resources contact:** Cathy Hartwell **Sales:** $57.3 million **Number of employees:** 20 **Number of employees for previous year:** 15 **Industry designation:** Oil & gas—exploration & production **Company type:** Public

Remington Oil & Gas (formerly Box Energy) is an independent energy company that explores for, develops, and produces oil and natural gas. The company owns interests in oil and gas leases in the Gulf of Mexico and on the Gulf Coast. The firm also has inland holdings in Alabama, Mississippi, New Mexico, and Texas. Three customers account for nearly all of Remington Oil & Gas' sales. The company has proved reserves of 4.5 million barrels of oil and 36.5 billion cu. ft. of natural gas. Through S-Sixteen Holding, Idaho spudillionaire J.R. Simplot owns 57% of the firm.

Rick's Cabaret International, Inc.

3113 Bering Dr., Houston, TX 77057

Telephone: 713-785-0444 **Fax:** 713-785-2593 **Metro area:** Houston, TX **Human resources contact:** Erich N. White **Sales:** $7.8 million **Number of employees:** 350 **Number of employees for previous year:** 160 **Industry designation:** Leisure & recreational services **Company type:** Public **Top competitors:** The Men's Club of Houston; Fantasy Nightclub; Caligula XXI

Rick's Cabaret International ain't "Casablanca," but it could be a Demi Moore movie. Rick's operates four topless bars (two in Houston, and one each in New Orleans and Minneapolis). The company caters to highbrow, visually-oriented partiers with dough to blow, and features VIP rooms for customers who pay a $250-$550 membership. The company's former employees include Playboy bunnies and models such as Anna Nicole Smith, who met her future husband, billionaire J. Howard Marshall, while working at the club. Rick's also owns Tantra, a Houston dance and pool hall. Through its 93% interest in Taurus Entertainment, Rick's operates the XTC Cabaret in Austin, Texas. CEO Robert Watters owns 27% of Rick's.

St. Luke's Episcopal Hospital

6720 Bertner Ave., Texas Medical Center, Houston, TX 77030

Telephone: 713-791-1000 **Fax:** 713-794-6182 **Metro area:** Houston, TX **Web site:** http://www.sleh.com **Human resources contact:** Irene Helsinger **Sales:** $640.2 million **Number of employees:** 4,700 **Number of employees for previous year:** 3,980 **Industry designation:** Hospitals **Company type:** Not-for-profit **Top competitors:** Harris County Hospital District; Sisters of Charity Health Care System; Memorial Hermann Healthcare System

St. Luke's Episcopal Hospital has been deep in the hearts of Texans. Opened in 1954 by the Episcopal Diocese of Texas, St. Luke's has some 950 beds and admits more than 27,000 patients annually. Its health care services also include home health care, outpatient surgery, and physical therapy. The Texas Heart Institute, under Dr. Denton Cooley, performed the first successful heart transplant in the US and the world's first total artificial heart transplant. A proposed alliance with Columbia/HCA Healthcare was derailed because St. Luke's land deed does not permit for-profit operations on its grounds.

Santa Fe Energy Resources, Inc.

1616 S. Voss, Ste. 1000, Houston, TX 77057

Telephone: 713-507-5000 **Fax:** 713-507-5341 **Metro area:** Houston, TX **Human resources contact:** Charles C. Hain **Sales:** $291 million **Number of employees:** 1,286 **Number of employees for previous year:** 1,209 **Industry designation:** Oil & gas—exploration & production **Company type:** Public **Top competitors:** Shell Oil Company; TOTAL SA; Exxon Corporation

Do you know the way, Santa Fe? Santa Fe Energy Resources explores for oil and natural gas fields that it develops into producing wells. Its land-based domestic operations are in the Texas Permian Basin and southeastern New Mexico; it also is involved in offshore projects in the Gulf of Mexico. Internationally, the firm's production and development interests are concentrated in Argentina, Gabon, and Indonesia. Santa Fe Energy has proved reserves of more than 170 million barrels of oil equivalent and approximately 253 billion cu. ft. of natural gas. The company has agreed to acquire Snyder Oil.

Sensus Drug Development Corporation

98 San Jacinto Blvd., Ste. 430, Austin, TX 78701

Telephone: 512-487-2000 **Fax:** 512-487-2045 **Metro area:** Austin, TX **Web site:** http://www.sensuscorp.com **Human resources contact:** Lisa White **Number of employees:** 19 **Number of employees for previous year:** 15 **Industry designation:** Drugs **Company type:** Private **Top competitors:** Genentech, Inc.; Novartis AG; Neurocrine Biosciences, Inc.

To Sensus Drug Development bigger isn't better. Sensus develops drugs to treat endocrine gland disorders, particularly acromegaly (gigantism), which causes abnormal growth as well as the enlargement of and abnormalities in the liver, spleen, heart, and other organs. Acromegalics also are prone to cancer, diabetes, and heart disease. Sensus's most advanced drug candidate, Trovert, which the company has licensed from Ohio University and biotech firm Genentech, inhibits the growth hormone causing acromegaly. The drug is in the final stages of clinical testing. Sensus also believes Trovert will be effective in treating blindness and kidney disease caused by diabetes. Contractors make test quantities of the drug.

Seven Seas Petroleum Inc.

1990 Post Oak Blvd., 3 Post Oak Central, Ste. 960, Houston, TX 77056

Telephone: 713-622-8218 **Fax:** 713-621-9770 **Metro area:** Houston, TX **Sales:** $800,000 **Number of employees:** 67 **Number of employees for previous year:** 33 **Industry designation:** Oil & gas—exploration & production **Company type:** Public

Seven Seas Petroleum explores and develops oil and gas properties, primarily in Colombia. The company owns interests in seven prospective oil-producing areas, including sites in Australia and Papua New Guinea. Seven Seas' main property is its 57% interest in the Dindal and Rio Seco association contracts in the Upper Magdalena Basin near Bogota, Colombia. The contracts for these zones were made with Colombia's national oil company, Ecopetrol. International financier George Soros owns about 8% of the company. All of Seven Seas' properties are in the initial stages of exploration and development.

Sheridan Energy, Inc.

1000 Louisiana, Ste. 800, Houston, TX 77002

Telephone: 713-651-7899 **Fax:** 713-651-3056 **Metro area:** Houston, TX **Human resources contact:** Sheryl Rowell **Sales:** $19.8 million **Number of employees:** 20 **Number of employees for previous year:** 14 **Industry designation:** Oil & gas—exploration & production **Company type:** Public

Sheridan Energy owns and operates oil- and natural-gas-producing properties in the Texas Panhandle, central Oklahoma, and Arkansas, and along the Gulf Coast of Texas and Louisiana. The company, which owns interests in about 600 wells, has proved reserves of 65 billion cu. ft. of natural gas and 2.2 million barrels of oil. Sheridan, a spinoff of TGX, has grown through acquisitions from Pioneer Natural Resources (interests in more than 430 wells) and Enron affiliate Grand Gulf Production (interests in 24 wells). Enron owns approximately 36% of Sheridan.

Silverleaf Resorts, Inc.

1221 Riverbend Dr., Ste. 120, Dallas, TX 75247

Telephone: 214-631-1166 **Fax:** 214-638-7256 **Metro area:** Dallas-Fort Worth, TX **Web site:** http://www.silverleafresorts.com **Sales:** $138.4 million **Number of employees:** 2,347 **Number of employees for previous year:** 1,602 **Industry designation:** Leisure & recreational services **Company type:** Public **Top competitors:** Fairfield Communities, Inc.; Vacation Break U.S.A., Inc.; Sunterra Corp.

Silverleaf Resorts owns and operates 23 time-share home resorts in 11 states, mostly in the East and South. The company's focus is on its "drive-to resorts," which are located near major metro areas (such as Chicago, Houston, New York City, and St. Louis) and encourage short-stay vacationers. In addition, the company owns "destination resorts" that are more luxurious and expensive. Each resort offers a variety of amenities including fishing, boating, tennis, golf, and horseback riding. Silverleaf's 61,000 time-share owners pay an average of about $8,000 for annual one-week stays. CEO Robert Mead owns 52% of the company.

Sisters of Charity Health Care System

2600 North Loop West, Houston, TX 77092

Telephone: 713-681-8877 **Fax:** 713-680-4896 **Metro area:** Houston, TX **Web site:** http://www.sch.org **Human resources contact:** Mary Lynch **Sales:** $2.1 billion **Number of employees:** 16,000 **Number of employees for previous year:** 15,000 **Industry designation:** Hospitals **Company type:** Not-for-profit **Top competitors:** Memorial Hermann Healthcare System; Columbia/HCA Healthcare Corporation; Harris County Hospital District

Sisters of Charity Health Care System is a Catholic, not-for-profit firm that operates 15 acute care hospitals, four long-term care centers, and seven long-term acute care facilities in Arkansas, Louisiana, Texas, Utah, and Ireland. The system also offers HealthPrompt, a free healthcare advice and referral telephone service, and Home Health Care, which provides therapy and healthcare for homebound patients. The Sisters of Charity runs an HMO through its partnership with the Memorial Hermann Healthcare System of Houston. The Sisters first organized in France in 1625 and opened their first US facility in 1867. Sisters of Charity is merging with San Antonio's Incarnate Word Health System, forming Christus Health.

SMART Technologies, Inc.

11701 Stonehollow Dr., Ste. 500, Austin, TX 78758

Telephone: 512-719-9100 **Fax:** 512-719-9167 **Metro area:** Austin, TX **Web site:** http://www.smartdna.com **Human resources contact:** Barbara Taylor **Sales:** $8.1 million (Est.) **Number of employees:** 160 **Number of employees for previous year:** 80 **Industry designation:** Computers—online services **Company type:** Private **Top competitors:** BroadVision, Inc.

Don't get caught in the Web. SMART Technologies makes software for companies that sell products and provide services through their Web pages. Its SMART DNA product integrates and delivers information over the Internet to customers, resellers, distributors, analysts, and the media. Web pages created with SMART's software are intended to provide a single interface to all aspects of a company, including sales, marketing, customer service, and technical support. The firm's major customers include Apple Computer, Compaq, Minolta, and Motorola. SMART was founded in 1995 by Jasiph Decoux, Mark Benson, and Jason Parish through a merger of MIS2 and NetTools.

Snyder Oil Corporation

777 Main St., Ste. 1400, Fort Worth, TX 76102

Telephone: 817-338-4043 **Fax:** 817-882-5899 **Metro area:** Dallas-Fort Worth, TX **Web site:** http://www.snyderoil.com **Human resources contact:** Roger B. Rice **Sales:** $141.1 million **Number of employees:** 306 **Number of employees for previous year:** 259 **Industry designation:** Oil & gas—exploration & production **Company type:** Public **Top competitors:** Barrett Resources Corporation; KCS Energy, Inc.; Royal Dutch/Shell Group

In a rocky market, Snyder Oil digs deep for profits. The company explores for and develops oil and gas properties. It operates about 1,500 wells, primarily in the Gulf of Mexico, northern Louisiana, and the Rocky Mountains. Snyder Oil also gathers, transports, and markets natural gas and holds about 700,000 undeveloped acres in the US. The company participates in international exploration through its 16% interest in Soco International, which is focused in Mongolia and Russia, and through its 7% stake in Cairn Energy, which has oil and gas operations on the Indian subcontinent. The company has agreed to be bought by Santa Fe Energy Resources.

Southern Foods Group Incorporated

3114 S. Haskell Ave., Dallas, TX 75223

Telephone: 214-824-8163 **Fax:** 214-824-0967 **Other address:** PO Box 279000, Dallas, TX 75227 **Metro area:** Dallas-Fort Worth, TX **Human resources contact:** Stuart Gibson **Sales:** $1.2 billion (Est.) **Number of employees:** 4,500 **Number of employees for previous year:** 2,500 **Industry designation:** Food—dairy products **Company type:** Private **Top competitors:** Dean Foods Company; Land O'Lakes, Inc.; Borden, Inc.

Business is mooving right along at Southern Foods Group, which has dairy processing and distribution operations in Alabama, Colorado, Hawaii, Idaho, Iowa, Louisiana, Mississippi, Montana, Nebraska, Oklahoma, Texas, and Utah. Founded in 1987, the company distributes milk, ice cream, fruit juices and drinks, whipping cream, half-and-half, cheese, yogurt, eggs, butter, margarine, and nondairy creamers under labels including the Foremost Dairy, Meadow Gold, Oak Farms Dairy, and Schepps-Foremost brand names. Southern Foods expanded beyond Texas, Louisiana, and Mississippi with the 1997 purchase of Borden's 17 Meadow Gold dairies. Dairy Farmers of America, the largest US dairy co-op, owns 50% of the company.

Southern Mineral Corporation

1201 Louisiana, Ste. 3350, Houston, TX 77002

Telephone: 713-658-9444 **Fax:** 713-658-9447 **Metro area:** Houston, TX **Web site:** http://www.somin.com **Human resources contact:** Margie Ewald **Sales:** $21.5 million **Number of employees:** 38 **Number of employees for previous year:** 27 **Industry designation:** Oil & gas—exploration & production **Company type:** Public

Southern Mineral is an oil and gas company that acquires, explores for, and produces oil and natural gas. The company does not operate any properties but participates as working interest owner in wells drilled and operated by other companies. It has interests in oil and gas wells primarily in Arkansas, Oklahoma, and the Gulf Coast, as well as in Canada and Ecuador. The company also owns mineral rights to approximately 385,000 gross acres, about half of which are in southern Mississippi. The company generally leases its acreage to other companies for exploration and development. Southern Mineral's purchase of Canadian energy concern Neutrino Resources will increase its proved reserves by more than 75%.

Sprint Paranet, Inc.

1776 Yorktown St., Ste. 300, Houston, TX 77056

Telephone: 713-626-4800 **Fax:** 713-626-4860 **Metro area:** Houston, TX **Web site:** http://www.paranet.com **Human resources contact:** Wendy Blaettner **Sales:** $66.2 million **Number of employees:** 818 **Industry designation:** Computers—services **Company type:** Subsidiary **Top competitors:** Stream International Inc.; REALTECH Systems Corporation

Not wanting to miss the boat, Sprint Corporation boarded the network management bandwagon with its 1997 acquisition of Paranet. The resulting company, Sprint Paranet, provides vendor-independent distributed network support and related services for large businesses. Services include LAN and WAN design and upgrades, integration, intranet implementation, disaster recovery planning, help desk support, and day-to-day management of large networks. Sprint Paranet also supplies personnel to handle peak loads and specific network problems. The company has about 30 branches in such cities as Atlanta, Chicago, Dallas, Houston, and Phoenix. Customers include American Express, Motorola, Siemens, and Texas Instruments.

Sterling Software, Inc.

300 Crescent Ct., Ste. 1200, Dallas, TX 75201

Telephone: 214-981-1000 **Fax:** 214-981-1215 **Metro area:** Dallas-Fort Worth, TX **Web site:** http://www.sterling.com **Human resources contact:** Steve Fallon **Sales:** $719.9 million **Number of employees:** 3,500 **Number of employees for previous year:** 7,050 **Industry designation:** Computers—corporate, professional & financial software **Company type:** Public **Top competitors:** Network Associates, Inc.; Computer Associates International, Inc.; International Business Machines Corporation

Sterling is pure software. Sterling Software makes applications development, computer network management, and information management software. The company boasts 20,000 customer sites worldwide (including 90 of the US's 100 largest industrial and service companies). Sterling Software also provides technical services to the US government (about 20% of sales), including such agencies as NASA and the Department of Defense. About 40% of the company's sales are outside North America. Sterling continues to expand its market presence through complementary acquisitions. The Wyly family, which includes two of the company's founders, owns 9% of Sterling Software.

Suiza Foods Corporation

2515 McKinney Ave., Ste. 1200, Dallas, TX 75201

Telephone: 214-303-3400 **Fax:** 214-303-3499 **Metro area:** Dallas-Fort Worth, TX **Human resources contact:** Jeff Dandurand **Sales:** $3.3 billion **Number of employees:** 16,716 **Number of employees for previous year:** 7,050 **Industry designation:** Food—dairy products **Company type:** Public **Top competitors:** Dean Foods Company

Suiza Foods produces milk, fruit drinks, and plastic packaging. Suiza makes and distributes dairy products through its Land-O-Sun Dairies, Swiss Farms, Velda Farms, and other subsidiaries in California, the Southeast, and the Midwest. Suiza-Puerto Rico is that island's largest fresh milk producer, and Suiza Fruit drinks are market leaders. Suiza plants make plastic bottles in 13 states, and its Continental Can subsidiary makes packaging in the US and Europe. Suiza has grown through more than 35 acquisitions since 1988, including its 1997 purchase of the MorningStar Group (Lactaid, Second Nature egg substitute). To focus on its dairy and plastic packaging businesses, Suiza has sold its Reddy Ice subsidiary.

Sun Energy Partners, L.P.

13155 Noel Rd., Dallas, TX 75240

Telephone: 972-715-4000 **Fax:** 972-715-3311 **Metro area:** Dallas-Fort Worth, TX **Human resources contact:** Frances G. Heartwell **Sales:** $523 million **Number of employees:** 1,046 **Number of employees for previous year:** 976 **Industry designation:** Oil & gas—exploration & production **Company type:** Public **Top competitors:** Unocal Corporation; Burlington Resources Inc.; Vastar Resources, Inc.

Sun Energy Partners doesn't want to hear about solar power. The company explores for and produces oil and gas, primarily in the Gulf of Mexico, through operating partnerships. It has proved reserves of an estimated 221 million barrels of oil and 1.2 billion cu. ft. of natural gas. In the Gulf of Mexico, Sun Energy has ownership interests in 38 producing platforms, 21 of which it operates. The company has interests in 60 onshore fields in five states, operating about 75% of the production. Sun Energy also has ownership interests in various offshore pipelines and facilities. Major customers include Sunoco, BP Amoco, Koch Oil, and ProEnergy. The company is controlled by Kerr-McGee.

Surrey, Inc.

13110 Trails End Rd., Leander, TX 78641

Telephone: 512-267-7172 **Fax:** 512-267-4864 **Metro area:** Austin, TX **Web site:** http://www.surreysoap.aa.psiweb.com **Sales:** $9.2 million **Number of employees:** 146 **Number of employees for previous year:** 72 **Industry designation:** Cosmetics & toiletries **Company type:** Public **Top competitors:** Johnson & Johnson; The Body Shop International PLC; The Dial Corporation

Soap gets Surrey in a lather. The company makes name-brand and private-label glycerin and cream soaps for retailers such as Elizabeth Arden, Avon, Wal-Mart, and Bath & Body Works. Surrey uses synthetic moisturizers rather than animal fat in its glycerin soaps, which it says makes them purer and harder. Surrey's branded products include Hill Country Soap Company glycerin and cream soaps, Surrey Men's Line shaving sets, Pure Pleasure soap-making kits and antibacterial liquid soap, and Simmer Scents potpourri. The company also makes traditional soap and scented candles. Chairman and CEO John van der Hagen, a co-founder, and his wife, Mary, own more than 35% of Surrey.

Swift Energy Company

16825 Northchase Dr., Ste. 400, Houston, TX 77060

Telephone: 281-874-2700 **Fax:** 281-874-2726 **Metro area:** Houston, TX **Web site:** http://www.swiftenergy.com **Human resources contact:** Charles Lopez **Sales:** $80.4 million **Number of employees:** 203 **Number of employees for previous year:** 194 **Industry designation:** Oil & gas—exploration & production **Company type:** Public **Top competitors:** Apache Corporation; Frontier Oil Corporation; Chesapeake Energy Corporation

No laggard, oil and gas exploration and production company Swift Energy has interests in more than 1,600 producing wells in 10 US states, primarily in Oklahoma, Texas, and Wyoming. The company's core production areas are the AWP Olmos Field in South Texas, which represents a majority of Swift Energy's proved reserves, and Texas' Austin Chalk Trend. Swift Energy employs development drilling and secondary recovery techniques on many of its properties. The company's proved reserves consist of more than 500 billion cu. ft. of natural gas equivalent.

Tanisys Technology, Inc.

12201 Technology Blvd., Ste. 125, Austin, TX 78727

Telephone: 512-335-4440 **Fax:** 512-257-5310 **Metro area:** Austin, TX **Web site:** http://www.tanisys.com **Human resources contact:** Richard R. Giandana **Sales:** $33.1 million **Number of employees:** 199 **Number of employees for previous year:** 143 **Industry designation:** Computers—peripheral equipment **Company type:** Public **Top competitors:** SMART Modular Technologies, Inc.; Micron Electronics, Inc.; Kingston Technology Company

They say memory is the first thing to go. Tanisys Technology makes off-the-shelf and build-to-order semiconductor memory modules and testers for OEMs that make custom electronics, digital cameras, PCs, personal digital assistants, and servers. The company makes DRAM, flash memory, and SRAM products and DarkHorse-branded memory module testers. It also licenses its proprietary Tanisys Touch sensor technology, which is used for touch pads on automation equipment, interactive kiosks, and monitors. Tanisys also offers support services such as assembly, integration, and testing. It sells its products directly and through independent representatives. Customers include Siemens (27% of sales) and LG Semicon (14%).

Tatham Offshore, Inc.

600 Travis St., Ste. 7400, Houston, TX 77002

Telephone: 713-224-7400 **Fax:** 713-224-7574 **Metro area:** Houston, TX **Human resources contact:** Melody Lanier **Sales:** $11.5 million **Number of employees:** 15 **Industry designation:** Oil & gas—exploration & production **Company type:** Public **Top competitors:** Global Marine Inc.; R&B Falcon Corporation; Diamond Offshore Drilling, Inc.

Tatham Offshore is staying in the water, but the company's focus has shifted from the Gulf of Mexico to the Atlantic Ocean off Canada. When former affiliate DeepTech was acquired by El Paso Energy, Tatham gave up its oil and gas producing properties in the Gulf and wound up with two semisubmersible drilling rigs. The rigs, Tatham's main operating assets, are managed by Schlumberger's Sedco Forex unit. In Atlantic Canada, Tatham is pursuing opportunities in natural gas development, production, gathering and transmission, and processsing, including a proposed pipeline that would run from Newfoundland to the eastern US coast. A group led by CEO Thomas Tatham owns 80% of the company.

Telescan, Inc.

5959 Corporate Dr., Ste. 2000, Houston, TX 77036

Telephone: 281-588-9700 **Fax:** 281-588-9797 **Metro area:** Houston, TX **Web site:** http://www.telescan.com **Human resources contact:** Judy Lucas **Sales:** $15.5 million **Number of employees:** 146 **Number of employees for previous year:** 134 **Industry designation:** Computers—online services **Company type:** Public **Top competitors:** Reuters Group PLC; The Thomson Corporation; Data Broadcasting Corporation

Telescan helps investors make dollars and sense out of financial data. The company develops and operates online database systems and Web sites (Wall Street City) that serve individual, corporate, and institutional investors. The Telescan family of online financial databases and software offer financial data and analysis tools. Telescan might spin off some discontinued operations such as its online and database services for publications, its Computer Sports Network (online interactive golf and baseball), and its interest in the Knowledge Express Data Systems LC database, which serves universities, corporations, and the US government. General Electric's NBC and GE Capital together own about 10% of the company.

TETRA Technologies, Inc.

25025 I-45 North, The Woodlands, TX 77380

Telephone: 281-367-1983 **Fax:** 281-364-2240 **Metro area:** Houston, TX **Web site:** http://www.tetratec.com **Human resources contact:** Linden Price **Sales:** $238.5 million **Number of employees:** 1,425 **Number of employees for previous year:** 1,290 **Industry designation:** Chemicals—diversified **Company type:** Public **Top competitors:** Halliburton Company; The Dow Chemical Company; Pool Energy Services Co.

TETRA Technologies is a foursquare provider of specialty inorganic chemical products, services, and process technologies to the oil and gas, agricultural, and environmental services markets. Its oil and gas division sells chemicals and fluids used in well completion, workover operations, and other drilling applications to customers such as Shell Oil, Texaco, and Unocal. TETRA also provides on-site fluid management and filtering services. Its agricultural group makes zinc-, manganese-, and calcium chloride-based products for animal and plant nutrition and sells ground-drying chemicals (DampRid). TETRA also offers chemicals used to treat wastewater, solid-waste streams, and refinery and petrochemical waste.

Texas Biotechnology Corporation

7000 Fannin St., Ste. 1920, Houston, TX 77030

Telephone: 713-796-8822 **Fax:** 713-796-8232 **Metro area:** Houston, TX **Web site:** http://www.tbc.com **Human resources contact:** Debbie Hedgepath **Sales:** $2.3 million **Number of employees:** 84 **Number of employees for previous year:** 79 **Industry designation:** Drugs **Company type:** Public **Top competitors:** Novartis AG; Biogen, Inc.; Hoechst Marion Roussel, Inc.

Development-stage Texas Biotechnology is roundin' up some medical breakthroughs. The biopharmaceutical firm develops small-molecule drugs to treat vascular disease. Its drug candidates include NOVASTAN, which is marketed in Japan; the drug is an anticoagulant with potential in cardiac and other treatments. Other products in development target cancer and inflammatory diseases. The company has also developed a computer-assisted small-molecule drug design system that helps it in drug-candidate identification. Texas Biotechnology's corporate partners—which include SmithKline Beecham, Mitsubishi Chemical, and Synthelabo—help it develop and commercialize its drugs.

Texas Health Resources

600 E. Las Colinas Blvd., Irving, TX 75039

Telephone: 214-818-4500 **Fax:** 214-818-4652 **Metro area:** Dallas-Fort Worth, TX **Web site:** http://www.texashealth.org **Human resources contact:** Bonnie Bell **Sales:** $1.3 billion **Number of employees:** 15,000 **Industry designation:** Hospitals **Company type:** Not-for-profit **Top competitors:** Columbia/HCA Healthcare Corporation; Parkland Health & Hospital System; Baylor Health Care System

The largest hospital system in North Texas, Texas Health Resources is a not-for-profit health care system with 16 hospitals, most of them in the Dallas-Fort Worth area. The system includes mental health centers, a retirement community and senior care centers, consulting and management services, and Harris Methodist Health Plan, an HMO with some 300,000 members. Texas Health Resources' alliance with Baylor Health Care System is on hold until its troubled HMO merges with Blue Cross and Blue Shield of Texas, creating the state's largest health insurance company. Its physician organization, Harris Methodist Select, may disband if neither Texas Health Resources nor Blue Cross (TX) accepts its 6,000 doctor contracts.

Texas Petrochemicals Corporation

3 Riverway, Ste. 1500, Houston, TX 77056

Telephone: 713-627-7474 **Fax:** 713-475-7761 **Metro area:** Houston, TX **Human resources contact:** Jim Rhodes **Sales:** $514.8 million (Est.) **Number of employees:** 328 **Number of employees for previous year:** 319 **Industry designation:** Chemicals—diversified **Company type:** Private **Top competitors:** Lyondell Chemical Company; Engelhard Corporation; Exxon Chemical Company

Texas Petrochemicals, maker of fossil fuel derived chemicals, lives up to the maxim "everything's bigger in Texas." The company is one of the foremost suppliers of butadiene, butene-1, high-purity isobutylene, diisobutylene, and isobutylene concentrate in the US. Its chemicals are used in the manufacture of synthetic rubber and alcohol, plastic resins, and lubricants. The company is also one of North America's largest makers of MTBE, an emission-reducing octane-booster. It even operates its own power plant to power its chemical facility, and sells the excess capacity to neighboring facilities. Texas Petrochemicals Holdings wholly owns Texas Petrochemicals.

Texoil, Inc.

110 Cypress Station Dr., Ste. 220, Houston, TX 77090

Telephone: 281-537-9920 **Fax:** 281-537-8324 **Metro area:** Houston, TX **Web site:** http://www.texoil.com **Sales:** $10.4 million **Number of employees:** 28 **Number of employees for previous year:** 16 **Industry designation:** Oil & gas—exploration & production **Company type:** Public

Texoil is involved in the acquisition, exploration, development, and production of oil and natural gas, primarily in the Texas Gulf Coast region and southern Louisiana. In addition to its exploration activities, Texoil purchases proved reserves and re-engineers older fields to increase production and reduce costs. The company has proved reserves of about 4.7 million barrels of oil and 11.6 million cu. ft. of natural gas. Its more than 270 gross oil wells and almost 85 gas wells produce approximately 255 thousand barrels of oil and 710 thousand cu. ft. of gas per year. Texoil sells its production to third parties, including Gateway Gathering, EOTT Energy, and Phillips.

Thermo Instrument Systems Inc.

860 W. Airport Fwy., Ste. 301, Hurst, TX 76504

Telephone: 781-622-1000 **Fax:** 781-622-1123 **Other address:** PO Box 2108, Santa Fe, NM 87504 **Metro area:** Killeen, TX **Web site:** http://www.thermo.com/subsid/thi.html **Human resources contact:** Fred Florio **Sales:** $1.7 billion **Number of employees:** 9,700 **Number of employees for previous year:** 9,398 **Industry designation:** Instruments—scientific **Company type:** Public **Top competitors:** Hewlett-Packard Company; The Perkin-Elmer Corporation; Beckman Coulter, Inc.

Thermo Instrument Systems makes equipment for determining the type and quantity of elements in gases, liquids, and solids. The company produces imaging equipment, mass spectrometers, and photonics through a number of subsidiaries that are spun off to sell minority stakes to outside investors. Thermo Instrument's equipment measures radioactivity, air pollution, complex chemical compounds, and toxic metals, and monitors other industrial processes. Thermo Instrument has facilities in the Europe and the US, and continues an acquisition expansion program. The company started as a subsidiary of Thermo Electron, which still owns an 84% interest.

ThermoLase Corporation

2055-C Luna Rd., Carrollton, TX 75006

Telephone: 972-488-0710 **Fax:** 972-241-9731 **Metro area:** Dallas-Fort Worth, TX **Web site:** http://www.thermo.com/subsid/tlz.html **Human resources contact:** Barbara Miller **Sales:** $40.1 million **Number of employees:** 486 **Number of employees for previous year:** 454 **Industry designation:** Cosmetics & toiletries **Company type:** Public **Top competitors:** ESC Medical Systems Ltd.; Alberto-Culver Company; Candela Corporation

ThermoLase wants to make its bucks in the beauty business. The company makes skin care products and operates spas that use a laser system it developed for cosmetic skin resurfacing and hair removal. The company's 11 Greenhouse spas across the US use its SoftLight laser system (similar to the lasers used to remove tattoos). ThermoLase has licensed SoftLight for use in doctors' offices. Subsidiary Creative Beauty Innovations makes lotions, shampoos, and other products (which account for 57% of sales) sold through department stores, company spas, upscale salons, and doctors. Tech-company incubator Thermo Electron, in part through subsidiary ThermoTrex, owns about 80% of ThermoLase.

Thousand Trails, Inc.

2711 LBJ Fwy., Ste. 200, Dallas, TX 75234

Telephone: 972-243-2228 **Fax:** 972-488-5008 **Metro area:** Dallas-Fort Worth, TX **Web site:** http://www.1000trails.com **Human resources contact:** David McCrum **Sales:** $76.5 million **Number of employees:** 1,355 **Number of employees for previous year:** 1,289 **Industry designation:** Leisure & recreational services **Company type:** Public **Top competitors:** Kampgrounds of America, Inc.; International Leisure Hosts, Ltd.; Rank America Inc.

Thousand Trails is making happy campers of the 111,000 members who use its 53 campsites in the US and British Columbia. Dues-paying members (half are senior citizens) can bring their own RVs and tents or rent trailers and cabins. The campgrounds offer amenities such as electricity, water, sewer connections, convenience stores, game machines, and laundry facilities. Member benefits also include a vehicle insurance program and a camping magazine. Subsidiary UST Wilderness Management manages 130 campgrounds for the US Forest Service, and subsidiary Resort Parks International offers a reciprocal program allowing members access to 325 recreational facilities. Director Andrew Boas controls 48% of the company.

Tidel Technologies, Inc.

5847 San Felipe, Ste. 900, Houston, TX 77057

Telephone: 713-783-8200 **Fax:** 713-783-6003 **Metro area:** Houston, TX **Web site:** http://www.tidel.com **Human resources contact:** Sue Weatherley **Sales:** $33.6 million **Number of employees:** 122 **Number of employees for previous year:** 96 **Industry designation:** Computers—corporate, professional & financial software **Company type:** Public **Top competitors:** NCR Corporation; Triton Systems, Inc.; Diebold, Incorporated

Idle hands need Tidel's cash. Tidel Technologies (formerly American Medical Technologies) makes automated teller machines (ATMs) and related software, money access systems, and environment monitoring equipment. Its ATM systems (AnyCard) come in both single and multi-cassette models. Its access cash controllers, which help reduce theft by serving as drop safes and cash dispensers, are used in gas stations, convenience stores, and other specialty retailers (including all 7-Eleven stores). Tidel also makes underground fuel storage monitors and leak detectors, but it is moving away from this business and is offering products to existing customers only. The company sells its products through distributors worldwide.

Titan Exploration, Inc.

500 W. Texas, Ste. 500, Midland, TX 79701

Telephone: 915-498-8600 **Fax:** 915-687-0192 **Metro area:** Odessa, TX **Sales:** $72.9 million **Number of employees:** 94 **Number of employees for previous year:** 30 **Industry designation:** Oil & gas—exploration & production **Company type:** Public **Top competitors:** Pioneer Natural Resources Company; Santa Fe Energy Resources, Inc.; Apache Corporation

Titan Exploration might not be a giant yet, but the company takes steps to make marks on the earth—primarily in the Permian Basin of West Texas and New Mexico, the Gulf Coast region, and the Gulf of Mexico, where it acquires and operates oil and gas properties. The company has estimated proved reserves of 30.3 million barrels of oil and 345.4 billion cu. ft. of natural gas. Titan Exploration operates more than 700 productive wells and has leasehold interests in nearly 700,000 developed and undeveloped acres. Enron and Western Gas Resources are the company's top customers.

Tom Brown, Inc.

500 Empire Plaza Bldg., Midland, TX 79701

Telephone: 915-682-9715 **Fax:** 915-682-9171 **Other address:** PO Box 2608, Midland, TX 79702 **Metro area:** Odessa, TX **Web site:** http://www.tombrown.com **Human resources contact:** B. Jack Reed **Sales:** $130.6 million **Number of employees:** 269 **Number of employees for previous year:** 158 **Industry designation:** Oil & gas—exploration & production **Company type:** Public **Top competitors:** Devon Energy Corporation; Chesapeake Energy Corporation; KCS Energy, Inc.

Tom Brown produces crude oil and natural gas in Colorado, New Mexico, Texas, and Wyoming, where it owns interests in about three million acres. The company has proved reserves of about 390 billion cu. ft. of gas equivalent, with more than 1,200 gross productive wells annually producing about 31.8 billion cu. ft. of gas and 1.2 million barrels of oil. Wildhorse (a subsidiary that primarily produces natural gas) owns almost 1,000 miles of gathering lines and two processing plants in the Rocky Mountains, where the company produces about half of its gas. Tom Brown sells its products under month-to-month contracts and at market prices.

Trilogy Software, Inc.

6034 W. Courtyard Dr., Austin, TX 78730

Telephone: 512-794-5900 **Fax:** 512-794-8900 **Metro area:** Austin, TX **Web site:** http://www.trilogy.com **Human resources contact:** Michelle Friesenhahn **Sales:** $150 million (Est.) **Number of employees:** 400 **Number of employees for previous year:** 340 **Industry designation:** Computers—corporate, professional & financial software **Company type:** Private **Top competitors:** Baan Company N.V.; Oracle Corporation; SAP AG

Trilogy Software (formerly Trilogy Development Group) makes Selling Chain, a suite of front office software that simplifies the selling process for everything from computers to airplanes. Many products have several customer-selected variables. Selling Chain ensures that the options are compatible, provides information on any additional products required, and calculates the cost of the order. Other functions include trade promotions and commissions and e-commerce management. Customers include Dell, AT&T, Compaq, Boeing, IBM, and Alcatel. Trilogy's majority-owned pcOrder.com sells computers over the Internet. Founder and CEO Joe Liemandt owns 55% of Trilogy.

UICI

4001 McEwen Dr., Ste. 200, Dallas, TX 75244

Telephone: 972-392-6700 **Fax:** 972-392-6721 **Metro area:** Dallas-Fort Worth, TX **Human resources contact:** Richard Hooton **Sales:** $955.8 million **Number of employees:** 3,400 **Number of employees for previous year:** 2,100 **Industry designation:** Insurance—accident & health **Company type:** Public **Top competitors:** Aon Corporation; Guarantee Trust Life Insurance Company; Atlantic American Corporation

UICI (formerly United Insurance Companies) sells health insurance to students and the self-employed and sells niche market life insurance through three subsidiaries. Its business units also offer credit cards to higher-risk clients and technical and service support for health care providers. Primarily an insurance marketing organization that finds leads and handles the paperwork, UICI pays its 5,000 agents on a straight commission basis. The company has acquired Insurdata (which processes health care transactions) and Education Finance Group, and it has agreed to acquire National Motor Club of America. Founder Ronald Jensen owns about 18% of the company.

Ultramar Diamond Shamrock Corporation

6000 N. Loop 1604 West, San Antonio, TX 78249

Telephone: 210-592-2000 **Fax:** 210-592-2195 **Other address:** PO Box 696000, San Antonio, TX 78269 **Metro area:** San Antonio, TX **Web site:** http://www.udscorp.com **Human resources contact:** Penelope R. Viteo **Sales:** $11.1 billion **Number of employees:** 23,000 **Number of employees for previous year:** 17,200 **Industry designation:** Oil refining & marketing **Company type:** Public **Top competitors:** Tosco Corporation; Texaco Inc.; USX-Marathon Group

Luck has nothing to do with ranking. Ultramar Diamond Shamrock, formed by the 1996 merger of Ultramar and Diamond Shamrock, is the #2 independent oil refining and marketing company in the US, behind Tosco. It owns seven refineries with a total capacity of 650,000 barrels per day. Ultramar Diamond Shamrock also has about 6,300 gas stations and operates petrochemical, home heating oil, natural gas liquids, and convenience store businesses. Most of its US and Canadian convenience stores operate under the Diamond Shamrock, Total, Ultramar, and Beacon names.

Union Pacific Resources Group Inc.

801 Cherry St., Fort Worth, TX 76102

Telephone: 817-321-6000 **Fax:** 817-321-7584 **Other address:** PO Box 7, Fort Worth, TX 76101 **Metro area:** Dallas-Fort Worth, TX **Human resources contact:** Anne M. Franklin **Sales:** $1.8 billion **Number of employees:** 2,900 **Number of employees for previous year:** 1,907 **Industry designation:** Oil & gas—exploration & production **Company type:** Public **Top competitors:** Sonat Inc.; Burlington Resources Inc.; Texaco Inc.

Union Pacific Resources Group, a spinoff of railroad giant Union Pacific, is an independent natural gas and oil exploration and production company. It has properties in the Austin Chalk trend in Texas and Louisiana and more than seven million acres (granted to Union Pacific by the federal government in the 19th century) in Colorado, Wyoming, and Utah. It also has major operations in western Canada, the Gulf of Mexico, Guatemala, and Venezuela. Union Pacific Resources, which has reserves equivalent to more than 1.2 billion barrels of oil, also has passive interests in trona (used to make soda ash) and coal mining. It markets its oil and gas to customers through subsidiary Union Pacific Fuels.

Union Texas Petroleum Holdings, Inc.

1330 Post Oak Blvd., Houston, TX 77056

Telephone: 713-623-6544 **Fax:** 713-968-2771 **Other address:** PO Box 2120, Houston, TX 77252 **Metro area:** Houston, TX **Web site:** http://www.uniontexas.com **Human resources contact:** Chris Dimick **Sales:** $909.4 million **Number of employees:** 1,300 **Number of employees for previous year:** 1,100 **Industry designation:** Oil & gas—exploration & production **Company type:** Subsidiary **Top competitors:** Exxon Corporation; Royal Dutch/Shell Group; Mobil Corporation

Texas isn't big enough to hold Union Texas Petroleum Holdings. Union Texas, a subsidiary of global integrated oil company Atlantic Richfield (ARCO), explores for and produces oil and gas, primarily in Indonesia, Pakistan, Venezuela, and the UK sector of the North Sea. Union Texas has proved reserves of more than 570 million barrels of oil equivalent. The company is developing projects in such areas as Alaska, Africa, Central Asia, and the Middle East. Union Texas also owns a 42% stake in the Geismar olefins plant in Louisiana, which produces ethylene.

United Dental Care, Inc.

13601 Preston Rd., Ste. 500 East, Dallas, TX 75240

Telephone: 972-458-7474 **Fax:** 972-458-7963 **Metro area:** Dallas-Fort Worth, TX **Web site:** http://www.uniteddental.com **Human resources contact:** Danielle Kendall **Sales:** $174 million **Number of employees:** 660 **Number of employees for previous year:** 507 **Industry designation:** Medical practice management **Company type:** Subsidiary **Top competitors:** SafeGuard Health Enterprises, Inc.

United Dental Care is a managed dental care company that operates prepaid dental benefits plans in 29 states, primarily Arizona, Colorado, Missouri, New Jersey, New Mexico, Oklahoma, and Texas. The company provides prepaid dental care alone, through contracts with HMOs, or through employers, and can also operate in combination with indemnity plans and preferred provider organizations (PPOs). United Dental serves almost two million members through a network of about 6,700 general and specialty dentists, though members may also use doctors outside the network. In 1998 Protective Life Corporation bought the company to add to its roster of specialty care providers.

U.S. Gas Transportation, Inc.

2711 Haskell Ave., Ste. 2050, Dallas, TX 75204

Telephone: 214-827-9464 **Fax:** 214-827-2718 **Metro area:** Dallas-Fort Worth, TX **Human resources contact:** Jett Rominger **Sales:** $375 million (Est.) **Number of employees:** 30 **Number of employees for previous year:** 28 **Industry designation:** Oil refining & marketing **Company type:** Private

U.S. Gas Transportation (USGT) is a natural gas marketing firm. The company sells gas to public utilities and other major companies in the US and other countries. U.S. Gas Transportation has rights to almost 30 pipelines. Proving that, in some things, size doesn't matter, the small regional company has been ranked as the second-best gas marketing firm to work with by North American gas producers (Public Service Electric & Gas Co. is #1; larger gas marketers finished much farther down the list). Founded by president Nanci Mackenzie and two partners in 1987, the company is now owned by Mackenzie.

U.S. Physical Therapy, Inc.

3040 Post Oak Blvd., Ste. 222, Houston, TX 77056

Telephone: 713-297-9050 **Fax:** 713-297-7090 **Metro area:** Houston, TX **Web site:** http://www.usphys.com **Human resources contact:** Kimberly Cox **Sales:** $44 million **Number of employees:** 716 **Number of employees for previous year:** 650 **Industry designation:** Health care—outpatient & home **Company type:** Public

U.S. Physical Therapy develops, owns, and operates outpatient physical and occupational therapy clinics. To attract and retain physical therapists, the company offers recruited therapists a minor partnership interest in new clinics. With 85 clinics operating in 25 states, treatment focuses on workers' compensation, sports/recreational, and postsurgical injuries. Business originates from physician referrals. Services are paid for by commercial health insurance, managed care programs, Medicare, workers' compensation insurance, or proceeds from personal injury cases. While U.S. Physical Therapy's strategy is to develop new centers, its competitors primarily acquire and consolidate existing clinics.

Valero Energy Corporation

7990 W. IH 10, San Antonio, TX 78230

Telephone: 210-370-2000 **Fax:** 210-370-2103 **Other address:** PO Box 500, San Antonio, TX 78292 **Metro area:** San Antonio, TX **Web site:** http://www.valero.com **Human resources contact:** Keith D. Booke **Sales:** $5.5 billion **Number of employees:** 2,500 **Number of employees for previous year:** 1,855 **Industry designation:** Oil refining & marketing **Company type:** Public **Top competitors:** Tosco Corporation; Sunoco, Inc.; Ultramar Diamond Shamrock Corporation

Having sold off its natural gas operations to West Coast utility company PG&E in 1997, Valero Energy is now focused on refining and marketing petroleum products. Valero refines low-cost residual oil into clean-burning, higher-margin products, including reformulated gasoline, low-sulfur diesel, and oxygenates. The company's five refineries in Texas, Louisiana, and New Jersey (three of which it picked up with its 1997 acquisition of Basis Petroleum) have a daily production capacity of 735,000 barrels. Valero is also expanding its alliances with gasoline marketers, especially in the Northeast and Texas.

Vastar Resources, Inc.

15375 Memorial Dr., Houston, TX 77079

Telephone: 281-584-6000 **Fax:** 281-584-3268 **Metro area:** Houston, TX **Web site:** http://www.vastar.com **Human resources contact:** Jeff Bender **Sales:** $941.1 million **Number of employees:** 1,122 **Number of employees for previous year:** 1,063 **Industry designation:** Oil & gas—exploration & production **Company type:** Public

Vastar Resources is an 82%-owned subsidiary of Atlantic Richfield that explores for, develops, produces, and markets natural gas, natural gas liquids, and crude oil. Its principal producing areas include the Texas and Louisiana Gulf Coast and the Gulf of Mexico; the San Juan/Rockies area in New Mexico, Colorado, and Wyoming; and the mid-Continent area, including Oklahoma, Arkansas, and Kansas. It markets its natural gas (64% of sales) through Southern Company Energy Marketing, a joint venture in which it owns a 40% stake (#1 US electricity provider Southern Company owns the other 60%). The company markets its crude oil and natural gas liquids directly.

Venus Exploration, Inc.

1250 NE Loop 410, Ste. 1000, San Antonio, TX 78209

Telephone: 210-930-4900 **Fax:** 210-930-4901 **Metro area:** San Antonio, TX **Sales:** $2.5 million **Number of employees:** 26 **Number of employees for previous year:** 21 **Industry designation:** Oil & gas—exploration & production **Company type:** Public

Venus Exploration explores for and develops oil and natural gas in 10 states, including Texas, Oklahoma, West Virginia, and Kansas. The company's properties incude interests in more than 49,000 gross developed and undeveloped acres. Venus Exploration has total proved reserves of 2.4 billion cu. ft. of natural gas equivalent and a daily net production of 2.45 million cu. ft. of gas equivalent. Production from its 105 oil and 120 gas wells is sold at the wellhead to oil and gas companies, including Dow Hydrocarbons & Resources, Stephens & Johnson Operating Co., and Flying J Oil & Gas. Chairman and CEO Eugene Ames and his family own more than 35% of the company.

VHA Inc.

220 E. Las Colinas Blvd., Irving, TX 75039

Telephone: 972-830-0000 **Fax:** 972-830-0012 **Other address:** 140909, Irving, TX 75014 **Metro area:** Dallas-Fort Worth, TX **Web site:** http://www.vha.com **Human resources contact:** Kim R. Alleman **Sales:** $254.2 million **Number of employees:** 1,100 **Number of employees for previous year:** 1,000 **Industry designation:** Hospitals **Company type:** Cooperative

Cooperative VHA, formerly Voluntary Hospitals of America, is keeping the US healthy through a nationwide network of community-owned health care organizations. With more than 1,600 members in 48 states and the District of Columbia, the co-op represents nearly one-quarter of US community-owned hospitals. VHA offers networking and education opportunities for health care workers, evaluation of medical software, and physician referral and demand management. VHA members purchase medical supplies from Novation, a joint venture with University HealthSystem Consortium. Subsidiary HealthCare Purchasing Partners International sells to more than 2,400 customers outside the VHA network.

Vista Energy Resources, Inc.

550 W. Texas Ave., Ste. 700, Midland, TX 79701

Telephone: 915-570-5045 **Fax:** 915-688-0589 **Metro area:** Odessa, TX **Human resources contact:** R. Cory Richards **Sales:** $6.6 million **Number of employees:** 28 **Number of employees for previous year:** 23 **Industry designation:** Oil & gas—exploration & production **Company type:** Public **Top competitors:** Abraxas Petroleum Corporation; The Wiser Oil Company; Santa Fe Energy Resources, Inc.

Vista Energy Resources has a clear view of its future—exploring for oil and gas in the Permian Basin. Vista Energy Resources uses 3-D seismic technology to explore for and develop domestic oil and gas properties, primarily in the Permian Basin of West Texas and southeastern New Mexico. The company has proved reserves of 14 million barrels of oil equivalent. Vista Energy Resources, which was formed by the merger of independent oil firms Vista Partnership and Midland Resources in 1998, operates more than 400 producing wells. NGP, an energy investment partnership, owns 52% of Vista Energy Resources.

Westbridge Capital Corp.

777 Main St., Fort Worth, TX 76102

Telephone: 817-878-3300 **Fax:** 817-878-3880 **Metro area:** Dallas-Fort Worth, TX **Human resources contact:** Tammy Haggard **Sales:** $166.1 million **Number of employees:** 388 **Number of employees for previous year:** 345 **Industry designation:** Insurance—accident & health **Company type:** Public

Westbridge Capital is an insurance holding company that primarily underwrites medical expense and supplemental health insurance products to self-employed individuals and small-business owners. The company's medical expense policies reimburse various medical and hospital costs and offer reduced deductibles and coinsurance payments when policyholders use company PPO providers. Critical care and specified disease products include indemnity policies for the treatment of specified diseases and lump sum payments upon diagnosis of internal cancer or other catastrophic diseases. Westbridge Capital sells its insurance through company-owned and independent agencies.

XTRA On-Line, Inc.

301 Market St., 5th Fl., Dallas, TX 75202

Telephone: 214-753-4000 **Fax:** 214-753-4001 **Metro area:** Dallas-Fort Worth, TX **Web site:** http://www.xtraonline.com **Human resources contact:** Gigi Brakey **Number of employees:** 52 **Industry designation:** Computers—corporate, professional & financial software **Company type:** Private **Top competitors:** The SABRE Group Holdings, Inc.; Microsoft Corporation; Travel Services International, Inc.

XTRA On-Line's PowerTrip travel reservation software works like an ATM for travel agencies: Customers conduct their business by computer, and the agency collects fees on the transaction. XTRA On-Line (XOL) licenses PowerTrip to more than 200 travel agencies. Corporate travelers use the service to make online reservations through a database of travel information provided by airlines, car rental companies, and hotels worldwide. PowerTrip also reports company policies for different positions within a company and tracks expenses for budgetary review before or after travel. President Richard Kumpf founded XOL in 1996 when he spun off his travel agency's software unit.

Zonagen, Inc.

2408 Timberloch Place, Ste. B-4, The Woodlands, TX 77380

Telephone: 281-367-5892 **Fax:** 281-363-8796 **Metro area:** Houston, TX **Web site:** http://www.zonagen.com **Human resources contact:** Tara Stewart **Sales:** $10.2 million **Number of employees:** 51 **Number of employees for previous year:** 39 **Industry designation:** Biomedical & genetic products **Company type:** Public **Top competitors:** Pfizer Inc

Zonagen develops treatments for human reproductive disorders. Product development focuses on fertility drugs, contraceptives, Vasomax (oral treatment for male erectile dysfunction), and Vasofem (for female sexual dysfunction). Drug firm Schering-Plough has licensed the marketing rights to Vasomax, which was approved in Mexico (under the name Z-Max) but still needs regulatory approval in the US. The firm researches other areas of reproductive health care, such as treatments for benign prostate hyperplasia and prostate cancer, and a product to enhance vaccine effectiveness. Subsidiary Fertility Technologies markets and distributes therapies to obstetricians/gynecologists, urologists, and fertility clinics.

Zydeco Energy, Inc.

1710 Two Allen Center, 1200 Smith St., Houston, TX 77002

Telephone: 713-659-2222 **Fax:** 713-659-2221 **Metro area:** Houston, TX **Web site:** http://www.znrg.com **Sales:** $400,000 **Number of employees:** 22 **Number of employees for previous year:** 17 **Industry designation:** Oil & gas—exploration & production **Company type:** Public **Top competitors:** Miller Exploration Company; XPLOR Energy, Inc.; Apache Corporation

Zydeco music has plenty of energy, but Zydeco Energy is looking for more than a lively tune. The independent oil and gas exploration company concentrates on the Louisiana Transition Zone in the Gulf of Mexico. It uses its proprietary Wavefield Imaging 3-D seismic technology to find new sources in this generally heavily surveyed and much-drilled oil patch. Zydeco Energy has proved reserves of about 2,600 barrels of oil and 104 million cu. ft. of gas. The company was formed in 1995 in a merger between independent oil and gas company Zydeco Exploration and acquisition vehicle TN Energy Services Acquisition.

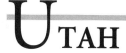

UTAH

Anesta Corp.

4745 Wiley Post Way, Ste. 650, Salt Lake City, UT 84116

Telephone: 801-595-1405 **Fax:** 801-595-1406 **Metro area:** Salt Lake City, UT **Web site:** http://www.anesta.com **Sales:** $700,000 **Number of employees:** 77 **Number of employees for previous year:** 73 **Industry designation:** Drugs **Company type:** Public

Anesta develops oral transmucosal (OT) drug delivery systems, which allow drugs to be quickly and painlessly absorbed into the bloodstream through the mouth's mucous membrane. Anesta's sedative and painkiller Fentanyl Oralet is approved by the US Food and Drug Administration (FDA) and is marketed in the US by Abbott Laboratories, which has extensively funded the company. Its Actiq has been approved for the treatment of cancer pain, and other OT-fentanyl products for smoking cessation, migraine headaches, and nausea are either being tested or are awaiting FDA approval. Anesta is entering the European market with Spanish pharmaceutical company Grupo Ferrer as its exclusive distributor in Spain and Portugal.

Ballard Medical Products

12050 Lone Peak Pkwy., Draper, UT 84020

Telephone: 801-572-6800 **Fax:** 801-572-6869 **Metro area:** Salt Lake City, UT **Web site:** http://www.bmed.com **Human resources contact:** Geri Stelling **Sales:** $150.1 million **Number of employees:** 1,336 **Number of employees for previous year:** 1,145 **Industry designation:** Medical instruments **Company type:** Public **Top competitors:** Becton, Dickinson and Company; Allegiance Corporation; Boston Scientific Corporation

Ballard Medical Products makes specialized medical products, including Trach Care endotracheal (respiratory) products (40% of sales). The firm also makes MIC enteral (feeding) products, foamers and solutions (Foam Care), endoscopy accessories, heat and moisture exchangers, and procedure trays. Ballard's products are used in hospital emergency rooms, intensive care units, respiratory therapy units, and hospital and outpatient surgical centers. Company subsidiaries include Mist Assist, Inc. (respiratory products) and Cardiotronics Systems (stimulation electrodes). Ballard sells its products in 66 countries, but only about 10% of sales come from outside the US. Kimberly-Clark is buying the firm.

Cyclopss Corporation

3646 W. 2100 South, Salt Lake City, UT 84120

Telephone: 801-972-9090 **Fax:** 801-972-9092 **Metro area:** Salt Lake City, UT **Web site:** http://www.cyclopss.com **Human resources contact:** Mondis Nkoy **Sales:** $1.2 million **Number of employees:** 25 **Number of employees for previous year:** 22 **Industry designation:** Pollution control equipment & services **Company type:** Public **Top competitors:** Hawkins Chemical, Inc.; STERIS Corporation; Ecomat, Inc.

Cyclopss has one eye on the power of ozone. The company designs, manufactures, and markets technologies that harness the naturally occurring gas for sterilization purposes. Ozone, through oxidation, acts as an environmentally sound alternative to chemical disinfectants. Through its subsidiaries, Cyclopss produces technological systems for use in food processing, textile care, and medical instrument sterilization and develops specialty chemicals for the aerospace and biotech industries. Its computerized VAC Soil Counting System automates garment inventory, billing, and work scheduling for large-scale laundry operations. Cyclopss markets through direct sales and is looking for contracts with distributors.

Dynatronics Corporation

7030 Park Centre Dr., Salt Lake City, UT 84121

Telephone: 801-568-7000 **Fax:** 801-568-7711 **Metro area:** Salt Lake City, UT **Web site:** http://www.dynatronics.com **Human resources contact:** Karen Morgan **Sales:** $12.3 million **Number of employees:** 131 **Number of employees for previous year:** 103 **Industry designation:** Medical products **Company type:** Public **Top competitors:** Henley Healthcare, Inc.; Empi, Inc.; Rehabilicare Inc.

Dynatronics makes medical equipment to keep active people on the go. Its products include electrotherapy and ultrasound therapy equipment; such medical supplies and soft goods as wraps, braces, and bandages, walking aids and training equipment; rehabilitation therapy tables and equipment; and the Synergie Lifestyle System, which combines massage therapy equipment (including a special table and body suit), nutritional supplements, and a diet program for cosmetic weight loss. Dynatronics has manufacturing facilities in South Carolina, Tennessee, and Utah, but also uses subcontractors. The company's products are sold through a catalog and dealers to doctors, therapists, and other medical specialists.

Huntsman Corporation

500 Huntsman Way, Salt Lake City, UT 84108

Telephone: 801-532-5200 **Fax:** 801-584-5781 **Metro area:** Salt Lake City, UT **Web site:** http://www.huntsman.com **Human resources contact:** William Chapman **Sales:** $4.8 billion (Est.) **Number of employees:** 9,550 **Number of employees for previous year:** 8,000 **Industry designation:** Chemicals—diversified **Company type:** Private **Top competitors:** BASF Aktiengesellschaft; The Dow Chemical Company; E. I. du Pont de Nemours and Company

Family-owned Huntsman Corporation is the largest privately held chemical business in the US. Huntsman makes a range of industrial chemicals, petrochemicals, and specialty chemicals used by the plastics, chemical, detergent, rubber, and packaging industries. Huntsman Chemical and Huntsman Corporation units make polypropylene, expandable polystyrenes, protective packaging, and surfactants. The company sold off its polystyrene and styrene monomer (the primary raw material used to make polystyrene, expandable resins, and a variety of rubber-based products) businesses to raise cash to pay down debt. Huntsman Packaging produces printed and laminated films used in food packaging, medical products, and other items.

Intermountain Health Care

36 S. State St., Salt Lake City, UT 84111

Telephone: 801-442-2000 **Fax:** 801-442-5652 **Metro area:** Salt Lake City, UT **Web site:** http://www.ihc.com **Human resources contact:** Gary Hart **Sales:** $2 billion **Number of employees:** 22,000 **Number of employees for previous year:** 20,000 **Industry designation:** Hospitals **Company type:** Not-for-profit **Top competitors:** Holy Cross Health System Corporation; Kaiser Foundation Health Plan, Inc.; Columbia/HCA Healthcare Corporation

Intermountain Health Care (IHC) is a full-service health care organization serving more than 425,000 members in Utah, Idaho, and Wyoming. It operates more than 20 hospitals and is affiliated with more than 2,500 physicians, including 400 employed by the IHC Physician Group. IHC Health Plans offers health insurance to individuals, families, businesses, and persons covered by Medicaid. The IHC Foundation donates heavily to support health programs in its communities. The company was formed in 1975 when the Mormons (Church of Jesus Christ of Latter Day Saints) decided to donate 15 of their hospitals to the communities they served.

Interwest Home Medical, Inc.

235 E. 6100 South, Salt Lake City, UT 84107

Telephone: 801-261-5100 **Fax:** 801-266-5319 **Metro area:** Salt Lake City, UT **Web site:** http://www.iwhm.com **Human resources contact:** Sherrie Eichenberger **Sales:** $28.6 million **Number of employees:** 300 **Number of employees for previous year:** 250 **Industry designation:** Medical services **Company type:** Public **Top competitors:** Integrated Health Services, Inc.; Apria Healthcare Group Inc.; American HomePatient, Inc.

Interwest Home Medical helps patients get back on their feet by keeping them comfy in bed. The company provides home health care products and services from nearly 30 locations in Alaska, California, Colorado, Idaho, Nevada, and Utah. The company's oxygen and respiratory care operations, which account for 55% of sales, include the training and monitoring patients who use oxygen equipment, ventilators, and other respiratory devices. Interwest also rents and sells rehabilitation equipment such as wheelchairs and vehicle adapters. The company's home medical product division offers canes, walkers, braces, lifts, hospital beds, and first aid and other supplies. Interwest has made nearly 20 acquisitions since 1996.

IOMED, Inc.

3385 W. 1820 South, Salt Lake City, UT 84104

Telephone: 801-975-1191 **Fax:** 801-972-9072 **Metro area:** Salt Lake City, UT **Web site:** http://www.iomed.com **Human resources contact:** Mary A. Crowther **Sales:** $10.3 million **Number of employees:** 80 **Number of employees for previous year:** 73 **Industry designation:** Medical products **Company type:** Public **Top competitors:** Novartis AG; Astra AB; Empi, Inc.

IOMED hopes to make fear of needles a thing of the past. The company's products deliver water-soluble ionic drugs through a patient's skin, via low levels of electricity. Advantages cited by IOMED include less-frequent and more programmable dosing, as well as potential patient self-administration. Physical therapists have used the system on more than 11 million patients to treat such conditions as tendinitis and carpal tunnel syndrome. The FDA has approved the delivery system for a local dermal anesthetic and an anti-inflammatory steroid. IOMED got a boost when its dermal anesthetic Numby Stuff was used in an episode of the TV series "ER." Elan International Services owns about 30% of IOMED.

Iomega Corporation

1821 W. Iomega Way, Roy, UT 84067

Telephone: 801-778-1000 **Fax:** 801-332-3804 **Metro area:** Salt Lake City, UT **Web site:** http://www.iomega.com **Human resources contact:** Kevin O'Connor **Sales:** $1.7 billion **Number of employees:** 4,865 **Number of employees for previous year:** 4,816 **Industry designation:** Computers—peripheral equipment **Company type:** Public **Top competitors:** Imation Corp.; Seagate Technology, Inc.; Sony Corporation

Iomega's data-storage devices—including the Zip drive, which has sold more than 16 million units worldwide—offer high storage capacity and portability. The company is working to boost sales by persuading computer makers such as Apple, Dell, Hewlett-Packard, and IBM to make Zip drives standard features in PCs. The company also makes Jaz, an up-to-2GB drive, and is making plans to release Clik , a disk-based storage product for use with handheld computers, cellular phones, and digital cameras. The company has sold off its Ditto product line (tape backup system). Iomega sells its products through distributors, original equipment manufacturers, and retailers.

Merit Medical Systems, Inc.

1600 W. Merit Pkwy., South Jordan, UT 84095

Telephone: 801-253-1600 **Fax:** 801-253-1687 **Metro area:** Salt Lake City, UT **Human resources contact:** Brent Bowen **Sales:** $68.4 million **Number of employees:** 989 **Number of employees for previous year:** 755 **Industry designation:** Medical products **Company type:** Public **Top competitors:** Maxxim Medical, Inc.; St. Jude Medical, Inc.; Pfizer Inc

Merit Medical Systems produces disposable medical products used in the diagnosis and treatment of cardiovascular disease. The company's products include control syringes, inflation devices, specialty syringes, high-pressure tubing and connectors, waste handling and disposal products, a disposable blood pressure transducer, disposable hemostasis valves, and contrast management systems. US sales, which make up about 60% of Merit Medical Systems' total sales, are made primarily to hospitals; foreign sales are largely made through independent dealers in Belgium; Canada, France, Germany, Ireland, the Netherlands, and the UK. Subsidiary Sentir makes silicon sensors.

Mining Services International Corporation

8805 S. Sandy Pkwy., Sandy, UT 84070

Telephone: 801-233-6000 **Fax:** 801-233-6004 **Metro area:** Salt Lake City, UT **Human resources contact:** Connie Bolda **Sales:** $27 million **Number of employees:** 95 **Number of employees for previous year:** 70 **Industry designation:** Chemicals—specialty **Company type:** Public **Top competitors:** Orica Limited

Mining Services International breaks big rocks into little rocks. The company's products include commercial mining explosives used to blast away rock encasing base metals and precious metals, coal, industrial minerals, and construction sites. The company also makes and sells liquid sodium cyanide through Cyanco, its 50-50 joint venture with Germany-based Degussa-Huls. The acid is used to extract gold from deposits, primarily in the western US. The company markets its products directly in the US and Canada and through distribution arrangements in Africa and the Middle East and around the Mediterranean.

Mrs. Fields' Original Cookies, Inc.

2855 E. Cottonwood Pkwy., Ste. 400, Salt Lake City, UT 84121

Telephone: 801-736-5600 **Fax:** 801-736-5970 **Metro area:** Salt Lake City, UT **Web site:** http://www.mrsfields.com **Human resources contact:** Chandra Leetham **Sales:** $133.6 million (Est.) **Number of employees:** 6,614 **Number of employees for previous year:** 4,007 **Industry designation:** Food—confectionery **Company type:** Private **Top competitors:** J & J Snack Foods Corp.; Triarc Companies, Inc.; Mr. Bulky Treats & Gifts

Any way these cookies crumble, it's sweet success for Mrs. Fields'. The company, which sells cookies, pretzels, brownies, and other baked goods in 12 countries, dominates the retail market for specialty cookies. It operates and franchises more than 1,300 stores under the Mrs. Fields', The Original Cookie Company, and Great American Cookie Company names, as well as more than 300 pretzel stores under the Pretzel Time and Hot Sam names. Founder Debbie Fields, who is a company director, opened her first store in 1977. Capricorn Investors owns the company.

Myriad Genetics, Inc.

320 Wakara Way, Salt Lake City, UT 84108

Telephone: 801-584-3600 **Fax:** 801-584-3640 **Metro area:** Salt Lake City, UT **Web site:** http://www.myriad.com **Human resources contact:** Barbara Berry **Sales:** $23.2 million **Number of employees:** 270 **Number of employees for previous year:** 197 **Industry designation:** Biomedical & genetic products **Company type:** Public **Top competitors:** Incyte Pharmaceuticals, Inc.; Millennium Pharmaceuticals, Inc.; The Perkin-Elmer Corporation

Mutants beware: Myriad Genetics hunts for mutant genes. The company's, well, myriad of technologies includes analyses of family histories to identify inherited risks for cancer, heart attacks, and other diseases; bioinformatic gene mapping; and protein interaction identification (a database called ProNet). The company's BRACAnalysis determines a woman's predisposition for breast or ovarian cancer; its CardiaRisk determines predisposition for other diseases. Myriad Genetics has research alliances with several pharmaceutical firms, which fund research in exchange for licenses to make and sell Myriad's tests. The company has discovered and sequenced several major human genes.

NACO Industries, Inc.

395 W. 1400 North, Logan, UT 84341

Telephone: 435-753-8020 **Fax:** 435-752-7041 **Metro area:** Salt Lake City, UT **Web site:** http://www.naco-industries.com **Sales:** $7.2 million **Number of employees:** 114 **Number of employees for previous year:** 100 **Industry designation:** Chemicals—plastics **Company type:** Public **Top competitors:** Formosa Plastics Corporation; NIBCO INC.; Eagle Pacific Industries, Inc.

NACO Industries' middle name should be PVC. The company's main products are polyvinyl chloride (PVC) pipe fittings and valves that are sold through wholesale distributors in the US to the irrigation, industrial, construction, and utility industries. Its pipe fittings and valves account for about 86% of revenues. The company's pipe fittings include couplers, elbows, end caps, reducers, and tees; valves include low-pressure butterfly valves and air-relief valves. NACO also makes fiberglass and composite products such as auto parts and decorative building parts. NACO's four manufacturing plants are in Utah, Kansas, and California.

Nu Skin Enterprises, Inc.

75 W. Center St., Provo, UT 84601

Telephone: 801-345-6100 **Fax:** 801-345-3099 **Metro area:** Salt Lake City, UT **Web site:** http://www.nuskin.net **Human resources contact:** Claire Averett **Sales:** $913.5 million **Number of employees:** 1,000 **Number of employees for previous year:** 900 **Industry designation:** Cosmetics & toiletries **Company type:** Public

Multilevel marketer Nu Skin Enterprises (formerly Nu Skin Asia Pacific) owns the rights to the Nu Skin name and trademarks and markets its personal care and nutritional products worldwide, except in North America. Its purchase of Nu Skin USA and other privately held owners of Nu Skin marketing rights will give it worldwide ownership. Nu Skin personal care items include cosmetics, fragrances, body and hair care, and related products. The Interior Design Nutritionals brand includes nutritional supplements, weight-loss products, snacks, and sports nutrition products. The firm, controlled by the Roney family, bought health supplement developer Pharmanex and plans to buy Internet company Big Planet.

Nutraceutical International Corporation

1400 Kearns Blvd., 2nd Fl., Park City, UT 84060

Telephone: 435-655-6000 **Fax:** 435-647-3802 **Metro area:** Salt Lake City, UT **Human resources contact:** Clyde Robbins **Sales:** $104.7 million **Number of employees:** 460 **Number of employees for previous year:** 430 **Industry designation:** Vitamins & nutritional products **Company type:** Public **Top competitors:** Herbalife International, Inc.; Rexall Sundown, Inc.; NBTY, Inc.

Nutraceutical International wants to pump you up and/or slim you down. The firm sells more than 1,000 nutritional supplements, vitamins and minerals, and diet/energy products in the US and abroad. It makes more than 90% of its products and sells them under such names as Solaray, NaturalMax, VegLife, KAL, Premier One, and Solar Green brand names (marketing many brands helps the firm gain more shelf space). Products include Beefense, Peaceful Planet, and Super DietMax. The company markets to more than 10,000 health foods stores in the US, with its Au Naturel unit handling marketing in about 30 other countries. Bain Capital owns more than 40% of the firm, which is buying nutritional products maker Futurebiotics.

OEC Medical Systems, Inc.

384 Wright Brothers Dr., Salt Lake City, UT 84116

Telephone: 801-328-9300 **Fax:** 801-328-4300 **Metro area:** Salt Lake City, UT **Web site:** http://www.oecmed.com **Human resources contact:** Susan Traenstrum **Sales:** $188.7 million **Number of employees:** 715 **Number of employees for previous year:** 635 **Industry designation:** Medical products **Company type:** Public **Top competitors:** Picker International, Inc.; Hologic, Inc.; Lunar Corporation

OEC Medical Systems develops computer-based X-ray and fluoroscopic imaging systems for hospitals, outpatient clinics, and surgical centers. Its intraoperative/interventional X-ray imaging systems combine radiographic and fluoroscopic imaging with digital image-processing capabilities to improve image quality, lower X-ray dosage, and reduce costs for a number of applications. Products include mobile X-ray imaging systems and stationary urological imaging systems. The company owns German medical equipment maker Barwig Medizinische Systeme and has wholly owned distribution subsidiaries in France, Germany, Italy, and Switzerland.

Paradigm Medical Industries, Inc.

1127 W. 2320 South, Ste. A, Salt Lake City, UT 84119

Telephone: 801-977-8970 **Fax:** 801-977-8973 **Metro area:** Salt Lake City, UT **Human resources contact:** Thomas F. Motter **Sales:** $500,000 **Number of employees:** 19 **Number of employees for previous year:** 15 **Industry designation:** Medical instruments **Company type:** Public **Top competitors:** Allergan, Inc.; Bausch & Lomb Incorporated; Alcon Laboratories, Inc.

Paradigm Medical Industries keeps baby blues seeing clearly with its ophthalmic surgical and diagnostic systems. A primary focus is cataract removal systems: The company makes the Precisionist Thirty Thousand, Precisionist 3000 Plus, and Ultrasonic Biometric Analyzer, all of which are ultrasound systems that help ophthalmologists remove cataracts. Paradigm Medical is also developing a laser system with Dixon Medical Laser Laboratory at the University of Utah. These systems can be integrated in the company's Photon Workstation with proprietary hardware and software. In addition to its cataract equipment, Paradigm Medical has developed the Blood Flow Analyzer, which can diagnose glaucoma.

Security National Financial Corporation

5300 S. 360 West, Ste. 310, Salt Lake City, UT 84123

Telephone: 801-264-1060 **Fax:** 801-265-9882 **Other address:** PO Box 57250, Salt Lake City, UT 84157 **Metro area:** Salt Lake City, UT **Human resources contact:** Diana C. Olson **Sales:** $28.5 million **Number of employees:** 186 **Number of employees for previous year:** 165 **Industry designation:** Insurance—life **Company type:** Public **Top competitors:** Southern Security Life Insurance Company; Service Corporation International; Zions Bancorporation

Life. Death. Mortgages. Security National Financial Corporation sells annuity products and life, accident, and health insurance through independent agents in 29 states. The company also owns about 60% of Florida-based Southern Security Life Insurance, which sells universal life policies. Security National also sells funeral plan policies primarily to low- and middle-income buyers and owns cemeteries and funeral homes in Arizona, California, and Utah. Other company subsidiaries make residential and commercial mortgage loans for new construction and existing homes primarily in the Salt Lake City area. Chairman and CEO George Quist controls the company.

Sento Corporation

808 E. Utah Valley Dr., American Fork, UT 84003

Telephone: 801-492-2000 **Fax:** 801-492-2100 **Other address:** PO Box 1970, Orem, UT 84059 **Metro area:** Salt Lake City, UT **Web site:** http://www.sento.com **Human resources contact:** Emily Knell **Sales:** $20.6 million **Number of employees:** 160 **Number of employees for previous year:** 76 **Industry designation:** Computers—services **Company type:** Public **Top competitors:** Arthur D. Little, Inc.; Control Data Systems, Inc.; UBICS, Inc.

Sento's into techno can-do. The information technology firm offers support wherever customers need it, specializing in training, consulting, and technical services. The company also provides systems integration, product support, help desk outsourcing, and software distribution, among other services, catering to midsized businesses and corporate divisions. The service emphasis is a change for Sento, a longtime distributor of other manufacturers' computer hardware and software. Sento continues to boost its consulting and training presence through acquisitions. Gary Godfrey, president of precursor Spire Technologies, owns 18% of Sento.

TenFold Corporation

180 W. Election Rd., Draper, UT 84020

Telephone: 801-495-1010 **Fax:** 801-495-0353 **Metro area:** Salt Lake City, UT **Web site:** http://www.10fold.com **Human resources contact:** Neil Morris **Sales:** $40.2 million (Est.) **Number of employees:** 318 **Industry designation:** Computers—services **Company type:** Private **Top competitors:** Computer Sciences Corporation; Andersen Consulting; Electronic Data Systems Corporation

TenFold is ratcheting up the competition in the information technology services industry by backing its large-scale applications development with a money-back guarantee. Offering services for a fixed price, TenFold uses its Universal Application technology to develop customized applications within a fixed period, usually four to eight months. TenFold also resells the applications it develops. Four of the company's customers (Crawford & Company, National Insurance Group, Provident Companies, and Unitrin) account for nearly 60% of its sales. Chairman, EVP, and chief technology officer Jeffrey Walker (a former Oracle EVP) founded TenFold in 1993. Walker and his family own about 59% of the company.

USANA, Inc.

3838 W. Parkway Blvd., Salt Lake City, UT 84120

Telephone: 801-954-7100 **Fax:** 801-956-9486 **Metro area:** Salt Lake City, UT **Web site:** http://www.usana.com **Sales:** $121.6 million **Number of employees:** 455 **Number of employees for previous year:** 359 **Industry designation:** Vitamins & nutritional products **Company type:** Public **Top competitors:** Amway Corporation; Herbalife International, Inc.; Nature's Sunshine Products, Inc.

USANA makes nutritional, personal care, and weight management products and sells them through a network of independent distributors in Australia, Canada, New Zealand, the UK, the US, and the Caribbean. Its nutritional supplements, including two top-selling products (USANA Essentials and Proflavanol), account for most of its sales. Additional products include USANA Sunscreen, Kids Choo-ables vitamins, shampoo and conditioners, and the LEAN (lifestyle management, education, activity, and nutrition) weight-loss program. Independent distributors, who build their sales from a network of other USANA distributors, account for all product sales. Founder Myron Wentz owns more than half of the company.

Utah Jazz

301 W. South Temple, Salt Lake City, UT 84101

Telephone: 801-325-2500 **Fax:** 801-325-2578 **Metro area:** Salt Lake City, UT **Web site:** http://www.nba.com/jazz **Human resources contact:** Jonette Jacobsmeyer **Sales:** $80.1 million (Est.) **Number of employees:** 75 **Industry designation:** Leisure & recreational services **Company type:** Private **Top competitors:** Minnesota Timberwolves; Houston Rockets; San Antonio Spurs, Ltd.

The Utah Jazz started out as the New Orleans Jazz in 1974 before moving to Salt Lake City in 1979. Despite rosters that included the likes of "Pistol" Pete Maravich, Darrel "Dr. Dunkenstein" Griffith, and Adrian Dantley, the team sang the post-season blues until 1984 when it made the playoffs for the first time (the team has returned to the playoffs every year since). The Jazz finally reached the NBA Finals in 1997 and 1998, but lost to the Chicago Bulls in both outings. All-time assist leader John Stockton and Karl "the Mailman" Malone make beautiful music together at the Delta Center, the Jazz's home court. Auto dealer Larry H. Miller bought the Jazz in 1985.

World InterNetWorks, Inc.

5152 N. Edgewood Dr., Ste. 250, Provo, UT 84604

Telephone: 801-426-1500 **Fax:** 801-762-0031 **Metro area:** Salt Lake City, UT **Human resources contact:** Steve Sager **Sales:** $7.8 million **Number of employees:** 61 **Number of employees for previous year:** 54 **Industry designation:** Computers—online services **Company type:** Public

Multilevel selling has come to the Internet. World InterNetWorks operates World Internet (WI) Mall, a virtual mall located at www.wimall.com. The company sells "storefronts" as well as merchandise to individuals for their own use or resale (although the merchandise is shipped from World InterNetWorks's own facilities). Storefront owners also receive a commission on sales made from the storefronts of people they have recruited. The company buys, imports, and warehouses most of the merchandise sold through the system. It also offers its distributors Web site development services. World InterNetWorks, Inc., was formerly known as Wealth International Inc., an import business.

ZEVEX International, Inc.

4314 ZEVEX Park Ln., Salt Lake City, UT 84123

Telephone: 801-264-1001 **Fax:** 801-264-1051 **Metro area:** Salt Lake City, UT **Human resources contact:** Dana Chisholm **Sales:** $10.5 million **Number of employees:** 155 **Number of employees for previous year:** 109 **Industry designation:** Medical products **Company type:** Public **Top competitors:** Siemens Corporation; Abbott Laboratories; Baxter International Inc.

Thanks to ZEVEX International, doctors suck—suck away cellulite and cataract fragments, that is. The company makes cataract removal systems, as well as handpieces used in ophthalmic surgery and in liposuction. It also makes air-bubble and liquid-level sensors used with such devices as intravenous systems, hemodialysis machines, and bypass surgery reservoirs. Most of its more than 100 products are designed and made for such medical device companies as Alaris Medical Systems, Allergan, Paradigm Medical Industries (its three largest customers), and Baxter Healthcare. Proprietary products include mobile enteral feeding pumps. Entities associated with investors Kirk Blosch and Jeff Holmes own about 26% of ZEVEX.

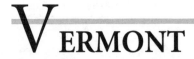

V ERMONT

Ben & Jerry's Homemade, Inc.

30 Community Dr., South Burlington, VT 05403

Telephone: 802-651-9600 **Fax:** 802-651-9646 **Metro area:** Burlington, VT **Web site:** http://www.benjerry.com **Human resources contact:** Richard Doran **Sales:** $209.2 million **Number of employees:** 751 **Number of employees for previous year:** 736 **Industry designation:** Food—dairy products **Company type:** Public **Top competitors:** Unilever; Diageo plc; Allied Domecq PLC

You're not eating ice cream because you like it, it's for charity! Ben & Jerry's Homemade is a top maker and marketer of super-premium ice cream, running scoop for scoop with Diageo's Haagen-Dazs. The quirky company sells ice cream and ice cream novelties, frozen yogurt, and sorbet with names like Cherry Garcia and Chunky Monkey. The company also franchises or owns about 170 Ben & Jerry's "scoop shops." In addition to creative flavors, Ben & Jerry's is known for social activism: The company donates almost 8% of pretax profits to philanthropic causes and seeks suppliers that minimize harmful social and agricultural practices. Ben & Jerry's products are available in the US, Canada, Japan, and in parts of Europe.

IDX Systems Corporation

1400 Shelburne Rd., South Burlington, VT 05403

Telephone: 802-862-1022 **Fax:** 802-862-9591 **Other address:** PO Box 1070, South Burlington, VT 05403 **Metro area:** Burlington, VT **Web site:** http://www.idx.com **Human resources contact:** Kim Murphy **Sales:** $321.7 million **Number of employees:** 1,833 **Number of employees for previous year:** 1,248 **Industry designation:** Computers—corporate, professional & financial software **Company type:** Public **Top competitors:** McKesson HBOC, Inc.; Shared Medical Systems Corporation

IDX Systems Corporation provides health care information systems to physician groups, management services organizations, health plans, hospitals, and integrated delivery networks. The company's software automates patient registration, billing and claim submittal, scheduling, and data management functions. It also provides physicians Internet access to patients' records. IDX's revenues come primarily from licensing its software products (at some 1,550 sites serving more than 96,000 physicians); installation, maintenance, and service fees; and the sale of hardware.

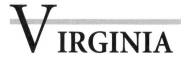

VIRGINIA

Advanced Engineering & Research Associates, Inc.

1919 S. Eads St., Ste. 400, Arlington, VA 22202

Telephone: 703-486-1993 **Fax:** 703-486-0795 **Metro area:** Washington, DC **Web site:** http://www.aera.com **Human resources contact:** Metta Vongsanghaier **Sales:** $25 million (Est.) **Number of employees:** 250 **Number of employees for previous year:** 225 **Industry designation:** Computers—services **Company type:** Private **Top competitors:** Metters Industries Inc.; Digital Systems International Corporation; CACI International Inc

Advanced Engineering & Research Associates (AERA) aims to improve efficiency in its clients' systems and employees. It provides services in information technology, acquisition logistics, systems engineering, interactive multimedia, and facilities engineering. AERA's areas of expertise include marine and aviation propulsion engineering, computer-based training, and electronic performance support systems (EPSS). Using support tools such as "applets" and "wizards," EPSS allows new users to easily navigate software. AERA first created these systems for NASA's Goddard Space Flight Center. The company's ten US offices serve government and commercial customers. Ned Daffan and three partners founded AERA in 1988.

American Safety Razor Company

One Razor Blade Ln., Verona, VA 24482

Telephone: 540-248-8000 **Fax:** 540-248-0522 **Web site:** http://www.thomasregister.com/olc/blades **Human resources contact:** Reginald B. Ryals **Sales:** $297.5 million **Number of employees:** 2,257 **Number of employees for previous year:** 2,100 **Industry designation:** Cosmetics & toiletries **Company type:** Public **Top competitors:** Warner-Lambert Company; Societe BIC S.A.; The Gillette Company

With single-digit market share, American Safety Razor (ASR) doesn't exactly give top stubblebuster Gillette a close shave. ASR's main products are value-priced shaving razors and blades. It also makes shaving soap, shaving cream, and aftershave; cotton products (cotton swabs, cotton balls, cosmetic pads, coils, pocket tissue, and foot care products); bladed hand tools (carpet knives, wall and floor strippers, and window scrapers); bar soap; and specialty industrial and medical blades. ASR sells its wares under such brand names as Personna, Burma Shave, GEM, Flicker, Bump Fighter, Blue Star, Pal, MBC, Royal, and Treet. Investment firm J. W. Childs is buying the company.

America Online, Inc.

22000 AOL Way, Dulles, VA 20166

Telephone: 703-448-8700 **Fax:** 703-918-1400 **Metro area:** Washington, DC **Web site:** http://www.aol.com **Human resources contact:** Mark Stavish **Sales:** $2.6 billion **Number of employees:** 8,500 **Number of employees for previous year:** 7,371 **Industry designation:** Computers—online services **Company type:** Public **Top competitors:** AT&T Corp.; Yahoo! Inc.; Microsoft Corporation

Its 16 million subscribers make America Online (AOL) the world's #1 provider of online services. AOL's 1998 acquisition of CompuServe (now subsidiary CompuServe Interactive Services), which has two million subscribers, boosted AOL's market share to 60%. AOL appeals to those seeking entertainment, but CompuServe is geared toward professionals and small-business owners. Its purchase of Netscape Communications in 1999 brought the popular Navigator Web browser and the Netcenter Internet portal into the AOL fold. AOL is looking beyond subscriber fees for revenues. It is working to sell advertising on its Web site and forging marketing agreements with other companies, collecting fees on sales to AOL subscribers.

BTG, Inc.

3877 Fairfax Ridge Rd., Fairfax, VA 22030

Telephone: 703-383-8000 **Fax:** 703-383-8999 **Metro area:** Washington, DC **Web site:** http://www.btg.com **Human resources contact:** Karen Wall **Sales:** $588.9 million **Number of employees:** 1,319 **Number of employees for previous year:** 1,168 **Industry designation:** Computers—services **Company type:** Public **Top competitors:** Science Applications International Corporation; Electronic Data Systems Corporation; Computer Sciences Corporation

BTG helps the government help itself. The company provides engineering, systems integration, and networking services to government agencies such as the US Department of Defense, US General Services Administration, and the Federal Aviation Administration. Its systems have been used in US military operations to track troop movement and other intelligence activity. More than 90% of its sales are from government contracts. Other services include e-commerce, Web development, network support, and distance learning. The company has sold its decreasingly profitable computer reselling business unit.

CACI International Inc

1100 N. Glebe Rd., Arlington, VA 22201

Telephone: 703-841-7800 **Fax:** 703-841-7882 **Metro area:** Washington, DC **Web site:** http://www.caci.com **Human resources contact:** William J. Clancy Jr. **Sales:** $326.1 million **Number of employees:** 3,700 **Number of employees for previous year:** 3,450 **Industry designation:** Computers—services **Company type:** Public **Top competitors:** Electronic Data Systems Corporation; PRC Inc.; Nichols Research Corporation

CACI International turns simulated processes into real profits. The company provides simulation technology for factory design, computer networks, communications systems, and the US Army's war games. It also supplies software and services for electronic commerce, digital document management, logistics, and year 2000 conversion. Nearly three-fourths of CACI's sales are to the US government, with the US Department of Defense alone accounting for nearly half of its sales. The company also serves commercial clients and state and local governments. Almost 90% of CACI's sales are within the US. The company has a UK-based subsidiary and offices in France and Germany.

Carilion Health System

1212 Third St., Roanoke, VA 24016

Telephone: 540-981-7900 **Fax:** 540-344-5716 **Other address:** P.O. Box 13727, Roanoke, VA 24036 **Metro area:** Roanoke, VA **Web site:** http://www.carilion.com **Human resources contact:** Houston L. Bell Jr. **Sales:** $780 million **Number of employees:** 8,728 **Number of employees for previous year:** 8,500 **Industry designation:** Hospitals **Company type:** Not-for-profit **Top competitors:** Columbia/HCA Healthcare Corporation; Mid Atlantic Medical Services, Inc.; Sentara Health System

As Virginia's largest health care network, Carilion Health System rings true. The system includes 11 hospitals, a nursing home, and a cancer center. Its Medical Center for Children in Roanoke serves as a regional pediatric referral site, and its Carilion Behavioral Health has become western Virginia's largest psychiatric service network. Through its 50%-owned, for-profit Carilion Health Plans subsidiary, the system now markets its own HMO and point-of-service health care plans and also two insurance plans. Carilion also offers hospice and home care services. Affiliated institutions include an athletic club and two wellness centers.

CEL-SCI Corporation

8229 Boone Blvd., Ste. 802, Vienna, VA 22182

Telephone: 703-506-9460 **Fax:** 703-506-9471 **Metro area:** Washington, DC **Web site:** http://www.cel-sci.com **Human resources contact:** Patricia B. Prichep **Sales:** $100,000 **Number of employees:** 39 **Number of employees for previous year:** 30 **Industry designation:** Biomedical & genetic products **Company type:** Public **Top competitors:** Progenics Pharmaceuticals, Inc.; Chiron Corporation; Cantab Pharmaceuticals plc

Development-stage CEL-SCI is working on immunotherapy drugs for cancer patients, and vaccines to prevent AIDS. The company's MULTIKINE product—made through a proprietary cell-culture technique—is being tested to treat head and neck cancer, prostate cancer, and HIV. CEL-SCI's LEAPS is a technology which may lead to synthetic vaccines for AIDS, tuberculosis, malaria, and herpes. The company's Viral Technologies subsidiary is testing potential AIDS vaccine HGP-30. CEL-SCI collaborates with other organizations, including Northeastern Ohio University, to fund research and develop applications for its products, which are in clinical tests in the US and other countries.

Commonwealth Biotechnologies, Inc.

911 E. Leigh St., Ste. G-19, Richmond, VA 23219

Telephone: 804-648-3820 **Fax:** 804-648-2641 **Metro area:** Richmond, VA **Web site:** http://www.cbi-biotech.com **Human resources contact:** Karen Hall **Sales:** $1.8 million **Number of employees:** 36 **Number of employees for previous year:** 33 **Industry designation:** Biomedical & genetic products **Company type:** Public **Top competitors:** Hyseq, Inc.; Genset; QIAGEN N.V.

Commonwealth Biotechnologies (CBI), working for the good of all, provides research and development services to biotechnology companies, academic institutions, and government agencies. Operating on both short- and long-term contractual bases, CBI serves more than 350 customers worldwide. Services consist of DNA analyses, genome and peptide/protein sequencing, compositional analyses, and other genetic research. Through its own proprietary research, funded through grants from such agencies as the National Institute of Health and the US Department of Agriculture, CBI is also developing anti-coagulation and other technologies for eventual licensing to other companies.

Deltek Systems, Inc.

8280 Greensboro Dr., McLean, VA 22102

Telephone: 703-734-8606 **Fax:** 703-734-0346 **Metro area:** Washington, DC **Web site:** http://www.deltek.com **Human resources contact:** Mary Burden **Sales:** $83.1 million **Number of employees:** 555 **Number of employees for previous year:** 353 **Industry designation:** Computers—corporate, professional & financial software **Company type:** Public **Top competitors:** PeopleSoft, Inc.; Oracle Corporation; SAP AG

Deltek Systems helps project-oriented companies manage, operate, and grow their businesses. Its client/server software includes Costpoint, an enterprisewide project accounting system; System 1, a DOS-based accounting and management program designed especially for businesses working with the federal government; Electronic Timesheet, an employee timekeeping system; and Allegro, a project and resource management tool. Software modules include accounting, human resources and payroll, materials management, and reporting tools. Deltek's more than 2,000 clients include Lockheed Martin, Raytheon, and Xerox. Co-founders Donald and Kenneth deLaski (chairman and CEO, respectively) together own almost 60% of Deltek.

Digital Systems International Corporation

4301 N. Fairfax Dr., Ste. 725, Arlington, VA 22203

Telephone: 703-522-6067 **Fax:** 703-522-6367 **Metro area:** Washington, DC **Web site:** http://www.dsint.com **Sales:** $106 million (Est.) **Number of employees:** 900 **Number of employees for previous year:** 821 **Industry designation:** Computers—services **Company type:** Private **Top competitors:** BTG, Inc.; Metters Industries Inc.; CACI International Inc

Founded in 1988, Digital Systems International offers a variety of information technology services primarily to federal organizations. The company provides enterprise resource planning, e-commerce, and procurement systems; installs and services communications networks and transaction processing systems; and designs and distributes secure document delivery systems (IFX, InPhase). Subsidiary Earl Industries repairs US Navy and commercial ships and provides related industrial services. Customers include the US Postal Service, the Navy, and the Department of Defense. Consulting, training, and support services are also available. CEO Willie Woods owns the company.

Doughtie's Foods, Inc.

2410 Wesley St., Portsmouth, VA 23707

Telephone: 757-393-6007 **Fax:** 757-399-3558 **Metro area:** Norfolk, VA **Human resources contact:** Sharon Stevens **Sales:** $85.2 million **Number of employees:** 211 **Number of employees for previous year:** 210 **Industry designation:** Food—meat products **Company type:** Public **Top competitors:** Hormel Foods Corporation; Thorn Apple Valley, Inc.; Foodbrands America, Inc.

It's a meat market at Doughtie's Foods—barbecue, chili, and deli meats. Formerly a meat and seafood processor, Doughtie's Foods has sold its manufacturing operations in order to focus on food distribution. The company's meats keep the Doughtie's brand name, but other companies now supply the products. From its Virginia distribution center, Doughtie's Foods also sells a variety of other items, including produce, eggs, dry and canned goods, and restaurant supplies. Customers include supermarkets, restaurants, schools, and hospitals in Delaware, the District of Columbia, Maryland, North Carolina, and Virginia. Family trusts established by late founder Robert Doughtie control half of the company.

Erols Internet, Inc.

7921 Woodruff Ct., Springfield, VA 22151

Telephone: 703-321-8000 **Fax:** 703-321-8707 **Metro area:** Washington, DC **Web site:** http://www.erols.com **Human resources contact:** Patty Perkins **Sales:** $10.9 million **Number of employees:** 293 **Industry designation:** Computers—online services **Company type:** Subsidiary **Top competitors:** CompuServe Interactive Services, Inc.; America Online, Inc.; AT&T Corp.

Like Errol Flynn's swashbuckler movies, Erols Internet plays well in the East. The Internet service provider (ISP) ranks #1 in its market, with more than 320,000 residential and business subscribers in the Boston-Washington, DC, corridor. Customers can get reduced rates by paying in advance for long-term contracts. Erols' services include dial-up and high-speed Internet access, Internet security, e-commerce support, and Web site design and hosting. The company provides news and entertainment content through a partnership with Planet Direct, a subsidiary of CMG Information Services. Telecommunications services provider RCN acquired Erols in 1998.

Fuisz Technologies Ltd.

14555 Avion at Lakeside, Chantilly, VA 20151

Telephone: 703-995-2400 **Fax:** 703-803-6460 **Metro area:** Washington, DC **Human resources contact:** Jale Osgood **Sales:** $61.2 million **Number of employees:** 411 **Number of employees for previous year:** 116 **Industry designation:** Drugs **Company type:** Public

Fuisz Technologies develops and manufactures its proprietary CEFORM and SHEARFORM technologies for oral drug delivery and food applications. The company's primary focus is on the commercialization of its rapid dissolving tablet and controlled release technologies, principally for over-the-counter pharmaceuticals. The company has applied its technology to develop two rapid dissolving tablets, FlashDose and EZ Chew. Fuisz Technologies intends to market its rapid dissolving tablets through licensing arrangements with third parties. Subsidiary FuiszDrugStore.com sells over-the-counter pharmaceuticals online. Fuisz has research and manufacturing facilities in the US and Ireland.

Guardian Technologies International

22570 Markey Ct., Dulles, VA 20166

Telephone: 703-444-7931 **Fax:** 703-444-9894 **Metro area:** Washington, DC **Web site:** http://www.guardiantech.com **Human resources contact:** Nancy Anderson **Sales:** $1.2 million **Number of employees:** 30 **Number of employees for previous year:** 21 **Industry designation:** Protection—safety equipment & services **Company type:** Public **Top competitors:** Bodycote International plc; DHB Capital Group Inc.; Armor Holdings, Inc.

Under heavy fire from financial fallout, Guardian Technologies may need to take refuge under its own products. Guardian Technologies markets body armor to US and foreign law enforcement agencies, private security firms, US military organizations, and foreign defense forces. The company manufactures and distributes bulletproof vests, shields, blankets, seat-cover liners, and other protective gear, including K-9 vests and men's and women's undergarments. The firm's auditors have issued a warning about its stability, and chairman Oliver North's salary has been slashed. North, a controversial figure, was once an aide to US President Ronald Reagan and gained notoriety in the 1980s for his role in illegal arms sales.

InfraCorps Inc.

7400 Beaufont Springs Dr., Ste 415, Richmond, VA 23225

Telephone: 804-272-6600 **Fax:** 804-272-1110 **Metro area:** Richmond, VA **Web site:** http://www.etsi-inc.com **Human resources contact:** Warren E. Beam Jr. **Sales:** $12.6 million **Number of employees:** 149 **Number of employees for previous year:** 89 **Industry designation:** Pollution control equipment & services **Company type:** Public **Top competitors:** ITEQ, Inc.; TRC Companies, Inc.; Aqua Alliance Inc.

InfraCorps, formerly ETS International, specializes in the installation and renovation of water, wastewater, and gas utility pipelines. Its wholly owned subsidiaries include InfraCorps of Virginia, a construction firm, and InfraCorps of Florida, which uses trenchless technologies to install and repair subsurface pipelines. The company sold its patents and licenses for its Limestone Emission Control (LEC) system to Christel Clear Technologies, a newly formed company owned by former company officers and directors. InfrCorps also sold its ETS Analytical Services to Q Enterprises, also owned by a former company officer. A prior contract to build LEC systems in China has placed InfraCorps at risk.

Inova Health System

2990 Telestar Ct., Falls Church, VA 22042

Telephone: 703-289-2000 **Fax:** 703-289-2070 **Metro area:** Washington, DC **Web site:** http://www.inova.com **Human resources contact:** Ellen Menard **Sales:** $915 million **Number of employees:** 13,000 **Number of employees for previous year:** 9,500 **Industry designation:** Hospitals **Company type:** Not-for-profit **Top competitors:** Columbia/HCA Healthcare Corporation; Helix/Medlantic; The Johns Hopkins Health System Corporation

Inova Health System is Virginia's largest not-for-profit health care provider. It provides acute and subacute care, long-term care, home health care, and mental health, obstetrics, and gynecological services in the Virginia suburbs of Washington, DC. Inova's network includes five hospitals, as well as assisted-living centers (for those needing less-constant care than nursing homes provide) and several family practice locations. The system maintains affiliations with about 3,500 physicians. Founded in 1956 as a country hospital in Fairfax, Virginia, the system has grown in sophistication and scope as metropolitan Washington, DC, has expanded into its area.

Mars, Inc.

6885 Elm St., McLean, VA 22101

Telephone: 703-821-4900 **Fax:** 703-448-9678 **Metro area:** Washington, DC **Web site:** http://www.mars.com **Sales:** $15 billion (Est.) **Number of employees:** 30,000 **Number of employees for previous year:** 28,500 **Industry designation:** Food—confectionery **Company type:** Private **Top competitors:** Nestle S.A.; Hershey Foods Corporation; Ralston Purina Company

Mars is the #2 US candy maker, after Hershey. It makes M&M's, the #1 chocolate candy in the world, 3 Musketeers, Dove, Milky Way, Skittles, Snickers, and Starburst candies. Other products include ice cream versions of several of its candy bars; Combos, Kudos, and Twix snacks; Uncle Ben's rice, the US market leader; and pet food under the names Kal Kan, Pedigree, Sheba, and Whiskas. It also manufactures drink vending equipment and electronic automated payment systems. Co-presidents and brothers John Mars and Forrest Mars Jr., their sister VP Jacqueline Mars Vogel, and father (Forrest Sr.), own the highly secretive $14 billion enterprise—making the Mars family one of the richest in the country.

Metro Information Services, Inc.

200 Golden Oaks Ct., Virginia Beach, VA 23450

Telephone: 757-486-1900 **Fax:** 757-306-0251 **Other address:** PO Box 8888, Virginia Beach, VA 23450 **Metro area:** Norfolk, VA **Web site:** http://www.metrois.com **Human resources contact:** Marilynn C. Moschel **Sales:** $213.9 million **Number of employees:** 2,469 **Number of employees for previous year:** 2,074 **Industry designation:** Computers—services **Company type:** Public

Metro Information Services fills employment gaps with information technology (IT) consulting and custom software development. These include application systems development and maintenance, IT architecture and engineering, systems consulting, project outsourcing, and general support services. The acquisitive company offers services in all major computer technology platforms to businesses in such industries as communications, financial services, health care, and manufacturing. The company has about 40 branches and 2,500 consultants. John Fain, who is the company's chairman, president, and CEO, owns nearly 60% of Metro Information Services.

Metters Industries Inc.

8200 Greensboro Dr., Ste. 500, McLean, VA 22102

Telephone: 703-821-3300 **Fax:** 703-821-3996 **Metro area:** Washington, DC **Web site:** http://www.metters.com **Human resources contact:** Fred Atkinson **Sales:** $37.8 million (Est.) **Number of employees:** 450 **Industry designation:** Computers—services **Company type:** Private **Top competitors:** PRC Inc.; Nichols Research Corporation; CACI International Inc

Samuel Metters left the service and joined the services. Metters is the founder, owner, and CEO of systems integrator Metters Industries. The company, which he started in the early 1980s after retiring from the US Army, also offers services such as Web page design, software and database development, training, logistics and other engineering support, and network consulting and integration. Metters Industries makes products such as document management software (OPTIX), military simulators, and microfilm scanners and other optics-based systems. The majority of its customers are defense and federal entities. Other clients include Federal Express, Marriott International, and Mobil.

Mobil Chemical Company

3225 Gallows Rd., Fairfax, VA 22037

Telephone: 703-846-3000 **Fax:** 703-846-4669 **Metro area:** Washington, DC **Web site:** http://www.mobil.com/business/chemical/index.html **Human resources contact:** Ron Schaefer **Sales:** $3.5 billion **Number of employees:** 4,100 **Industry designation:** Chemicals—diversified **Company type:** Subsidiary

If you need to orient your polypropylene or catalyze your zeolites, Mobil Chemical may be able to oblige. Mobil Chemical's 30 facilities turn petroleum into a wide variety of petrochemical products and base stocks, from fuel additives and lubricants to toys and Frito packages. Its petrochemical division makes olefins and aromatics, which are used to make various "enes" —ethylene, propylene, and polyethylene. The films division produces oriented polypropylene films for food packaging and other uses. The company's chemical products operation makes fuel additives, synthetic lubricant base stocks, zeolite catalysts, and other products. Mobil Chemical is a subsidiary of Mobil Corporation.

The Motley Fool, Inc.

123 N. Pitt St., Alexandria, VA 22314

Telephone: 703-838-3665 **Fax:** 703-684-3603 **Metro area:** Washington, DC **Web site:** http://www.fool.com **Human resources contact:** Julie Tammenin **Sales:** $2 million (Est.) **Number of employees:** 130 **Number of employees for previous year:** 105 **Industry designation:** Computers—online services **Company type:** Private **Top competitors:** TheStreet.com, Inc.; Market Guide Inc.; Yahoo! Inc.

The jokers at the Motley Fool, a free online financial advice service, say their mission is "to inform, amuse, and enrich" investors. Founded as a newsletter by brothers David and Tom Gardner in 1993, the Motley Fool Web site attracts over one million visitors a month. It offers financial news, research, and analysis, as well as a message board where investors can share information. The company also publishes a series of books and produces a syndicated weekly column that appears in more than 145 newspapers across the US. Other media ventures include "The Motley Fool Radio Show" (a joint venture with Cox Radio), commentary on "Marketplace Radio," and an international Web site (Motley Fool UK).

Network Solutions, Inc.

505 Huntmar Park Dr., Herndon, VA 20170

Telephone: 703-742-0400 **Fax:** 703-742-3386 **Metro area:** Washington, DC **Web site:** http://www.netsol.com **Human resources contact:** Carla Leavelle **Sales:** $93.7 million **Number of employees:** 260 **Number of employees for previous year:** 220 **Industry designation:** Computers—online services **Company type:** Public **Parent company:** Science Applications International Corporation **Top competitors:** Andersen Worldwide; International Network Services; International Business Machines Corporation

Network Solutions is—for now, at least—the exclusive registrar of Internet addresses ending in domains .com, .org, .net, and .edu. The company, which earns more than 85% of its sales from registration services, has registered over three million addresses. Network Solutions also provides intranet development and network security services. The company's exclusive registration contract with the US government, which was set to expire in 1998, has been extended while the transition to a not-for-profit administrative body and an openly competitive registration system is set. Research and development powerhouse Science Applications International owns 45% of Network Solutions and controls 90% of the voting power.

Online Resources & Communications Corporation

7600 Colshire Dr., McLean, VA 22102

Telephone: 703-394-5100 **Fax:** 703-394-5105 **Metro area:** Washington, DC **Web site:** http://www.orcc.com **Human resources contact:** Beth Nettuno **Sales:** $4.3 million (Est.) **Number of employees:** 171 **Industry designation:** Computers—services **Company type:** Private **Top competitors:** Integrion Financial Network LLC; Microsoft Corporation; CheckFree Holdings Corporation

Regional and community financial institutions looking for a Web commerce presence can take Online Resources & Communications' systems to the bank. The company's turnkey Opus system enables such financial services as remote banking, electronic bill payment, and investment management. Online Resources also offers Web site design and hosting services and an Internet portal site (Financial Service Center) that provides access to Web banking, insurance, and investment services. The company serves more than 300 banks and credit unions across the US. Online Resources was co-founded in 1989 by CEO Matthew Lawlor, a former venture capitalist and Chemical Bank executive who owns nearly 20% of the company.

PHP Healthcare Corporation

11440 Commerce Park Dr., Reston, VA 20191

Telephone: 703-758-3600 **Fax:** 703-758-7249 **Metro area:** Washington, DC **Web site:** http://www.phphealthcare.com **Human resources contact:** John Bucur **Sales:** $400.1 million **Number of employees:** 3,300 **Number of employees for previous year:** 3,100 **Industry designation:** Health care—outpatient & home **Company type:** Public **Top competitors:** Aetna Inc.; UnitedHealth Group; Humana Inc.

PHP Healthcare Corporation provides managed health care services to government agencies, the US military, and large corporations such as GTE and Bethlehem Steel. The company offers primary and specialty medical care and services through its networks of affiliated physicians and hospitals. In markets with large enough clients, PHP operates its own medical centers. It has two divisions: one to provide service to commercial clients and one to serve government agencies. PHP manages more than 80 health care operations in 29 states, the District of Columbia, Puerto Rico, and Panama. Retired founder Charles Robbins retains some 17% of the company, which has filed for Chapter 11 bankruptcy protection.

Pittston Brink's Group

1000 Virginia Center Pkwy., Glen Allen, VA 23058

Telephone: 804-553-3600 **Fax:** 804-553-3750 **Other address:** PO Box 4229, Glen Allen, VA 23058 **Metro area:** Richmond, VA **Web site:** http://www.brinks.com **Human resources contact:** Frank T. Lennon **Sales:** $1.5 billion **Number of employees:** 41,800 **Number of employees for previous year:** 22,400 **Industry designation:** Protection—safety equipment & services **Company type:** Public **Top competitors:** Borg-Warner Security Corporation; Protection One, Inc.; Tyco International Ltd.

For Pittston Brink's Group, crime pays. The company has two major businesses: Brink's and Brink's Home Security. Brink's provides armored car services, currency and deposit processing, ATM servicing, and air courier services worldwide. Brink's Home Security installs, maintains, and monitors electronic home security systems in the US and Canada and has more than 500,000 subscribers to its security monitoring system. Pittston Brinks is one of three separately traded stocks that make up the Pittston Company. The other two are Pittston BAX Group (airfreight) and Pittston Minerals Group (mining).

PRC Inc.

1500 PRC Dr., McLean, VA 22102

Telephone: 703-556-1000 **Fax:** 703-556-1174 **Metro area:** Washington, DC **Web site:** http://www.prc.com **Human resources contact:** Walter Goodlett **Sales:** $834 million **Number of employees:** 5,800 **Number of employees for previous year:** 5,600 **Industry designation:** Computers—services **Company type:** Subsidiary **Parent company:** Litton Industries, Inc. **Top competitors:** Computer Sciences Corporation; Andersen Consulting; Electronic Data Systems Corporation

Uncle Sam wants to become automated, and PRC wants to help. A subsidiary of Litton Industries, PRC offers information technology (IT) services such as systems integration and desktop outsourcing to government entities and commercial customers. Using its Flexible Information Technology (FlexIT) development tool, the company creates and implements customized systems that have the cost and schedule advantages associated with mass-produced systems. Benefiting from growing public-sector demand for IT services, PRC is the lead contractor for the General Services Administration's PC operations outsourcing program. The company has more than 175 offices worldwide.

Pro-Football, Inc.

21300 Redskins Park Dr., Ashburn, VA 20147

Telephone: 703-478-8900 **Fax:** 703-729-7605 **Metro area:** Washington, DC **Web site:** http://www.nfl.com/redskins/index.html **Sales:** $115.1 million (Est.) **Number of employees:** 100 **Industry designation:** Leisure & recreational services **Company type:** Private **Top competitors:** Arizona Cardinals; New York Giants; Dallas Cowboys Football Club, Ltd.

Pro-Football, Inc. is one of Washington, DC's most recognizable institutions—the Washington Redskins. The team dates to 1932, when it was known as the Boston Braves. It changed its name in 1933 and moved to Washington, DC, four years later. The team, which moved to Jack Kent Cooke Stadium in 1997, holds an NFL record for 30 consecutive sold-out seasons. As part of the nation's most-watched sports league, the Redskins expect to get almost $80 million a year from a new NFL TV contract. A new ownership group that includes banking brothers Howard and Edward Milstein (45% owners of the NHL's New York Islanders), and Daniel Snyer (CEO of Snyer Communications) is buying the team for a record $750 million

Proxicom, Inc.

11600 Sunrise Valley Dr., Reston, VA 20191

Telephone: 703-262-3200 **Fax:** 703-262-3201 **Metro area:** Washington, DC **Web site:** http://www.proxicom.com **Human resources contact:** Brenda Wagner **Sales:** $42.4 million (Est.) **Number of employees:** 380 **Number of employees for previous year:** 245 **Industry designation:** Computers—online services **Company type:** Private **Top competitors:** Organic Online, Inc.; iXL Enterprises, Inc.; USWeb/CKS

Point and purchase. Proxicom brings e-commerce to Web sites that link organizations to consumers and other businesses in the energy, telecommunications, retail, manufacturing, and financial services markets. The company also designs intranets for internal corporate communications. Services include consulting, marketing, application development, systems and network design, and legacy and third-party software integration. Proxicom's largest customers are Pacific Gas and Electric (15% of sales) and General Electric (14%). Founder, chairman, and CEO Raul Fernandez owns about 45% of the company, which plans to provide Web consulting services in Italy through a joint venture with Ericsson.

PSINet Inc.

510 Huntmar Park Dr., Herndon, VA 20170

Telephone: 703-904-4100 **Fax:** 703-904-4200 **Metro area:** Washington, DC **Web site:** http://www.psi.net **Human resources contact:** William P. Cripe **Sales:** $259.6 million **Number of employees:** 775 **Number of employees for previous year:** 515 **Industry designation:** Computers—online services **Company type:** Public **Top competitors:** MCI WorldCom, Inc.; Sprint Corporation; AT&T Corp.

PSINet is big in the business of linking big business to the Internet. The company offers a variety of access services, Web-site design and hosting, electronic commerce, and security programs. PSINet has offices in 11 countries and serves 26,500 corporate customers. Many Internet service companies are being acquired by large telecommunications companies, but PSINet remains independent, focusing instead on its own expansion. The company is no longer an Internet service provider (ISP) for individual consumers, but it does allow other consumer-based ISPs to use its networks for a fee. IXC Communications owns a 20% stake in the company in exchange for giving PSINet access to IXC's high-speed digital phone lines.

RBX Corporation

5221 Valleypark Dr., Roanoke, VA 24019

Telephone: 540-561-6100 **Fax:** 540-561-6141 **Metro area:** Roanoke, VA **Human resources contact:** Mark T. Dobbins **Sales:** $281.7 million (Est.) **Number of employees:** 2,272 **Number of employees for previous year:** 2,036 **Industry designation:** Rubber & plastic products **Company type:** Private **Top competitors:** Sekisui Chemical Co., Ltd.; Carpenter Co.

RBX Corporation and its subsidiaries have a solid grip on the rubber foam market. The company makes generic and custom-mixed closed-cell rubber foam, polyethylene foam, and mixed rubber compounds. Closed-cell rubber foam is used to make insulation, wetsuits, beverage can insulators, computer mouse pads, and other products; polyethylene foam is used to make packaging and marine buoys. The company's custom-mixed rubber polymers are sold to original equipment manufacturers for making auto tires, car parts, and agricultural tools. The company is 99%-controlled by American Industrial Partners, including president and CEO Theodore Rogers and chairman Tom Barrett (a former chairman of Goodyear).

Sentara Health System

6015 Poplar Hall Dr., Ste. 300, Norfolk, VA 23502

Telephone: 757-455-7000 **Fax:** 757-455-7964 **Metro area:** Norfolk, VA **Web site:** http://www.sentara.com **Human resources contact:** Vicki Humphries **Sales:** $900.9 million **Number of employees:** 8,190 **Number of employees for previous year:** 7,734 **Industry designation:** Hospitals **Company type:** Not-for-profit **Top competitors:** Carilion Health System; Bon Secours Health System, Inc.; Riverside Health System

Health care's a beach for Sentara Health System. The not-for-profit organization operates more than 70 facilities throughout southeastern Virginia and northeastern North Carolina. The system has six hospitals, nine assisted-living centers, about 40 health care centers, an integrated outpatient health care campus, and a fitness center. Additionally, Sentara offers health coverage (including HMOs) for more than 270,000 people. The company also provides home health services, ground and air medical transport, community health education programs, and mobile diagnostic vans. After merging with rival Tidewater Health Care, Sentara owns Virginia Beach's two hospitals (Virginia Beach General and Sentara Bayside).

Smithfield Foods, Inc.

200 Commerce St., Smithfield, VA 23430

Telephone: 757-365-3000 **Fax:** 757-365-3017 **Metro area:** Norfolk, VA **Human resources contact:** Tom Ross **Sales:** $3.9 billion **Number of employees:** 19,500 **Number of employees for previous year:** 17,500 **Industry designation:** Food—meat products **Company type:** Public **Top competitors:** Cargill, Incorporated; ConAgra, Inc.; IBP, inc.

Smithfield Foods is the largest fresh-pork processor in the US, with #2 IBP right on its curly tail. The vertically integrated company has interests in hog research and hog farms (its acquisition of Carroll's Foods will make it the top US hog producer as well). Its products include fresh pork and processed meats sold under the John Morrell, Lykes, Patrick Cudahy, Fleetwood, Schneider, and Smithfield names. Its flagship fresh-pork brand, Smithfield Lean Generation Pork, is distributed nationally. Smithfield Foods sells its products to grocery stores, food distributors, and food service operators. It distributes nationally and in Japan and Mexico, and it is making major moves into Canada and Europe.

Sunrise Assisted Living, Inc.

9401 Lee Hwy., Ste. 300, Fairfax, VA 22031

Telephone: 703-273-7500 **Fax:** 703-273-7501 **Metro area:** Washington, DC **Web site:** http://www.sunrise-al.com **Human resources contact:** Christine Braccio **Sales:** $170.7 million **Number of employees:** 5,190 **Number of employees for previous year:** 3,377 **Industry designation:** Nursing homes **Company type:** Public **Top competitors:** Genesis Health Ventures, Inc.; Emeritus Assisted Living; Sun Healthcare Group, Inc.

Sunrise Assisted Living provides alternatives to nursing homes primarily to higher-income senior citizens at about 70 facilities in 13 states. The company's facilities, each designed to resemble a Victorian manor, feature single- and double-occupancy suites and offer assistance with such daily living activities as bathing, eating, and dressing; medication management and Alzheimer's care can also be arranged. Sunrise facilities contract with outside providers for services such as infusion therapy. Sunrise often sells its facilities as part of its business plan but stays on to manage them. It operates in the Atlantic states from New York to Florida but also has facilities in California, Colorado, and Washington.

Trigon Healthcare, Inc.

2015 Staples Mill Rd., Richmond, VA 23230

Telephone: 804-354-7000 **Fax:** 804-354-3399 **Metro area:** Richmond, VA **Web site:** http://www.trigon.com **Human resources contact:** Ann Odehnal **Sales:** $2.2 billion **Number of employees:** 3,740 **Number of employees for previous year:** 3,583 **Industry designation:** Health maintenance organization **Company type:** Public

Virginia's largest managed health care company, Trigon Healthcare, serves about 1.8 million members (more than 25% of the state's population) through provider networks. Its network consists of HMOs, PPOs, and participating provider networks. It offers both fully insured arrangements (Trigon provides specified services for a fixed fee) and self-funded programs (the customer bears all or a portion of the risk). It also offers specialty products such as dental, wellness, and disability insurance coverage and provides employee benefits and workers' compensation administration and health management services. Products are marketed to groups and individuals under the Blue Cross/Blue Shield name in Virginia.

User Technology Associates, Inc.

950 N. Glebe Rd., Ste. 100, Arlington, VA 22203

Telephone: 703-522-5132 **Fax:** 703-522-6457 **Metro area:** Washington, DC **Web site:** http://www.utanet.com/main.htm **Human resources contact:** Paul Bonolis **Sales:** $57 million (Est.) **Number of employees:** 800 **Industry designation:** Computers—services **Company type:** Private

User Technology Associates (UTA) provides computer and support services such as software development, information technology, telecommunications engineering, logistics, and acquisitions management. Some of its core disciplines include space operations software (enlisted for Pathfinder and Voyager missions), law enforcement software, and year 2000 solutions. The company has 18 sites in Washington, DC, another 18 across the US, and overseas offices in the UK and South Korea. UTA is a prime contractor and subcontracts at 30 federal agencies, including the Defense Nuclear Agency and the FDIC. President and CEO Yong Kim founded the company in 1985.

UUNET WorldCom

3060 Williams Dr., Fairfax, VA 22031

Telephone: 703-206-5600 **Fax:** 703-206-5601 **Metro area:** Washington, DC **Web site:** http://www.uu.net **Human resources contact:** Diana E. Lawrence **Sales:** $265 million **Number of employees:** 1,400 **Number of employees for previous year:** 306 **Industry designation:** Computers—online services **Company type:** Subsidiary **Parent company:** WorldCom, Inc. **Top competitors:** GTE Corporation; Sprint Corporation; AT&T Corp.

I am he as U are he as U are me and we are all together on the Internet ... and many of us get there through UUNET WorldCom, one of the world's largest Internet service providers (ISPs). A subsidiary of telecom titan MCI WorldCom, UUNET provides Internet access over its backbone network for businesses, small ISPs, and both America Online and the Microsoft Network. The company owns and operates Internet networks in Canada, the US, and nine European countries; UUNet also maintains connections with ISPs in the Asia/Pacific region.

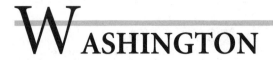

W ASHINGTON

Advanced Digital Information Corporation

11431 Willows Rd. N.E., Redmond, WA 98052

Telephone: 425-881-8004 **Fax:** 425-881-2296 **Other address:** P.O. Box 97057, Redmond, WA 98073 **Metro area:** Seattle, WA **Web site:** http://www.adic.com **Human resources contact:** Judy Porterfield **Sales:** $114.6 million **Number of employees:** 566 **Number of employees for previous year:** 208 **Industry designation:** Computers—peripheral equipment **Company type:** Public **Top competitors:** International Business Machines Corporation; Quantum Corporation; Hewlett-Packard Company

Tape it to the limit, one more time. Advanced Digital Information Corporation (ADIC) makes automated tape libraries. The company buys tape drives from other manufacturers and outfits them with robotic arms. These arms select a tape from a multi-tape unit, then add or access data. Units range from desktop-size to large, stand-alone units. ADIC also sells accessories such as tape media, cables, and mounting kits. ADIC's largest customers, distributors Ingram Micro and Tech Data, account for 22% and 15% of sales, respectively. About a fourth of the company's sales are international, generated primarily in Europe.

ARIS Corporation

2229 112th Ave. NE, Bellevue, WA 98004

Telephone: 425-372-2747 **Metro area:** Seattle, WA **Web site:** http://www.aris.com **Sales:** $115.8 million **Number of employees:** 593 **Number of employees for previous year:** 371 **Industry designation:** Computers—services **Company type:** Public **Top competitors:** Admiral plc; Computer Learning Centers, Inc.; PLATINUM technology, inc.

ARIS teaches clients how to get the most from their Oracle, Microsoft, and Sun Microsystems software. It provides training and consulting services for packaged software, integrated systems, and customized applications (geared to clients' particular needs) in the US and the UK. ARIS also develops supplementary software (ARIS DFRAG and NoetixViews) for Oracle database and packaged applications and offers course titles that cover Java and Internet/intranet and other network technologies. Founder and CEO Paul Song and his wife, human resources director Tina Song, own 45% of ARIS. Consulting represents 54% of sales, and clients include Boeing, the IRS, and Lockheed Martin.

Cell Therapeutics, Inc.

201 Elliott Ave. West, Ste. 400, Seattle, WA 98119

Telephone: 206-282-7100 **Fax:** 206-284-6206 **Metro area:** Seattle, WA **Web site:** http://www.cticseattle.com **Human resources contact:** Vonni Sytsma **Sales:** $13.2 million **Number of employees:** 179 **Number of employees for previous year:** 106 **Industry designation:** Drugs **Company type:** Public **Top competitors:** SunPharm Corporation; SUGEN, Inc.; AXYS Pharmaceuticals, Inc.

Cell Therapeutics is a toxic avenger. The development-stage company researches small-molecule drugs for the treatment of cancer, inflammatory diseases, and immune diseases. Lisofylline, its lead product, is being developed to combat serious or fatal infections in cancer patients undergoing radiation or chemotherapy. The drug, being developed with Johnson & Johnson, may also help prevent acute lung injury and death from mechanical ventilation. Other drugs under development include a treatment for multi-drug resistant tumors and an agent to make tumors more sensitive to radiation. The company's joint venture with City of Hope National Medical Center focuses on finding new treatments for diabetes.

Concur Technologies, Inc.

6222 185th Ave. NE, Redmond, WA 98052

Telephone: 425-702-8808 **Fax:** 425-702-0674 **Metro area:** Seattle, WA **Web site:** http://www.concur.com **Human resources contact:** John A. Prumatico **Sales:** $17.2 million **Number of employees:** 231 **Number of employees for previous year:** 179 **Industry designation:** Computers—corporate, professional & financial software **Company type:** Public **Top competitors:** Clarus Corporation; Trilogy Software, Inc.; PeopleSoft, Inc.

Hate filling out expense reports and purchase requests? Concur Technologies (formerly Portable Software) hopes its Xpense Management Solution software will make those tasks easier. The Web-based application tracks travel and entertainment expenses, prepares reports, and submits them. Concur's CompanyStore software automates front office requisition and order processes. The company also offers consulting, customer support, and training services. Customers include American Airlines, AT&T, Hewlett-Packard, and Pfizer. Concur sells its products directly and has referral arrangements with American Express (which owns a minority stake in the company) and payroll giant Automatic Data Processing.

Corixa Corporation

1124 Columbia St., Ste. 200, Seattle, WA 98104

Telephone: 206-754-5711 **Fax:** 206-754-5715 **Metro area:** Seattle, WA **Web site:** http://www.corixa.com **Human resources contact:** Bernie Paul **Sales:** $18.3 million **Number of employees:** 132 **Number of employees for previous year:** 104 **Industry designation:** Drugs **Company type:** Public

Corixa focuses on T-cell vaccines for treating and preventing cancer and infectious diseases. Its vaccines for the treatment of breast, prostate, ovarian, lung, and other cancers are in research, preclinical studies, and Phase I clinical trials. Corporate partners on vaccines are SmithKline Beecham and Biologicals S.A.; it has partnered with Pasteur Merieux Connaught in preclinical studies of a vaccine additive to boost immune response for infectious diseases. The company is also working with Abbott Laboratories to develop diagnostics for tuberculosis. Its purchase of GenQuest and Anergen gave it expertise in non-vaccine gene therapies and rheumatoid arthritis treatment, respectively.

Data Dimensions, Inc.

411 108th Ave. NE, Ste. 2100, Bellevue, WA 98004

Telephone: 425-688-1000 **Fax:** 425-688-1099 **Metro area:** Seattle, WA **Web site:** http://www.data-dimensions.com **Human resources contact:** Diana Wong **Sales:** $114.5 million **Number of employees:** 791 **Number of employees for previous year:** 450 **Industry designation:** Computers—services **Company type:** Public **Top competitors:** Cap Gemini S.A.; Andersen Worldwide; International Business Machines Corporation

Data Dimensions, Inc. (DDI) makes money fixing the year 2000 problem (Y2K) caused by most date-dependent software programs that use a two-digit year code and thus are unable to differentiate between 1900 and 2000. DDI designs solutions to this problem, primarily for large corporations and government agencies, and offers tools such as Ardes 2k, a Web-site or CD-ROM guide to recognizing and resolving Y2K, and Interactive Vendor Review, a Y2K vendor-compliance database. The company is using its Y2K cures as an inroad to other computer-consulting needs of its clients. DDI licenses its services internationally and markets them in Europe through a UK-based subsidiary. About 6% of the company's sales are outside the US.

Emeritus Assisted Living

3131 Elliott Ave., Ste. 500, Seattle, WA 98121

Telephone: 206-298-2909 **Fax:** 206-301-4500 **Metro area:** Seattle, WA **Web site:** http://www.emeritus.com **Human resources contact:** Kristina Pfeil **Sales:** $151.5 million **Number of employees:** 4,106 **Number of employees for previous year:** 3,299 **Industry designation:** Nursing homes **Company type:** Public

Emeritus Assisted Living (formerly Emeritus Corporation) runs assisted-living homes for senior citizens who do not want skilled nursing care, but who may want supervision and assistance with daily activities. The company holds interests in about 130 communities in 26 states and Canada. Emeritus has a joint venture with Sanyo Electric to provide assisted-living services in Japan and owns a 31% interest in Alert Care Corporation, a Canada-based assisted-living company. Emeritus has a close relationship with Holiday Retirement, a private company that owns more than 200 retirement homes in the US, Canada, and Europe. Chairman and CEO Daniel Baty, who owns almost 30% of Emeritus, is also Holiday's chairman.

fine.com International Corporation

1525 Fourth Ave., Ste. 800, Seattle, WA 98101

Telephone: 206-292-2888 **Fax:** 206-292-2889 **Metro area:** Seattle, WA **Web site:** http://www.fine.com **Human resources contact:** Mark Herbold **Sales:** $3.4 million **Number of employees:** 43 **Number of employees for previous year:** 24 **Industry designation:** Computers—online services **Company type:** Public **Top competitors:** The Leap Group, Inc.; K2 Design, Inc.; USWeb/CKS

As a developer of Internet and intranet Web sites for corporate clients, fine.com International is paving the information superhighway. Not simply a Web site creator, fine.com also hosts Web sites and offers maintenance and analytical services. Using primarily Microsoft products, the company has designed more than 100 Web sites for clients including FTD, Kellogg, and McDonald's. fine.com's rapid growth has included a joint project with Mitsui & Co. in Japan, as well as the acquisitions of Web site creators Pacific Analysis & Computing and Meta4 Digital Designs. The family of founder and CEO Daniel Fine owns about 35% of the company, which has offices in the US, the UK, and Japan.

Go2Net, Inc.

999 Third Ave., Ste. 4700, Seattle, WA 98104

Telephone: 206-447-1595 **Fax:** 206-447-1625 **Metro area:** Seattle, WA **Web site:** http://www.go2net.com **Human resources contact:** Laurie Likai **Sales:** $4.8 million **Number of employees:** 69 **Number of employees for previous year:** 23 **Industry designation:** Computers—online services **Company type:** Public **Top competitors:** Excite, Inc.; America Online, Inc.; Yahoo! Inc.

Internet surfers catch a wave on the Go2Net virtual beach each day. Offering branded Web sites in areas such as personal finance, Web searching, commerce, and games, Go2Net's collection of eight Web destinations includes Silicon Investor (financial discussions), MetaCrawler (search service), and HyperMart (free Web hosting). The sites can be accessed through the Go2Net portal and are all technology-driven. The company generates more than 70% of its revenue from advertising, but it also makes money through subscription services on the Silicon Investor and HyperMart Web sites, selling its advertisers' products, and licensing its Web technology. Microsoft co-founder Paul Allen is buying a majority stake in Go2Net.

Group Health Cooperative of Puget Sound

521 Wall St., Seattle, WA 98121

Telephone: 206-326-3000 **Fax:** 206-448-5439 **Metro area:** Seattle, WA **Web site:** http://www.ghc.org **Human resources contact:** John Nagelmann **Sales:** $1 billion **Number of employees:** 8,300 **Number of employees for previous year:** 7,179 **Industry designation:** Health maintenance organization **Company type:** Not-for-profit **Top competitors:** Foundation Health Systems, Inc.; Adventist Health; PacifiCare Health Systems, Inc.

Group Health Cooperative of Puget Sound is a not-for-profit managed health care group serving more than 30 counties in Washington and five counties in Idaho. Members may participate in HMO, PPO, or point-of-service health plans. The co-op, which is governed by an 11-member board, controls Group Health Northwest. Group Health Cooperative of Puget Sound has allied with Virginia Mason Medical Center to share medical centers and hospitals. Despite strong market share, the cooperative had experienced less-than-stellar financial performance in years past, prompting its 1997 affiliation with Kaiser Permanente, the nation's largest health care delivery system. The organization is owned by its nearly 700,000 members.

ICOS Corporation

22021 20th Ave. SE, Bothell, WA 98021

Telephone: 425-485-1900 **Fax:** 425-489-0356 **Metro area:** Seattle, WA **Web site:** http://www.icos.com **Human resources contact:** Michelle Yetman **Sales:** $110.8 million **Number of employees:** 312 **Number of employees for previous year:** 252 **Industry designation:** Drugs **Company type:** Public

ICOS Corporation researches and develops drugs for chronic inflammatory diseases such as asthma, atherosclerosis, and multiple sclerosis and for conditions such as hypertension and diabetes. It explores the inflammatory process at the molecular level, then identifies therapeutic agents able to treat the disease. Potential products include Hu23F2G, which is in clinical trials to treat patients with chronic progressive multiple sclerosis; PDE inhibitor-A, which is in preclinical stages as an asthma treatment; and IC351, an anti-impotence pill. ICOS has collaborative agreements with drugmakers Abbott Labs, Glaxo Wellcome, and UK-based Cambridge Antibody Technology. Microsoft's Bill Gates owns 13% of ICOS.

Immunex Corporation

51 University St., Seattle, WA 98101

Telephone: 206-587-0430 **Fax:** 206-587-0606 **Metro area:** Seattle, WA **Web site:** http://www.immunex.com **Human resources contact:** Kathy J. Spencer **Sales:** $243.5 million **Number of employees:** 1,007 **Number of employees for previous year:** 886 **Industry designation:** Biomedical & genetic products **Company type:** Public **Top competitors:** Amgen Inc.; Bristol-Myers Squibb Company; Merck & Co., Inc.

Immunex develops and manufactures biopharmaceutical products to treat cancer, autoimmune disorders, and infectious diseases. The company's primary approved products are Leukine, which is used to treat bone marrow transplant patients, and Novantrone, which is used to treat acute non-lymphocytic leukemia and to ease pain associated with prostate cancer. The FDA has approved Immunex's Enbrel, a rheumatoid arthritis treatment that has the potential to be a financial mother lode. Immunex is also developing drugs that treat asthma, leukemia, and certain cancers. Pharmaceutical research giant American Home Products owns 54% of Immunex.

InfoSpace.com, Inc.

15375 90th Ave. NE, Redmond, WA 98052

Telephone: 425-882-1602 **Fax:** 425-869-7501 **Metro area:** Seattle, WA **Web site:** http://www.infospace.com **Human resources contact:** Randy Massengale **Sales:** $9.4 million **Number of employees:** 76 **Number of employees for previous year:** 36 **Industry designation:** Computers—online services **Company type:** Public **Top competitors:** infoUSA Inc.; Banyan Systems Incorporated; Yahoo! Inc.

InfoSpace.com provides content to more than 800 Web sites, including America Online, Deja News, and go2net. The company also offers national Yellow and White Pages directories, integrated with related city guides, maps, news, and classified advertisements to create a complete package. It owns the rights to content from about 75 third-party providers. In addition to serving Internet portals and destination sites, InfoSpace.com provides information to suppliers of cellular phones, digital pagers, and other Internet access devices. The company, which is expanding in Europe, generates virtually all of its sales from national and local advertising. Founder and CEO Naveen Jain owns about 50% of InfoSpace.com.

INTERLINQ Software Corporation

11980 NE 24th St., Bellevue, WA 98005

Telephone: 425-827-1112 **Fax:** 425-827-0927 **Metro area:** Seattle, WA **Web site:** http://www.interlinq.com **Human resources contact:** Diane Harter **Sales:** $18.3 million **Number of employees:** 154 **Number of employees for previous year:** 133 **Industry designation:** Computers—corporate, professional & financial software **Company type:** Public **Top competitors:** SS&C Technologies, Inc.; CFI ProServices, Inc.; New Era of Networks, Inc.

INTERLINQ Software makes software for granting residential and construction loans. Its MortgageWare Enterprise line (52% of sales) manages the flow of qualifying borrowers, originating and processing applications, closing and tracking loans, and examining in-process loans to meet secondary-market commitments. INTERLINQ sells its products directly and through other software developers, system integrators, and OEMs. Its FlowMan software integrates computer systems and routes data throughout an organization. INTERLINQ also offers consulting and training services. Longtime shareholder William Hambrecht (formerly with IPO specialist Hambrecht & Quist) is planning to take INTERLINQ private through a leveraged buyout.

Key Tronic Corporation

4424 N. Sullivan Rd., Spokane, WA 99216

Telephone: 509-928-8000 **Fax:** 509-927-5555 **Other address:** PO Box 14687, Spokane, WA 99214 **Metro area:** Spokane, WA **Web site:** http://www.keytronic.com **Human resources contact:** Ken C. Clement **Sales:** $170.1 million **Number of employees:** 2,685 **Number of employees for previous year:** 2,434 **Industry designation:** Computers—peripheral equipment **Company type:** Public **Top competitors:** The Cherry Corporation; Cybex Computer Products Corporation; Fujitsu Limited

Key Tronic tap-tap-taps out computer keyboards. About 85% of the company's sales come from its customized and standard keyboard designs. Key Tronic sells its products to more than 140 original equipment manufacturers. Hewlett-Packard, Microsoft, and Toshiba together account for more than 50% of sales. The company has added other types of advanced input devices to its line—including fingerprint recognition products—in an effort to overcome a spotty record of profits. Key Tronic also performs contract manufacturing of electronics, molding, and liquid crystal display items.

Medtronic Physio-Control Inc.

11811 Willows Rd. NE, Redmond, WA 98052

Telephone: 425-867-4000 **Fax:** 425-881-2405 **Metro area:** Seattle, WA **Web site:** http://www.physio-control.com **Human resources contact:** V. Mark Droppert **Sales:** $175.3 million **Number of employees:** 840 **Number of employees for previous year:** 830 **Industry designation:** Medical instruments **Company type:** Subsidiary

Medtronic Physio-Control, a subsidiary of Medtronic, makes an integrated line of noninvasive emergency cardiac defibrillator and vital sign assessment devices, disposable electrodes, and data management software. The company's products are used in both out-of-hospital and hospital settings for the early detection and treatment of life-threatening events including trauma, heart attack, and the acute heart rhythm disturbances of ventricular fibrillation, tachycardia, and bradycardia. The firm has developed a full line of products under the LIFEPAK and FIRST MEDIC names. Users include emergency medical technicians, paramedics, critical care nurses, and physicians.

Nintendo of America Inc.

4820 150th Ave. NE, Redmond, WA 98052

Telephone: 425-882-2040 **Fax:** 425-882-3585 **Metro area:** Seattle, WA **Web site:** http://www.nintendo.com **Human resources contact:** Bev Mitchell **Industry designation:** Computers—peripheral equipment **Company type:** Subsidiary **Parent company:** Nintendo Co., Ltd. **Top competitors:** SEGA Enterprises, Ltd.; Hasbro, Inc.; Sony Corporation

Nintendo of America promotes good hand-eye coordination. The company is the North American base for Japanese parent Nintendo Corp., which sells video game systems such as Nintendo 64 (N64) and the popular Game Boy as well as software (it created the beloved Mario Brothers). Nintendo of America is battling #1 Sony (PlayStation) and #3 SEGA for video game market share. Nintendo has decided to stay with a cartridge format rather than switching to cheaper CD-ROMs. Recent offerings include a color Game Boy, a Game Boy camera and printer, and a handheld game called "Pokemon" (Pocket Monsters). Nintendo of America provides equipment and space to DigiPen, a video game design school, and gets first dibs on its graduates.

ONYX Software Corporation

310 120th Ave. NE, Bellevue, WA 98005

Telephone: 425-451-8060 **Fax:** 425-990-3343 **Metro area:** Seattle, WA **Web site:** http://www.onyx.com **Sales:** $35.1 million **Number of employees:** 281 **Industry designation:** Computers—corporate, professional & financial software **Company type:** Public **Top competitors:** SAP AG; The Vantive Corporation; PeopleSoft, Inc.

ONYX Software has Microsoft running through its veins. The company makes customer management tools for the Redmond giant's BackOffice corporate resource planning software. Its main product, ONYX Customer Center, combines client marketing, sales, and service data so users across a corporation can track service histories, manage support queries, and generate sales prospect lists from a single database. Sierra Health Services and Cincinnati Bell are among ONYX's customers. ONYX's three founders, all ex-Microsoft employees, together own more than 40% of the company. Its culture mirrors Gates-ville's, with generous benefits and open internal communication.

Optiva Corporation

13222 SE 30th St., Bellevue, WA 98005

Telephone: 425-957-0970 **Fax:** 425-401-4838 **Metro area:** Seattle, WA **Web site:** http://www.optiva.com **Human resources contact:** Judy M. Loucks **Sales:** $103 million (Est.) **Number of employees:** 468 **Number of employees for previous year:** 338 **Industry designation:** Cosmetics & toiletries **Company type:** Private **Top competitors:** The Gillette Company; Conair Corporation; Allegheny Teledyne Incorporated

Optiva makes a powered toothbrush that uses patented sonic technology, fluid dynamics, and electromechanical design to aid in removing plaque bacteria from between teeth and at the gumline. The company intends to develop additional consumer oral care products to complement its toothbrush, which is sold under the sonicare name. The company sells its products in the US through warehouse clubs (Costco and Sam's Club), drugstores (Eckerd and Walgreen), mass merchandisers (Target and Wal-Mart), specialty retailers (The Sharper Image), and department stores (Sears). Optiva also distributes its products in Japan and the UK.

ORCA Technologies, Inc.

24000 35th Ave. SE, Ste. 200, Bothell, WA 98021

Telephone: 425-354-1600 **Fax:** 425-354-1625 **Metro area:** Seattle, WA **Human resources contact:** Kathleen Mikos **Number of employees:** 47 **Number of employees for previous year:** 25 **Industry designation:** Computers—online services **Company type:** Public **Top competitors:** America Online, Inc.; Northwest Pacifica, Inc.; SBC Communications Inc.

The mighty ORCA conquered the MONITRx and the TeleVar, gobbled the BOSS, then ate DNA and restructured itself. The result of these acquisitions—Jungle Street, BOSS Internet Group, and Digital Network Associates—and others is ORCA Technologies, which provides Internet and long-distance phone service in the Pacific Northwest. Concentrating on small communities and rural areas, ORCA has become a regional Internet service provider with about 16,000 customers in Idaho, Oregon, and Washington. Its services are sold by about 40 resellers, including community agencies. More than 90% of ORCA's sales are from Internet access fees, but it also offers computer networking, proprietary software, and Web design and services.

PathoGenesis Corporation

201 Elliott Ave. West, Seattle, WA 98119

Telephone: 206-467-8100 **Fax:** 206-270-3313 **Metro area:** Seattle, WA **Web site:** http://www.pathogenesis.com **Human resources contact:** Kent J. DeLucenay **Sales:** $400,000 **Number of employees:** 159 **Number of employees for previous year:** 115 **Industry designation:** Drugs **Company type:** Public **Top competitors:** Spiros Development Corporation II, Inc.; Discovery Laboratories, Inc.; Genentech, Inc.

Bacteria, beware. PathoGenesis is on your trail. The company develops drugs and delivery systems for treating lung diseases. Its primary product is TOBI (tobramycin solution for inhalation), the first FDA-approved inhaled antibiotic solution for targeting the "Pseudomonas" bacterium responsible for most infections in cystic fibrosis (CF) patients. The company is developing TOBI for treatment of tuberculosis (TB) and similar infections, and is also working on PA-1648, an oral antibiotic treatment for TB. PathoGenesis owns the rights to TOBI, but will pay Children's Hospital in Seattle a royalty on drug sales. Its PathoGenesis Limited subsidiary was formed to oversee European approval and marketing of TOBI.

Pope Resources

19245 10th Ave. NE, Poulsbo, WA 98370

Telephone: 360-697-6626 **Fax:** 360-697-1156 **Other address:** PO Box 1780, Poulsbo, WA 98370 **Metro area:** Seattle, WA **Human resources contact:** Marsha Royer **Sales:** $43 million **Number of employees:** 135 **Number of employees for previous year:** 45 **Industry designation:** Agricultural operations **Company type:** Public **Top competitors:** MAXXAM Inc.; U.S. Timberlands Company, L.P.; IP Timberlands, Ltd.

At Pope Resources money really does grow on trees. The partnership raises trees, Douglas fir primarily, on its 76,000-acre tree farm near Seattle, Washington (all of the partnership's properties are within a 50-mile radius of Seattle). Pope sells its timber in the US and abroad, primarily to Japan. The partnership also develops real estate, primarily single-family homes, building lots, and income producing properties. Some of the partnership's income producing properties include water and sewer facilities, a golf course, a marina, and an RV park.

ProCyte Corporation

8511 154th Ave. NE, Bldg. A., Redmond, WA 98052

Telephone: 425-869-1239 **Fax:** 425-869-8901 **Metro area:** Seattle, WA **Web site:** http://www.procyte.com **Sales:** $2.6 million **Number of employees:** 37 **Number of employees for previous year:** 28 **Industry designation:** Drugs **Company type:** Public **Top competitors:** Bristol-Myers Squibb Company; L'Oreal; Johnson & Johnson

ProCyte develops and makes copper-peptide products used to treat wounds and care for skin and hair. A C. R. Bard subsidiary is marketing and distributing ProCyte's Iamin and OsmoCyte lines of chronic wound care products in North America. ProCyte also makes products used to treat patients following chemical peels, dermabrasion, liposuction, and hair-restoration surgery. Another firm will market ProCyte's Blue Copper anti-aging cream at cosmetic counters in such stores as Saks and Neiman Marcus. While ramping up its own product lines, ProCyte has performed contract manufacturing for select clients, an activity that accounts for about three-fourths of its sales.

RealNetworks, Inc.

1111 Third Ave., Ste. 2900, Seattle, WA 98101

Telephone: 206-674-2700 **Fax:** 206-674-2699 **Metro area:** Seattle, WA **Web site:** http://www.real.com **Human resources contact:** Karen Schlemmer **Sales:** $64.8 million **Number of employees:** 326 **Number of employees for previous year:** 278 **Industry designation:** Computers—online services **Company type:** Public **Top competitors:** VocalTec Communications Ltd.; Macromedia, Inc.; Xing Technology Corporation

RealNetworks (formerly known as Progressive Networks) pioneered the streaming software that allows audio and video broadcasters to deliver their products over the World Wide Web in real time. The company's RealPlayer software is used by more than 30 million Web surfers who download the software for free. Software license fees from broadcasters account for more than 75% of RealNetworks' sales. Companies that have purchased the company's broadcasting tools and services include ABC, At Home (Internet services), Dow Jones, and NBC. Almost 75% of RealNetworks' sales are in North America. Founder and CEO Robert Glaser owns nearly half of the company.

SeaMED Corporation

14500 NE 87th St., Redmond, WA 98052

Telephone: 425-867-1818 **Fax:** 425-867-0622 **Metro area:** Seattle, WA **Web site:** http://www.seamed.com **Human resources contact:** Gene Gerrard **Sales:** $70 million **Number of employees:** 508 **Number of employees for previous year:** 317 **Industry designation:** Medical instruments **Company type:** Public **Top competitors:** General Electric Company; Colorado MEDtech, Inc.; Mallinckrodt Inc.

SeaMED Corporation makes sure medical technology companies aren't up a creek without a paddle. The company manufactures consoles, control modules and other electronic devices (about 60% of sales) for such companies as United States Surgical Corporation, Eastman Kodak, Johnson & Johnson, and C.R. Bard. It also provides engineering and regulatory expertise to help customers commercialize their instruments. SeaMED can design and manufacture an instrument or make one to its customers' specifications. SeaMED also makes coins-for-bills machines for Coinstar, which accounts for about 25% of its sales. The company, which is being acquired by Plexus Corp., has five plants in Washington.

The Seattle Mariners Professional Baseball Organization

83 King St., 3rd Fl., Seattle, WA 98104

Telephone: 206-346-4000 **Fax:** 206-346-4100 **Other address:** PO Box 4100, Seattle, WA 98104 **Metro area:** Seattle, WA **Web site:** http://www.mariners.org **Human resources contact:** Marianne Short **Sales:** $89.8 million (Est.) **Number of employees:** 85 **Industry designation:** Leisure & recreational services **Company type:** Private **Top competitors:** Anaheim Angels Baseball Club, Inc.; The Athletics Investment Group; Texas Rangers Baseball

The Seattle Mariners baseball team has struggled to keep its sinking ship afloat. It joined Major League Baseball in 1977, but didn't post a winning season until 1991. The team no longer habitually loses games, but it still loses money. After several owners left rather than risk losses, a group of local investors (backed by Japan's Nintendo Corp.) purchased the company in 1992. Amid controversy, the deal was structured so the team would be operated by the American investors. Owners hope the team, which attracts record numbers of fans, will see a profit for the first time in a decade in 1999 when it moves into the new Safeco Field (the nation's most expensive ball park, built for almost $500 million).

Seattle Seahawks

11220 NE 53rd St., Kirkland, WA 98033

Telephone: 425-827-9777 **Fax:** 425-893-5108 **Metro area:** Seattle, WA **Web site:** http://www.seahawks.com **Human resources contact:** Cindy Kelley **Sales:** $77.1 million (Est.) **Number of employees:** 130 **Number of employees for previous year:** 110 **Industry designation:** Leisure & recreational services **Company type:** Private **Top competitors:** The Denver Broncos Football Club; Oakland Raiders; Kansas City Chiefs

A Seattle Seahawks fan can buy a game ticket for a miserly $10—the lowest price in the National Football League (NFL). But, some would argue, that's about what the team is worth. Billionaire Paul Allen, co-founder of Microsoft, thinks otherwise, having bought the team in 1997 from Ken Behring. Among his first changes was selling some game tickets for $10. He also plans to demolish the Kingdome in 2000 and move the team into a new open-air stadium. The Seahawks, which joined the league as an expansion team in 1976, haven't made the NFL playoffs since 1988. However Seattle hopes its chances improve for the 1999-2000 season when former Green Bay Packers coach Mike Holmgren takes the helm.

Sisters of Providence Health System

520 Pike St., Seattle, WA 98101

Telephone: 206-464-3355 **Fax:** 206-464-3038 **Other address:** PO Box 11038, Seattle, WA 98111 **Metro area:** Seattle, WA **Web site:** http://www.providence.org **Human resources contact:** Sue Byington **Sales:** $2.3 billion **Number of employees:** 21,800 **Number of employees for previous year:** 20,368 **Industry designation:** Hospitals **Company type:** Not-for-profit **Top competitors:** Adventist Health; Tenet Healthcare Corporation; Columbia/HCA Healthcare Corporation

Sisterhood is powerful in health care. The order of the Sisters of Providence runs a health care network (the Sisters of Providence Health System) that spans the West Coast from California to Alaska. The system consists of the PeaceHealth PPO and HMO programs, with more than one million members; 11 hospitals; two health resource centers; and two physician networks (one, Medalia Health Network, in cosponsorship with the Franciscan Health System) that focus on primary care. In addition to providing medical and related services for the poor, the organization—whose roots go back to the 1840s—also fulfills its charitable mission by operating housing projects for the poor and elderly and a high school.

SonoSite, Inc.

19807 N. Creek Pkwy., Ste. 200, Bothell, WA 98011

Telephone: 425-951-1200 **Fax:** 425-951-1201 **Other address:** PO Box 3020, Bothell, WA 98041 **Metro area:** Seattle, WA **Web site:** http://www.sonosite.com **Sales:** $1 million **Number of employees:** 61 **Number of employees for previous year:** 30 **Industry designation:** Medical products **Company type:** Public

SonoSite (formerly SonoSight), a development-stage company, makes handheld ultrasonic imaging devices used to examine patients in emergency care and other situations. Physicians and other medical personnel can use the company's primary imaging technology at the examining table, at the bedside, or in the field. The company expects to introduce a working model of its product in late 1998. SonoSite plans to use third-party manufacturers and distributors to market its products to clinical specialists such as emergency, cardiology, and military doctors. The US Navy is partially funding the company's research.

U.S. Timberlands Company, L.P.

1301 Fifth Ave., Ste. 3725, Seattle, WA 98101

Telephone: 206-652-5000 **Fax:** 206-405-2940 **Metro area:** Seattle, WA **Web site:** http://www.ustimberlands.com **Sales:** $77.3 million **Number of employees:** 32 **Number of employees for previous year:** 30 **Industry designation:** Agricultural operations **Company type:** Public **Top competitors:** Crown Pacific Partners, L.P.; Hampton Affiliates; Georgia-Pacific Corporation

U.S. Timberlands isn't stumped—it's a lumber company. The company owns about 633,000 fee acres of timberland and 3,000 additional acres of cutting rights east of the Cascade Range in Oregon. Its total estimated merchantable timber volume is about 2.1 billion board feet. In addition, U.S. Timberland owns about 180,000 acres of managed tree farms and a seed orchard that produces five million conifer seedlings a year, half of which are sold to other forest product companies. Its Ponderosa Pine, Douglas Fir, and Lodgepole Pine logs are processed for sale as plywood, lumber, and other wood products by third-party conversion companies such as Collins Products, Crown Pacific Partners, and Boise Cascade.

Visio Corporation

2211 Elliott Avenue, Seattle, WA 98121

Telephone: 206-956-6000 **Fax:** 206-956-6001 **Metro area:** Seattle, WA **Web site:** http://www.visio.com **Human resources contact:** Susan Slaton **Sales:** $166 million **Number of employees:** 555 **Number of employees for previous year:** 355 **Industry designation:** Computers—corporate, professional & financial software **Company type:** Public **Top competitors:** Corel Corporation; Autodesk, Inc.; Micrografx, Inc.

Visio wants its customers to get the big picture. The company makes Windows-based drawing and diagramming software used by nearly 2.8 million people to create everything from space plans to network designs. About half of Visio's sales come from business diagramming and technical drawing software; the other half comes from information technology (IT) design and documentation tools. Visio's software line includes business diagramming tool Visio Standard, technical drawing tools Visio Technical and IntelliCAD, and IT design tool Visio Professional. Ingram Micro accounts for more than a third of the company's sales. Visio also counts Hewlett-Packard and Boeing among its customers.

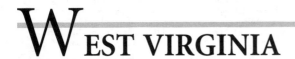

WEST VIRGINIA

Petroleum Development Corporation

103 E. Main St., Bridgeport, WV 26330

Telephone: 304-842-3597 **Fax:** 304-842-0913 **Human resources contact:** Ersel Morgan **Sales:** $83 million **Number of employees:** 81 **Number of employees for previous year:** 75 **Industry designation:** Oil & gas—exploration & production **Company type:** Public **Top competitors:** Cabot Oil & Gas Corporation; Newstar Resources Inc.; Mitchell Energy & Development Corp.

The hills are alive for Petroleum Development, which produces natural gas primarily in the West Virginia and Pennsylvania portions of the Appalachian Basin and in Michigan. The company also has interests in producing properties in Ohio and Tennessee; its proved reserves consist of 57 billion cu. ft. of natural gas and 45,000 barrels of oil. Petroleum Development sells natural gas to utilities and industrial end-users. It markets its own natural gas and that of other Appalachian Basin producers through subsidiary Riley Natural Gas. Subsidiary Paramount Natural Gas is a regulated natural gas distribution utility in Ohio, and Petroleum Development's Paramount Transmission unit markets nautal gas in Ohio.

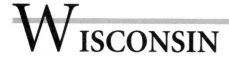

WISCONSIN

Alternative Living Services, Inc.

450 N. Sunnyslope Rd., Ste. 300, Brookfield, WI 53005

Telephone: 414-789-9565 **Fax:** 414-789-9592 **Metro area:** Milwaukee, WI **Web site:** http://www.assisted.com **Human resources contact:** Janice Teuscher **Sales:** $244.4 million **Number of employees:** 5,935 **Number of employees for previous year:** 2,103 **Industry designation:** Nursing homes **Company type:** Public **Top competitors:** Emeritus Assisted Living; Beverly Enterprises, Inc.; HCR Manor Care, Inc.

Alternative Living Services (ALS) is no hippie commune. The company operates assisted-living residences that offer services to the frail and elderly and to Alzheimer's sufferers who don't require full nursing home care. ALS has more than 325 residences operating in about 25 states. The company offers personal care, health care, and support services to its residents, with specialized facilities designed for people ranging from those with memory loss to the relatively independent. Each ALS residence is designed to have a home-like environment. The company is expanding its resident capacity with more facilities in preparation for retiring baby boomers.

ARI Network Services, Inc.

330 E. Kilbourn Ave., Milwaukee, WI 53202

Telephone: 414-278-7676 **Fax:** 414-283-4357 **Metro area:** Milwaukee, WI **Web site:** http://www.arinet.com **Human resources contact:** Mary Pierson **Sales:** $8 million **Number of employees:** 106 **Number of employees for previous year:** 77 **Industry designation:** Computers—services **Company type:** Public **Top competitors:** Sterling Commerce, Inc.; Electronic Data Systems Corporation; Harbinger Corporation

ARI Network Services provides e-commerce software and services to the agribusiness, equipment, transportation, and publishing industries. The company's products include ARISE (sales automation software), Meppel (software that reports product movement), Newsfinder (a news stories database), PLUS (an electronic parts catalog for equipment dealers), and TradeRoute (software that handles documents for product ordering and warranties). ARI also offers support services such as telecommunications networking, database management, online catalog production, application development, training, and consulting. Its two largest customers are the Association of American Railroads and Roche Vitamins.

Bone Care International, Inc.

One Science Ct., Madison, WI 53711

Telephone: 608-236-2500 **Fax:** 608-236-2525 **Metro area:** Madison, WI **Sales:** $100,000 **Number of employees:** 27 **Number of employees for previous year:** 15 **Industry designation:** Drugs **Company type:** Public **Top competitors:** NPS Pharmaceuticals, Inc.; Chugai Pharmaceutical Co., Ltd.; Hoffmann-La Roche, Inc.

Marrow-minded Bone Care International is a development-stage company working on improved D-hormones for treating kidney disease, osteoporosis, psoriasis, prostate cancer, breast cancer, and hyperparathyroidism. The company is awaiting FDA approval for Hectoral's use in preventing excessive hormone production in the kidneys of renal-disease patients; Hectoral may also have uses in treating osteoporosis and prostate cancer. Another product under development is intended to treat advanced prostate, colon, and breast cancers. Bone Care International plans to market its products directly in the US, and through distribution agreements worldwide. Founder and chairman Richard Mazess owns 30% of the company.

Century Foods International

915 Hoeschler Dr., Sparta, WI 54656

Telephone: 608-269-1900 **Fax:** 608-269-1910 **Metro area:** La Crosse, WI **Sales:** $85 million (Est.) **Number of employees:** 165 **Industry designation:** Food—dairy products **Company type:** Private **Top competitors:** Kraft Foods, Inc.; Groupe Danone; Land O'Lakes, Inc.

If "Eat light" is the next century's motto, Century Foods International is ready. This maker of dairy goods (mostly light varieties) supplies food companies with its brand-name products, including Ready Cheese (pasteurized cheese spread), Pizazz! (fat-free), and Lacey Delite. Products are sold to more than 400 food processors in 45 countries. Century Foods' big cheese, president and CEO Michael Otten, started the company in 1991 with two other former employees of Ridgeview, which was bought out by Dutch DMV International. Otten is the majority owner of Century Foods.

GE Technical Products and Services

PO Box 414, Milwaukee, WI 53201

Telephone: 800-626-2004 **Metro area:** Milwaukee, WI **Human resources contact:** Marc J. Saperstein **Sales:** $4.9 billion **Number of employees:** 16,000 **Industry designation:** Medical products **Company type:** Division **Parent company:** General Electric Company **Top competitors:** Elcom International, Inc.; Picker International, Inc.; AT&T Corp.

You "can" get technical with GE Technical Products and Services, a division of General Electric composed of GE Medical Systems and GE Information Services (GEIS). GE Medical Systems is a major global maker of such diagnostic imaging equipment as magnetic resonance, ultrasound, and computed tomography (CT) scanners, with units in France, Japan, and India. GEIS leads the charge for electronic commerce with electronic data interchange (EDI), Internet, risk management, and other services. GEIS provides EDI technology for such clients as J. C. Penney, Kmart, and Dayton Hudson and is merging its communications network with that of MCI WorldCom. GE Technical accounts for about 5% of General Electric's total sales.

The Green Bay Packers, Inc.

1265 Lombardi Ave., Green Bay, WI 54304

Telephone: 920-496-5700 **Fax:** 920-496-5738 **Other address:** PO Box 10628, Green Bay, WI 54307 **Metro area:** Green Bay, WI **Web site:** http://www.packers.com **Sales:** $82.8 million **Number of employees:** 92 **Number of employees for previous year:** 90 **Industry designation:** Leisure & recreational services **Company type:** Not-for-profit **Top competitors:** Tampa Bay Buccaneers; Detroit Lions; Minnesota Vikings Football Club

The Green Bay Packers are the National Football League's oldest team and the only original franchise still in its original city. The Packers are organized as a not-for-profit corporation and are publicly owned by about 110,000 shareholders. Its shares do not appreciate and pay no dividends. In the first offering since 1950, Green Bay sold more than 100,000 new shares ($200 each) to finance renovation efforts at Lambeau Field. Since the team plays in the NFL's smallest market, it relies heavily on TV revenues, which account for more than half of the company's sales. The Green Bay Packers won the 1997 Super Bowl and returned to the big game in 1998, when they were defeated by the Denver Broncos.

Lawter International, Inc.

One Terra Way, 8601 95th St., Kenosha, WI 53142

Telephone: 414-947-7300 **Fax:** 414-947-7539 **Metro area:** Milwaukee, WI **Human resources contact:** Tina Lennertz **Sales:** $212.8 million **Number of employees:** 613 **Number of employees for previous year:** 549 **Industry designation:** Chemicals—specialty **Company type:** Public

Lawter International makes ink stick. The company manufactures specialty chemicals that allow inks and coatings to be quickly and accurately applied to a variety of surfaces. Its products include printing ink vehicles that enable ink to hold color, slip additives that give extra surface resistance to ink, and synthetic and hydrocarbon resins that improve ink's durability and drying speed. Lawter manufactures and markets its chemicals in North America, Europe, and the Pacific Rim. Its top customers are Coates/Lorilleux, Dianippin Ink and Chemicals, Flint Ink, Sakata, and Toyo.

Lunar Corporation

313 W. Beltline Hwy., Madison, WI 53713

Telephone: 608-274-2663 **Fax:** 608-274-5374 **Metro area:** Madison, WI **Web site:** http://www.lunarcorp.com **Human resources contact:** Tamra Klongland **Sales:** $79.7 million **Number of employees:** 314 **Number of employees for previous year:** 265 **Industry designation:** Medical instruments **Company type:** Public **Top competitors:** OEC Medical Systems, Inc.; Hologic, Inc.; Norland Medical Systems, Inc.

If you're dense, Lunar Corporation will know it. The company develops and sells bone densitometers, X-ray or ultrasound scanning machines that measure bone density as a way of diagnosing osteoporosis and other metabolic bone disease. The DPX-IQ, Lunar's flagship product, uses X-rays to measure bone density of various regions, while its Achilles ultrasound device measures bone density through the heel. Other products include scanners that diagnose injuries to knees, wrists, and other extremities. Lunar is the exclusive US distributor of the Artoscan Extremity Magnetic Resonance Imaging (MRI) scanner, made by Italian medical device company ESAOTE Biomedica. Founder Richard Mazess owns 33% of the company.

Marathon Cheese Corporation

304 East St., Marathon, WI 54448

Telephone: 715-443-2211 **Fax:** 715-443-3843 **Other address:** PO Box 185, Marathon, WI 54448 **Metro area:** Wausau, WI **Sales:** $525 million (Est.) **Number of employees:** 1,200 **Number of employees for previous year:** 1,000 **Industry designation:** Food—dairy products **Company type:** Private **Top competitors:** Kraft Foods, Inc.; Great Lakes Cheese Company, Inc.; Schreiber Foods, Inc.

Which firm has a reason to say "cheese" and mean it? Marathon Cheese, the world's #1 independent cheese packager. The company buys and packages cheese from such clients as Kraft Foods, Land O'Lakes, and Schreiber Foods, then resells it in the US and internationally. Marathon Cheese also acts as a contract packager for cheese processors who make more cheese than they can handle. It offers sizes from shredded and cubed cheese for consumer convenience to 22-pound blocks, packaging about five million pounds per week of cheddar, Swiss, and other varieties. Ray and Marie Goldbach started the company in their basement in 1952.

Milwaukee Brewers Baseball Club

County Stadium, 201 S. 46th St., Milwaukee, WI 53214

Telephone: 414-933-4114 **Fax:** 414-933-5474 **Other address:** PO Box 3099, Milwaukee, WI 53201 **Metro area:** Milwaukee, WI **Web site:** http://www.milwaukeebrewers.com **Human resources contact:** Thomas Gausden **Sales:** $46.9 million (Est.) **Number of employees:** 130 **Number of employees for previous year:** 70 **Industry designation:** Leisure & recreational services **Company type:** Private **Top competitors:** Chicago National League Ball Club, Inc.; St. Louis Cardinals, L.P.; Houston Astros Baseball Club

Realignment's not a dirty word to the Milwaukee Brewers; in fact, it makes them downright ecstatic. As part of Major League Baseball's realignment plan, the club, formed with the 1970 purchase of the Seattle Pilots franchise, is the first major-league team since 1900 to change leagues. Now a member of the National League Central Division, Milwaukee joins five other teams—Chicago, Cincinnati, Houston, Pittsburgh, and St. Louis. And the change doesn't stop there: In 2000 the Brewers' new stadium, Miller Park, will open for play. Wendy Selig-Prieb took over as team CEO after Bud Selig, her father, placed his ownership of the Brewers into a trust in order to become Major League Baseball's commissioner.

Milwaukee Bucks

1001 N. Fourth St., Bradley Center, Milwaukee, WI 53203

Telephone: 414-227-0500 **Fax:** 414-227-0543 **Metro area:** Milwaukee, WI **Web site:** http://www.nba.com/bucks **Sales:** $42.7 million (Est.) **Number of employees:** 38 **Industry designation:** Leisure & recreational services **Company type:** Private **Top competitors:** Charlotte Hornets; Chicago Bulls; Atlanta Hawks, Ltd.

The Milwaukee Bucks entered the NBA in 1968 and soon cashed in. After finishing the 1968-69 season last in their division, the Bucks drafted Lew Alcindor (later Kareem Abdul-Jabbar), who wasted no time in leading the team to the NBA Championship in 1971. Abdul-Jabbar left for Los Angeles in a 1975 trade, and although the Bucks were somewhat successful in the late 1970s and 1980s under coach Don Nelson, the team hasn't won a championship since. Now led by coach Chris Ford and forward Glen Robinson (the #1 overall pick in the 1994 NBA draft), the Bucks play in Milwaukee's Bradley Center. Senator Herb Kohl of Wisconsin owns the team.

Northland Cranberries, Inc.

800 First Ave. South, Wisconsin Rapids, WI 54495

Telephone: 715-424-4444 **Fax:** 715-422-6800 **Other address:** PO Box 8020, Wisconsin Rapids, WI 54495 **Metro area:** Wausau, WI **Web site:** http://www.northlandcran.com **Human resources contact:** David J. Lukas **Sales:** $112.8 million **Number of employees:** 212 **Number of employees for previous year:** 203 **Industry designation:** Agricultural operations **Company type:** Public **Top competitors:** Ocean Spray Cranberries, Inc.; The Coca-Cola Company; Tropicana Products, Inc.

A breakaway from Ocean Spray, Northland Cranberries hopes to chip away at its former parent's domination of the cranberry market. Northland, with 25 marshes in Massachusetts and Wisconsin, considers itself the world's largest cranberry grower, but Ocean Spray's over 700 member-growers still grow 70% of all North American cranberries. Northland processes its berries into concentrate and bottles it under private labels, its own brand, and its Minot brand. It bought Seneca's juice division (apple, grape, and citrus juices) in 1998 and now owns its TreeSweet and Awake brands and an exclusive license for the Seneca name for juices. Northland also sells juice and fruit products to industrial and wholesale customers.

The Northwestern Mutual Life Insurance Company

720 E. Wisconsin Ave., Milwaukee, WI 53202

Telephone: 414-271-1444 **Fax:** 414-299-7022 **Metro area:** Milwaukee, WI **Web site:** http://www.northwesternmutual.com **Human resources contact:** Susan A. Lueger **Sales:** $12.3 billion **Number of employees:** 3,818 **Number of employees for previous year:** 3,513 **Industry designation:** Insurance—life **Company type:** Mutual company **Top competitors:** Metropolitan Life Insurance Company; John Hancock Mutual Life Insurance Company; The Prudential Insurance Company of America

If you listen carefully, you might hear The Quiet Company at work. Northwestern Mutual Life Insurance is a diversified insurance and financial services company and one of the top 10 US life insurers. Owned by its nearly three million policyholders, the company sells more individual life insurance than any other US firm and also sells health and retirement products, fixed and variable annuities, and mutual funds. It markets its wares via a network of some 7,500 agents and is renowned for employee training practices. It is also a major direct lender for commercial real estate projects. It owns Robert W. Baird & Co., a regional investment bank based in Milwaukee, and pension manager Frank Russell Company.

Ophidian Pharmaceuticals, Inc.

5445 E. Cheryl Pkwy., Madison, WI 53711

Telephone: 608-271-0878 **Fax:** 608-277-2395 **Metro area:** Madison, WI **Web site:** http://www.ophidian.com/ **Human resources contact:** Sue Maynard **Sales:** $300,000 **Number of employees:** 33 **Number of employees for previous year:** 32 **Industry designation:** Drugs **Company type:** Public **Top competitors:** Astra AB; IgX Corp.; Eli Lilly and Company

It's a good thing hen's eggs are more common than hen's teeth, or Ophidian Pharmaceuticals might have a problem. The development-stage company is using eggs to create an antitoxin treatment for a serious bowel infection commonly associated with broad-spectrum antibiotic use. The drug is undergoing animal trials. Ophidian (the name means "snake-like," and that's no yolk) is also researching applications of its technology for gastrointestinal infections and inflammatory bowel disease. The company has licensing agreements and alliances with other companies, researchers, and government agencies; however, its partnership with Eli Lilly was terminated in 1998.

ProVantage Health Services, Inc.

13555 Bishops Ct., Ste. 201, Brookfield, WI 53005

Telephone: 414-784-4600 **Fax:** 414-641-3947 **Metro area:** Milwaukee, WI **Web site:** http://www.provantageinc.com **Human resources contact:** Jane Koontz **Sales:** $500.9 million **Number of employees:** 387 **Industry designation:** Health maintenance organization **Company type:** Subsidiary **Top competitors:** Advance Paradigm, Inc.; MedPartners, Inc.; Express Scripts, Inc.

If knowledge is power, then ProVantage Health Services is a democracy. The company offers pharmacy benefit management (PBM) and health information technology (HIT) services to some 3,500 health organizations. ProVantage's PBM services include a retail pharmacy network, a mail-order pharmacy system, and vision benefits management. Its ATI program keeps records of patients' prescriptions to prevent drug interactions. HIT programs include RationalMed software (outcomes assessment), ProVQuery (pharmaceutical decision support software), ProVMed (health care data software), and ProVCOR (outcomes analysis software). ShopKo Stores is spinning off ProVantage, but it will retain majority ownership after the IPO.

Sargento Foods Inc.

One Persnickety Place, Plymouth, WI 53073

Telephone: 920-893-8484 **Fax:** 920-893-8399 **Metro area:** Milwaukee, WI **Web site:** http://www.sargento.com/1999.03/home.asp **Human resources contact:** Ed Sturzel **Sales:** $330 million (Est.) **Number of employees:** 1,000 **Industry designation:** Food—dairy products **Company type:** Private **Top competitors:** Marathon Cheese Corporation; Saputo Group Inc.; Kraft Foods, Inc.

Sargento Foods doesn't actually milk the cows or stir the curds, but it does shred, package, and market mozzarella, cheddar, and other cheeses made to its own specifications and those of retail customers. By turning cheese into value-added products, such as "recipe ready" shredded cheese blends, its popular MooTown Snacks (aimed at kids), and sliced cheeses for sandwiches, Sargento has been successful in the shadow of cheese giant Kraft Foods. Its food service product line includes frozen appetizers such as breaded cheese sticks. Historically innovative (it was the first to package shredded cheese), Sargento was founded in 1953 and is owned and operated by the Gentine family; it sells its products worldwide.

S.C. Johnson & Son, Inc.

1525 Howe St., Racine, WI 53403

Telephone: 414-260-2000 **Fax:** 414-260-2133 **Metro area:** Milwaukee, WI **Web site:** http://www.scjohnsonwax.com **Human resources contact:** Gayle P. Kosterman **Sales:** $5 billion (Est.) **Number of employees:** 13,200 **Number of employees for previous year:** 12,500 **Industry designation:** Soap & cleaning preparations **Company type:** Private **Top competitors:** Unilever; The Procter & Gamble Company; The Clorox Company

S.C. Johnson & Son helped consumers move from the flyswatter to the spray can. One of the world's largest makers of consumer chemical products, the company makes products for household cleaning, storage, and insect control, including Drano drain cleaner, Dow bathroom cleaner, Glade air freshener, Johnson floor wax, OFF! insect repellent, Windex window cleaner, and Ziploc plastic bags. It has sold many of its personal-care lines. It was the first to sell an indoor/outdoor insecticide (Raid, 1956). Family-owned S.C. Johnson operates in more than 50 countries and has interests in sanitation services and commercial pest control. Chairman Samuel Johnson, great-grandson of the founder, owns about 60% of the firm.

STRATTEC SECURITY CORPORATION

3333 W. Good Hope Rd., Milwaukee, WI 53209

Telephone: 414-247-3333 **Fax:** 414-247-3329 **Metro area:** Milwaukee, WI **Human resources contact:** Chuck Snyder **Sales:** $186.8 million **Number of employees:** 2,680 **Number of employees for previous year:** 2,665 **Industry designation:** Protection—safety equipment & services **Company type:** Public **Top competitors:** Directed Electronics, Inc.; The Eastern Company; Code-Alarm, Inc.

STRATTEC SECURITY might very well have made the key you locked inside your car or truck the other day. It makes all of DaimlerChrysler's US auto and truck locks and keys and most of those used by Ford and General Motors. Other customers include truck manufacturers Kenworth, Mack, Freightliner, and Peterbilt. STRATTEC's key products include not only mechanical and electromechanical locks, but electronic locks featuring radio-frequency identification and other sophisticated security features. The company's big three US OEM customers account for about 85% of sales. STRATTEC also makes precision zinc die castings for the transportation, security, and small-engine industries.

Sybron International Corporation

411 E. Wisconsin Ave., Milwaukee, WI 53202

Telephone: 414-274-6600 **Fax:** 414-274-6561 **Metro area:** Milwaukee, WI **Web site:** http://www.sybron.com **Human resources contact:** Eileen A. Short **Sales:** $960.7 million **Number of employees:** 7,900 **Number of employees for previous year:** 6,300 **Industry designation:** Medical & dental supplies **Company type:** Public **Top competitors:** Corning Incorporated; Millipore Corporation; Becton, Dickinson and Company

Sybron International makes laboratory and dental products for markets in the US and abroad. More than 60% of the company's sales come from three subsidiaries that make lab products: Nalge Nunc International (plastic labware, biopharmaceutical packaging products, and plastic tubing), Erie Scientific (microscope slides, cover glass, supplies used in clinical labs), and Barnstead Thermolyne (laboratory apparatuses, water purification systems). Its Sybron Dental Specialties subsidiary makes dentistry products and appliances and other materials and instruments used in the course of orthodontic treatment; subsidiary Samco Scientific makes plastic pipettes and specimen containers.

United Wisconsin Services, Inc.

401 W. Michigan St., Milwaukee, WI 53203

Telephone: 414-226-6900 **Fax:** 414-226-6229 **Metro area:** Milwaukee, WI **Web site:** http://www.uwz.com **Human resources contact:** Sue Fiegel **Sales:** $656.9 million **Number of employees:** 1,236 **Industry designation:** Health maintenance organization **Company type:** Public **Top competitors:** UnitedHealth Group; Aetna Inc.; Humana Inc.

Cheeseheads aren't the only ones turning to United Wisconsin Services, Inc. (UWSI) for health insurance. A managed health care and employee benefits provider, the company covers more than 1.6 million people nationwide. Its HMOs include Compcare, Compcare Northwest, Northwoods, Unity, and Valley Health Plans. The company also provides consulting services; a dental HMO; pharmaceutical services; and life, disability, and other employee benefit insurance coverages. Blue Cross & Blue Shield United of Wisconsin, which formed UWSI in 1983, owns 38% of the firm.

EMPLOYER-SPONSORED DESCRIPTIONS

The CNA Corporation

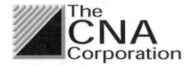

Description of Organization: The nation's oldest civilian organization engaged in operations research and systems analysis in support of government agencies. CNAC is a not-for-profit corporation.

Number of Employees: 525, including 240 research analysts

Headquarters Location: Alexandria, Virginia

Academic Fields of Recruitment Interest: Applied mathematics, economics (health, human capital, environment, labor, econometrics, I/O, and other micro fields), operations research, political science (quantitative specialties preferred), statistics

Major Entry-Level Opportunities for New Graduates: Empirical research and policy analysis

BACKGROUND AND OPERATIONS

The operation that evolved into The CNA Corporation (CNAC) was launched during World War II as the Anti-Submarine Warfare Operations Research Group. This organization brought together many of the nation's top civilian scientists and analysts in an urgent effort to solve one of the most pressing problems of the day: combating the Nazi submarines that threatened the supply lines of the European allies. Many of the young academics who participated in these early efforts maintained lifelong associations with CNAC and helped foster a corporate culture based on analytic excellence.

Today, CNAC is an independent, not-for-profit organization that undertakes analysis on a wide range of issues for a variety of clients, in addition to the Navy and Marine Corps. Of the 240 analysts on the research staff, most are young—on average, they are less than ten years out of graduate school, and almost all hold the Ph.D. or the terminal degree in their field. A principal objective in CNAC's hiring is to identify researchers who can work independently and who can manage significant responsibility. Within a few years of joining CNAC, an analyst

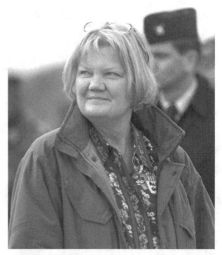

Dr. Aline Quester, CNAC Research Analyst, at USMC Base, Camp Lejeune.

is likely to be providing direct research support to the senior staff of a government agency. A second but equally important objective is identifying candidates who share a commitment to building good collegial relationships among coworkers and fostering diversity in the workplace.

Because CNAC recruits researchers with unusually strong capabilities, it offers attractive salaries and benefits (see "The Organization as Employer" section). In addition to the monetary and professional rewards of working at CNAC, many researchers enjoy having the opportunity to take field assignments outside the Alexandria, Virginia, headquarters. At some point in their careers, many choose to take a two-year field placement. At present, CNAC

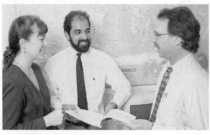

CNA analysts celebrating publication of research.

has research staff members working in Europe, Asia, and Hawaii and along the Pacific and mid-Atlantic coasts.

EMPLOYMENT OPPORTUNITIES

The People CNAC Is Seeking. CNAC hires an average of 20 to 30 research analysts per year. With rare exceptions, staff positions are restricted to those who have received, or are about to receive, the terminal degree in their field. CNAC has expanded its client base and is now recruiting in the following disciplines:
• Applied mathematics
• Economics–health, human capital, environment, labor, econometrics, I/O, and other micro fields
• Operations research
• Political science (quantitative specialties preferred)
• Statistics

The Work CNAC Is Doing. Over the last few years, CNAC has worked on research projects sponsored by the Navy, the Federal Aviation Administration, the Veterans Administration, the Marine Corps, the Carnegie Corporation of New York, and several other agencies and institutions. Among the questions that analysts have considered are the following:
• How can the FAA reduce operational errors among private and commercial aircraft in U.S. airspace?
• Does the Veterans' Health Administration distribute resources among its regions in an appropriate fashion?
• What are the best methods for the Navy to attract and retain high-quality people?
• How can CNAC best assist officers in the Russian military to make the transition to civilian life?
• What would be the costs to the Department of Defense in offering enhancements in medical insurance coverage to Medicare-eligible military retirees?
• How can the Marine Corps improve its humanitarian operations, such as those it has undertaken in northern Iraq, Bangladesh, Somalia, and Haiti?
• How have the health-care reform initiatives recently introduced by the Department of Defense affected military readiness and the quality of peacetime medical services?
• What savings can the Navy realize by outsourcing various operations and functions to the private sector?
• What investments in information systems would most improve the quality of combat medical care?

THE ORGANIZATION AS EMPLOYER

Research Infrastructure and Support. New analysts frequently comment that "CNAC seems to have things wired right." Researchers are supported by a programming staff, extensive computer facilities, an in-house group of professional editors and graphic artists, and comprehensive library services.

Salaries and Fringe Benefits. CNAC pays competitive salaries to recruit the best research analysts and offers an unusually liberal benefits package. Employees are provided with medical, life, and long-term disability insurance. In addition to ten paid holidays, new staff members receive three weeks of paid vacation per year (this increases to four weeks after three years of service). CNAC offers a matching retirement plan with TIAA/CREF or Fidelity: new employees who contribute 5 percent of their pretax income receive a 9 percent matching contribution from CNAC, a far more generous matching plan than that made by most public or private employers.

The Career Path. Analysts are assigned progressively more challenging research problems and increasing responsibilities in project oversight.

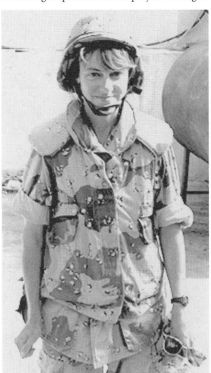

Dr. Katherine McGrady, Director of CNAC's Marine Corps Program, on maneuvers.

Some researchers who establish a strong track record in directing projects eventually assume a formal position in research management. Others choose to remain directly involved in analysis and progress through CNAC by taking on work that is more challenging or more critical to senior policy makers.

Local Amenities. CNAC is less than 10 minutes from downtown Washington, D.C., one of the most livable, diverse, and culturally rich cities in the world. It would take years to explore the capital's theaters, museums, performing arts centers, restaurants, parks, bike trails, and historical attractions. There are several excellent local universities for those who wish to continue their education or establish professional relationships.

APPLICATION AND INFORMATION

CNAC accepts resumes and employment inquiries throughout the year. Normally, candidates who are invited for interviews are asked to demonstrate their ability to conduct an independent investigation or analysis and to present material clearly by giving a presentation on a subject of their own choice.

Applicants selected are subject to a security investigation and must meet eligibility requirements for access to classified information. U.S. citizenship is required.

Direct inquiries to:

Ms. Carolyn P. Williams, Manager of
    Employment
The CNA Corporation
4401 Ford Avenue
Alexandria, Virginia 22302-8268
Fax: 703-824-2740
E-mail: resumes@cna.org
World Wide Web: http://www.cna.org

Veterans Health Administration
Department of Veterans Affairs

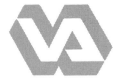

Description of Organization: The largest component of the Department of Veterans Affairs (VA); provides medical, surgical, psychiatric, nursing, and specialty care and also conducts research studies

Number of Employees: More than 200,000

Headquarters Location: Washington, D.C.

Fields of Recruitment Interest: Physicians and non-physician primary care providers such as advanced practice nurses (nurse practitioners), occupational therapists, pharmacists, physical therapists, physician assistants, and others who comprise a variety of primary care-based teams

BACKGROUND AND OPERATIONS

The Veterans Health Administration (VHA) is the largest integrated health-care provider in the nation with more than 200,000 employees and an annual medical care budget of more than $17 billion. VHA treats nearly one million patients on an inpatient basis and provides care on an outpatient basis at a rate of more than 30 million visits annually at more than 950 health-care facilities located throughout the country.

VHA provides medical, surgical, psychiatric, and nursing care as well as specialty care, such as hemodialysis, organ transplant, spinal cord injury, substance abuse treatment, ambulatory care, critical care, and long-term care. It also conducts research studies on AIDS, diabetes, drug addiction, epilepsy, nerve regeneration, Alzheimer's disease, and other problems associated with aging.

Technological advances, economic factors, demographic changes, and the rise of managed health care, among other things, are causing a dramatic shift away from inpatient care and a corresponding increase in ambulatory care. VHA is adapting its service delivery to align with the changes occurring in the larger, overall health-care environment.

The blueprint for this transformation is a new VHA infrastructure that has eliminated the previous four-region nationwide structure, replacing it with 22 smaller, more autonomous networks of facilities called Veteran's Integrated Service Networks, or VISNs. These entities have shifted focus from independent medical facilities to groups of centers working collaboratively to provide efficient, accessible care to the veteran population served in their areas. Primary care is the central focus of patient treatment in both outpatient and inpatient settings of the "new" VHA.

EMPLOYMENT OPPORTUNITIES

Entry-Level and Experienced Personnel

VA offers unparalleled opportunities for career growth to non-physician primary care providers and associated allied health professionals.

Under a unique federal personnel system, VA facilities may directly appoint physicians, advanced practice nurses (nurse practitioners) physician assistants, physical therapists, occupational therapists, pharmacists, registered or certified respiratory therapists, and expanded-function dental auxiliaries to positions for which no civil service examination is required.

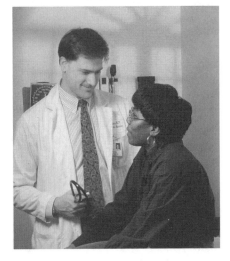

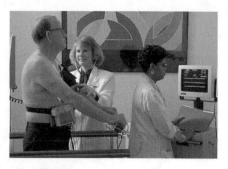

THE ORGANIZATION AS EMPLOYER

VA's mission is to provide the best possible care for the nation's veterans. In recognition of the contributions made by physicians and non-physician primary care providers and associated allied health professionals in achieving this goal, VA offers extensive and competitive employment benefits and educational opportunities. These health-care professionals at VA earn thirteen to twenty-six days of paid vacation (thirty days for physicians) and personal leave each year. They also earn thirteen days of sick leave annually (fifteen days for physicians), with no limit on accumulation. Military leave is authorized up to fifteen days per year for active reservists and members of the National Guard. There are also ten paid federal holidays.

VA offers a variety of group health insurance plans, with premiums partially paid by the federal government. Term life insurance, with coverage based on salary, is available, with the cost shared by the federal government. Family and additional coverage options are available. Newly hired non-physician primary care providers and associated allied health professionals are covered by the Federal Employees' Retirement System (FERS). FERS is a three-tier retirement plan composed of Social Security benefits, FERS basic benefits, and the Thrift Savings Plan, which is a tax-deferred savings plan similar to 401(k) plans offered in the private sector.

Numerous other benefits are offered by VA, including mobility between facilities, liability protection, cash awards for adopted suggestions, smoke-free and drug-free workplaces, employee wellness programs, credit unions, dining facilities, free parking at most facilities, and child care at some facilities.

The Family and Medical Leave Act and the Family Friendly Leave Act allow employees to balance their work and family lives by taking reasonable amounts of leave for medical reasons, for the birth or adoption/foster care of a child, and for the care of a child, spouse, or parent who has a serious health problem. The Voluntary Leave Transfer Program allows other federal employees to donate annual leave for a medical emergency of an employee or family member.

In general, starting salaries for VA health-care professionals are based on education and experience and can vary by location. Therefore, applicants should directly contact the facility where they would like to work for specific information about salaries currently being offered.

VA recognizes the importance of ongoing education and the benefit it provides to both veteran patients and VA employees. Opportunities are available through specialized programs for qualifying staff and students, tuition support for job-related and continuing education courses, VA national and regional education programs, and paid time off for approved continuing education programs.

APPLICATION AND INFORMATION

VA health-care facilities have specialized medical care programs and range in size from 110 to more than 1,400 beds. As such, a variety of opportunities are available for physicians and other health-care professionals. To gain a first-hand view of VA health care, interested individuals are encouraged to arrange to visit VA facilities in their area by calling or writing for an appointment. Telephone numbers are listed in local directories under "U.S. Government." Correspondence may also be addressed to the Human Resources Management Service.

Physicians, advanced practice nurses (nurse practitioners), physician assistants, physical therapists, occupational therapists, and pharmacists are invited to write or call:

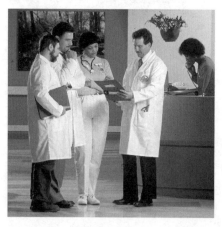

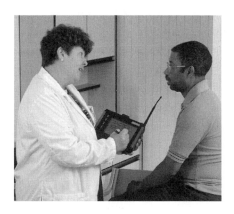

Healthcare Staff Development and Retention
  Office
VA Placement Service
1555 Poydras Street, Suite 1971
New Orleans, Louisiana 70112
800-949-0002 (toll-free)
World Wide Web: http://vacareers.va.gov

INDEXES

Company Index

Primary Industry Index

Computers—engineering, scientific & CAD-CAM software

Computers—online services

Cosmetics & toiletries

Drugs

Medical & dental supplies

Medical instruments

Medical practice management

Medical products

Medical services

Optical character recognition

Paints & related products

Photographic equipment & supplies

Pollution control equipment & services

Protection—safety equipment & services

Metropolitan Area Index

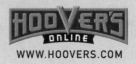

PETERSON'S—YOUR ONLINE GUIDE TO THE FUTURE!

The Education Supersite℠ at petersons.com gives you the tools and the help you need to find and win the job of your dreams. You can:

- Search for career opportunities
- Find helpful articles to steer your search
- Get advice on building a portfolio

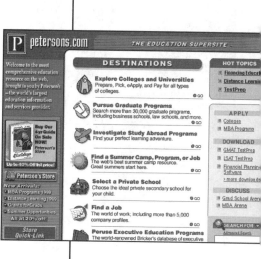

And if you're looking for advice on finding the right graduate program, look no further than the **Enrollment Message Center** at **petersons.com**!

- Explore program options by discipline
- E-mail program contacts for more information
- Best of all? It's **FREE**

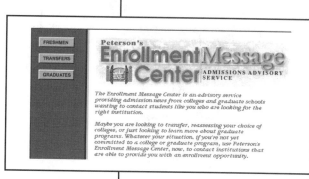

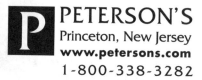

PETERSON'S
Princeton, New Jersey
www.petersons.com
1-800-338-3282

Wait! There's more!➔

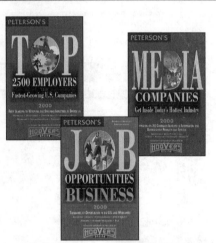
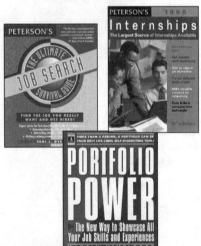
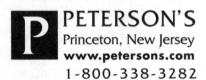